Nutritional Influences
on Illness
A Sourcebook of Clinical Research

SECOND EDITION

Also by Melvyn R. Werbach

Nutritional Influences on Mental Illness: A Sourcebook of Clinical Research

Third Line Medicine: Modern Treatment for Persistent Symptoms

SECOND EDITION

Nutritional Influences on Illness

A sourcebook of clinical research

Melvyn R. Werbach, M.D.
Assistant Clinical Professor
School of Medicine, UCLA
Los Angeles, California

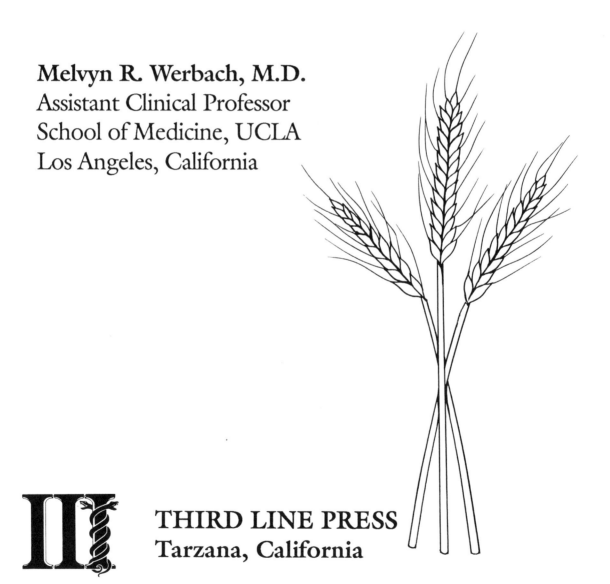

THIRD LINE PRESS
Tarzana, California

Although the author has exhaustively researched all sources to ensure the accuracy and completeness of the information contained in this book, we assume no responsibility for errors, inaccuracies, omissions or any inconsistency herein.

The treatment of illness must be supervised by a physician or other licensed health professional. The information presented in this book is intended for education only and does not contain treatment recommendations for the public.

Second Printing

Printed in the United States of America

ISBN 0-9618550-3-7

Library of Congress Catalog Card Number: 92-93557

To my wife, Gail,
and my sons, Kevin and Adam,
for their love and support
which made this book possible.

NUTRITIONAL INFLUENCES ON ILLNESS:
A SOURCEBOOK OF CLINICAL RESEARCH
SECOND EDITION

TABLE OF CONTENTS

PART II: APPENDICES

INTRODUCTION

As nutritional science has developed, so have the clinical applications. Clinical nutrition was initially limited to treating general malnutrition and specific nutritional deficiency states. In the past two decades, the field has gradually broadened to include the treatment of subclinical deficiencies and dependencies, as well as the provision of nutrients in massive doses as pharmacologic agents. Unfortunately, early work in this area drew strong criticism due to the premature advocacy of certain treatments despite the lack of adequate scientific validation.

Scientific justification for an expanded definition of clinical nutrition has been considerably strengthened since then. Laboratory tests can provide evidence of inadequate nutriture despite the lack of clinical findings of classical nutritional deficiency syndromes. Even in the absence of laboratory validation of nutritional deficiencies, numerous studies utilizing rigorous scientific designs have demonstrated impressive benefits from nutritional supplementation. It is now well established, for example, that nutritional factors are of major importance in the pathogenesis of both atherosclerosis and cancer, the two leading causes of death in Western countries, and studies validating their importance in the pathogenesis of many other diseases continue to be published.

It is hoped that the material presented in this book will enable all health care professionals to better utilize nutritional science in their practices by summarizing the available data. *Nutritional Influences on Illness* covers the field of nutritional medicine, while its companion book, *Nutritional Influences on Mental Illness*, covers nutritional psychiatry. The bulk of the text consists of a series of chapters covering the major illnesses for which a reasonable amount of nutritional literature exists. Basic dietary factors are discussed first, then vitamins, minerals, other nutritional factors and, finally, other related factors, with special attention to the influence of food sensitivities on illness.

Each chapter presents a series of statements concerning relevant nutrients, with each statement being followed by selected abstracts from the literature which either substantiate or refute it. (*These statements are not therapeutic recommendations!*) Whenever possible, randomized, controlled clinical trials are presented; because such studies are often lacking, however, observational (epidemiologic) studies, open trials, animal experiments and even informal clinical observations are also included. Clinicians must decide for themselves how strong they believe the scientific evidence must be before utilizing a particular nutrient. In order to assist you in reaching decisions, abstracts of review articles are included to provide the advice of acknowledged experts.

Abstracts are presented in the order of their year of publication, with the latest papers listed first. As it is not possible to include all studies, preference has been given to the best, the most relevant, and the most recent.

Seven appendices are included. Their suggested use is as follows:

Common Nutritional Deficiencies: Provides an "index of suspicion" since, the more common a deficiency, the more likely it is that it contributes to the patient's symptomatology.

Dangers of Nutritional Supplementation: Should be consulted routinely before initiating nutritional supplementation for information concerning possible adverse effects, especially when the dosages suggested are in the pharmacologic range.

Laboratory Methods for Nutritional Evaluation: A guide to choosing the best available laboratory method to appraise nutritional status for each major nutrient. Methods are listed in rough order of preference.

Nutrient Bioavailability and Interactions: Should be consulted routinely when evaluating specific nutrients in order to identify factors that may be affecting their current levels or which could be utilized to modify such levels.

Signs and Symptoms of Abnormal Tissue Nutrient Levels: Provides a brief listing of many of the signs and symptoms of nutrient deficiencies and toxicities. Should be consulted to discover whether the patient's presentation is consistent with that of a suspected deficiency or toxicity.

Signs and Symptoms of Heavy Metal Toxicity: Provides a brief listing of many of the signs and symptoms of heavy metal toxicities.

How to Rule Out Food Sensitivities: A guide to the various methods of evaluating a patient for the presence of food sensitivities that may contribute to the illness.

A useful sequence for reaching a decision regarding the role of nutrients both as causative factors and as potential therapeutic agents is as follows:

1. Include the patient's dietary history and current eating patterns when taking a medical history.
2. Examine the patient for signs of nutritional deficiencies as part of the medical examination.
3. Review the specific chapters relating to the patient's complaints and/or diagnosis.
4. Review the relevant appendices.
5. If indicated, perform selective evaluative laboratory testing.

All patients deserve appropriate trials of well-validated nutritional interventions. How early in the course of treatment these trials should be undertaken depends upon how they compare to the other therapeutic options in regard to:

1. the evidence that nutritional factors play a causative or a curative role in the illness;
2. their demonstrated safety and efficacy;
3. their cost; and
4. patient preference.

In addition, patients who have failed to respond to well-validated treatments should be considered for appropriate trials of poorly-validated but reasonably safe nutritional interventions.

> *NOTE: The treatment of such patients is discussed in: Werbach, MR.* **Third Line Medicine: Modern Treatment for Persistent Symptoms.** *London & New York. Arkana Paperbacks, 1986. (See the order form at the end of this book.)*

While clinical nutrition provides a complex, highly sophisticated approach to understanding and treating illness, it is also a young and still primitive field with an often disappointingly inadequate scientific literature. It is hoped that the reader will come away from this book with a deeper appreciation of the state of this rapidly evolving field as it exists today — and will be better able, not only to utilize nutrition in practice, but to answer the many questions concerning nutrition being asked of health professionals by an increasingly sophisticated public.

PART ONE

ILLNESSES AND THE EFFECTS OF NUTRIENTS, TOXIC METALS AND ENVIRONMENTAL SENSITIVITIES

ACNE ROSACEA

VITAMINS

<u>Vitamin A</u>:

Oral administration of <u>isotretinoin</u> (13-*cis*-retinoic acid), a stereoisomer of all-*trans*-retinoic acid, may be beneficial.

> **Experimental Study:** Following treatment with isotretinoin, the inflammatory papules, pustules, and nodules were curtailed, while the vasomotor lability and telangiectasia were unchanged (*Plewig G et al. Action of isotretinoin in acne rosacea and gram-negative folliculitis. <u>J Invest Dermatol</u> 86:390-93, 1986*).

<u>Vitamin B complex</u>:

Supplementation may be beneficial (*Tulipan L. Acne rosacea: A vitamin B complex deficiency. <u>Arch Dermatol Syphilol</u> 56:589, 1947; Gross P. Non-pellagrous eruptions due to deficiency of the vitamin B-complex. <u>Arch Dermatol Syphilol</u> 43:504, 1941*).

- <u>Niacin</u>:

Supplementation may be beneficial.

> **Clinical Observation:** Daily IV injections of nicotinamide 20 cg rapidly improves skin lesions. The day after the first injection the lesions are already less intense. After some days this improvement is very marked. They subsequently remain stationary and never completely disappear despite the continuation of treatment (*Daïnow I. Recherches cliniques sur certaines propriétés anti-allergiques de la nicotinamide. <u>Z Vitaminforsch</u> 15:245-50, 1944*).

- <u>Vitamin B6</u>:

Supplementation may be beneficial.

> **Experimental Study:** 2 pts. with both acne rosacea and vulgaris were supplemented with riboflavin 10 mg daily and pyridoxine 50 mg daily. There was slight improvement which was not greater than that attainable by topical treatment. When the riboflavin was stopped, the improvement persisted, but after pyridoxine was stopped, it promptly worsened (*Stillians AW. Pyridoxine in treatment of acne vulgaris. <u>J Invest Dermatol</u> 7:150-51, 1946*).

- <u>Riboflavin</u>:

Deficiency in rats is associated with corneal vascularization (similar to rosacea keratitis) which remits with riboflavin supplementation (*Bessey OA, Wolbach SB. Vascularization of the cornea of the rat in riboflavin deficiency, with a note on corneal vascularization in vitamin A deficiency. <u>J Exper Med</u> 69:1, 1939; Eckardt RE, Johnson LV. Nutritional cataract and relation of galactose to appearance of senile suture line in rats. <u>Arch Ophthalmol</u> 21:315, 1939*).

Supplementation may be beneficial.

> **Experimental Study:** 32/36 pts. with rosacea keratitis had prompt healing following small doses (1-4.5 mg daily orally or by injection) of riboflavin. 9 of these pts. also had cutaneous rosacea and 4 of them improved (*Johnson L, Eckardt R. Rosacea keratitis and conditions with vascularization of the cornea treated with riboflavin. <u>Arch Ophthalmol</u> 23:899, 1940*).

- -

OTHER FACTORS

Rule out hydrochloric acid deficiency.

> *Note: While gastric anacidity had been reported in the past to be a relatively common condition which was associated with acne rosacea and a number of other illnesses, the presence of achlorhydria is no longer accepted unless a potent parietal-cell stimulant (such as histamine) is employed in gastric analysis. More recent studies suggest that histamine-fast anacidity is uncommon before the fifth decade of life and, although it probably does not occur in a normal stomach, its presence is not necessarily associated with symptoms (Rappaport EM. Achlorhydria: Associated symptoms and response to hydrochloric acid. N Engl J Med 252(19):802-5, 1955).*

Deficiency may be associated with vitamin B malabsorption (*Allison JR. Effect of hydrochloric acid on absorption of B-complex. South Med J 38:235, 1945*).

> **Observational Study:** Of 30 pts. with subacute or chronic conditions which had resisted all forms of local treatment, 12 (40%) had no HCl and only 4 (13%) had normal HCl levels. The severity of the condition seemed to correlate with the extent of the the HCl deficiency and also seemed to be associated with signs of vitamin B complex deficiency (*Allison JR. The relation of hydrochloric acid and vitamin B complex deficiency in certain skin diseases. South Med J 38:235-241, 1945*).

> **Observational Study:** 2 pts. with rosacea keratitis who had a history of adequate dietary riboflavin failed to improve with the addition of riboflavin to their diet. Analysis of their gastric contents after administration of 3 mg histamine failed to show any free hydrochloric acid. In addition, 5/9 pts. with cutaneous rosacea who failed to improve with riboflavin also were achlorhydric following histamine stimulation (*Johnson L, Eckardt R. Rosacea keratitis and conditions with vascularization of the cornea treated with riboflavin. Arch Ophthalmol 23(5):899-907, 1940*).

If deficient, supplementation may be beneficial.

- with vitamin B complex:

> **Experimental Study:** Of 30 pts. with subacute or chronic conditions which had resisted all forms of local treatment, improvement of the HCl deficient pts. followed treatment with supplemental HCl and vitamin B complex (*Allison JR. The relation of hydrochloric acid and vitamin B complex deficiency in certain skin diseases. South Med J 38:235-241, 1945*).

Pancreatic enzymes:

Serum lipase concentrations may be deficient.

> **Observational Study:** Pancreatic function was studied in 21 pts. and 21 controls by means of the cerulein infusion test. Compared to controls, pts. had significantly lower lipase concentration and output (with the decrease ranging from 18.5-66% of normal) despite normal flow rate and normal bicarbonate and chymotrypsin concentration and output, suggesting that deficient lipase secretion could be responsible, at least partly, for the clinical manifestations of rosacea (*Barba A et al. Pancreatic exocrine function in rosacea. Dermatologica 165:601-6, 1982*).

Supplementation may be beneficial.

> **Clinical Observation:** When pts. complain of digestive symptoms, the administration of pancreatic extracts may ameliorate both the dyspepsia and the skin lesions (*Barba A et al. Pancreatic exocrine function in rosacea. Dermatologica 165:601-6, 1982*).

ACNE VULGARIS

DIETARY FACTORS

General:

The Western diet is associated with an increased incidence of acne (*Rosenberg EW, Kirk BS. Acne diet reconsidered. Arch Dermatol 117:193-95, 1981*).

Observational Study: Far less acne was found among the black population in Kenya eating traditional diets than among young blacks in the U.S. (*Rosenberg EW, Kirk BS. Acne diet reconsidered. Arch Dermatol 117:193-95, 1981; Verhagen ARHB. Skin diseases, in LC Vogel et al, Eds. Health and Diseases in Kenya. Nairobi, Kenya, East African Literature Bureau, 1974, pp. 499-507*).

Observational Study: Far less acne was found among the black population in Zambia eating traditional diets than among young blacks in the U.S. (*Rosenberg EW, Kirk BS. Acne diet reconsidered. Arch Dermatol 117:193-95, 1981; Ratnam AV, Jayaraju K. Skin diseases in Zambia. Br J Dermatol 101:449-53, 1979*).

Observational Study: After World War II, Eskimos who changed to Western diets developed a number of new diseases including acne (*Bendiner E. Disastrous trade-off: Eskimo health for white civilization. Hosp Pract 9:156-89, 1974*).

Observational Study: Acne disappeared in Europe during the starvation years of World War II, but returned as soon as the diet returned to normal (*Lobitz WC. The structure and function of the sebaceous glands. Arch Dermatol 76:162-71, 1957*).

Low fat diet.

Dietary fat is associated with increased sebum production. Normals have a moderate increase, while male acne pts. have a marked increase (*Lobitz WC. The structure and function of the sebaceous glands. Arch Dermatol 76:162-71, 1957; Lorincz AL, Rothman S. Acne Med Clinics N A March, 1958, pp. 497-504*).

Low carbohydrate diet.

Dietary carbohydrate is associated with increased sebum production. Normals have a moderate increase, while male acne pts. have a marked increase (*Lobitz WC. The structure and function of the sebaceous glands. Arch Dermatol 76:162-71, 1957; Lorincz AL, Rothman S. Acne Med Clinics N A March, 1958, pp. 497-504*).

High fiber diet.

Clinical Observation: Several pts. showed rapid clearing following supplementation with 1 oz daily of an all-bran cereal, perhaps due to correction of the effects of constipation (*Kaufman WF. The diet and acne. Letter. Arch Dermatol 119(4):276, 1983*).

Avoid refined carbohydrates:

Observational Study: In a study of over 1000 physicians, dentists and their wives, five parameters of refined carbohydrate consumption were found to be significantly related ($p<0.01$ to <0.001) to the incidence of skin signs and symptoms of dermatoses. Those subjects reporting one or more symptoms and signs consumed a significantly greater quantity of refined carbohydrate compared to those reporting none as measured by each parameter: total calories, calories from refined carbohydrate, percentage of calories from refined carbohydrate, gms. of refined carbohydrate, and tsps. of sugar (*Ringsdorf WM Jr, Cheraskin E. Diet and dermatosis. South Med J 69(6):732 & 734, 1976*).

Negative Observational Study: The sucrose intake of 9 male and 7 female pts. aged 15-27 was not significantly different from that of controls (*Bett DGG et al. Sugar consumption in acne vulgaris and seborrhoeic dermatitis. Br Med J 3:153-55, 1967*).

Experimental Study and Theoretical Discussion: While a literature review suggests that there is no metabolic derangement of carbohydrate or glucose metabolism in the blood or skin of pts., prolonged or repeated hyperglycemia may aggravate acne. Because, in this study, a post-prandial refractory period was found, desserts eaten following meals will not affect acne adversely. "Sweets," however, were found to produce sharp elevations of blood sugar in fasting individuals; thus eating sweets between meals can aggravate acne (*Mullins JF, Naylor D. Glucose and the acne diathesis: An hypothesis and review of the literature. Tex Rep Biol Med 20:161-75, 1962*).

VITAMINS

Folic Acid:

Supplementation may be beneficial.

Experimental Study: 8 pts. with acne vulgaris were given oral synthetic folic acid 5-10 mg daily. 6 were "much improved" and 1 was "improved" (*Callaghan TJ. The effect of folic acid on seborrheic dermatitis. Cutis 3:583-88, 1967*).

Vitamin A:

WARNING: Because of the potential toxicity of high doses, close medical supervision is necessary

General Review Article: *Leyden JJ. Retinoids and acne. J Am Acad Dermatol 19(1 Pt 2):164-68, 1988*

Serum levels of retinol and retinol-binding protein may be lower in patients than in controls.

Observational Study: Compared to 37 controls, mean serum concentrations of retinol and retinol-binding protein were significantly decreased in pts. (p<0.01) (*Rollman O, Vahlquist A. Vitamin A in skin and serum: Studies of acne vulgaris, atopic dermatitis, ichthyosis vulgaris and lichen planus. Br J Dermatol 113(4):405-13, 1985*).

Skin vitamin A levels may be decreased.

Observational Study: Compared to the skin of 37 controls, mean retinol concentration was decreased in both involved and uninvolved acne skin (p<0.05), probably due to diminished supply of vitamin A from the blood (*Rollman O, Vahlquist A. Vitamin A in skin and serum: Studies of acne vulgaris, atopic dermatitis, ichthyosis vulgaris and lichen planus. Br J Dermatol 113(4):405-13, 1985*).

Supplementation with vitamin A may be beneficial.

Experimental Study: 136 pts. were treated in 1 study, and 30 pts. were treated in a second study. Doses below 300,000 IU daily were ineffective. Retinol in doses of 300,000 IU for women and 4-500,000 IU for men was highly efficacious; 85% of pts. treated with 300,000 IU daily achieved a good (50% or more decrease in inflammatory lesions) to excellent (75%) response within 3-4 months. Serum vitamin A levels rose steadily during the 12-wk. period as did serum triglyceride levels. Cheilitis, xerosis, headaches, nose bleeding, telogen effluvium, and abnormal liver function studies frequently occurred, demonstrating that the margin of therapeutic efficacy to toxicity was narrow (*Kligman AM et al. Oral vitamin A in acne vulgaris. Int J Dermatol 20(4):278-85, 1981; Kligman AM et al. Oral vitamin A (retinol) in acne vulgaris, in CE Orfanos et al, Eds. Retinoids: Advances in Basic Research and Therapy. New York, Springer-Verlag, 1981:245-53*).

Negative Double-blind Experimental Study: After 3 mo., administration of vitamin A 150,000 IU daily showed little or no beneficial effect compared to placebo when evaluated by a panel viewing color photographs in a trial involving 61 patients. Results did suggest, however, that deterioration may have been lessened by vitamin A since only 2/13 pts. whose skin worsened were in the experimental group (results not significant) (*Anderson JAD, Stokoe IH. Vitamin A in acne vulgaris. Br Med J 2:294-96, 1963*).

- with <u>Vitamin E</u>:

Vitamin E affects the biologic utilization of vitamin A, and vitamin A absorption is markedly impaired in vitamin E-deficient animals (*Ames SR. Factors affecting absorption, transport and storage of vitamin A. Am J Clin Nutr 22:934, 1969*).

Supplementation may be beneficial.

Experimental Study: Over 100 pts. had conditions which were successfully controlled with ave. daily doses of 100,000 IU of vitamin A and 800 IU of vitamin E. Most responded within weeks and maintenance of control was obtained with lower doses (*Ayres S Jr., Mihan R. Acne vulgaris and lipid peroxidation: New concepts in pathogenesis and treatment. Int J Dermatol 17:305, 1978*).

Oral administration of <u>isotretinoin</u> (13-*cis*-retinoic acid), a stereoisomer of all-*trans*-retinoic acid, may increase epidermal retinol levels.

Experimental Study: While oral isotretinoin failed to affect serum levels of retinol, retinol-binding protein, or prealbumin (transthyretin), epidermal retinol levels increased by an ave. of 53% (p<0.01), and dehydroretinol levels decreased by 79% (<0.001), in acne pts. following 3 mo. of treatment (*Rollman O, Vahlquist A. Oral isotretinoin (13-cis-retinoic acid) therapy in severe acne: Drug and vitamin A concentrations in sebum and skin. J Invest Dermatol 86(4):384-89, 1986*).

Oral administration of <u>isotretinoin</u> (13-*cis*-retinoic acid) may be beneficial.

WARNING: Compared to retinol, the safety profile of tretinoin is not significantly better. Teratogenic effects are most important, and mucocutaneous side-effects occur in nearly all patients. Other side-effects include skeletal hyperostoses, problems with dark adaptation, Staph aureus infections and aggravation of inflammatory bowel disease (*Leyden JJ. Retinoids and acne. J Am Acad Dermatol 19(1 Pt 2):164-68, 1988*).

Review Article: Isotretinoin has proved to be quite effective in the treatment of severe recalcitrant cystic acne under conditions in which toxicity is manageable (*Bushnell DE et al. The retinoids in acne. Am Fam Physician 29(3):221-26, 1984*).

Experimental Study: Doses of 1 mg/kg/d and higher of isotretinoin produced profound improvement with prolonged periods of remission in pts. with acne conglobata (*Peck GL et al. Prolonged remissions of cystic and conglobate acne with 13-cis-retinoic acid. N Engl J Med 300:329-33, 1979*).

Topical application of <u>isotretinoin</u> may be beneficial.

Experimental Double-blind Study: In a multi-centered trial, topical application of a 0.05% isotretinoin gel formulation was clearly effective in the treatment of moderately severe acne. Significant reduction in inflammatory lesions occurred after 5 wks. of twice daily treatment, and a significant reduction in noninflammatory lesions occurred after 8 weeks. Irritant reactions were infrequently observed (*Chalker DK et al. Efficacy of topical isotretinoin 0.05% gel in acne vulgaris. Results of a multicenter, double-blind investigation. J Am Acad Dermatol 17:251-54, 1987*).

<u>Tretinoin</u> (vitamin A acid; retinoic acid) is a metabolite of retinol which is found in the blood in a concentration approximately 2 orders of magnitude lower than that of retinol (*Emerick RJ et al. Formation of retinoic acid from retinol in the rat. Biochem J 102:606-11, 1967*). Although it is too toxic for systemic use (*Schumacher A et al. Zur lokalbehandlung von keratosen mit vitamin-A saure. Dermatologia 124:65-80, 1962*), topical application may be beneficial.

WARNING: May cause skin irritation.

Negative Experimental Blinded Study: Although topical retinoic acid reduced the number of comedones and inflammed lesions and improved the disease, a similar improvement was found with placebo (*Christiansen JV et al. Topical tretinoin, vitamin A acid (Airol) in acne vulgaris. Dermatologica 148:82-89, 1974*).

Vitamin B6:

Supplementation may be beneficial, especially for premenstrual acne flares.

WARNING: May worsen acne vulgaris or cause an acneiform exanthema.

Observational Study: Deterioration of acne vulgaris or eruption of an acneiform exanthema could be established during treatment with vitamin B_6 and/or vitamin B_{12} in 14 patients. Females were by far the more frequently affected. Characteristic is the appearance of lesions outside the typical age gp. affected by acne vulgaris. Lesions consisted of loosely disseminated small papules or papulopustules on the face (especially on the forehead and chin), on the upper parts of the back and chest and spreading to the upper arm and usually faded shortly after B_6 or B_{12} was stopped (*Braun-Falco O, Lincke H. [The problem of vitamin B6/B12 acne. A contribution on acne medicamentosa. MMW 118(6):155-60, 1976*).

Experimental Single-blind Study: 72 pts. aged 16-29 with acne for 1-10 yrs. alternately received either pyridoxine 25 mg twice daily (which was raised to 50 mg 5 times daily if improvement was not seen) or placebo. None had anatomical evidence of B-vitamin deficiency or conditions known to affect the requirement or utilization of vitamin B complex. 9/37 treated pts. (24.3%) showed complete clearing of the lesions, 19/37 (51.5%) showed definite improvement, and 6/37 were unchanged. Among controls, 0/35 showed complete clearing, 7/35 showed improvement, and 19 were unchanged. Nine in the control gp. dropped out compared to 3 in the treated group. In 3 unimproved control pts., pyridoxine was substituted without their knowledge after 4, 6, and 7 mo., respectively. There was complete clearing of the lesions in 1 and 3 mo. in 2 of these patients. All treated pts. also reported a considerable decrease in skin oiliness, even in some cases to the point of actual dryness and scaling, perhaps because of improvement in the metabolism of unsaturated fatty acids (*Joliffe N et al. Effects of pyridoxine (vit. B6) on resistant adolescent acne. J Invest Dermatol 5:143, 1942*).

Vitamin B12:

WARNING: May worsen acne vulgaris or cause an acneiform exanthema.

Observational Study: Deterioration of acne vulgaris or eruption of an acneiform exanthema could be established during treatment with vitamin B_6 and/or vitamin B_{12} in 14 patients. Females were by far the more frequently affected. Characteristic is the appearance of lesions outside the typical age group affected by acne vulgaris. Lesions consisted of loosely disseminated small papules or papulopustules on the face (especially on the forehead and chin), on the upper parts of the back and chest and spreading to the upper arm and usually faded shortly after B_6 or B_{12} was stopped (*Braun-Falco O, Lincke H. [The problem of vitamin B6/B12 acne. A contribution on acne medicamentosa. MMW 118(6):155-60, 1976*).

- -

MINERALS

Iodine:

WARNING: Excess supplementation may cause or exacerbate acneiform eruptions (*Hitch JM. Acneform eruptions induced by drugs and chemicals. JAMA 200:879-80, 1967*).

Note: Kelp as a dietary supplement (Fischer AA. Contact Dermatitis. Third Edition. Philadelphia, Lea and Febiger, 1986:593) or fast foods (How nutritious are fast-foods? Consum Rep 40:278-81, 1975) may contain sufficient iodine for this adverse effect.

Selenium:

- with Vitamin E:

RBC glutathione peroxidase levels may be reduced. If so, levels may normalize with supplementation.

Observational Study: 47 male acne pts. had significantly decreased erythrocyte glutathione peroxidase levels compared to controls, while the levels of 47 female pts. not on oral contraceptives did not differ from those of controls (*Michaëlsson G, Edqvist L. Erythrocyte glutathione peroxidase activity in acne vulgaris and the effect of selenium and vitamin E treatment. Acta Derm Venereol (Stockh) 64(1):9-14, 1984*).

Patients with low RBC glutathione peroxidase levels and pustular acne respond best to supplementation.

Experimental Study: 29 pts. with severe acne received selenium ($Na_2 SeO_3$) 200 μg and vitamin E (tocopheryl succinate) 10 mg twice daily for 6-12 wks. with "good" results, especially in those with pustular acne and low glutathione peroxidase activity, and improvement was usually paralleled by a slow rise in glutathione peroxidase activity (*Michaëlsson G, Edqvist L. Erythrocyte glutathione peroxidase activity in acne vulgaris and the effect of selenium and vitamin E treatment. Acta Derm Venereol (Stockh) 64(1):9-14, 1984*).

Zinc: 90 - 135 mg. daily with meals (results in 1 - 3 months)

Serum levels may be reduced (*Pohit J et al. Zinc status of acne vulgaris patients. J Appl Nutr 37(1):18-25, 1985*).

Hair zinc may be reduced (*Pohit J et al. Zinc status of acne vulgaris patients. J Appl Nutr 37(1):18-25, 1985*).

Nail zinc may be reduced (*Pohit J et al. Zinc status of acne vulgaris patients. J Appl Nutr 37(1):18-25, 1985*).

Epidermal zinc levels may be reduced.

Observational Study: Pts. had reduced epidermal zinc levels despite normal serum zinc concentrations, suggesting zinc deficiency. There was no correlation between epidermal, dermal and serum zinc (*Michaëlsson G, Ljunghall K. Patients with dermatitis herpetiformis, acne, psoriasis and Darier's disease have low epidermal zinc concentrations. Acta Derm Venereol (Stockh) 70(4):304-8, 1990*).

Supplementation may be beneficial.

Note: Effervescent zinc sulfate, which was used in some of the studies, provides zinc as zinc citrate and zinc tartrate, not as zinc sulfate (Jaffe L. Zinc in acne. Letter. J Am Acad Dermatol 61:269, 1982).

Experimental Double-blind Study: Pts. with inflammatory acne received zinc gluconate 200 mg/d (30 mg elemental zinc). Following treatment, the inflammatory score in the zinc gp. was significantly lower than that of controls (p<0.02) (*Dreno B et al. Low doses of zinc gluconate for inflammatory acne. Acta Derm Venereol (Stockh) 69(6):541-3, 1989*).

Review Article: "The use of oral zinc . . . has gotten mixed reviews" (*Dobson RL, Nelson PF. What's new: A review of advances in therapy. J Am Acad Dermatol 5:323-27, 1981*).

— —

OTHER NUTRITIONAL FACTORS

Omega-6 Essential Fatty Acids:

Patients have a low concentration of linoleic acid in their sebum, and EFA deficiency in the pilosebaceous epithelium might account for follicular hyperkeratosis in acne (*Downing DT et al. Essential fatty acids and acne vulgaris. J Am Acad Dermatol 14:221-25, 1986*).

Observational Study: Acyl ceramides recovered from comedones contain much lesss linoleic acid than those from normal epidermis, suggesting that a localized insufficiency of linoleic acid in the follicular epithelium is an etiologic factor in comedogenesis (*Wertz PW et al. The composition of ceramides from human stratum corneum and from comedones. J Invest Dermatol 84:410-12, 1985*).

Observational Study: Levels of linoleic acid in sebum decrease progressively as the severity of acne increases (*Morello AM, Downing DT, Strauss JS. Octadecadienoic acids in the skin surface lipids of acne patients and normal subjects. J Invest Dermatol 66:319-23, 1976*).

All known nonantibiotic antiacne agents reduce sebum formation and thus are likely to increase the concentration of linoleic acid in sebum (*Horrobin DF. Essential fatty acids in clinical dermatology. J Am Acad Dermatol 20:1045-53, 1989*).

- with a low fat diet:

Supplementation may be beneficial.

Experimental Study: Supplementation with corn oil (which is rich in linoleic acid) appeared to improve the clinical course in acne pts. on low-fat diets (*Hubler WR. Unsaturated fatty acids in acne. Arch Dermatol 79:644, 1959*).

- -

OTHER FACTORS

Rule out food sensitivities.

General:

Negative Experimental Study: 120 pts. underwent intracutaneous allergen testing with 23 of the most important food antigens. Test results on 83/120 (69.2%) were negative. 9 pts. (7.4%) showed an immediate reaction on 4 or more extracts. Almonds showed the most positive reactions (11.6%), then malt (10%), cheese, mustard, red pepper (8.3% each), and wheat flour (7.5%). Pts. were placed on an elimination diet based on the results of skin testing, placed on an "acne diet," or told to follow no diet. After 3 mo. 45 pts. were evaluated and no statistical difference was found between the 3 groups. Although diet is generally not very significant, it can be possibly useful in some cases (*Wuthrich B, Much T. [Acne vulgaris: Results of food allergen tests and a controlled elimination diet.] Dermatologica 157(5):294-95, 1978 (in German)*

Review Article: "There is no well-documented study proving that foods aggravate acne. There are, however, statements of belief that this is so" (*Rasmussen JE. Diet and acne. Int J Dermatol 16:488-92, 1977*).

Negative Experimental Study: Over a 6 yr. period, each new pt. was questioned about prohibited foods and his actual experience linking diet to exacerbations of the acne. 8-10% of pts. claimed chocolate as a cause and 3-4% blamed nuts, cola or milk. Most of the pts. reporting associations believed that their acne worsened substantially within 36 hrs. after eating the prohibited food, worsened in proportion to the amt. of food eaten, and the acne flare lasted 3-5 day afterwards. Gps. of 4-8 subjects, all sensitive to the same food, ate large amts. of that food daily for 1 wk. and changes in the appearance of their acne were objectively recorded. Absolutely no major flares of acne were produced by the foods. While 1/3 of subjects developed new lesions during the 10 days of the tests, these were within the expected variation for control patients, and almost half of the pts. showed slight improvement (*Anderson PC. Foods as a cause of acne. Am Fam Physician 3(3):102-03, 1971*).

Chocolate:

Review Article: Although there are specific contraindications to the ingestion of chocolate by selected individuals, these do not apply to the general population with high frequency (*Fries JH. Chocolate: A review of published reports of allergic and other deleterious effects, real or presumed. Ann Allergy 41(4):195-207, 1978*).

Experimental Double-blind Study: Of 500 allergy pts., 16.2% believed that chocolate caused allergic symptoms, but only 10 manifested very specific allergic symptoms within a predictable time after eating chocolate. 8 of these ten were fed both placebos and defatted chocolate in capsule form. In 3/8, the reported clinical symptoms were reproduced after ingestion of the cocoa capsules, but not after the placebos. Only 1 of these 3 had a positive skin test to chocolate (*Maslansky L, Wein G. Effect of chocolate on acne vulgaris. Letter. JAMA 211(11):1856, 1970*).

Negative Experimental Double-blind Study: 65 adolescents were feed either unusually large amts. of chocolate or a placebo bar of candy. Evaluation was made in measurement of quantity, composition and comedogenic potency of sebum. Results suggested that "ingestion of high amounts of chocolate did not materially affect the course of acne vulgaris or the output or composition of sebum" (*Fulton JE et al. Effect of chocolate on acne vulgaris. JAMA 210:2071, 1969*).

> *Note: This study has been criticized because the placebo candy bar did not differ sufficiently from chocolate in its fat and sugar content, and the adverse effects of chocolate may be due, in fact, to its high content of molecular carbons, enhanced by the content of sugar and xanthines, which are said to cause diminished fluidiy of sebum (Acne, soap, and chocolate. Editorial. Med J Aust 1:584, 1975; Mackie BS, Mackie LE. Chocolate and acne. Aust J Dermatol 15:103-09, 1974).*

Milk:

Has been said to aggravate acne due either to its progesterone content or to its animal fat content.

> **Negative Observational Study:** Sex hormones known to produce acne were not detectable in bovine milk when analyzed by methods capable of detecting concentrations less than 10 µg of testosterone and androsterone and 15 µg of estradiol glucuronides/liter, suggesting that milk ingestion could not be the cause of acne based on its conjugated hormone content (*Brewington CR et al. Evidence for the absence of the conjugates of acne-causing hormones in cow's milk. Proc Soc Exp Biol Med 139(3):745-48, 1972*).

Azelaic Acid:

A natural product of Pityrosporum ovale.

Topical application may be beneficial.

> **Experimental Double-blind Study:** 40 pts. received topically either 20% azelaic acid in a cream base or the cream base alone. After 1,2 and 3 mo., azelaic acid was significantly better than placebo in terms of overall acne grade and inflamed lesions. Side effects were minimal. When compared to benzoyl peroxide, retinoic acid and oral tetracycline in an 8 mo. study involving 859 pts., it caused significantly less dermatitis than either benzoyl peroxide or retinoic acid (*Norris J et al. Azelaic acid really does work in acne - a double-blind national and international study. Br J Dermatol 32(Suppl):34, 1987*).

> **Experimental Double-blind Study:** 45 male pts. received either topical azelaic acid or oral tetracycline. After 6 mo., both treatments were beneficial, with tetracycline slightly more effective. Azelaic acid caused few side-effects and considerably reduced the number of cutaneous microorganisms (*Bladon PT et al. Topical azelaic acid and the treatment of acne: A clinical and laboratory comparison with oral tetracycline. Br J Dermatol 114:493, 1986*).

High-Chromium yeast: 1 tsp. 2 times daily (≈400 µg chromium)

Skin glucose tolerance (but **not** oral glucose tolerance) is significantly impaired in acne vulgaris (*Abdel KM et al. Glucose tolerance in blood and skin of patients with acne vulgaris. Int J Dermatol 22:139-49, 1977*).

Supplementation with high chromium yeast improves oral glucose tolerance and enhances insulin sensitivity, probably due to its chromium content (*Offenbach E Pistunyer F. Beneficial effect of chromium-rich yeast on glucose tolerance and blood lipids in elderly patients. Diabetes 29:919-25, 1980*).

The benefits of high-chromium yeast may be due to the effect of insulin on essential fatty acid metabolism, since insulin induces delta-6-desaturase synthesis which is required for conversion of linoleic acid to prostaglandins (*McCarty M. High chromium yeast for acne? Med Hypotheses 14:307-10, 1984*).

Supplementation may be beneficial.

> **Experimental Study:** 10 pts. rapidly improved following supplementation with high-chromium yeast ("Chromax") 2 tsp daily providing 400 µg chromium (*Rubin D - reported in McCarty M. High chromium yeast for acne? Med Hypotheses 14:307-10, 1984*).

- -

COMBINED TREATMENT

Experimental Study: 98 pts. with acne of varying severity were treated. 31/98 had had acne for at least 10 years, and many of them had been unsuccessfully treated with oral antibiotics. On the following regime, 90/98 (92%) had a good to excellent response, 2 (2%) had a poor response and 42 (43%) had 90-100% clearing of their condition in 2 mo. or less:

1. Avoid inorganic iron (inactivates vitamin E).
2. Avoid female hormones (antagonistic to vitamin E).
3. Avoid extra iodine (can aggravate acne).
4. Avoid commencial soft drinks with brominated vegetable oils (can aggregate acne).
5. Avoid over 1 glass milk daily (hormones can aggravate acne).
6. Avoid vitamin B$_{12}$ (can produce or aggravate acne).
7. Vitamin A (water-soluble) 50,000 IU twice daily before meals.
8. Vitamin E (d,alpha-tocopheryl acetate or succinate) 400 IU twice daily before meals.
9. Pyridoxine 50 mg once or twice daily for premenstrual and menstrual acne.
10. Benzoyl peroxide 5% gel applied at night after washing gently with nonmedicated soap.
11. Well balanced diet, low in fat and sugars.

(Ayres S, Mihan R. Acne vulgaris: Therapy directed at pathophysiologic defects. Cutis 28:41-2, 1981)

ACQUIRED IMMUNODEFICIENCY SYNDROME (A.I.D.S.)

See Also: CANDIDIASIS
IMMUNODEFICIENCY
INFECTION

DIETARY FACTORS

Prevent and treat malnutrition.

The development of protein-energy malnutrition (PEM) is multifactorial and includes alterations in nutrient intake, absorption, and metabolism, all of which are potentially treatable. While the development of PEM has important ramifications for immune and cognitive function, and "quality of life," its effect upon the development and progression of AIDS is yet unknown. Recent studies have demonstrated the ability of AIDS pts. to replete body mass as a result of enteral or parenteral therapies or to respond favorably to appetite stimulants (*Kotler DP. Management of nutritional and disease gastroenterological problems in the acquired immunodeficiency syndrome. Abstract. J Am Coll Nutr 8(5):453, 1989*).

NUTRITIONAL FACTORS

General Review Article: Nutritional deficiencies can impair immunity and so influence susceptibility to infectious agents, including ones that are common and relatively virulent in AIDS. A variety of nutrients affect several of the immune functions that are defective in HIV-infected individuals. For example, beta-carotene increased the number of CD4$^+$ cells; vitamin D decreased the CD4$^+$/CD8$^+$ ratio; vitamin E decreased the number of CD8$^+$ cells and increased the CD4$^+$/CD8$^+$ ratio; and iron increased the number of peripheral lymphocytes in human receiving supplementation. Furthermore, nutritional deficiencies can influence GI function, while infectious diseases can influence nutrient requirements by altering the efficiency of absorption and the rate of tissue metabolism. Malnutrition, depressed serum zinc levels, and intestinal nutrient malabsorption have been found in AIDS patients. These findings suggest that dietary manipulations might diminish the immune defects in HIV infection and enhance resistance to opportunistic infections; however, dietary alterations in immune defects are generally not well quantified and may be small relative to the magnitude of the defects observed in AIDS patients. Because conflicting or adverse effects have been reported for some nutrients, recommendations for dietary supplementation in HIV-infected pts. are premature and possibly hazardous (*Moseson M et al. The potential role of nutritional factors in the induction of immunologic abnormalities in HIV-positive homosexual men. J Acquir Immune Defic Syndr 2(3):235-47, 1989*).

VITAMINS

Folic Acid:

Levels may be reduced.

Observational Study: 74 HIV-infected pts. aged 17-68 were studied using microbiological assays. Controls consisted of healthy seronegative individuals. For people not supplemented with folic or folinic acid and not taking antifolate drugs, serum and RBC folate was significantly decreased. Folate deficiency, evidenced by a significant decrease in serum and/or RBC folate, was frequent, being found in 64% and 57%, respectively, of the HIV-infected, nonsupplemented patients. This deficiency was observed at all stages of HIV infection. Of the unsupplemented pts., none had a raised serum or RBC folate while, in the supplemented gp., 56% had a raised serum folate and none had a decreased serum or RBC folate level. Because many of the drugs used to treat opportunistic infections function via an antifolate mechanism, their use in this population could be a major cause of hematological side-effects (*Poudes P et al. Folate, vitamin B12, and HIV infection. Letter. Lancet 335:1401-02, 1990*).

Negative Observational Study: 58% of 100 homosexual HIV-positive men who were asymptomatic except for lymphadenopathy had significantly elevated plasma and RBC folate levels by microbiological assay as compared to 300 controls. While many pts. were taking multivitamin supplements, these supplements frequently did not contain folate and no pt. was taking >400 μg folate, the recommended daily intake. As the pharmacologic agents employed to treat the opportunistic infections that frequently plague the HIV-infected pt. function through an antifolate mechanism, there may be a relationship between the elevated levels and the illness (*Beach RS et al. Altered folate metabolism in early HIV infection. JAMA 259(4):519, 1988*).

> *Note: It is possible that pts. with elevated plasma and RBC folate levels were vitamin B12-deficient since, in B12 deficiency, serum folate levels (as measured as 5-methyl tetrahydrofolate) are elevated. This is because vitamin B12 is needed for the demethylation of 5-methyl tetrahydrofolate, a substance which is not available for cellular DNA synthesis. Also, significant cell destruction in a catabolic state can cause transient elevation of extracellular nutrients (Tilkian SM et al. Altered folate metabolism in early HIV infection. Letter. JAMA 259:3128-29, 1988).*

Deficiency may cause neurological degeneration.

Case Reports: 2 children aged 2 1/2 yrs. presented with neurological disease due to congenital infection with HIV and were found to have reduced concentrations of total folates in cerebrospinal fluid in the range associated with progressive demyelination. Plasma and RBC folate was low in one of the pts., who was also anemic. There were no megaloblastic changes on peripheral blood films. One pt. had areas of low attenuation in the subcortical white matter on computerized tomography, while the other had bilateral calcification in the basal ganglia. Similar lesions have been seen in children with defective folate metabolism (*Smith I et al. Folate deficiency and demyelination in AIDS. Lancet 2:215, 1987*).

Thiamine:

Neuropathological changes characteristic of Wernike's encephalopathy, which results from thiamine deficiency, have been repeatedly described post-mortem in non-alcoholic AIDS patients (*Davtyan DG, Vinters HV. Wernicke's encephalopathy in AIDS patient treated with zidovudine. Letter. Lancet 1:919-20, 1987; Foresti V, Confalonieri F. Wernike's encephalopathy in AIDS. Letter. Lancet 1:1499, 1987; Lindboe CF, Loberg EM. Wernicke's encephalopathy in non-alcoholics: an autopsy study. J Neurol Sci 90:125-9, 1989; Schwenk J et al. Wernicke's encephalopathy in two patients with acquired immunodeficiency syndrome. J Neurol 7:445-7, 1990*).

May be deficient.

Observational Study: 39 pts. with AIDS or AIDS-related complex were studied at various stages of the disease. In no case was there a history of alcohol abuse or any neurological symptoms suggestive of Wernicke's encephalopathy. 9/39 (23%) pts., 8 of whom were receiving zidovudine, had a thiamine pyrophosphate % activation (TPP effect) of >15%, indicating a moderate-to-severe thiamine deficiency (*Butterworth RF et al. Thiamine deficiency in AIDS. Letter. Lancet 338:1086, 1991*).

Vitamin A:

Supplementation may be beneficial.

Theoretical Discussion and Review Article: It is hypothesized that supplemental vitamin A or β-carotene may both decrease tumor incidence and mortality rates and prevent the enhancement of mortality rates due to trauma, cytotoxic agents, chemicals, radiation, etc. In one study, topical retinoic acid reversed "hairy" leukoplakia in an AIDS pt. while, in another study, the morbidity and mortality of mice which developed an AIDS-like syndrome following inoculation with a murine leukemic virus was reduced by supplemental vitamin A (*Kanofsky JD et al. Is there a role for vitamin A or β-carotene in HIV therapy? Poster presentation at the 31st Annual Meeting, American College of Nutrition, October 13-15, 1990*).

Vitamin B₁₂:

Metabolism may be abnormal and associated with both peripheral neuropathy and myelopathy.

Observational Study: 20% of a gp. of HIV-infected pts. referred for neurological evaluation tested for vitamin B₁₂ status showed abnormal vitamin B₁₂ metabolism. This abnormality was associated with both peripheral neuropathy and myelopathy (*Kieburtz K et al. Abnormal vitamin B₁₂ metabolism in human immunodeficiency virus infection. Arch Neurol 48:312-14, 1991*).

Plasma/serum levels may be reduced.

Observational Study: 74 HIV-infected pts. aged 17-68 were studied using microbiological assays. Controls consisted of healthy seronegative individuals. For people not supplemented with vitamin B₁₂, the mean plasma B₁₂ was significantly reduced. Vitamin B₁₂ deficiency, evidenced by decreased plasma vitamin B₁₂ levels, was present in 10% of the pts. (mainly in CDC stage IV disease), while a slightly increased B₁₂ level was present in 29% of the patients. Because low B₁₂ levels may be associated with an increased risk of hematological toxic effects in pts. on zidovudine, and because folic acid treatment may cause neurological injury when given to patients with B₁₂ deficiency, assays for serum vitamin B₁₂ are advised for HIV-infected patients (*Poudes P et al. Folate, vitamin B₁₂, and HIV infection. Letter. Lancet 335:1401-02, 1990*).

Observational Study: 3/11 (27%) AIDS pts. had low serum vitamin B₁₂ levels and 8/11 (73%) had abnormal Schilling test results. In addition, 15% of 121 unselected AIDS pts. and 7% of 27 pts. without AIDS but who were seropositive for HIV-1 had low serum vitamin B₁₂ levels (*Harriman GR et al. Vitamin B₁₂ malabsorption in patients with acquired immunodeficiency syndrome. Arch Intern Med 149(9):2039-41, 1989*).

If metabolism is abnormal, supplementation may reverse neurological signs and symptoms.

Experimental Study: HIV-infected pts. with abnormal vitamin B₁₂ metabolism and peripheral neuropathy or myelopathy showed a therapeutic response to treatment with vitamin B₁₂. Vacuolar myelopathy was especially responsive (*Kieburtz K et al. Abnormal vitamin B₁₂ metabolism in human immunodeficiency virus infection. Arch Neurol 48:312-14, 1991*).

- and/or Folic Acid:

Supplementation may reduce the toxicity of azidothymidine (AZT) (*Herzlich BC et al. Synergy of inhibition of DNA synthesis in human bone marrow by azidothymidine plus deficiency of folate and/or vitamin B₁₂? Am J Hematology 33:177-83, 1990*).

Vitamin C:

Plasma level may be reduced.

Observational Study: 17 pts. with mild or severe ARC, 7 with AIDS, and 6 asymptomatic HIV-positive pts. were studied. In this gp., 8 had experienced 10 or more lbs. of weight loss in the the past 6 mo. and 93% were anergic to skin test antigens. 27% had below normal plasma ascorbate concentrations (*Bogden JD et al. Micronutrient status and human immunodeficiency virus (HIV) infection. Ann N Y Acad Sci 587:189-95, 1990*).

Supplementation may be beneficial.

In vitro Experimental Study: Ascorbate was found to mediate an anti-HIV effect by diminishing viral protein production in infected cells and reverse transcriptase stability in extracellular virions (*Harakeh S, Jariwalla RJ, Pauling L. Suppression of human immunodeficiency virus replication by ascorbate in chronically and acutely infected cells. Proc Natl Acad Sci U S A 87(18):7245-9, 1990*).

In vitro Experimental Study: Continuous exposure of HIV-infected T-lymphocyte culture lines to non-cytotoxic ascorbate concentrations physiologically obtainable in blood plasma resulted in significant inhibition of both virus replication in chronically infected cells and multinucleated giant-cell formation in acutely infected cells (*Harakeh

S et al.   Suppression of human immunodeficiency virus replication by ascorbate in chronically and acutely infected cells.   J Nutr Med 1:345-6, 1990).

Clinical Observation: Preliminary clinical evidence based on experience with over 250 HIV-positive pts. is that massive doses of ascorbate (20-200 gms/24 hrs) can suppress symptoms and markedly reduce the tendency for secondary infections. Pts. are instructed to titrate the dose until it relieves the toxic symptoms or almost produces diarrhea. The depletion of CD4$^+$ T-cells is slowed, stopped, or sometimes reversed for several yrs. when doses close to tolerance are maintained. In addition, a topical vitamin C paste can be very effective in the treatment of herpes simplex and, to a lesser extent, some Kaposi's lesions (*Cathcart RF 3rd. Glutathione and HIV infection. Letter. Lancet 1:235, 1990; Cathcart RF 3rd. Vitamin C in the treatment of acquired immune deficiency syndrome (AIDS). Med Hypotheses 14(4):423-33, 1984*).

Clinical Observations: AIDS pts. were treated with an "ascorbate flush and fill" technique as follows: Treatment was initiated with 1/4 to 1 level tsp. of sodium ascorbate 2-3 times daily with an increase in the frequency to every 6 hrs., every 4 hrs., and then even every 2 hrs. until the development of diarrhea (the level of the "ascorbate flush"). Since higher therapeutic levels can be achieved during acute stresses (such as following cytotoxic drug therapy or a severe bout of influenza), attempts must continue to be made to further increase the ascorbate intake to obtain an 'ascorbate fill,' the level at which the tissues are saturated. The addition of massive doses of IV ascorbate (up to 250 gm in 24 hrs.) helps to achieve such a 'fill.' After improvement, the IV program is gradually scaled down. With the use of the 'flush and fill' technique, killer T cell activity and the T helper/T suppressor ratio were improved. The lesions of Kaposi's sarcoma were suppressed and even in some cases eliminated (*Brighthope I. AIDS - Remissions using nutrient therapies and megadose intravenous ascorbate. Int Clin Nutr Rev 7(2):53-75, 1987*).

- with N-acetyl-L-cysteine or glutathione:

In vitro Experimental Study: The effects of nontoxic concentrations of ascorbic acid (AA), its calcium salt, and 2 thiol-based reducing agents, glutathione (GSH) and N-acetyl-L-cysteine (NAC) against HIV-1 replication in chronically infected T lymphocytes were compared. Calcium ascorbate reduced extracellular HIV reverse transcriptase (RT) activity by about the same magnitude as AA. Long-term experiments showed that continuous presence of AA was necessary for HIV suppression. NAC caused less than twofold inhibition of HIV RT and conferred a synergistic effect (about 8-fold inhibition) when tested simultaneously with AA. In contrast, nonesterified GSH had no effect on RT concentrations and did not potentiate the anit-HIV effect of AA (*Harakeh S, Jariwalla RJ. Comparative study of the anti-HIV activities of ascorbate and thiol-containing reducing agents in chronically HIV-infected cells. Am J Clin Nutr 54:1231S-5S, 1991*).

Vitamin E:

Supplementation may be beneficial.

Theoretical Discussion: Among the possible effects of the HIV virus on T-cells in AIDS is the cell membrane distortion of the T4 cell protein receptor for Genetically Related Macrophage Factor (GRF). The integrity of this specific T-cell receptor takes on profound significance due to its relationship to soluble antigen. Alpha-tocopherol has been shown to assist in the maintenance of cell membrane structure and may have application in a strategy of membrane restoration (*Hollins TD. T4 cell receptor distortion in acquired immune deficiency syndrome. Med Hypotheses 26(2):107-11, 1988*).

- -

MINERALS

Calcium:

Plasma levels may be reduced (*Bogden JD et al. Micronutrient status and human immunodeficiency virus (HIV) infection. Ann N Y Acad Sci 587:189-95, 1990*).

Germanium:

Administration of germanium sesquioxide may be beneficial.

Experimental Placebo-controlled Study: 20 Mexican volunteers with AIDS were given germanium or placebo together with standard treatment. After 18 mo., the health of 80% of the germanium gp. improved (*Germanium. Artsenkrant Belgium 20:397, 1988*).

Conference Report: Organic germanium is one of the six medications recommended for intensive clinical testing on AIDS pts. It is considered to be somewhat effective for those who are infected with AIDS for the purpose of preventing them from falling into CDC gps. 3 or 4 and has been found to have a low toxicity (*Report from the International AIDS Treatment Conference, Tokyo, Japan, February 13-14, 1987*).

Magnesium:

Plasma levels may be reduced (*Bogden JD et al. Micronutrient status and human immunodeficiency virus (HIV) infection. Ann N Y Acad Sci 587:189-95, 1990*).

Potassium:

May be deficient (*Kotler DP et al. Body composition studies in patients with the acquired immunodeficiency syndrome. Am J Clin Nutr 42(6):1255-65, 1985*).

Selenium:

May be deficient (*Dworkin BM et al. Selenium deficiency in the acquired immunodeficiency syndrome. J Parenter Enteral Nutr 10(4):405-07, 1986*).

Zinc: Up to 150 mg daily for 3-6 mo. to correct marginal deficiencies (<0.9 µg/g serum)
(*Shambaugh GE Jr. Zinc and AID S. J Appl Nutr 40(20):138-39, 1989*).

Zinc is an important element for immune system functioning (*see "IMMUNODEFICIENCY"*).

Multiple ejaculations of semen, with its high zinc content, might theoretically increase the risk of zinc deficiency (*Prasad AS. Ann Rev Nutr 5:341, 1985*).

Serum levels may be reduced (*Bogden JD et al. Micronutrient status and human immunodeficiency virus (HIV) infection. Ann N Y Acad Sci 587:189-95, 1990; Falutz J et al. Zinc as a cofactor in human immunodeficiency virus-induced immunosuppression. Letter. JAMA 259(19):2850-51, 1988*).

Low zinc levels may be responsible for the reduced thymic secretory function seen in patients with AIDS and AIDS-related complex.

Observational Study: Serum zinc levels and plasma concentrations of active thymulin and of total zinc-saturable thymulin were measured in 7 AIDS pts., 12 lymphadenopathy syndrome (LAS) pts., 10 healthy controls and 9 age-matched drug users who were uninfected with HIV. AIDS pts. showed significantly reduced serum zinc concentrations (p<0.001) and nearly undetectable levels of circulating thymulin (p<0.001) but normal levels of total zinc-saturable thymulin when compared to healthy controls. LAS pts. had values between those recorded for healthy controls and those of AIDS patients. These findings demonstrate that the reduced thymulin level is due to decreased zinc saturation at the peripheral level, which probably depends on a concomitant zinc deficiency. The low values of zinc and thymulin in AIDS pts., which approach those found in the most severe congenital zinc deficiency (acrodermatitis enteropathica), raise the question of whether some of the immunologic defects observed in AIDS and LAS might depend on concomitant alterations in zinc, and suggest that zinc supplementation may prevent or correct the immune derangement seen in the course of HIV infection (*Fabris N et al. AIDS, zinc deficiency, and thymic hormone failure. Letter. JAMA 259(6):839-40, 1988*).

– –

OTHER NUTRITIONAL FACTORS

<u>Amino Acids</u>:

- <u>Arginine</u>:

Supplementation may enhance natural killer cell activity.

Experimental Study: Arginine 30 g/d for 3 days increased the number of circulating $CD56^+$ cells by a median of 32% (p<0.01) in 8 volunteers. This increase was associated with a mean rise of 91% in natural killer (NK) cell activity (p=0.003) and of 58% in the cell activity of their activated counterparts, lymphokine-activated-killer (LAK) cells, (p=0.001) in 13 volunteers. The substantial enhancement of human NK and LAK cell activity by arginine could be useful in many immunosuppressed states, such as AIDS and HIV infection, in which depressed NK cell activity is an important component of the disease process (*Park KGM et al. Stimulation of lymphocyte natural cytotoxicity by L-arginine. Lancet 337:645-6, 1991*).

- <u>Cysteine</u>:

Precursor to glutathione.

(*See also "<u>Glutathione</u>" below*)

Plasma levels may be reduced (*Jarstrand C et al. Glutathione and HIV infection. Letter. Lancet 1:234-36, 1990*).

N-acetyl cysteine (NAC), because of the addition of an acetyl group, is a more stable form of cysteine and is more active biologically (*Issels RD et al. Promotion of cystine uptake and its utilization for glutathione biosynthesis induced by cysteamine and N-acetylcysteine. Biochem Pharmacol 37:881, 1988; Saez G et al. The production of free radicals during the auto-oxidation of cysteine and their effect on isolated rat hepatocytes. Biochim Biophys Acta 719:24, 1982*).

Administration of N-acetyl cysteine (NAC) may be beneficial.

In vitro Experimental Study: In a study using the chronically infected monocytic U1 cell line as a cellular model for HIV latency, NAC suppressed the induction of HIV expression mediated by PMA, TNF-α, and IL-6. Reverse transcriptase activity was decreased 80-90% after pretreatment with NAC, and the accumulation of HIV mRNA was substantially suppressed (*Kalebic T et al. Suppression of human immunodeficiency virus expression in chronically infected monocytic cells by glutathione, glutathione ester, and N-acetyl cysteine. Proc Natl Acad Sci U S A 88:986-90, 1991*).

Clinical Observation: Pts. most likely to benefit from administration of NAC are those with cachexia. They rapidly feel better and then regain weight (*James JS. AIDS Treatment News, Issue #88, October 6, 1989*).

Note: NAC is available in Europe as Fluimucil and is usually taken as 600 mg (1 tablet) 3 times daily or 400 mg (1 packet of powder) 4 times daily. It is not available for oral use in the US (*James JS. AIDS Treatment News, Issue #88, October 6, 1989*).

- <u>Cystine</u>:

Plasma level may be reduced (*Dröge W et al. Abnormal amino-acid concentrations in the blood of patients with acquired immunodeficiency syndrome (AIDS) may contribute to the immunological defect. Biol Chem Hoppe-Seyler 369:143-48. 1988*).

- Methionine:

Plasma level may be reduced (*Dröge W et al. Abnormal amino-acid concentrations in the blood of patients with acquired immunodeficiency syndrome (AIDS) may contribute to the immunological defect. Biol Chem Hoppe-Seyler 369:143-48. 1988*).

Beta-carotene:

Plasma level may be reduced (*Bogden JD et al. Micronutrient status and human immunodeficiency virus (HIV) infection. Ann N Y Acad Sci 587:189-95, 1990*).

Choline:

Plasma level may be reduced (*Bogden JD et al. Micronutrient status and human immunodeficiency virus (HIV) infection. Ann N Y Acad Sci 587:189-95, 1990*).

Chondroitin Polysulfate:

Supplementation may be beneficial.

In vitro Experimental Study: 3 chondroitin sulfates and 5 chondroitin polysulfates were evaluated *in vitro* for inhibition of HIV-1 replication and compared to results obtained with compounds of known antiretroviral activity. Chondroitin polysulfate with a molecular weight of 9000 daltons (CPS 9000) was the most effective polyanionic compound studied. In contrast with zidovudine, it was not toxic for MT-4 cells up to a concentration of 500 µg/ml (*Jurkiewicz E et al. In vitro anti-HIV-1 activity of chondroitin polysulphate. AIDS 3(7):423-27, 1989*).

Coenzyme Q$_{10}$:

Supplementation may be beneficial.

Experimental and Observational Study: Compared to controls, blood levels of CoQ$_{10}$ in both AIDS and ARC (AIDS-related complex) patients were significantly lower (p<0.001), with AIDS pts. having lower levels than ARC patients (p<0.01). 7 pts. with AIDS or ARC were treated with CoQ$_{10}$ 200 mg daily. One was lost to follow-up and one expired after stopping CoQ$_{10}$. The other 5 pts. improved symptomatically and had no opportunistic infections after 4-7 months. T$_4$/T$_8$ ratios increased in 3/5 pts., and became normal in 1 case. There were no side effects (*Folkers K et al. Biochemical deficiencies of coenzyme Q$_{10}$ in HIV-infection and exploratory treatment. Biochem Biophys Res Commun 153:888-96, 1988*).

Essential Fatty Acids:

Theoretical Discussion: Gamma-linolenic acid (an omega-6 fatty acid) and/or eicosapentaenoic acid (an omega-3 fatty acid) and their derivatives may be the source of natural endogenous agents against AIDS by preventing the spread of viral infection (due to their ability to destroy enveloped viruses), by controlling cancer development either directly (due to their cytostatic and cytotoxic effects on cancer cells) or indirectly (by modulating the immune response and by protecting from genetic damage). Supplementation with these polyunsaturated fatty acids should be considered in the prevention, and possibly the treatment, of AIDS (*Bëgin ME, Das UN. A deficiency in dietary gamma-linolenic and/or eicosapentaenoic acids may determine individual susceptibility to AIDS. Med Hypotheses 20(1):1-8, 1986*).

- Omega-3 Fatty Acids:

Supplementation may be beneficial.

Theoretical Discussion: The dietary ratio of omega-6 fatty acids (linoleic acid) to omega-3 fatty acids (linolenic acid, EPA, DHA) for all of human history prior to the 19th century has been estimated to be about 1:1. Currently the ratio in industrialized nations hovers around 5:1. Japan, with its heavy fish consumption and low animal and vegetable fat intake, is an exception. In Japan, AIDS is extremely rare, suggesting that excessive linoleic acid consumption in other industrialized nations may promote AIDS by activating macrophages and suppressing lymphocytes (*Smith RS. Is fish oil protective against AIDS? J Orthomol Med 6:2, 64-66*).

Theoretical Discussion: Critical concentrations of prostaglandin E (which is derived from the essential fatty acids) may be needed for the HIV virus to facilitate its entry into a lymphocyte. If so, lowering PGE levels in high risk gps. using aspirin, alone or in combination with eicosapentaenoic acid (an omega-3 fatty acid), would stop the ability of HIV to attack helper T cells and so prevent multiplication of the virus (*Vaddadi KS, Das UN. HIV virus, prostaglandins and essential fatty acids; a suggested mechanism for T helper cell penetration. Med Hypotheses 26:229-30, 1988*).

- Omega-6 Fatty Acids:

Supplementation may be beneficial.

Theoretical Discussion: Repeated viral infections may disrupt the biosynthesis of prostaglandin E_1 (PGE$_1$) which plays an important role in the regulation of T lymphocyte function and thus may contribute to the risk of developing acquired immunodeficiency syndrome. In order to restore PGE$_1$ synthesis, the author suggests supplementation with gammalinolenic acid in addition to:
1. Pyridoxine (assists in the conversion of GLA to DGLA)
2. Ascorbic acid IV along with L-lysine (assists in the conversion of DGLA to PGE$_1$ and enhances interferon production and phagocytic activity)
3. Zinc (assists in the conversion of DGLA to PGE$_1$)
4. Eicosapentaenoic acid (inhibits the conversion of DGLA to arachidonic acid)
5. Niacin (assists in the synthesis of the anti-oxidant NADPH)
6. Riboflavin (assists in the synthesis of glutathione reductase).
(*Marcus SH. Breakdown of PGE₁ synthesis is responsible for the acquired immunodeficiency syndrome. Med Hypotheses 15:39-46, 1984*).

- Omega-3 Fatty Acids and
  Omega-6 Fatty Acids:

Combined supplementation may be beneficial.

Experimental Double-blind Crossover Study: 18 ARC pts. were randomized with regard to AZT treatment status and received either 240 GLA, an omega-6 fatty acid, and 960 mg EPA, an omega-3 fatty acid, divided into 16 capsules daily (OmegaSyn™) or placebo. After 6 mo., pts. rated themselves on a "quality of life" scale. The scale was significantly higher ($p \leq 0.0005$) for the experimental gp. vs. the placebo group; it also was significantly higher ($p \leq 0.025$) for experimental pts. on AZT vs. placebo pts. on AZT. In both instances, the "quality of life" improved for experimental pts., while it worsened for placebo patients. Pts. on placebo were then switched to the experimental regimen. After 5 mo., their ave. "quality of life" ratings were better than at the start of the study 11 mo. earlier ($p \leq 0.01$). The sub-gp. of pts. on AZT showed similar gains, but the results were not significant. Further data analysis suggests that the reduction of fatigue was the major factor influencing the improvement in quality of life ratings. It is hypothesized that the fatgue associated with ARC may be caused by an essential fatty acid deficiency causing reduced oxgen transfer to muscle cells (*OmegaSyn™ as a dietary intervention in ARC patients. Unpublished study. BioSyn, 21 Tioga Way, Marblehead, MA 01945, 1989*).

Glutathione:

(*See also "Cysteine" above*)

A tripeptide composed of the amino acids cysteine, glutamic acid and glycine.

Important to cellular defense against the damaging effects of free radicals.

May be deficient in HIV-seropositive individuals.

Observational Study: Total and reduced glutathione concentrations in venous plasma of symptom-free HIV-seropositive pts. were about 30% of those of normals, while total and reduced glutathione concentrations in lung epithelial lining fluid were about 60% of those of normals. Since glutathione enhances immune function, glutathione deficiency may contribute to the progressive immune dysfunction of HIV infections (*Buhl R et al. Systemic glutathione deficiency in symptom-free HIV-seropositive individuals. Lancet 2:1294-97, 1989*).

Supplementation may be beneficial.

In vitro Experimental Study: Glutathione (GSH), glutathione ester (GSE), and N-acetylcysteine (NAC) suppressed in a dose-dependent fashion the induction of HIV expression in a chronically infected monocytic cell line (as mediated by PMA, TNF-alpha, and IL-6) in the absence of cytotoxic or cytostatic effects. Reverse transcriptase activity, inducible by PMA, TNF-alpha, and IL-6, was decreased 80-90% by pretreatment with GSH, GSE or NAC. The accumulation of HIV mRNA was substantially suppressed after pretreatment with NAC but to a lesser extent after pretreatment with GSH or GSE. These findings suggest that therapy with thiols may be of value in the treatment of HIV infection (*Kalebic T et al. Suppression of human immunodeficiency virus expression in chronically infected monocytic cells by glutathione, glutathione ester, and N-acetylcysteine. Proc Natl Acad Sci U S A 88(3):986-90, 1991*).

Administration of N-acetylcysteine (NAC) may increase glutathione levels in patients by serving as a nutritional precursor for glutathione synthesis (*Corcoran GB, Wong BK. Role of glutathione in prevention of acetaminophen-induced hepatotoxicity by N-acetyl-L-cysteine in vivo: Studies with N-acetyl-D-cysteine in mice. J Pharmacol Exp Ther 238:54-61, 1986; Lauterburg BH et al. Mechanism of action of N-acetylcysteine in the protection against the hepatotoxicity of acetaminophen in rats in vivo. J Clin Invest 71:980-91, 1983*).

- -

OTHER FACTORS

Egg Lipid Extract (AL 721): 10g daily after an overnight fast

A potent membrane fluidizer extracted from egg yolks, which operates by extracting cholesterol from the cell membrane, consisting of 70% neutral lipids, 20% phosphatidylcholine and 10% phosphatidylethanolamine (*Lyte M, Shinitzky M. A special lipid mixture for membrane fluidization. Biochim Biophys Acta 812:133-38, 1985*).

Note: The phosphatidylethanolamine (PE) content is most relevant because PE is virtually the sole source of arachidonic acid in the product, and arachidonic acid is essential for supporting the signal transduction functions of cell membranes, as well as being the major source of secondary messenger molecules that interact with the immune system. Four commercial formulas were assayed; the percent of PE is as follows: HNLEL®, Lucas Meyer GmbH, Hamburg: 6%; Houba, Premier: 4%; PE9+/Prem. Ovalectin, Nutri-cology: 4%; AL-721, Ethigen: 2% (Kidd PM, Huber W. One good dinner per month. Letter. Townsend Letter for Doctors December, 1989).

Extraction of cholesterol from HIV with egg lipid extract may decrease its infectivity.

In vitro Experimental Study: Extraction of HIV cholesterol with AL 721 induced a marked reduction, or even complete abolishment, of its infectivity (*Crews FT et al. J Cell Biochem Suppl 11D:304, 1987*).

Administration may be beneficial.

Review Article: In antigen-negative and asymptomatic pts., AL 721 seems to arrest the disease at the asymptomatic stage and to prevent further development to antigenemia. In antigen-positive asymptomatic pts., the antigen level is reduced in most cases and is retained at the basal level as long as AL 721 treatment continues. However, AL 721 is practically ineffective in pts. with a high load of HIV. Marked improvements in overt clinical and personal parameters like fever, diarrhea, weight, appetite, physical and social activities, were observed in virtually all pts. receiving AL 721. As all studies have been uncontrolled, the placebo effect may play a role. The observed effect of treatment on leukocyte count was positive but marginal (*Shinitzky M et al. Lipid regimens for the treatment of AIDS, in RR Watson, Ed. Cofactors in HIV-1 Infection and AIDS. Boca Raton, FL, CRC Press, 1990*).

Experimental Study: 16 HIV sero-positive pts., 7 of whom were antigen-negative and asymptomatic and the other 9 of whom were antigen-positive and virtually asymptomatic, received AL 721 10 g daily in a fat-free breakfast for up to 16 months. The presence of HIV antigens in the serum was monitored by enzyme immunoassay. In 5/9 antigen-positive pts., HIV antigen concentration was reduced to a basal level after about 3 months. 3

of these pts. were asymptomaic, 1 suffered by PGL and 1 had Kaposi's sarcoma. In one of the antigen-positive pts. who did not respond, the addition of AZT to the treatment resulted in a marked decrease in antigen level. In another AIDS pt., this combination from the onset resulted in a similar decrease. The 2 other non-responding pts. were at the stage of full-blown AIDS. These results suggest that AL 721, an innocuous compound, may be effective in reducing the serum HIV level in pts. at the pre-clinical stage (*Yust I et al. Reduction of circulating HIV antigens in seropositive patients after treatment with AL-721. Isr J Med Sci 26(1):20-6, 1990*).

Negative Experimental Study: 7 homosexual men (5 with AIDS, 1 with ARC) who had declined zidovudine received AL 721 15 g twice daily. After 12 wks., there was no clinical or laboratory evidence of benefit (*Peters BS et al. Ineffectiveness of AL721 in HIV disease. Letter Lancet 335:545-46, 1990*).

Proteolytic Enzymes:

Administration may be beneficial.

Theoretical Discussion: Hydrolytic enzyme combinations such as Wobe-Mugos® or Wobenzym® (Mucos-Pharma, Geretsried, Germany) may possibly reduce immune deficiency and support immune defenses by mobilizing and eliminating tissue-bound and circulating HIV-induced immune complexes (*Stauder G et al. The use of hydrolytic enzymes as adjuvant therapy in AIDS/ARC/LAS patients. Biomed Pharmacother 42:31-34, 1988*).

Rule out food and chemical sensitivities:

Clinical Observation: Food and chemical sensitivities occur frequently in pts. and may aggravate symptoms considered to be part of the syndrome (*Cathcart RF 3rd. Vitamin C in the treatment of acquired immune deficiency syndrome (AIDS). Med Hypotheses 14(4):423-33, 1984*).

ALCOHOLISM

See Also: HEPATITIS   MYOPATHY
        "HYPOGLYCEMIA"   NEURALGIA & NEUROPATHY

> *KEY:*   *C* = *may affect craving for alcohol*
>   *T* = *may affect alcohol toxicity*
>   *W* = *may affect symptoms of alcohol withdrawal*

OVERVIEW

There are many nutritional deficiencies which may be caused by excessive alcohol ingestion, and deficient nutrient intake is commonly associated with alcoholism. By improving nutritional status, not only may it be possible to prevent some of the diseases associated with alcoholism, but there is preliminary evidence that both alcohol craving and the symptoms of alcohol withdrawal may be ameliorated.

1. Reducing toxicity.

   Many of the toxic effects of alcoholism are due, not to alcohol, but to the associated nutritional deficiencies. A well-balanced, nutritionally adequate is often protective. However, due to impairments in utilizing ingested nutrients, nutritional supplementation is often required. Protective nutrients include vitamin A, vitamin B complex, vitamin C, vitamin E, magnesium, selenium, and zinc. In addition, some accessory nutrients such as amino acids, carnitine, catechin, choline, gamma-linolenic acid, glutathione and pantethine may protect the liver from damage due to alcohol.

2. Reducing the craving for alcohol.

   Research is this area is limited, but several preliminary studies suggest that alcohol craving is associated with poor nutrition. Normals placed on a diet particularly high in raw foods began to spontaneously avoid alcohol (and tobacco), while chronic alcoholics placed on a nutritious diet along with a multivitamin supplement did far better at follow-up in abstaining from alcohol than did controls. Studies with rats have had similar results: In one study, a "junk food" diet, especially when coffee was included, led to increased alcohol consumption. Other studies have found that the animals increased their alcohol consumption when they were made deficient in the vitamin B complex or zinc.

   Supplementation with certain specific nutrients may reduce craving although, once again, confirmatory studies are needed. Nicotinic acid and pantethine are said to be beneficial due to their ability to reduce acetaldehyde, and there is early evidence that gamma-hydroxy butyric acid, glutamine and tryptophan may also be effective. Also, pharmacologic doses of lithium may have some efficacy, not only due to lithium's antidepressant effect, but also because of other, yet unidentified, mechanisms.

   Hypoglycemia may stimulate alcohol consumption, while alcohol consumption can induce hypoglycemia. Food sensitivities have also been accused of causing alcohol craving, but scientific evidence is lacking.

3. Reducing the severity of alcohol withdrawal syndromes.

   Hypophosphatemia, which may develop 2-4 days into withdrawal, can be easily mistaken for delerium tremens and possibly fosters its development. Early studies suggest that supplementation with evening primrose oil, gamma-hydroxybutyric acid, or taurine may lessen or even prevent withdrawal syndromes.

DIETARY FACTORS

<u>Well-balanced, nutritionally adequate diet</u>.
(C,T)

Review Article (T): "Current evidence suggests that excessive ethanol consumption is itself probably responsible for most of the medical disorders associated with alcohol abuse, and that malnutrition potentiates the adverse effects of ethanol" (*Diamond I. Alcoholic myopathy and cardiomyopathy. Editorial. <u>N Engl J Med</u> 320(7):458-59, 1989*).

Experimental Controlled Study (T): 7 normal subjects were fed 3 different diets which were high or low in protein and/or calories and then challenged with alcohol. Low calorie intake and low protein intake each impaired ethanol excretion (*Wissel PS. <u>Drug-Nutrient Interactions</u> 5:161, 1987*).

Review Article (T): Malnutrition is common in chronic alcoholics which is only partly due to inadequate protein intake in the face of alcohol ingestion as alcohol, despite its high theoretical calorific value, is relatively ineffective as a source of calories. This situation is often compounded by increased mucosal permeability which may lead to leakage of nutrients from the blood to the gut lumen, increased gut motility with increased transit times, and impaired salt and water absorption. In addition, alcohol inhibits absorption of vitamins and nutrients by active transport processes (*World MJ et al. Alcoholic malnutrition and the small intestine. <u>Alcohol Alcohol</u> 20(2):89-124, 1985*).

Animal Experimental Study (C): One gp. of rats which was fed a typical teenage "junk food" diet continuously increased its alcohol consumption during the study, while another gp. which received a well-balanced control diet maintained a low level of alcohol intake. When supplemented with either caffeine or coffee, both gps. significantly increased their alcohol intake. Results suggest that "metabolic controls to drinking exist which are sensitive to dietary factors" (*Register UD et al. Influence of nutrients on intake of alcohol. <u>J Am Diet Assoc</u> 61(2):159-62, 1972*).

<u>Increase consumption of <u>raw foods</u></u>.
(C)

Experimental Study (C): 32 hypertensives ingested an average of 62% of their calories as uncooked food for a mean of 6.7 months. 80% of those who smoked or drank alcohol abstained spontaneously (*Douglass J et al. Effects of a raw food diet on hypertension and obesity. <u>South Med J</u> 78(7):841, 1985*).

Consume <u>fructose</u> before ethanol ingestion.
(T)

Experimental Study (T): 10 male volunteers were injected with ethanol to maintain a steady blood alcohol level. The rate of ethanol metabolism was monitored prior to and following oral fructose 100 mg by measuring the amt. of ethanol required to maintain the steady state. Prior fructose ingestion increased ethanol metabolism by 80% in some subjects. Significant variations among subjects were attributed to differences in their plasma fructose concentrations. However, blood lactate increased after fructose ingestion, increasing the lactate/pyruvate ratio and suggesting that the assumption that fructose increases ethanol metabolism by consuming NADH to allow faster dissociation of the alcohol dehydrogenase-NADH complex may be invalid (*Mascord D et al. The effect of fructose on alcohol metabolism and on the [lactate]/[pyruvate] ratio in man. <u>Alcohol Alcohol</u> 26:53-9, 1991*).

- -

VITAMINS

<u>Vitamin A</u>:
(T)

WARNING: Although 5 times the daily vitamin A requirement has no detectable adverse effects when given alone, when combined with alcohol there is striking leakage of the mitrochondrial enzyme glutamic dehydrogenase into the bloodstream and potentiation of fibrinogenesis. Thus, in heavy drinkers, vitamin A supplementation might hasten rather than alleviate the development of liver disease (*Lieber CS. Biochemical and molecular basis of alcohol-induced injury to liver and other tissues. <u>N Engl J Med</u> 319(25):1639-50, 1988*).

May be deficient (*Majumdar SK et al. Vitamin A utilization status in chronic alcoholic patients. Int J Vitam Nutr Res 53(3):273-79, 1983*).

May be depressed in <u>alcoholic myopathy</u> (*Ward RJ et al. Reduced antioxidant status in patients with chronic alcoholic myopathy. Biochem Soc Trans 16:581, 1988*).

Vitamin A plus zinc deficiencies are said to cause such alcoholic disorders as <u>night blindness, cirrhosis, impaired immune function</u>, etc. (*Scholmerich J et al. Zinc and vitamin A deficiency in liver cirrhosis. Hepatogastroenterology 30:1333-8, 1982*).

Supplementation may be beneficial.

Review Article (T): Vitamin A supplementation should be given to the alcoholic pt. not only to correct <u>night blindness</u> and <u>sexual inadequacies</u>, but also to alleviate potential <u>liver dysfunction</u> (*Lieber CS. Biochemical and molecular basis of alcohol-induced injury to liver and other tissues. N Engl J Med 319(25):1639-50,1988*).

Experimental and Observational Study (T): 11/37 pts. who demonstrated <u>diminished taste and olfactory detection</u> compared to controls were deficient in both zinc and vitamin A. All 37 received oral doses of vitamin A 10,000 mg daily. After 4 wks. of treatment, both those with and without zinc deficiency demonstrated a higher degree of taste and olfactory sensitivity (*Garrett-Laster M et al. Impairment of taste and olfaction in patients with cirrhosis: The role of vitamin A. Hum Nutr Clin Nutr 38C:203-214, 1984*).

<u>Vitamin B Complex</u>:   100 mg. daily
(C,T)

Often deficient in alcoholics (esp. thiamine, pyridoxine and vitamin B_{12} and folate) due both to inadequate intake and impairment in absorption (*Baines M. Detection and incidence of B and C vitamin deficiency in alcohol-related illness. Ann Clin Biochem 15:307-12, 1978*).

Deficiency may increase the craving for alcohol.

Animal Experimental Study (C): Rats made deficient in B vitamins were more likely to choose alcohol than water - but supplementation reversed their tastes (*Norton VP. Interrelationships of nutrition and voluntary alcohol consumption in experimental animals. Br J Addiction 72(3):205-12, 1977*).

- <u>Folic Acid</u>:

Alcohol may reduce folate absorption (*Blocker DE et al. Am J Clin Nutr 46:503, 1987*).

Alcohol ingestion may increase urinary folate excretion (*McMartin KE et al. Cumulative excess urinary excretion of folate in rats after repeated ethanol treatment. J Nutr 116:1316-25, 1986; Russell RM et al. Am J Clin Nutr 38:64-70, 1983*).

Plasma/serum levels may be reduced (*Majumdar SK et al. Blood vitamin status (B_1, B_2, B_6, folic acid and B_{12}) in patients with alcoholic liver disease. Int J Vitam Nutr Res 52(3):266-71, 1982; Thornton WE, Pray BJ. Lowered serum folate and alcohol withdrawal syndromes. Psychosomatics December 1977, pp. 32-36*).

Reduced plasma/serum folate may be related to <u>depression</u>.

Observational Study (T): The plasma folate of 41 pts. (6.9 ± 0.5 ng/ml) did not differ from that of a control gp. of 60 normal subjects with no history of alcoholism or psychiatric illness (7.0 ± 0.3 ng/ml). However, by dividing the pts. into those with a folate level ≥7 ng/ml and below the mean (<7 mg/ml), a striking difference in depressive morbidity was revealed. The mean morbidity scores (Beck Depression Inventory) for the low folate gp. was approx. twice as high as that for the high folate gp, while the Severity of Dependence Questionnaire scores did not differ significantly and there was no difference in liver function tests (*Merry J et al. Alcoholism, depression and plasma folate. Letter. Br J Psychiatry 141:103-04, 1982*).

- <u>Niacin:</u>   250 mg twice daily (1 month trial)
  (C,T,W)

May be deficient.

> **Experimental Study:** In 20 alcoholic pts., evidence of pellagra was found at autopsy. Typically, these pts. had entered the hospital confused, disoriented and agitated. Pellagrin skin lesions were absent. Treatment with antibiotics and vitamins B_1, B_6, B_{12} and C was unsuccessful. Later diarrhea occurred which failed to respond to treatment and they died of bronchopneumonia. Subsequently, when 4 pts. presented similarly, niacin was added to the treatment regimen and all 4 recovered (*Ishii N, Nishihara Y. Pellagra among chronic alcoholics: Clinical and pathological study of 20 necropsy cases. J Neurol Neurosurg Psychiatry 44:209-15, 1981*).

Supplementation may reduce craving and toxicity.

> **Clinical Observation (C):** Drug and alcohol craving was successfully treated in pts. by giving 500-1000 mg/d of time-release niacin over 3-4 weeks. When niacin was stopped, the craving returned (*Cleary JP. Niacinamide and addictions. Letter. J Nutr Med 1:83-84, 1990*).

> **Theoretical Discussion (C):** There is evidence that the degradation of ethanol to acetaldehyde is accelerated in chronic alcoholics while the second step in the degradation of acetaldehyde is slowed down; thus acetaldehyde is elevated. Acetaldehyde has been shown to condense with dopamine in the brain to form tetrahydro - papoveroline, a morphine-like substance, which has been postulated to cause alcohol addiction (*Davis BE, Walsh MJ. Alcohol, amines and alkaloids: A possible biochemical basis for alcohol addiction. Science 167:1005-1007, 1970*). Nicotinic acid oxidizes alcohol to reduce acetaldehyde levels and also saturates NAD brain receptors to abolish a possible deficiency of NAD which would cause irritability and restlessness (*Cleary JP. The NAD deficiency diseases. J Orthomol Med 1(3):149-57, 1986*).

> **Experimental Study (C,T):** 507 alcoholics were treated with nicotinic acid 3 gms or more daily for 5 years. Results suggested that 30% of alcoholics, and 50-60% of "organic" alcoholics, benefit from supplementation both by symptom reduction and reduced recidivism (*Smith RF. Status report concerning the use of megadose nicotinic acid in alcoholics. J Orthomol Psychiatry 7(1), 1978; Smith RF. A five-year trial of massive nicotinic acid therapy of alcoholics in Michigan. J Orthomol Psychiatry 3:327-31, 1974*).

> **Experimental Study (T):** Nicotinic acid supplementation reduced mortality from 90% to 14% in a large series of pts. who were admitted with severe impairment of consciousness or delirium, and cogwheel rigidity of the limbs with uncontrollable grasping and sucking reflexes, half of whom showed evidence of niacin deficiency (*Jolliffe N et al. Nicotinic acid deficiency encephalopathy. JAMA 114:307-12, 1940*).

Supplementation may reduce alcohol withdrawal symptoms.

> **Experimental Study (W):** Alcoholics in withdrawal noted immediate abolition of almost all physical withdrawal symptoms while receiving up to 1 gm daily of diphosphopyridine nucleotide (NAD), the coenzyme form of niacin, by slow drip IM injection for 4 days. (*O'Holleran P. West J Surg Obstet Gynecol May-June, 1961, pp. 101-04*).

- <u>Pantothenic Acid:</u>

Urinary excretion may be reduced (*Tao HG, Fox HM. Measurements of urinary pantothenic acid excretions of alcoholic patients. J Nutr Sci Vitaminol (Tokyo) 22(4):333-37, 1976*).

- <u>Riboflavin:</u>

Blood levels may be deficient (*Baines M. Detection and incidence of B and C vitamin deficiency in alcohol-related illness. Ann. Clin. Biochem. 15(6):307-12, 1978; Majumdar SK et al. Blood vitamin status (B_1, B_2, B_6, folic acid and B_{12}) in patients with alcoholic liver disease. Int J Vitam Nutr Res 52(3):266-71, 1982*).

- Thiamine:
  (C,T)

Blood levels may be deficient (*Baines M. Detection and incidence of B and C vitamin deficiency in alcohol-related illness. Ann Clin Biochem 15:307-12, 1978; Hoyumpa AM Jr. Alcohol and thiamine metabolism. Alcoholism Clin Exp Res 7:11-14, 1983; Majumdar SK et al. Blood vitamin status (B_1, B_2, B_6, folic acid and B_{12}) in patients with alcoholic liver disease. Int J Vitam Nutr Res 52(3):266-71, 1982*).

Thiamine deficiency is due not only to inadequate intake, but also to the interference of ethanol with both the gastrointestinal absorption of thiamine and its utilization for the synthesis of coenzyme and thiamine-dependent haloenzymes (*Leevy CM. Thiamin deficiency and alcoholism. Ann N Y Acad Sci 378:316-26, 1982*) as well as to reduced hepatic storage due to fatty metamorphosis (*Huyumpa AM Jr. Mechanisms of thiamin deficiency in chronic alcoholism. Am J Clin Nutr 33(12):2750-61, 1980*).

Thiamine deficiency appears to be responsible for Wernicke's Syndrome and Korsakoff's Psychosis (*Dreyfus PM, Victor M. Effects of thiamine deficiency on the central nervous system. Am J Clin Nutr 9:414-25, 1971*), while alcoholic polyneuropathy may be due either to deficiency or to a defect in thiamine utilization.

Observational Study (T): Plasma thiamine levels in 30 pts. with peripheral neuropathy were comparable to those of normal subjects, although RBC transketolase activity was lower. In pts. with Wernike's-Korsakoff's Syndrome, both measures were lower than those of normals. Results suggest that, in peripheral neuropathy, pts. have a defect in thiamine utilization rather than a lack of thiamine itself (*Paladin F, Russo Perez G. The haematic thiamine level in the course of alcoholic neuropathy. Eur Neurol 26(3):129-33, 1987*).

Experimental Study (T): 12 pts. with alcoholic polyneuropathy were deprived of alcohol and given only a vitamin B-free diet. After a maximum of 5 days, neuritic symptoms worsened in most of the patients. With the addition of thiamine, there was improvement in all cases. After a maximum of 2 wks., the improvement was purely symptomatic with no measurable effect on the neuritic signs in 10/12 patients. In 2 pts. who were maintained on a vitamin B-deficient diet plus thiamine alone for 8 full wks., a definite improvement occurred in motor and sensory signs and there was a return of ankle jerks. 4 of the 10 pts. who improved suffered a worsening of symptoms and signs initially for the first 2-3 days after the addition of thiamine (*Victor M, Adams RD. On the etiology of the alcoholic neurologic diseases. Am J Clin Nutr 9(4):379-97, 1961*).

Supplementation may reduce drinking behavior.

Animal Experimental Study (C): Rats were given diets containing different levels of thiamine. For the first wk., they were first given ethanol as their only drinking fluid. Subsequently they could choose between ethanol and water. During the free-choice period, rats on the high-thiamine diet containing 20 mg thiamine HCl/kg drank only 1/5 as much ethanol as the rats given the optimum diet with 4 mg thiamine HCl/kg. Rats on a thiamine-deficient diet containing no measurable thiamine showed a significant tendency to increase ethanol drinking when intake was expressed relative to total energy intake, but ethanol intake on a g/kg body-weight basis was about the same as that of the optimum diet group. These differences in voluntary alcohol consumption cannot be explained by changes in the ethanol elimination rate or acetaldehyde accumulation in blood during ethanol oxidation (*Eriksson K, Pekkanen L, Rusi M. The effects of dietary thiamin on voluntary ethanol drinking and ethanol methabolism in the rat. Br J Nutr 43(1):1-13, 1980*).

If deficient, supplementation may benefit alcoholic psychosis.

Case Report: A 36 year-old female was brought to the psychiatric emergency room after stabbing herself in the chest. On examination she was extremely agitated and appeared to be responding to hallucinations. Nystagmus was present. Despite neuroleptic medication, her condition deteriorated and she experienced a grand mal seizure so the neuroleptic was discontinued. She had normal levels of calcium and magnesium, vitamin B_{12} and folic acid. A history of alcohol abuse was elicited, so she was started on diazepam and another neuroleptic was added before diazepam was gradually withdrawn. She remained delusional and confused and continued to experience hallucinations. Thiamine 100 mg/day was added and, in 24 hrs., there was partial clearing of her psychosis; in 48 hrs., she had no evidence of psychosis (*Bakhai YD, Muqtadir S. Thiamine deficiency and psychosis. Letter. Am J Psychiatry 144(5):687-88, 1987*).

- <u>Vitamin B$_6$</u>:

A functional deficiency is common (*Majumdar SK et al. Blood vitamin status (B$_1$, B$_2$, B$_6$, folic acid and B$_{12}$) in patients with alcoholic liver disease. <u>Int J Vitam Nutr Res</u> 52(3):266-71, 1982*) due to impaired conversion to pyridoxal-5-phosphate (the active form) and enhanced degradation (*Lumeng L. The role of acetaldehyde in mediating the deleterious effect of ethanol on pyridoxal-5-phosphate metabolism. <u>J Clin Invest</u> 62:286-93, 1978*).

Pyridoxal-5-phosphate acts as co-enzyme for a wide variety of metabolic transformations of amino acids, as well as for the enzymatic steps in the metabolism of tryptophan, tyrosine, sulfur-containing amino acids and other hydroxyaminoacids. The decarboxylase enzymes which require it as essential co-enzyme are important for the biosynthesis of dopamine, serotonin (5HT), γ-amino-n-butryric acid (GABA) and taurine. Deficiency of pyridoxal-5-phosphate could thus lead to a deficiency of all these neurotransmitters (*Thomson AD. Alcohol and nutrition. <u>Clin Endocrinol Metab</u> 7(2):405-28, 1978*).

- <u>Vitamin B$_{12}$</u>:
(T)

May be deficient despite normal or elevated serum levels in <u>alcoholic hepatitis</u>, since the diseased liver is unable to absorb serum B$_{12}$ normally.

Observational Study: Compared to normals, liver content of cobalamin in 27 alcoholics was low while serum cobalamin and RBC cobalamin analogues were high, confirming earlier work which suggested that, in alcoholism and liver disease, cobalamin depletion in tissues may be masked by normal to high serum cobalamin and analogue levels. The failure of damaged liver to take up from the serum cobalamin and analogues, compounded by the release of these compounds and their binders from damaged liver into the serum, can account for these findings (*Kanazawa S, Herbert V. Total corrinoid, cobalamin (viamin B$_{12}$), and cobalamin analogue levels may be normal in serum despite cobalamin in liver depletion in patients with alcoholism. <u>Lab Invest</u> 53(1):108-10, 1985*).

Plasma vitamin B$_{12}$ levels may serve as an indicator of the severity of alcoholic hepatitis and a predictor of mortality.

Observational Study (T): 320 pts. and 212 controls were tested for plasma B$_{12}$ levels along with liver function studies. There was a positive corrrelation between high plasma B$_{12}$ levels and liver function tests consistent with liver damage, and plasma B$_{12}$ levels rose as death from alcoholic hepatitis approached (*Baker H et al. Plasma vitamin B$_{12}$ titres as indicators of disease severity and mortality of patients with alcoholic hepatitis. <u>Alcohol Alcoholism</u> 22(1):15, 1987*).

<u>Vitamin C</u>:
(T)

May be deficient (*Baines M. Detection and incidence of B and C vitamin deficiency in alcohol-related illness. <u>Ann Clin Biochem</u> 15:307-12, 1978*).

Supplementation may reduce the effects of ethanol toxicity by improving ethanol clearance.

Experimental Controlled Study (T): 17 healthy males subjects who were occasional drinkers and nonsmokers and were not on vitamin C supplementation were studied. Each subject served as his own control and was studied with no ascorbic acid supplementation, after 2 g ascorbic acid given 1 hr. before alcohol consumption, and after supplementation with 500 mg ascorbic acid daily for 2 wks. prior to alcohol consumption. At both 0.5 and 0.8 g/kg body weight, short-term as well as long-term pretreatment with ascorbic acid significantly enhanced the clearance of plasma alcohol, with no significant difference between short- and long-term pretreatments (*Chen MF et al. Effect of ascorbic acid on plasma alcohol clearance. <u>J Am Coll Nutr</u> 9(3):185-89, 1990*).

Experimental Placebo-controlled Study (T): 20 healthy male subjects received either 5 gm of time-release ascorbic acid or placebo for 2 wks. prior to ethanol consumption. Following ethanol consumption, ascorbic acid pretreatment resulted in significant enhancement in blood ethanol clearance, improved motor coordination and color discrimination and an increase in serum triglyceride levels, all in half the subjects. Impairment in intellectual function and elevation in blood lactate/pyruvate ratios, however, were unchanged (*Susick RL Jr, Zannoni VG.*

Effect of ascorbic acid on the consequences of acute alcohol consumption in humans. Clin Pharmacol Ther 41(5):502-09, 1987).

When taken before or during alcohol ingestion, supplementation may prevent fatty infiltration of the liver (*DiLuzio NR. A mechanism of the acute ethanol-induced fatty liver and the modification of liver injury by antioxidants. Lab Invest 15:50-61, 1966*).

Vitamin D:

Serum levels may be reduced, even despite normal dietary intake (*Bjorneboe GE et al. Calcium status and calcium-regulating hormones in alcoholics. Alcoholism (N Y) 12(2):229-32, 1988*).

Vitamin E:
(T)

Plasma/serum levels may be reduced (*Bjorneboe G et al. Diminished serum concentrations of vitamin E in alcoholics. Ann Nutr Med 32:56-61, 1988; Tanner AR et al. Depressed selenium and vitamin E levels in an alcoholic population: Possible relationship to hepatic injury through increased lipid peroxidation. Dig Dis Sci 31:1307-12, 1986; Ward RJ et al. Antioxidant status in alcoholic liver disease in man and experimental animals. Biochem Soc Trans 17:492, 1989*).

Chronic heavy alcohol intake may reduce hepatic vitamin E levels.

Animal Experimental Study: Chronic alcohol ingestion in rats decreased alpha tocopherol in the liver, in part by increased conversion of alpha tocopherol to tocopheryl quinone, thereby enhancing the vitamin E requirement (*Kawase T et al. Lipid perioxidation and antioxidant defense systems in rat liver after chronic ethanol feeding. Hepatology 10:815-21, 1989*).

May be depressed in alcoholic myopathy.

Observational Study: 2/3 of chronic alcoholics develop atrophy of type II skeletal muscle. In this study, 10/21 chronic alcoholic pts. showed atrophy of the type II fibers in their quadriceps muscle on biopsy. The mean plasma alpha tocopherol concentration was significantly lower in alcoholics with myopathy than in those with normal muscle structure or in non-alcoholic controls. Plasma vitamin E and vitamin A levels were significantly correlated, and the mean plasma selenium level was significantly reduced in alcoholics with myopathy compared to those with normal muscle structure and to normal controls, suggesting impaired antioxidant status (*Ward RJ et al. Reduced antioxidant status in patients with chronic alcoholic myopathy. Biochem Soc Trans 16:581, 1988*).

When taken before or during alcohol ingestion, supplementation may prevent fatty infiltration of the liver.

Animal Experimental Study (T): Chronic alcohol ingestion in rats, when accompanied by low dietary intake of vitamin E, was found to promote lipid peroxidation which, in turn, may contribute to the development of hepatic injury (*Kawase T et al. Lipid peroxidation and antioxidant defenses systems in rat liver after chronic ethanol feeding. Hepatology 10:815-21, 1989*).

May protect against the cardiotoxic effects of alcohol.

Animal Experimental Study (T): Mice pretreated with vitamin E by injection prior to injection of a large dose of alcohol exhibited much less evidence of myocardial cell damage than control mice (*Redetzki JE et al. Amelioration of cardiotoxic effects of alcohol by vitamin E. J Toxicol Clin Toxicol 20(4):319-31, 1983*).

- -

MINERALS

Calcium:
(T)

Serum levels may be reduced (*Bjorneboe GE et al. Calcium status and calcium-regulating hormones in alcoholics. Alcoholism (N Y) 12(2):229-32, 1988*).

Hypocalcemia is caused primarily by hypoalbuminemia but can result also from deficient intake, malabsorption, excessive renal losses, hypomagnesemia (*Pitts TO, Thiel DH. Disorders of divalent ions and vitamin D metabolism in chronic alcoholism. Recent Dev Alcohol 4:357-77, 1986*) and acute pancreatitis (*Thomson AD. Alcohol and nutrition. Clin Endocrinol Metab 7(2):405-28, 1978*).

Supplementation may be beneficial.

- with potassium and sodium:

> **Clincal Observations (T):** "Intensive calcium" (Calmonose, Atlas Chemical Co.) is a combination of calcium, sodium lactate, dextrose, and the chlorides of sodium and potassium, so prepared that calcium is about 30% colloidal in character to protect against calcium toxicity. Since IV intensive calcium was introduced to the author's alcoholism treatment program, hospitalizations have been reduced to an all-time low, rehabilitation results have been most gratifying, and the prognosis for the most difficult cases, such as combined alcohol and drug abuse, has been considerably improved (*O'Brien CC. Experimental evidence in the treatment of alcoholism by intensive calcium therapy. J Am Osteopath Assoc 51(8):393-94,428, 1952*).

Lithium:
(C)

Administration of a pharmacologic dosage may reduce alcohol intake.

> **Review Article (C):** While lithium has been shown to reduce depression in alcoholics, there is preliminary evidence that it also causes a decline in alcohol consumption through other mechanisms. However, the negative results of a recent large-scale double-blind study suggest that lithium is of limited efficacy (*Backlage NE, Jefferson JW. Alternative uses of lithium in psychiatry. Psychosomatics 28(5):239-56, 1987; Jefferson JW. Lithium: The present and the future. J Clin Psychiatry 51:8(Suppl):4-8, 1990*).

Magnesium:
(T,W)

Hypomagnesemia, which is common in hospitalized alcoholics, results from deficient intake, malabsorption, excessive renal losses, and reduced cellular uptake (*Pitts TO, Thiel DH. Disorders of divalent ions and vitamin D metabolism in chronic alcoholism. Recent Dev Alcohol 4:357-77, 1986*).

> **Observational Study:** Higher alcohol intake was associated with lower serum magnesium in a study of 48 males subjects whose ave. daily alcohol intake was 120 gm (4 oz) and 37 female subjects whose ave. daily alcohol intake was 32 gm (1 oz). Subjects did not have overt dietary deficiencies (*Kärkkäinen P et al. Alcohol intake correlated with serum trace elements. Alcohol Alcohol 23:279-82, 1988*).

Hypomagnesemia is associated with hypocalcemia which can be reversed by magnesium administration (*Pall HS et al. Hypomagnesaemia causing myopathy and hypocalcaemia in an alcoholic. Postgrad Med J 63:665-67, 1987; Thomson AD. Alcohol and nutrition. Clin Endocrinol. Metab 7(2), 405-28, 1978*).

Intracellular magnesium depletion can cause cardiomyopathy (*Burch GE, Giles TD. The importance of magnesium deficiency in cardiovascular disease. Am Heart J 94:649-57, 1977*) as well as a myopathy which responds rapidly to supplementation (*Pall HS et al. Hypomagnesaemia causing myopathy and hypocalcaemia in an alcoholic. Postgrad Med J 63:665-67, 1987*).

Serum magnesium may be low before and during the early stages of delirium tremens, although it does not appear that low magnesium provokes the syndrome.

> **Observational Study (W):** In a study of 41 male pts., mean age 49, hospitalized with the diagnosis of delerium tremens, stepwise multiple regression based on 46 quantitative and dummy variables (the latter used to represent the presence of various concomitant diseases) pointed to serum magnesium concentration as the most important factor in predicting the duration of delerium tremens (*Stendig-Lindberg G, Rudy N. Stepwise regression analysis of an intensive 1-year study of delirium tremens. Acta Psychiatr Scand 62:273-97, 1980*).

Observational Study (W): Plasma magnesium was low in 9 pts. with delirium tremens during the first days of the acute state and then spontaneously normalized, while normal plasma magnesium was consistently seen among 11 pts. with impending delerium tremens. RBC and CSF magnesium was normal for both groups. Findings suggest that disturbances in magnesium metabolism do not play a role in the etiology or pathogenesis of delerium tremens, although they may contribute to the development of alcoholic encephalopathy (*Kramp P et al. Magnesium concentrations in blood and cerebrospinal fluid during delirium tremens. Psychiatry Res 1(2):161-71, 1979*).

Phosphorus:
(T,W)

Hypophosphatemia, which is common in hospitalized alcoholics, results from deficient intake, malabsorption, excessive renal losses, and reduced cellular uptake (*Pitts TO, Thiel DH. Disorders of divalent ions and vitamin D metabolism in chronic alcoholism. Recent Dev Alcohol 4:357-77, 1986; Stein JH, Smith WO, Ginn HE. Hypophosphatemia in acute alcoholism. Am J Med Sci 252:78-83, 1966*).

Hypophosphatemia may develop in alcoholics 2 to 4 days after hospitalization and, when severe, its neurological features are similar to those of delerium tremens (*Knochel JP. The pathophysiology and clinical characteristics of severe hypophosphatemia. Arch Intern Med 137:203-20, 1977*). When severe, it may be associated with visual hallucinations (*Barbe B et al. Visual hallucinations related to severe hypophosphataemia. Letter. Lancet 338:1083, 1991; Treloar A et al. Hypophosphataemia, hallucinations, and delerium tremens. Letter. Lancet 338:1467-8, 1991*).

It is possible (but unproven) that delerium tremens may be fostered by hypophosphatemia; if so, then phosphate supplementation may be an appropriate adjunctive treatment for alcohol withdrawal (*Larner AJ. Hypophosphataemia, hallucinations, and delerium tremens. Letter. Lancet 338:1467, 1991*).

Potassium:
(W)

Plasma levels may be depressed in patients with delirium tremens (*Blay SL et al. [Plasma electrolyte changes in chronic alcoholic patients with and without delirium tremens.] Acta Psiquiatr Psicol Am Lat 27(4-5):311-14, 1981*).

Selenium:
(T)

Essential for the activity of glutathione peroxidase which protects against alcohol-induced liver damage.

Whole blood, plasma, serum and red blood cell levels may be reduced, especially in patients with liver damage (*Dworkin B, Rosenthal W. Letter. Lancet 1:1015, 1984; Kärkkäinen P et al. Alcohol intake correlated with serum trace elements. Alcohol Alcohol 23:279-82, 1988*).

May be depressed in alcoholic myopathy (*Ward RJ et al. Reduced antioxidant status in patients with chronic alcoholic myopathy. Biochem Soc Trans 16:581, 1988*).

- and Vitamin E:

The combined antioxidant effect of selenium and vitamin E may protect against free radical damage and consequent alcoholic liver disease.

Observational Study (T): Serum selenium and vitamin E levels of alcoholics were compared to those of controls. Liver disease activity, as judged by transaminase (AST) levels, was more markedly abnormal in pts. with combined serum vitamin E and selenium deficiency. Serum lipid peroxides were elevated in those with combined deficiencies and the values correlated significantly with serum transaminases (p=0.03) (*Tanner AR et al. Depressed selenium and vitamin E levels in an alcoholic population: Possible relationship to hepatic injury through increased lipid peroxidation. Dig Dis Sci 31:1307-12, 1986*).

Observational Study (T): 36 pts. were studied using measurement of an amino-terminal collagen type III peptide (PIIP) as an indicator of liver inflammation. Selenium and vitamin E deficiency were associated with elevated PIIP levels, suggesting that these nutrients may protect the liver of alcoholics from free radical damage leading to liver disease (*Lu W et al. Aminoterminal procollagen III peptide elevation in alcoholics who are selenium and vitamin E deficient. Clinica Chimica Acta 154:165-70, 1986*).

Sodium:

Plasma levels may be depressed in patients with delirium tremens (*Blay SL et al. [Plasma electrolyte changes in chronic alcoholic patients with and without delirium tremens.] Acta Psiquiatr Psicol Am Lat 27(4-5):311-14, 1981*).

Zinc:
(C,T)

Chronic alcohol consumption may be associated with zinc deficiency (*McClain CJ, Su L-C. Zinc deficiency in the alcoholic: A review. Alcoholism: Clin Exp 7:5, 1983; Wu CT et al. Serum zinc, copper, and ceruloplasmin levels in male alcoholics. Biol Psychiatry 19:1333-8, 1982*).

Deficiency may be associated with increased alcohol consumption.

Animal Experimental Study (C): Zinc-deficient rats showed a significantly greater voluntary alcohol intake as compared with pair-fed controls (*Collipp PJ et al. The effects of dietary zinc deficiency on voluntary alcohol drinking in rats. Alcoholism (N Y) 8(6):556-59, 1984*).

Deficiency impairs ethanol metabolism, thus increasing the risk of liver damage (*Das I, Burch RE, Hahn HK. Effects of zinc deficiency on ethanol metabolism and alcohol and aldehyde dehydrogenase activities. J Lab Clin Med 104(4):610-17, 1984; Milne DB, Johnson P, Gallagher S. Effect of short-term dietary zinc intake on ethanol metabolism in adult men. Clin Res 39:A652, 1991*).

Supplementation may be beneficial in preventing alcohol toxicity.

- with Vitamin C:

Animal Experimental Study (T): *Yunice AA, Lindeman RD. Effect of ascorbic acid and zinc sulphate on ethanol toxicity and metabolism. Proc Soc Exp Biol Med 154:146-50, 1977*

OTHER NUTRITIONAL FACTORS

Amino Acids:
(T)

Supplementation with mixed freeform amino acids may be beneficial in alcoholic hepatitis.

Experimental Controlled Study (T): 17/35 pts. with alcoholic hepatitis randomly received amino acids 70-85 gm IV daily. All 35 had similar clinical and biochemical features and received a 3000 kcal 100 gm protein diet. After 28 days, ascites and encephalopathy tended to improve more in the study group. Serum bilirubin and albumin improved only in the study group. 4 pts. died in the control gp., but none in the study gp. (*Nasrallah SM, Galambos JT. Aminoacid therapy of alcoholic hepatitis. Lancet 2:1276-7, 1980*).

- Branched Chain (leucine, isoleucine, valine):

May be depressed in the plasma.

Review Article: Depression in branched chain amino acids is due to multiple factors including dietary deficiency and liver disease causing portal-systemic shunting, hyperinsulinemia and hyperglucagonemia (*Shaw S, Lieber CS. Plasma amino acids in the alcoholic: Nutritional aspects. Alcoholism (N Y) 7(1):22-27, 1983*).

- <u>Glutamine</u>: 2 grams (1/2 tsp.) daily in divided doses.
  (C)   *(Powder may also be licked off teaspoon when craving alcohol.)*

    Supplementation may affect the craving for alcohol.

        Experimental Double-blind Crossover Study (C): 7 men and 3 women with long histories of excessive drinking took 5 capsules daily in divided doses with meals of either 0.2 g L-glutamine or lactose placebo. After 6 wks. on L-glutamine, 9/10 subjects as well as their friends and relatives stated that glutamine diminished the desire to drink, decreased anxiety and improved sleep. 2 or 3 subjects continued to do well after placebo substitution, but no subjects responded to placebo unless they had first responded to glutamine *(Rogers LL, Pelton RB. Q J Stud Alcohol 18(4):581-7, 1957).*

        Animal Experimental Study (C): Administering 100 mg/d glutamine to rats diminished their voluntary alcohol consumption by 34%, while administering 100 mg/d of glutamic acid, monosodium glutamate, asparagine or glycine led to an increase in alcohol consumption *(Rogers LL et al. Voluntary alcohol consumption by rats following administration of glutamine. J Biol Chem 220(1):321-3, 1956).*

- <u>Taurine</u>:
  (T,W)

    A potent *in vitro* activator of yeast aldehyde dehydrogenase *(Watanabe A et al. Lowering of liver acetaldehyde but not ethanol concentrations by pretreatment with taurine in ethanol-loaded rats. Experientia 41(11):1421-22, 1985).*

    Supplementation may reduce acetaldehyde concentrations following ethanol ingestion.

        Animal Experimental Study (T): A rise in blood and liver acetaldehyde concentrations following ethanol loading was significantly reduced when rats were pretreated orally with taurine which produced a 4-fold increase in liver taurine content *(Watanabe A et al. Lowering of liver acetaldehyde but not ethanol concentrations by pretreatment with taurine in ethanol-loaded rats. Experientia 41(11):1421-22, 1985).*

    Supplementation may reduce the symptoms of <u>alcohol withdrawal</u>.

        Experimental Study (W): Taurine 3 g daily for 7 days successfully ameliorated symptoms of alcohol withdrawal *(Ikeda H. Effects of taurine on alcohol withdrawal. Letter. Lancet 2:509, 1977).*

- <u>Tryptophan</u>:
  (C,T)

    Serum level following an oral load may be reduced.

        Experimental Study: There were no differences in serum tryptophan levels between alcoholics and controls under fasting conditions. Following an oral tryptophan load, however, alcoholics currently drinking or under treatment with disulfiram (Antabuse) had below normal serum tryptophan levels, while there were no differences between treated alcoholics not receiving disulfiram and normal controls *(Hjorth M et al. Serum tryptophan levels in alcoholics. Drug Alcohol Depend 7(2):157-61, 1981).*

    Transport into the brain may be impaired, causing a relative serotonin deficit.

        Observational Study: Compared to all alcoholics in the study, the ratio of tryptophan over other amino acids competing for brain entry was found to be lowest one day after cessation of drinking and to increase progressively over the following 2-3 weeks. When the population was divided into 2 gps. according to whether pts. started abusing alcohol before or after age 20, associations between a low tryptophan ratio and depressive and aggressive tendencies were significant only in the subgroup of pts. with an early onset of alcoholism. Results suggest that pts. with an early onset of alcoholism may have a preexisting serotonin deficit that could manifest itself by an increased alcohol intake early in life and by an increased vulnerability to fluctuations in precursor availability *(Buydens-Branchey L et al. Age of alcoholism onset. II. Relationship to susceptibility to serotonin precursor availability. Arch Gen Psychiatry 46(3):213-36, 1989).*

Negative Observational Study: Alcoholics were found to have elevated tryptophan levels in the cerebrospinal fluid as compared to healthy controls even after abstention from ethanol for several weeks, while acute ethanol consumption by healthy volunteers led to a decrease in tryptophan levels during intoxication (*Beck O et al. Tryptophan levels in human cerebrospinal fluid after acute and chronic ehtanol consumption. Drug Alcohol Depend 12(3):217-22, 1983*).

A decreased ratio of tryptophan to other amino acids competing for brain transport may be due to enhanced tryptophan catabolism following drinking cessation.

Observational Study: Urinary kynurenine (which reflects tryptophan oxygenase activity) was measured following an oral tryptophan load in 5 alcoholics both shortly after hospital admission and 1 mo. later. Results are consistent with significantly enhanced tryptophan oxygenase activity shortly after cessation of drinking. This enhancement may be due to a rise in glucocorticoids since plasma cortisol, measured hourly for 6 h after the start of the experiment, was higher shortly after cessation of drinking than 1 mo. later (*Buydens-Branchey L et al. Increase in tryptophan oxygenase activity in alcoholic patients. Alcoholism (NY) 12(1):163-67, 1988*).

A decreased ratio of tryptophan to other amino acids competing for brain transport may be associated with depression.

Observational Study (T): The ratio of tryptophan and its competitors was significantly lower in the plasma of depressed alcoholics than in nondepressed alcoholics and normal controls. The decreased ratio was due primarily to decreased tryptophan and increased tyrosine and phenylalanine values (*Branchey L et al. Relationship between changes in plasma amino acids and depression in alcoholic patients. Am J Psychiatry 141(1):1212-15, 1984*).

A decreased ratio of tryptophan to other amino acids competing for brain transport may be especially associated with aggression and suicide among depressed alcoholics.

Observational Study (T): A significant association was found between histories of aggression and depression among alcoholics and a decreased ratio of tryptophan to other amino acids competing for brain transport, and depressed pts. having a history of aggression had the lowest tryptophan ratio values. These values differed significantly from those found in depressed pts. with no aggression history and pts. with no history of aggression and depression. 2/3 suicide attempters in the study fell also in the gp. of pts. with a history of aggression (*Branchey L et al. Depression, suicide and aggression in alcoholics and their relationship to plasma amino acids. Psychiatry Res 12(3):219-26, 1984*).

Decreased plasma tryptophan may be associated with memory impairment and blackouts.

Observational Study (T): Plasma tryptophan values were significantly lower in male pts. who had experienced blackouts than in pts. who had not, while no significant differences between the 2 pt. gps. were observed for the other amino acids sharing with tryptophan the same brain transport carrier. Drinking history variables did not differentiate among the 2 pt. groups (*Branchey L et al. Association between low plasma tryptophan and blackouts in male alcoholic patients. Alcoholism (NY) 9(5):393-95, 1985*).

Decreased plasma and cerebrospinal fluid tryptophan may be associated with alcoholic epilepsy.

Observational Study (T): Compared to normal controls, alcoholic pts. with epilepsy showed a highly significant decrease in cerebrospinal fluid levels and in both free and total tryptophan plasma levels (*Marion JL et al. [Alcoholic epilepsy. Decrease of tryptophan levels in the blood and cerebrospinal fluid.] Presse Med 14(12):681-83, 1985*) (in French).

Supplementation may reduce impairment of mental function following alcohol ingestion.

Experimental Study (T): Alcohol-induced impairment of facial recognition, but not of verbal recall, was attenuated by pretreatment with oral tryptophan (*Westrick ER et al. Dietary tryptophan reverses alcohol-induced impairment of facial recognition but not verbal recall. Alcoholism (N Y) 12(4):531-33, 1988*).

Supplementation may reduce alcohol craving.

> **Animal Experimental Study (C):** In cats unrestrictedly selecting alcohol and water during 5 mo. to 4.5 yrs. under normal feeding, intraperitoneal injection of L-tryptophan lowered alcohol intake (*Baskina NF, Lapin IP. [Changes in alcohol choice by chronically alcoholized cats as affected by tryptophan, its metabolites and preparations affecting its metabolism.] Farmacol Toksikol 45(1):70-76, 1982*).

Beta-Carotene:
(T)

Plasma levels may be inversely correlated with the severity of liver disease (*Ward RJ et al. Antioxidant status in alcoholic liver disease in man and experimental animals. Biochem Soc Trans 17:492, 1989*).

Carnitine:
(T)

Supplementation may inhibit alcohol-induced fatty liver, perhaps by facilitating the oxidation of the increased fatty acid load produced by alcohol ingestion.

> **Animal Experimental Study (T):** Rats fed ethanol as 36% of total calories developed typical hepatic steatosis (accumulation of total lipids, triglycerides, cholesterols, phospholipids and free fatty acids). Supplementation of the ethanol diet with 1% D,L carnitine, 0.05% L-lysine and 0.2% L-methionine (carnitine precursors) significantly lowered ethanol-induced increases of various lipid fractions except for free fatty acids. The lipid-lowering effect of carnitine was superior to that of its precursors and their effect together was no greater than that of carnitine alone. The results suggest that a deficiency of functional carnitine may exist in chronic alcoholics (*Sachan DS et al. Ameliorating effects of carnitine and its precursors on alcohol-induced fatty liver. Am J Clin Nutr 39:738-44, 1984*).

Choline:
(T)

Supplementation may reduce <u>liver damage</u> due to alcohol.

> **Negative Animal Experimental Study (T):** Massive choline supplementation failed to prevent liver fibrosis due to ethanol in baboons but did cause liver toxicity (*Lieber CS et al. Choline fails to prevent liver fibrosis in ethanol-fed baboons but causes toxicity. Hepatology 5(4):561-72, 1985*).

> **Negative Experimental Study (T):** Massive choline supplementation failed to prevent the fatty liver produced by alcohol in normal subjects (*Lieber CS, Rubin E. Alcoholic fatty liver. N Engl J Med 280(13):705-08, 1969*).

- with additional <u>protein</u>:

> **Animal Experimental Study (T):** The liver damage induced by alcohol in rhesus monkeys could be prevented by increasing dietary protein and choline (*Rogers AE et al. Acute and chronic effects of ethanol in non human primates, in KC Hayes, Ed. Primates in Nutritional Research. New York, Academic Press, 1979:249-89*).

Supplementation may foster healing of <u>fatty liver</u> changes.

> *Note: Supplementation is ineffective in patients with alcoholic liver injury who continue to drink (Phillips GB GB, Davidson CS. Arch Intern Med 94:585-603, 1954; Post J et al. Gastroenterology 20:403-10, 1952; Volwiler W et al. Gastroenterology 11:164-82, 1948).*

> **Experimental Study (T):** After 8-10 days, 3 alcoholic pts. with fatty livers failed to respond to purified diets consisting of glucose solution (1,600 kcal) containing vitamin and mineral supplements either clinically, in liver function tests, or in liver fat content as estimated from liver biopsy. When choline dihydrogen citrate 6.5 g/d was added to this diet for 10 days, 2/5 similar pts. responded. Serum bilirubin concentration, bromsulphalein retention, urine urobilinogen and liver size decreased, while serial liver biopsies, which initially showed a marked degree of fatty change, demonstrated rapid improvement (*Phillips GB, Davidson CS. Nutritional aspects of cirrhosis in*

alcoholism - effect of a purified diet supplemented with choline. Ann N Y Acad Sci 57:812, 1954; Phillips GB et al. Comparative effects of a purified and an adequate diet on the course of fatty cirrhosis in the alcoholic. J Clin Invest 31:351, 1952).

Gamma-Hydroxybutyric Acid: 50 mg/kg daily
(W)

A constituent of the mammalian brain which is found in the highest concentrations in the hypothalamus and basal ganglia.

Supplementation may reduce symptoms of alcohol withdrawal.

> WARNING: Adverse effects have included coma and tonic-clonic seizure-like activity.   Acute effects resolve within 7 hrs. (*Dyer JE. gamma-Hydroxybutyrate: a health-food product producing coma and seizurelike activity. Am J Emerg Med 9(4):321-4, 1991*).   Other reported acute symptoms are abrupt drowsiness, dizziness, a "high," headache, and nausea and vomiting.   Following discontinuation of the supplement, there is full recovery.   No clear dose-response effect has been observed (*Chin MY, Kreutzer RA, Dyer JE. Acute poisoning from gamma-hydroxybutyrate in California. West J Med 156(4):380-4, 1992*).

> **Experimental Double-blind Study (W):**   23 pts. randomly received either GHB 50 mg/kg orally in a syrup preparation or the syrup alone.   Active treatment led to a prompt reduction of withdrawal symptoms including tremors, sweating, nausea, depression, anxiety, and restlessness.   Dizziness was the only side effect (*Gallimberti L et al. Gamma-hydroxybutyric acid for treatment of alcohol withdrawal syndrome. Lancet 2:787-89, 1989*).

Glutathione: 300 mg. daily
(T)

May protect from alcohol-induced liver damage.

> **Animal Experimental Study (T):**   Results of experiments on the ethane expiration of rats after treatment with carbon tetrachloride suggest that lipid peroxidation may be involved in the toxic process induced by ethanol within the hepatocytes.   The increased formation of lipid peroxides could overload the peroxide inactivating capacities of glutathione peroxidase by depleting glutathione in the hepatocytes which is released as oxidized glutathione.   The increased amt. of lipid peroxides could then damage the cell (*Kappus H et al. Lipid peroxidation induced by ethanol and halogenated hydrocarbons in vivo as measured by ethane exhalation, in H Sies, A Wendel Eds. Functions of Glutathione in Liver and Kidney. Berlin, Springer-Verlag, 1978*).

Omega-6 Fatty Acids: Example: Evening Primrose Oil: 1/2 - 1 gram three times daily
(C,T,W)

linoleic acid $\rightarrow$ gamma-linolenic acid $\rightarrow$ DGLA $\rightarrow$ PGE$_1$

Alcohol blocks the conversion of linoleic acid to gamma-linolenic acid and enhances the conversion of dihom-mogamma-linolenic acid to prostaglandin E$_1$; the result is a deficiency in GLA which can be replaced by primrose oil. Supplementation with EPO may theoretically prevent alcohol toxicity and, by preventing the development of tolerance due to DGLA depletion, the development of alcohol addiction (*Horrobin DF. A biochemical basis for alcoholism and alcohol-induced damage including the fetal alcohol syndrome and cirrhosis: Interference with essential fatty acid and prostaglandin metabolism. Med Hypotheses 6:929-42, 1980*).

May reduce the severity of alcohol withdrawal.

> **Experimental Double-blind Study (T,W):**   21 pts. undergoing alcohol detoxification received either EPO or placebo along with diazepam as needed for 3 weeks.   Compared to controls, 1.) there was a significantly faster return of liver enzymes towards normal; 2.) the amount of diazepam needed to ease withdrawal symptoms in treated pts. was significantly reduced; 3.) there was a modest but consistent lowering of the score for measures of withdrawal severity; and 4.) cognitive function on one of the psychomotor tests significantly improved. 34 pts. were then randomly chosen for a 6-month trial.   Again there was some recovery in cognitive function although there were no significant differences in test results (*Glen I et al. Possible pharmacological approaches to the prevention and treatment of alcohol-related CNS impairment: Results of a double blind trial of essential fatty*

acids, in G Edwards, J Littleton, Eds. Pharmacological Treatments for Alcoholism. London, Croom, Helm, 1984, pp. 331-50).

Animal Experimental Study (W): Evening primrose oil, but not olive oil, was able to inhibit withdrawal symptoms in alcohol-treated rats (*Karpe F et al. The effect of dietary primrose oil on ethanol withdrawal in the rat. Acta Pharmacol Toxicol (Copenh) 53(Suppl 2):18P, 1983*).

May prevent liver damage due to high alcohol intake.

Animal Experimental Study (T): When rats were supplemented with gamma linolenic acid during 10 days of ethanol administration, the high hepatic triglyceride levels and histological evidence of fatty liver were partially mitigated (*Segarnick DJ et al. Gamma-linolenic acid inhibits the development of the ethanol-induced fatty liver. Prostaglandins Leukotrienes Med. 17:277-82, 1985*).

Pantethine: 300 mg 2-3 times daily
(C,T)

A metabolic intermediate which is the stable disulfide form of pantetheine, a derivative of pantothenic acid and a precursor of Coenzyme A.

Acetaldehyde, the primary metabolite of alcohol, may promote alcohol addiction by combining with monamine metabolites to form addicting morphine-like alkaloids (*Myer RD. Tetrahydroisoquinolines in the brain: The basis of an animal model of addiction. Alcohol Clin Exp Res 2:145, 1978; Cohen G, Collins MA. Alkaloids from catecholamines in adrenal tissue: Possible role in alcoholism. Science 167:1749-51, 1970; Davis VE, Walsh MJ. Alcohol, amines, and alkaloids: a possible biochemical basis for alcohol addiction. Science 167:1005-7, 1970*).

Acetaldehyde has also been implicated in the pathogenesis of alcoholic liver disease and alcoholic cardiomyopathy and may play a role in the development of atherosclerosis as related to ethanol ingestion (*Watanabe A et al. Lowering of blood acetaldehyde but not ethanol concentrations by pantethine following alcohol ingestion: Different effects in flushing and non-flushing subjects. Alcohol Clin Exp Res 9:272, 1985; Sprince H et al. Protection against acetaldehyde toxicity in the rat by L-cysteine, thiamin and L-2-methylthiazolidine-4-carboxylic acid. Agents Actions 4(2):125-30, 1974*).

Supplementation with pantethine may reduce the adverse effects of acetaldehyde by increasing the activity of aldehyde dehydrogenase, the enzyme which metabolizes it.

Note: Pantethine will not be effective in pts. who flush after alcohol ingestion, probably due to a lack of hepatic low Km aldehyde dehydrogenase enzyme (Watanabe A et al. Lowering of blood acetaldehyde but not ethanol concentrations by pantethine following alcohol ingestion: Different effects in flushing and nonflushing subjects. Alcoholism (N Y) 9(3):272-76, 1985).

Experimental Study (T): Administration of pantethine prior to alcohol ingestion reduced acetaldehyde levels in the blood of human volunteers and in the liver of experimental animals. Since ethanol levels were unaffected, this reduction is believed to have been due to an increase in aldehyde dehydrogenase activity (*Watanabe A et al. Lowering of blood acetaldehyde but not ethanol concentrations by pantethine following alcohol ingestion: Different effects in flushing and non-flushing subjects. Alcohol Clin Exp Res 9:272, 1985*).

In vitro Experimental Study (T): Pantethine increased aldehyde dehydrogenase activity by as much as 71% (*Watanabe A et al. Lowering of blood acetaldehyde but not ethanol concentrations by pantethine following alcohol ingestion: Different effects in flushing and non-flushing subjects. Alcohol Clin Exp Res 9:272, 1985*).

- -

COMBINED NUTRITIONAL TREATMENT

Nutritious diet plus multivitamin supplementation:
(C)

> **Experimental Controlled Study (C):** Chronic alcoholics who averaged 13 oz. alcohol daily for 15-20 yrs. were studied. While the control gp. only received the standard hospital diet, the experimental gp. also followed a special diet plan which included foods such as wheat germ and unsweetened fruit as well as decaffeinated coffee and avoided all snacks except for nuts, cheese, peanut butter and milk. In addition, they attended a nutrition education class and were placed on a multivitamin supplement which they were asked to continue for 6 mo. after discharge. At the 6 mo. follow-up 81% of the experimental gp. was still sober compared to 38% of the control gp. (*Guenther RM. Role of nutritional therapy in alcoholism treatment. Int J Biosoc Res 4(1):5-18, 1983*).

- -

OTHER FACTORS

Rule out food sensitivities.
(C,T)

> **Observational Study (T):** Compared to controls, 36 pts. who consumed 80-150 gm (3-5 oz) of ethanol daily for 3 yrs. or more showed increased excretion of oral chromium 51-labeled EDTA (suggesting abnormally high intestinal uptake) which decreased the longer they remained abstinent until it reached the level of the controls for most of the patients. The small bowel was found to be the site of the increased intestinal permeability. It is suggested that the increased permeability to toxic "non-absorbable" compounds of <5000 molecular weight may account for some of the extra-intestinal tissue damage seen in alcoholics (*Bjarnason I et al. The leaky gut of alcoholism: Possible route of entry for toxic compounds. Lancet 1:179-82, 1984*).

> **Experimental Study:** The ingestion of either grain alcohol or whiskey increased the size, intensity and duration of the allergic skin wheal, regardless of the subjects' clinical sensitivity to alcoholic beverages. This effect was unrelated to the absolute blood alcohol level. Results suggest that, in those who are sensitive to alcohol, alcohol ingestion merely brings to a clinical level a subclinical allergic reaction, and food or inhalant allergens unrelated to the contents of the brew may become potent enough to cause symptoms, or the alcoholic medium could enhance the small quantities of allergens which it contained to a level sufficient to produce an allergic reaction (*Dees SC. An experimental study of the effect of alcohol and alcoholic beverages on allergic reactions. Ann Allergy 7:185, 1949*).

Rule out reactive hypoglycemia.
(C)

May be induced by alcohol.

> **Review Article:** The increase in gastric acidity which follows alcohol ingestion might cause excessive release of gut secretagogues which augment beta-cell responsiveness to glucose fluctuations, leading to excessive insulin release (*Freinkel N, Getzger BE. Oral glucose tolerance curve and hypoglycemias in the fed state. N Engl J Med 280:820-8, 1969*).

May stimulate alcohol consumption.

> **Animal Experimental Study (C):** When insulin production was decreased by administering alloxan (which destroys pancreatic beta cells), the animals stopped drinking alcohol. Alcohol consumption resumed when insulin was administered and increased as the frequency of the insulin dose increased (*Forander et al. Q J Stud Alcohol. 19:379, 1958*).

ALLERGY
(ALTERED REACTIVITY)

See Also: BRONCHIAL ASTHMA
URTICARIA (CHRONIC)

OVERVIEW

1. Plasma ascorbate levels are negatively correlated with blood histamine levels, and ascorbate supplementation may lower elevated blood histamine levels. Moreover, in a recent double-blind crossover study, vitamin C supplementation prevented inhaled histamine from impairing pulmonary function in patients with allergic rhinitis.

2. There is early scientific evidence that calcium supplementation may reduce allergic reactions.

3. Chronic magnesium deficiency may increase allergic reactions.

4. Several other nutrients may reduce allergic reactions, but their efficacy has yet to be proven. These include niacin, pantothenic acid, vitamin B$_{12}$, vitamin E, zinc, essential fatty acids oleic acid and certain bioflavonoids.

5. Foods may provoke a wide variety of symptoms by multiple mechanisms.

6. MSG sensitivity may possibly be reduced by nutrients. Vitamin B$_6$ was shown to do so in a double-blind study, and vitamin C reduced the neurotoxicity of MSG administered intra-peritoneally in an animal study.

7. Sulfite sensitivity may be blocked by vitamin B$_{12}$ administration. While it may be related to molybdenum deficiency, the benefits of molybdenum supplementation are unproven.

8. Formaldehyde sensitivity may possibly be reduced by pantethine supplementation, but controlled clinical trials are lacking.

- -

VITAMINS

Niacin:

May inhibit mast cell degranulation and histamine release.

Animal Experimental Study: In guinea pigs given nicotinamide intra-peritoneally, then exposed to histamine aerosols, appearance of the first symptoms of dyspnea was delayed (p<0.01), and the number of animals developing anaphylactic shock diminished significantly. Nicotinamide, which itself produces a slight bronchial constriction in isolated guinea pig lungs, not only protects against histamine constriction, but relaxes histamine-induced bronchial constriction after 3-4 minutes (*Bekier E, Maslinski CZ. Antihistaminic action of nicotinamide. Agents Actions 4(3):196, 1974*).

In vitro Experimental Study: Nicotinamide was found to exert an antihistaminic action on the isolated guinea pig ileum (*Halpern BN et al. Le role des mediateurs chimiques dans la regulation de l'eosinophilie sanguine. Bull Soc Pathol Exot Filiales 55:489-99, 1962*).

Supplementation may be beneficial in seasonal allergic rhinitis

Case Reports: IM or IV administration of 10-20 cg of nicotinamide resulted in rapid improvement in pts. with hay fever (*Daïnow I. Recherches cliniques sur certaines propriétés anti-allergiques de la nicotinamide. Z Vitaminforsch 15:245-50, 1944*).

Pantothenic Acid:

Supplementation may reduce allergic reactions.

> *Note: Too large a dose of pantothenic acid is suspected of producing dryness of the nasal mucosa (Martin W. On treating allergic disorders. Letter. Townsend Letter for Doctors Aug/Sept, 1991:670-1).*

Clinical Observation: The majority of over 100 pts. with allergic rhinitis who took pantothenic acid 250 mg twice daily had almost instant relief (*Martin W. On treating allergic disorders. Letter. Townsend Letter for Doctors Aug/Sept, 1991:670-1*).

Clinical Observation: A physician with allergies took 100 mg at bedtime and found that his nasal stuffiness cleared in less than 15 min. and that he stopped awakening at 4 or 5 AM with cough and mucous secretion. He subsequently found that many of his patients also noted significant relief of nasal congestion from supplementation (*Crook WG. Letter. Ann Allergy 49:45-46, 1987*).

Clinical Observation: Observations were made in our laboratory indicating that pantothenic acid could be used to combat allergy. Subsequently a pharmaceutical house found that, while it was somewhat effective, it was not superior to certain available antihistaminics (*Williams RJ. The expanding horizon in nutrition. Texas Rep Biol Med 19(2):245-58, Summer, 1961*).

Vitamin B_6:

Supplementation may be beneficial for MSG sensitivity.

Experimental Double-blind Study: 12/27 unsupplemented students who were fasted and then challenged in sequence with either a large dose of monosodium glutamate (MSG) or placebo showed characteristic symptoms. There were no significant differences in red blood cell glutamic-oxaloacetic transaminase activity between reactive and non-reactive subjects. These 12 received pyridoxine 50 mg daily or placebo. After 12 wks. they were rechallenged with MSG. 8/9 who proved on decoding to have received pyridoxine now showed no response to MSG. Of the 3 who had received placebo, all were still MSG-responsive. A probability of error of <0.01 was calculated for a real difference in these 2 gps. of 9 and 3, respectively (*Folkers K et al. Biochemical evidence for a deficiency of vitamin B6 in subjects reacting to monosodium-L-glutamate by the chinese restaurant syndrome. Biochem Biophys Res Commun 100:972-7, 1981*).

Vitamin B_{12}:

Supplementation may be beneficial.

Case Reports: 1000 µg IM once weekly for 4 weeks. Results:
        Intractable asthma: 18/20 improved
        Chronic urticaria: 9/10 improved
        Chronic contact dermatitis: 6/6 improved.
        Atopic dermatitis: 1/10 greatly improved;
                    5/10 moderately improved
(*Simon SW. Vitamin B12 therapy in allergy and chronic dermatoses. J Allergy 2:183-5, 1951*)

Supplementation may reduce sulfite sensitivity.

Experimental Single- and Double-blind Study: 24 pts. were studied who had a history of one or more of the following symptoms following ingestion of sulfite-containing foods: nasal and sinus congestion, rhinitis, postnasal drip, frontal headache, and bronchospasm. 18/24 were proven to be sulfite-sensitive by single-blind challenge and were re-challenged following pre-medication with 2000 µg of sub-lingual vitamin B_{12}. 17/18 were effectively blocked of their adverse reactions to sulfites, and 6 of the 17 were then challenged with sulfite-containing wine in a single-blind fashion following 2 days of abstension from B_{12} and known sulfite-blocking drugs. The results were then compared with challenge following pre-medication with B_{12}. (4 of the 6 pts. were challenged in a double-blind fashion with a placebo candy which appeared and tasted similar to B_{12}.) 2/6 had a significant (at least 15%) drop in FEV_1, during the initial sulfite challenge, and both pts. were blocked of these pulmonary changes after B_{12}. pre-medication. During the wine challenge, one pt. had a 53% drop in FEV_1 which was also blocked after B_{12} pre-medication. In addition, all 6 pts. had one or more of the following symptoms following sulfite and wine challenges which were blocked by pre-medication with B_{12}: rhinorrhea, nasal blockage, frontal headache, itchy throat and wheezing (except for 2 pts. for whom B_{12} failed to block symptoms following the wine challenge). Pts. experienced no significant changes in symptoms following challenge with sulfite-free vodka, suggesting that they were not alcohol-sensitive. Blood level of B_{12} indicated that sublingual B_{12} becomes available as early as 15 min. after administration and is still elevated at 24 hrs., suggesting that a once-daily dose of 2-4000 μg would be an effective prophylactic measure (*Bhat NK - Presentation at the 43rd Annual Meeting, American Academy of Allergy and Immunology, 1987*).

Vitamin C:

Supplementation may reduce <u>MSG sensitivity</u>.

> **Animal Experimental Study:** Injections of ascorbic acid prior to intra-peritoneal injection of MSG 2.5 g/kg in 500 chickens prevented the paralysis and convulsions that would have occurred. Similarly the adverse effects of MSG when given to guinea pigs and monkeys fed a low ascorbate diet were abolished when they were given ascorbate by intra-peritoneal injection, suggesting that the addition of ascorbic acid together with MSG to foods may prevent MSG-induced toxic reactions in man (*Ahmad K, Jahan K. Studies on the preventive and curative action of ascorbic acid on the neurological toxicity of monosodium glutamate. Food Nutr Bull 7(1):51-3, 1985*).

Elevations of circulating histamine occur as the result of marginal ascorbic acid status (*Caldwell EJ et al. Histamine and ascorbic acid: A survey of women in labor at term and significantly before term. Int J Vitam Nutr Res 58(3):319-25, 1988*).

> **Observational Study:** For 437 normal subjects, when the plasma-reduced ascorbic acid level was below 1 mg/100 ml, the whole blood histamine level increased exponentially as the ascorbic acid level decreased. For subjects with ascorbic acid levels below 0.7 mg/100 ml, the increase in blood histamine was highly significant. Oral administration of ascorbic acid 1 g/day for 3 days to 11 volunteers resulted in a reduction of the blood histamine level in every instance (*Clemetson CA. Histamine and ascorbic acid in human blood. J Nutr 110(4):662-68, 1980*).

Supplementation may reduce blood histamine levels.

> **Experimental Study:** When 11 normals with either low vitamin C levels or high blood histamine levels were given ascorbic acid 1 gm x 3 days, blood histamine levels fell in all 11 subjects (*Clemetson CA. Histamine and ascorbic acid in human blood. J Nutr 110(4):662-68, 1980*).

Supplementation may protect against <u>systemic anaphylaxis</u>.

> **Animal Experimental Studies:** Supplementation with ascorbic acid provided a significant degree of protection against fatal anaphylactic shock in passively sensitized guinea pigs (*Feigen GA et al. Enhancement of antibody production and protection against systemic anaphylaxis by large doses of vitamin C. Res Commun Chem Pathol Pharmacol 38(2):313-33, 1982; Pavlovic S, Fraser R. Effects of different levels of vitamin C on the vitamin C concentration of guinea pigs plasma and the effect of vitamin C intake on anaphylaxis. Med Interne 26(3):235-44, 1988*).

Supplementation may reduce the symptoms of <u>seasonal allergic rhinitis</u>.

> **Experimental Double-blind Crossover Study:** 16 pts. with allergic rhinitis received a single dose of vitamin C 2 gm and placebo in either order. In the placebo gp., histamine inhalation caused a significant decrease in the maximal expiratory flow (MEF_{50}), indicating impaired pulmonary function. In contrast, histamine inhalation failed to decrease MEF_{50} in the treated gp. (*Bucca C et al. Effect of vitamin C on histamine bronchial responsiveness of patients with allergic rhinitis. Ann Allergy 65:311-14, 1990*).

Negative Experimental Double-blind Study: 24 pts. with seasonal allergic rhinitis were studied by anterior rhinomanometry to evaluate nasal respiratory efflux. 4 pts. were excluded because of non-specific nasal reactivity. The other 20 pts. were randomly treated with either ascorbic acid 2 gm or placebo. Both gps. successfully reduced nasal respiratory efflux after histamine challenge; there were no significant differences between the 2 gps. (*Bellioni P et al. La provocazione istaminica in soggetti allergici. Il ruolo dell'acido ascorbico. Eur Rev Med Pharm Sci 9:419-22, 1987*).

Negative Experimental Double-blind Study: The skin wheal and flare response to histamine and the nasal response to allergens were evaluated in 8 pts. with seasonal allergic rhinitis 3 days after receiving ascorbic acid 2 gm daily and again after 3 days on placebo. In a second study, 6 subjects received either placebo or 1,2 or 4 gm ascorbic acid daily. In both studies, there were no differences between placebo and ascorbic acid, which suggests that ascorbic acid in doses up to 4 gm daily will not suppress the histamine skin response and would have no beneficial effect on symptoms resulting from allergen exposure (*Fortner BR Jr et al. The effect of ascorbic acid on cutaneous and nasal response to histamine and allergen. J Allergy Clin Immunol 69(6): 484-488, 1982*).

Vitamin E:

May possess antihistaminic properties.

Experimental Study: Volunteers injected with histamine showed far less swelling around the injection site when pretreated with vitamin E for 5-7 days (*Kamimura M. Antiinflammatory activity of vitamin E. J Vitaminol 18(4):204-9, 1972*).

- -

MINERALS

Calcium:

Supplementation may reduce atopic allergic responses.

Experimental Double-blind Crossover Study: 25 pts. with allergic rhinitis received 9 mmol calcium IV or a placebo in a double-blind crossover design. They were then given increasing intranasal doses of an allergen. The dosage of an allergen required to induce an allergic reaction (defined as a 50% decrease in nasal air flow) was 170% after calcium administration as compared to after placebo administration (p=0.021) (*Bachert C et al. [Decreased reactivity in allergic rhinitis after intravenous application of calcium. A study on the alteration of local airway resistance after nasal allergen provocation.] Arzneimmittelforsch 40:984-7, 1990*).

- with Vitamin D_2:

Experimental Double-blind Crossover Study: 12 pts. with allergic bronchial asthma and airway obstruction received oral calcium in combination with vitamin D_2 (calciferol). Within 60 min., in comparison to placebo, a statistically significant reduction in airway resistance and intrathoracic gas volume, as well as an increase of forced expiratory one second volume and forced inspiratory one second volume, was observed (*Utz G, Hauck AM. [Oral application of calcium and vitamin D_2 in allergic bronchial asthma.] MMW 118(43):1395-8, 1976*).

Magnesium:

Chronic magnesium deficiency may produce Gell and Coombs type 1 allergic manifestions (*Durlach J Repports experimentaux et cliniques entre magnésium et hypersensibilite. Rev Fr Allergo 15:133-46, 1975*).

Animal Experimental Study: In a study using rats, there was a clear synergism of antigen challenge and severe magnesium deficiency on blood and urinary histamine levels, suggesting that severe magnesium deficiency could aggravate diseases which are caused by abnormal histamine release after exposure to an IgE-stimulating antigen (*Wei W, Kranz KB. A synergism of antigen challenge and severe magnesium deficiency on blood and urinary histamine levels in rats. J Am Coll Nutr 9(6):616-22, 1990*).

Molybdenum:

The trace element contained in the enzyme sulfite oxidase which detoxifies sulfite to the inert and harmless sulfate.

Deficient or absent in the majority of people with sulfite sensitivity (*Papaioannou R, Pfeiffer CC. Sulfite sensitivity - unrecognized threat:. Is molybdenum the cause? J Orthomol Psychiatry 13(2):105-110, 1984*).

If deficient, sulfite oxidase activity is impaired (*Abumrad NN et al. Amino acid intolerance during prolonged total parenteral nutrition reversed by molybdate therapy. Am J Clin Nutr 34:2551-59, 1981*) and supplementation may be beneficial.

> **Case Report:** 53 year-old female asthmatic was found to have 10-20 ppm urinary sulfite in a 24 hour urine. She was treated with molybdenum IV for 3 mo. starting with 250 μgm twice weekly for 6 injections, then 500 μgm twice weekly, and finally with 750 μgm for the last 4 injections. During treatment urinary sulfite output dropped to 2-6 ppm, her wheezing considerably lessened, she discontinued theophylline and prednisone and reduced her use of inhalers from 4 times daily to twice daily (*Wright J, Littleton K. Defects in sulphur metabolism. Int Clin Nutr Rev 9(3):118-19, 1989*).

Zinc:

Erythrocyte zinc levels may be low in patients with chemical sensitivities (*Rogers SA. Zinc deficiency as model for developing chemical sensitivity. Int Clin Nutr Rev 10(1):253-59, 1990*).

May inhibit the release of histamine from basophils and mast cells.

> **In vitro Experimenal Study:** Preincubation of human basophils and lung mast cells with zinc chloride caused dose-related inhibition of histamine and peptide leukotriene C4 release induced by anti-IgE (*Marone G et al. Physiological concentrations of zinc inhibit the release of histamine from human basophils and lung mast cells. Agents Actions 18(1-2):103-06, 1986*).

If low, supplementation may reduce chemical sensitivities.

> - with a multivitamin, multimineral supplement:

> > **Case Report:** A 53 year-old female had an 11 yr. history of headaches along with leg aches, insomnia, periorbital edema and a shakey, jittery feeling. She had worked for 15 yrs. in a factory where she shaped wax forms with a hot tool before they were used near her station to cast plastic parts. Medical evaluation including a computerized axial tomography (CAT) scan failed to reveal pathology, and immunotherapy was ineffective. Single-blind chemical testing provoked her headache and, when trichloroethylene was tested, the neutralizing dose terminated it. A blood level of trichloroethylene after a day of work was elevated (26.1 vs. population ave. of 1.1 ng/dL). The headaches were less severe at home, but persisted for 8 mo. after she remained out of work, and worsened if she went into certain stores or offices or returned to the place of employment to visit. At this time, her RBC zinc level was 870 μg/dL (normal range: 880-1600 μg/dL). She was placed on 105 mg zinc gluconate daily in divided doses as well as on multiple vitamins and other minerals. Within 2 mo. her serum zinc level was normal (1060 μg/dL) and she reported that she was markedly improved. Her seum tetachloroethylene level had dropped to 1.3 ng/dL. One mo. later, she was tested double-blind to trichloroethylene; again the chemical resulted in a headache which could be neutralized, while normal saline had no effect (*Rogers SA. Zinc deficiency as model for developing chemical sensitivity. Int Clin Nutr Rev 10(1):253-59, 1990*).

- -

OTHER NUTRITIONAL FACTORS

Bioflavonoids:

Like the drug disodium chromoglycate, the bioflavonoids possess a benzopyrone nucleus.

May inhibit histamine release from mast cells and basophils as well as a number of other mediators of allergic response when stimulated by antigens and other ligands (*Middleton E Jr et al. The effects of citrus flavonoids on human basophil and neutrophil function. Planta Medica 53:325-28, 1987*).

- Catechin:

A naturally occurring flavonoid.

May inhibit histadine decarboxylase, the enzyme responsible for the conversion of histadine to histamine.

Experimental Study: Pts. with urticaria and food allergies who received catechin prior to administration of food antigens were protected from an increase of histamine in the gastric mucosa in response to the antigens (*Wendt P et al. The use of flavonoids as inhibitors of histadine decarboxylase in gastric diseases: Experimental and clinical studies. Naunyn Schmiedebergs Arch Pharmacol (Suppl.) 313:238, 1980*).

- Quercetin: 1 - 2 gm daily divided into 3-6 doses

A flavonoid believed to reduce allergic processes due to its ability to:

1. stabilize mast cells and basophils, thereby inhibiting degranulation and subsequent release of histamine and other inflammatory mediators (*Ogasawara H, Middleton E Jr. Effect of selected flavonoids on histamine release (HR) and hydrogen peroxide (H_2O_2) generation by human leukocytes. J Allergy Clin Immunol 75:184, 1985*).

2. inhibit several enzymes (e.g. lipoxygenase, phospholipases, cyclic nucleotide phosphodiesterase) through its interaction with calmodulin to dampen the inflammatory response (*Neshino H. Quercetin interacts with calmodulin, a calcium regulatory protein. Experientia 40(2):184-5, 1984*).

3. decrease leukotriene formation by inhibiting various steps in eicosanoid metabolism (*Yoshimoto T et al. Flavonoids: Potent inhibitors of arachidonate 5-lipoxygenase. Biochem Biophys Res Commun 116:612-18, 1983*).

Fatty Acids:

Allergic individuals may demonstrate reduced delta-6-desaturase activity causing impairment in the desaturation of alpha-linolenic (omega-3 series) and linoleic (omega-6 series) essential fatty acids. Results of preliminary clinical trials suggest that supplementation with appropriate fatty acids may alleviate a broad range of allergic inflammatory symptoms in certain individuals (*Galland L. Increased requirements for essential fatty acids in atopic individuals: A review with clinical descriptions. J Am Coll Nutr 5(2):213-28, 1986*).

- Oleic Acid:

An omega-9 fatty acid found in high quantities in olive oil.

Supplementation may inhibit histamine release (*Tasaka K et al. Anti-allergic constituents in the culture medium of Ganoderma lucidum. (I). Inhibitory effect of oleic acid on histamine release. Agents Actions 23(3-4):153-56, 1988*).

- Omega-3 Fatty Acids (Fish Oil):

Review Article: "A fish oil enriched diet has the potential to modulate the humoral and inflammatory components of the allergic response by inhibiting the generation of pro-inflammatory lipid mediators and by suppressing the responses of target cells and tissues. However, the modulating influence of alternative fatty acid substrates on arachidonic acid metabolism may not always be beneficial . . ." (*Lee TH, Arm JP. Modulation of the allergic response by fish oil lipids and eicosatrienoic acid. Prog Clin Biol Res 297:57-69, 1989*).

- Omega-6 Fatty Acids:

linoleic acid $\rightarrow$ gamma-linolenic acid $\rightarrow$ DGLA $\rightarrow$ PGE_1

Atopic patients may have a block in the conversion of linoleic acid to prostaglandin E_1.

Observational Study: In the plasma phospholipids of 50 pts. with atopic eczema, cis-linoleic acid was elevated and gamma-linolenic acid (GLA) as well as the prostaglandin precursors DGLA and arachidonic acid were decreased. This suggests that atopics have a defect in the functioning of delta-6-desaturase which converts linoleic acid to gamma-linolenic acid (*Manku MS et al. Reduced levels of prostaglandin precursors in the blood of atopic patients: Defective delta-6-desaturase function as a biochemical basis for atopy. Prostaglandins Leukotrienes Med 9(6):615-28, 1982*).

Pantethine:

A metabolic intermediate which is the stable disulfide form of pantetheine, a derivative of pantothenic acid and a precursor of Coenzyme A.

Increases the activity of aldehyde dehydrogenase, the enzyme which metabolizes aldehydes (*Watanabe A et al. Lowering of blood acetaldehyde but not ethanol concentrations by pantethine following alcohol ingestion: Different effects in flushing and non-flushing subjects. Alcohol Clin Exp Res 9:272, 1985*). This could be of value to patients hypersensitive to formaldehyde.

Note: Pantethine will probably not be effective in pts. who flush after alcohol ingestion, probably due to a weak aldehyde dehydrogenase enzyme (Watanabe A et al. Lowering of blood acetaldehyde but not ethanol concentrations by pantethine following alcohol ingestion: Different effects in flushing and non-flushing subjects. Alcohol Clin Exp Res 9:272, 1985).

Case Report: A man with moderately severe formaldehyde sensitivity received 300 mg pantethine twice daily. Within 1 wk. he reported a marked reduction in sensitivity (*Pantethine: possible treatment for formaldehyde sensitivity. Ecological Formulas, 1061-B Shary Circle, Concord, CA 94518, 1986*).

- -

OTHER FACTORS

Lactobacillus Acidophilus and
Bifidobacteria:

Deficiency may be associated with food allergies.

Observational Study: All cases of a group of children suffering from symptoms of food allergies showed evidence of deficiencies of Lactobacillus and Bifidobacteria combined with Enterobacteriaceae overgrowth (*Kuvaeva I et al. The microecology of the gastrointestinal tract and the immunological status under food allergy. Nahrung 28(6-7):689-93, 1984*).

Rule out food sensitivities.

(See also "Rule out food sensitivities" in other chapters.)

Experimental Study: 142 pts. with perennial allergic rhinitis underwent evaluation. 41/47 with a "positive food allergy history" developed 65 (90%) positive nasal responses as measured by rhinomanometry during 72 food ingestion challenges. 54/95 pts. with an "unknown food allergy history" developed 68 (50%) positive nasal responses during 132 food ingestion challenges. Responses included isolated immediate (within 3 hrs.), isolated late (6-24 hrs.), isolated delayed (28-52 hrs.) and combinations of immediate and either late or delayed responses. Results suggest that foods are more commonly involved in allergic rhinitis than usually expected (*Pelikan Z. Nasal response to food ingestion challenge. Arch Otolaryngol Head Neck Surg 114(5):525-30, 1988*).

Experimental Study: 197 pts. with perennial allergic rhinitis were tested by both skin prick and IgE RAST for the main seasonal and perennial inhalant allergens in that area; if results were negative and environmental control did not relieve symptoms, they were given an elimination diet restricted to rice, olive oil, turkey, lettuce, peeled pears, salt, sugar, water and tea. Those that improved within 3 wks. were challenged with foods and received skin prick tests and IgE RAST for food allergens. When the results of skin prick tests, IgE RAST and food challenges correlated, a diagnosis of of IgE-mediated allergy was made; when such a correlation was not present, a diagnosis of "food intolerance" was made.   When food challenges were negative or equivocal and skin pricks and IgE RAST were negative, chemical additive oral challenges were performed.   52/197 (26.4%) had food "intolerance," 19.8% house dust mite allergy, 18.8% seasonal or perennial inhalent allergy, 3.6% cat allergy, 1.5% mold allergy and 23% remained undiagnosed.   24 pts. (12.2%) had hypersensitivity to food additives; 25% of them to acetyl salicylic acid, 8.3% sodium salicylate, 16.6% tartrazine, 16.6% sodium bisulfite and 8% BHT-BHA.   The results suggest a surprisingly high incidence of non-IgE-mediated food intolerance as well as hypersensitivity to food additives (*Pastorello E et al. Evaluation of allergic etiology in perennial rhinitis. Ann Allergy 55:854-56, 1985*).

Experimental Study: 322 children under 1 yr. of age with respiratory allergy and negative inhalent skin tests were studied.   320 (99%) had symptoms of allergic rhinitis and 273 (85%) had bronchial asthma.   They were placed on a six-week hypoallergenic diet consisting of Meat Base Formula (Gerber), carrots, broccoli and apricots.   292 (91%) showed significant improvement of respiratory symptom scores.   On subsequent oral food challenge, symptoms were reproduced in only 51% of the children.   The most common allergens in decreasing order of importance were milk, egg, chocolate, soy, legumes and cereals.   Skin tests with food allergens rarely correlated with challenge reults.   117 (40%) later developed inhalent respiratory allergy.   Only 6% studied 5 yrs. or longer showed any evidence of food sensitivity.   Results suggest that (1) infants with respiratory allergy will respond to an hypoallergenic diet, (2) symptoms may or may not reappear on food challenge, (3) food allergy tends to be "outgrown," (4) many "grow into" inhalant respiratory allergy (*Ogle KA, Bullock JD. Children with allergic rhinitis and/or bronchial asthma treated with elimination diet: A five-year follow-up. Ann Allergy 44:273-8, 1980*).

Experimental Study: 4 pts. with urticaria, rhinitis and/or asthma went into remission after they were placed on additive-free diets (*Freedman BJ. A diet free from additives in the management of allergic disease. Clin Allergy 7:417-21, 1977*).

ANEMIA

See Also: CELIAC DISEASE

VITAMINS

Folic Acid:

Deficiency is well-known to be associated with a megaloblastic anemia which is corrected by supplementation.

May be deficient in sickle cell anemia (*Pierce LE, Rath CE. Evidence for folic acid deficiency in the genesis of anemic sickle cell crisis. Blood 20:19, 1962*).

Supplementation may be beneficial in sickle cell anemia.

> **Review Article:** "Numerous case reports describing an exacerbation of the chronic anemia that was reversed by folic acid therapy led to routine folate supplementation. More recent studies have shown, however, that clinically significant folic acid deficiency occurs only in a small minority of sickle cell patients" (*Reed JD et al. Nutrition and sickle cell disease. Am J Hematol 24(4):441-45, 1987*).

> **Case Report and Review Article:** A pt. with sickle-cell anemia developed a megaloblastic bone marrow at age 27 due to folic acid deficiency. Only after 1000 μg of folic acid did the bone marrow become normoblastic and the serum folate normal, with a concomitant fall in urinary formiminoglutamic acid (*Lindenbaum J et al. Folic acid deficiency in sickle-cell anemia. N Engl J Med 269(17):875-82, 1963*).

If deficient, supplementation may be beneficial in aplastic anemia.

> **Case Report:** A young man with an extensive family history of leukemia, pancytopenia, and neutropenia developed severe aplastic anemia. His red cells showed megaloblastic changes and treatment with high doses of folate resulted in striking clinical improvement even though RBC folate levels remained low. Further studies revealed a genetically induced abnormality of folate uptake (*Branda RF et al. Folate-induced remission in aplastic anemia with familial defect of celular folate uptake. N Engl J Med 298(9):469-75, 1978*).

Pantothenic Acid:

If deficient, supplementation may be beneficial.

> **Case Report:** 53 year-old black female was admitted with anorexia, weight loss, lethargy, incontinence and hypochromic anemia with increased iron storage in the bone marrow. After an unsuccessful trial of pyridoxine, all symptoms and signs improved dramatically following administration of pantothenic acid (pantothenyl alcohol 50-200 mg IM daily). Several years later, a similar clinical picture developed and there was a clinical, but probably not a hematologic, response to a multi-vitamin preparation containing large amts. of pantothenic acid, suggesting that lethargic psychotic pts. with iron-loaded hypochromic anemia unresponsive to pyridoxine might benefit from a trial of pantothenic acid (*McCurdy PR. Is there an anemia responsive to pantothenic acid? J Am Geriatr Soc 21(2):88-91, 1973*).

Riboflavin:

Deficiency may be associated with a normochromic, normocytic anemia and reticulocytopenia which responds to supplementation.

Experimental Study: Riboflavin deficiency was induced in 8 adult males, each of whom developed an anemia which was reversed by riboflavin administration (*Lane M, Alfrey CP, Jr. The anemia of human riboflavin deficiency. Blood 25(4):432-42, 1965*).

May be deficient in sickle cell anemia.

Observational and Experimental Study: 90% of 41 vitamin E-deficient pts. were also riboflavin-deficient. Supplementation with the RDA level of riboflavin for 3 mo. failed to raise riboflavin levels to the normal range (*Sindel LJ et al. Nutritional deficiencies associated with vitamin E deficiency in sickle cell patients: the effect of vitamin supplementation. Nutr Res 10:267-73, 1990*).

Thiamine:

Deficiency may be associated with a megaloblastic anemia.

Case Report: A 3 month-old girl presented with symptoms of severe anemia, diabetes, deafness and severe cardiac and neurological distubances which, despite normal blood transketolase, responded to 100 mg daily thiamine and reappeared when treatment was suspended, suggesting that every patient with unexplained anemia deserves a therapeutic trial with high dose thiamine (*Mangel H et al. Thiamine-dependent beriberi in the "thiamine-responsive anemia syndrome." N Engl J Med 311:836-8, 1984*).

Case Report: A case of megaloblastic anemia failed to respond to B$_{12}$ or folic acid but responded to supplementation with oral thiamine 20 mg daily. When, on 2 occasions, the supplementation was stopped, the anemia recurred (*Rogers LE et al. Thiamine-responsive megaloblastic anemia. J Pediatr 74(4):494-504, 1969*).

Vitamin A:

Deficiency is associated with anemia due to impaired hemoglobin synthesis which is reversible with supplementation.

Observational Study: In a gp. of 148 Iranians, low plasma vitamin A levels were correlated with reduced hemoglobin values (*Bozorgmehr B. A study of possible relationship between vitamin A and some hematopoietic factors. Am J Clin Nutr 46:531, 1987*).

Experimental Study: 8 middle-aged males gradually developed anemia several months after being placed on a vitamin-A deficient diet. The decline in serum hemoglobin began well before the loss of night vision or the attainment of "deficient" serum vitamin A values. Repletion with either carotene or vitamin A led to a prompt and complete hematologic recovery (*Hodges RE et al. Hematopoietic studies in vitamin A deficiency. Am J Clin Nutr 31:876-85, 1978*).

May be deficient in sickle cell anemia.

Observational and Experimental Study: 76% of 41 vitamin E-deficient pts. were also vitamin A-deficient. Supplementation with the RDA level of vitamin A for 3 mo. failed to raise vitamin A levels to the normal range (*Sindel LJ et al. Nutritional deficiencies associated with vitamin E deficiency in sickle cell patients: the effect of vitamin supplementation. Nutr Res 10:267-73, 1990*).

Vitamin B$_6$:

Deficiency may be associated with a microcytic anemia despite adequate dietary intake and no other evidence of systemic B$_6$ deficiency (*Bernat I. Pyridoxine responsive anemias, in Iron Metabolism. New York, Plenum Press, 1983, pp. 313-14; Horrigan DL, Harris JW. Pyridoxine-responsive anemias in man. Vitam Horm 26:549-68, 1968*).

If deficient, supplementation may be beneficial.

Experimental Study: 18/34 pts. with sideroblastic anemia unresponsive to vitamin B$_6$ and folate had subnormal concentrations of serum and RBC pyridoxal phosphate (PLP) and *in vitro* evidence of defective phosphorylation of pyridoxine and pyridoxal to PLP. Treatment of these pts. with parenteral PLP 25-50 mg 4 times daily for 8-10 days produced significant elevation of hemoglobin in 11 cases (*Hines JD, Love D. Abnormal vitamin B$_6$ metabolism in sideroblastic anemia: Effect of pyridoxal phosphate therapy. Clin Res 23:403A, 1975*).

Experimental Study: 3 pts. who had failed to respond to iron supplementation were given 100 mg B6 daily which resolved the anemia (*Hines JD, Harris JW. Pyridoxine-responsive anemia: Description of three patients with megaloblastic erythropoiesis. Am J Clin Nutr 14:137-46, 1964*).

May be of therapeutic benefit in sickle cell anemia.

Experimental Study: 5 pts. with SCA had below normal levels of pyridoxal phosphate, and an increased ratio of RBC to plasma PLP. Treatment with pyridoxine 50 mg twice daily for 8 mo. to 2 yrs. was associated with fewer painful crises, increased hemoglobin levels, a general increase in well-being, and a trend towards normalization of the RBC to plasma PLP ratio (*Natta CL. Painful crises due to sickle-cell anemia: Effect of vitamin B6 supplementation. IM 7(10):132-40, 1986*).

Experimental Controlled Study: 16 pts. with SCA had signficantly lower plasma pyridoxal phosphate than controls while their RBC pyridoxal phosphate was significantly elevated, possibly reflecting a greater affinity of PLP to the sickle Hb beta chain than to the normal beta chain. Oral supplementation of 5 pts. with 50 mg. vitamin B6 twice daily for 2 mo. resulted in increased plasma and red cell PLP levels and a slight, insignificant increase in erythrocyte cell number, hemoglobin concentration and hematocrit. One subject also experienced reduction in the frequency and duration of painful crises (*Natta CL, Reynolds RD. Apparent vitamin B6 deficiency in sickle cell anemia. Am J Clin Nutr 40:235-9, 1984*).

Vitamin B12:

Deficiency is well-known to produce pernicious anemia, a megaloblastic anemia.

Supplementation may reverse the neurologic changes due to pernicious anemia (*Berk L et al. Effectiveness of vitamin B12 in combined system disease. N Engl J Med 239:328, 1948*).

Vitamin C:

Deficiency is occasionally associated with a normochromic, normocytic or macrocytic anemia. Less commonly, a megaloblastic anemia has been reported. While the megaloblastosis is believed to be due to a dietary deficiency of folic acid or to an impaired metabolism of folic acid, some pts. have responded to ascorbic acid supplementation alone, probably because ascorbic acid appears to assist in preventing oxidation of tetrahydrofolates to 10-formylfolic acid which would remove them from the metabolic pool (*Sauberlich HE. Ascorbic acid, in Nutrition Reviews' Present Knowledge in Nutrition, Fifth Edition. Washington, D.C., The Nutrition Foundation, Inc., 1984*).

Markedly enhances non-heme iron absorption for the prevention and treatment of iron-deficiency anemia (*Monsen ER. Ascorbic acid: An enhancing factor in iron absorption, in Nutritional Bioavailability of Iron. American Chemical Society, 1982:85-95*).

May be reduced in in beta-thalassemia.

Observational Study: Compared to controls, 52 pts. with heterozygous beta-thalassemia showed a moderate reduction in mean vitamin C platelet levels (*Giuberti M et al. Plasma vitamin E, platelet vitamin C and plasma ferritin levels in heterozygous beta-thalassemia. Nutr Rep Int 35(6):1141-50, 1987*).

Supplementation may stimulate hemopoiesis.

Experimental Study: Healthy young women were supplemented with either 50 or 100 mg of ascorbic acid daily. After 8 wks., they were found to have significantly higher hemoglobin and hematocrit levels, as well as higher erythrocyte counts. These values returned to baseline 10 wks. after the cessation of supplementation (*Ajayi OA, Nnaji UR. Effect of ascorbic acid supplementation on haematological response and ascorbic acid status of young female adults. Ann Nutr Metab 34:32-6, 1990*).

Vitamin E:

Deficiency may be associated with anemia which responds to supplementation.

Review Article: Vitamin E should be viewed as a potential erythropoietic factor for humans, and it should receive trials in pts. with anemia of obscure etiology, particularly in those with erythroid hyperplasia and unexplained ineffective erythropoiesis (*Drake JR, Fitch CD. Status of vitamin E as an erythropoietic factor. Am J Clin Nutr 33:2386-93, 1980*).

Experimental Study: Red cell survival was studied using ^{51}Cr-tagged cells in 8 vitamin-E deficient subjects. Before vitamin E therapy, the T 1/2 for ^{51}Cr in all 8 subjects ranged from 10-28 days (mean 19.2 days). Following therapy, the values ranged from 19-30 days (mean 24.9 days), a significant difference (p<0.025) (*Leonard PJ, Losowsky MS. Effect of alpha-tocopherol administration on red cell survival in vitamin E-deficient human subjects. Am J Clin Nutr 24:388-93, 1971*).

The anemia associated with <u>cystic fibrosis</u> and other causes of <u>pancreatic insufficiency</u> may respond to vitamin E supplementation.

Experimental and Observational Study: Cystic fibrosis pts. showed a significant reduction in RBC half-life compared to controls. When treated with vitamin E, RBC survival time approached normal (*Farrell PM et al. J Clin Invest 60:233-41, 1977*).

The anemia associated with <u>Mediterranean-type G$_6$PD deficiency</u> may respond to vitamin E supplementation.

Experimental Study: 23 pts. were treated for 90 days with 800 IU oral vitamin E. Compared to baseline values, RBC survival and hemoglobin concentration increased significantly, while reticulocytosis decreased significantly (*Corash L et al. Reduced chronic hemolysis during high-dose vitamin E administration in Mediterranean type glucose-6-phosphate dehydrogenase deficiency. N Engl J Med 303:416-20, 1980*).

Levels may be low in <u>sickle cell anemia</u> which may respond to supplementation.

Observational and Experimental Study: 53/77 pts. (69%) were deficient in vitamin E. Daily supplementation with 800 IU of vitamin E over a 6 mo. period resulted in a progressive increase in serum vitamin E levels (*Sindel LJ et al. Nutritional deficiencies associated with vitamin E deficiency in sickle cell patients: the effect of vitamin supplementation. Nutr Res 10:267-73, 1990*).

Experimental Study: Following administration of 450 IU daily oral vitamin E for 6-35 wks., 6 pts. showed an ave. decrease of 44% in the number of irreversibly sickled cells (*Natta CL et al. A decrease in irreversibly sickled erythrocytes in sickle cell anemia patients given vitamin E. Am J Clin Nutr 33:968-71, 1980*)

See Also:

Negative Experimental Study: *Chiu D et al. Peroxidation, vitamin E, and sickle-cell anemia. Ann N Y Acad Sci 393:323-35, 1982*

Plasma levels may be low in <u>beta-thalassemia</u>.

Observational Study: Compared to controls, 52 pts. with heterozygous beta-thalassemia showed a moderate reduction in mean vitamin E plasma levels (*Giuberti M et al. Plasma vitamin E, platelet vitamin C and plasma ferritin levels in heterozygous beta-thalassemia. Nutr Rep Int 35(6):1141-50, 1987*).

- -

MINERALS

<u>Copper:</u>

Deficiency is associated with a hypochromic, microcytic anemia.

Case Report: A 35-year-old Caucasian woman ingested 110-165 mg elemental zinc as zinc sulfate for 10 months. She developed a slowly worsening microcytic-hypochromic anemia found to be due to copper deficiency. Zinc supplementation was eliminated and she was supplemented with 2 mg copper daily. After 2 mo., her anemia was unchanged. She received 10 mg copper chloride IV over a period of 5 days, and responded (*Hoffman HN et al. Zinc-induced copper deficiency. Gastroenterology 94:508-12, 1988*).

Review Article: Nutritional copper deficiency is well documented in both the newborn undergoing rapid growth on a copper-poor diet and in the pt. on total parenteral nutrition for long periods without copper supplementation. In both situations, anemia and neutropenia are the most striking hematologic abnormalities (*Williams DM. Copper deficiency in humans. Semin Hematol 20(2):118-28, 1983*).

Copper deficiency, due to its effects on ceruloplasmin, may cause an iron-deficiency anemia which can only be corrected with copper supplementation as it impairs iron absorption and reduces heme synthesis while increasing iron accumulation in storage tissues (*Watts DL. The nutritional relationships of copper. J Orthomol Med 4(2):99-108, 1989*).

Iron:

Deficiency is believed to be the most frequent cause of anemia and responds well to supplementation (*Bernat I. Iron deficiency, in Iron Metabolism. New York, Plenum Press, 1983:215-74*).

- and Vitamin A:

Combined supplementation may be beneficial.

Experimental Placebo-controlled Study: 99 anemic Guatemalan children aged 1-8 yrs. were supplemented with vitamin A, iron, vitamin A plus iron, or placebo. After 2 mo., vitamin A and iron supplementation alone each produced significant increases in hemoglobin, hematocrit, erythrocytes and percent transferrin saturation; however, simultaneous administration of both nutrients resulted in a better response of serum iron and percent transferrin saturation than either nutrient alone, suggesting that vitamin A may be involved in iron metabolism (*Mejia LA, Chew F. Hematological effect of supplementing anemic children with vitamin A alone and in combination with iron. Am J Clin Nutr 48:595-600, 1988*).

Often deficient in patients with pernicious anemia.

Observational Study: Iron deficiency coexisted in 25/121 (20.7%) PA pts., while another 27/121 (22.3%) developed iron deficiency 1 mo. to 14 yrs. later. Results suggest that pts. with PA are at high risk for iron deficiency (*Carmel R et al. Iron deficiency occurs frequently in patients with pernicious anemia. JAMA 257(8):1081-83, 1987*).

Deficiency is known to be a relatively common occurrence in sickle cell anemia, especially in children and pregnant women (*Reed JD et al. Nutrition and sickle cell disease. Am J Hematol 24(4):441-55, 1987*).

Deficiency may be secondary to celiac disease (*Depla AC et al. Anemia: monosymptomatic celiac disease: A report of 3 cases. Hepatogastroenterology 37(1):90-1, 1990*).

The hypoferremia of inflammation is not identical to iron deficiency; rather it is a redistribution of iron in the face of normal or increased iron stores, and thus may have the advantages of reducing the iron supply to pathogens without adverse effects on host resistance (*Hershko C et al. Iron and infection. Br Med J 296:660-64, 1988*).

Zinc:

WARNING: Pharmacologic doses of zinc ($\approx$100-300 mg daily) for several months can produce a severe copper deficiency causing a sideroblastic anemia with hypocupremia, anemia, leukopenia and neutropenia (*Copper deficiency induced by megadoses of zinc. Nutr Rev 43(5):148-49, 1985; Broun RE et al. Excessive zinc ingestion: a reversible cause of sideroblastic anemia and bone marrow depression. JAMA 264:1441-3, 1990; Forman WB et al. Zinc abuse: an unsuspected cause of sideroblastic anemia. West J Med 152:190-2, 1990; Hoffman HN II et al. Zinc-induced copper deficiency. Gastroenterology 94:508-12, 1988; Patterson WP et al. Zinc-induced copper deficiency: megamineral sideroblastic anemia. Ann Intern Med 103:385, 1985; Prasad AS et al. Hypocupremia induced by zinc deficiency in adults. JAMA 240:2166-8, 1978*).

Plasma levels may be low in <u>sickle cell anemia</u>.

Observational Study: 10% of 41 vitamin E-deficient pts. were also zinc-deficient (*Sindel LJ et al. Nutritional deficiencies associated with vitamin E deficiency in sickle cell patients: the effect of vitamin supplementation. <u>Nutr Res</u> 10:267-73, 1990*).

Review Article: Although studies on the role of zinc in sickle cell disease are generally small, most do support a relationship between sickle cell anemia and zinc deficiency (*Reed JD et al. Nutrition and sickle cell disease. <u>Am J Hematol</u> 24(4):441-45, 1987*).

Supplementation may be beneficial.

Experimental Study: Supplementation of 41 zinc-deficient pts. with the RDA level of zinc for 3 mo. raised plasma zinc levels significantly to the normal range (*Sindel LJ et al. Nutritional deficiencies associated with vitamin E deficiency in sickle cell patients: the effect of vitamin supplementation. <u>Nutr Res</u> 10:267-73, 1990*).

Experimental Study: 30 pts. with homozygous sickle cell anemia were found to have serum zinc levels which were significantly below normal; their electrokinetic potential (a measure of membrane stability) was also low. Following administration of zinc sulfate 200 mg 3 times daily (about 50 mg elemental zinc) for 4 mo., a significant improvement in serum zinc and electrokinetic potential was seen. 18 mo. after zinc was discontinued, there was a greater than 50% reduction in sickle cell crises, with comparable reductions in days in the hospital and days out of work (*Gupta VL et al. Efficacy of oral zinc therapy in the management of sickle cell crises. <u>Indian J Med Res</u> 86:803-07, 1987*).

- -

COMBINED SUPPLEMENTATION

<u>Folic Acid</u>,
<u>Vitamin B12</u> and
<u>Iron</u>:

Supplementation may be beneficial in <u>anemia of pregnancy</u>.

Experimental Study: Hemoglobin concentration rose in all pregnant pts. given iron, but declined in those given no iron. Those given folic acid and vitamin B12 in addition to iron showed an even greater rise in mean hemoglobin concentration than those given iron only (*Sood SK et al. <u>J Trop Med Hyg</u> 77:177, 1974*).

Experimental Study: 3 gps.of pregnant pts. took daily doses of iron 100 mg, iron 100 mg and folate 300 µg, or folate 300 µg. 96% of the women receiving iron and folate showed a rise in hemoglobin, while only 26% of those receiving iron or folate alone showed such a rise. When a program was instituted in which iron and folate were given to all pregnant women in a selected community, anemia was reduced from over 50% to below 6% (*Izak G et al. <u>Scand J Haematol</u> 11:236, 1973*).

<u>Vitamin C</u>,
<u>Vitamin E</u>,
<u>Zinc</u> and
<u>Essential Fatty Acids</u>:

Combined supplementation may be beneficial in <u>sickle cell anemia</u>.

Experimental Study: 13 pts. (aged 0.7-17.9 y) with homozygous sickle cell disease were supplemented with a daily dose of α-tocopherol acetate 460 mg, vitamin C 600 mg, zinc 109 mg and soybean oil (11 g linoleic acid; 1.5 g linolenic acid) for 8 mo. (suppl 1) and α-tocopherol, vitamin C, and fish oil 180 mg EPA; 120 mg DHA) for 7 months (suppl 2). Suppl 1 decreased irreversibly sickled cells by 37.5%, decreased RBC protoporphyrin and urinary porphyrins, and increased the RBC total fatty acid/cholesterol ratio. Suppl 2 decreased plasma triglycerides, moderately increased the RBC double-bond index, but decreased the RBC total fatty acid/cholesterol ratio. The supplements did not change hemoglobin concentrations, RBC age, or number of aplastic and vasoocclusive crises. Results suggest that zinc reduces irreversibly sickled cells. Augmentation of RBC antioxidant status by α-tocopherol and vitamin C, and incorporation of ω3 fatty acids into RBC's, do not affect the hemolytic component, while effects on the vasoocclusive component are unclear (*Muskiet FAJ et al. Supplementation of patients with homozygous sickle cell disease with zinc, a-tocopherol, vitamin C, soybean oil, and fish oil. Am J Clin Nutr 54:736-44, 1991*).

- -

OTHER FACTORS

Rule out hydrochloric acid deficiency.

If deficient, iron absorption is significantly impaired in iron-deficiency anemia.

Experimental Study: In pts. with iron-deficiency anemia, iron absorption was found to be related to the maximal acid output of the stomach following a histamine infusion (*Jacobs A et al. Gastric acidity and iron absorption. Br J Haematol 12:728-36, 1966*).

If deficient, the survival of ingested bacteria may be increased, leading to intestinal bacterial overgrowth (*Giannella RA et al. Influence of gastric acidity on bacterial and parasitic enteric infections. Ann Intern Med 78:271-76, 1973*).

Patients with sickle cell anemia may have intestinal bacterial overgrowth which can be associated with nutritional deficiencies (*Heyman MB et al. Elevated fasting breath hydrogen and abnormal hydrogen breath tests in children with sickle cell disease: a preliminary report. Am J Clin Nutr 49:654-57, 1989*); this overgrowth, in turn, could theoretically be secondary to hydrochloric acid deficiency.

If deficient, supplementation may be beneficial in iron-deficiency anemia.

Experimental Study: 24 pts. with histamine-fast achlorhydria were given iron 5 mg in 300 ml water or in 300 ml 0.05 N HCl. Both ferric chloride and ferrous ascorbate were better absorbed with acid, although acid failed to increase the absorption of hemoglobin iron (*Jacobs A et al. Role of hydrochloric acid in iron absorption. J Appl Physiol 19(2):187-8, 1964*).

Experimental Study: 25 diabetic pts. with blood counts 4.2 million or less who were under good diabetic control were randomly selected to receive glutamic acid HCl 5 gr 3 times daily before meals which, at the end of 1 month, was replaced by ferrous carbonate 6 3/4 gr 3 times daily. At the end of another month, both supplements were prescribed concomitantly. Following the first month, the RBC increased significantly from 4.06 to 4.56 million, while iron supplementation failed to be followed by a significant change. Following combined supplementation, RBC again increased significantly by 1/4 million. The experiment was replicated with similar results (*Rabinowich IM. Achlorhydria and its clinical significance in diabetes mellitus. Am J Dig Dis 16:322-32, 1949*).

See Also:

> *Jacobs A, Rhodes J. Gastric factors influencing iron absorption in anaemic patients. Scand J Hematol 4:105, 1967*

Rule out milk sensitivity in infants.

May cause the loss of 1-5 ml of blood daily in the stool (which can be detected by tests for occult blood) leading to iron-deficiency anemia. Half the iron deficiency in infants in the US is estimated to result from milk-induced GI bleeding (*Oski FA. Don't Drink Your Milk! Syracuse, Mollica Press, 1983*).

See Also:

> *Bahna SL, Heiner DC. Allergies to Milk. New York, Grune and Stratton, 1980*

APHTHOUS STOMATITIS

(CANKER SORES)

NUTRIENTS

<u>Folic Acid</u>,
<u>Vitamin B$_{12}$</u>, and/or
<u>Iron</u>:

May be deficient and, if deficient, may respond to supplementation.

Case Report: A women with repeated episodes of AS had moderately low serum levels of <u>vitamin B$_{12}$</u> which were untreated. 2 yrs. later, she was treated with colchicine and reported some improvement in oral ulcers, but little improvement in the concurrent glossitis. Symptoms worsened and the dosage was increased. Although some symptoms temporarily improved, in time symptoms worsened again and the dosage was increased once more until she discontinued treatment. At that time her serum B$_{12}$ levels had fallen to 50 pg/ml (normal range: 200-1000), she was absorbing <1% of dietary intake of the vitamin, and showed no intrinsic factor activity. IM injections of vitamin B$_{12}$ 1000 μg/d for the first wk., twice weekly for 1 mo., and then monthly, produced immediate improvements, with complete and lasting remission of all oral ulcerations, glossitis, and anemia. Results suggest that vitamin B$_{12}$ status should always be considered for pts. with this disorder, and especially if they are receiving colchicine (*Palopoli J, Waxman J. Recurrent aphthous stomatitis and vitamin B$_{12}$ deficiency. <u>South Med J</u> 83:475-77, 1990*).

Observational Study: In a study of 69 pts. with recurrent aphthous stomatitis, hemoglobin levels and RBC indices were normal; however, there was a small minority of pts. with deficiencies of <u>iron</u> (low serum ferritin), <u>folate</u> (low RBC folate), or <u>vitamin B$_{12}$</u> (low serum levels) that would have remained undetected if only hemoglobin and RBC indices were done. Therapeutic studies are needed to establish the frequency with which deficiencies actually predispose to this condition (*Porter SR et al. Hematologic status in recurrent aphthous stomatitis compared to other oral disease. <u>Oral Surg Oral Med Oral Pathol</u> 66(1):41-4, 1988*).

Negative Observational Study: Compared to 23 healthy controls, only 3/90 pts. proved to have abnormalities when CBC, serum <u>iron</u> and total iron-binding capacity, serum <u>vitamin B$_{12}$</u>, and serum or RBC <u>folate</u> were measured. There were no statistically significant differences between the pt. and control populations, and no one in either gp. had abnormal serum vitamin B$_{12}$ or serum or RBC folate assays (*Olson JA et al. Serum vitamin B$_{12}$, folate, and iron levels in recurrent aphthous ulceration. <u>Oral Surg Oral Med Oral Pathol</u> 54(5):517-20, 1982*).

Experimental and Observational Study: 21/100 children with recurrent aphthous ulcerations (RAU) showed some hematological abnormality. Of these, 5 had <u>iron</u> deficiency anemia, 13 had iron deficiency without anemia, 2 had low RBC <u>folate</u> levels (1 of whom had a decreased serum folate), and 4 had borderline folate levels. (The 2 children with established folate deficiency also had decreased serum iron levels.) One child had a borderline <u>vitamin B$_{12}$</u> level which became normal on retesting. 4 of the children with iron deficiency anemia received iron supplements; 6 mo. later 2/4 reported dramatic improvement in RAU and 1/4 reported a slight improvement. All 3 had normal hemoglobin and serum iron on retesting. The fourth child, who was folate deficient and anemic, still had low iron and folate levels 6 mo. later despite folate supplementation and stated that her ulcers had worsened. The other girl with established folate deficiency and low serum iron levels was given both folate and iron supplements and reported a marked improvement 6 mo later; her iron and folate levels were normal on retesting. 6/9 children with iron deficiency but no anemia who returned for follow-up 6 mo. after starting iron supplementation had normal serum iron levels. 5 of these 6 children reported some improvement in RAU. The remaining 3 children still had below normal levels of serum iron after 6 mo. of supplementation but reported a slight improvement in RAU (*Field EA et al. Clinical and haematological assessment of children with recurrent aphthous ulceration. <u>Br Dent J</u> 163:19-22, 1987*).

Experimental and Observational Study: In a gp. of 330 pts., 23 were deficient in iron, 6 in vitamin B$_{12}$, 7 in folic acid, and 11 in 2 or more of these nutrients, for a total of 47 pts. (14.2%). Pts. with an associated glossitis or angular cheilitis were more likely to suffer from a deficiency. After 33 of the pts. with proven nutritional deficiencies received supplementation for 6 months (oral iron for 6 mo., B$_{12}$ IM every 2 mo., folic acid 5 mg 3 times daily), 23/33 (70%) had a complete remission, 11/33 (33%) improved, and 5/33 (15%) were not helped (*Wray D et al. Nutritional deficiencies in recurrent aphthae. J Oral Pathol 7(6):418-23, 1978*).

Experimental and Observational Study: In a gp. of 130 pts., 15 were deficient in iron, 5 in vitamin B$_{12}$, 7 in folic acid, and 4 in 2 or more of these nutrients for a total of 23/130 (17.7%) compared to 11/130 (8.5%) controls matched for age and sex. After 1 yr., 15/23 (65%) pts. on replacement therapy showed complete remission and 8/23 (35%) definite improvement, while only 33/107 (31%) pts. with no deficiency who received local symptomatic treatment had a remission or were improved, a significant difference (p<0.001). Most pts. with vitamin B$_{12}$ or folic acid deficiency improved rapidly; those with iron deficiency showed a less dramatic response (*Wray D et al. Recurrent aphthae: Treatment with vitamin B$_{12}$, folic acid, and iron. Br Med J 2:490-93, 1975*).

Zinc:

Supplementation may be beneficial, especially if levels are low.

Experimental Study: In a gp. of 159 pts., 10 ml of 1% zinc sulfate syrup orally 2-3 times daily together with local application of a 1% zinc sulfate paste produced good results in 81% both after 6 mo. and after 1 yr. (*Wang SW et al. [The trace element zinc and aphthosis. The determination of plasma zinc and the treatment of aphthosis with zinc.] Rev Stomatol Chir Maxillofac 87(5):339-43, 1986*) (*in French*).

Negative Experimental Double-blind Crossover Study: In a 3 mo. study of 25 pts. with recurrent AS, supplementation resulted in a small but statistically insignificant improvement. 4 pts. had to discontinue zinc because of side-effects. The results fail to confirm the beneficial effects of zinc (*Wray D. A double blind trial of systemic zinc sulfate in recurrent aphthous stomatitis. Oral Surg 53(5):469-72, 1982*).

Experimental Study: In a series of 32 pts., 8 with initial serum zinc levels >110 µg/dL, and 9 with initial levels <110 µg/dL received zinc sulfate supplementation up to a total of 660 µg/d. All pts. with initial zinc levels <110 µg/dL showed improvement (50-100% reduction in the frequency of episodes), while only 3/8 pts. with initial levels >110 µg/dL improved, suggesting that a local or general zinc deficiency, or a defect in zinc metabolism, may be one of the causes of recurrent AS (*Merchant HW et al. Zinc sulfate supplementation for treatment of recurring oral ulcers. South Med J 70(5):559-61, 1977*).

OTHER FACTORS

Rule out food sensitivities.

Review Article: Despite the many anecdotal reports, there are no systematic studies demonstrating a causal relationship between foods and canker sores (*Bock SA. Do certain foods cause canker sores? Questions and answers. JAMA 257(3):379, 1987*).

Experimental Study: 5/12 pts. improved on a strict elimination diet and were found to be reactive to milk, cheese, wheat, tomato, vinegar, lemon, pineapple and mustard. In 4 of these 5 pts., a particular food was identified which, when eliminated from the normal diet, led to either marked improvement or resolution (*Hay KD, Reade PC. The use of an elimination diet in the treatment of recurrent aphthous ulceration of the oral cavity. Oral Surg Oral Med Oral Pathol 57(5):504-7, 1984*).

Experimental Double-blind and In vitro Study: 18/60 (30%) pts. with recurrent AS were atopic with a history of respiratory allergy which was confirmed by an *in vitro* histamine release assay. The nonatopic pts. had a significantly higher incidence of *in vitro* histamine release to foods than did controls. The leukocytes from 23 pts. (38%) released histamine to food antigens. In a double-blind trial, pts. eliminated foodstuffs to investigate the correlation between *in vitro* histamine release and the development of AS. Only 30% of pts. had a decreased incidence of ulcers after eliminating foods which had induced *in vitro* histamine release. On rechallenge, 30% of the foods which caused histamine release also correlated to increased incidence of oral lesions. In 8 pts., ingestion of certain foodstuffs was correlated to oral ulceration by food diaries and elimination-rechallenge in an open trial; however, dietary manipulation did not completely eliminate ulcerations in any of them, suggesting that food sensitivities may play a minor role (*Wray D et al. Food allergens and basophil histamine release in recurrent aphthous stomatitis. Oral Surg Oral Med Oral Pathol 54(4):388-95, 1982*).

Negative Experimental and Observational Study: In a survey of 218 students, no significant relationship was found between recurrent AS and a history of an allergic diathesis. When RAS-positive and RAS-negative subjects were challenged with tomatoes, strawberries and walnuts, the results failed to document any causative effect (*Eversole RL et al. Effects of suspected foodstuff challenging agents in the etiology of recurrent aphthous stomatitis. Oral Surg Oral Med Oral Pathol 54(1):33-38, 1982*).

Experimental Study: 5/20 (25%) pts. in whom celiac disease had been excluded responded to removal of gluten and had a positive gluten challenge (*Wray D. Gluten-sensitive recurrent aphthous stomatitis. Dig Dis Sci 26(8):737-40, 1981*).

Observational Study: 56% of 61 atopic pts. had a history of AS and 18% could associate the development of aphthous ulcers with the ingestion of specific foods (*Wilson CWM. Food sensitivities, taste changes, aphthous ulcers and atopic symptoms in allergic disease. Ann Allergy 44(5):302-07, 1980*).

Lactobacillus acidophilus:

Oral administration along with local application may be beneficial.

Negative Experimental Double-blind Study: 80 mental retardates with oral ulcerations received Bacid, a viable human strain of L. acidophilus in 100 mg of carboxymethylcellulose base, 2 caps 4 times daily for 10 days or placebo during a 12-mo. study. The contents were mixed with 2 oz milk, held in the mouth for a few minutes, and then swallowed. About 90% of the lesions were clinically judged to be canker sores; the balance were cold sores (herpes simplex). 18/80 pts. had repeat episodes of oral ulcerations during the study; they were then switched to the alternative treatment. Bacid failed to affect the duration of healing of the lesions; its effect on pain could not be studied, however, as the majority of the pts. were unable to communicate responsibly with respect to the degree of pain experienced (*Gertenrich RL, Hart RW. Treatment of oral ulcerations with Bacid (Lactobacillus acidophilus). Oral Surg 30(2):196-200, 1970*).

Experimental Study: Pts. were routinely instructed to break open a capsule of Lactobacillus acidophilus and apply the powder to the ulcerated areas several times daily. They were also instructed to swallow 2 capsules daily for 1 week. All pts. reported immediate pain relief, complete clearing of lesions in about 10 days, and no early recurrence (*James APR. Common dermatologic disorders. CIBA Clinical Symposia. 19(2):38-64, 1967*).

- with Lactobacillus bulgaricus:

Experimental Study: When given during the early burning or itching stage to 22 pts. with recurrent AS, viable yogurt cultures containing L. acidophilus and L. bulgaricus blocked eruption of blisters in all pts. (*Abbott PL. J Oral Surg vol. 19, 1961*).

Case Reports: 6 pts. are described who benefited by dissolving 2 tablets containing Lactobacillus acidophilus and Lactobacillus bulgaricus in their mouths 4 times daily (*Weekes DJ. N Y State J Med 58(16), August 15, 1958*).

ATHEROSCLEROSIS
(including CORONARY HEART DISEASE)

See Also: **CARDIAC ARRHYTHMIA**
CEREBROVASCULAR DISEASE
PERIPHERAL VASCULAR DISEASE

KEY: *A = concerns angina pectoris*
           C = concerns total cholesterol
           G = concerns atherogenesis
           H = concerns HDL cholesterol
           L = concerns LDL cholesterol
           M = concerns CVD mortality and MI
           P = concerns platelet adhesiveness and/or aggregation
           R = concerns plaque regression
           T = concerns triglycerides

OVERVIEW

1. To prevent the development of atherosclerosis.

   Reduction of <u>dietary cholesterol</u> may be beneficial for those whose serum cholesterol levels are affected by it. Atherogenesis appears to be associated with the dietary intake of <u>fat</u>. However, specific fatty acids vary in their effects. Certain <u>saturated fatty acids</u> are atherogenic while, in general, <u>monounsaturates</u> and <u>polyunsaturates</u> tend to decrease coronary risk factors. (When polyunsaturates are hydrogenated, they become at least as atherogenic as saturated fatty acids.)

   A <u>high fiber diet</u> may combat atherogenesis by improving the lipid profile. <u>Vegetables</u> appear to be the best source of protein, and the consumption of <u>complex carbohydrates</u> as opposed to <u>refined sugars</u>, should be encouraged. <u>Coffee</u> intake should be restricted. The contribution of <u>alcohol</u> may depend upon inake, with a minimum of 2 drinks daily being beneficial, and higher consumption having adverse effects.

   Epidemiologic studies suggest that the consumption of <u>cold water fish</u> (which have a high concentration of omega-3 fatty acids) may beneficial, and studies suggests that this may be due to the positive effects on lipid metabolism, platelet aggregation and blood viscosity.

   Deficiencies of <u>folic acid</u>, <u>vitamin B6</u>, <u>vitamin B12</u>, <u>vitamin C</u>, <u>vitamin E</u>, <u>calcium</u>, <u>chromium</u>, <u>copper</u>, <u>magnesium</u>, <u>selenium</u>, <u>beta-carotene</u>, <u>coenzyme Q10</u>, or <u>linoleic acid</u> appear to increase the risk of atherosclerosis and/or mortality from atherosclerosis. Even when they are not deficient, supplementation with certain of these nutrients may still be beneficial, as may supplementation with <u>niacin</u>, <u>chondroitin sulfate A</u>, <u>pantethine</u> or <u>taurine</u>.

2. To promote regression of atherosclerotic plaques.

   Scientific literature showing specific nutrients to induce plaque regression in humans is lacking, although the addition of <u>chromium</u> or soya <u>lecithin</u> to the diet has modified arterial lesions in rabbits with cholesterol-induced atherogenesis.

3. To reduce angina pectoris.

Magnesium deficiency may adversely affect cardiac function and is not uncommon among angina patients. L-carnitine has been shown to be effective. Several other nutrients may also be beneficial, but the evidence is less convincing.

-- --

DIETARY FACTORS

Avoid obesity.
(C,G,T)

Review Article (C,G,T): In the overweight pt., calorie restriction can improve tissue sensitivity to insulin. Insulin resistance and hyperinsulinemia are associated with hypertension and an atherogenic lipid profile. Elevated plasma insulin concentrations enhance VLDL synthesis, leading to hypertriglyceridemia. Progressive elimination of lipid and apolipoproteins from the VLDL particle leads to an increased formation of intermediate-density and low-density lipoproteins, both of which are atherogenic. Last, insulin, independent of its effects on blood pressure and plasma lipids, is known to be atherogenic (*DeFronzo RA, Ferrannini E. Insulin resistance. A multifaceted syndrome responsible for NIDDM, obesity, hypertension, dyslipidemia, and atherosclerotic cardiovascular disease. Diabetes Care 14(3):173-94, 1991*).

Negative Review Article (G): "Inconsistent results with regard to the nature, strength, and linearity of the association between obesity and atherosclerosis do not support the hypothesis that obesity causes atherosclerosis, despite its biological plausibility" (*Barrett-Connor EL. Obesity, atherosclerosis, and coronary artery disease. Ann Intern Med 103 (6 Pt 2):1010-9, 1985*).

Low fat diet (below 30% of calories).
(C,G,H,T)

> *Note: Depending upon their fatty acid and cholesterol contents, low fat diets may reduce HDL cholesterol (Judd JT et al. Effects of diets varying in fat in P/S ratio on blood pressure and blood lipids in adult men. Prog Lipid Res 20:571-74, 1982; Grundy SM. Comparison of monounsaturated fatty acids and carbohydrates for lowering plasma cholesterol. N Engl J Med 314(2):745-48, 1986).*

> *Note: Even a low-fat diet can increase the risk of atherosclerosis if the fat is primarily saturated (Mendis K, Kumarasunderam R. The effect of daily consumption of coconut fat and soya-bean fat on plasma lipids and lipoproteins on young normolipidaemic men. Br J Nutr 63:547-52, 1990).*

Experimental Placebo-controlled Study (G): 162 nonsmoking men aged 40-59 with progressive atherosclerosis who had undergone coronary bypass surgery randomly received either a diet which was focused on reduction in the intake of fats and cholesterol or a standardized placebo diet in which dietary goals were for total fat calories to provide 26% of energy, <5% of energy from saturated fat, 10% of energy from polyunsaturated fat, 10% of energy from monounsaturated fat, and >250 mg cholesterol per day. Each quartile of increased consumption of total fat and polyunsaturated fat was associated with a significant increase in risk of new lesions. Subjects in whom new lesions did not develop increased dietary protein to compensate for reduced intake of fat. Results indicate that protein and carbohydrate, rather than monounsaturated or polyunsaturated fat, should be substituted for fat calories when total and saturated fat intakes are reduced to currently recommended levels (*Blankenhorn DH et al. The influence of diet on the appearance of new lesions in human coronary arteries. JAMA 263(12):1646-52, 1990*).

Negative Case Reports (C,H,T): Due to multiple food sensitivities, 7 pts. with hypercholesterolemia were placed on a diet in which over 90% of calories came from beef fat along with nutritional supplementation. No sucrose, milk or grains were permitted. Total cholesterol dropped from an ave. of 263 mg/dl to 189 mg/dl, HDL cholesterol rose from 21% of total cholesterol to 34%, and triglycerides dropped from 113 mg/dl to 74 mg/dl. Only 2 pts. had a weight loss of >10 lb. Results suggest that elevated serum cholesterol levels may be caused by some factor in grains, sucrose, or milk that interferes with cholesterol metabolism (*Newbold HL. Reducing the serum cholesterol level with a diet high in animal fat.. South Med J 81(1):61-63, 1988; Newbold HL. The reduction of serum cholesterol while feeding a high animal fat diet. Int J Vitam Nutr Res 56(2):190, 1986*).

Review Article (C): There is limited scientific evidence that a reduction in total fat calories will reduce total plasma cholesterol levels in most people. Studies do suggest that some individuals have a cholesterol-lowering benefit from reducing total fat calories; yet, in these studies, often two variables have been changed, fat quantity and quality, which complicates interpretation of the results (*McNamara DJ. The diet-heart question: How good is the evidence? Contemp Nutr 12(4), 1987*).

"Mediterranean" diet.
(C,H,L)

Roughly 30-40% of energy from fat which is largely from olive oil, a rich source of the monounsaturate oleic acid.

> **Review Article (C,H,L):** The disadvantage of a low-fat diet is that, not only does LDL cholesterol decrease, but HDL cholesterol also decreases. Also, fats in this diet often come from polyunsaturated fatty acids which lower HDL levels. Currently, there is insufficient evidence that the lowering of HDL by a reduction in fat intake is innocuous; thus the traditional Mediterranean diet, which uses monounsaturates as a major source of energy, may be preferable. Monounsaturates do not lower HDL levels, and populations that follow this diet have rates of coronary diesase as low as populations consuming very-low-fat diets (*Sacks FM, Willett WW. More on chewing the fat: The good fat and the good cholesterol. Editorial. N Engl J Med 325(24):1740-2, 1991*).

Choose poly- and monounsaturated oils as the major source of dietary fat.
(C,G,H,L,M,P,T)

Saturated fat may increase coronary risk factors, while poly- and monounsaturates may decrease them (*Dreon DM et al. The effects of polyunsaturated fat vs monounsaturated fat on plasma lipoproteins. JAMA 263(18):2462-66, 1990*).

> WARNING: High blood levels of polyunsaturated fatty acids may increase the risk of developing atherosclerosis unless there is adequate antioxidant protection (*Kok F et al. Do antioxidants and polyunsaturated fatty acids have a combined association with coronary atherosclerosis? Atherosclerosis 86:85-90, 1991*).

> *Note: While palmitic acid (16:0), myristic acid (14:0) and, to a lesser extent, lauric acid (12:0), are implicated, not all saturated fatty acids have been shown to be atherogenic. Medium-chain saturated fatty acids of C:12:0 (lauric acid) and shorter chain length do not enter into the prostaglandin cascade; coconut oil, for example, has not been shown to raise LDL cholesterol or to foster atheroscleorsis (Blackburn GL, Babayan VK. Letter. J Am Coll Nutr 8(3):253-4, 1989). In fact, stearic acid, a long-chain saturated fatty acid which is abundant in cocoa butter and animal fat, does not appear to raise LDL cholesterol (Bonanome A, Grundy SM. Effect of dietary stearic acid on plasma cholesterol and lipoprotein levels. N Engl J Med 318:1244-8, 1988; Denke MA, Grundy SM. Effects of fats high in stearic acid on lipid and lipoprotein concentrations in men. Am J Clin Nutr 54:1036-40, 1991).*

> *Note: At least when margarine is compared to butter, while a high polyunsaturated to saturated fat ratio may lower LDL cholesterol as well as apolipoprotein B, significant decreases in protective subfractions of HDL, namely HDL_2 and lipoprotein A-I, may occur which could cancel the benefits (Fumeron F et al. Lowering of HDL_2-cholesterol and lipoprotein A-I particle levels by increasing the ratio of polyunsaturated to saturated fatty acids. Am J Clin Nutr 53:655-9, 1991).*

> *Note: Saturated fat intake is at least as closely related to arterial and venous thrombosis as it is to atherosclerosis and is more closely related to the clotting activity of platelets and their response to thrombin than serum cholesterol (Renaud S. Dietary fatty acids and platelet function. Proc Nutr Soc Aust 10:1-13, 1985).*

Polyunsaturates are about half as powerful in lowering total serum cholesterol as saturated fats are in raising it (*Keys A, Parlin RW. Serum cholesterol response to changes in dietary lipids. Am J Clin Nutr 19:175, 1966; Hagsted DM et al. Quantitative effects of dietary fat on serum cholesterol in man. Am J Clin Nutr 17:281, 1985*).

Saturated fat intake may be negatively correlated with HDL cholesterol levels (*Fehily AM et al. Dietary determinants of lipoproteins, total cholesterol, viscosity, fibrinogen, and blood pressure. Am J Clin Nutr 36(5):890-6, 1982*), while polyunsaturates, when provided at normally consumed levels, do not appear to affect HDL cholesterol concentrations (*Iacono JM, Dougherty RM. Lack of effect of linoleic acid on the high-density-lipoprotein cholesterol fraction of plasma proteins. Am J Clin Nutr 53:660-4, 1991*).

Monounsaturates appear superior to polyunsaturates in their effects on lipid metabolism (*Mata P et al. Effects of long-term monounsaturated- vs polyunsaturated-enriched diets on lipoproteins in healthy men and women. Am J Clin Nutr 55:846-50, 1992*).

Oleic acid, a monounsaturate, may be superior to linoleic acid, a polyunsaturate, in reducing susceptibility to peroxidative damage (*Reaven P et al. An oleate rich diet in man reduces susceptibility of LDL to oxidative modification. Clin Res 39:61A, 1991*).

A high monounsaturate, low cholesterol diet may be superior to a low fat, low cholesterol, high carbohydrate diet in regard to its effects on serum lipids (*Grundy SM et al. Comparison of monounsaturated fatty acids and carbohydrates for reducing raised levels of plasma cholesterol in man Am J Clin Nutr 47(6):965-69, 1988*).

Low cholesterol diet.
(C,G,H,L,T)

> *Note: After corrections for differences in body weight and the proportion of dietary cholesterol absorbed, only about one-fourth of the the population will be sensitive to dietary cholesterol and have a significant increase in serum cholesterol levels in response to an increase in dietary cholesterol (McNamara DJ. Dietary cholesterol: effect on lipid metabolism. Curr Opin Lipidology 1:18-22, 1990; McNamara DJ. The diet-heart question: How good is the evidence? Contemp Nutr 12(4), 1987).*

Dietary cholesterol may be directly related to serum cholesterol level.

> *Note: Hyper-response to dietary cholesterol does not appear to occur in individuals following a low-fat, high-fiber diet; in this situation, reduction in dietary cholesterol below 400 mg/d produces no further substantial cholesterol lowering (Edington JD et al. Serum lipid response to dietary cholesterol in subjects fed a low-fat, high-fiber diet. Am J Clin Nutr 50:58-62, 1989; Edington J et al. Effect of dietary cholesterol on plasma cholesterol concentration in subjects following reduced fat, high fibre diet. Br Med J 294:333-36, 1987).*

Negative Experimental Controlled Study (C,H,L,T): 18 normolipidemic males were fed 6 different species of shellfish. Each portion was equal in protein to that in animal foods in the normal diet; however, <1/2 the amt. of fat normally eaten in animal foods was allowed for their preparation. Oyster, clam, crab, and mussel diets (low in cholesterol and high in omega-3 fatty acids), lowered VLDL triglycerides and cholesterol and, except for the mussel diet, LDL and total cholesterol. Squid and shrimp diets (higher in cholesterol and lower in omega-3 fatty acids) did not change blood lipids. The LDL/HDL radio was decreased in the oyster and mussel diets. Oyster, mussel, and squid diets increased HDL_2 cholesterol. Cholesterol absorption was decreased on the oyster, clam, and mussel diets. When consumed with moderate dietary fat restriction, oysters, clams, mussels, and crab appear to be useful in hypolipidemic diets for normolipidemic men (*Childs MT et al. Effects of shellfish consumption on lipoproteins in normolipidemic men. Am J Clin Nutr 51:1020-27, 1990*).

Negative Experimental Double-blind Crossover Study (C,H): 25 healthy men with an ave. plasma cholesterol of 5.3 mmol/L failed to show significant elevations in mean plasma concentrations of cholesterol, LDL cholesterol or apolipoprotein B following the addition of dietary cholesterol equal to about 2 eggs daily either while on a high saturated fat diet or on a diet modified in fat and fatty acid composition. Although the mean HDL cholesterol concentration did not change, the proportion of HDL_2 particles increased significantly, especially in subjects who did not show a rise in plasma cholesterol, suggesting that this may represent a means of clearing dietary cholesterol (*Kestin M et al. Effect of dietary cholesterol in normolipidemic subjects is not modified by nature and the amount of dietary fat. Am J Cin Nutr 50:528-32, 1989*).

Observational Study (C): In a cohort of 1824 middle-aged men followed for 25 yrs., intake of dietary cholesterol was associated with risk of death from ischemic heart disease, from other cardiovascular diseases combined, from all cardiovascular diseases combined, and from all causes combined. As this effect was partly independent of total serum cholesterol, results suggest that the intake of dietary cholesterol should be low even in those without overt hyperlipidemia (*Shekelle RB, Stamler J. Dietary cholesterol and ischaemic heart disease. Lancet 1:1177-79, 1989*).

> *Note: This study has been criticized on the following grounds:*
> *1. No difference in mortality from CHD or from all causes was found in men in the first and fourth quartile of cholesterol intake, which suggests the absence of a correlation between dietary and serum cholesterol and raises doubts about the causal role of dietary cholesterol (Skrabanek P. Dietary cholesterol and heart disease. Letter. Lancet 2:110-11, 1989).*
> *2. Only by pooling CHD with "other cardiovascular diseases" was statistical significance achieved (Skra-*

banek P. Dietary cholesterol and heart disease. Letter. Lancet 2:110-11, 1989).

3. Diet recall and death certificates are notoriously unreliable methods of data collection (Skrabanek P. Dietary cholesterol and heart disease. Letter. Lancet 2:110-11, 1989).

4. Age-adjusted all-cause mortality was higher in the first (219-502 mg cholesterol/d) than in the second (505-578 mg/d) quintile (Goldstein MR. Dietary cholesterol and heart disease. Letter. Lancet 2:111, 1989).

5. The reported association between dietary cholesterol and mortality could be due to any number of dietary or environmental risk factors. While dietary cholesterol may indeed raise serum cholesterol and be athero-genic in animals, these animals, mostly herbivores, have guts that are not adapted to deal with more than a minimal amt. of dietary cholesterol. When pigs - a more appropriate model - are used, the results are inconclusive (Totman R. Dietary cholesterol and heart disease. Letter. Lancet 2:111, 1989).

Review Article (C): Over the usual range of cholesterol intakes (0-400 mg/1000 kcal) the usual serum cholesterol response is approximately linear, each 1 mg/100 kcal resulting in an expected increase of serum cholesterol of approx. 0.1 mg/dl. Thus, with a 2500 kcal diet, an increase of 100 mg/day would be expected to increase cholesterol by approx. 4 mg/dl. However, very large differences in response have been reported for similar changes in cholesterol intake (*Hegsted DM. Serum cholesterol response to dietary cholesterol: A re-evaluation. Am J Clin Nutr 44(2):299-305, 1986*).

Experimental Double-blind Crossover Study (H,L): 17 college-aged lactovegetarians who usually consumed an ave. of 3 eggs/wk. were randomly assigned to either a 1 egg/ day diet or an identical-looking, egg-free diet. The egg diet was significantly correlated with raised LDL cholesterol and apolipoprotein B levels compared to the control diet, while HDL cholesterol levels were unchanged (*Sacks E et al. Ingestion of egg raises plasma low-density lipoproteins in free-living subjects. Lancet 2:647-9, 1984*)

Negative Observational Study (C): In a study of 912 subjects, results suggested that "differences in egg consumption usually observed in a free-living U.S. population, consuming large amounts of fats and cholesterol from other sources, are unrelated to intrapopulation differences in blood cholesterol level." The data fail to show, however, the effect of egg consumption upon people who consume negligible amounts of cholesterol from other dietary sources (*Dawber T et al. Eggs, serum cholesterol and coronary heart disease. Am J Clin Nutr 36:617-25, 1982*).

> *Note: Although eggs are rich in cholesterol, half the fat in eggs is monounsaturated. This may explain why the ingestion of eggs may fail to elevate serum cholesterol.*

Plasma cholesterol levels are more sensitive to saturated fat intake than to dietary cholesterol (*Truswell AS. ABC of nutrition. Reducing the risk of coronary heart disease. Br Med J 291:34-37, 1985*).

Experimental Studies (C): In 69% of 75 12-wk. studies, subjects compensated for increased cholesterol intake by decreasing cholesterol fractional absorption and/or endogenous cholesterol synthesis. When plasma cholesterol did increase, measurement of sterol synthesis in isolated blood mononuclear leukocytes suggested a failure to suppress endogenous cholesterol synthesis. Plasma cholesterol levels were more sensitive to dietary fat quality than to cholesterol quantity (*McNamara DJ et al. Heterogeneity of cholesterol homeostasis in man: Response to changes in dietary fat quality and cholesterol quantity. J Clin Invest 79(6):1729-39, 1987*).

The effect of increasing dietary cholesterol appears dependent upon the polyunsaturate to saturate (P/S) ratio. As the ratio increases, the impact of dietary cholesterol diminishes (*Nestel PJ. Fish oil attenuates the cholesterol-induced rise in lipoprotein cholesterol. Am J Clin Nutr 43:752, 1986; Pyorala K. Dietary cholesterol in relation to plasma cholesterol and coronary heart disease. Am J Clin Nutr 45:1176-84, 1987; Schonfeld G et al. Effect of dietary cholesterol and fatty acids on plasma lipoproteins. J Clin Invest 69:1072, 1982*).

The predictive value of increased cholesterol intake as related to long-term coronary heart disease deaths may be independent of plasma cholesterol level (*Pyorala K. Dietary cholesterol in relation to plasma cholesterol and coronary heart disease. Am J Clin Nutr 45:1176-84, 1987; Shekelle RB et al. Diet, serum choleterol, and death from coronary heart disease: the Western Electric Study. N Engl J Med 304:65-70, 1981*).

In experimental animals, including primates, cholesterol-free diets have resulted in regression of atherosclerosis (*Malknow MR. Experimental models of atherosclerosis regression. Atherosclerosis 48:105, 1983*).

Avoid <u>hydrogenated vegetable oils</u>.
(C,G,H,L,M)

Examples: margarine; vegetable shortenings

Hydrogenated vegetable oils appear to be as atherogenic as animal fats; whether they are <u>more</u> atherogenic is as of yet unclear.

A. Dietary intake of hydrogenated vegetable oils is associated epidemiologically with atherosclerosis, just as is dietary intake of animal fats (*Martin W. Margarine (not butter) the culprit? Letter. <u>Lancet</u> 2:407, 1983; Kummerow FA. Nutrition imbalance and angiotoxins as dietary risk factors in coronary heart disease. <u>Am J Clin Nutr</u> 32:58-83, 1979*).

B. The combined results of numerous experimental studies suggest that replacement of hydrogenated fat with unhydrogenated fat is of little value in reducing serum lipid levels (*Emken EA. Nutrition and biochemistry of trans and positional fatty acid isomers in hydrogenated oils. <u>Annu Rev Nutr</u> 4:339-76, 1984*).

C. Hydrogenated vegetable oils have a higher content of *trans* fatty acids which may <u>elevate</u> cholesterol (*Mensink RP, Katan MB. Effect of dietary trans fatty acids on high-density and low-density lipoprotein cholesterol levels in healthy subjects. <u>N Engl J Med</u> 323(7):439-45, 1990*), perhaps because of their anti-essential fatty acid action (*Hill EG et al. Intensification of essential fatty acid deficiency in the rat by dietary trans-fatty acids. <u>J Nutr</u> 109:1759-67, 1979*), and the accumulation of *trans* fatty acids in adipose tissue may be positively correlated with the risk of death from coronary heart disease (*Thomas LH et al. Concentration of trans unsaturated fatty acids in the adipose body tissue of decedents dying of ischaemic heart disease compared with controls. <u>J Epidemiol Community Health</u> 37(1):22-24, 1983; Thomas LH et al. Concentration of 18:1 and 16:1 transunsaturated fatty acids in the adipose body tissue of decedents dying of ischaemic heart disease compared with controls: Analysis by gas liquid chromatography. <u>J Epidemiol Community Health</u> 37(1):16-21, 1983*).

Avoid <u>deep frying</u> and otherwise <u>minimize heating of fats.</u>
(C,G)

Fat which has been used to deep fry chicken or fish can contain as much as 214 mg cholesterol per 100 gm (*Kummerow FA. Nutrition imbalance and angiotoxins as dietary risk factors in coronary heart disease. <u>Am J Clin Nutr</u> 32:58-83, 1979*).

Heating of fat is believed to oxidize cholesterol to form 25-hydroxy cholesterol which has been shown to accelerate degeneration of smooth muscle cells in arterial tissue (*Imai H et al. Angiotoxicity and arterioscleosis due to contaminants of USP-grade cholesterol. <u>Arch Pathol Lab Med</u>, 100:565, 1976*), thus setting the stage for the development of atherosclerosis (*Alexander JC. Chemical and biological properties related to toxicity of heated fats. <u>J Tox Env Health</u> 7:125-38, 1981; Kummerow FA. Nutrition imbalance and angiotoxins as dietary risk factors in coronary heart disease. <u>Am J Clin Nutr</u> 32:58-83, 1979*).

Note: Heating foods in a microwave would minimize the formation of 25-hydroxy cholesterol (Kummerow FA. Nutrition imbalance and angiotoxins as dietary risk factors in coronary heart disease. <u>Am J Clin Nutr</u> 32:58-83, 1979).

High <u>fiber</u> diet.
(C,H,L,T)

May improve lipid metabolism.

Note: Soluble fibers (such as pectins or gums) may be more effective than insoluble fibers in reducing serum cholesterol levels (Borel P et al. Wheat bran and wheat germ: Effect on digestion and intestinal absorption of dietary lipids in the rat. <u>Am J Clin Nutr</u> 49:1192-1202, 1989).

Review Article (C,H,L,T): While the Am. Heart Assoc. diet lowers serum cholesterol only 3-7%, diets rich in soluble fiber lower serum cholesterol 20-30% Carefully controlled clinical studies indicate <u>guar</u> supplements lower cholesterol about 8%, <u>pectin</u> supplements lower cholesterol about 15%, and <u>psyllium</u> supplements lower cholesterol about 16% over the short term. Incorporating <u>oat bran</u> or <u>beans</u> into the diet lowers cholesterol 19%

over a short-term period. Long-term studies indicate prudent diets including soluble fiber from oat and bean sources lower serum cholesterol more than 20% and sustain these lower values for at least 2 yrs. for hypercholesterolemic men. LDL-cholesterol values remain about 25% lower and HDL-cholesterol values increase more than 10% for these men during this follow-up period (*Anderson JW, Tietyen-Clark J. Dietary fiber: Hyperlipidemia, hypertension, and coronary heart disease. Am J Gastroenterol 81(10):907-19, 1986*).

Negative Experimental Crossover Study (C,H,T): 3 gps. of 10 normals received pectin 12 gm daily, cellulose 15 gm daily or lignin 12 gm daily in 8-wk. randomized crossover studies. Dietary records showed that diet was otherwise unchanged. None of the 3 fibers altered total cholesterol, HDL cholesterol, triglycerides or the ratio of HDL cholesterol to total cholesterol (*Hillman LC et al. The effects of the fiber components pectin, cellulose and lignin on serum cholesterol levels. Am J Clin Nutr 42(2):207-13, 1985*).

SPECIFIC FIBERS:

- Beans:

WARNING: Legumes may increase the risk of cholesterol gallstones by fostering the supersaturation of bile with cholesterol (*Nervi F et al. Influence of legume intake on biliary lipids and cholesterol saturation in young Chilean men. Gastroenterology 96:825-30, 1989*).

Canned dried beans: May lower serum cholesterol and triglyceride levels (*Anderson JW et al. Serum lipid response of hypercholesterolemic men to single and divided doses of canned beans. Am J Clin Nutr 51:1013-19, 1990*).

Guar Gum: May lower serum cholesterol levels (*Turner P et al. Metabolic studies on the hypolipidaemic effect of guar gum. Atherosclerosis 81:145-50, 1990*).

- Carrots:

Calcium pectate, found in carrot fiber, binds bile acids to prevent their resorption. Just 2 carrots daily may lower elevated cholesterol levels by 10-20% (*Hoagland PD, Pferrer PE. J Agric Food Chem May/June, 1987*).

- Cereal fibers:

General (comparisons):

Experimental Double-blind Crossover Study (H,L,T): 24 mildly hypercholesterolemic men had 11.8 g dietary fiber/d from each of 3 cereal brans (wheat, rice and oat) added to a low-fiber diet for 4 wks. each. Plasma total- and LDL cholesterol were significantly lowered only by oat bran. Compared with wheat bran, the ratios of plasma HDL cholesterol to total cholesterol and of apolipoprotein A-I to B were significantly increased with oat bran (both by 4.7%, $p<0.05$), and rice bran (2.3%, $p<0.05$, ns 3.9%, $p<0.05$, respectively) (*Kestin M et al. Comparative effects of three cereal brans on plasma lipids, blood pressure, and glucose metabolism in mildly hypercholesterolemic men. Am J Clin Nutr 52:661-6, 1990*).

Experimental Crossover Study (L,T): 12 hypercholesterolemic men randomly received either a typical American diet containing 56 g of oat-bran cereal (25 g oat bran) or the same diet with corn flakes substituted for oat bran. After 2 wks., pts. completed 2 wks. on the alternate diet. Compared with corn flakes, the oat bran diet lowered serum total cholesterol and LDL cholesterol significantly by 5.4% ($p<0.05$) and 8.5% ($p<0.025$), respectively (*Anderson JW et al. Oat-bran cereal lowers serum total and LDL cholesterol in hypercholesterolemic men. Am J Clin Nutr 52:495-99, 1990*).

Negative Experimental Double-blind Crossover Study (C,H,L): 20 healthy subjects aged 23-49 consumed isocaloric supplements of high-fiber oat bran (87 g/d) and a low-fiber refined-wheat product in either order for 6 wks. each. Mean serum total, low-density lipoprotein and high-density lipoprotein cholesterol levels were not significantly different during the high-fiber and low-fiber periods. However, both types of supplements lowered the mean baseline serum cholesterol level by 7-8%. The subjects ate less saturated fat and cholesterol and more polyunsaturated fat during both periods of supplementation than at baseline. Those changes in dietary fats were sufficient to explain all the reduction in serum cholesterol levels caused by the high-fiber and low-fiber diets (*Swain JF et al. Comparison of the effects of oat bran and low-fiber wheat on serum lipoprotein levels and blood pressure. N Engl J Med 322(3):147-52, 1990*).

Note: This study has been criticized as:
1. 18/20 pts. were able to ascertain when they were receiving the high fiber supplements;
2. the high-fiber gp. received 15% more total fat than the low-fiber gp.,
3. the low-fiber gp., as compared to the high-fiber gp., had an increase in cardiac risk (due to a lower HDL/total cholesterol ratio)
(Milliman WB. In reply to NEJM study on oat bran. Letter. Townsend Letter for Doctors May, 1990).

Oat bran:

Negative Experimental Controlled Study (C,L): 40 hypercholesterolemic men and women added 30, 60, and 90 g oat bran/d or no oat bran to their usual diet (which was relatively high in saturated fatty acids) for 1 mo. periods. No differences in plasma total or LDL cholesterol were found (*Leadbetter J, Ball MJ, Mann JI. Effects of increasing quantities of oat bran in hypercholesterolemic people. Am J Clin Nutr 54:841-5, 1991*).

Experimental Controlled Study (C): 236 healthy volunteers followed the Am. Heart Assoc. fat-modified dietary guidelines. After 4 wks., their total cholesterol levels had dropped about 11 mg/dl. They were then randomly split into 2 groups. Gp. 1 added 2 oz (dry wt.) of oatmeal daily in the form of cereal, muffins or other oatmeal-containing foods, while gp. 2 avoided oat products. After 8 wks., both gps. had further reduced their cholesterol levels; however, cholesterol dropped more among those eating oatmeal. Those who started with the highest blood cholesterol levels had the greatest reductions (*Van Horn L. Serum lipid response to a fat-modified, oatmeal-enhanced diet. Prev Med 17(3):1988*).

Wheat bran:

Experimental Study (C,H,L): 8 hypercholesterolemic men consumed a control diet (15% protein, 55% carbohydrate, 30% fat, 450 mg cholesterol, 15 g total dietary fiber) for 1 wk. followed by a similar diet which was higher in fiber for 3 weeks.. In the test diet, a minimum of 50% of the soluble fiber was derived from refined wheat products (waffles, bread, crackers, hamburger buns). Neither diet contained oats or legumes. Total serum cholesterol averaged 225 and 202 mg/dL after the control and test diet period, respectively. Serum cholesterol reductions ranged from 1.5-22.3%, with the ave. reduction of 9.8% (p<0.01) after the test diet. LDL-cholesterol decreased 12.7% (p<0.005) between control (153 mg/dL) and test phase (133 mg/dL). Serum triglycerides, HDL-cholesterol and body weight did not change significantly. Results suggest that the inclusion of refined wheat-based bakery products in a prudent diet may improve serum lipid profiles (*Anderson JW et al. Wheat-based bakery products selected for high soluble fiber content lower serum cholesterol or hypercholesterolemic men. Abstract. J Am Coll Nutr 8(5):445, 1989*).

Negative Experimental Study (C,T): 82 male pts. with a previous MI received wheat bran 70-80 gm daily as part of an anti-atherosclerotic diet. There was no evidence of a hypolipidemic action (*Meshcheryakova A et al. Effect of wheat bran included in an anti-atherosclerotic diet on some lipid metabolism parameters in patients with coronary heart disease. Vopr Pitan 1985, pp. 9-13*).

Experimental Double-blind Crossover Study (C,H,L): After 8 wks., wheat fiber (purified) 10.5 gm daily, when added to a lipid-lowering diet, significantly increased HDL cholesterol in 12 hypercholesterolemic men, but was associated with non-significant decreases in LDL and VLDL cholesterol, and total cholesterol was unchanged (*Lindgärde F, Larsson L. Effects of concentrated bran fibre preparation on HDL-cholesterol in hypercholesterolaemic men. Hum Nutr Clin Nutr 38(1):39-45, 1984*).

- Pectin:

Experimental Double-blind Crossover Study (C,H,L): 27 pts. (aged 32-65) with a mean cholesterol level of 275 ml/dl took a 5 gm capsule of grapefruit pectin or placebo 3 times daily. After 8 wks., while pts. on placebo failed to demonstrate changes in lab values, serum cholesterol levels in experimental pts. had dropped a mean of 7.6%, LDL by 10.8%, and the LDL/HDL ratio by 9.8%. 1/3-1/2 of pts. demonstrated improvements greater than 10% and up to 20% in these parameters (*Cerda JC et al. The effect of grapefruit pectin on patients at risk for coronary heart diseases without altering diet or lifestyle. Clin Cardiol 11(9):589-94, 1988*).

Experimental Study (C): 2-3 apples daily (1 mo. trial) were effective in lowering total blood cholesterol levels for 24/30 healthy subjects whose diets were otherwise uncontrolled. Since 2-3 gm pectin-in-apple produces the same effect as 6-50 gm of purified pectin, other components of apples may also be involved (*Sable-Amplis R et al. Further studies on the cholesterol-lowering effect of apple in humans. Nutr Res 3:325-8, 1983*).

In vitro Experimental Study (L): Grapefruit pectin was found to interact specifically with low-density lipoprotein, suggesting a biochemical basis by which it may cause lowering of serum and/or tissue cholesterol levels (*Baig MM, Cerda JJ. Pectin: Its interaction with serum lipoproteins. Am J Clin Nutr 34:50-53, 1981*).

- Psyllium: psyllium hydrophilic mucilloid 1 tsp 3 times daily

Experimental Placebo-controlled Study (C,L): 96 hypercholesterolemic pts. were fed either 5.1 g psyllium daily or placebo in conjunction with a "prudent" diet. After 16 wks., psyllium supplementation was associated with a 5.6% reduction in total cholesterol and a 8.6% reduction in LDL cholesterol. HDL cholesterol levels, which initially decreased, had returned to their original levels and triglyceride levels were unchanged (*Leven EG et al. Comparison of psyllium hydrophilic mucilloid and cellulose as adjuncts to a prudent diet in the treatment of mild to moderate hypercholesterolemia. Arch Intern Med 150:1822-7, 1990*).

Choose vegetables as a source of protein rather than animal products.
(C,G,H,L,T)

Not only are vegetables low in fat and cholesterol-free, but saponins decrease cholesterol absorption by competing for cholesterol binding sites (*Potter JD, et al. Soya, saponins and plasma cholesterol. Lancet 1:223-4, 1979*). A vegetarian diet may also be beneficial for other reasons, including its high fiber content.

Observational Study (C,H,L): Total and LDL cholesterol concentrations were higher in meat eaters than vegans, with vegetarians and fish eaters (who avoid meat) having similar intermediate values. HDL cholesterol was highest in the fish eaters but did not differ among the other groups. These differences suggest that the incidence of coronary heart disease may be 24% lower in lifelong British vegetarians and 57% lower in lifelong vegans than in meat eaters (*Thorogood M et al. Plasma lipids and lipoprotein cholesterol concentrations in people with different diets in Britain. Br Med J 295:351-53, 1987*).

Experimental Study (C,H): 21 vegetarians received their usual diet for 2 wks., a diet in which 250 gm beef was added isocalorically for 4 wks., and their usual diet for 2 more weeks. HDL cholesterol was unchanged, while total cholesterol rose significantly by 19% during the meat-eating period and systolic BP increased 3% (*Sacks FM et al. Effect of ingestion of meat on plasma cholesterol of vegetarians. JAMA 246:640-4, 1981*).

Compared to vegetable protein, animal protein raises serum lipid levels.

Negative Experimental Controlled Study (C,L): 10 healthy subjects (5 males & 5 females) received a very-low fat (9% energy from fat) lean-beaf (500 g/d) diet to which beef drippings (high in fat) were added in a stepwise manner in wks. 4 and 5. Total cholesterol concentrations fell significantly within 1 wk. of commencing the diet and rose the beef drippings were added. These changes were almost entirely due to changes in LDL cholesterol. Results suggest that it is the beef fat, not the beef itself, that is associated with elevations in serum cholesterol concentrations (*O'Dea K et al. Cholesterol-lowering effect of a low-fat diet containing lean beef is reversed by the addition of beef fat. Am J Clin Nutr 52:491-94, 1990*).

Negative Experimental Study (C,H,L,T): 10 normolipidemic women received alternate 3-wk. controlled feedings of similar low-fat diets containing either tofu (soy protein) or cheese. Plasma total cholesterol and LDL-cholesterol were significantly lower (p<0.010 and p<0.001, respectively) following consumption of the tofu compared to the cheese diet. There were no significant differences in HDL cholesterol or triglycerides. When 5 additional women received alternate 3-wk. controlled feedings in which the amt. and type of dietary fat were equilibrated, plasma lipid responses were similar, suggesting that the high ratio of polyunsuaturates to saturates of tofu, rather than the protein source, was responsible for the beneficial effects of tofu on serum lipids (*Meredith L et al. Alterations in plasma lipid levels resulting from tofu and cheese consumption in adult women. J Am Coll Nutr 8(6):573-79, 1989*).

Review Article (C): Animal studies have shown that animal proteins, most notably casein, increase plasma total cholesterol concentrations compared with vegetable proteins such as soy, which has been shown to be hypocholesterolemic in rats, swine, primates, and rabbits. While vegetarians have lower plasma cholesterol concentrations than omnivores, it is unclear whether this effect results specifically from the animal or the vegetable nature of the protein. In human experiments, substituting soy protein for mixed protein reduces plasma total cholesterol in hypercholesterolemic subjects. The mechanism responsible for the effects of different proteins on plasma cholesterol has not been established (*Forsythe WA et al. Dietary protein effects on cholesterol and lipoprotein concentrations: A review. J Am Coll Nutr 5(6):533-49, 1986*).

Review Article (G): Individuals consuming a diet high in animal protein whose plasma lysine to arginine ratio is 3.5 to 1 or higher have a significantly increased AS risk due to excessive dietary lysine. Animal protein has a L/A ratio of 3-4/1, while plant protein has a L/A ratio of 1-1.25/1. Compared to omnivores, individuals consuming a vegetarian diet have a significant reduction in the incidence of AS (*Sanchez A. Nutr Rep Int 28:497, 1983*).

Increase complex carbohydrates.
(C,H,L,M)

A high complex carbohydrate diet may be protective against coronary heart disease.

Observational Study (M): A prospective study analyzed the diets of 3 gps. in 1959 and surveyed subsequent mortality in 1982: men born and living in Ireland, men born in Ireland who migrated to Boston, and men born in Boston to Irish immigrants. When all gps. were combined, those who died of CHD were more likely to have significantly less total carbohydrate and fiber intake (as well as starch and vegetable protein). Cholesterol intake and the ratio of saturated to unsaturated fats were likely to be higher. The authors suggest that the nutritional change most closely linked to the increased mortality rate from CHD (which began to rise in the 1920s) was a decrease in complex carbohydrates rather than changes in the consumption of dietary lipids (*Kushi LH et al. Diet and 20-year mortality from coronary heart disease. The Ireland-Boston Diet-Heart Study. N Engl J Med 312(13):811-18, 1985*).

While both a high complex carbohydrate diet and a high-monounsaturated oil diet both lower total and LDL cholesterol, the high carbohydrate diet may lower HDL cholesterol, while the high-monounsaturate diet may increase it (*Mensiunk R et al. Effects of monounsaturated fatty acids versus complex carbohydrates on serum lipoproteins and apoproteins in healthy men and women. Metabolism 38:172-78, 1989*).

Restrict refined carbohydrates.
(G)

Theoretical Discussion (G): The high correlation between dietary lipid and heart disease mortality may be largely secondary to the high correlation that refined carbohydrates have with dietary lipids, on the one hand, and with CHD on the other. This becomes apparent only when examples are found of a weak or negative correlation between dietary lipids and refined carbohydrates. It is suggested that dietary lipids are only of secondary importance, while refined carbohydrate consumption is of primary importance (*Temple NJ. Coronary heart disease: Dietary lipids or refined carbohydrates? Med Hypothesis 10(4):425-35, 1983*).

Restrict refined sugar to below 10% of calories.
(C,G,H,P,T)

Sugar may promote atherogenesis.

Review Article (C,P,T): Results of studies suggest that high sugar diets correlate with higher plasma triglyceride concentrations and, to a lesser extent, cholesterol concentrations. In about 30% of subjects, a high sugar diet can result in an increase in insulin in fasting blood and an increase in corticosteroid concentration, platelet adhesiveness and platelet agglutination (*Yudkin J. Metabolic changes induced by sugar in relation to coronary heart disease and diabetes. Nutr Health 5(1/2):5-8, 1987*).

Observational Study (G): Yemenites who have lived in Israel for over 25 yrs. have a significantly greater prevalence of ischemic heart disease. While no sugar was eaten in Yemen, about 20% of carbohydrates ingested by Yemenites in Israel is in the form of sucrose. Fat consumption in Yemen was mainly of animal origin and its quantity was much the same as the total of animal fat and margarine consumed by Jews living in Israel, although Yemenites in Israel also consume about 16 g of soya, olive, and sesame oil. There is no significant difference in the amt. of protein consumption, nor in the total amt. of carbohydrate consumption or in the proportion of calories derived from carbohydrates (*Cohen AM et al. Change of diet of Yemenite Jews in relation to diabetes and ischaemic heart-disease. Lancet 2:1399-401, 1961*).

Sugar may increase urinary chromium loss, and chromium deficiency is a risk factor for ASHD (*see "Chromium" below*) (*Kozlovsky AS et al. Effects of diets high in simple sugars on urinary chromium losses. Metabolism 35:515, 1986*).

A high sugar intake is associated with increased total cholesterol and triglycerides (*Miyoshi T et al. Effects of a high sugar diet on the serum constituents in healthy subjects. Igaku to Seibutsugaku 105(4):265-7, 1982; Reiser S et al. Blood lipids, lipoproteins, apoproteins, and uric acid in men fed diets containing fructose or high-amylose cornstarch. Am J Clin Nutr 49:832-39, 1989; Reiser S et al. Isocaloric exchange of dietary starch and sucrose in humans. I. Effects on levels of fasting blood lipids. Am J Clin Nutr 32(8):1659-69, 1979*).

A high sugar intake is associated with decreased HDL cholesterol (*Yudkin J et al. Effects of high dietary sugar. Br Med J 281:1396, 1980*).

Sugar may promote atherosclerosis only in people with "sucrose-induced hyperinsulinism."

Observational Study (P): A gp. of 27 male pts. with peripheral vascular disease was compared to a matched control gp. consuming a similar amount of sugar (ave. 120 g/d). Both the platelet adhesiveness and insulin level were higher in the pts. and, only in the pts., sugar intake was significantly correlated with platelet adhesiveness and insulin levels measured before and after oral glucose (*Yudkin J, Szanto S. The relationship between sucrose intake, plasma insulin and platelet adhesiveness in men with and without occlusive vascular disease. Proc Nutr Soc 29(1):Suppl:2A-3A, 1970*).

Experimental Study (P): A gp. of young men were given a high-sucrose diet for 10 days and their level of immuno-reactive insulin was measured before and after. Three subjects demonstrating "sucrose-induced hyperinsulinism" (SIH) and three controls were selected to be given a high-sucrose diet while their electrophoretic platelet motility was monitored. Following 14 days, only the platelets of the 3 subjects with SIH showed a pattern of electrophoretic behavior in the presence of ADP that is characteristic of individuals with atherosclerosis. This pattern reverted towards normal 14 days after the end of the high-sucrose diet (*Szanto S, Yudkin J. Dietary sucrose and the behaviour of blood platelets. Proc Nutr Soc 29(1):Suppl:3A, 1970*).

Experimental Study (G,P,T): 19 men ages 21-44 followed high-sucrose, no-sucrose and "normal" diets for alternating 2 wk. periods. On the high sucrose diet, there was no change in cholesterol, triglycerides rose in all 19, and 6/19 demonstrated an increase in insulin levels, platelet adhesiveness and body weight. It is suggested that the effect of sucrose in producing hyperinsulinism may be more relevant than its effect on blood lipids, and that only individuals who show sucrose-induced hyperinsulinism are susceptible to the development of ischemic heart disease by dietary sucrose (*Szanto S, Yudkin J. The effect of dietary sucrose on blood lipids, serum insulin, platelet adhesiveness and body weight in human volunteers. Postgrad Med J 45:602-7, 1969*).

Sucrose may be inferior to glucose in regard to its effects on serum lipids.

Review Article (G): Long term consumption of sugars such as sucrose and fructose rather than starch and other glucose-based carbohydrates has, according to many studies, enhanced risk factors associated with the development of heart disease; thus pts. known to have high triglyceride and insulin levels may benefit from reducing their intake of fructose and sucrose (*Reiser S. Effect of dietary sugars on metabolic risk factors associated with heart disease. Nutr Health 3:203-16, 1985*).

Experimental Study (C): 18 subjects were confined to a locked institution and were placed on a chemically defined diet containing 17 amino acids, a little fat, vitamins, essential minerals and glucose. Serum cholesterol dropped rapidly for each of the subjects. Their initial ave. was 227 mg/dl. After 2 wks. it had dropped to 173 mg/dl, and after another 2 wks. to 160 mg/dl. One quarter of the glucose in the diet was then replaced by sucrose. Within 1 wk., the ave. cholesterol concentration had risen to 178, and after 2 more wks. to 208. The sucrose was then replaced again by glucose and, within 1 wk., the ave. cholesterol concentration had dropped to 175 and continued to drop until it leveled off at 150 mg/dl (*Winitz M et al. Studies in metabolic nutrition employing chemically defined diets. I. Extended feeding of normal human adult males. Am J Clin Nutr 23:525-45, 1970; Winitz M et al. Effect of dietary carbohydrate on serum cholesterol levels. Arch Biochem Biophys 108:576-79, 1964*).

Avoid coffee.
(C,G,L,M,P,T)

> **Review Article (C,G,L,M):** It has become increasingly clear that drinking coffee brewed by mixing coffee grounds with hot or boiling water raises the serum cholesterol concentration, an effect that is substantially reduced by filtering. However, a recent Norwegian study *(Tverdal A et al. Br Med J 300:566-9, 1991)* showed that coffee consumption strongly predicts coronary death, beyond what could be explained by its cholesterol raising effect. Moreover, in the Kaiser Permanente study *(Klatsky AL et al. Am J Epidemiol 132:479-88, 1990)*, an increase in coronary risk was seen after prolonged follow-up, whereas in the health professional follow up study, an increase was seen only for decaffeinated coffee *(Grobbee DE et al. N Engl J Med 323:1026-32, 1990)*. While different study designs may explain part of the descrepancy, longer studies with multiple assessments of exposure to decaffeinated and caffeinated coffee are needed before we can decide whether decaffeinated coffee increases the risk of heart disease *(Thelle DS. Coffee, cholesterol, and coronary heart disease: The secret is in the brewing. Br Med J 302:804, 1991)*.

The epidemiologic link between coffee consumption, hyperlipidemia and atherosclerosis may be at least partly due to an association between coffee consumption and the consumption of saturated fats, rather than to the effects of coffee.

> **Observational Study:** Male heavy coffee drinkers were found to eat approximately 24% more saturated fats than non-coffee drinkers *(Haffner SM et al. Coffee consumption, diet and lipids. Am J Epidemiol 122(1):1-12, 1985)*.

Abstention from coffee may reduce serum cholesterol levels.

> **Experimental Controlled Study (C):** 25/33 hypercholesterolemic men abstained from coffee for 5 weeks. Compared to controls, total serum cholesterol levels fell significantly an average of 10% in all abstainers. After 10 wks., the 9 who continued to abstain showed a 13% ave. decrease, while those who returned to coffee exhibited a gradual increase to baseline levels. This effect was independent of the use of sugar, cream, tea or cigarettes *(Førde OH et al. The Tromsø heart study: Coffee consumption and serum lipid concentrations in men with hypercholesterolaemia: A randomised intervention study. Br Med J 290:893-5, 1985)*.

Caffeine ingestion may increase platelet reactivity.

> **Experimental Study (P):** 12 healthy volunteers ingested 100 mg caffeine. There was a four-fold rise in plasma beta-thromboglobulin, a platelet-specific protein and an measure of platelet reactivity *(Ammaturo V et al. Caffeine stimulates in vivo platelet reactivity. Acta Med Scand 224:245-47, 1988)*.

Drink alcoholic beverages in moderation.
(G,H,L,M,P)

> (Moderate drinking is defined as no more than 2 drinks daily. One drink is defined as 1-1.5 oz of 80-proof whiskey, 3.5-5 oz wine, or 12 oz beer.)
>
> WARNINGS:
> 1. Risk of cirrhosis increases with 2 drinks/d for women, 4 drinks/d for men.
> 2. Women who drink 1.5 drinks/d increase their risk of breast cancer by 60%.
> 3. Risk of hypertension increases starting with 2 drinks/d.
> 4. 2-3 drinks/d is associated with a higher incidence of hemorrhagic stroke
> 5. Toddlers sustain slight damage to motor development when their mothers consume 1-4 drinks/d while breast-feeding *(Nat. Research Council, US Dept. of Health and Human Services; Am. Heart Assoc. - reported in the Los Angeles Times, October 17, 1989)*.

The effect of alcohol on CHD risk is controversial in regard to moderate drinking, although heavy drinking is clearly detrimental *(Regan TJ. Alcohol and the cardiovascular system. JAMA 264(3):377-81, 1990)*.

A. Evidence for a beneficial effect from moderate drinking:

> **Observational Study (G):** The association between self-reported alcohol intake and coronary disease was studied prospectively among 51,529 male health professionals. 350 confirmed cases of coronary disease occurred during the study period. After adjustment for coronary risk factors, including dietary intake of cholesterol, fat, and

dietary fiber, increasing alcohol intake was inversely related to coronary disease incidence (p for trend <0.001). Exclusion of 10,302 current non-drinkers or 16,342 men with disorders potentially related to coronary disease which might have led men to reduce their alcohol intake, did not substantially affect the relative risks (*Rimm EB et al. Prospective study of alcohol consumption and risk of coronary disease in men. Lancet 338:464-8, 1991*).

Review Article (G): The consistency, strength and independence of the inverse relationship between moderate alcohol consumption and coronary artery disease argues persuasively for a causal association. A plausible and likely mechanism is the effect of moderate alcohol consumption on lipoprotein and apolipoprotein levels (*Moore RD, Pearson TA. Moderate alcohol consumption and coronary artery disease. A review. Medicine 65(4):242-67, 1986*).

Alcohol, when taken with a meal high in saturated fat, reduces platelet aggregation.

Experimental Study (P): In a study using healthy volunteers, a 5-oz glass of white wine did not inhibit platelet aggregation unless it were taken with a meal high in saturated (but not a meal high in unsaturated) fat (*Fenn CG, Littleton JM. Interactions between ethanol and dietary fat in determining human platelet function. Thrombosis Haemostas 51(1):50-53, 1984*).

Moderate alcohol consumption is associated with increased diameter of the coronary arteries.

Observational Study (M): 20/31 males aged 20-66 without angiographic evidence of coronary artery disease were non-drinkers or low alcohol consumers, while 11/31 were moderate drinkers drinking an ave. of 1 drink daily. Based on coronary angiography, moderate alcohol consumption was independently associated with an ave. 26% increase in the cross-sectional area of the left main coronary artery and an ave. 31% increase in the size of the left anterior descending artery (*Fried LP et al. Long-term effects of cigarette smoking and moderate alcohol consumption on coronary artery diameter. Mechanisms of coronary artery disease independent of atherosclerosis or thrombosis? Am J Med 80(1):37-44, 1986*).

B. Evidence against a beneficial effect from moderate drinking:

Observational Study (M): In examining the health status of a gp. of middle-aged men, 70% of the abstainers were ex-drinkers who had drifted from heavy or moderate drinking into the non-drinking category as a result of accumulating ill-health. In 7 yrs. of follow-up, the non-drinkers had higher total and cardiovascular mortality than the light/occasional drinkers as a large proportion were already chronically ill (*Shaper AG et al. Alcohol and mortality in British men: explaining the U-shaped curve. Lancet 2:1267-73, 1988*).

Review Article (G,H): Epidemiologic data suggest that alcohol does not protect against coronary heart disease. Although longitudinal and cross-sectional studies have shown an association between moderate alcohol ingestion and decreased risk of coronary AS, they may be biased because the light drinkers include people who are generally more health-conscious and/or those who drink very rarely or very small amounts. Moderate alcohol ingestion, which raises HDL cholesterol, does not raise HDL_2 levels (which have been epidemiologically correlated with reduced incidence of coronary AS), but raises HDL_3 levels (which are believed to be unrelated to the incidence of coronary AS). In addition, alcohol ingestion has a detrimental effect on blood pressure, body weight and glucose tolerance, all of which relate to CHD risk. Thus the influence of alcohol is detrimental to the prevention of CHD (*Eichner ER. Alcohol versus exercise for coronary protection. Am J Med 79(2):231-40, 1985*).

Consume dairy products, especially those which are low in fat.
(A,C,H,L,T)

Note: There are arguments that milk, even if the butterfat is removed, is atherogenic (*Freed DLJ, Ed. Health Hazards of Milk. London, Baillière Tindall, 1984*).

GENERAL

Negative Observational Study (H,L): When compared to strict vegetarians, the LDL cholesterol levels of lactovegetarians were 24% higher and the HDL cholesterol levels were 7% higher. Analysis within and among vegetarian populations suggests that ingestion of fatty dairy products raises LDL cholesterol on a percentage basis about 3 times more than it raises HDl cholesterol level (*Sacks FM et al. Plasma lipoprotein levels in vegetarians. The effect of ingestion of fats from dairy products. JAMA 254(10):1337-41, 1985*).

Observational Study (C,H,L,T): Gps. of 10-13 healthy volunteers were provided supplements of 2% butterfat milk, whole milk, skim milk, yogurt, buttermilk, and sweet acidophilus milk daily. After 3 wks., despite caloric increases on all supplements, no significant increases were found in total, LDL and HDL cholesterol levels. There were significant increases in triglycerides only in the gps. taking yogurt and acidophilus, and only these 2 gps. had significant weight gains (*Thompson LU et al. The effect of fermented and unfermented milks on serum cholesterol. Am J Clin Nutr 36(6):1106-11, 1982*).

MILK

Experimental Study (C): 82 volunteers aged 30-70 added 1 qt. of skim milk to their normal daily diet. Those whose cholesterol levels were above 230 mg/dl experienced drops averaging 8% after 8 wks., while those with lower initial levels experienced little change (*Arun Kilara, associate professor of food science, Pennsylvania State University, USA - reported in Med World News January 11, 1988, p. 39*).

Experimental Study (C): 54 volunteers who received 2% butterfat milk for 1 wk. demonstrated slightly reduced serum cholesterol levels; triglycerides were unaffected (*Hepner G et al. Hypocholesterolemic effect of yogurt and milk. Am J Clin Nutr 32(1):19-24, 1979*).

Skim milk from cows immunized against human intestinal bacteria may be more beneficial than ordinary skim milk.

Experimental Double-blind Crossover Study (C,L): 11 pts. with primary hypercholesterolemia randomly received skim milk (90 g powder) from immunized cows or control skim milk in either order for 8 wks. each. After 8 wks., pts. ingesting skim milk from immunized cows showed an 8% decrease in serum total cholesterol (p<0.025), a 4% decrease in LDL cholesterol (n.s.) and an 8% decrease in the atherogenic index (total cholesterol/HDL cholesterol) (p<0.05) compared to placebo treatment (*Golay A et al. Cholesterol-lowering effect of skim milk from immunized cows in hypercholesterolemic patients. Am J Clin Nutr 52:1014-9, 1990*).

YOGURT

Experimental Study (C): 5 men and 6 women ate 3 cups yogurt daily. After the first week, their ave. cholesterol level had decreased from 252-230 (5-10% reduction) where it stayed for the remaining 11 wks. of the study; serum triglycerides were unaffected (*Hepner G et al. Hypocholesterolemic effect of yogurt and milk. Am J Clin Nutr 32(1):19-24, 1979*).

- -

COMBINED DIETARY PROGRAMS

"Cardiovasoprotective diet" (high in complex carbohydrates, dietary fiber, vegetable proteins, polyunsaturates, high P:S
(C,G,M,T)   ratio, high potassium, magnesium and vitamin C, low in saturated fat and cholesterol).

Experimental Single-blind Study (C,G,M,T): 422 high risk pts. received either a "cardiovasoprotective diet" or a usual diet. After 1 yr., there was a significant decrease in the total risk factors (25.3%) in the experimental gp. compared to controls (p<0.02). Mean serum cholesterol (9.2%), triglyceride (13%) and fasting blood sugar (15.2%) were significantly lowered. There was a significant decrease in total cardiovascular complications in the experimental group. Also, fatal and non-fatal MI and sudden death, overall complications and mortality due to ischemic heart disease were less in the experimental gp. (results not significant) (*Singh RB et al. Risk factor intervention through dietary modification. J Nutr Med 1:267-75, 1990*).

Experimental Single-blind Study (A,C,M,T): 260 pts. with acute MI randomly received either a cardiovasoprotective diet (Gp. A) or a usual diet (Gp. B) 72 hrs. after infarction. After 6 wks., overall mortality was higher in Gp. B (10.1%) than Gp. A (6.0%). Complications such as angina and arrhythmias requiring treatment, reinfarction, left ventricular strain and chronic left ventricular failure were significantly more common in Gp. B compared to Gp. A (p<0.001). Mean serum cholesterol and triglyceride levels were significantly reduced (p<0.05) compared to initial levels only in Gp. A (*Singh RB et al. Nutritional intervention in acute myocardial infarction. J Nutr Med 1:179-86, 1990*).

High carbohydrate, high fiber, low fat diet.
(C,G,H,T)

    Review Article (C,G,T): High carbohydrate, high fiber diets lower serum cholesterol and triglyceride levels about 20%, theoretically reducing risk for coronary artery disease by 40% (*Anderson JW, Gustafson NJ. High-carbohydrate, high-fiber diet: Is it practical and effective in treating hyperlipidemia? Postgrad Med 82(4):40-55, 1987*).

    Experimental Controlled Study (C,H,T): The effects of 4 different diets (Western reference diet with 40% energy from fat & P/S ratio 0.27, low-fat diet with 27% energy from fat & P/S ratio 1.0 and reduced cholesterol content, low-fat diet supplemented with fiber and a diet with 40% energy from fat with fiber supplementation) on 12 normal males were evaluated. The effects of fat modification and fiber supplementation (reduced serum cholesterol, LDL cholesterol and serum triglycerides) were strongly additive (*Lewis B et al. Towards an improved lipid-lowering diet: Additive effects of changes in nutrient intake. Lancet December 12, 1981*).

Low fat, cholesterol-free diet with a high ratio of polyunsaturated to saturated fats.
(C,L)

    Experimental Study (C,L): 7 pts. with heterozygous familial hypercholesterolemia responded well to an 11 day cholesterol-free diet with with a high ratio of polyunsaturates to saturates (3:1). Dietary fat, carbohydrate and protein comprised 18.0%, 69.2%, and 12.8% of calories, respectively. After 11 days, the mean plasma cholesterol dropped from 8.37 to 7.17 mmol/L and LDL cholesterol from 5.93 to 4.90 mmol/L (17.5%) (*Mokuno H et al. Cholesterol-free diet with a high ratio of polyunsaturated to saturated fatty acids in heterozygous familial hypercholesterolaemia: significant lowering effect on plasma cholesterol. Horm Meta Res 22:246-51, 1990*).

Total parenteral nutrition.
(C,R)

    Experimental Study (C,R): A fat-free total parenteral nutrion (TPN) formula was evolved based on the ability of the formula to lower cholesterol and cause plaque regression in rabbits. This formula consists of 18 L-amino acids formulated in ratios and quantities that are optimal for decreasing plasma cholesterol in each pt. along with dextrose for non-protein caloric requirements, vitamins, minerals and trace elements. Modifications in the amino acid dosages are made depending upon plasma and urine amino acid concentrations. This formula was utilized successfully in 13 pts. with severe cardiovascular disease. In addition to improvements in blood lipids, all pts. improved clinically as manifested by improved cardiovascular function, improved levels of physical activity, decreased or absent symptoms, increased strength and sense of well being, and ability to reduce significantly or omit the dosages of cardiovascular medictions they had been taking. In most pts., significant regression of the coronary artery atherosclerotic lesions were documented on repeat angiography (*Dudrick SJ et al. Experimental and clinical atherosclerosis: Their experimental reversal. Trans Stud Coll Physicians Phila 10(1-4):35-61, 1988*).

- -

VITAMINS

Folic acid: 5 mg daily (14 day trial)
(G)

    Coenzyme in the conversion of homocysteine, an atherogenic amino acid (*see discussion under "Vitamin B6" below*), to methionine.

    Low levels may be inversely correlated with homocysteine levels (*Brattström L et al. Impaired homocysteine metablism in early-onset cerebral and peripheral occlusive arterial disease. Effects of pyridoxine and folic acid treatment. Atherosclerosis 81(1):51-60, 1990; Israelsson B et al. Homocysteine and myocardial infarction. Atherosclerosis 71(2-3):227-33, 1988*).

    Supplementation may reduce homocysteine concentrations.

        Experimental Study: Folic acid 5 mg daily for 14 days significantly reduced total plasma homocysteine levels in 11/13 normal subjects (p<0.01). Vitamin B12 (cyanocobalamin) 1 mg or pyridoxine 40 mg was ineffective. Results are consistent with the hypothesis that excess folate enhances the remethylation of homocysteine to methionine (*Brattström LE et al. Folic acid - An innocuous means to reduce plasma homocysteine. Scand J Clin Lab Invest 48:215-21, 1988*).

Supplementation may be beneficial.

Animal Experimental Study (G): Rats given an atherogenic diet showed a decrease in lipoprotein lipase activity in the aorta and plasma. After administration of folic acid, there was a significant increase in lipoprotein lipase activity. Activity of this enzyme is known to be somehow associated with atherosclerosis and there is evidence that it has a protective effect against lipid infiltration (*Povoa H Jr et al. Folic acid and lipoprotein lipase from aorta and blood plasma of atherosclerotic rats. Biomed Biochim Acta 43(2):241-44, 1984*).

Experimental Study (G): 15/17 elderly pts. with diffuse, chronic arteriosclerosis given 5-7.5 mg folic acid daily developed increased capillary blood flow and improved vision (*Kopjas TL. Effect of folic acid on collateral circulation in diffuse chronic arteriosclerosis. J Am Geriatr Soc 14(11):1187-92, 1966*).

Niacin: Take up to 3 gm. daily in divided doses.
(C,H,L,M,T)   Start with 100 mg 3 times daily with meals;
    increase as needed by 100 mg 3 times daily
    each week (niacinamide is ineffective).

(*See Also: "Inositol Nicotinate" below*)

WARNING: May have significant side-effects; treatment should be under medical supervision. (*See "Appendix B: Dangers of Nutritional Supplementation".*)

WARNING: Not recommended as a first-line hypolipidemic drug in type II diabetics as it may result in deterioration of glycemic control and increase plasma uric acid (*Garg A, Grundy SM. Nicotinic acid as therapy for dyslipidemia in non-insulin-dependent diabetes mellitus. JAMA 264(6):723-26, 1990*).

Recommended as the "first drug to be used" when dietary intervention fails to adequately reduce elevated LDL cholesterol levels (*Hoeg JM et al. Special communication: An approach to the management of hyperlipoproteinemia. JAMA 255(4):512-21, 1986*).

Experimental Placebo-controlled Study (C,H,L,T): In a randomized study, pts. with elevated LDL cholesterol consumed either 2, 1.5, 1.25 or 1 gm/d niacin in a wax-matrix sustained-release form and were compared to placebo and diet-treated groups. Pts. who consumed niacin in doses of 1.5 g or more showed significant reductions in LDL cholesterol. Total cholesterol dropped 18.4% and 13.3%, and the ratio of total cholesterol to HDL cholesterol dropped 20.4% and 19.4% in the 2 g and 1.5 g gps., respectively. Improvements were also noted in HDL cholesterol and triglyceride levels. Several liver enzymes, including AST, lactate dehydrogenase and alkaline phosphatase, increased as LDL cholesterol decreased, but only in the pts. receiving niacin, suggesting that the liver may be the site of niacin's effects on lipids. Side effects were minimal, with a drop-out rate of only 3.4% (*Keenan J et al. Niacin revisited: A randomized, controlled trial of wax-matrix sustained-release niacin in hypercholesterolemia. Arch Intern Med 151:1424-32, 1991*).

Review Article (C,H,L,T): Effective in decreasing triglycerides, total cholesterol and LDL cholesterol and in increasing HDL cholesterol (*The Medical Letter Vol. 27, No. 695, August 30, 1985*).

Supplementation may reduce the risk of myocardial infarction and of death from myocardial infarction.

Experimental Placebo-controlled Study (M): Beginning in 1969, 1119 men aged 30-64 were randomized to receive niacin 3 g/d at entry, and 2789 men were randomized to receive placebo. At the end of the first stage of the study (1975), the niacin-treated gp. showed a lower incidence of MI. At follow-up (1981), there were 69 fewer deaths in the men who had been previously randomized to the niacin gp. than were expected on the basis of mortality in the placebo group (p=0.0004). In addition, men with initially higher cholesterol values experienced the greatest benefit from niacin therapy (*Berge K, Canner P. Coronary Drug Project: Experience with niacin. Eur J Clin Pharmacol 40:S49-51, 1991*).

Supplementation may reduce serum lipoprotein Lp(a), an independent risk factor for ischemic heart disease, in hyperlipidemic subjects.

Experimental Study (G,L): 31 hyperlipidemic pts. received 4 gm nicotinic acid daily. After 6 wks., the serum levels of Lp(a) were significantly reduced. The decrease was 38% (95% confidence interval of 28-47%). There was a linear relationship between the percentage decrease of Lp(a) and that of LDL cholesterol (r=0.88), suggesting that there may be inhibition of apolipoprotein B synthesis which is a protein common to the two lipoproteins (*Carlson LA et al. Pronounced lowering of serum levels of lipoprotein Lp(a) in hyperlipidaemic subjects treated with nicotinic acid. J Intern Med 226:271-76, 1989*).

Low-dose niacin may increase HDL cholesterol levels and improve the total cholesterol/HDL cholesterol ratio with less side effects.

Experimental Study (H,L,T): 55 pts. werre given long-acting niacin 1 g/d. After 6.7 mo., total cholesterol and triglyceride levels failed to change significantly; however HDL cholesterol rose 31% and total cholesterol/HDL cholesterol ratio was reduced 27%. 40% of pts. left the study mainly because of adverse side effects. Apart from 1 pt. who developed overt diabetes, of questionable relationship to niacin, no pt. developed serious side effects such as jaundice or peptic ulcer (*Luria MH. Effect of low-dose niacin on high-density lipoprotien cholesterol and total cholesterol/high density lipoprotein cholesterol ratio. Arch Intern Med 148:2493-95, 1988*).

<u>Vitamin B6</u>:   40 mg. daily
(C,G,M,P,T)

Animal studies have repeatedly shown that a vitamin B6-deficient diet results in atherosclerotic lesions that are widely distributed in all vessels of all calibres (*Rinehart JF, Greenberg LD. Vitamin B6 deficiency in the Rhesus monkey. Am J Clin Nutr 4:318-25, 1956; Rinehart JF, Greenberg LD. Arteriosclerotic lesions in pyridoxine deficient monkeys. Am J Pathol 25:481-96, 1949*).

Vitamin B6 levels may drop during the acute phase of myocardial infarction.

Observational Study (M): The vitamin B6 status of 84 pts. with acute MI was compared with that of 84 controls. Mean pyridoxal-5[1]-phosphate (PLP) plasma levels were significantly lower in pts. than in controls. RBC PLP levels were also lower, but not significantly. Basal activity and total potential activity of the B6-dependent enzyme aspartate aminotransferase also suggested the presence of B6 deficiency. The relative risk of acute MI in pts. int he lowest quartile of plasma PLP was 5 times greater than in those in the highest quartile (*Kok FJ et al. Low vitamin B6 status in patients with acute myocardial infarction. Am J Cardiol 63:513-16, 1989*).

Supplementation may inhibit platelet aggregation and prolong clotting time.

Review Article (P): Because of its relation to atherosclerosis and thrombosis, vitamin B6 is one of the most promising prospects in the search for agents which will inhibit platelet activation and intravascular coagulation. "If thrombin and fibrin formation in addition to platelet activation are important in the pathogenesis and progress of atherosclerotic lesions, then moderate doses of vitamin B6 (say 40 mg a day) may suffice to alter the natural history of such a process" (*Is vitamin B6 an antithrombotic agent? Lancet 1:1299-1300, 1981*).

Experimental Study (P): In healthy volunteers IV pyridoxine 5[1]-phosphate (PALP) not only inhibited platelet aggregation but also prolonged the whole-blood clotting time and thrombin clotting time. The clotting time of PALP-bound fibrinogen was 2-3 times longer than the control value (*Subbarao K et al. Pyridoxal 5[1]-phosphate - a new physiological inhibitor of blood coagulation and platelet function. Biochem Pharmacol 28:531-34, 1979*).

There is considerable evidence that the amino acid <u>homocysteine</u> may initiate arteriosclerotic changes. Homocysteine is normally converted to the non-toxic cystathionine; however, the incidence of heterozygous homocystinuria due to B6-dependent cystathionine synthase deficiency is about 1 in 70 and deficiencies of nutrients involved in homocysteine metabolism may raise plasma homocysteine levels.

Observational Study (G): Hyperhomocysteinemia was detected in 16/38 pts. with cerebrovascular disease (42%), 7/25 pts. with peripheral vascular disease (28%), and 18/60 pts. with coronary vascular disease (30%) compared to none of 27 normal controls. After adjustment for the effects of conventional risk factors, the lower 95% confidence limit for the odds ratio for vascular disease among pts. with hyperhomocysteinemia as compared to normals was 3.2. The geometric-mean peak serum homocysteine level was 1.33 times higher in pts. with all vascular disease than in normals (p=0.002). The presence of cystathionine beta-synthase deficiency was confirmed in 18/23 pts. with vascular disease who had hyperhomocysteinemia. Results suggest that hyperhomocysteinemia is an independent risk factor for vascular disease, including coronary disease, which is probably due in most instances to cystathionine beta-synthase deficiency (*Clarke R et al. Hyperhomocysteinemia: an independent risk factor for vascular disease. N Engl J Med 324(17):1149-55, 1991*).

> *Note: The authors also found an inverse relation between both RBC folate and serum vitamin B₁₂ levels and hyperhomocysteinemia. They believe that there are probably multiple mechanisms involved in the pathogenesis of hyperhomocysteinemia and suggest that the relative contributions of genetic and nutritional factors require further study (Clarke R et al. Homocysteinemia: a risk factor for vascular disease. Letter. N Engl J Med 325(13):966-7, 1991).*

Observational Study (G): 72 pts. below age 55 with occlusive arterial disease of cerebral, carotid, or aorto-iliac vessels were studied. 20 pts. (36%) had basal homocysteinemia. Also, 20 pts. (36%) had abnormal increases of plasma homocysteine after peroral methionine loading, reaching levels which exceeded the highest value for 46 comparable controls and were within the range for 20 obligate heterozygotes for homocystinuria due to pyridoxal-5-phosphate-dependent cystathionine beta-synthase deficiency. Basal plasma homocysteine content was strongly and negatively correlated to vitamin B₁₂ and folate concentrations. Plasma pyridoxal-5-phosphate (PLP) was depressed in most pts. but there was no correlation between PLP and homocysteine levels (*Brattström L et al. Impaired homocysteine metablism in early-onset cerebral and peripheral occlusive arterial disease. Effects of pyridoxine and folic acid treatment. Atherosclerosis 81(1):51-60, 1990*).

Observational Study (C,T): In a study of 52 males aged 30-60, plasma homocysteine levels were correlated with total cholesterol (p<0.001) and triglyceride (p<0.010) levels (*Olszewski AJ et al. Reduction of plasma lipid and homocysteine levels by pyridoxine, folate, cobalamin, choline, riboflavin, and troxerutin in atherosclerosis. Scand J Clin Lab Invest 48(3):215-21, 1988*).

Observational Study (G): Compared to 26 healthy males of the same age, the plasma proteins of 26 male survivors of MI 2-3 mo. after the acute phase were found to contain a high concentration of homocysteine which was about 25 times the quantity found in the control group (*Olszewski AJ, Szostak WB. Homocysteine content of plasma proteins in ischemic heart disease. Atherosclerosis 69(2-3):109-13, 1988*).

Negative Observational Study (G): The risk of heart attack or stroke was not increased in parents of homozygous homocystinurics (heterozygous for homocystinuria) (*Mudd SH et al. A study of cardiovascular risk in heterozygotes for homocystiuria. Am J Hum Genet 33:883-93, 1981*).

Vitamin B₆ is coenzyme for the conversion of homocysteine to cystathionine; thus a B₆ deficiency is theorized to cause arterial damage due to the accumulation of homocysteine, and supplementation may reduce elevated homocysteine levels.

> *Note: See also "Folic acid" above and "Vitamin B₁₂" and 'Betaine' below.*

Experimental Study: Supplementation with pyridoxine improved abnormal homocysteine metabolism in 10/11 pts. with heterozygous homocystinuria due to cystathionine beta-synthase deficiency, and homocysteine metabolism became normal in 6 out of the 11 pts. (*Boers GHJ et al. Heterozygosity for homocystinuria in premature peripheral and cerebral occlusive arterial disease. N Engl J Med 313:709, 1985*).

Experimental Study (G): In a retrospective study of 629 pts. with homocystinuria due to cystathionine beta-synthase deficiency, initial thromboembolic events and mortality occurred earlier in untreated B₆-responsive pts. than in treated B₆-responsive patients, while pyridoxine treatment of late-detected B₆-responsive pts. retarded the rate of occurrence of initial thromboembolic events (*Mudd SH et al. The natural history of homocystinuria due to cystathionine beta-synthase deficiency. Am J Hum Genet 37(1):1-31, 1985*).

Animal Experimental Study (G): Arteriosclerotic plaques were found in the aorta and arteries of rabbits given homocysteine thiolactone, methionine or homocysteic acid. Pyridoxine prevented thrombosis and pulmonary embolism but did not prevent arteriosclerotic plaques (*McCully KS, Wilson RB. Homocysteine theory of arteriosclerosis. Atherosclerosis 22(2):215-27, 1975*).

- with <u>Folic Acid</u>:

> **Experimental Study:** 20 pts. below age 55 with occlusive arterial disease of cerebral, carotid, or aorto-iliac vessels found to have impaired homocysteine metabolism were treated with pyridoxine hydrochloride 240 mg/d and folic acid 10 mg/d. After 4 wks., fasting homocysteine was reduced by a mean of 53%, and the increase in plasma homocysteine after methionine loading was reduced by a mean of 39%, suggesting that the impaired metabolism can be improved easily and without side effects (*Brattström L et al. Impaired homocysteine metablism in early-onset cerebral and peripheral occlusive arterial disease. Effects of pyridoxine and folic acid treatment. <u>Atherosclerosis</u> 81(1):51-60, 1990*).

<u>Vitamin B$_{12}$</u>:
(G)

Deficiency is associated with elevated homocysteine levels (*see discussion of homocysteine under "<u>Vitamin B$_6$</u>" above*).

> **Observational Study:** Total plasma homocysteine was twice as high in 20 asymptomatic vitamin B$_{12}$-deficient subjects as in 21 controls (p<0.0001), and higher than in 14 heterozygotes for homocysteinuria due to cystathionine beta-synthase deficiency (p<0.01). Eight (40%) B$_{12}$-deficient subjects had significant homocysteinemia (>+2 SD for controls) (*Brattström LE et al. Higher total plasma homocysteine in vitamin B$_{12}$ deficiency than in heterozygosity for homocystinuria due to cystathionine beta-synthase deficiency. <u>Metabolism</u> 37(2):175-78, 1988*).

When vitamin B$_{12}$ is deficient, supplementation may decrease elevated homocysteine levels.

> **Experimental Study:** Elevated total plasma homocysteine levels in 20 asymptomatic subjects decreased to normal following supplementation with hydroxycobalamin (*Brattström LE et al. Higher total plasma homocysteine in vitamin B$_{12}$ deficiency than in heterozygosity for homocystinuria due to cystathionine beta-synthase deficiency. <u>Metabolism</u> 37(2):175-78, 1988*).

- with <u>Choline</u>, <u>Folic Acid</u>, , <u>Riboflavin</u>, <u>Troxerutin</u>, and <u>Vitamin B$_6$</u>:

Combined supplementation may be beneficial.

> **Experimental Study (C,T):** A gp. of 12 male survivors of MI was given pyridoxine, folate, coabalamin, choline, riboflavin, and troxerutin. After 21 days, the plasma concentrations of homocysteine declined to 57% of the pretreatment values, and cholesterol, triglycerides, and LDL apolipoprotein B declined to 79% (p<0.001), 68% (p<0.01) and 63% (p<0.001) of the pretreatment values, respectively (*Olszewski AJ et al. Reduction of plasma lipid and homocysteine levels by pyridoxine, folate, cobalamin, choline, riboflavin, and troxerutin in atherosclerosis. <u>Scand J Clin Lab Invest</u> 48(3):215-21, 1988*).

<u>Vitamin C</u>:   1 gram three times daily (3 wk. trial)
(A,C,F,G,H,L,P,T)

Leukocyte and plasma concentrations of ascorbate are significantly decreased in coronary heart disease (*Horsey J et al. Ischaemic heart disease and aged patients: Effects of ascorbic acid on lipoproteins. <u>J Hum Nutr</u> 35:53-58, 1981; Ramirez J, Flowers NC. Leukocyte ascorbic acid and its relationship to coronary artery disease in man. <u>Am J Clin Nutr</u> 33:2070-87, 1980; Vallance BD et al. Reassessment of changes in leucocyte and serum ascorbic acid after acute myocardial infarction. <u>Br Heart J</u> 4:64-68, 1978*), possibly because of increased degradation and excretion due to the greatly enhanced rates of oxidation of ascorbate in inflammation by activated neutrophils (*Roberts P et al. Vitamin C and inflammation. <u>Med Biol</u> 62:88, 1984*).

A marginal vitamin C deficiency may contribute to atherosclerosis as:

1. <u>Cholesterol-7-alpha-hydroxylase</u>, which is utililzed in synthesizing bile acids from cholesterol, is vitamin C-dependent. When, in guinea pigs, a marginal vitamin C deficiency slows this reaction, it causes cholesterol accumulation in the liver, blood plasma and arteries, an increase in the total cholesterol to HDL cholesterol ratio, prolongation of plasma cholesterol half-life, an increase in the cholesterol to bile acids ratio in bile, cholesterol gallstone formation and atheromatous changes in coronary arteries.
2. Vitamin C stimulates plasma <u>lipoprotein lipase</u> which is required in the catabolism of triglycerides;

3. Vitamin C is required in the <u>hydroxylation of proline</u> for collagen formation, and thus influences arterial wall integrity.
(*Ginter E et al. Vitamin C in the control of hypercholesterolemia in man. <u>Int J Vitam Nutr Res</u> Suppl 23:137-52, 1982; Turley S et al. Role of ascorbic acid in the regulation of cholesterol metabolism and the pathogenesis of atherosclerosis. <u>Atherosclerosis</u> 24:1-18, 1976*).

Plasma vitamin C levels may be inversely correlated with the risk of angina pectoris (*Riemersma RA et al. Risk of angina pectoris and plasma concentrations of vitamins A, C and E and carotene. <u>Lancet</u> 337:1-5, 1991*).

Plasma vitamin C levels may be inversely correlated with indicators of cardiovascular disease risk.

Observational Study (G): Plasma ascorbic acid was measured in 148 male and 93 female healthy elderly Chinese-Americans. The difference in risk factors associated with a one standard deviation increase in plasma ascorbic acid was as follows:
Systolic BP: -5.5 mm Hg (p<0.002)
Diastolic BP: -2.9 mm Hg (p<0.002)
log HDL cholesterol: +4.1% (p<0.02)
Fasting blood glucose: -38 mmol/L (p<0.04)
(*Choi ESK et al. Correlation of plasma ascorbic acid with cardiovascular risk factors. Abstract. <u>Am J Clin Nutr</u> 51:511, 1990*).

Plasma vitamin C levels may be directly correlated with HDL cholesterol levels (*Esk C et al. Correlation of plasma ascorbic acid with cardiovascular risk factors. <u>Clin Res</u> 38:A747, 1990; Hallfrisch J et al. High plasma vitamin C associated with increased plasma HDL- and HDL$_2$ - cholesterol. <u>Clin Res</u> 39:A203, 1991*).

If deficient, supplementation may lower elevated total cholesterol, LDL cholesterol, triglycerides and total lipids, while raising HDL cholesterol levels, increasing fibrinolytic activity and decreasing platelet aggregation.

Review Article (C,G,H): The concept that ascorbic acid protects against coronary heart disease developed in the late 1970s when vitamin C intakes in industrialized nations were lower than at present. Supplementation was then shown to lower plasma total cholesterol and, among some elderly men, to raise HDL cholesterol. However, among people in initially good vitamin C nutriture, these effects are usually not seen (*Trout DL. Vitamin C and cardiovascular risk factors. <u>Am J Clin Nutr</u> 53:322S-5S, 1991*).

Review Article (C): In most hypercholesterolemic persons with low vitamin C status, ascorbic acid 500-1000 mg daily lowers total cholesterol in blood plasma. The maximum drop is after about 6 mo. and sometimes it may rise again - probably because, as it accelerates the conversion of cholesterol to bile acids recycling through the liver, a feedback system slows down the reaction. However, if a cholesterol-binding agent such as pectin is given along with vitamin C, the decline in cholesterol is striking and sustained (*Ginter E et al. Vitamin C in the control of hypercholesterolemia in man. <u>Int J Vitam Nutr Res Suppl</u> 23:137-52, 1982*).

Review Article (C): "It has been repeatedly demonstrated that ascorbic acid does not affect the plasma cholesterol level in subjects with an initial blood cholesterol value of under 200 mg%, or even slightly raises it. There is likewise little hope of success in hyperlipidemic patients with a continuous good supply of vitamin C, because in that case some other factor, and not ascorbate deficiency, is reponsible for impaired lipid metabolism" (*Ginter E. Chronic marginal vitamin C deficiency: biochemistry and pathophysiology. <u>Wld Rev Nutr Diet</u> 33:104-41, 1979*).

<u>Vitamin D:</u>
(C,G,M)

WARNING: Animal studies suggest that excess intake may accelerate the frequency of degenerated smooth muscle cell death in the intima of arterial tissue. The resulting lesions appear under electron microscopy to be identical to those in thoracic aortic tissue obtained during coronary bypass surgery. It seems judicious to reduce this risk factor by eliminating vitamin D$_2$ and D$_3$ from all vitamin supplements, from all food and cereal products and from the diet of livestock 1 mo. before slaughter so that the intake of vitamin D is no larger than the 400 IU/quart in milk which is necessary to prevent rickets in children (*Kummerow FA. Nutrition imbalance and angiotoxins as dietary risk factors in coronary heart disease. <u>Am J Clin Nutr</u> 32:58-83, 1979*).

Animal Experimental Study (G,M): Grossly normal areas of the aorta from weanling swine fed vitamin D3 25,000 IU/lb. of basal ration for 3 mo. had a higher frequency of degenerated smooth muscle cells under electron microscopy than similar areas of control swine. Similarly, weanling piglets fed 12,500 IU/lb. developed identical lesions and developed extensive lipid deposits and coronary occlusion by age 6 months (*Taura M et al. Coronary atherosclerosis in normo-cholesterolemic swine artery. Arter Wall 4:395, 1978; Huang WY et al. The influence of vitamin D on plasma and tissue lipids and atherosclerosis in swine. Artery 3:439, 1977*).

Observational Study (C): Out of a gp. of 100 farmers aged 35-55, the 25 who were taking vitamin D preparations (roughly 700-2500 IU daily) had a significantly higher ave. serum cholesterol (266 mg/100 ml) than the other 75 (243 mg/100 ml) (*Dalderup LM. Vitamin D, cholesterol, and calcium. Lancet 1:645-6, 1968*).

Vitamin E: 600 IU daily
(A,G,H,L,M,P,T)

> WARNING: High dosages are not recommended for people with hypertension, rheumatic heart disease or ischemic heart disease except under close medical supervision.

Plasma level may be inversely correlated with mortality from ischemic heart disease (*Gey KF et al. Inverse correlation between plasma vitamin E and mortality from ischemic heart disease in cross-cultural epidemiology. Am J Clin Nutr 53:326S-34S, 1991*).

Plasma level may be inversely correlated with the risk of angina pectoris (*Riemersma RA et al. Risk of angina pectoris and plasma concentrations of vitamins A, C and E and carotene. Lancet 337:1-5, 1991*).

May regulate endothelial cell proliferation and repair as well as protect these cells against oxidative injury (*Boscobionik D, Szewczyk A, Azzi A. Alpha-tocopherol (vitamin E) regulates vascular smooth muscle cell proliferation and protein kinase C activity. Arch Biochem 286:264-9, 1991; Hennig B et al. Protective effects of vitamin E in age-related endothelial cell injury. Int J Vitam Nutr Res 59:273-79, 1989*).

Supplementation may inhibit platelet adhesiveness (*Steiner M. Influence of vitamin E on platelet function in humans. J Am Coll Nutr 10(5):466-73, 1991*) and aggregation (*Creter D et al. Effect of vitamin E on platelet aggregation in diabetic retinopathy. Acta Hematol. 62:74, 1979*).

Supplementation may increase HDL cholesterol.

Experimental Study (H): 8 subjects were given vitamin E 800 IU daily. After 6 wks., 3/8 had similar increases in HDL cholesterol, HDL-apolipoprotein A, total apolipoprotein A, and the HDL/LDL cholesterol ratio. Lipid changes in the other subjects fell within the range of random variation and showed no significant trends. Results suggest that vitamin E "responders" and "non-responders" exist which may explain the contradictory outcomes of studies on the effect of vitamin E upon plasma lipids (*Muckle T, Hazir D. Variation in human blood high-density lipoprotein response to oral vitamin E megadosage. Am J Clin Pathol 91:165-71, 1989*).

Experimental Double-blind Study (H): 60 hypercholesterolemic but otherwise healthy pts. received 500 IU vitamin E or placebo. After 90 days, experimental pts. had statistically significant increases in HDL cholesterol, apolipoprotein A and the apo A to apo B ratio, while the total cholesterol to HDL cholesterol ratio decreased (*Cloarec MJ et al. Alpha-tocopherol: Effect on plasma lipoproteins in hypercholesterolemic patients. Isr J Med Sci 23(8):869-72, 1987*).

Negative Experimental Double-blind Study (H): 78 volunteers received alpha tocopherol 728 mg or placebo. No consistent effect on HDL cholesterol levels was observed either at 4 wks. or at 6 months. Further analysis indicated that there were no significant changes in HDL cholesterol in subjects with low initial levels (*Kalbfleisch JH et al. Alpha-tocopherol supplements and high-density-lipoprotein-cholesterol levels. Br J Nutr 55(1):71-78, 1986*).

Supplementation may prevent the oxidation of low-density lipoprotein.

Experimental Study (G): 12 healthy adults volunteers received various doses of natural-source vitamin E supplements for 21 days. The resistance of LDL from subjects to copper-mediated oxidation was significantly higher during supplementation; however, the effectiveness of vitamin E in protecting LDL from oxidation varied from person to person (*Dieber-Rotheneder M et al. Effect of oral supplementation with D-alpha-tocopherol on the vitamin E concent of human low density lipoproteins and resistance to oxidation. J Lipid Res 32:1325-32, 1991*).

Supplementation may reduce the size of a myocardial infarct.

Animal Experimental Study (M): Using acute coronary ligation and reperfusion as an animal model of MI in rabbits, following 1 hr. ischemia and 6 hrs. reperfusion, the percentage necrosis of the heart region at risk (infarct size) was 30.5% in controls compared to none in rabbits pretreated with dietary vitamin E 200 IU/gk/d for 10 days. After 3 hrs. ischemia and 6 hrs. reperfusion, the controls had 74.1% necrosis compared to 23.1% in the supplemented rabbits (*Axford-Gatley RA, Wilson GJ. Reduction of experimental myocardial infaract size by oral administration of alpha-tocopherol. Cardiovasc Res 25:89-92, 1991*).

Supplementation may prevent the peroxidation of membrane lipids leading to endothelial injury and capillary leaking following coronary bypass surgery.

Experimental Controlled Study (G): For 10 pts. pretreated with vitamin E 2000 IU 12 hrs. before cardiac bypass surgery, free radical levels did not increase significantly during or after surgery. However, free radical levels progressively increased during surgery for 20 pts. in the control group. Following surgery, blood vitamin E levels were significantly reduced only in the controls, suggesting that vitamin E was consumed during surgery (*Cavarocchi NC et al. Superoxide generation during cardiopulmonary bypass: Is there a role for vitamin E? J Surg Res 40:519-27, 1986*).

- with Vitamin A:

Experimental Controlled Study (G): Half of a gp. of 16 pts. scheduled for coronary artery bypass graft surgery received vitamin E 400 mg and vitamin A 100,000 IU daily for 5 days prior to surgery. Based on tissue samples analyzed for hydroperoxide-initiated damage, there was oxidative stress to the preischemic heart tissue in the control gp. prior to the ischemic period which increased substantially during the reperfusion period. Although oxidative stress was noted in the supplemented gp., the damage was significantly less severe (*Ferreira R et al. Antioxidant action of vitamins A and E in patients submitted to coronary bypass surgery. Vasc Surg 25:191-5, 1991*).

- -

MINERALS

GENERAL:

Drink hard rather than soft water.
(H,G,L,M)

Observational Study (M): A study of 27 municipalities in Sweden has confirmed the existence of an inverse relationship between water hardness and mortality from cardiovascular causes, and particularly confirmed the cardioprotective benefits of high magnesium levels in drinking water (*Rylander R, Bonevik H, Rubenowitz E. Magnesium and calcium in drinking water and cardiovascular mortality. Scand J Work Environ Health 17:91-4, 1991*).

Observational Study (M): All 23 hearts examined at autopsy in 1986 following death from acute MI at The George Washington U. Hospital (GWUH) in Washington, D.C. (where drinking water magnesium is low and the death rate from acute MI is high) were compared to 23 consecutive hearts following death from acute MI at the Salt Lake VA Medical Center (SLVA) (where drinking water magnesium is high and the acute MI death rate is low). There were 15 instances of cadiac myocyte calcification among the GWUH cases, but none among the SLVA cases (p<0.00002). When only white males were considered, the difference remained significant (p<0.0004). Some of these calcified cells were far removed from any infarction. Findings suggest that myocyte calcium deposition may be a factor in the increased risk of MI death in regions with low magnesium levels in the drinking water (*Bloom S, Peric-Golia L. Myocardial calcification, acute infarction, and Mg in drinking water: Salt Lake City vs Washington DC. Abstract. J Am Coll Nutr 8(5):455, 1989*).

Animal Experimental Study (H,L): Rabbits given hard water had lower serum total, VLDL, and LDL cholesterol and higher HDL cholesterol than those given deionized water (*Porter LP et al. Effects of water hardness upon lipid and mineral metabolism in rabbits. Nutr Res 8:31-45, 1988*).

Review Article (G): Since absorption of elements in drinking water is usually twice that of foods (as there are no chelating agents present), they may have a greater influence than if in foods. Water hardness is usually caused by dissolved calcium and magnesium although, in a few areas, hardness may also result from iron or aluminum salts. The concentrations of these elements is usually small in relation to that in the food. In areas where drinking water is hard, the incidence of hypertension, cardiovascular disease and stroke are often less than in soft water areas. The beneficial influence of water hardness may be from alkalinity or from competition between divalent ions. Toxic elements, such as lead and cadmium, may be leached from pipes in soft water areas because of low pH; also, the intestinal absorption of lead and cadmium may be retarded by the presence of competing ions in hard water, i.e. calcium and magnesium. In several studies, animals reared in hard water areas showed less atherosclerotic lesions at autopsy than animals reared in soft water areas. When rabbits were fed a ration resulting in hypercholesterolemia, atherosclerotic lesions were more severe when they were given hard water than when given soft water (*Borgman RF. Dietary factors in essential hypertension. Prog Food Nutr Sci 9:109-47, 1985*).

Calcium: 1.5 gram daily
(C,G,P,T)

Intracellular calcium may play a role in atherogenesis.

Review Article (G): Evidence concerning the hypothesis that cell calcium is causally related to atherogenesis is reviewed, including:
1. arterial calcium is increased in atherosclerosis;
2. this increase in tissue calcium content is largely intracellular;
3. the increased intracellular calcium content is caused by increased plasma membrane calcium permeability;
4. the increased calcium content is causally related to atherogenesis;
5. many of the cell physiological, cell biological, biochemical, and molecular biological processes, known to function abnormally in atherosclerosis, are also known to be calcium-regulated;
6. these processes are activated or inactivated in atherosclerosis in a manner consistent with increased cell calcium (*Phair RD. Cellular calcium and atherosclerosis: A brief review. Cell Calcium 9(5-6):275-84, 1988*).

Calcium deficiency may be a cause of atherosclerosis.

Theoretical Discussion (G): In old age, low calcium and vitamin D intake, short solar exposure, decreased intestinal absorption, and falling renal function with insufficient 1,25-dihydroxyvitamin D synthesis all contribute to calcium deficiency, secondary hyperparathyroidism, bone loss and possibly calcium shift from the bone to soft tissue, and from the extracellular to the intracellular compartment, blunting the sharp concentration gap between these compartments. Consequences may include arteriosclerosis and hypertension due to the increase of calcium in the vascular wall (*Fujita T. Aging and calcium as an environmental factor. J Nutr Sci Vitaminol (Tokyo) 31 Suppl S15-9, 1985*).

Increased serum calcium concentrations may be associated with hypercholesterolemia.

Observational Study (C): In a screening survey of 18,000 adults, serum calcium concentrations were positively related to serum cholesterol concentrations over a wide range of the distribution along with systolic and diastolic BP and serum glucose, suggesting that changes in calcium metabolism are related to a metabolic syndrome of hyperlipidemia, hypertension and impaired glucose tolerance (*Lind L et al. Relation of serum calcium concentration to metabolic risk factors for cardiovascular disease. Br Med J 297:960-63, 1988*).

Supplementation may decrease total cholesterol and triglycerides and inhibit platelet aggregation.

Experimental Double-blind Crossover Study (C): 43 hypertensive and 27 normotensive subjects randomly received 1000 mg of elemental calcium or placebo. After 8 wks., mildly hyperlipidemic normotensive pts. on calcium supplementation had a significant decrease in total cholesterol (p<0.05), but no significant changes in plasma lipids occurred with calcium supplementation in hypertensive subjects. Triglycerides were unchanged (*Karanja N et al. Plasma lipids and hypertension: response to calcium supplementation. Am J Clin Nutr 45(1):60-5, 1987*).

Animal Experimental Study (C,G,P,T): Rabbits were fed a high (45%) saturated fat diet containing either a basic amount of calcium and magnesium (group I) or increased calcium (group II). After 6 mo., gp. II rabbits demonstrated significant prolongation of clotting time, decrease in platelet aggregation, and decrease in plasma total cholesterol, with a less significant decrease in plasma triglycerides. In addition the excretion of fecal lipids and saturated fatty acids was greatly increased. Compared to gp. I, rabbits in gp. II demonstrated significantly less severe atherosclerosis and significantly less accumulation of cholesterol in the aorta (*Renaud S et al. Protective effects of dietary calcium and magnesium on platelet function and atherosclerosis in rabbits fed saturated fat. Atherosclerosis 47:187-98, 1983*).

Experimental Studies (C): 4 men with normal total serum cholesterol levels were fed 3,370 mg calcium daily (710 mg from dietary sources; 2,660 mg from supplements). After 4 days, serum cholesterol decreased by an ave. of 14 mg. Another gp. of volunteers were then given a total intake of 1,600 mg calcium daily. After 3 wks., both serum calcium and triglycerides decreased, with the major decrease within the first wk. of the study. Fat excretion in the feces increased, suggesting that calcium combined with fatty acids in the gut to cause the excretion of calcium soaps (*Yacowitz H. Br Med J May, 1965*).

<u>Chromium:</u>   200 µg daily
(C,G,H,M,R,T)

Chromium deficiency is a risk factor for ASHD (*Nutr Rev 41:307-10, 1983; Simonoff M et al. Low plasma chromium in patients with coronary artery and heart diseases. Biol Trace Element Res 6:431-9, 1984*).

Observational Study (G): In a study of 32 subjects in whom coronary artery disease was assessed by cineangiography, serum chromium levels were significantly lower in subjects with coronary heart disease than in the sera of normal individuals. Only subjects free of CHD had chromium concentrations $\geq$5.5 µg Cr/L (*Newman HA et al. Serum chromium and angiographically determined coronary artery disease. Clin Chem 24(4):541-44, 1978*).

Observational Study (M): Postmortem analysis of aortic tissue from people who died of coronary heart disease showed lower chromium content when compared to samples taken from accident victims (*Schroeder HA et al. Chromium deficiency as a factor in atherosclerosis. J Chronic Dis 23:123-42, 1970*).

Chromium supplementation may reduce total cholesterol and triglycerides and raise HDL cholesterol (*Lefavi RG. Has chromium been overlooked as a hypolipidemic agent? Nutr Rep 9(9), Sept. 1991*).

See also: "<u>Brewer's Yeast</u>" below

Experimental Double-blind Crossover Study (G,L): 28 volunteers with untreated hypercholesterolemia (220-330 mg/dl) randomly received chromium 200 µg/d as chromium tripicolinate 1.6 mg and placebo in either order with a 2-wk. wash-out period between trials. After 6 wks. of treatment, total cholesterol decreased 7%, LDL cholesterol decreased 10%, apolipoprotein A-I rose 11%, and apolipoprotein B decreased 16%. All of these changes were highly statistically significant. An upward trend in HDL cholesterol was not significant and no change was seen in triglyceride levels. In contrast, the only significant change following placebo was a 12% increase in apolipoprotein B. There were no side effects (*Press RI, Geller J, Evans GW. The effect of chromium picolinate on serum cholesterol and apolipoprotein fractions in human subjects. West J Med 152:41-5, 1990*).

Negative Experimental Double-blind Crossover Study (C,H,L,T): 10 noninsulin-dependent diabetics (aged 37-68) received inorganic trivalent chromium 200 µg daily. After 6 wks., serum total cholesterol and triglycerides and their high-density, low-density and very low-density lipoprotein fractions showed no change as compared to the placebo period (*Uusitupa MI et al. Effect of inorganic chromium supplementation on glucose tolerance, insulin response, and serum lipids in noninsulin-dependent diabetics. Am J Clin Nutr 38(3):404-10, 1983*).

Chromium supplementation retards the development of experimental atherosclerosis and may result in plaque regression in experimental animals (*Abraham AS et al. The effect of chromium on cholesterol-induced atherosclerosis in rabbits. Atherosclerosis 41:371-79, 1982*).

- with <u>Niacin:</u>

Combined supplementation, using a dose of niacin much lower than that found effective when given alone, may lower total cholesterol.

Experimental Double-blind Study (C):   34 college-age male athletes with normal cholesterol levels recieved either 200 μg of niacin-bound chromium (chromium polynicotinate containing 2 mg niacin), 800 μg of niacin-bound chromium (8 mg niacin) or placebo. After 8 wks., the ave. serum cholesterol in the 200 μg gp. dropped 14%, that of the 800 μg gp. dropped 18%, and that of the control gp. was unchanged (*Lefavi R. Lipid-lowering effects of a dietary nicotinic acid-chromium (III) complex in male athletes.   FASEB J 5(6):A1645, 1991*).

Note: This oxygen-coordinated complex of niacin-bound chromium was found to be 18 times more biologically active than other chromium-niacin complexes tested, possibly because its shape resembles "the part of the GTF structure which is recognized by the receptors or enzymes involved in the expression of the biological effect" (Cooper J et al. Structure and biological activity of nitrogen and oxygen coordinated nicotinic acid complexes of chromium. Inorganica Chemica Acta 91:1-9, 1984).

Case Reports (C):   One subject had a cholesterol level of 10.33 mmol/L (399 mg/dL). After 4 wks. of supplementation with nicotinic acid 100 mg daily and chromium chloride 200 μg daily, total cholesterol decreased to 8.86 mmol/L (342 mg/dL). After 4 mo., total cholesterol was 7.25 mmol/L (280 mg/dL). The other subject had a cholesterol level of 8.73 mmol/L (337 mg/dL) which decreased after 4 wks. of supplementation to 6.73 mmol/L (260 mg/dL) (*Urberg M et al. Hypochlesterolemic effect of nicotinic acid and chromium supplementation. J Fam Pract 27(6):603-06, 1988*).

Copper:
(C,G,H,L)

WARNING: Copper may promote free radical reactions and lipid peroxidation.

Observational Study (G,L): In a study of 126 middle-aged men, the mean increase in the maximal common carotid intima media thickness after 2 yrs. was greater in men with high serum copper concentrations. Moreover, raised serum LDL cholesterol concentration was associated with accelerated progression of atherosclerosis only in men with higher than median serum copper concentrations, especially in men with serum selenium concentrations below the median value (*Salonen JT et al. Interactions of serum copper, selenium, and low density lipoprotein cholesterol in atherogenesis. Br Med J 302:756-60, 1991*).

Copper deficiency may be associated with increased total cholesterol and decreased HDL cholesterol levels.

Experimental Study (H,L): 24 healthy males (with a mean pre-test copper consumption about 60% of the US RDA of 2 mg) were fed low-copper diets. After 11 wks., LDL cholesterol was significantly higher and HDL cholesterol was significantly lower. After supplementing them with 3 mg copper daily, LDL was 8% lower and HDL was 15% higher than the pre-test period (*Reiser S et al. Effect of copper intake on blood cholesterol and its lipoprotein distribution in men. Nutr Rep Int 36(3):641-50, 1987*).

Dietary cholesterol may lower liver copper (at least in rabbits), suggesting that dietary cholesterol may contribute to coronary heart disease by depleting liver copper levels (*Klevay LM. Dietary cholesterol lowers liver copper in rabbits. Biol Trace Element Res 16:51-57, 1988*).

Iron:
(G)

WARNING: It is possible that even relatively low levels of dietary iron may contribute to the risk of atherosclerosis (*McCord J. Is iron sufficiency a risk factor in ischemic heart disease? Circulation 83:1112-14, 1991; Sullivan JL. The iron paradigm of ischemic heart disease. Am Heart J 117:1177-88, 1989*).

Magnesium: 400 mg daily
(A,C,G,H,L.M,P,T)

May be deficient.

Experimental Study (M): 38 pts. with ischemic heart disease admitted to a coronary care unit with suspected MI were compared to controls using an IV magnesium loading test. Mean magnesium retention was 34% compared to 5% in controls, and there was no significant difference between those with confirmed MI and those without MI. Also, in a gp. of 9 pts. with chronic ischemic heart disease, mean magnesium retention was 57% Pts. receiving diuretics retained more magnesium than those not receiving them, although the latter gp. had a significantly greater magnesium retention than controls, suggesting that diuretics contribute to magnesium deficiency but are not the only cause (*Rasmussen HS et al. Magnesium deficiency in patients with ischemic heart disease with and without acute myocardial infarction uncovered by intravenous loading test. Arch Intern Med 148:329-32, 1988*).

Experimental Study (M): 5 pts. with acute myocardial infarction and 6 healthy controls underwent a magnesium retention test together with a biopsy of the quadriceps lateralis muscle to assay tissue magnesium levels. Magnesium retention was 42% in the MI gp. and 22% in the control group (p<0.01); muscle magnesium content was also lower in the MI gp. compared to controls (*Jeppesen BB. Magnesium status in patients with acute myocardial infarction: A pilot study. Magnesium 5(2):95-100, 1986*).

Observational Study (M): During the first 32 hrs., 13 pts. with acute MI had significant reductions in serum magnesium level, while no increase in urinary magnesium was seen, suggesting that hypomagnesemia during acute MI is caused by a shift of the mineral from the extracellular to the intracellular space (*Rasmussen HS. Magnesium and acute myocardial infarction. Arch Intern Med 146:872, 1986*).

Review Article: "Chronic, low grade magnesium deficiency may be much more common than is conventionally considered since magnesium is not studied regularly in clinical medicine, as are sodium, potassium, and chloride. . . . The need in clinical medicne to measure serum concentration of magnesium in all patients with heart disease . . . cannot be overemphasized" (*Burch GE, Giles TD. The importance of magnesium deficiency in cardiovascular disease. Am Heart J 94:649-57, 1977*).

Magnesium deficiency is associated with increased risk of coronary artery disease, sudden cardiac death, myocardial infarction and ventricular tachyarrhythmias (*Lauler DP, Ed. A symposium: Magnesium deficiency - pathogenesis, prevalence, and strategies for repletion. Am J Cardiol 16(14):G1G-46G, 1989; Shattock M et al. The ionic basis of anti-ischemic and anti-arrhythmic properties of magnesium in the heart. J Am Coll Nutr 6:27-33, 1987*).

Supplementation may reduce risk the of cardiac arrhythmias, vasospastic angina and death following myocardial infarction.

Experimental Study: 17 pts. on their first day following coronary bypass surgery were studied. IV magnesium was found to help prevent the BP-raising effects of epinephrine without affecting heart rate or function, suggesting that small doses of magnesium after coronary bypass surgery may be beneficial in preventing arrhythmias and coronary artery constriction (*Prielipp RC et al. Magnesium inhibits the hypertensive but not the cardiotonic actions of low-dose epinephrine. Anesthesiology 74:973-9, 1991*).

Review Article (M): An overview of the data from controlled studies of IV magnesium in myocardial infarction amounting to about 1300 pts. suggests that the reduction of early arrhythmias and deaths in magnesium-treated pts. is real and substantial (*Teo K et al. Effect of intravenous magnesium on mortality in myocardial infarction. Circulation 82:III-393, 1990*).

Experimental Study (A): 15 pts. with variant angina were injected IV with 10 ml of 20% magnesium sulfate during each anginal episode. While, untreated, each episode lasted 5-15 min., treated attacks lasted 1/2 - 2 minutes. Pretreatment with parenteral magnesium sulfate in 4 of these pts. prevented further attacks (*Cohen L, Kitzes R. Magnesium sulfate in the treatment of variant angina. Magnesium 3:46-49, 1984*).

Supplementation may prevent calcification of blood vessels and the development of atherosclerosis (*Seelig MS, Heggtveit HA. Magnesium interrelationships in ischemic heart disease: A review. Am J Clin Nutr 27(1):59-79, 1974*).

Animal Experimental Study (G,T): Rabbits consumed either a standard or a 1% cholesterol diet. In addition, some of the rabbits on the 1% cholesterol diet consumed varying amts. of magnesium. Results showed the magnesium-supplemented diets reduced the extent of aortic lesions and the cholesterol content of the aorta in a dose-dependent manner. Although magnesium had no effect on lowering the cholesterol-induced rise in serum total cholesterol and HDL-cholesterol, it decreased the elevation in triglyceride levels. Magnesium may reduce atherosclerotic lesions by modulating cholesterol accumulation in the aortic wall, possibly by preventing the formation of foam cells, protecting the vascular endothelial cells, or by some unknown effect related to the reduction in serum triglycerides (*Ouchi Y et al. Effect of dietary magnesium on development of atherosclerosis in cholesterol-fed rabbits. Atherosclerosis 10:732-7, 1990*).

Supplementation may reduce total cholesterol, raise HDL cholesterol and inhibit platelet aggregation.

Experimental Study (C,H,L):   16 pts. with abnormally low HDL cholesterol levels (also elevated LDL and VLDL cholesterol) received enteric-coated magnesium chloride (400 mg elemental magnesium) for a mean of 4 months.   Total plasma cholesterol significantly decreased from 297 to 257; HDL cholesterol significantly increased from 35.2 to 46.7; and VLDL and LDL cholesterol significantly decreased from 262 to 210 mg/dl. These results suggest that magnesium therapy should be considered a first-choice option in the treatment of lipid abnormalities since it is safer than drugs in current use (*Davis WH et al. Monotherapy with magnesium increases abnormally low high density lipoprotein cholesterol: A clinical essay. Curr Ther Res 36:341, 1984*).

In vitro Experimental Study (P): While sodium and potassium failed to affect platelet clumping and blood-clotting, these effects were both highly correlated with the concentration of added magnesium (*Hughes A, Tonks RS. Platelets, magnesium, and myocardial infarction. Lancet 1:1044-6, 1965*).

- and Potassium:

When the level of either magnesium or potassium is deficient, administration of the combination may be more effective than either alone due to the inability of the heart muscle to hold on to potassium in the absence of magnesium (*Dychner T, Wester PO. Magnesium and potassium in serum and muscle in relation to disturbances of cardiac rhythm, in Magnesium in Health and Disease. Spectrum Publishing Company, 1980:551-7; Rayssiguier Y. Role of magnesium and potassium in the pathogenesis of arteriosclerosis. Magnesium 3(4-6):226-38, 1984*).

Selenium:
(C,G,M,P)

Serum, erythrocyte and toenail selenium levels may be negatively correlated with the risk of atherosclerosis and myocardial infarction.

Observational Study (M): Compared to 84 controls, 84 pts. with acute MI had significantly lower mean concentrations of erythrocyte and toenail selenium and non-significantly lower mean plasma selenium concentrations. A positive trend in the risk of acute MI from high to low toenail selenium levels was observed, which persisted after adjustment for other risk factors. Because toenail selenium level reflects blood levels up to 1 yr. before sampling, these findings suggest that a low selenium status was present before the infarction and, thus, may be of etiologic relevance. By contrast, RBC glutathione peroxidase activity was significantly higher in cases than in controls, possibly as a defense against increased oxidant stress either preceding or following the acute event (*Kok FJ et al. Decreased selenium levels in acute myocardial infarction. JAMA 261(8):1161-4, 1989*).

Negative Observational Study (M): In a 9-year prospective Dutch study, no significant association between serum selenium and cardiovascular mortality was observed before or after multivariate analysis (*Kok FJ et al. Serum selenium, vitamin antioxidants, and cardiovascular mortality: A 9-year follow-up study in the Netherlands. Am J Clin Nutr 45(2):462-8, 1987*).

Observational Study (C,G,M): In a sample of 1110 men aged 55-74, serum selenium levels were negatively correlated with age and positively correlated with hemoglobin levels and serum cholesterol. Men with coronary heart disease or claudication exhibited levels below 45 µg/l significantly more frequently. Levels below 45 µg/l were significantly associated with increased risk of death from all causes including cardiovascular disease, but only in individuals with evidence of coronary heart disease. In the entire population, death from stroke was responsible for more than half of the increased mortality associated with low selenium levels (*Virtamo J et al. Serum selenium and the risk of coronary heart disease and stroke. Am J Epidemiol 122:276-82, 1985*).

The positive correlation between low serum selenium and risk of cardiovascular disease may be due to a correlation between selenium and polyunsaturated fatty acid levels.

Observational Study (G): A longitudinal case-control study of 33 pts. with 1 or more risk factors for CHD and 64 controls showed that the serum selenium concentration was not associated with development of clinical manifestations of CHD during a follow-up of 5-7 years. Polyunsaturated acid content, especially eicosapentaenoic acid, in serum cholesterol esters and phospholipids was positively correlated with selenium concentration. As a low content of polyunsaturates in serum lipids was an independent risk factor in these pts., it is hypothesized that the high coronary risk in subjects wih a very low serum selenium (<45 μg/L) might be due not to selenium deficiency but to a coexisting low concentration of polyunsaturated fatty acids in serum (*Miettinen TA et al. Serum selenium concentration related to myocardial infarction and fatty acid content of serum lipids. Br Med J 287:517-19, 1983*).

The positive correlation between low serum selenium and risk of cardiovascular disease may be due to the antioxidant effect of selenium

Observational Study (G,L): In a study of 126 middle-aged men, the mean increase in the maximal common carotid intima media thickness after 2 yrs. was greater in men with low serum selenium concentrations. Moreover, raised serum LDL cholesterol concentration was associated with accelerated progression of atherosclerosis only in men with higher than median concentrations of serum copper (a pro-oxidant), especially in men with serum selenium concentrations below the median value (*Salonen JT et al. Interactions of serum copper, selenium, and low density lipoprotein cholesterol in atherogenesis. Br Med J 302:756-60, 1991*).

Deficiency may be associated with increased LDL cholesterol.

Animal Experimental Study (L): Rats were placed on a diet which was high in polyunsaturated fat, very low in cholesterol and selenium-deficient or supplemented with selenium. After 20 wks., rats on the deficient diet had significantly higher LDL cholesterol levels (*Stone WL et al. Effects of dietary selenium and vitamin E on plasma lipoprotein cholesterol levels in male rats. Ann Nutr Metab 30:94-103, 1986*).

Supplementation may reduce platelet aggregation (by increasing prostacyclin production).

Experimental Study (P): Elderly nursing home residents received high selenium yeast containing 200 μg selenium daily. After 5 wks., plasma levels of both platelet factor 4 and thromboglobulin had fallen significantly, indicating a reduction of platelet aggregation (*Stead NW et al. Selenium (Se) balance in the dependent elderly. Am J Clin Nutr 39:677, 1984*).

Experimental Study (P): In 6 human volunteers given supplementary selenium 10 μg/kg for 6 wks., bleeding time nearly doubled. (*Schiavon R et al. Selenium enhances prostacyclin production by cultured epithelial cells: Possible explanation for increased bleeding times in volunteers taking selenium as a dietary supplement. Thrombosis Res 34:389, 1984*).

Supplementation may improve prognosis following acute myocardial infarction.

Experimental Double-blind Study (M): Following an acute MI, 81 pts. randomly received, in addition to conventional therapy, 100 μg/d of selenium from selenium-rich yeast or placebo. 89% had pretreatment levels <100 μg/L, a level below which platelet glutathione peroxidase activity has been shown to be submaximal. After 6 mo., there were 4 cardiac deaths and 2 non-fatal reinfarctions in the placebo gp. compared to no deaths and 1 non-fatal reinfarction in the experimental group (results not significant) (*Korpela H et al. Effect of selenium supplementation after acute myocardial infarction. Res Commun Chem Pathol Pharmacol 65:249-52, 1989*).

Selenium and
Vitamin E:
(A,L)

Deficiency may be associated with increased LDL cholesterol.

Animal Experimental Crossover Study (L): Rats were placed on a diet which was high in polyunsaturated fat, very low in cholesterol and either selenium- and vitamin E-deficient or supplemented with selenium and vitamin E. After 20 wks., rats on the deficient diet had significantly higher LDL cholesterol levels. Results could be reversed in the two gps. by switching their diets for 55 wks. As the alteration of rat lipoprotein profiles was a slow process, it is suggested that the effects of selenium and vitamin E supplementation in humans be studied for much longer periods than 6 weeks (*Stone WL et al. Effects of dietary selenium and vitamin E on plasma lipoprotein cholesterol levels in male rats. Ann Nutr Metab 30:94-103, 1986*).

Supplementation may reduce anginal pains.

> **Experimental Double-blind Crossover Study (A):** 22/24 pts. receiving selenium 1 mg and vitamin E 200 IU daily reported reduced angina compared to 3/24 pts. on placebo (*cited in Frost DV, Lish PM. Selenium in biology. Ann Rev Pharm 18:259, 1975*).

Zinc:
(C,H,L,T)

The association between zinc nutriture and atherosclerosis is poorly understood:

A. Plasma and tissue zinc levels are reduced in atherosclerotic patients (*Halsted JA, Smith JC, Jr. Plasma zinc in health and disease. Lancet 1:322-24, 1970; Netsky MG et al. Tissue zinc and human disease. Relation of zinc content of kidney, liver, and lung to atherosclerosis and hypertension. Am J Clin Pathol 51:358-65, 1969; Volkov NF. Cobalt, manganese and zinc content in the blood of atherosclerotic patients. Fed Proc 22:T897-99, 1963*).

B. Despite animal studies suggesting a positive correlation between zinc intake and HDL cholesterol (*Koo SI, Williams DA. Relationship between the nutritional status of zinc and cholesterol concentration of serum lipoproteins in adult male rats. Am J Clin Nutr 34(11):2376-81, 1981*), zinc intake has been shown in other studies to be <u>negatively</u> correlated with HDL cholesterol without a relationship to total cholesterol, LDL cholesterol or triglycerides(*Black MR et al. Zinc supplements and serum lipids in young adult white males. Am J Clin Nutr 47:970-75, 1988; Umoren J. Serum total cholesterol and HDL-cholesterol levels as associated with copper and zinc intake in physically active and sedentary elderly men and women. Adv Exp Med Biol 258:171-81, 1989*).

C. In addition, minimal zinc supplementation (>15 mg daily) in humans has been shown to prevent the exercise-related increase in HDL cholesterol (*Crouse SF et al. Zinc ingestion and lipoprotein values in sedentary and endurance-trained men. JAMA 252:755-87, 1984; Goodwin JS et al. Relationship between zinc intake, physical activity and blood levels of high density lipoprotein cholesterol in a healthy elderly population. Metabolism 34(6):519-23, 1985*).

D. It has been suggested that these contradictory findings are due to the fact that, while improved zinc nutriture has a beneficial effect on HDL cholesterol, higher levels of zinc supplementation may lower body <u>copper</u> levels, and the resultant copper deficiency could account for the adverse effects on cholesterol metabolism. Copper supplementation may therefore be indicated when supplemental zinc is provided (*Fischer P et al. The effect of dietary copper and zinc on cholesterol metabolism. Am J Clin Nutr 33:1019-25, 1980; Katya-Katya M et al. The effect of zinc supplementation on plasma cholesterol levels. Nutr Res 4:633-38, 1984; Klevay LM. Interactions of copper and zinc in cardiovascular disease. Ann N Y Acad Sci 355:140-151, 1980; Medeiros D et al. Serum lipids and glucose as associated with hemoglobin levels and copper and zinc intake in young adults. Life Sci 32(16):1897-904, 1983*).

E. Zinc supplementation may be beneficial by increasing alpha-lipoproteins and decreasing beta-lipoproteins.

> **Experimental Placebo-controlled Study (C):** 20 pts. received either 200 mg zinc sulfate 3 times daily or placebo. After 1 mo., the experimental gp. showed a significant decrease in total serum cholesterol and beta-lipoproteins, and a significant increase in alpha-lipoproteins (*Shah DR et al. Effect of oral zinc sulphate on serum lipids and lipoproteins in human subjects. Indian J Physiol Pharmacol 32(1):47-50, 1988*).

- -

OTHER NUTRITIONAL FACTORS

N-Acetylcysteine:
(G)

L-cysteine and reduced glutathione are thiol metabolites of N-acetylcysteine.

Administration may reduce lipoprotein(a).

Note: Lipoprotein(a) is a cholesterol-rich complex of low-density lipoprotein linked by disulfide bridges with the large glycoprotein apo(a). At very high plasma concentrations, it is associated with atherosclerotic disease (Berg K. Lp(a) lipoprotein: an overview, in AM Scanu, Ed. Lipoprotein(a). San Diego, Academic Press, 1989).

Negative In vitro Experimental Study: NAC was found to decrease the immunoreactivity of Lp(a), but failed to change total plasma cholesterol or total protein, suggesting that the changes in plasma Lp(a) noted by other investigators may have been due to attenuation of antibody reactivity and not to actual changes in Lp(a) mass (*Scanu AM. N-acetylcysteine and immunoreactivity of lipoprotein(a). Letter. Lancet 337:1159, 1991*).

Experimental Study: 12 pts. with high Lp(a) and 7 volunteers with normal Lp(a) levels received NAC 1.2-2.4 g/d. In the volunteers, plasma lipoprotein levels were unaffected by NAC administration, and side effects were limited to abdominal complaints in 2 of them. In pts. with plasma Lp(a) levels >40 mg/dl, NAC produced only a small, but significant, reduction in Lp(a) levels, suggesting that it is too early to consider NAC as a powerful agent to lower Lp(a) concentrations (*Stalenhoef AFH et al. N-acetylcysteine and lipoprotein. Letter. Lancet 337:491, 1991*).

In vitro Experimental Study: Plasma samples from a pt. with a high Lp(a) concentration were incubated with increasing amts. (0-40 mg/ml) of NAC. Significant dissociation of apo(a) from Lp(a) was achieved only with higher doses. Together with these results, the 10% bioavailability and its large distribution volume suggest that very high oral doses would be necessary to dissociate apo(a) from the low-density lipoprotein particle (*Stalenhoef AFH et al. N-acetylcysteine and lipoprotein. Letter. Lancet 337:491, 1991*).

Case Reports: NAC 2 g/d as a 5% solution mixed with soda or juice was administered to 2 pts. with high lipoprotein(a) levels for 4 wks. followed by 4 g/d for 4 weeks. The extent of Lp(a) reduction (70%) has not been seen with any other treatment. Clinical studies of the effect of Lp(a) reduction on atherosclerotic and thrombotic disease are suggested (*Gavish D, Breslow JL. Lipoprotein(a) reduction by N-acetylcysteine. Lancet 337:203-4, 1991*).

L-Arginine:
(G)

(*See Also: "Lysine to Arginine Ratio"*)

Supplementation may correct endothelial dysfunction in coronary microcirculation.

Experimental Controlled Study (G): Hypercholesterolemia impairs endothelial function, possibly by interference with the intracellular formation of endothelium-derived relaxing factor from its precursor L-arginine. 8 hypercholesterolemic pts. and 7 age-matched controls received graded intracoronary infusions of the endothelium-dependent agent acetylcholine (AC). In controls, AC induced a moderate dose-dependent constriction of the epicardial artery segment of the left anterior descending artery and increased coronary blood flow. In pts., the vasoconstrictive effect of AC on epicardial segments was similar, but the increase in coronary blood flow was significantly attenuated. L-arginine restored the AC-induced increase in blood flow in pts. but did not affect coronary blood flow in controls, suggesting that hypercholesterolemia impairs endothelium-dependent dilatation of the coronary microcirculation and that this impairment can be restored by short-term administration of L-arginine (*Drexler H et al. Correction of endothelial dysfunction in coronary microcirculation of hypercholesterlaemic patients by L-arginine. Lancet 338:1546-50, 1991*).

Aspartic Acid:
(M)

- with Magnesium and Potassium:

Administration of magnesium and potassium aspartate (1 gm of each twice daily) may be beneficial.

Review Article (M): Potassium/magnesium aspartate is useful in the treatment of myocardial infarction, cardiac arrhythmias and congestive heart failure. Aspartates speed the onset of the therapeutic effects of digitalis while reducing both its maintenance dosage and potential cardiotoxic effects. Hyperkalemia is the only significant contraindication (*Grujic M, Perinovic M.   [Treatment of acute myocardial infarction and chronic heart failure with K-Mg aspartate.]   Med Welt 25 (50):2124-6, 1974) (in German).*

Beta-carotene:
(A,M)

Plasma concentration may be inversely correlated with the risk of angina pectoris (*Riemersma RA et al.   Risk of angina pectoris and plasma concentrations of vitamins A, C and E and carotene.   Lancet 337:1-5, 1991*).

Supplementation may reduce the risk of cardiovascular events in patients with coronary artery disease.

Experimental Placebo-controlled Study (M): 160/333 male physicians with a history of angina or revascularization, a subgroup of the 20,000 participant Physicians' Health Study, were randomly selected to receive beta-carotene 50 mg every other day.   After several yrs. of follow-up, compared to placebo controls, that gp. had a significant 54% reduction in major coronary events and a 54% reduction in major vascular events.   In addition, the combination of beta-carotene with aspirin seemed to have an additive effect, but the numbers were too small for statistical verification (*J Michael Gaziano, cardiology fellow, Harvard U. - presented at the Am. Heart Assoc. scientific session, Dallas - reported in Med World News, January, 1991*).

Betaine: 6 gm daily
(G)

The oxidative product of choline.

Supplementation may be beneficial for patients with homocystinuria.

Note: See "Vitamin B6" above for a discussion of homocystinuria.

Experimental Study: The effects on plasma amino acids of a methionine load were assessed for 6 pyridoxine-responsive homocystinuric patients both before and after adding betaine 6 gm daily to the treatment regimen of pyridoxine and folic acid.   Prior to betaine, all pts. had higher plasma methionine and homocysteine and lower cysteine than 17 controls during the 24 hrs. after challenge.   After betaine, these responses were reduced to near normal (*Wilcken DE et al.   Homocystinuria due to cystathionine beta-synthase deficiency — the effects of betaine treatment in pyridoxine-responsive patients.   Metabolism 34(12):1115-21, 1985*).

Experimental Study: 10 pyridoxine-unresponsive homocystinuric pts. and 1 pt. with homocystinuria due to a defect in cobalamin metabolism were treated with betaine 6 gm daily in addition to conventional therapy.   All pts. had a substantial decrease in plasma total homocysteine levels (p<0.001) and an increase in total cysteine levels (p<0.001).   Changes in plasma methionine were variable.   Fasting levels of plasma amino acids became normal in 2 pts., and in 6 there was immediate clinical improvement.   There were no adverse side effects (*Wilcken DE et al. Homocystinuria - the effects of betaine in the treatment of patients not responsive to pyridoxine.   N Engl J Med 309(8):448-53, 1983*).

Bioflavonoids:
(P)

Supplementation with flavones may reduce platelet adhesiveness (*Robbins RC.   Flavones in citrus exhibit antiadhesive action on platelets.   Int J Vitam Nutr Res 58:418-21, 1988*).

Supplementation with anthocyanosides may reduce platelet aggregation (*Pulliero G et al.   Ex vivo study of the inhibitory effects of Vaccinium myrtillus (Bilberry) anthrocyanosides on human platelet aggregation.   Fitoterapia 60(1):69-75, 1989*).

Note: Anthocyanosides are the flavonoid component of plants belonging to the genus Vaccinium, such as bilberry, black current and grape.

Carnitine: DL: 1500 mg. twice daily (1 month trial)
(A,C,H,T)   L: 750 mg. twice daily

Supplementation may allow the ischemic heart increased energy expenditure before coronary insufficiency develops by increasing its ability to oxidize fatty acids.

Experimental Controlled Study (A): 16 subjects with effort-induced angina and 14 controls received L-carnitine 3 g/d orally for 30 days. A bicycle ergometer exercise test that initially revealed a 1.5 mm (mean) depression of the ST-T segment in the angina subjects after pharmacological wash-out, revealed only a 1 mm depression in the same subjects following carnitine treatment. M-code echocardiography showed positive changes in a number of ventricular function parameters in the angina subjects and also, to a lesser extent, in the healthy controls (*Canale C et al. Bicycle ergometer and echocardiographic study in healthy subjects and patients with angina pectoris after administration of L-carnitine: Semiautomatic computerized analysis of M-mode tracing. Int J Clin Pharmacol Ther Toxicol 26(4):221-24, 1988*).

Experimental Double-blind Crossover Study (A): 44 men with chronic stable effort-induced angina randomly received either L-carnitine 1 gm twice daily or placebo. After 4 wks., the exercise workload was increased, onset of angina was delayed, and ST segment depression at maximum workload was reduced in the pts. receiving L-carnitine compared to controls (*Cherchi A et al. Effects of L-carnitine on exercise tolerance in chronic, stable angina: A multicenter, double-blind, randomized, placebo controlled crossover study. Int J Clin Pharmacol Ther Toxicol 23(10):569-72, 1985*).

Supplementation may improve lipid metabolism.

Experimental Study (C,T): 20 diabetics received 1 mg/kg DL-carnitine for 10 days. There was a significant reduction of total serum lipids, triglycerides and cholesterol (*Abdel-Aziz MT et al. Effect of carnitine on blood lipid pattern in diabetic patients. Nutr Rep Int 29:1071, 1984*).

Experimental Study (H,T): 2 pts. with low HDL cholesterol but otherwise normal levels of cholesterol and triglycerides received 1 gm carnitine daily. HDL cholesterol substantially increased along with an increase in the HDL/total cholesterol ratio, while triglycerides decreased (*Rossi CS, Silliprandi N. Effect of carnitine on serum HDL cholesterol: Report of two cases. Johns Hopkins Med J 150:51-4, 1982*).

Coenzyme A:
(C,H,T)

Derived from pantethine which, at a dosage of 300 mg 3 times daily, has been shown in several controlled studies to improve lipid metabolism (*see "Pantethine" below*).

Supplementation may improve lipid metabolism.

Experimental Study (C,H,T): 14 pts. with type II or type IV hyperlipidemia received injections of coenzyme A daily. After 20, days, mean total serum cholesterol fell about 10%, triglycerides fell 36.5%, and HDL cholesterol increased by 23% (*Ghidini O et al. Effects of short-term treatment with coenzyme A or sulodexide on plasma lipids in patients with hypertriglyceridemia (type IV) or mixed hyperlipemia (type IIb). Int J Clin Pharmacol Ther Toxicol 24:390, 1986*).

Coenzyme Q10 (ubiquinone):   30-150 mg. daily in divided doses   (4 - 20 wk. trial)
(A,G)

Suggested as a physiologically important lipid-soluble antioxidant (*Frei B, Kim MC, Ames BN. Ubiquinol-10 is an effective lipid-soluble antioxidant at physiological concentrations. Proc Natl Acad Sci U S A 87:4879-83, 1990*).

Found in LDL fractions in the plasma (*Yuzuriha T, Takada M, Katayama K. Transport of [^{14}C]coenzyme Q10 from the liver to other tissues after intravenous administration to guinea pigs. Biochim Biophys Acta 759:286-91, 1983*).

May protect against atherogenesis.

Observational Study (G): In a comparison of 72 pts. to 245 normal subjects, the plasma total and LDL cholesterol levels and the triglyceride level were higher, and the plasma ubiquinone level was lower, in pts. than in normals. In addition, the ratio of total to HDL cholesterol and the ratio of LDL cholesterol to ubiquinone were higher in the pt. group. The correlation between plasma ubiquinone and LDL cholesterol in the pt. group was significant (p<0.05), and the increase in ubiquinone associated with an increase in LDL cholesterol was lower in pts. than in normals. There was a greater difference in the ratio of LDL cholesterol to ubiquinone (43%) than in the ratio of total to HDL cholesterol (17%) between the pts. and the normal subjects. Results suggest that the ratio of LDL cholesterol to ubiquinone may be an indicator of the risk of atherogenesis and that ubiquinone may have an important role in the prevention of atherosclerosis (*Hanaki Y, Sugiyama S, Ozawa T. Ratio of low-density lipoprotein cholesterol to ubiquinone as a coronary risk factor. Letter. N Engl J Med 325(11):814-15, 1991*).

Supplementation may reduce anginal episodes and improve cardiac function.

Experimental Double-blind Study (A): 10 men and women with stable angina pectoris received in random order 150 mg CoQ10 daily or placebo. After 4 wks., subjects as compared to controls experienced a 53% reduction in the frequency of anginal episodes (1.25 vs. 2.65/wk; not statistically significant). Treadmill tolerance time (i.e. before angina) was significantly increased from 345 to 406 seconds, and the time until 1 mm of ST-segment depression occurred increased significantly from 196-284 seconds (*Kamikawa T et al. Effects of coenzyme Q10 on exercise tolerance in chronic stable angina pectoris. Am J Cardiol 56:247, 1985*).

Experimental Controlled Study (A): After 1-3 mo. of supplementation with 30 mg daily of CoQ10, 12 pts. showed improvement vs. controls in functional class, exercise-induced S-T segment depression and exercise tolerance (128% increase in exercise tolerance after 4 wks., 184% increase after 8-12 wks.) (*Awata N et al. The effects of coenzyme Q10 on ischemic heart disease evaluated by dynamic exercise test, in Biomedical and Clinical Aspects of Coenzyme Q. Vol. 2. Amsterdam, Elsevier/North Holland Biomedical Press, 1980, pp. 247-54*).

Supplementation may reduce blood viscosity.

Experimental Study: 12 pts. (mean age 49 ± 16 yrs.) received 20 mg CoQ10 3 times daily. After 2 mo., blood viscosity was reduced at each of 4 shear rates and yield shear stress decreased significantly (*Kato T et al. Reduction of blood viscosity by treatment with coenzyme Q10 in patients with ischemic heart disease. Int J Clin Pharmacol Ther Toxicol 28(3):123-6, 1990*).

Supplementation may protect the myocardium during coronary artery bypass surgery.

Experimental Study: 60 pts. undergoing coronary artery bypass grafting receiving CoQ10 5 mg/kg IV 2 hr. prior to the onset of the bypass (which was performed using saphenous vein associated with cold cardioplegia in the standard fashion) and results were compared retrospectively with those of 18 controls. Heart rate, mean arterial pressure, and cardiac index showed no significnat difference between the CoQ and control groups. However, compared to controls, left ventricular stroke work index was significantly elevated at 6 and 10 hrs. of reperfusion following bypass in the CoQ-treated gp. and serum MB-CK was lower at 0 and 6 hrs. of reperfusion. Results suggest that pretreatment with IV CoQ is effective in preventing left ventricular depression in early reperfusion and in minimizing myocardial cellular injury during bypass followed by reperfusion (*Sunamori M et al. Clinical experience of coenzyme Q10 to enhance intraoperative myocardial protection in coronary artery revascularization. Cardiovasc Drugs Ther 5 Suppl 2:297-300, 1991*).

Glycosaminoglycans: 1200 mg. three times daily
(C,G,M,P,T)

Chondroitin sulfate is a constituent of acidic glycosaminoglycans found in arterial walls. These substances have anti-coagulant, anti-lipemic and anti-thrombogenic properties in addition to facilitating wound healing. They appear to form complexes with VLDL and LDL lipoproteins *in vitro* and *in vivo*. It has been suggested that the binding of LDL to glycosaminoglycans plays a significant role in the promotion of atheroma by causing a breakdown in the integrity of the extracellular collagen matrix components and an increased affinity for cholesterol (*Kostner GM et al. The interaction of human plasma low density lipoproteins with glycosamino-glycans: Influence of the chemical composition. Lipids 21:24-8, 1985*).

Experimental Controlled Study (C,P,T): Half of 46 elderly pts. received 3 gm chondroitin polysulfate daily while the other half received placebo. After 6-64 mo., serum cholesterol in the treated gp. fell to 10-20% lower and serum triglycerides fell to 27% lower than controls. After 3 mo., mean clotting time was prolonged by 50%. It is suggested that CPS acts similarly to heparin, but is much safer as no side-effects were reported (*Nakazawa K, Murata K. The therapeutic effect of chondroitin polysulphate in elderly atherosclerotic patients. J Int Med Res 6(3):217-25, 1978*).

Experimental Controlled Study (C,M,P): Of 120 EKG-demonstrated CHD pts. followed for 6 yrs., those receiving chondroitin-4-sulfate showed significantly fewer abnormal cardiac events (10%) vs. those in the control gp. (70%). There was also a highly significant difference in the death rate (7% vs. 23%) and treated pts. showed significant prolongation of thrombus formation time and reduced serum cholesterol levels. 10 gm pure C-4-S was given 3 times daily for 3 mo., then 1.5-3 gm daily for 4.5 yrs., and 0.75-1.5 gm daily for the rest of the study (*Izuka K, Murata K. Experientia 29:255-7, 1973*).

Experimental Controlled Study (M): 60/120 pts. with proven CHD were randomly selected to receive chondroitin sulfate A daily for 6 yrs. in addition to conventional treatment, while 60 received only conventional treatment. Whereas 42 controls experienced coronary incidents, only 6 pts. receiving CSA experienced incidents (p<0.001). Similarly, whereas 14 controls died of MI, only 4 pts. receiving CSA died of MI (p<0.001) (*Morrison LM, Enrick L. Coronary heart disease: Reduction of death rate by chondroitin sulfate A. Angiology 24:269-87, 1973*).

Inositol:
(C,T)

(*See Also: "Inositol nicotinate" below*)

A lipotropic agent.

Supplementation may help to protect against increases in total cholesterol and fatty acids in the liver (*Gavin G, McHenry EW. Inositol as a lipotropic agent. J Biol Chem 148:275, 1944*).

Inositol Hexanicotinate:
(C)

Inositol hexanicotinate combines the properties of both inositol and nicotinic acid.

Absorbed intact and hydrolyzed slowly to release inositol and niacin (*Harthon L, Brattsand R. Enzymatic hydrolysis of pentaerythritol tetranicotinate and meso-inositol hexanicotinate in blood and tissues. Arzneimittelforsch 29:1859-62, 1979*).

Side effects are reduced compared to those of niacin (*Hotz W. Nicotinic acid and its derivatives: A short survey. Adv Lipid Res 20:195-217, 1983*).

Has both anticholesterolemic and antilipemic effects which are more pronounced than those of niacin.

Animal Experimental Study (C): Administration of inositol hexanicotinate to hypercholesterolemic rabbits significantly reduced elevated serum lipid fractions. The hypocholesterolemic effect of IHN was more pronounced than that of nicotinic acid. The hypolipemic effect may be attributed to its action in inhibiting lipolysis, improving peripheral glucose utilization, and reducing the level of glycolysis products in serum (*El-Enein AAM et al. The role of nicotinic acid and inositol hexanicotinate as anti-cholesterolemic and antilipemic agents. Nutr Rep Int 28(4):899-911, 1983*).

Experimental Study (C): Inositol hexanicotinate was more effective in reducing hypercholesterolemia than was nicotinic acid (*Kruse W et al. Nocturnal inhibition of lipolysis in man by nicotinic acid and derivatives. Eur J Clin Pharmacol 16(1):11, 1979*).

Experimental Study (C): 16 hypercholesterolemic pts. received inositol hexanicotinate 200 mg 3 or 4 times daily. After 4 wks., mean serum cholesterol values were reduced. After 12 wks., the reduction became statistically significant. There were no side effects (*Dorner VG, Fischer FW. The influence of m-inositol hexanicotinate ester on serum lipids and lipoproteins. Arzneimittelforsch 11:110-13, 1961*).

<u>Lecithin</u>:   example: soya lecithin 12 gm daily
(C,G,H,L,P,R,T)

There is no evidence for a specific effect of lecithin on serum cholesterol independent of its <u>linoleic acid</u> content (*Knuiman JT et al. Lecithin intake and serum cholesterol. <u>Am J Clin Nutr</u> 49(2):266-8, 1989*).

Supplementation may normalize lipoproteins and reduce platelet aggregation.

Experimental Study (C,H,L,P,T): 9 pts. with type IIa hypolipoproteinemia and 9 pts. with type IV hyperlipoproteinemia were given soya lecithin 12 g/day. After 3 mo., plasma cholesterol and triclycerides were reduced by 15 and 23%, respectively, and HDL cholesterol increased by 16% in the hypercholesterolemic patients. Platelet function was unchanged. In the hypertriglyceridemic pts., total cholesterol fell by 14% and there was a 27% reduction in platelet aggregation (p<0.01). 17 hypertriglyceridemic pts. then received increasing doses of soya lecithin for 1-mo. periods; the optimal lipoprotein-lowering effect was achieved with 12 g/d. LDL and VLDL lipoprotein levels were reduced, and HDL and apolipoprotein A-I concentrations were increased. Platelet aggregation was significantly reduced in parallel with the reduction in triglyceride level (*Brook JG et al. Dietary soya lecithin decreases plasma triglyceride levels and inhibits collagen- and ADP-induced platelet aggregation. <u>Biochem Med Metab Biol</u> 35(1):31-39, 1986*).

Experimental Double-blind Crossover Study (C,H,L): 35 gm. daily of lecithin (53% phosphatidyl choline) significantly lowered total cholesterol and LDL cholesterol and raised HDL cholesterol after 2-3 mo. in 10 Alzheimer's pts. (*Vroulis G et al. Reduction of cholesterol risk factors by lecithin in patients with Alzheimer's disease. <u>Am J Psychiatry</u> 139(12):1633-34, 1982*).

<u>Lysine</u> to
<u>Arginine</u> ratio:
(C,G)

Lowering the lysine/arginine ratio may reduce the risk of atherosclerosis.

Review Article (G): Individuals consuming a diet high in animal protein whose plasma lysine to arginine ratio is 3.5 to 1 or higher have a significantly increased AS risk due to excessive dietary lysine. Compared to omnivores, individuals consuming a vegetarian diet have a significant reduction in the incidence of AS. Animal protein has a L/A ratio of 3-4/1, while plant protein has a L/A ratio of 1-1.25/1. (*Sanchez A. <u>Nutr Rep Int</u> 28:497, 1983*).

Lowering the lysine/arginine ratio may affect serum cholesterol concentrations.

Animal Experimental Study (C): The effect of varying the compositions of dietary proteins on the relative cholesterolemic effects of animal and vegetable proteins was investigated in rabbits. It was concluded that the lysine/arginine ratio is not the major determinant of the cholesterolemic properties of proteins, but that the overall amino acid composition is primarily concerned (*Gibney MJ. The effect of dietary lysine to arginine ratio on cholesterol kinetics in rabbits. <u>Atherosclerosis</u> 47(3):263-70, 1983*).

<u>Omega-3 Fatty Acids</u>:
(A,C,F,G,H,L,M,P,T)

Eicosapentaenoic acid (EPA) and docosahexaenoic acid (DHA).

Highest in cold water fish (herring, salmon, bluefish, tuna, etc.).

Suggested dosage: 3 grams daily of a combination of EPA and DHA

Experimental Controlled Study (H,T): 45 healthy normotriglyceridemic volunteers randomly received either 0, 1.5, 3 or 6 g/d of EPA and DHA as capsules of a marine-lipid concentrate, each of which provided 300 mg EPA and 200 mg DHA as their ethyl esters with 1 mg vitamin E (SuperEPA, Pharmacaps, Inc., UK). After 12 wks., serum triglycerides and HDL_3-cholesterol concentrations showed a dose-dependent reduction (p<0.05) and HDL_2 cholesterol increased (p<0.05). No dose-dependent effects were observed in the VLDL-, LDL-, and total HDL-cholesterol subfractions. Significant dose-related increases of the omega-3 fatty acids 20:5, 22:5, and 22:6 were found, corresponding roughly to decreases of the omega-6 fatty acids 18:2 and 20:4 (p<0.001). Results for 3 and

6 g dosages were similar, suggesting that 3 g of omega-3 ethyl fatty acids appears to be the appropriate supplementation dose in humans, at least regarding lipid-profile changes and the ability to incorporate such fatty acids in the plasma phospholipids (*Blonk MC et al. Dose-response effects of fish-oil supplementation in healthy volunteers. Am J Clin Nutr 52:120-27, 1990*).

WARNING: Supplementation of omega-3 fatty acids may require additional <u>vitamin E</u> intake to prevent increased membrane peroxidation and cellular damage (*Laganiere S, Fernandes G. High peroxidizability of subcellular membrane induced by high fish oil diet is reversed by vitamin E. <u>Clin Res</u> 35:A565, 1987*) and for optimal therapeutic results:

Experimental Double-blind Crossover Study: 12 healthy subjects received 30 mL/d of fish oil supplemented with either 0.31 IU/g or 1.5 IU/g vitamin E. While the low vitamin E gp. showed only modest reductions in serum triglycerides and no changes in fibrinogen, the high vitamin E gp. had marked decreases in serum triglycerides (48%) and fibrinogen (11%). The low vitamin E gp. also had a 9% decrease in serum vitamin E levels and a 122% increase in malondialdehyde levels, while these values normalized when they consumed the high-vitamin-E containing oil (*Haglund O et al. The effects of fish oil on triglycerides, cholesterol, fibrinogen, and malondialdehyde in humans supplemented with vitamin E. <u>J Nutr</u> 121:165-9, 1991*).

General Review Article:

"In summary . . . , the available evidence indicates theat the n-3 PUFA components of seafoods are effective in lowering plasma TGs and reducing eicosanoid-mediated reactions. Thus, fish oils may be useful for diabetics and subjects with familial hypertriglyceridemia. Consumption of seafoods as a regular dietary practice would appear to be prudent for prophylactic effects, whereas, for therapeutic purposes, ingestion of fish oil enriched with n-3 PUFAs on a frequent basis may be beneficial" (*Kinsella JE et al. Dietary n-3 polyunsaturated fatty acids and amelioration of cardiovascular disease: possible mechanisms. <u>Am J Clin Nutr</u> 52:1-28, 1990*).

Platelet levels may be inversely correlated with the presence of coronary heart disease.

Observational Study (A,M): In a study of several hundred randomly selected middle-aged subjects, platelet membrane levels of eicosapentaenoic acid made a significant and independent contribution to the explanation of angina pectoris but not to acute myocardial infarction, while platelet levels of docosahexaenoic acid did not differ between cases and controls. The estimated relative risk of angina pectoris was inversely related to the level of platelet membrane eicosapentaenoic acid. Omega-3 fatty acids were not found in adipose tissue (*Wood DA et al. Linoleic and eicosapentaenoic acids in adipose tissue and platelets and risk of coronary heart disease. <u>Lancet</u> 1:177-83, 1987*).

Note: The finding that platelets harvested soon after an acute myocardial infarction did not contain less EPA than the platelets of healthy men may be explained by the fact that the population studied consumed hardly any EPA, and thus differences would be unlikely to be found (Akos K. Eicosapentaenoic acid. Letter. <u>Lancet.</u> May 9, 1987, p. 1083).

Intake may be inversely correlated with subsequent mortality from coronary heart disease.

Review Article (M): Various cohort and epidemiological studies have found that eating fish once or twice a wk. (about 30 g/d) decreases mortality from heart disease by 50%. While this does not vary up to an intake of 150 g/d, the very high intake of the Eskimos (400 g/d) decreases the risk still further (*Kromhout D. n-3 fatty acids and coronary heart disease. <u>B N F Nutr Bull</u> 15:93-102, 1990*).

Experimental Controlled Study (M): 2033 men who had recovered from MI were allocated to receive or not receive advice on each of 3 dietary factors: a reduction in fat intake and an increase in the ratio of polyunsaturated to saturated fat, an increase in fatty fish intake (to 2-3 portions per wk.), and an increase in cereal fiber intake. The advice on fat was not associated with any difference in mortality. The subjects advised to eat fatty fish had a 29% reduction in 2 yr. all-cause mortality compared with those not so advised. This effect, which was significant, was not altered by adjusting for 10 potential confounding factors. Subjects given fiber advice had a slightly higher mortality than other subjects (not significant). The 2 yr. incidence of reinfarction plus death from ischemic heart disease was not affected by any of the 3 dietary regimens (*Burr ML et al. Effects of changes in fat, fish, and fibre intakes on death and myocardial reinfarction: diet and reinfarction trial (DART). <u>Lancet</u> 2:757-61, 1989*).

Observational Study (M): Fish consumption of almost 11,000 Swedes in 1967-8 was classified as high, moderate, low or none. All subjects with prior histories of cardiovascular symptoms were excluded. Subsequent mortality from CHD and myocardial infarction from 1969-82 was found to show a dose-response relation, with the lowest risk for those who had high fish consumption. The pattern of risks was similar for men and women As there were few subjects who never consumed fish, subjects with low fish consumption were included in the "unexposed" gp. and thus the strength of the inverse correlation may have been underestimated (*Norell SE et al. Fish consumption and mortality from coronary heart disease. Br Med J 293:426, 1986*).

Observational Study (M): The fish consumption and mortality from coronary heart disease were studied over 20 yrs. regarding 872 men residing in a town in the Netherlands. An inverse dose-response relation was observed between fish consumption in 1960 and CHD during 20 yrs. of follow-up, with mortality more than 50% lower among those who consumed at least 30 g of fish daily. As little as 1-2 fish dishes per wk. may help to prevent CHD (*Kromhout D et al. The inverse relation between fish consumption and 20-year mortality from coronary heart disease. N Engl J Med 312:1205-9, 1985*).

Supplementation may protect against the progression of atherosclerosis during ingestion of an atherogenic diet.

Animal Experimental Study (G): Rhesus monkeys were fed diets containing 2% cholesterol and either 25% coconut oil (Gp. I), 25% fish oil (Menhaden)/coconut oil (1:1) (Gp. 2), or 25% fish oil/coconut oil (3:1) (Gp. III). After 12 mo., ave. serum cholesterol levels were 987 mg/dl for Gp. 1, 463 mg/dl for Gp. II, and 405 mg/dl for Gp. III. An ave. of 79% of the aortic intima was involved in AS in Gp. I, 48% in Gp. II, and 36% in Gp. III. The aortas of both fish-oil gps. contained significantly less cholesterol and, microscopically, the aortic and carotid artery lesions were smaller in cross-sectional area and in thickness, and contained less macrophages in the fish-oil gps. (*Davis HR et al. Fish oil inhibits development of atherosclerosis in rhesus monkeys. Arteriosclerosis 7(5):441-49, 1987*).

Supplementation may decrease blood viscosity.

Experimental Double-blind Study: 30 healthy subjects received fish oil capsules containing 1.26 or 2.52 g ω-3 fatty acids daily or placebo. After 5 wks. at the high dosage, systolic BP, plasma viscosity and RBC rigidity were significantly decreased (p<0.01). Vitamin E concentration was reduced only in the low dosage gp. (p<0.01) (*Bach R et al. Effects of fish oil capsules in two dosages on blood pressure, platelet functions, haemorheological and clinical chemistry parameters in apparently healthy subjects. Ann Nutr Metab 33:359-67, 1989*

Supplementation may reduce postprandial lipemia.

Experimental Study (H,T): 16 normal volunteers took 2.2 g omega-3 fatty acids/d from fish oils. Oral fat loads were given once at the start and end of the study and the rise in chylomicron triglyceride and omega-3 fatty acid levels were measured. After 4 wks., supplementation was associated with a 36% decrease in chylomicron triglyceride levels (p<0.01) and a 26% decrease in fasting triglyceride levels (p<0.05). HDL cholesterol levels increased by 13% (p<0.01) due entirely to an increase in the HDL$_2$ subfraction. There were no differences between subjects who received fish oil capsules and those who received fish oil emulsion (*Harris WS, Windsor SL. N-3 fatty acid supplements reduce chylomicron levels in healthy volunteers. J Appl Nutr 43(1):5-15, 1991*).

Supplementation may reduce total cholesterol and increase HDL cholesterol. In addition, fish oils are the only polyunsaturated oils which may lower triglycerides.

Note: In some studies, fish oil administration has raised LDL cholesterol levels. As long as these levels are not elevated, however, there is no reason to avoid their use. When high triglyceride levels are lowered by weight loss, diet, or medications, LDL cholesterol increases because pts. with high triglyceride levels have abnormally low LDL levels and these low levels increase to normal when triglyceride levels normalize (Davidson MH. Fish oil vs. total lipid profile. Letter. Med World News February 22, 1988, p. 10). It seems likely that fish oils, by lowering high triglyceride levels, raise LDL cholesterol by the same mechanism.

Note: Not all omega-3 rich fish oils have the same effect, possibly due to differences in their EPA:DHA ratios:

Fish Oil	EPA:DHA
Pollack	3.8
MaxEPA (North Sea fish)	1.6
Salmon	0.8
Tuna	0.35

Experimental Controlled Study (C,H,L,T): 8 normolipidemic men were fed three 36%-fat diets containing primarily butter, EPA-rich pollock, or DHA-rich tuna or salmon-blend oils. Compared to the butter diet, VLDL triglycerides decreased equally (71-78%) with all diets; LDL cholesterol and apolipoprotein B decreased 16% and 13%, respectively, on the tuna and salmon-blend oil but did not change (-1%) and increased 19% with the pollack diet; HDL cholesterol and lipoproteins A-I and A-II decreased with all diets but more with the pollack diet than with the tuna and salmon diets. The 23-31% decrease in total cholesterol on the tuna and salmon diets resulted mostly from decreased LDL-C, whereas the 16% decrease on pollack oil resulted mostly from decreased HDL-C (*Childs MT et al. Divergent lipoprotein responses to fish oils with various ratios of eicosapentaenoic acid and docosahexaenoic acid. Am J Clin Nutr 52:632-39, 1990*).

Negative Experimental Controlled Crossover Study (L): 21 normotriglyceridemic males received diets containing 200 g of Dover sole (low in ω-3 fatty acids), Chinnock Salmon (higher in ω-3 fatty acids) or sablefish (higher in ω-3 fatty acids) as part of a Western diet for 18-day dietary periods. Concentrations of serum LDL-C and apolipoprotein B rose on the salmon and sablefish diets as compared with the sole diet, suggesting that consumption of fish with moderate amts. of ω-3 fatty acids may cause a deleterious rise in LDL-C and apo B concentrations in normotriglyceridemic males (*Gerhard GT et al. Comparison of three species of dietary fish: effects on serum concentrations of low-density-lipoprotein cholesterol and apolipoprotein in normotriglyceridemic subjects. Am J Clin Nutr 54:334-9, 1991*).

Experimental Controlled Crossover Study (H,L,T): 36 healthy young males randomly and successively received fat-controlled diets, with and without a fish-oil supplement (MaxEPA 6 g/d), for 3 wks. each. Total calorie, fat, and cholesterol intakes were similar in the two diets. Triglycerides in serum and VLDL lipoproteins were lower and HDL$_2$ was higher in the omega-3 supplemented diet, and platelet aggregation decreased significantly. However, LDL cholesterol and plasminogen-activator-inhibitor (PAI) activity significantly increased (although PAI activity remained in the normal range) (*Fumeron F et al. n-3 polyunsaturated fatty acids raise low-density lipoproteins, high-density lipoprotein 2, and plasminogen-activator inhibitor in healthy young men. Am J Clin Nutr 54:118-22, 1991*).

Experimental Double-blind Crossover Study (H,T): 27 Israeli hyperlipidemic pts. randomly received either supplementation with fish oil 15 g/d (EPAGIS, Agis Ltd, Tel Aviv) containing 5.2 g ω-3 PUFAs/d and a vegetable oil mixture supplying linoleic and α-linolenic acid in either order. Despite the habitual high linoleic acid intake of the study population, ingestion of fish oil resulted in a 40% decrease in triglyceride concentration, a 12% increase in HDL cholesterol, and a significant decrease in plasma viscosity, whereas the vegetable oil placebo had no effect (*Green P et al. Effect of fish-oil ingestion on cardiovascular risk factors in hyperlipidemic subjects in Israel: a randomized, double-blind crossover study. Am J Clin Nutr 52:1118-24, 1990*).

Review Article (C,L,T): Fish oil supplements have proven effective in lowering plasma triglycerides, but available data have not shown that they lower LDL or HDL cholesterol in normolipidemic or hypercholesterolemic individuals. These findings, coupled with the lack of information on long-term safety of large amts. of fish oils, suggest that supplementation with fish oil capsules cannot be recommended (*Margolis S, Dobs AS. Nutritional management of plasma lipid disorders. J Am Coll Nutr 8 Suppl S:33S-45S, 1989*).

Supplementation may lower plasma lipids even despite high cholesterol intake.

Experimental Study (C,H,L,T): 6 pts. with heterozygous familial hypercholesterolemia were placed on 2 diets at 4-wk. intervals which supplied similar calorie, fat and fish oil (22 gms/1000 kcal with a 30% omega-3 fatty acid concentration) contents; however, the first diet was low in cholesterol, while the second was high in cholesterol (200 mg/1000 kcal). Both the low- and high-cholesterol diets lowered plasma lipids, including total cholesterol, VLDL-cholesterol, LDL-cholesterol, HDL-cholesterol, and triglycerides. The ratio of total cholesterol to HDL-cholesterol, which was poor at entry, failed to improve (*Hatcher L et al. Dietary fish oil in familial hypercholesterolemia: Response to added cholesterol.* Clin Res *35:A772, 1987*).

Experimental Study (C): A diet rich in ω-3 fatty acids ameliorated the effect of added dietary cholesterol on the plasma cholesterol (*Nestel PJ. Fish oil attenuates the cholesterol-induced rise in lipoprotein cholesterol.* Am J Clin Nutr *43:752, 1986*).

Supplementation may inhibit the development of atherosclerosis by inhibiting the production of a protein similar to platelet-derived growth factor (PDGF). PDGF is believed to be involved in the exchange of information and materials between the blood and arterial walls, a process which, in turn, may relate to the development of atherosclerosis.

In vitro Experimental Study (G): Fish oils (MaxEPA) were incubated with bovine aortic endothelial cells; this resulted in a significant reduction in production of a PDGF-like protein by these cells which was independent of total protein production. Safflower oil had only 1/10th to 1/20th of the effect and peanut oil had none. Antioxidants interfered with the action of fish oils on production of this protein (*Fox PL, Dicorieto PE. Fish oils inhibit endothelial cell production of platelet-derived growth factor-like protein.* Science *241:453-56, 1988*).

Supplementation may reduce tissue damage from acute ischemia.

Animal Experimental Study (M): Following coronary artery ligation, there was a significant reduction in the loss of creatine kinase in rats fed 5% menhaden oil compared to rats fed 5% corn oil (*Hock CE et al. Effect of dietary fish oil on myocardial phospholipids and myocardial ischemic damage.* Am J Physiol *252(3 Pt. 2):H554-60, 1987*).

Animal Experimental Controlled Study (M): Following coronary artery ligation, 25% of the left ventricle was damaged in controls compared to only 3% damage in dogs fed omega-3 fatty acids (*Culp BR et al.* Prostaglandins *20:1021, 1980*).

Supplementation may reduce anginal pain and improve exercise tolerance.

Experimental Study (A,C,H,L,T): 107 subjects with either heart disease, hyperlipidemia or no symptoms received 3.6 gm. daily of EPA (MaxEPA) for up to 2 years. At the end, those with angina reported fewer episodes of pain and needed less nitroglycerin. Triglycerides, cholesterol, bleeding times and VLDL and LDL lipoproteins decreased, while HDL increased significantly (*Saynor R et al. The long-term effect of dietary supplementation with fish lipid concentrate on serum lipids, bleeding time, platelets and angina.* Atherosclerosis *50:3-10, 1984*).

Experimental Study (A,C,H,T): 150 ASHD pts. and normal volunteers were supplemented with fish oils (MaxEPA) for up to 3 years. Long term patients were able to reduce nitrate therapy and exhibited increased exercise tolerance while taking the supplement. After 2 years, triglycerides, which fell sharply during the first few weeks, remained low. Total cholesterol was significantly lower and HDL cholesterol was significantly higher. Bleeding time increased when the daily dose was 20 ml. (3.6 gm.) of EPA but not when it was 10 ml. (1.8 gm) (*Saynor R, Verel D. Eskimos and their diets. Letter.* Lancet *1:1335, 1983*).

Supplementation may be effective in the prevention and treatment of thrombotic disorders by reducing platelet aggregation and improving blood flow dynamics.

Experimental Crossover Controlled Study (P): 23 healthy, young males received diets containing 200 g of Dover sole (low in ω-3 fatty acids), Chinnock Salmon (higher in ω-3 fatty acids) or sablefish (higher in ω-3 fatty acids) as part of a Western diet for 18-day dietary periods. Bleeding time increased moderately when salmon diets were consumed (p=0.06). Platelet aggregation decreased with collagen as an agonist on sablefish diets (p=0.03) and with ADP as an agonist on salmon and sablefish diets (p=0.04). Thromboxane B_2 concentrations decreased moderately on sablefish and salmon diets (p=0.06). Results suggest that certain species of fish, when consumed in reasonable amts. as part of a Western diet, may cause modestly positive effects on platelet function (*Wander RC, Patton BD. Comparison of three species of fish consumed as part of a Western diet: effects on platelet fatty acids and function, hemostasis, and production of thromboxane.* Am J Clin Nutr *54:326-33, 1991*).

Supplementation may reduce the risk of thrombus formation by reducing plasma fibrinogen concentration.

Experimental Double-blind Crossover Study (F): Following a 6-wk. run-in period, 10 pts. with hyperlipoprote-inemia types IIb or IV received 4.6 g/d of n-3 fatty acids from fish oil, or corn oil supplying 5.3 g/d of linoleic acid, for 8 wks. each in random order, with a 4-wk. washout period in between during which they received olive oil "placebo" capsules. Plasma fibrinogen levels showed statistically significant reductions during both the fish oil and corn oil treatment periods (*Radack K et al. The comparative effects of n-3 and n-6 polyunsaturated fatty acids on plasma fibrinogen levels: A controlled clinical trial in hypertriglyceridemic subjects. J Am Coll Nutr 9(4):352-57, 1990*).

Experimental Double-blind Study (F): 64 men aged 35-40 were randomly assigned to receive either 14 gm fish oil concentrate (Apothekernes Laboratorium AS, Norway) or 14 gm olive oil daily. After 3 wks., there was a 13.2% decrease in plasma fibrinogen concentrations in men taking fish oil so that this value was significantly lower than that of men receiving olive oil (p<0.05); after 6 wks. there were no further changes (*Flaten H et al. Fish-oil concentrate: effect on variables related to cardiovascular disease. Am J Clin Nutr 52:300-306, 1990; Høstmark AT et al. Fish oil and plasma fibrinogen. Br Med J 297:180-81, 1988*).

Supplementation may improve cardiac function.

Experimental Double-blind Crossover Study (A): 8 pts. with stable coronary artery disease and positive exer-cise stress tests received 3.2 gm EPA and 2.2 gm DHA daily. After 12 wks., the ω-3 fatty acids caused significant reductions in BP, heart rate, and the product of systolic arterial pressure and heart rate, especially in response to exercise. There were also positive, but non-significant, trends towards greater exercise times to ST depression, reduced angina frequency, and reduced nitroglycerin usage (*Mehta JL et al. Dietary supplementation with omega-3 polyunsaturated fatty acids in patients with stable coronary heart disease. Am J Med 84:45-52, 1988*).

Supplementation may inhibit restenosis after percutaneous transluminal coronary angioplasty (PTCA).

Experimental Double-blind Study (G): 205 pts. undergoing a first PTCA received 15 caps/d containing 1 g of either fish oils (MaxEPA) or olive oil starting 3 wks. prior to surgery and continuing for 6 mo. afterwards. Pts. on MaxEPA had a statistically significant (p=0.03) lower frequency of restenosis than those on olive oil. After controlling for treatment, a lower frequency of restenosis was observed among pts. with higher omega-3 fatty acid intake (p=0.003) (*Meyer F et al. Effects of fish oil supplements and fish consumption in the prevention of resteno-sis after coronary angioplasty. Abstract. Am J Clin Nutr 53:P-24, 1991*).

Negative Experimental Double-blind Study (G): In a randomized study of 204 pts., the treatment gp. received 6 g/d of omega-3 fatty acids starting 5.4 (SD 3.2) days before PTCA and continuing for 6 months. The incidence of angiographic restenosis was 34% in the fish oil gp. and 23% in the controls who received an olive oil placebo. Lack of benefit was not influenced by length of pretreatment, compliance or plasma EPA concentrations (*Reis GJ et al. Randomised trial of fish oil for prevention of restenosis after coronary angioplasty. Lancet 2:177-81, 1989*).

> *Note: This study has been criticized as the "placebo" used was olive oil which is high in monounsaturates, and diets high in monounsaturates may be of benefit in preventing atherosclerosis (Milner MR. Fish oil for preventing coronary restenosis. Letter. Lancet 2:693, 1989).*

Low erucic acid rapeseed oil (LEAR), which contains 10% α-linolenic acid, may be an effective source of omega-3 fatty acids.

Experimental Study: 10 type II hyperlipidemic pts. received LEAR as a replacement for the edible oils in their usual diet. After 5 mo., RBC ω-3 fatty acids increased from 2 to 50%. Total serum cholesterol decreased from 272 to 258 (p<0.05), LDL decreased from 191 to 177 (not significant), HDL decreased from 58 to 57 (not significant), and triglycerides decreased from 142 to 123 (not significant). HDL_2 decreased from 22 to 17 (p<0.02), while HDL_3 increased from 36 to 40 (p<0.05). Other significant findings were increased serum calcium, decreased uric acid, decreased tocopherol, and decreased β-carotene. Results suggest that LEAR may be an alter-native source of omega-3 fatty acids to fish oil; however, vitamin supplementation may be needed to provide adequate anti-oxidation (*Bierenbaum ML et al. Low erucic acid rapeseed oil (LEAR) in hyperlipidemia. Abstract. J Am Coll Nutr 8(5):445, 1989*).

Fish oils appear to be equally effective as fish in producing lipid and lipoprotein changes, but not as effective in improving hemostatic factors (*Cobiac L et al. Lipid, lipoprotein, and hemostatic effects of fish vs fish oil n-3 fatty acids in mildly hyperlipidemic males. Am J Clin Nutr 53:1210-16, 1991*).

Omega-6 Fatty Acids:
(C,G,M,P)

Linoleic acid $\rightarrow$ GLA $\rightarrow$ DGLA $\rightarrow$ Prostaglandin E_1

Several oils are rich in linoleic acid, while evening primrose oil is one of the richest sources of gammalinolenic acid (GLA). When, due to such factors as aging, the intake of *trans* fatty acids, pyridoxine, magnesium or zinc deficiencies, excessive alcohol consumption, etc., the conversion of linoleic acid to GLA is inhibited, primrose oil is superior to most oils as a PGE_1 precursor (*Horrobin DF. The importance of gamma-linolenic acid and prostaglandin E_1 in human nutrition and medicine. J Holistic Med 3:118-139, 1981*).

> *Note: Borage and blackcurrent oils are higher in GLA than evening primrose oil, although it is not known how they compare therapeutically.*

> WARNING: High blood levels of polyunsaturates, especially the omega-6 fatty acids, may increase the risk of atherosclerosis unless there is adequate antioxidant protection.

> **Observational Study (G):** Pts. with >85% stenosis in one or more coronary blood vessels were compared to controls with <50% stenosis in all coronary vessels. Serum polyunsaturated fatty acid levels were similar in both groups. However, plasma selenium levels were lower in pts. than in controls and the ratios of selenium to linoleic acid (an omega-6 fatty acid), selenium to total polyunsaturates, and selenium to total omega-6 fatty acids were lower in patients. These differences were most pronounced in pts. with low serum alpha tocopherol levels. In this sub-gp., the ratio of selenium to polyunsaturated fatty acids was lower in the pts. than in the controls for all fatty acids as well as for EPA and DHA (omega-3 fatty acids) (*Kok F et al. Do antioxidants and polyunsaturated fatty acids have a combined association with coronary atherosclerosis? Atherosclerosis 86:85-90, 1991*).

Tissue levels may be inversely correlated to the risk of coronary heart disease.

> **Observational Study (G):** When the fatty acid composition of total RBC lipids were compared in 20 men presenting with acute myocardial infarction with that of healthy controls, pts. had significantly lower linoleic acid levels. Levels of DGLA and arachidonic acid, however, were not significantly different (*Rapley CH et al. Fatty acid pattern and ischaemic heart disease. Lancet 1:1202, 1987*).

> **Negative Observational Study (G):** Plasma linoleic acid levels of acute MI pts. 8 mo. after their attack were no different than those of healthy controls. Platelet linoleic acid was 8.2% in the healthy controls compared to 3.9% in the Greenland Eskimo, even though the incidence of acute MI is lower in the Eskimo. Finally, the linoleic acid content of ave. Danish food is twice that of the Eskimo. These findings suggest that the ratio between the omega-6 and the omega-3 fatty acids in food and tissue lipids may be a better predictor of the risk of ischemic heart disease than measures of linoleic acid (*Bang HO, Dyerberg J. Fatty acid pattern and ischaemic heart disease. Lancet 1:663, 1987*).

> **Observational Study (A,G,M):** In a study of several hundred randomly selected middle-aged men, there was a progressive inverse relationship between adipose linoleic acid and the estimated relative risk of angina pectoris. This relationship was independent of traditional risk factors. There was also a progressive inverse relationship between adipose tissue linoleic acid and the estimated relative risk of acute myocardial infarction, but it was confounded by smoking habit as smokers consumed less linoleic acid than non-smokers (*Wood DA et al. Linoleic and eicosapentaenoic acids in adipose tissue and platelets and risk of coronary heart diseae. Lancet 1:176-82, 1987*).

Serum levels of omega-6 fatty acids may be inversely correlated with the risk of myocardial infarction.

> **Observational Study (G,M):** In a secondary prevention study of postinfarction middle-aged men, linoleic acid in serum total lipids was the first variable in the stepwise regression analysis of metabolic, nutritional and cardiovascular factors. When the dependent variable was cardiovascular death, it was the only fatty acid entering the

regression and was followed by previous myocardial infarction, heart volume index and hyperlipoproteinemia. Unlike other fatty acids, it was distinguished by its low percentage of accumulation of deaths. The decreased percentage of linoleic acid was also evident in the comparison of fatty acid patterns of cardiovascular deaths in age- and triglyceride-matched men free from ischemic heart disease. Results confirm prospective associations found in previously healthy men and suggest conclusions about the relevance of low serum linoleic acid to long-term prognosis after MI (*Välek J et al. Serum linoleic acid and cardiovascular death in postinfarction middle-aged men. Atherosclerosis 54(1):111-8, 1985*

Administration of evening primrose oil (rich in gamma-linolenic acid) may lower plasma cholesterol.

Experimental Placebo-controlled Study (C): 84 pts. received 4 gm evening primrose oil daily x 12 weeks. Afterwards, cholesterol was significantly decreased in pts. whose cholesterol had been >192 mg% (*Horrobin DF, Manku MS. How do poly-unsaturated fatty acids lower plasma cholesterol levels? Lipids 18:558-62, 1983*).

Administration of omega-6 fatty acids may decrease platelet aggregability.

Experimental Study (C,P): 6 healthy volunteers received safflower oil 60 mg. daily as a source of linoleic acid. After 2 wks., there was decreased platelet aggregation to ADP in addition to decreased cholesterol. Fibrinolysis and bleeding times were unaltered (*Challen AD et al. The effect of aspirin and linoleic on platelet aggregation, platelet fatty acid composition and haemostatis in man. Hum Nutr Clin Nutr 37(3):197-208, 1983*).

Administration of omega-6 fatty acids may reduce plasma fibrinogen concentration.

Experimental Double-blind Crossover Study (F): Following a 6-wk. run-in period, 10 pts. with hyperlipoprotein-emia types IIb or IV received 4.6 g/d of n-3 fatty acids from fish oil, or corn oil supplying 5.3 g/d of linoleic acid, for 8 wks. each in random order, with a 4-wk. washout period in between during which they received olive oil "placebo" capsules. Plasma fibrinogen levels showed statistically significant reductions during both the fish oil and corn oil treatment periods (*Radack K et al. The comparative effects of n-3 and n-6 polyunsaturated fatty acids on plasma fibrinogen levels: A controlled clinical trial in hypertriglyceridemic subjects. J Am Coll Nutr 9(4):352-57, 1990*).

Omega-3 vs. Omega-6 Fatty Acids:

The polyunsaturated fatty acids (PUFAs) of vegetable oils, containing mostly linoleic acid [omega-6], are effective in counteracting the effects of dietary saturated acids, but the omega-3 PUFAs of fish oils may be equally or more hypolipidemic (*Kinsella JE et al. Dietary n-3 polyunsaturated fatty acids and amelioration of cardiovascular disease: possible mechanisms. Am J Clin Nutr 52:1-28, 1990*).

Omega-3 vs. Omega-6 vs. Omega-9 Fatty Acids:
(C,L)

May be equally effective in lowering total, LDL and VLDL cholesterol concentrations in plasma (*Chan JK et al. Dietary α-linolenic acid is as effective as oleic acid and linoleic acid in lowering blood cholesterol in normolipidemic men. Am J Clin Nutr 53:1230-4, 1991*).

Omega-6 vs. Omega-9 Fatty Acids:
(P)

Substituting linoleic acid (omega-6) for oleic acid (omega-9) may raise the threshold for platelet aggregation (*Burri BJ et al. Platelet aggregation in humans is affected by replacement of dietary linoleic acid with oleic acid. Am J Clin Nutr 54:359-62, 1991*).

A diet rich in oleic acid (omega-9) may reduce the susceptibility of low-density lipoprotein to oxidative modification.

Note: Oxidized low-density lipoprotien is more atherogenic than native LDL.

Experimental Study: After 5 wks., oxidation of the LDL isolated from subjects consuming an oleate-enriched diet generated significantly less conjugated dienes and at a slower rate than LDL from subjects on a linoleate-enriched diet. After incubation with endothelial cells, LDL from the oleate gp. underwent less degradation by macrophages. These results suggest that the diet can be altered so as not to increase LDL cholesterol concentrations while decreasing the susceptibility of LDL to oxidative modification (*Reaven P et al. Feasibility of using an oleate-rich diet to reduce the susceptibility of low-density lipoprotein to oxidative modification in humans. Am J Clin Nutr 54:701-6, 1991*).

Pantethine: 300 mg 2-4 times daily with food
(C,H,L,P,T)   Changes in cholesterol may take 1-2 months.
                          Maximal effect may require 4 or more months.

The active form of pantothenic acid (the fundamental moiety of coenzyme A). (*See "Coenzyme A" above.*)

Supplementation may decrease serum triglyceride and cholesterol levels.

Experimental Study (C,H,T): 24 pts. (mean age 51 yrs.) with Types IIA, IIB or IV hyperlipidemia received pantethine 300 mg 3 times daily. After 1 yr., there was a highly significant ($p<0.001$) reduction of about 17% in mean serum cholesterol levels which had become evident within 1 month and persisted thereafter. Mean HDL cholesterol levels increased by about 15% (results not significant) and mean triglyceride levels fell by 48% ($p<0.01$). There were no significant side effects (*Arsenio L et al. Effectiveness of long-term treatment with pantethine in patients with dyslipidemia. Clin Ther 8:537-45, 1986*).

Experimental Double-blind Crossover Study (C,H,L,T): 29 pts. (11 with type IIB hyperlipoproteinemia, 15 with type IV, 3 with an isolated reduction of HDL cholesterol) received pantethine 300 mg 3 times daily or placebo. After 8 wks., type IIB pts. demonstrated a highly significant lowering of plasma total and LDL cholesterol (-13.5% for each) and HDL cholesterol increased about 10%. Switching to placebo was associated with a rapid return to baseline measures. Both in type IIB and type IV pts., plasma triglyceride levels were reduced about 30% when pantethine was given first; when it was given after placebo reductions were less striking (-17.8% for type IIB and -13% for type IV). In type IV pts. and those with an isolated HDL cholesterol reduction, HDL cholesterol levels failed to increase. In type IV pts., LDL cholesterol levels showed a variable response; they tended to increase when below 132 mg/dl prior to treatment, and to reduce when above this level (*Gaddi A et al. Controlled evaluation of pantethine, a natural hypolipidemic compound, in patients with different forms of hyperlipoproteinemia. Atherosclerosis 50(1):73-83, 1984*).

Negative Experimental Double-blind Study (C): Supplementation was ineffective for pts. who had previously failed to respond to a combined drug/diet regime (*Da Col PG et al. Pantethine in the treatment of hyper-cholesterolemia: A randomized double-blind trial versus tiadenol. Curr Ther Res 36:314, 1984*).

Supplementation may increase microsomal lipoprotein lipase which is positively correlated with HDL cholesterol levels (*Noma A et al. Effect of pantethine on post-heparin plasma lipolytic activities and adipose tissue lipoprotein lipase in rats. Horm Met Res 16:233-6, 1984*).

Supplementation may inhibit platelet aggregation.

Experimental Study (P): Following 28 days of supplementation with pantethine 300 mg 4 times daily, hyperlipidemic pts. demonstrated inhibition of platelet aggregation and thromboxane A_2 production (*Prisco D et al. Effect of pantethine treatment on platelet aggregation and thromboxane A_2 production. Curr Ther Res 35:700, 1984*).

Phytosterols: beta-sitosterol 300 mg - 1 g per meal
(C,H,L,T)   immediately before or after meals (2 wk. trial)

Cholesterol analogs found in vegetables.

Administration may decrease cholesterol absorption by displacing cholesterol from bile salt (taurocholate) micelles (*Ikeda I et al. Inhibition of cholesterol absorption in rats by plant sterols. J Lipid Res 29(12):1573-82, 1988*).

Note: Approximately twice the amount of phytosterol as the amount of cholesterol ingested is required for optimal efficacy (Beveridge JMR et al. Magnitude of the hypocholesterolemic effect of dietary sitosterol in man. J Nutr 83:119, 1964).

- <u>Beta Sitosterol</u>:

Experimental Study (C):   Ingestion of beta-sitosterol 1 g along with a meal containing 500 mg cholesterol decreased cholesterol absorption by 42% (*Mattson FH et al. Optimizing the effect of plant sterols on cholesterol absorption in man. <u>Am J Clin Nutr</u> 35(4):697-700, 1982*).

- <u>Gamma Oryzanol</u>:

A mixture of several sterols, especially cycloartenol, combined with ferulic acid (which may also have a cholesterol-lowering effect).

Rice bran is a rich source.

Administration may be improve the lipid profile.

Experimental Study (C,H,L,T):   67 pts. with type IIA (n=35), type IIB (n=19), or type IV (n=13) hyperlipoproteinemia received 300 mg/d of gamma-oryzanol for 3 months. Mean plasma cholesterol in type IIA and IIB pts. decreased significantly from the second month (-8% and -12%, respectively) due to a fall in LDL cholesterol levels. Mean plasma triglyceride levels of all pts. decreased significantly (-14%) by the third month. HDL cholesterol increased significantly after 3 mo. in the type IIB subjects (*Yoshino G et al. Effects of gamma-oryzanol on hyperlipidemic subjects. <u>Curr Ther Res</u> 45:543-52, 1989*).

Experimental Study (C,H):   14 normals, 3 hyperlipidemic pts. and 7 pts. with gallstones received gamma oryzanol 600 mg daily. After 4 wks., cholesterol absorption was shown to be inhibited, and both HDL cholesterol and apolipoprotein A1 were increased (*Kawamoto T et al. The effects of ursodeoxycholic acid, gamma oryzanol and beta sitosterol on serum lipids and apolipoprotein A1. <u>Med J Hiroshima Univ</u> 33(5):919, 1985*).

See Also:

Experimental Single-blind Study (C): *Orimo H. Lipid-lowering effect of gamma oryzanol in man - a single blind study. <u>Sixth Int Sympos Atherosclerosis</u> 1982:236*

<u>Saponins</u>:
(C)

A structurally diverse group of naturally occurring compounds, found mainly in plants, consisting of a steroid or triterpene group linked to one or more sugar molecules. Most saponin-containing plants are legumes, with the greatest dietary intake most likely to come from alfalfa sprouts, chickpeas, green peas, lentils, soya beans, peanuts, navy beans, mung beans, kidney beans and broad beans (*Oakenfull D, Sidhu GS. Could saponins be a useful treatment for hypercholesterolaemia? <u>Europ J Clin Nutr</u> 44:79-88, 1990*).

Supplementation may reduce cholesterol levels.

Review Article (C):   There is now a substantial body of evidence that dietary saponins can lower plasma cholesterol concentrations. They act either directly, by inhibiting absorption of cholesterol from the small intestine, or indirectly, by inhibiting the reabsorption of bile acids (*Oakenfull D, Sidhu GS. Could saponins be a useful treatment for hypercholesterolaemia? <u>Europ J Clin Nutr</u> 44:79-88, 1990*).

<u>Taurine</u>:
(C,G,M,P)

General Review Article: *Huxtable RJ, Sebring LA. Cardiovascular actions of taurine. <u>Prog Clin Biol Res</u> 125:5-37, 1983*

Arrhythmias characteristic of acute myocardial ischemia may be partly due to loss of intracellular taurine (*Crass MF, Lombardini JB. Release of tissue taurine from the oxygen-deficient perfused rat heart. <u>Proc Soc Exp Biol Med</u> 157:486-8, 1978*).

Observational Study (M): Blood samples from 97 consecutive pts. admitted for chest pains were analyzed for taurine concentrations. The mean maximum taurine concentrations in whole blood from acute MI pts. were greater than that of pts. without acute MI. By contrast, there was no difference in plasma taurine in the 2 gps., indicating that a cellular component(s) of whole blood was sequestering taurine. A myocardial source for the blood taurine rise is probable, and there is evidence that the myocardium selectively leaks taurine but not other amino acids (*Lombardini JB, Cooper MW. Elevated blood taurine levels in acute and evolving myocardial infarction. J Lab Clin Med 98(6):849-59, 1981*).

Supplementation may stabilize platelets against aggregation.

Experimental Study (P): Platelets from healthy subjects with normal taurine status demonstrated increased resistance to aggregation by 30-70% when the subjects were supplemented with taurine at 400 mg/d for 14 days or 1600 mg/d for 8 days, respectively (*Hayes KC et al. Taurine modulates platelet aggregration in cats and humans. Am J Clin Nutr 49:1211-16, 1989*).

Supplementation may improve cholesterol metabolism.

Negative Experimental Study (C): 4 healthy males received taurine 3.2 g/d for 2 wks., while another 5 healthy males were administered cholesterol 1 g/d for 2 wks. followed by taurine and cholesterol simultaneously for 2 weeks. Taurine administration alone did not alter either serum or biliary lipid composition, although taurine-conjugated bile acids were increased. When taurine and cholesterol were administered together, both LDL cholesterol and the bile lithogenic index were increased (*Tanno N et al. Effect of taurine administration on serum lipid and biliary lipid composition in man. Tohoku J Exp Med 159(2):91-100, 1989*).

Animal Experimental Study (C): Taurine suppressed elevation in serum cholesterol levels in rats placed on a diet containing 0.5% cholesterol, 1% cholic acid and omega-aminosulfonic acids. Serum triglyceride levels were unaffected. Taurine also inhibited intestinal absorption of cholesterol (*Yamada J et al. Effects of omega-aminosulfonic acids on lipid metabolism in dietary hyperlipidemic rats. J Pharmacobiodyn 6(6):373-80, 1983*).

Supplementation may combat atherogenesis.

Animal Experimental Study (G): Mice receiving nicotine along with vitamin D_3 developed severe myocardial and aortic calcinosis within 4 days. Treatment with taurine increased the survival rate and reduced the elevation of calcium content in both aorta and myocardium, suggesting that taurine, which is capable of regulating calcium flux, may also prevent the progression of arteriosclerosis (*Yamauchi-Takihara K et al. Taurine protection against experimental arterial calcinosis in mice. Biochem Biophys Res Commun 140(2):679-83, 1986*).

- -

MICROORGANISMS

Brewer's yeast: 20 gm. daily (8 week trial)
(C,H,L,T)

Administration may lower LDL cholesterol while raising HDL cholesterol.

Experimental Study (C,H): 46 healthy volunteers were classified as either normolipidemic or hyperlipidemic and supplemented with brewer's yeast. After 8 wks., triglycerides were unchanged but serum cholesterol was reduced for 8/15 hyperlipidemic subjects and 10/11 normolipidemic subjects, while HDL cholesterol increased for both gps. (*Elwood JC et al. Effect of high-chromium brewer's yeast on human serum lipids. J Am Coll Nutr 1:263-74, 1982*).

Experimental Single-blind Study (C): 24 elderly pts. (4 of whom were hypercholesterolemic) who received chromium-rich brewer's yeast for 8 wks. improved glucose tolerance and significantly decreased serum cholesterol (especially in the hypercholesterolemic pts.) and total lipids, while the findings on controls who received chromium-poor tortula yeast were unchanged (*Offenbachaer EG, Pi-Sunyer FX. Beneficial effect of chromium-rich yeast on glucose tolerance and blood lipids in elderly subjects. Diabetes 29:919-25, 1980*).

Experimental Study (H,L): Subjects received 7 gm GTF-rich brewer's yeast (15 μg chromium). After 6 wks. there was a significant increase (ave. 17.6%) in HDL cholesterol levels. HDL to LDL ratios improved from an ave. of 0.413 to 0.596, an improvement of 44% (*Riales R. Chromium in Nutrition and Metabolism. North-Holland Biomedical Press, 1979:199-212*).

- -

TOXIC MINERALS

Cadmium:

Deaths from cardiovascular diseases appear to be strongly correlated with high concentrations of airborne cadmium and cadmium in milk (*Carroll RE. JAMA 198:267, 1966; Gunn SA et al. Bull Pathol 8:42, 1967; Schroeder HA. Ecologist 1:11, 1971*).

- -

OTHER FACTORS

Activated Charcoal:
(C,H,L,T)

Supplementation may reduce triglycerides and LDL cholesterol while raising HDL cholesterol.

Negative Double-blind Experimental Study (C,T): 12 mainly primary hypercholesterolemic pts. randomly recieved either 15 gm activated charcoal or 15 gm non-activated charcoal in granulated form as placebo. After 12 wks., the same pts. were randomized again to receive either 30 gm activated charcoal or 30 gm non-activated charcoal. Mean serum cholesterol levels in pts. treated with activated charcoal failed to decrease significantly although, in both gps. during treatment with activated charcoal, 1 pt. had a significant decrease in serum cholesterol level. No decrease in serum triglycerides was observed in 3 hypertriglyceridemic patients (*Hoekstra JBL, Erkelens DW. Effect of activated charcoal on hypercholesterolaemia. Letter. Lancet 2:455, 1987*).

Experimental Study (C,H,L): 7 pts. with hypercholesterolemia who had responded only marginally to 10 yrs. of treatment with clofibrate, gemfibrozil and/or nicotinic acid received activated charcoal 8 gm 3 times daily. After 4 wks., plasma total cholesterol decreased by 41%, LDL cholesterol decreased by 25%, and HDL cholesterol increased by 8%. Except for black stools, there were no side effects (*Kuusisto R et al. Effect of activated charcoal on hypercholesterolaemia. Lancet 2:366-67, 1986*).

AUTO-IMMUNE DISORDERS (GENERAL)

See Also: LUPUS   RAYNAUD'S SYNDROME
              MULTIPLE SCLEROSIS   RHEUMATOID ARTHRITIS
              MYOPATHY   SCLERODERMA
              NEUROMUSCULAR DEGENERATION VASCULITIS

DIETARY FACTORS

Low fat diet.

Animal Experimental Study: Phagocytosis by periotoneal macrophages and natural killer cell activity were markedly reduced in mice fed high saturated fat diets. The results of this study performed on lupus-prone mice suggest that diets high in fat may influence immune responses and thus may affect the onset and severity of auto-immune disease, and that a low-fat diet can reduce the development of the disease by maintaining normal immune responses. The data also suggest that unsaturated fats may influence T helper cell activity and therefore antibody production, whereas saturated fats may affect cellular immune responses which are dependent on membrane contact (*Morrow J et al. Dietary fat and immune function. J Immunol 135(6):3857, 1985*).

- -

VITAMINS

Vitamin C:

Spleen weight, an index of autoimmune progression, may be inversely related to spleen vitamin C levels in humans, guinea pigs and mice (*Leibovitz B, Siegel BV. Ascorbic acid and the immune response. Adv Exp Med Biol 135:1-25, 1981*).

Vitamin E:

Supplementation may be beneficial.

> WARNING: Pts. with hypertension, coronary heart disease or diabetes mellitus should be started on no more than 100 IU initially and need to be carefully monitored by their physician.

Case Reports: Pts. are described with various autoimmune diseases (2 with porphyria cutanea tarda, 4 with discoid lupus erythematosus, 3 with scleroderma, 3 with morphea, 2 with Raynaud's phenomenon, 5 with vasculitis-type eruptions, 1 with polymyositis) who improved following months of supplementation with D-alpha-tocopherol acetate or succinate 800-1600 IU daily (*Ayres S, Mihan R. Is vitamin E involved in the autoimmune mechanism? Cutis 21:321-25, 1978*).

Case Reports: 4 pts. with porphyria improved following supplementation with 100 IU water-miscible alpha-tocopheryl acetate per day, and urinary excretion of coproporphorins and uroporphorins declined to normal levels (*Nair PP et al. Vitamin E and porphorin metabolism in man. Arch Intern Med 128:411-15, 1971*).

Animal Experimental Study: Estrogen administration to dogs produced thrombocytopenic purpura which was cured by large doses of vitamin E and could be prevented by prior administration of vitamin E (*Skelton F et al. Science 163:762, 1946*).

MINERALS

<u>Selenium</u>:

- with <u>Vitamin E</u>:

Supplementation may be beneficial.

Experimental Double-blind Study: 81 pts. with disabling muscular pain, stiffness and aching of long duration, some of whom had connective tissue diseases, received sodium selenite (140 µg Se) and α-tocopherol 100 mg daily or placebo. Following supplementation, glutathione peroxidase levels increased in 75% of the patients. Mean pain score reduction was significantly more frequent and more marked among pts. whose glutathione peroxidase levels increased than among those whose levels decreased. While pain score reduction was more pronounced among treated pts., the reduction as compared to pts. on placebo was not significant (*Jameson S et al. Pain relief and selenium balance in patients with connective tissue disease and osteoarthrosis: A double-blind selenium tocopherol supplementation study. Nutr Res Suppl 1:391-97, 1985*).

OTHER NUTRITIONAL FACTORS

<u>Omega-3 Fatty Acids (Fish Oils)</u>:

Eicosapentaenoic acid (EPA) and docosahexaenoic acid (DHA).

Highest in cold water fish. Available in a refined form as "MaxEPA" (18% EPA).

Suggested MaxEPA dosage: 3 - 9 grams daily in divided doses (or 10 ml concentrate twice daily)

WARNING: Supplementation may require additional vitamin E intake to prevent increased membrane peroxidation and cellular damage (*Laganiere S, Fernandes G. High peroxidizability of subcellular membrane induced by high fish oil diet is reversed by vitamin E. Clin Res 35:A565, 1987*).

May change the balance of prostaglandins and leukotrienes (which are powerful mediators of inflammation and immune responses).

Experimental Study: The diets of 7 normal subjects were supplemented with 3.2 gm EPA or 1.8 gm MaxEPA daily for 6 weeks. EPA in neutrophils was increased 7 fold without any increase in arachidonic acid. When the neutrophils were activated, there was a 37% reduction in the release of arachidonic acid and a 48% reduction in the inflammatory products of this pathway. In addition, the adherence of neutrophils to bovine epithelial cells as monolayers treated with leukotriene B-4 was completely inhibited. The results suggest that diets enriched with fish oil-derived fatty acids have anti-inflammatory effects by inhibiting the 5-lipoxygenase pathway, thus causing a reduction in the release of leukotrienes along with a reduction in the release of superoxide from neutrophils (*Lee TH et al. N Engl J Med 312:1217, 1985*).

Shown in animal models of autoimmune disease to help delay disease-onset, prevent kidney destruction and prolong life.

Animal Experimental Study: The development of autoimmune disease in lupus-prone mice was dramatically slowed by feeding them a diet containing fish oil (*Alexander NJ et al. The type of dietary fat affects the severity of autoimmune disease in NZB/NZW mice. Am J Pathol 127(1):106-21, 1987*).

Animal Experimental Study: Dietary supplementation of fish oil as the exclusive source of lipid was found to suppress autoimmune lupus in mice, delaying the onset of renal disease and prolonging survival (*Kelley VE et al. A fish oil diet rich in eicosapentaenoic acid reduces cyclooxygenase metabolites, and suppresses lupus in MRL-lpr mice. J Immunol 134(3):1914-19, 1985*).

Omega-6 Fatty Acids:

Prostaglandin E₁ is said to be a key determinant of T-suppressor cell activity and thus excessive PGE₁ formation would be associated with excess suppressor function in the immune system. However, since stores of PGE₁ precursor di-homo-gammalinolenic acid are limited, excess PGE₁ formation may be followed by depletion of DGLA and a fall in PGE₁ leading to failure of T-suppressor function with autoimmune attack. Evening primrose oil, a source of gamma linolenic acid (the DGLA precursor), may thus be beneficial in recurrent and relapsing auto-immune disorders such as multiple sclerosis, rheumatoid arthritis, familial Mediterranean fever, asthma, migraine and inflammatory disorders of the skin and bowel (*Horrobin DF. A biochemical basis for the actions of lithium on behavior and on relapsing and remitting disorders of inflammation and immunity. Med Hypotheses 7(7):891-906, 1981*).

Animal Experimental Study: Experimental allergic encephalomyelitis was induced in guinea pigs. Dietary supplementation with linoleic acid both before and during the time in which clinical signs normally appeared was effective in reducing clinical signs of the disease, weight loss, frequency of perivascular lesions in the CNS and ability of isolated lymph node cells to respond to myelin basic protein *in vitro* (*Meade CJ et al. Reduction by linoleic acid of the severity of experimental allergic encephalomyelitis in the guinea pig. J Neurol Sci 35(2-3):291-308, 1978*).

Animal Experimental Study: PGE₁ successfully controlled the auto-immune inflammatory disease, including kidney damage, which develops spontaneously in NZB/W mice (*Zurier RB et al. Prostaglandin E treatment in NZB/W mice, I. Arthritis Rheum 20:723-8, 1977; Krakauer K et al. Prostaglandin E₁ treatment of NZB/W mice, III. Clin Immunol Immunopathol 11:256, 1978*).

BENIGN BREAST DISEASE

See Also: CANCER
PREMENSTRUAL SYNDROME

DIETARY FACTORS

Low fat diet.

Observational Study: Dietary patterns of 854 biopsied cases of benign breast disease and of matched controls were analyzed. Women with atypical lesions reported a higher intake of all types of foods which was due primarily to foods containing ≥10% fat. Odds ratios associated with the highest fat consumption quartile were close to 3.0, and there was a trend for increasing saturated fatty acid consumption with increasing ductal atypica. The association with fat intake was strengthened by adjusting for hormonal and demographic confounders (*Lubin F et al. Nutritional factors associated with benign breast disease etiology: a case-control study. Am J Clin Nutr 50:551-56, 1989*).

Experimental Controlled Study: 21 pts. with severe persistent cyclical mastopathy of at least 5 years' duration randomly received either general dietary advice or were taught how to reduce dietary fat to 15% of calories while increasing complex carbohydrate consumption to maintain caloric intake. After 6 mo., there was a significant reduction in the intervention gp. in the severity of premenstrual breast tenderness and swelling. Physical exam showed reduced breast swelling, tenderness, and nodularity in 6/10 pts. in the intervention gp. and in 2/9 pts. in the control gp. (*Boyd NF et al. Effect of a low-fat high-carbohydrate diet on symptoms of cyclical mastopathy. Lancet 2:128-32, 1988*).

Avoid methylxanthines (found in coffee, tea, chocolate, cola).

> *Note: The results of some studies suggest that total abstention may sometimes be necessary to obtain clinical benefits. (Minton JP, Aboud-Issa H. Nonendocrine theories of the etiology of benign breast disease. World J Surg 13(6):680-84, 1989*).

Observational Study: Daily methylxanthine ingestion was assessed for 102 women who visited a radiologist for mammograms. Fibrocystic breast disease was found to be positively correlated with both caffeine and total methylxanthine ingestion (*Bullough B, Hindi-Alexander M, Fetouh S. Methylxanthines and fibrocystic breast disease: a study of correlations. Nurse Pract 15(3):36-8, 43-4, 1990*).

Experimental Study: 138 pts. with symptoms of fibrocystic breast disease, including breast pain, were counseled to abstain from or reduce caffeine consumption. After 1 yr., 113 pts. (81.9%) had reduced their caffeine intake substantially and, of those, 69 (61%) reported a decrease or absence of breast pain (*Russell LC. Caffeine restriction as initial treatment for breast pain. Nurse Pract 14(2):36-37,40, 1989*).

Observational Study: 383 pts. with biopsy-confirmed benign proliferative epithelial disorders (BPED) of the breast were compared to 192 controls whose biopsy did not show epithelial proliferation, and 383 unbiopsied community controls. Overall, there was relatively little variation in BPED risk with total methylxanthine intake, or with intake of caffeine or theophylline, while there was a positive association between theobromine intake and BPED risk, but only when cases were compared with biopsy controls. Total methylxanthine intake was positively associated with risk of BPED showing severe atypia, but the trend in risk was significant only when compared to community controls (*Rohan TE et al. Methylxanthines and benign proliferative epithelial disorders of the breast in women. Int J Epidemiol 18(3):626-33, 1989*).

Negative Review Article: In its 1986 report, toxicologists at the U. S. Food and Drug Administration concluded that recent, more reliable studies have failed to show any relationship between benign breast disease and coffee consumption (*Lecos CW. Caffeine jitters: Some safety questions remain. FDA Consumer 12/87-1/88*).

Negative Observational Study: In a case-control study of 2300 Israeli women, no association was found between fibrocystic breast disease and the intake of caffeine-containing beverages (*Lubin F et al. A case-control study of caffeine and methylxanthines in benign breast disease. JAMA 253(16):2388-92, 1985*).

Observational Study: In a study of 634 women with fibrocystic breast disease and 1066 controls, the occurrence of disease was positively associated with the ave. daily consumption of caffeine. Women who consumed 31-250 mg of caffeine/day had a 1.5-fold increase in odds of disease, while those who drank over 500 mg/day had a 2.3-fold increase. The association was particularly high among women with atypical lobular hyperplasia and sclerosing adenosis with concomitant papillomatosis or papillary hyperplasia, both of which have been associated with an increased breast cancer risk. There was no association with fibroadenoma or other forms of benign breast disease (*Boyle CA et al. Caffeine consumption and fibrocystic breast disease: A case-control epidemiologic study. JCNI 72(5):1015-19, 1984*).

- -

VITAMINS

Vitamin A:

Supplementation may be beneficial.

> WARNING: High doses of vitamin A can be toxic and should only be given under close medical supervision.

Experimental Study: 10/12 women with moderate to severe breast pain which had not responded to mild pain-killers or caffeine withdrawal reported reduction in breast pain following supplementation with 150,000 IU vitamin A daily. In 5 pts. breast masses decreased at least 50%. Two pts. had to stop supplementation due to severe headaches and 3 had mild reactions, while five had no side effects. Pts. who responded showed continued benefit at follow-up 8 mo. later, and side effects were rapidly reversed (*Band PR et al. Treatment of benign breast disease with vitamin A. Prev Med 13:549-54, 1984*).

Vitamin E: 400 - 600 IU daily (3 month trial)

Supplementation may be beneficial.

Negative Experimental Double-blind Crossover Study: Women with mammographic evidence of benign breast disease randomly received alpha-tocopherol acetate 600 mg and placebo in either order for 3 mo. each. 37/86 (43%) pts. reported subjective improvement in breast symptoms after supplementation compared to 19/85 (22%) after placebo. 19% of pts. improved mammographically on supplementation vs. 12% on placebo. No significant subjective or objective effects after treatment were observed, possibly reflecting the small sample size (*Meyer EC et al. Vitamin E and benign breast disease. Surgery 107(5):549-51, 1990*).

Negative Experimental Double-blind Study: In a randomized trial, 128 women with confirmed mammary dysplasia received placebo or 150, 300 or 600 IU daily of D,L-alpha tocopherol. After 2 mo., just over half reported benefits from placebo and from the highest dose of vitamin E. Vitamin E had no significant effects on any of the hormones measured (*London RS et al. The effect of vitamin E on mammary dysplasia: A double-blind study. Obstet Gyn 65:104-6, 1985*).

Experimental Placebo-controlled Study: 22/26 pts. responded to 600 IU of D,L alpha-tocopheryl acetate in 8 wks. following an initial placebo trial. Cystic lesions and tenderness disappeared in 10, and 12 had a decrease in the number and size of the lesions with or without pain relief (*London RS et al. Mammary dysplasia: Endocrine parameters and tocopherol therapy. Nutr Res 2:243-47, 1982*).

Experimental Double-blind Study: 17 pts. with mammary dysplasia and 6 age-matched controls received placebo for one menstrual cycle followed by D,L-alpha-tocopheryl acetate 600 IU daily for two cycles. 15/17 pts. (88%) showed a clinical response. The ratio of progesterone to estradiol, which is abnormal in mammary dysplasia pts., rose from 30 to 53 in pts. and was unchanged in controls, while elevated LH and FSH levels were decreased to normal levels (*London RS et al. Endocrine parameters and alpha-tocopherol therapy of patients with mammary dysplasia. Cancer Res 41 (9 Pt 2):3811-13, 1981; Sundaram GS et al. Serum hormones and lipoproteins in benign breast disease. Cancer Res 41 (9 Pt 2):3814-16, 1981*).

Experimental Placebo-controlled Study: 26 women with middle-stage mammary dysplasia were given a placebo for 4 wks. followed by vitamin E 600 IU daily. After 8 wks., 10/29 pts. experienced complete regression of breast lumps and marked clinical improvement (*Gonzalez ER. Vitamin E relieves most cystic breast disease; may alter lipids, hormones. JAMA 244:1077, 1980*).

- -

MINERALS

Iodine:

Deficiency may be associated with the development of fibrocystic breast disease.

Animal Experimental Study: Iodine-deficient rats developed lesions which resembled histologically human fibrocystic breast disease. This finding was more notable on older rats (*Krouse TB et al. Age-related changes resembling fibrocystic disease in iodine-blocked rat breasts. Arch Pathol Lab Med 103:631-34, 1979*).

Supplementation may be beneficial.

Review Article: Several publications report that the hyperplasia associated with fibrocystic breast disease clears substantially in chronic cases with the administration of inorganic iodides (example: Lugol's solution of KI and NaI) or caseoiodine (iodine caseinate), and that symptomatology improves in >90% of the treated group. However, the fibrosis remains and, when substantial, may be considered ominous with a precancerous potential (*Ghent WR, Eskin BA. Elemental iodine supplementation in clinical breast dysplasia. Abstract. Proc Annu Meet Am Assoc Cancer Res 27:189, 1986*).

Note: Over 90% of women will have recurrences within 9 months if treatment is stopped (Bernard Eskin, professor of ob-gyn, Medical College of Pennsylvania, USA, and William Ghent, professor of surgery, Queen's University, Kingston, Ontario, Canada - reported in Med World News, January 11, 1988, p. 25).

- Aqueous (diatomic) iodine:

Experimental Study: 715 pts. received diatomic iodine. Relief was typically noted 2-8 wks. later, depending upon the severity of the condition. After 4 mo., all pts. were cyst-free and about 70% were completely pain-free. While fibrosis tended to persist, within 1 yr., the condition and the associated pain resolved in 95% of patients. Long-standing fibrosis, however, took as long as 3 yrs. to resolve. The major side effect was a transient aggravation of breast pain starting 3 wks. to 6 mo. after treatment commenced and lasting 1-3 wks. coinciding with breast shrinkage and softening of breast lumps (*Bernard Eskin, professor of ob-gyn, Medical College of Pennsylvania, USA, and William Ghent, professor of surgery, Queen's University, Kingston, Ontario, Canada - reported in Med World News, January 11, 1988, p. 25*).

Experimental Study: 299 pts. who complained of chronic mastodynia with lumpy or swollen breasts were evaluated by thermography, mammography and breast examination. After confirmation of a benign process, an oral dose of aqueous iodine (Iomech Ltd., Toronto) 3-6 mg/d was given. Pts. on caseoiodine (iodine caseinate) were transferred to aqueous iodine therapy. After 12 wks., fibrosis was well-controlled in both new pts. and those transferred from caseoiodine therapy; thus, while all iodine compounds ameliorate the pain and cyst formation of benign breast dysplasia, aqueous iodine reduces or clears the significant fibrosis seen in these tissues (*Ghent WR, Eskin BA. Elemental iodine supplementation in clinical breast dysplasia. Abstract. Proc Annu Meet Am Assoc Cancer Res 27:189, 1986*).

- Iodine Caseinate:

Experimental Study: 90% of 588 pts. had good to excellent results following supplementation with iodine caseinate. 43% had complete pain relief, while 44% had some persistent discomfort which was associated with persistent fibrosis (*Bernard Eskin, professor of ob-gyn, Medical College of Pennsylvania, USA - reported in Med World News January 11, 1988, p. 25*).

OTHER NUTRITIONAL FACTORS

Omega-6 Fatty Acids:

> Example: Evening primrose oil 1500 mg twice daily.

Administration may be beneficial in mastalgia.

> **Experimental Study:** Using danazol, bromocriptine or evening primrose oil, a clinically useful improvement in pain can be anticipated in 77% of pts. with cyclical mastalgia and 44% with non-cyclical mastalgia (*Gately CA, Mansel RE. Management of the painful and nodular breast. Br Med Bull 47(2):284-94, 1991*).

> **Experimental Placebo-controlled Study:** 291 pts. with severe persistent breast pain in whom breast cancer had been excluded were treated with evening primrose oil 3 g/d for 3-6 months. Following treatment, 45% of 92 pts. with cyclical mastalgia had either no residual pain or residual pain which was easily bearable compared to 19% of pts. on placebo. For non-cyclical mastalgia, 27% of 33 pts. responded compared to 9% of pts. on placebo. Side effects were minimal (*Pye JK et al. Clinical experience of drug treatments for mastalgia. Lancet 2:373-77, 1985*).

> **Experimental Double-blind Study:** 73 pts. with mastalgia with or without lumpiness randomly received evening primrose oil 3 g/d or placebo. 19 pts. dropped out within the first 3 mo., 16 of whom were on placebo. After 3 mo., pain and tenderness were significantly reduced in both cyclical and non-cyclical groups as compared to baselines, while controls failed to significantly improve. Nodularity was reduced only in pts. with cyclical symptoms (*Pashby NL et al. A clinical trial of evening primrose oil in mastalgia. Br J Surg 68:801-24, 1981*).

Administration does not appear to be beneficial in recurrent breast cyst formation.

> **Experimental Double-blind Study.** 200 women with proven breast cysts randomly received evening primrose oil (Efamol) 3 g/d or placebo. After 1 yr., there were no significant differences in the total number of recurrent cysts nor in the number of pts. developing cysts between the 2 groups (*Mansel RE et al. Effect and tolerability of n-6 essential fatty acid supplementation in patients with recurrent breast cysts - a randomized double-blind placebo-controlled trial. J Nutr Med 1:195-200, 1990; Mansel RE et al. A randomized trial of dietary intervention with essential fatty acids in patients with categorized cysts. Ann N Y Acad Sci 586:288-94, 1990*).

BENIGN PROSTATIC HYPERPLASIA

MINERALS

<u>Selenium</u>:

May protect against cadmium-induced growth stimulation of prostatic tissue (*see "Cadmium" below*).

In vitro Experimental Study: While cadmium was found to stimulate the growth of human prostatic epithelium, selenium (at proper concentrations) inhibited the growth stimulation induced by cadmium (*Webber MM. Selenium prevents the growth stimulatory effects of cadmium on human prostatic epithelium. Biochem Biophy Res Commun 127(3):871-77, 1985*).

<u>Zinc</u>:

The prostate contains a higher concentration of zinc than any other organ in the body.

Plasma levels may be elevated (*Bandlish U, Prabhakar BR, Wadehra PL. Plasma zinc level estimation in enlarged prostate. Indian J Pathol Microbiol 31(3):231-4, 1988*).

Erythrocyte levels may be normal (*Feustel A, Wennrich R. Zinc and cadmium plasma and erythrocyte levels in prostatic carcinoma, BPH, urological malignancies, and inflammations. Prostate 8(1):75-9, 1986*).

Prostatic zinc concentration correlates inversely with the amount of prostatic fibromuscular stroma (*Gonick P et al. Atomic absorption spectrophotometric determination of zinc in the prostate. Invest Urol 6:345-7, 1969*). While, in BPH, prostatic zinc is elevated, the elevation is in prostatic fluid rather than within cells (*Schrodt GR et al. The concentration of zinc in diseased human prostate glands. Cancer 17:1555-66, 1964*) due to decreased tissue binding (*Györkey F et al. Zinc and magnesium in human prostate gland: Normal, hyperplastic and neoplastic. Cancer Res 27:1348-53, 1967; Györkey F, Sato CS. In vitro ^{65}zinc-binding capacities of normal, hyperplastic and carcinomatous human prostate gland. Exp Mol Pathol 8:216-24, 1968*).

Prolactin increases testoterone uptake by the prostate (*Farnsworth WE et al. Interaction of prolactin and testosterone in the human prostate. Urol Res 9:79-88, 1981*). Zinc inhibits prolactin secretion by the pituitary (*Judd AM et al. Zinc acutely, selectively and reversibly inhibits pituitary prolactin secretion. Brain Res 294:190-2, 1984*). While it increases prolactin uptake into the prostate, zinc reduces the specific binding of prolactin to the receptor (*Leake A et al. Interaction between prolactin and zinc in the human prostate gland. J Endocrinol 102(1):73-6, 1984*).

Inhibits the activity of 5-alpha-reductase, the enzyme that irreversibly converts testosterone to dihydrotestosterone (*Leake A et al. The effect of zinc on the 5-alpha-reduction of testosterone by the hyperplastic human prostate gland. J Steroid Biochem 20:651-5, 1984*).

Inhibits the specific binding of androgens to the prostatic cytosol and nuclear androgen receptors (*Leake A et al. Subcellular distribution of zinc in the benign and malignant human prostate: Evidence for a direct zinc androgen interaction. Acta Endocrinol 105:281-8, 1984*).

Supplementation may be beneficial.

Experimental Study: Zinc supplementation reduced the size of the prostate and BPH symptomatology in the majority of patients (*Fahim MS et al. Zinc treatment for the reduction of hyperplasia of the prostate. Fed Proc 35:361, 1976*).

Experimental Study: 19 pts. took zinc sulfate 150 mg (34 mg elemental zinc) daily for 2 mo. followed by 50-100 mg (11-23 mg elemental zinc) daily. All pts. reported symptomatic improvement and 14/19 had shrinkage of the prostate, as determined by rectal palpation, X-ray and endoscopy. Compared to baseline, semen zinc levels were increased (*Irving M. Bush and associates, Cook County Hospital, Chicago. Zinc and the prostate. Presented at the annual meeting of the Am. Med. Assoc., Chicago, 1974*).

- -

OTHER NUTRITIONAL FACTORS

Amino Acids:

Supplementation with the combination of L-glutamic acid, L-alanine and glycine (two 6-gr caps 3 times daily for 2 wks. following by 1 cap 3 times daily) may be beneficial.

Experimental Double-blind Study: Pts. randomly received either (1) L-glutamic acid, L-alanine and glycine, (2) L-glutamic acid and L-alanine, or (3) L-glutamic acid alone. Outcomes showed a significant difference between the reduction in subjective symptoms in the gp. receiving all 3 agents versus the 2 control groups. However, in none of the pts. was satisfactory improvement observed on rectal palpation or x-ray examination (*Shimaya M, Sugiura H. [Double blind test of PPC for prostatic hyperplasia.] Hinyokika Kiyo 16(5):231-36, 1970*).

Experimental Placebo-controlled Study: 45 pts. were supplemented with glutamic acid, alanine and glycine in the form of 6 gr capsules at a dosage of 2 caps 3 times daily for 2 wks. followed by 1 cap 3 times daily, while 40 pts. received placebo. After 3 mo., nocturia was relieved or reduced in 56% of treated pts. compared to 15% of controls, urgency was reduced in 66% compared to 11% of controls (exacerbated in 7% of controls), frequency was reduced in 43% compared to 15% of controls, and delayed micturition was alleviated in 50% compared to none of the controls. 11% of treated pts. had a reduction in prostatic enlargement, and 5% an increase, compared to 5% and 2.5%, respectively, of the controls (results n.s.). There were no side effects (*Dumrau F. Benign prostatic hyperplasia: Amino acid therapy for symptomatic relief. Am J Geriatr 10:426-30, 1962*).

Experimental Placebo-controlled Crossover Study: 32/40 men with non-cancerous prostate enlargement were treated with glycine, alanine and glutamic acid, while the other 8 served as controls. In the treated gp., prostate size decreased in 92% and returned to its normal size in 32%, while the control gp. showed no improvement (*Feinblatt HM, Gant JC. Palliative treatment of benign prostatic hypertrophy: Value of glycine, alanine, glutamic acid combination. J Maine Med Assoc 46:99-102, 1958*).

Essential Fatty Acids:

Nutritional precursors to prostaglandins.

A prostaglandin deficiency may be a cause of BPH.

Theoretical Discussion: Experimental data suggest that, when testosterone enters the prostate cell, it both converts to dihydrotestosterone (which enters the cell nucleus and stimulates protein synthesis and growth), and stimulates prostaglandin synthesis and release. The released prostaglandins, in addition to their role in male reproductive physiology, inhibit further testosterone binding to the prostate. With aging, PG synthesis may become less efficient, resulting in a decline of the putative inhibitory effect of PG on cell growth and an increase in testosterone binding to prostatic cells. The combined effects might produce unrestrained protein synthesis and cell growth resulting in BPH (*Klein LA, Stoff JS. Prostaglandins and the prostate: An hypothesis on the etiology of benign prostatic hyperplasia. Prostate 4(3):247-51, 1983*).

Review Article: "The importance of PGs in inflammatory changes in the prostate gland and the therapeutic possibilities for these clinical symptoms which may result from influencing PGs can be seen from some studies, but it is not yet possible to draw a final conclusion at this point in time" (*Bach D, Walker H. How important are prostaglandins in the urology of man? Urol Int 37(3):160-71, 1982*).

Supplementation may be beneficial.

Experimental Study: 19 pts. were supplemented with a total of 60 mg/d of linoleic, linolenic, and arachidonic acids. After 3 days, the dosage was reduced to 40 mg/d and, after several wks., they were given a maintenance dosage of 10-20 mg/d. Upon evaluation following several wks. of treatment, all 19 had a reduction in the size of the prostate, an increase in the force of the urine stream and a diminution of residual urine. 12/19 no longer had any residual urine, and 13/19 no longer had nocturia (*Hart JP, Cooper WL. Vitamin F in the treatment of prostatic hyperplasia. Report Number 1, Lee Foundation for Nutritional Research, Milwaukee, Wi., 1941*).

- -

OTHER FACTORS

Rule out cadmium toxicity.

Cadmium exposure may cause prostatic hyperplasia.

Animal Experimental Study: Cadmium chloride was injected into the rt. ventral prostatic lobe of 100 12-mo.-old male rats. 270 days after the injection, simple hyperplasia was found in 38, atypical hyperplasia in 29, atypical hyperplasia with severe dysplasia in 11 and invasive prostatic carcinoma in 5 (*Hoffman L et al. Carcinogenic effects of cadmium on the prostate of the rat. J Cancer Res Clin Oncol 109(3):193-99, 1985*).

Prostatic cadmium levels may be elevated.

Negative Observational Study: In a study of cadmium levels of prostatic tissue, there was no evidence of high cadmium concentrations in hypertrophic and carcinomatous prostatic tissue (*Lahtonen R. Zinc and cadmium concentrations in whole tissue and in separated epithelium and stroma from human benign prostatic hypertrophic glands. Prostate 6(2):177-83, 1985*).

Observational Study: Prostatic cadmium concentrations in BPH were measured by atomic absorption spectroscopy and were found to be considerably higher than in normal tissue (23.11 ± 3.28 vs. 5.25 ± 0.62 nmol/g). Prostatic dihydrotestosterone levels were directly proportional to the cadmium concentrations (*Habib FK et al. Metal-androgen interrelationships in carcinoma and hyperplasia of the human prostate. J Endocrinol 71(1):133-41, 1976*).

BRONCHIAL ASTHMA

See Also: ALLERGY

OVERVIEW

1. Certain asthmatics may be provoked by specific food challenges.

2. Caffeine appears to be as effective a bronchodilator as theophylline although, due to its adverse effects, its use should be limited to acute situations.

3. Early studies suggest that asthmatics may be deficient in niacin, vitamin B6 and vitamin C. There is also early evidence that supplementation with these vitamins may be effective. Perhaps supplementation is beneficial only when it remedies a pre-existing deficiency, but this hypothesis needs to be further validated.

4. Intravenous vitamin B12 has repeatedly been shown to be effective in open trials.

5. Both inhalation and IV administration of magnesium have been shown in double-blind studies to improve pulmonary function in asthmatics.

6. There may be a correlation between sodium intake and the severity of asthmatic symptoms.

- -

DIETARY FACTORS

Restrict salt:

> The bronchial reactivity to histamine is related to the severity of asthmatic symptoms (*Juniper EF, Frith PA, Hargreave FE. Airways responsiveness to histamine and methacholine: Relationship to minimum treatment to control symptoms of asthma. Thorax 36(8):575-9, 1981*).

Sodium intake may be correlated with the bronchial response to histamine.

> **Experimental Double-blind Crossover Study:** 36 subjects on a low sodium diet were supplemented with slow sodium 80 mmol/d and placebo in random order. A significant association between sodium excretion and bronchial response to histamine was found (*Burney PG et al. The effect of changing dietary sodium on the bronchial response to histamine. Thorax 44(1):36-41, 1989*).

> **Experimental Study:** 6 male and 4 female pts. aged 18-63 (5/10 were atopic) doubled their salt intake. After 1 mo., there was a significant increase in bronchial reactivity to histamine in 9/10 pts. (*Javaid A et al. Effect of dietary salt on bronchial reactivity to histamine in asthma. Br Med J 297:454 , 1988*).

> **Observational Study:** In a study of 138 men, salt intake, as measured by 24 hr. urinary sodium excretion, was strongly related to bronchial reactivity to inhaled histamine, suggesting that a high sodium diet may potentiate bronchial reactivity (*Burney PG et al. Response to inhaled histamine and 24 hour sodium excretion. Br Med J 292:1483-86, 1986*).

> **Observational Study:** Sales of table salt in the different regions of England and Wales were found to be independently correlated with mortality from asthma for men and for children, but not for women (*Burney PG et al. Response to inhaled histamine and 24 hour sodium excretion. Br Med J 292:1483-86, 1986*).

Alcohol:

Alcohol is a modest bronchodilator, but it can also be a potent bronchoconstrictor, usually due to congeners in a particular beverage, probably by inducing absorption of allergic macromolecules through the gut mucosa (*Ayres JG. Alcohol and asthma. Immunol Allergy Pract 10(11):423-34, 1988*).

Caffeine:

Theophylline is a metabolic product of caffeine.

　WARNING: May be toxic when combined with theophylline.

May be effective as a mild bronchodilator (but is not recommended on a regular basis due to its potential for side-effects).

Experimental Placebo-controlled Crossover Study: 10 pts. with bronchial asthma received caffeine 3.5 mg/kg and 7 mg/kg and placebo 2 hrs. before exercise. Caffeine significantly improved baseline FEV_1 and prevented exercise-induced bronchoconstriction only at a dose of 7 mg/kg and was well tolerated (*Kivity S et al. The effect of caffeine on exercise-induced bronchoconstriction. Chest 97(5):1083-5, 1990*).

Experimental Double-blind Study: Pts. received three 6-oz cups of brewed coffee, each containing 150 mg caffeine. Even a single cup was found to produce as much as a 15% increase in FEV_1. The effect was 40% as potent as that of theophylline (*Gong H Jr et al. Bronchodilator effects of caffeine in coffee. A dose-response study of asthmatic subjects. Chest 89(3):335-42, 1986*).

Experimental Double-blind Study: 23 pts. on continuous bronchodilator therapy whose forced expiratory flow from 25-75% of vital capacity (FEF 25-75) was less than 50% of normal received either caffeine 10 mg/kg (equivalent to 2 strong cups of coffee for a 50 kg person) or theophylline 5 mg/kg. The effects of the 2 drugs were very similar and minor side effects of headache, dizziness and tremor were noted with both (*Becker AB et al. The bronchodilator effects and pharmacokinetics of caffeine in asthma. N Engl J Med 310(12):743-46, 1984*).

- -

VITAMINS

Niacin:　　100 mg daily

Intake may be inversely correlated with the incidence of wheezing.

Observational Study: 24-hr. dietary recalls were obtained from 9074 white and black adults aged 30 and older in the second US National Health and Nutrition Examination Survey. Nutrient-specific logistic regression from these data controlling for age, race, sex and pack-years of cigarette smoking revealed that increased dietary niacin was associated with a reduced rate of wheezing. Individuals in the 16th percentile of niacin intake had 25% more wheezing than those in the 84th percentile (*Schwartz J, Weiss ST. Dietary factors and their relation to respiratory symptoms. The Second National Health and Nutrition Examination Survey. Am J Epidemiol 132(1):67-76, 1990*).

Blood levels may be deficient.

Observational Study: In a study of 124 pts. (59 males & 65 females), 83% were deficient in nicotinic acid, especially in the winter and spring. Asthma treatments failed to ameliorate the deficiency (*Rozanov EM et al. [Vitamin PP and C allowances and their correction in the treatment of bronchial asthma patients.] Vopr Pitan (6):21-24, 1987*).

Serum levels may be inversely associated with the incidence of wheezing.

Observational Study: In a study of 9074 white and black adult Americans aged 30 yrs. and older, after controlling for age, race, sex, calories, and pack-years of cigarette smoking, the serum niacin level was negatively associated with wheezing (*Schwartz J, Weiss ST. Dietary factors and their relation to respiratory symptoms. The Second National Health and Nutrition Examination Survey. Am J Epidemiol 132(1):67-76, 1990*).

Supplementation may inhibit mast cell degranulation and histamine release.

Animal Experimental Study: In guinea pigs given nicotinamide intra-periotoneally, then exposed to histamine aerosols, appearance of the first symptoms of dyspnea was delayed (p<0.01), and the number of animals developing anaphylactic shock diminished significantly. Nicotinamide, which itself produces a slight bronchial constriction in isolated guinea pig lungs, not only protects against histamine constriction, but relaxes histamine-induced bronchial constriction after 3-4 minutes (*Bekier E, Maslinski CZ. Antihistaminic action of nicotinamide. Agents Actions 4(3):196, 1974*).

In vitro Experimental Study: Nicotinamide was found to exert an antihistaminic action on the isolated guinea pig ileum (*Halpern BN et al. Le role des médiateurs chimiques dans la régulation de l'éosinophilie sanguine. Bull Soc Pathol Exot Filiales 55:489-99, 1962*).

Supplementation may be beneficial.

Animal Experimental Study: Prior treatment of guinea pigs with injections of nicotinamide 50 mg IM daily diminished the symptoms of experimental bronchial asthma. Nicotinamide also inhibited anaphylactic mast cell degranulation in mice and histamine release from rat-isolated peritoneal mast cells (*Bekier E et al. The inhibitory effect of nicotinamide on asthma-like symptoms and eosinophilia in guinea pigs, anaphylactic mast cell degranulation in mice, and histamine release from rat isolated peritoneal mast cells by compound 48/80. Int Arch Allergy 47:737-48, 1974*).

Experimental Study: IM or IV administration of nicotinamide 100-200 mg resulted in rapid improvement in pts. with bronchial asthma (*Daïnow I. Recherches cliniques sur certaines propriétés anti-allergiques de la nicotinamide. Z Vitaminforsch 15:245-50, 1944*).

Experimental Single-blind Study: Acute asthmatic paroxysms were definitely improved in 16/19 pts. following treatment of 50-100 mg IM of nicotinic acid, while 2/19 pts. had marked exacerbations. Control injections of sterile water were usually much less effective. The frequency and severity of asthmatic attacks were definitely reduced in 16/30 pts., many of whom had severe and frequent paroxysms not controlled by ephedrine or stramonium, and slightly reduced in another 10/30 pts. who received nicotinic acid 50-100 mg 2 or 3 times daily on a regular basis. Those who improved frequently relapsed when it was discontinued or when citric acid placebo was substituted for nicotinic acid, although 2/9 pts. did as well on placebo. Flushing and other side effects were common, and 2 pts. abandoned treatment due to adverse effects (*Melton G. Treatment of asthma by nicotinic acid. Br Med J May 15, 1943, pp. 600-01*).

Experimental Study: Severe asthmatic paroxysms were controlled in 16/21 pts. by IV injection of 100 mg of nicotinic acid. Relief occurred within 3-5 min., seemed to coincide with the appearance of the flush and lasted from a few hrs. up to 15 hours. Also, 5/9 pts. improved following oral ingestion of 200 mg nicotinic acid daily before meals and upon retiring. 11/18 pts. who responded to IV therapy also responded to oral therapy following a series of 1-3 IV injections (*Maisel FE, Somkin E. Treatment of asthmatic paroxysm with nicotinic acid. J Allergy 13:397-403, 1942*).

Vitamin B6:

Plasma and red blood cell levels may be reduced (*Delport R et al. Vitamin B6 nutritional status in asthma: The effect of theophylline therapy on plasma pyridoxal-5[1]-phosphate and pyridoxal levels. Int J Vitam Nutr Res 58(1):67-72, 1988; Reynolds RD, Natta CL. Depressed plasma pyridoxal phosphate concentrations in adult asthmatics. Am J Clin Nutr 41:684-8, 1985*).

Administration of theophylline may lower plasma pyridoxal-5[1]-phosphate levels while plasma pyridoxal levels are unchanged (*Delport R et al. Vitamin B6 nutritional status in asthma: The effect of theophylline therapy on plasma pyridoxal-5[1]-phosphate and pyridoxal levels. Int J Vitam Nutr Res 58(1):67-72, 1988; Ubbink JB et al. The relationship between vitamin B6 metabolism, asthma, and theophylline therapy. Ann N Y Acad Sci 585:285-94, 1990*).

Supplementation may be beneficial.

Experimental Controlled Study: 7 pts. and 6 controls received 50 mg pyridoxine twice daily. Both plasma and RBC pyridoxal phosphate levels only increased significantly in the controls; however, all asthmatics reported a dramatic decrease in the frequency, duration and severity of asthmatic attacks, and wheezing ceased in about 1 week (*Reynolds RD, Natta CL. Depressed plasma pyridoxal phosphate concentrations in adult asthmatics. Am J Clin Nutr 41:684-8, 1985*).

Experimental Study: 76 asthmatic children who received pyridoxine 200 mg daily demonstrated significant symptom improvement and a reduction in dosage of bronchodilators and cortisone required to relieve symptoms (*Collip PJ et al. Pyridoxine treatment of childhood bronchial asthma. Ann Allergy 35:93-7, 1975*).

Vitamin B_{12}:

Supplementation may be beneficial.

Experimental Study: When given preceeding a sulfite challenge, oral vitamin B_{12} (cyanocobalamin) was more effective than pharmacologic agents in blocking asthmatic reactions and was effective over a longer period of time (*Simon RA et al. Sulfite-sensitive asthma. Res Instit Scripps Clin Scientif Rep 39:57-58, 1982-83*).

Experimental Study: 85 pts. up to 60 yrs. old received vitamin B_{12} 1000 µg first weekly and then less frequently at intervals of up to 4 weeks. Of the pts. aged 0-10, 5/6 (83%) showed a moderate to marked improvement; of those aged 10-20, 14/19 (74%) improved; of those aged 20-30, 10/15 (67%) improved; of those aged 30-40, 13/25 (52%) improved; of those aged 40-50, 5/13 (38%) improved; and of those aged 50-60, 1/7 (14%) improved (*Crocket JA. Cyanocobalamin in asthma. Acta Allergologica XI:261-68, 1957*).

Experimental Study: 12 adult asthmatics received vitamin B_{12} IV daily for 15-20 days. 10/12 were completely relieved of wheezing. One had a recurrence after 3 mo.; another had a recurrence after 8 months. Both responded to repeat treatment. The asthma in the 2 pts. who failed to improve was associated with emphysema and hypertensive atherosclerosis (*Caruselli M. [Upon therapy for asthma using vitamin B12.] Riforma Medica (Naples) 66:841-64) (in Italian) (abstracted in JAMA 150(17):1731, 1952*).

Experimental Study: 18/20 pts. improved following IM injections of vitamin B_{12} 1000 µg once weekly for 4 weeks. Improvements included reduced wheezing and improvement in exertional dyspnea, sleep, or general condition (*Simon SW. Vitamin B12 therapy in allergy and chronic dermatoses. J.Allergy 22:183-5, 1951*).

Vitamin C: 2 grams daily; 4 -8 grams during reactions

Intake may be negatively correlated with rates of bronchitis and wheezing.

Observational Study: 24-hr. dietary recalls were obtained from 9074 white and black adults aged 30 and older in the second US National Health and Nutrition Examination Survey. Nutrient-specific logistic regression from these data controlling for age, race, sex and pack-years of cigarette smoking revealed that increased vitamin C intake (200 mg/d more than the 98 mg/d average) was associated with a 30% lower incidence of active bronchitis and wheezing (*Schwartz J, Weiss ST. Dietary factors and their relation to respiratory symptoms. The Second National Health and Nutrition Examination Survey. Am J Epidemiol 132(1):67-76, 1990*).

Serum levels may be negatively correlated with the incidence of wheezing (*Schwartz J, Weiss ST. Dietary factors and their relation to respiratory symptoms. The Second National Health and Nutrition Examination Survey. Am J Epidemiol 132(1):67-76, 1990*).

Plasma levels may be negatively correlated with blood histamine levels (*Clemetson CA. Histamine and ascorbic acid in human blood. J Nutr 110(4):662-68, 1980*).

Plasma/serum and leukocyte levels may be reduced (*Olusi SO et al. Plasma and white blood cell ascorbic acid concentrations in patients with bronchial asthma. Clinica Chimica Acta 92(2):161-66, 1979*).

Supplementation probably modifies airway reactivity by promoting prostanoid synthesis. These products may then modulate neurotransmission in the airway smooth muscle where reflex cholinergic bronchoconstriction is a major regulator of airway tone and reactivity (*Mohsenin V, DuBois AB. Vitamin C and airways. Ann N Y Acad Sci 498:259-68, 1987*).

Supplementation may reduce histamine levels.

Experimental Study: When 11 normals with either low vitamin C levels or high blood histamine levels were given ascorbic acid 1 gm. x 3 days, blood histamine levels fell in all 11 subjects (*Clemetson CA. Histamine and ascorbic acid in human blood. J Nutr 110(4):662-68, 1980*).

Supplementation may decrease the tendency to develop bronchoconstriction.

Experimental Double-blind Crossover Study: 16 pts. with allergic rhinitis received a single dose of vitamin C 2 g and placebo in either order. Histamine inhalation caused a significant decrease in the maximal expiratory flow rate only in the placebo gp. (*Bucca C et al. Effect of vitamin C on histamine bronchial responsiveness of patients with allergic rhnitis. Ann Allergy 65:311-14, 1990*).

Experimental Study: Pretreatment of normal subjects with vitamin C 500 mg was found to prevent nitrogen dioxide (NO_2) exposure from producing airway hyperresponsiveness to methacholine challenge (*Mohsenin V. Effect of vitamin C on NO_2-induced airway hyperresponsiveness in normal subjects. Am Rev Respir Dis 136:1408-11, 1987*).

Negative Experimental Double-blind Crossover Study: 16 adult asthmatics failed to show significant changes in FEV_1 and FVC following histamine inhalation after ascorbic acid 2 gm as compared with placebo, suggesting that it has no acute bronchodilator effect and does not alter bronchial responsiveness to histamine in asthmatic adults (*Malo JL et al. Lack of acute effects of ascorbic acid on spirometry and airway responsiveness to histamine in subjects with asthma. J Allergy Clin Immunol 78(6):11532-58, 1986*).

Experimental Study: Bronchoconstriction brought on by methacholine challenge in 14 mild asthmatics was inhibited by 1 gram oral ascorbic acid. The effects of ascorbic acid were blocked by indocin, suggesting that ascorbic acid exerts its effect via alteration of arachidonic acid metabolism (*Mohsenin V et al. Effect of ascorbic acid on response to methacholine challenge in asthmatic subjects. Am Rev Respir Dis 127:143-7, 1983*).

Experimental Double-blind Study: In a study of 41 Nigerian children, those receiving ascorbic acid 1000 mg daily for 14 wks had fewer than one-fourth as many asthmatic attacks as those receiving placebo and the attacks were significantly less severe. A few wks. after vitamin C was discontinued, the frequency of asthmatic attacks in the 2 gps. once again became similar (*Anah CO et al. High dose ascorbic acid in Nigerian asthmatics. Tropical Geograph Med 32:132-7, 1980*).

Supplementation may reduce exercise-induced bronchospasm.

Experimental Double-blind Study: 12 pts. with exercise-induced bronchospasm randomly received ascorbic acid 500 mg daily or placebo. After 2 days, pretreatment with ascorbic acid led to significant attenuation of the bronchospasm seen 5 min. after exercise compared to placebo (*Schachter EN, Schlesinger A. The attenuation of exercise-induced bronchospasm by ascorbic acid. Ann Allergy 49(3):146-51, 1982*).

- and Niacin:

Combined supplementation may be beneficial.

Experimental Study: In a study of 124 pts. (59 males & 65 females), rational doses of both nicotinic acid and vitamin C were determined with vitamin loadings in order to provide pts. with these vitamins during exacerbations. 90-110 mg of nicotinic acid and 275-300 mg of ascorbic acid was determined to be the appropriate supplementary dosage, depending upon the severity of their exacerbations. Supplementation with the 2 vitamins was found to intensify treatment effectiveness and to reduce the length of inpatient treatment (*Rozanov EM et al. [Vitamin PP and C allowances and their correction in the treatment of bronchial asthma patients.] Vopr Pitan (6):21-24, 1987*).

- -

MINERALS

<u>Calcium:</u>

- and <u>Vitamin D2</u>:

Supplementation may be beneficial.

Experimental Double-blind Crossover Study: 12 pts. with allergic bronchial asthma and airway obstruction received oral calcium in combination with vitamin D2 (calciferol). Within 60 min., in comparison to placebo, a statistically significant reduction in airway resistance and intrathoracic gas volume, as well as an increase of forced expiratory one second volume and forced inspiratory one second volume, was observed (*Utz G, Hauck AM. [Oral application of calcium and vitamin D2 in allergic bronchial asthma.] MMW 118(43):1395-8, 1976*).

<u>Magnesium:</u>

Blood levels may be reduced.

Negative Observational Study: 23 asthmatics age 18-50 presenting to the emergency dept. in acute exacerbation were matched for age, sex, race, and socioeconomic status with 15 controls. Serum magnesium levels were not significantly different and were not clinically useful for predicting the severity of disease (*Falkner D, Glauser J, Allen M. Serum magnesium levels in asthmatic patients during acute exacerbations of asthma. Am J Emerg Med 10(1):1-3, 1992*).

Negative Observational Study: In a gp. of 126 pts. with allergic/infectious asthma aged 16-58 (ave. 38.5), hypermagnesemia was established with statistical significance. The alteration covaried with the stage and severity of the disease and was favorably influenced by proper drug treatment (*Petrov D, Stoeva N. [Sodium, potassium, calcium and magnesium metabolism in patients with allergic-infectious bronchial asthma.] Vutr Boles 23(1):85-90, 1984*) (in Bulgarian).

Observational Study: 28 pts. with atopic asthma were studied both during an exacerbation and when asymptomatic and were compared to 3 healthy controls. During an asthma attack, blood and RBC magnesium decreased. The extent of the decrease was inversely correlated with the rise in histamine level and the number of eosinophils in the blood. This relationship was less marked in non-atopic asthma (*Chyrek-Borowska S, Obrzut D, Hofman J. The relation between magnesium, blood histamine level and eosinophilia in the acute stage of the allergic reactions in humans. Arch Immunol Ther Exp (Warsz) 26(1-6):709-12, 1978*).

Observational Study: Compared to controls, serum magnesium was depressed in 16/66 pts. (24%). When serum magnesium was measured on 26 of these pts. during acute asthmatic attacks, 13/26 (50%) were hypomagnesemic (*Haury VG. Blood serum magnesium in bronchial asthma and its treatment by the administration of magnesium sulfate. J Lab Clin Med 26:340-4, 1940*)

Supplementation may be beneficial.

Negative Experimental Controlled Study: 58/120 consecutive pts. aged 18-65 with acute asthma unresponsive to a single albuterol treatment randomly received 2 gm IV magnesium sulfate infused over 20 min. in addition to standard treatment while the rest of the gp. received only standard treatment. Magnesium therapy failed to alter the need for hospitalization, duration of emergency department treatment for pts. who could be discharged, or peak expiratory flow (*Green SM, Rothrock SG. Intravenous magnesium for acute asthma: failure to decrease emergency treatment duration or need for hospitalization. Ann Emerg Med 21(3):260-5, 1992*).

Experimental Double-blind Study: 38 pts. suffering from acute exacerbations of moderate to severe asthma randomly received either 1.2 g of magnesium sulfate or placebo after β-agonist therapy failed to produce significant improvement in peak expiratory flow rate (PEFR). The treatment gp. demonstrated an increased in PEFR from 225 to 297 L/min as compared to 208 to 216 L/min in the placebo group. In addition, the number admitted vs. discharged was significantly lower for the treatment gp. (7 vs. 12) than the placebo gp. (15 vs. 4) (*Skobeloff EM et al. Intravenous magnesium sulfate for the treatment of acute asthma in the emergency department. JAMA 262(9):1210-13, 1989*).

Experimental Double-blind Study: Parenterally-administrated magnesium significantly improved pulmonary function of asthmatic patients. The degree of improvement was positively correlated with serum magnesium levels (*Brunner EH et al. Effect of parenteral magnesium on pulmonary function, plasma cAMP, and histamine in bronchial asthma. J Asthma 22:3-11, 1985*).

Molybdenum:

The trace element contained in the enzyme sulfite oxidase which detoxifies sulfite to the inert and harmless sulfate.

Deficient or absent in the majority of people with sulfite sensitivity (*Papaioannou R, Pfeiffer CC. Sulfite sensitivity - unrecognized threat:. Is molybdenum the cause? J Orthomol Psychiatry 13(2):105-110, 1984*).

If deficient, supplementation may be beneficial.

Case Report: 53 year-old female asthmatic was found to have 10-20 ppm urinary sulfite in a 24 hour urine. She was treated with molybdenum IV for 3 mo. starting with 250 µgm twice weekly for 6 injections, then 500 µgm twice weekly, and finally with 750 µgm for the last 4 injections. During treatment urinary sulfite output dropped to 2-6 ppm, her wheezing considerably lessened, she discontinued theophylline and prednisone and reduced her use of inhalers from 4 times daily to twice daily (*Wright J, Littleton K. Defects in sulphur metabolism. Int Clin Nutr Rev 9(3):118-19, 1989*).

Selenium:

Whole blood and plasma/serum levels. as well as platelet glutathione activity, may be reduced (*Flatt A et al. Reduced selenium in asthmatic subjects in New Zealand. Thorax 45(2):95-9, 1990; Hasselmark L et al. Lowered platelet glutathione peroxidase activity in patients with intrinsic asthma. Allergy 45:523-7, 1990*).

Sodium:

The bronchial reactivity to histamine is related to the severity of asthmatic symptoms (*Juniper EF, Frith PA, Hargreave FE. Airways responsiveness to histamine and methacholine: Relationship to minimum treatment to control symptoms of asthma. Thorax 36(8):575-9, 1981*).

Sodium intake may be correlated with the bronchial response to histamine.

Experimental Double-blind Crossover Study: 36 subjects on a low sodium diet were supplemented with slow sodium 80 mmol/d and placebo in random order. A significant association between sodium excretion and bronchial response to histamine was found (*Burney PG et al. The effect of changing dietary sodium on the bronchial response to histamine. Thorax 44(1):36-41, 1989*).

Observational Study: In a study of 138 men, salt intake, as measured by 24 hr. urinary sodium excretion, was strongly related to bronchial reactivity to inhaled histamine, suggesting that a high sodium diet may potentiate bronchial reactivity (*Burney PG et al. Response to inhaled histamine and 24 hour sodium excretion. Br Med J 292:1483-86, 1986*).

Observational Study: Sales of table salt in the different regions of England and Wales were found to be independently correlated with mortality from asthma for men and for children, but not for women (*Burney PG et al. Response to inhaled histamine and 24 hour sodium excretion. Br Med J 292:1483-86, 1986*).

Zinc to Copper ratio:

May be inversely associated with the incidence of wheezing.

Observational Study: In a study of 9074 white and black adult Americans aged 30 yrs. and older, after controlling for age, race, sex, calories, and pack-years of cigarette smoking, the serum zinc to copper ratio was negatively associated with wheezing (*Schwartz J, Weiss ST. Dietary factors and their relation to respiratory symptoms. The Second National Health and Nutrition Examination Survey. Am J Epidemiol 132(1):67-76, 1990*).

- -

OTHER NUTRITIONAL FACTORS

Cysteine:

N-acetyl cysteine, given by inhalation, is a well-known and effective mucolytic agent (*Millman M et al. Use of acetylcysteine in bronchial asthma - another look. Ann Allergy 54(4):294-96, 1985*).

WARNING: May inhibit the usual decreasing bronchial reactivity to allergen after repeated allergen inhalation challenges ("allergen tachyphylaxis") (*Dorsch W et al. Adverse effects of acetylcysteine on human and guinea pig bronchial asthma in vivo and on human fibroblasts and leukocytes in vitro. Int Arch Allergy Appl Immunol 82(1):33-39, 1987*).

N-acetyl cysteine may also be given orally (200 mg three times daily); however it was ineffective in a recent double-blind trial (*Bylin G et al. No influence of acetylcysteine on gas exchange and spirometry in chronic asthma. Eur J Respir Dis 71(2):102-07, 1987*).

N-acetyl cysteine is converted to cysteine which may also have a mucolytic action.

Case Reports: Two asthmatics were able to reduce their use of medications after starting L-cysteine 500 mg twice daily (*Braverman ER, Pfeiffer CC. The Healing Nutrients Within. New Canaan, Conn., Keats Publishing Co., 1987*).

Omega-3 Fatty Acids (Fish Oils):

Most important member: eicosapentaenoic acid (EPA) which is particularly high in cold water fish.

Available in a refined form as "MaxEPA" (18% EPA) (R.P. Scherer)

Suggested MaxEPA dosage: 3 - 9 grams daily in divided doses (or 10 ml. concentrate twice daily)

WARNING: Supplementation may require additional vitamin E intake to prevent increased membrane peroxidation and cellular damage (*Laganiere S, Fernandes G. High peroxidizability of subcellular membrane induced by high fish oil diet is reversed by vitamin E. Clin Res 35:A565, 1987*).

Dietary fish intake is inversely associated with bronchitis and wheezing.

Observational Study: 24-hr. dietary recalls were obtained from 9074 white and black adults aged 30 and older. Nutrient-specific logistic regression from these data controlling for age, race, sex and pack-years of cigarettes smoking revealed that increased dietary fish intake was associated with reduced rates of active bronchitis and wheezing (*Schwartz J, Weiss ST. Dietary factors and their relation to respiratory symptoms. The Second National Health and Nutrition Examination Survey. Am J Epidemiol 132(1):67-76, 1990*).

The results of studies in which fish oil supplementation was provided to asthmatics have been contradictory.

Experimental Study: Supplementation of pts. with EPA led to changes in leukocyte mediator generation and chemotactic responses as well as a significant attenuation of the late asthmatic response to inhaled antigens (*Arm JP et al. Allergy Proc 10(3):185-87, 1989*).

Negative Experimental Double-blind Crossover Study: Pts. received either 15-20 ml of fish oil or olive oil placebo in either order. After 10 wks., plasma PGE_2 levels increased and there were no differences between regimens in regard to peak flow rates, symptoms or drug consumption (*Stenius-Aarniala B et al. Ann Allergy 62(6):534-47, 1989*).

Negative Experimental Single-blind Study: 10 pts. with aspirin-intolerant asthma received a control diet for 6 wks. followed by a fish oil diet. There were no significant changes in symptom scores during either diet. Peak expiratory flow values, however, were significantly lower, and bronchodilator usage was greater, during the fifth and sixth week of the fish oil diet than during the control diet (*Picado C et al. Effects of a fish oil enriched diet on aspirin intolerant asthmatic patients: A pilot study. Thorax 43(2):93-97, 1988*).

Negative Double-blind Experimental Study: 20 aspirin-intolerant subjects with mild asthma were studied. 12 received 3.2 gm eicosapentaenoic acid and 2.2 gm of docosahexaenoic acid daily, while 8 received placebo. After 10 wks., there was no significant change in airway responsiveness to histamine or any change in any of the clinical measurements. Also, in the experimental subjects only, neutrophil function was substantially suppressed. It is possible that the deleterious effects are limited to aspirin-intolerant asthmatics (*Arm JP et al. Effect of dietary supplementation with fish oil lipids on mild asthma. Thorax 43(2):84-92, 1988*).

Experimental Blinded Study: Pts. consumed capsules contained with 3.2 gm EPA and 2.2 gm DHA daily or placebo. After 10 wks., the usual shortness of breath observed in the late phase of the asthmatic response (the inflammatory component) following inhalation of an antigen decreased 36.6% in treated subjects, compared to 7.7% in controls (*Arm J et al. The effects of dietary supplementation with fish oil on asthmatic responses to antigen. J Clin Allergy 81:183, 1988*).

Omega-6 Fatty Acids:

Evening primrose oil is a rich source of gamma linolenic acid.

Administration of evening primrose oil has not been shown to be beneficial.

Experimental Double-blind Crossover Study: Pts. received either 15-20 ml of evening primrose oil or olive oil placebo in either order. After 10 wks., there were no differences between regimens in regard to peak flow rates, symptoms or drug consumption (*Stenius-Aarniala B et al. Ann Allergy 62(6):534-47, 1989*).

Experimental Study: 30 adult pts. received evening primrose oil 20 ml daily. After 10 wks., no differences were observed with respect to either symptoms or peak flow measurements (*Stenius-Aarniala B et al. Symptomatic effects of evening primrose oil, fish oil, and olive oil in patients with bronchial asthma. Abstract. Ann Allergy 55:330, 1985*).

Omega-9 Fatty Acids:

Administration of olive oil, rich in the omega-9 fatty acid oleic acid, has not been shown to be beneficial.

Experimental Study: 30 adult pts. received olive oil 20 ml daily. After 10 wks., no differences were observed with respect to either symptoms or peak flow measurements (*Stenius-Aarniala B et al. Symptomatic effects of evening primrose oil, fish oil, and olive oil in patients with bronchial asthma. Abstract. Ann Allergy 55:330, 1985*).

L-Tryptophan.

WARNING: May aggravate bronchial asthma; thus a low-tryptophan diet may be beneficial.

Experimental Double-blind Crossover Study: 18 pts. with endogenous asthma received either a normal amt. of tryptophan (1200 mg) in their diet or a low-tryptophan diet (200 mg). After 1 mo., 12 pts. felt better on the low tryptophan diet, 4 felt better on the normal diet and 2 noted no difference (p<0.05). The highest mean peak flow was greater for 14 pts. after the low-tryptophan diet, and for 4 pts. after the normal diet (p<0.02) (*Urge G et al. Tryptophan and endogenous asthma. Europ J Respir Dis Suppl. 136 65:175-76, 1984; Urge G et al. Effect of dietary tryptophan restrictions on clinical symptoms in patients with endogenous asthma. Allergy 38:211-2, 1983*).

Experimental Study: 8 pts. with endogenous asthma were prescribed a diet restricting tryptophan to 350 milligrams. After 4 wks., all had decreased symptoms; also 6/8 had improvements in peak flow while 2 had worsening (*Unge G et al. Tryptophan and endogenous asthma. Europ J Respir Dis Suppl. 136 65:175-76, 1984*).

- -

OTHER FACTORS

Rule out food sensitivities.

Experimental Study: 76 adult pts. with celiac disease were compared to 81 controls with non-inflammatory bowel diseases. There was a significantly increased prevalence (p<0.05) in CD pts. of airway obstruction in 21 cases (28%), positive skin-prick tests to both inhalents and foods in 34 (45%) and asthma in 15 (20%). 10 of the asthma pts. were provoked with 30 gm gluten per day over a 3 wk. period; 2 had reproducible gluten-induced wheezing. Results suggest that occult CD should be considered in every pt. who presents with disabling symptoms from chronic allergic disorders (*Williams AJ. Coeliac disease and allergic manifestations. Letter. Lancet 1:808, 1987*).

Experimental Double-blind Study: 107 pts. with bronchial asthma with an allergic component of a perennial type underwent 143 food ingestion challenges. 15/21 pts. with a "positive food history" developed bronchus-obstructive responses following 15 (71%) food challenges, while 45/86 pts. with an "unknown food history" developed bronchus-obstructive responses following 68 (56%) food challenges. Of these responses, 23 were within 2 hrs., 11 were 4-24 hrs. following challenge, 34 were both within 2 hrs. and 4-24 hrs. following challenge, 6 were 28-56 hrs. following challenge, and 9 were both within 2 hrs. and 28-56 hrs. following challenge. In 22 pts., a double-blind ingestion challenge with the same foods was also performed 6 days later. The bronchial responses recorded after the open challenge and those after the double-blind challenge did not demonstrate any statistically significant differences (p<0.05). According to the patients' reports, avoidance for 8-12 mo. of the individual foods causing a positive bronchial response of any type led to a distinct decrease in bronchial complaints in 93% (*Pelikan Z, Pelikan-Filipek M. Bronchial response to the food ingestion challenge. Ann Allergy 58(3):164-72, 1987*).

Experimental Double-blind Study: Of 300 pts. (aged 7 mo. to 80 yrs.), only 25 had either a history or RAST results suggestive of food allergy. 20 of these pts. had interpretable food challenges; food challenge caused asthma in 6 and caused GI symptoms and atopic dermatitis in 5. Pretreatment with disodium chromoglycate 300 mg 30 min. prior to challenge blocked asthmatic responses in 4/5. Pts. with asthma and food allergy were generally young, had a current or past history of atopic dermatitis, and high total serum IgE levels (*Onorato J et al. Placebo-controlled double-blind challenge in asthma. J Allergy Clin Immunol 78(6):1139-46, 1986*).

Experimental Double-blind Study: For 2 wks., 21 adult pts. with active but stable bronchial asthma received an elemental diet (Vivasorb) along with mineral water and glucose, while 17 matched controls received regular hospital food blended to approximate the elemental diet in taste and texture. All 38 pts. also received standard medical treatment for their asthma. 9/21 pts. receiving the elemental diet improved (3 dramatically) and none deteriorated, while only 1/17 receiving hospital food clearly improved, and 5 deteriorated markedly. Outcome differences were significant both clinically and statistically. Results suggest that specific food sensitivities are likely to be important for many pts. with perennial asthma and thus they "should be tried with an antigen-free diet, preferably for 2-3 wks., even if the patients present with little or no evidence of extrinsic aetiology" (*Hoj L et al. A double-blind controlled trial of elemental diet in severe, perennial asthma. Allergy 36:257-62, 1981*).

Rule out hydrochloric acid deficiency.

Diminished hydrochloric acid may impair digestion and thus increase the potential allergenicity of foods.

Note: While gastric anacidity had been reported in the past to be a relatively common condition which was associated with a number of illnesses, the presence of achlorhydria is no longer accepted unless a potent parietal-cell stimulant (such as histamine) is employed in gastric analysis. More recent studies suggest that histamine-fast anacidity is uncommon before the fifth decade of life and, although it probably does not occur in a normal stomach, its presence is not necessarily associated with symptoms (Rappaport EM. Achlorhydria: Associated symptoms and response to hydrochloric acid. N Engl J Med 252(19):802-5, 1955).

Observational Study: The gastric secretion of hydrochloric acid following a standardized meal was studied in 200 asthmatic children (ages 6 mo. to 12 yrs.) and compared to a control gp. of pediatric surgical cases, non-asthmatic medical cases, and normal children. 80% of the asthmatic children had sub-normal levels of gastric acidity, compared to less than 10% of the controls. Hypochlorhydria was more prevalent in children below the age of 7, and gastric acid levels tended to rise towards puberty, perhaps reflecting the fact that spontaneous remissions are common around this age (*Bray GW. The hypochlorhydria of asthma of childhood. Quart J Med 24:181-97, 1931*).

If deficient, administration of hydrochloric acid may be beneficial.

Experimental Study: 160 asthmatic children found to have sub-normal levels of hydrochloric acid following a test meal received HCl before or during meals in addition to continued exclusion of foods to which they were known to be sensitive. There were immediate improvements in appetite, weight, sleep and asthmatic attacks - which became shorter in duration and lesser in intensity. If, based on skin tests, the chief offending antigens are removed, there is immediate freedom from attacks. If not, the attacks cease after 3 or more mo., depending upon the initial severity of the asthma (*Bray GW. The hypochlorhydria of asthma of childhood. Quart J Med 24:181-97, 1931*).

– –

COMBINED INTERVENTIONS

Vitamin B$_6$,
Vitamin B$_{12}$,
Magnesium,
Gastric re-acidification, and
Food allergy management:

Case Reports and Theoretical Discussion: It is suggested that cow's milk (and possibly other food antigens) may cause severe allergic gastritis which may result in hypochlorhydria, low pepsin secretion, and possible failure of 'intrinsic factor' production. Hypochlorhydria and low pepsin production result in incomplete digestion and macromolecular absorption, increasing both the number and severity of food allergies, while simultaneously impairing micronutrient nutrition, while failure of 'intrinsic factor' production results in vitamin B$_{12}$ malabsorption and possible defective B$_{12}$ utilization. The result is asthmatic wheezing in susceptible children (*Wright JV. Treatment of childhood asthma with parenteral vitamin B$_{12}$, gastric re-acidification, and attention to food allergy, magnesium and pyridoxine: Three case reports with background and an integrated hypothesis. J Nutr Med 1:277-82, 1990*).

CANCER

See Also: **CERVICAL DYSPLASIA**
BENIGN BREAST DISEASE
"HYPERESTROGENISM"

OVERVIEW

The National Academy of Sciences (US) estimates that 60% of women's cancers and 40% of men's cancers are related to nutritional factors. The cancers most closely associated with nutritional factors are breast and endometrial cancer in women, prostate cancer in men, and gastrointestinal cancer.

The value of a low fat, high fiber, high complex carbohydrate diet in cancer prevention is well-documented. Alcohol abuse increases cancer risk. Avoidance of smoked, pickled and salt-cured foods (due to their nitrosamine content) has been shown in both epidemiologic and animal studies to be beneficial in preventing cancers of the GI tract.

For several nutrients, the lower their intake, the greater the risk of developing certain cancers. Although the levels of many nutrients are lower in cancer patients than in healthy controls, it remains unclear whether these differences have causal implications. There is, however, early evidence that certain precancerous changes may be reversible with supplementation. Cervical dysplasia, for example, may possibly be reversed with folic acid supplementation, especially if folic acid is deficient, and calcium supplementaion may reduce the number of rapidly proliferating cells in the colonic epithelium in patients with family histories of colon cancer and elevated numbers of such cells compared to controls. Vitamin A or beta-carotene reduces the percent of genetically-damaged cells inside the cheek when betel quid, a tobacco-like plant mixture, is chewed regularly, while vitamin C reduces nitrosamine levels in the stomach and therefore may reduce the risk of gastric cancer.

There is little scientific literature on the efficacy of nutritional supplementation in reversing established cancers. Vitamin A may be of limited value, and studies recently completed or currently under way are examining the efficacy of its synthetic analogues. The efficacy of vitamin C is controversial. An "anti-angiogenesis" factor extracted from animal cartilage is showing early promise, but remains to be scientifically validated; similarly, the alkoxylglycerols appear promising but controlled studies have yet to be completed.

While the literature is only preliminary, nutrients appear to have some efficacy as adjuvants to standard treatments. Vitamin E and the combination of calcium and vitamin D may possibly enhance the effects of chemotherapy, while niacin, vitamin C, vitamin E, selenium, cysteine, coenzyme Q10 and superoxide dismutase show promise in reducing its toxicity. Similarly, the therapeutic effects of radiotherapy may possibly be enhanced by vitamin C, while glutamine, superoxide dismutase and Lactobacillus acidophilus may mitigate its damage to healthy tissue.

- -

DIETARY FACTORS

GENERAL:

Treat malnutrition.

Median survival may be shorter in patients with weight loss (*Dewys WD et al. Prognostic effect of weight loss prior to chemotherapy in cancer patients. Am J Med 69:491-97, 1980*).

Nutritional repletion is associated with return of immunocompetence, a reduction in sepsis, proper wound healing, and an apparent increase in tumor response to chemotherapy (*Copeland EM 3rd, Daly JM, Dudrick SJ. Nutrition and cancer. Int Adv Surg Oncol 4:1-13, 1981*).

Avoid <u>obesity</u>.

> **Review Article:** The link between obesity and cancer incidence was established over 40 yrs. ago and has been upheld consistently since. Similarly, obesity increases the rate of progression of malignant disease (*Kearney R. Promotion and prevention of tumour growth: Effects of endotoxin, inflammation and dietary lipids.* <u>Int Clin Nutr Rev</u> *7(4):157-68, 1987*).

<u>Low fat diet</u>.

> *(See Also: "<u>Fatty Acids</u>" below)*

May reduce cancer incidence and mortality.

> *Note: There is some question whether the association between fat intake and cancer is actually due to the influence of fat upon total caloric intake (DM Klurfeld & D Kritchevsky, Wistar Institute, Philadelphia - quoted in <u>Med World News</u> April 25, 1988).*

General:

> **Review Article:** "Evidence relating dietary fat to cancer at sites such as the breast and colon is provided by experiments showing that animals fed high-fat diets develop cancer at these sites more readily than do animals fed low-fat diets and by epidemiological data from different countries showing strong positive correlations between cancer incidence and mortality, and level of dietary fat. Experiments on animals have indicated that polyunsaturated vegetable oils promote cancer more effectively than do saturated fats or polyunsaturated fish oils, whereas in the epidemiological data, total dietary fat correlates with cancer incidence and mortality at least as well as does any particular type of fat. Case-control and cohort studies have not shown strong indications of a relationship between dietary fat and cancer, perhaps because of methodological difficulties inherent in such studies. The weight of evidence continues to indicate that long-term adherence to a low-fat diet can reduce the risk of some common types of cancer" (*Carroll KK. Dietary fats and cancer.* <u>Am J Clin Nutr</u> *53:1064S-7S, 1991*).

Breast Cancer:

> **Review Article:** In a review of data from 12 case-controlled studies, about 25% of postmenopausal breast cancers could be prevented with diet. In reviewing data from around the world, saturated fat and possibly monounsaturated fat increased risk. Reducing saturated fat intake from the recommended 10% of calories to 9% would lower breast cancer rates in the US alone by 10%. No association was found between fat intake and increased breast cancer rates in premenopausal women (*Howe G et al. Dietary factors and risk of breast cancer: Combined analysis of 12 case-control studies.* <u>J Natl Cancer Inst</u> *82:561-9, 1990*).

> **Review Article:** Data from animal experiments and human correlation studies strongly support the dietary fat-breast cancer hypothesis, and a causal relation between the two is biologically plausible. While some recent epidemiologic studies have had negative findings, the narrow range of dietary fat inake among subjects and the substantial measurement error in dietary assessment argue against drawing more than limited conclusions from these studies (*Schatzkin A et al. The dietary fat-breast cancer hypothesis is alive.* <u>JAMA</u> *261(22):3284-87, 1989*).

Intestinal Cancer:

> **Observational Study:** In a prospective study of 88,751 women 34-59 yrs. old and without a history of cancer, inflammatory bowel disease, or familial polyposis, 150 cases of colon cancer developed. After adjustment for total energy intake, animal fat was positively associated with the risk of colon cancer (p=0.01). The relative risk for the highest as compared with the lowest quintile was 1.89 (95% confidence interval, 1.13-3.15). No association was found for vegetable fat. The relative risk of colon cancer in women who ate beef, pork, or lamb as a main dish every day was 2.49 (95% confidence interval, 1.24-5.03), as compared to those reporting consumption less than once a month. Processed meats and liver were also significantly associated with increased risk, whereas fish and chicken without skin were related to decreased risk. The ratio of the intake of red meat to the intake of chicken and fish was particularly strongly associated with an increased

incidence of colon cancer (p=0.0005); the relative risk for women in the highest quintile of this ratio as compared with those in the lowest quintile was 2.49 (95% confidence interval, 1.50-4.13). A low intake of fiber from fruits appeared to contribute to the risk of colon cancer, but this relation was not statistically independent of meat intake (*Willett WC et al. Relation of meat, fat, and fiber intake to the risk of colon cancer in a prospective study among women. N Engl J Med 323:1664-72, 1990*).

Observational Study: Past lifestyle habits of 906 Chinese colorectal cancer pts. and over 2000 controls were analyzed. The strongest association was with saturated fat intake; cancer risk increased 4-fold from the lowest to the highest intake of saturated fat (*Whittemore A et al. Diet, physical activity, and colorectal cancer among Chinese in North America and China. J Natl Cancer Inst 82:915-26, 1990*).

Lung Cancer:

Observational Study: In a case-control study which included 5 ethnic gps. (Japanese, Caucasian, Chinese, Filipino, and Hawaiian), the attributable risk of a high saturated fat intake in regard to lung cancer, based on the assumption that all subjects reduced their saturated fat intake to the lowest 25th percentile of the population, ranged from 28% to 62% (*Zhao LP et al. Effects of saturated fat on lung, prostate, and breast cancer in five ethnic groups of Hawaii. Abstract. Am J Clin Nutr 53:P-31, 1991*).

Ovarian Cancer:

Observational Study: Dietary histories of 455 Italian women with ovarian cancer were compared with histories of 1385 controls. A high fat diet, especially from meat or butter, elevated the risk, while a diet high in fish, green vegetables, carrots and while grains provided the lowest risk (*Calvert RJ et al. J Natl Cancer Inst 79(4):875, 1987*).

Prostatic Cancer:

Observational Study: In a case-control study which included 5 ethnic gps. (Japanese, Caucasian, Chinese, Filipino, and Hawaiian), the attributable risk of a high saturated fat intake in regard to prostate cancer, based on the assumption that all subjects reduced their saturated fat intake to the lowest 25th percentile of the population, ranged from 24% to 74% (*Zhao LP et al. Effects of saturated fat on lung, prostate, and breast cancer in five ethnic groups of Hawaii. Abstract. Am J Clin Nutr 53:P-31, 1991*).

Urothelial Cancer:

Observational Study: Dietary intake data were collected on several hundred people in Sweden with and without urothelial cancer. People who consumed a high-fat diet showed a dose-response relative risk of 1.7 (*Steineck G et al. Vitamin A supplements, fried foods, fat and urothelial cancer. A case-referent study in Stockholm in 1985-87. Int J Cancer 45:1006-11, 1990*).

May enhance immune function, possibly by increasing natural killer cell activity.

Experimental Study: 17 healthy, normal-weight young males lowered their fat intake to <30% of calories as fat. After 3 mo., the paired t test showed a marked increase in natural killer cell activity from baseline (p=0.0002). Results of a general linear model showed an effect of lowering total dietary fat on increased NK-cell activity (~0.53% increase for each absolute % of calories as fat, p=0.14) for all men, and a highly significant effect in a subset of men who ate >25% of calories as fat at baseline (~1.22% increase, p=0.009) (*Barone J et al. Dietary fat and natural-killer-cell activity. Am J Clin Nutr 50:861-67, 1989*).

Low protein diet.

Gastric Cancer:

Observational Study: 1,016 pts. with gastric cancer were studied along with 1,159 population-based controls in high and low risk areas in Italy. Risk of gastric cancer increased with increasing consumption of protein (*Buiatti E et al. A case-control study of gastric cancer and diet in Italy: association with nutrients. Int J Cancer 45:899-901, 1990*).

Pancreatic Cancer:

Observational Study: In a German study involving 50,000 households, there was a positive association for both men and women between high protein intake and the risk of pancreatic cancer (*Böing H et al. Regional nutritional pattern and cancer mortality in the Federal Republic of Germany.* Nutr Cancer *7(3):121-30, 1985*).

Low fat, low protein diet.

There may be a positive correlation between the risk of non-Hodgkin's lymphoma and consumption of fat and protein.

Observational Study: The diet histories of 208 NHL Italian pts. and 401 hospital controls were compared. The consumption of milk, liver, butter and oil (primarily unsaturated) were all positively correlated with a higher risk of NHL while whole-grain bread and pasta were negatively correlated (*Franceschi S et al. Dietary factors and non-Hodgkin's lymphoma: a case-control study in the north-eastern part of Italy.* Nutr Cancer *12:333-41, 1989*).

Low cholesterol diet.

Cancer risk may be positively associated with dietary cholesterol.

Observational Study: Data from 188 males with lung cancer and 294 controls were adjusted for age, ethnicity, cigarette smoking and exposure to lung carcinogens. Dietary cholesterol was found to be positively and significantly associated with lung cancer risk (*Hinds MW et al.* Am J Clin Nutr *37:192-3, 1983*).

Cancer risk may be positively associated with serum cholesterol levels (which are influenced by both fat and cholesterol intake.)

Review Article: Low levels of serum cholesterol, particularly when at the lowest decile, are associated with increased cancer risk. Since that risk attentuates over time, it may be an early sign of an established cancer rather than a risk factor (*Sherwin RW et al. Serum cholesterol levels and cancer mortality in 361,662 men screened for the multiple risk factor intervention trial.* JAMA *257(7):943-48, 1987*).

Observational Study: In a study of 5125 men and 7363 women followed for a median of 10 yrs., men in the lowest cholesterol quintile had nearly double the risk of those in the highest quintile for both incidence and mortality. Among women a similar relation was seen for cancer mortality, but cancer incidence in the lowest quintile was only 1.2 times that of women in the highest quintile. The inverse cholesterol-cancer relation in men was present for cholesterol determinations made 6 or more years before the diagnosis of cancer, suggesting that it may not be merely a preclinical cancer marker (*Schatzkin A et al. Serum cholesterol and cancer in the NHANES epidemiologic followup study.* Lancet *2:298-301, 1987*).

Avoid eggs and fried foods.

Ovarian Cancer:

Observational Study: In a study of over 16,000 Seventh-Day Adventist women, those who ate eggs (fried or otherwise) at least 3 times weekly had a 3 times greater risk of fatal ovarian cancer than did women who ate eggs less than once weekly, while fish, chicken and potatoes were also positively associated with fatal ovarian cancer when they were fried. Consumption of fried eggs showed the strongest association with fatal ovarian cancer, perhaps due to interference with cholesterol biosynthesis and consequently the manufacture of ovarian hormones from the production of cytotoxic oxidation products of cholesterol (*Snowdon DA. Letter.* JAMA *254(3):356-7, 1985*).

Urothelial Cancer:

Observational Study: Dietary intake data were collected on several hundred people in Sweden with and without urothelial cancer. Increased risk for urinary tract cancer was observed in people who frequently consumed fried foods, such as fried meat and fried potatoes. These subjects had a relative risk of 2.4. No association between diet and cancer was noted for lean meat other than fried (*Steineck G et al. Vitamin A supplements, fried foods, fat and urothelial cancer. A case-referent study in Stockholm in 1985-87.* Int J Cancer *45:1006-11, 1990*).

Avoid <u>hydrogenated vegetable oils</u>.

Literature suggesting that they <u>are</u> carcinogenic:

Review Article: *Trans*-9, *trans*-12-octadecadienoic acid causes various toxicological and physiological aberrations (*Kinsella JE et al. Metabolism of trans fatty acids with emphasis on the effects of trans, trans-octadecadienoate on lipid composition, essential fatty acid, and prostaglandins: An overview. <u>Am J Clin Nutr</u> 34:2307, 1981*).

Note: This isomer is the only trans fatty acid which may have a toxic effect. As the thermodynamics of hydrogenation permit only insignificant amounts to be formed in hydrogenated fats, and relatively high dietary levels are required for it to have adverse effects, it poses no threat to human health at the levels now found in dietary fats (Hunter JE, Applewhite TH. Isomeric fatty acids in the US diet: Levels and health perspectives. <u>Am J Clin Nutr</u> 44(6):707-17, 1986).

Review Article: Partially-hydrogenated oils contain a relatively high percent of the un-natural *trans* form of fatty acids (up to 17% of processed vegetable oils, 47% of margarines and 58% of vegetable shortening). Since there are positive correlations of mortality from cancer with intake of total fat and vegetable fat, but not with animal fat or with total or individual unsaturated fatty acids in vegetable fats, *trans* fats may be a major contributor to the carcinogenic effect of fats (*Enig MG et al. Dietary fat and cancer trends - A critique. <u>Fed Proc</u> 37:2215-20, 1978*).

Note: This suggestion is subject to the criticism that epidemiological correlation does not demonstrate cause-and-effect relationships (Hunter JE, Applewhite TH. Isomeric fatty acids in the US diet: Levels and health perspectives. <u>Am J Clin Nutr</u> 44(6):707-17, 1986).

Animal Experimental Study: Mice fed 20% (by weight) olive oil diets containing 50% trielaidin or trilinoelaidin had a higher incidence of liver tumors than did controls (*Khan NA, Siddiqui KA. Carcinogenesis by ingestion of trans isomers from fatty acid esters and glycerides in place of natural cis isomers. <u>Bangladesh Pharm J</u> 6:19-20, 1977*).

Note: A number of other experiments testing the tumorigenicity of trans isomers under various circumstances with animal models have provided negative results (Brown RR. <u>Cancer Res</u> 41:3741-42, 1981; Erickson KC et al. <u>J Nutr</u> 114:1834-42, 1984; Reddy BS et al. <u>J Natl Cancer Inst</u> 75:791-98, 1985; Selenskas SL et al. <u>Cancer Res</u> 44:1321-26, 1984; Sugano M et al. <u>Nutr Cancer</u> 12(2):177-87, 1989; Watanabe M et al. <u>Am J Clin Nutr</u> 42:475-84, 1985).

Literature suggesting that they are <u>not</u> carcinogenic:

Review Articles: Reliable data do not support concerns about possible relationships of *trans* fatty acids to the development of cancer. *Trans* fatty acids do not pose any harm to humans consuming a balanced diet containing adequate linoleic acid (*Hunter JE, Applewhite TH. Isomeric fatty acids in the US diet: Levels and health perspectives. <u>Am J Clin Nutr</u> 44(6):707-17, 1986; Hunter JE et al. Isomeric fatty acids and tumorigenesis: A commentary on recent work. <u>Nutr Cancer</u> 7(4):199-209, 1985*).

High <u>fiber</u> diet.

Breast Cancer:

Review Article: Evidence from epidemiological studies suggests that dietary fiber may affect breast cancer risk. Fiber may have a protective role because of its influence on estrogen metabolism and excretion or because of the endocrine effects of the lignans, a family of compounds formed in the intestine from fiber-associated precursors (*Rose DP. Dietary fiber and breast cancer. <u>Nutr Cancer</u> 13:1-8, 1990*).

Review Article: For Western women, dietary fiber may be important in the prevention of breast cancer, and both the early onset of menarche and a high fat diet are risk factors in breast cancer. Breast cancer may be estrogen-dependent and dietary fiber may increase the fecal excretion of estrogen. Perhaps high fat diets are necessarily low in fiber and low fiber intake rather than high fat intake is the reason why high dietary fat is a risk factor (*Hughes RE. Hypothesis: A new look at dietary fiber. Hum Nutr Clin Nutr 40C:81-86, 1986*).

Colon and Rectal Cancer:

Experimental Study: Pts. with a history of resected colon or rectal cancer consumed 13.5 g wheat bran for 8 wks. followed by a 1-mo. period where only 2 g wheat bran were included in the diet. 6/8 pts. with initially high 24-hr. outgrowth labeling indices showed significant decreases in rectal mucosa biopsy specimens after treatment with wheat bran. An overall decrease of 22% was noted in rectal mucosa biopsy specimens obtained with inclusion of wheat bran in the diet, which was tolerated with no side effects. Wheat bran is believed to inhibit DNA synthesis and rectal mucosa cell proliferation in high-risk populations (*Alberts D et al. Effects of dietary wheat bran fiber on rectal epithelial cell proliferation in patients with resection for colorectal cancers. J Natl Cancer Inst 82:1280-5, 1990*).

In vitro Experimental Study: Several fibers (alpha-cellulose, lignin, psyllium, pectin, lupin, potato starch) were incubated with bile acids (chenodeoxycholic acid, deoxycholic acid) for 24 hrs., after which DNA was added to the medium and incubation continued for another 16 hours. Cellulose reduced the damaging effect of bile acids on DNA 408-fold. To a much lesser extent, psyllium reduced damage caused by DOC but not CDOC, and the other fibers had negligible effects. Results suggest that cellulose might promote polyesterification of bile acid to a biologically inactive form (*Cheah P, Bernstein H. Colon cancer and dietary fiber: Cellulose inhibits the DNA-damaging ability of bile acids. Nutr Cancer 13:51-57, 1990*).

Review Article: The international studies and most of the epidemiologic case-control studies show a protective benefit of foods containing fiber and none shows harm, suggesting that a variety of fiber-containing foods be eaten to protect against colon cancer (*Greenward P, Lanza E. Dietary fiber and colon cancer. Contemp Nutr 11(1), 1986*).

Dietary fiber may inhibit the development of large bowel neoplasia in patients with familial adenomatous polyposis by reducing the development of polyps.

Experimental Double-blind Study: In a 4-yr. study, 58 pts. with familial adenomatous polyposis randomly received ascorbic acid 4 g/d plus alpha-tocopherol 400 mg/d either with a low-fiber cereal or with a grain fiber supplement (Kellogg's All-Bran 22.5 g/d), or received placebo capsules and a low-fiber cereal. After 6 mo., pts. on the high-fiber diet showed shrinkage in the size and number of rectal polyps. While analysis by intent to treat suggested that fiber had a limited effect, adjustment for patient compliance showed a stronger benefit from the high-fiber supplement during the middle 2 yrs. of the trial. At month 24, the median polyp ratio (change from baseline) was 0.50 for the high-fiber gp. compared to 1.0 for the vitamin-only gp. and 1.16 for the control group. Vitamins C and E showed virtually no effect. Results provide evidence for inhibition of benign large bowel neoplasia by grain fiber supplements in excess a 11 g/d in this population and are consistent with the hypothesis that dietary grain fiber and total dietary fat act as competing variables in the genesis of large bowel neoplasia (*DeCosse JJ et al. Effect of wheat fiber and vitamins C and E on rectal polyps in patients with familial adenomatous polyposis. J Natl Cancer Inst 81(17):1290-97, 1989*).

Various hypotheses have attempted to explain the anti-carcinogenic effect of fiber upon colorectal cancer:

1. Fiber may serve as a bulking agent to reduce the concentration of mutagens or carcinogens in the lumenal contents (*Burkitt DP. Epidemiology of cancer of the colon and rectum. Cancer 28:3-13, 1971*).

2. Fiber may increase the rate of intestinal transit and reduce the contact time between the potentially harmful constituents and the mucosa (*Reddy BS et al. Metabolic epidemiology of large bowel cancer. Fecal bulk and constituents of high-risk North American and low-risk Finnish populations. Cancer 42:2832-38, 1978*).

3. Fibers are fermented by intestinal microbes. Fermentation products, such as short-chain fatty acids, acidify the lumenal contents; this acidic environment inhibits microbial enzymes that are able to modify endogenous constituents, such as bile acids, to produce mutagenic or carcinogenic compounds (*Dexter DL et al. Sodium butyrate-induced alteration of growth properties and glycogen levels in cultured human colon carcinoma cells. Histochem J 16:137-49, 1984; Hill MJ, Drasar BS. The normal colonic bacterial flora. Gut 16:318-23, 1975; Thornton JR. High colonic pH promotes colorectal cancer. Lancet 1:1081-82, 1981*).

Panceatic Cancer:

Observational Study: Consumption of fiber from fruits, vegetables, and whole grain products was inversely linked to pancreatic cancer risk, with a relative risk of 0.22 vs. 0.78 in the highest versus lowest quartile for fiber intake (*Howe G et al. Dietary factors and risk of pancreatic cancer: Results of a Canadian population-based case-control study. Int J Cancer 45:604-08, 1990*).

Prostate Cancer:

Observational Study: In a study of Seventh-Day Adventist men, vegans consumed and excreted more fiber than did lacto-ovo-vegetarians and nonvegetarians, while lacto-ovo-vegetarians consumed and excreted more fiber than did non-vegetarians. The more fiber a person consumed (especially lignin and the water-insoluble fibers such as cellulose), the greater was the binding to estrogen and testosterone, thus reducing the amt. of these hormones in the body and possibly decreasing prostate cancer risk (*Ross J et al. Dietary and hormonal evaluation of men at different risks for prostate cancer: Fiber intake, excretion, and composition, with in vitro evidence for an association between steroid hormones and specific fiber components. Am J Clin Nutr 51:365-70, 1990*).

Vegetarian diet.

Benefits may be due to such factors as its low fat content, high fiber content, its high carotenoid content and/or other factors.

Observational Study: Compared to age- and sex-matched omnivorous controls, male vegetarians aged 28-50 had significantly higher levels of carotene (but not of vitamins A, E or K). Cytotoxicity of peripheral blood lymphocytes was twice as high in vegetarians as in controls (*Malter M et al. Natural killer cells, vitamins and other blood components of vegetarian and omnivorous men. Nutr Cancer 12(3):271-78, 1989*).

Theoretical Discussion: Most vegetables lack delta-6-desaturase which converts linoleic to arachidonic acid. Human cells have this enzyme and thus humans do not need to eat the higher polyunsaturated fatty acids found in animal tissues. Many neoplastic cells, however, have lost the activity of 6D, and thus a vegetarian diet would deprive these cells of higher-chain fatty acids and inhibit the activity of 6D. Without higher-carbon fatty acids, neoplastic cell membranes would have altered fluidity and thus altered transport properties, receptor activity, sensitivity to external molecules, ability to reproduce, resistance to external agents, and overall survival. These alterations would make the cells easier prey for the self-defense of the body or for attack with therapeutic agents (*Siguel EN. Cancerostatic effect of vegetarian diets. Nutr Cancer 4(4):295-91, 1983*).

May decrease the risk of breast cancer by lowering estrogen levels.

Observational Study: 10 vegetarian premenopausal women were found to excrete 2-3 times as much estrogen as 10 non-vegetarian controls and have lower serum estrogen levels, suggesting that the fiber present in a whole-grain, whole-vegetable diet absorbs estrogen and removes it via fecal excretion (*Goldin BR et al. Estrogen excretion patterns and plasma levels in vegetarian and omnivorous women. N Engl J Med 307:1542-47, 1982*).

May decrease the risk of colon cancer, perhaps by reducing the levels of proximal carcinogens.

Review Article: Compared to breast cancer, there is stronger epidemiological evidence that the intake of animal fat or meat is associated with the risk of colon cancer. Although total energy intakes may also be a factor, the intake of vegetable fat was inversely related to the risk of colon cancer in recent studies (*Galli C, Butrum R. dietary ω3 fatty acids and cancer: an overview, in AP Simopoulos et al, Eds. Health Effects of ω3 Polyunsaturated Fatty Acids in Seafoods. World Rev Nutr Diet 66:3446-61, 1991*).

Experimental Study: Compared to vegetarians, omnivores eating a "Western-type" diet had higher levels of beta-glucuronidase, nitroreductase, azoreductase, and steroid 7-alpha-dehydroxylase in their fecal microflora. All of these enzymes are known to catalyze reactions that may result in the formation of proximal carcinogens. Removal of red meat from the diet of omnivores for 30 days resulted in reduced fecal steroid 7-alpha-dehydroxylase activity, but failed to reduce the activity of the other enzymes (*Goldin BR et al. Effect of diet and Lactobacillus acidophilus supplements on human fecal bacterial enzymes. J Natl Cancer Inst 64(2):255-61, 1980*).

May reduce the risk of gastric cancer by inhibiting nitrosamine formation (*Barale R et al. Vegetables inhibit, in vivo, the mutagenicity of nitrite combined with nitrosable compounds.* Mutation Res *120:145, 1983*).

Emphasize dark green and yellow vegetables.

Consumption may be negatively correlated with cancer risk.

General:

Observational Study: The association between consumption of carotene-containing vegetables and subsequent 5 yr. mortality from cancer was examined for 1271 subjects 66 yrs. of age or older. After controlling for age and smoking, those in the highest quintile of intake had a cancer mortality risk of 30% that of those in the lowest quintile. However, since salads, carrots and squash consumption was unrelated to risk of cancer mortality, and consumption of tomatoes or strawberries was most strongly correlated with low cancer risk, some other factor besides beta-carotene may be responsible (*Colditz GA et al. Increased green and yellow vegatable intake and lowered cancer deaths in an elderly population.* Am J Clin Nutr *41(1):32-6, 1985*).

Observational Study: A large scale, 20-year study found a negative correlation between eating green-yellow vegetables daily and the risk of lung, stomach and other cancers. Ex-smokers who ate green-yellow vegetables daily also decreased their risk of lung cancer. Among those who increased their vegetable consumption, there was a more than 25% reduction in the number of deaths from stomach cancer (*Dietary Aspects of Carcinogenesis September, 1983*).

Bladder Cancer:

Observational Study: In a case-control study of 163 cases of bladder cancer and 181 controls hospitalized for other acute conditions, the frequency of consumption of green vegetables and carrots was lower in the cases (*LaVecchia C et al. Dietary factors in the risk of bladder cancer.* Nutr Cancer *12:93-101, 1989*).

Breast Cancer:

Observational Study: In a case-control study of 1,108 histologically confirmed breast cancer pts. and 1,281 controls hospitalized for other acute conditions, a reduced risk was associated with a more frequent green vegetable consumption (*LaVecchia C et al. Dietary factors and the risk of breast cancer.* Nutr Cancer *10:205-14, 1987*).

Cervical Cancer:

Observational Study: When compared to 227 controls, dietary histories from 189 women aged 20-74 with diagnosed cervical cancer showed that frequent consumption of dark green and yellow vegetables and fruit juices was associated with reduced risk of cervical cancer (*Verreault R et al. A case-control study of diet and invasive cervical cancer.* Int J Cancer *43:1050-54, 1989*).

Endometrial Cancer:

Observational Study: The diets of 168 women with endometrial cancer were compared to those of 334 controls. Cancer risk was lower among women who consumed either carrots, spinach, broccoli, cantaloupe, or lettuce (all containing carotenes) at least once daily (*Barbone F et al. Diet and endometrial cancer. Abstract.* Am J Epidemiol *132:783, 1990*).

Lung Cancer:

Observational Study: 763 white male pts. with lung cancer and 900 controls were asked about their usual frequency of consumption 4 yrs. earlier of 44 food items which provide 83% of the vitamin A in the US diet and about vitamin supplements. Although men in the lowest quartile of carotenoid intake had a relative risk of 1.3 compared to those in the highest quartile after adjusting for smoking, the intake of vegetables, dark green vegetables, and especially dark yellow-orange vegetables showed stronger associations than did the carotenoid index. Consumption of dark yellow-orange vegetables was consistently more predictive of reduced risk than consumption of any other food gp. or total carotenoid index, possibly because of the high content of beta-carotene relative to other carotenoids in this particular food group. The protective effect of vegetables was limited to current and recent cigarette smokers, suggesting that vegetable intake prevents a late-stage event of carcinogenesis (*Ziegler RG et al. Carotenoid intake, vegetables, and the risk of lung cancer among white men in New Jersey. Am J Epidemiol 123(6):1080-93, 1986*).

Vulvar Cancer:

Observational Study: Diets of 201 cancer pts. and 342 controls were compared.   There was a definite association between a decreased intake of deep yellow-orange vegetables and alpha-carotene and cancer risk (*Ziegler R et al. Diet and the risk of vulvar cancer. Am J Epidemiol 132:778, 1990*).

Emphasize soy products.

Soy products lower the risk of several forms of cancer, over and above their low-fat, high-fiber content. They contain several anti-cancer compounds, including phytoestrogens such as isoflavones, protease inhibitors, phytosterols and saponins (*Messina M, Barnes S. The role of soy products in reducing risk of cancer. J Natl Cancer Inst 83:541-6, 1991*).

Avoid alcohol.

May be associated with an increased cancer risk.

General Review Article: Although alcohol has never been labeled a chemical carcinogen, and animal studies have never been able to produce cancer with alcohol, it has been implicated in many human cancers as confirmed by epidemiological studies. Cancer experts at an international meeting in France concluded that the "occurrence of malignant tumour of the oral cavity, pharynx, larynx, oesophagus, and liver, is causally related to the consumption of alcoholic beverages" (*Tuyns A. Alcohol and cancer. Proc Nutr Soc 49:145-51, 1990*).

General Review Article: Alcohol abuse is a recognized risk factor in the development of several cancers, including cancers of the upper alimentary and respiratory tracts, breast, pancreas, large bowel, and stomach. Its most well-known effect is the increased risk for oral and esophageal cancers due to combined alcohol and tobacco use. Alcohol probably has a cocarcinogenic effect which is active with a variety of chemical cocarcinogens, including the polycyclic aromatic hydrocarbons in tobacco and benzo(a)pyrenes in barbecued foods. Alcohol may also affect carcinogenesis indirectly by inducing other marginal vitamin and mineral deficiencies associated with increased cancer risk. When combined with vitamin A deficiency, alcohol abuse depletes liver vitamin A levels by mobilizing the vitamin from the liver to other organs and by stimulating the breakdown of retinol and retinoic acid, thus increasing cancer risk by reducing the protective effect of vitamin A. Alcohol may also increase lipid peroxidation (*Garro A, Lieber C. Alcohol and cancer. Ann Rev Pharmacol Toxicol 30:219-49, 1990*).

Breast Cancer:

Review Article: "Clearly alcohol can be linked to cancers of the oropharynx, larynx, oesphagus, and liver, but it may be premature to include breast cancer" (*Lowenfels AB. Alcohol and breast cancer. Letter. Lancet 335:1216, 1990*).

Review Article: All but 3 of the approximately 17 cohort and case-control studies that have investigated an association between alcohol intake and breast cancer have shown a 40-60% increase in risk with only moderate drinking (*Graham S. Editorial: Alcohol and breast cancer. N Engl J Med 316(19):1211-13, 1987*).

Colorectal Cancer:

Observational Study: A 17-yr. follow-up study of 265,118 Japanese adults aged 40 yr. and above revealed a close association between cancer of the sigmoid colon (n=91) and alcohol consumption: relative risk for drinkers vs. non-drinkers was 4.38 in men and 1.92 in women. In men, attributable risk was 74%, and relative risks in non-, infrequent, occasional, and daily drinkers were 1.00, 2.03, 3.83, and 5.42, respectively. Relative risks of daily consumption vs. non-consumption in men for cancers of the mouth, pharynx, esophagus, stomach, proximal colon, sigmoid colon, and rectum were 2.27, 2.44, 2.29, 0.92, 0.98, 5.42, and 1.39, respectively (*Hirayama T. Association between alcohol consumption and cancer of the sigmoid colon: Observations from a Japanese cohort study. Lancet 2:725-28, 1989*).

Observational Study: An analysis of time trends in cancer mortality since 1921 in the U.S., England and Wales, Australia and New Zealand, in relation to changes in per capita consumption of food stuffs and alcohol revealed that, for rectal cancer, and to a lesser extent colon cancer, beer consumption is the most consistent correlate in comparisons across time, and between place, sex, and age-group (*McMichael AJ et al. Time trends in colo-rectal cancer mortality in relation to food and alcohol consumption: United States, United Kingdom, Australia and New Zealand. Int J Epidemiol 8(4):295-303, 1980*).

Esophageal Cancer:

Observational Study: In a study of 178 pts., >50 alcoholic drinks/mo. represented a 3-fold increase in cancer risk (*Graham S et al. Nutritional epidemiology of cancer of the esophagus. Am J Epidemiol 131:454-67, 1990*).

Lung Cancer:

Review Article: Four correlation studies have shown a relationship between alcohol, particularly beer, consumption and lung cancer, and beer consumption was a risk factor in one case-control study. 8/10 prospective studies show alcoholics and high alcohol consumers to be at greater risk of lung cancer. There is also some animal evidence which supports the effects of alcohol on the likelihood of developing lung cancer (*Potter JD, McMichael AJ. Alcohol, beer and lung cancer: A meaningful relationship? Int J Epidemiol 13(2):240-42, 1984*).

Stomach Cancer:

Observational Study: In a German study involving 50,000 households, there was a significant positive association for both men and women between high alcohol intake and the risk of stomach cancer (*Böing H et al. Regional nutritional pattern and cancer mortality in the Federal Republic of Germany. Nutr Cancer 7(3):121-30, 1985*).

Upper Aerodigestive Tract (larynx, pharynx, mouth, esophagus):

Review Article: Of 23 published studies on upper aerodigestive tract cancer, 2 prospective cohorts showed a significantly increased risk at high levels of alcohol consumption. The remaining 21 were case-control studies, 17 of which showed an association with alcohol consumption; in 15 of these studies, the association was dose-related (*Alcohol and cancer. Editorial. Lancet 1:634-35, 1990*).

Avoid smoked, pickled and salt-cured foods.

Contain nitrosamines and polycyclic aromatic hydrocarbons which cause cancer in animals; they are also linked in epidemiologic studies with cancers of the stomach and esophagus (*The National Academy of Sciences. Nutrition, Diet and Cancer. 1982*).

Observational Study: 1,016 pts. with gastric cancer were studied along with 1,159 population-based controls in high and low risk areas in Italy. Risk of gastric cancer increased with increasing consumption of nitrites. The findings were consistent with the hypothesis that N-nitroso comopounds are involved in gastric cancer risk, as elevated risks were apparent for agents (nitrites, protein) that promote nitrosation, while decreased risks were found for nutrients (vitamin C and vitamin E) which inhibit the process (*Buiatti E et al. A case-control study of gastric cancer and diet in Italy: association with nutrients. Int J Cancer 45:899-901, 1990*).

Negative Observational Study: Nitrates and nitrites were measured in the saliva of 2 populations who differed in their risk of developing gastric cancer. The levels of both ions were significantly higher in the low-risk group, suggesting that, at least in Great Britain, nitrates are not an important cause of gastric cancer (*Forman D et al. Nitrates, nitrites and gastric cancer in Great Britain. Nature 313(6004):620-25, 1985*).

Observational Study: Decreasing gastric cancer rates have been linked to decreasing consumption of nitrates and nitrites, since americans now eat 1/4 the nitrates and nitrites they did in 1925 and there has been a three-fold decrease in stomach cancer mortality since that year. In addition, other countries where more nitrates are eaten have a higher stomach cancer rate (*Environ Med vol. 5, 1983*).

Avoid sugar.

Harmful effects may be either direct or indirect (for example, high sucrose intake is associated with a low intake of fiber).

Breast Cancer:

Animal Experimental Study: Mice which usually have a 50% death rate from breast cancer following injection with an aggressive mammary tumor were split into 3 gps. and given amts. of dietary sugar designed to produce 3 different glycemic levels prior to injection with the tumor. After 70 days, 16/24 (66%) of the mice in the high sugar gp. (ave. blood sugar: 115 mg/dl) died, 8/24 (33%) of mice in the "normal" sugar gp. (ave. blood sugar: 100 mg/dl) died, and only 1/20 (0.05%) of mice in the low sugar gp. (ave. blood sugar: 80 mg/dl) died (p<0.005) (*Santisteban GA et al. Glycemic modulation of tumor tolerance in a mouse model of breast cancer. Biochem Biophys Res Commun 132(3):1174-79, 1985*).

Observational Study: An epidemiologic survey of 21 countries has suggested that high sucrose intake is a major risk factor for the development of breast cancer in women over 45 yrs. of age (*Seely S, Horrobin DF. Diet and breast cancer: The possible connection with sugar consumption. Med Hypotheses 11(3):319-27, 1983*).

Animal Experimental Study: Rats on high sugar diets developed significantly more mammary tumors than those on a high starch diet (*Hoehn SK, Carroll KK. Effects of dietary carbohydrate on the incidence of mammary tumors induced in rats by 7,12-dimethylbenz(a)-anthracene. Nutr Cancer, 1(3):27-30, Spring, 1979*).

Review Article: Human breast cancer mortality shows a positive correlation with dietary sugar, and a negative correlation with complex carbohydrates in the diet (*Carroll KK. Dietary factors in hormone-dependent cancers, in M Winick, Ed. Current Concepts in Nutrition. Volume 6: Nutrition and Cancer. New York, John Wiley & Sons, 1977, pp. 25-40*).

Colorectal Cancer:

Experimental Study: Subjects were placed on a 2-wk. baseline diet followed by a test diet of the same composition, but with an added 120 gm sugar. With the addition of sugar, fecal bile acid concentrations increased and the oro-anal transit time decreased. Bacterial fermentation activity also increased, which was thought to partially explain the increase in total and secondary bile acids in the feces. Since these alterations in colonic activity are associated with elevated risk for colon cancer, sugar may increase the disease risk (*Kruis W et al. Influence of diets high and low in refined sugar on stool qualities, gastrointestinal transit time and fecal bile acid excretion. Gastroenterology 92:1483, 1987*).

Observational Study: The diets of 453 colonic and 365 rectal cancer cases were compared with those of 2,851 population controls. There were no significant differences in the ave. intake of the major nutrients, with the exception of carbohydrates; pts. had a larger intake, limited to oligosaccharides (sugar) (*Tuyns AJ et al. Colorectal cancer and the intake of nutrients: Oligosaccharides are a risk factor, fats are not. A case-control study in Belgium. Nutr Cancer 10:181-96, 1987*).

Observational Study: In comparing the diets of 50 colorectal cancer pts. with those of 50 very closely matched healthy controls, the cancer pts. were found to ingest 14% more energy (p<0.001), mostly in the form of carbohydrate (21% increase; p<0.001) and fat (14% increase; p<0.001). The extra carbohydrate was largely in the form of fiber-depleted sugar (40% increase; p<0.005) and the extra fat as fat/sugar combinations (36% increase; p<0.02). No difference was found in daily intakes of total dietary fiber, cereal fiber, vegetable fiber, natural sugar, or vitamins A,C and D. Energy intake per gm. of dietary fiber was 23% higher in cancer pts. (p<0.0005), suggesting a more refined diet. Thus fiber-depleted foods, especially sugar, may predispose to the development of large bowel cancer (*Bristol JB. Sugar, fat and the risk of colorectal cancer. Br Med J 291:1457, 1985; Bristol JB et al. Colorectal cancer and diet: A case-control study with special reference to dietary fibre and sugar. Proc Am Assoc Cancer Res 26:206, March, 1985*).

Stomach Cancer:

Observational Study: In a German study involving 50,000 households, there was a significant positive association for both men and women between high disaccharide intake and the risk of stomach cancer (*Böing H et al.

Regional nutritional pattern and cancer mortality in the Federal Republic of Germany. Nutr Cancer 7(3):121-30, 1985).

Avoid coffee.

The results of numerous observational studies are contradictory, and it remains unclear whether coffee consumption increases cancer risk.

Review Article: Caffeine has been found to both increase and decrease malignant cell development depending on the carcinogen it is used with, the type of host cell, and the stage of the cell cycle in which it is introduced. No causal relationship has been established between coffee intake and a variety of cancers (*Pozniak PC. The carcinogenicity of caffeine and cancer: A review. J Am Diet Assoc 85(9):1127-33, 1985).*

Intake of milk and dairy products has had both positive and negative associations with cancer.

Positive Association:

Observational Study: The reported milk consumption habits of 3334 pts. and 1300 comparable controls were studied. As a gp., cancer pts. more often reported frequent whole milk consumption; control pts. were more likely to report never drinking whole milk. Some associations were observed for a computed index of milk fat intake, but the overall pattern of effects was not fully explained by variations in fat content (*Mettlin CJ et al. Patterns of milk consumption and risk of cancer. Nutr Cancer 13:89-99, 1990).*

Observational Study: In a case-control study of 235 white women with epithelial ovarian cancer and 239 controls, the relative risk for ovarian cancer was 1.7 for the regular ingestion (≥monthly) of dairy products with prehydrolyzed lactose: yogurt (p=0.01) and 1.4 for cottage cheese (p=0.08); the regular ingestion of other dairy products did not distinguish cases from controls. Yogurt was consumed at least monthly by 49% of cases and 36% of controls. In the upper range of lactose consumption, 22% of cases consumed ≥22 g/d of lactose compared to 16% of controls. The mean RBC galactose-1-phosphate uridyl transferase activity of cases was significantly lower than that of controls, and cases had a mean lactose consumption to transferase activity (L/T) ratio of 1.17 compared to 0.98 for controls. In addition, there was a highly significant trend for increasing ovarian cancer risk with increasing L/T ratio. Since there is evidence that hypergonadotropic hypogonadism is associated with galactose consumption and metabolism, results are compatible with the model of ovarian cancer as a consequence of hypergonadotropic hypogonadism (*Cramer DW et al. Galactose consumption and metabolism in relation to the risk of ovarian cancer. Lancet 2:66-71, 1989).*

Note: This study has been criticized as other striking risk factors were not controlled for: never being pregnant (risk factor 1.86); Jewish (1.7); never married (1.56); and having 4 or more pregnancies (0.58). If marital status and parity are considered, the case-control gp. chosen for comparison cannot differentiate between the effect of yogurt consumption on cancer risk. Also, the differences in blood transferase activity were so small to be of doubtful biological meaning, and there are no data to indicate that ovarian cancer is more common in galactosemic women (Reichlin S. Galactose consumption and risk of ovarian cancer. Letter. Lancet 2:565, 1989).

Negative Association:

Review Article: Epidemiological and experimental studies suggest that dietary milk products may exert an inhibitory effect on the development of several types of tumors. For example, various types of cheeses and yogurt were recently found to suppress the growth of several experimental tumors in mice. Recent studies have also shown improvement in cases of cancer of the oral cavity, stomach, rectum, lung and cervix with increased milk consumption. Experiments suggest that the anti-tumor activity of dairy products is in the whey protein component of the milk which may have both anti-tumor and anti-carcinogenesis effects. Since whey protein is very rich in substrate for glutathione synthesis, whey protein diets result in increased glutathione concentration in certain tissues. Glutathione may have an anti-tumor effect because of its important role in immune enhancement. It may also have an anti-carcinogenic effect by detoxifying potential carcinogens (*Bounous G, Batist G, Gold P. Whey proteins in cancer prevention. Cancer Lett 57:91-4, 1991).*

- -

COMBINED DIETARY FACTORS

"Western-type" diet:

High in fat and protein; low in complex carbohydrate and fiber.

General:

The Western-type diet, rich in proteins and fat and poor in complex carbohydrates and fiber, is associated with high total and nonprotein bound androgens and low sex-hormone-binding globulin, a hormonal pattern which is accentuated in women with breast cancer. This suggests that the increased risk of breast cancer in Western countries could be mediated by effects of diet on hormone levels (*Adlercreutz H et al. Diet and plasma androgens in postmenopausal vegetarian and omnivorous women and postmenopausal women with breast cancer. Am J Clin Nutr 49:433-42, 1989*).

Colorectal Cancer:

Observational Study: Compared to Chinese in the People's Republic of China, Chinese-Americans of similar ages in San Francisco County, California had a 4-fold higher risk of colorectal cancer. The findings suggest that the high-fat, high-protein, low-carbohydrate diet consumed by the Chinese-Americans increases risk, while consumption of the high-carbohydrate diet consumed by the Chinese decreases the risk. In addition, the "westernized" diet was associated with high levels of cholesterol and bile acids in the stool and increased urinary excreton of 3-methylhistidine and malonaldehyde, evidence that perioxidzed fats and meats were consumed (*Yeung K et al. Comparisons of diet and biochemical characteristics of stool and urine between Chinese populations with low and high colorectal cancer rates. J Natl Cancer Inst 83:46-50, 1991*).

- -

VITAMINS

Folic Acid:

Folate deficiency may present a blood picture and bone marrow appearance which can be mistaken for leukemia (*Dokal IS et al. Vitamin B-12 and folate deficiency presenting as leukaemia. Br Med J 300:1263-64, 1990*).

Cervical Cancer

Localized deficiency in cervical epithelial cells may promote cervical dysplasia which may progress to carcinoma of the cervix.

Observational Study: 73% of 57 cervicovaginal smears diagnosed as showing changes characteristic of folic acid deficiency revealed evidence of cervical intraepithelial neoplasia (CIN stage I or II). 40% of the cervical biopsies from the 57 women taken within 2 wks. of the smears revealed focal folic acid deficiency-like changes, and 63% of the biopsies were positive for CIN I-III. Since papilloma-virus cytopathic effects were also present in 52% of the smears, and the folic acid deficiency-like changes in the biopsies were almost always in close proximity to papillomavirus cytopathic changes (which were found in 63%), it is suggested that changes thought to be specific for folic acid deficiency may also be seen in the setting of papillomavirus infection, often with concomitant CIN (*Fekete PS, Hammami A. Folic acid deficiency-like changes in cervicovaginal smears: a possible manifestation of papillomavirus infection? Abstract. Acta Cytologica 31(5):697, 1987*).

Plasma folate levels may be reduced (*Orr JW Jr et al. Nutritional status of patients with untreated cervical cancer. II. Vitamin assessment. Am J Obstet Gynecol 151(5):632-35, 1985*).

Supplementation may reverse megaloblastic changes in cervical epithelial cells despite the lack of evidence of systemic folate deficiency.

Experimental Study: Cervical epithelial cells of women using oral contraceptive agents showed megaloblastic features consistent with folic acid deficiency. Despite the lack of evidence of systemic folate deficiency, these changes disappeared with oral folate supplementation (*Whitehead N et al. Megaloblastic changes in the cervical epithelium: Association with oral contraceptive therapy and reversal with folic acid. JAMA 226:1421-24, 1973*).

Supplementation may reverse dysplastic changes in cervical epithelial cells, at least in women with reduced folate levels.

Experimental Double-blind Study: 47 young women on combination-type birth control pills with mild or moderate dysplasia received either 10 mg oral folate daily or placebo. After 3 mo., cervical biopsies showed significant improvement only in the women receiving folate. Pre-treatment folate levels were lower among contraceptive users than among non-users, and even lower among users with dysplasia. Morphological features of megaloblastosis were associated with dysplasia. The dysplasia completely disappeared in 7 women receiving folate, while 4 women on placebo showed progression to carcinoma *in situ*. Morphological features of megaloblastosis also improved with folate supplementation (*Butterworth CE Jr et al. Improvement in cervical dysplasia associated with folic acid therapy in users of oral contraceptives. Am J Clin Nutr 35(1):73-82, 1982*).

Rectal Cancer

Folic acid intake may inversely correlate with the risk of rectal cancer (*Freudenheim J et al. Folate intake and carcinogenesis of the colon and rectum. Int J Epidemiol 20:368-74, 1991*).

Niacin:

Supplementation may reduce the cardiotoxicity of adriamycin.

Animal Experimental Study: Niacin reduced the cardiotoxicity of adriamycin in mice without interfering with its antitumor activity (*Schmitt-Gräff A, Scheulen ME. Prevention of adriamycin cardiotoxicity by niacin, isocitrate or N-acetyl-cysteine in mice. A morphological study. Pathol Res Pract 181(2):168-74, 1986*).

- and Aspirin:

Combined administration may reduce thrombogenic complications or radiotherapy.

Experimental Controlled Study: 106 pts. with bladder carcinoma (stage T3NxMo) were followed for 3 yrs. after treatment with surgery along with pre- and post-operative gamma-beam radiation therapy. 51/106 also received nicotinic acid and aspirin at common doses to prevent thrombogenic complications, while the other 55 pts. served as controls. Relapses were noted in 33.3% of the experimental gp. compared to 72.5% of the controls. The 5-yr. survival in the treatment gp. was 72.5% compared to 27.4% in the control gp. (*Popov AI. [Effect of the nonspecific prevention of thrombogenic complications on late results in the combined treatment of bladder cancer.] Med Radiol (Mosk) 32(2):42-45, 1987*).

Riboflavin:

Intake may inversely correlate with the risk of prostate cancer (*Kaul L et al. The role of diet in prostate cancer. Nutr Cancer 9:123-28, 1987*).

Blood riboflavin level may inversely correlate with the risk of esophageal cancer (*Guo W et al. Correlations of dietary intake and blood nutrient levels with oesphageal cancer mortality in China. Nutr Cancer 13:121-27, 1990*).

Thiamine:

Intake may inversely correlate with the risk of prostate cancer (*Kaul L et al. The role of diet in prostate cancer. Nutr Cancer 9:123-28, 1987*).

Vitamin A:

Intake may inversely correlate with cancer risk (*see also "Vitamin A and Beta-Carotene" below*).

General Review Article: The association of high retinoid intake with decreased cancer risk may be due to immuno-suppression during vitamin A deficiency or immuno-enhancement during extremely high intakes. High dietary vitamin A enhances macrophage functioning, while retinol suppresses T-lymphocyte function *in vitro* (*Watson R et al. Cancer prevention by retinoids: Role of immunological modification. Nutr Res 5:663-75, 1985*).

Bladder Cancer: *Michalek AM et al. Vitamin A and tumor recurrence in bladder cancer. Cancer 9:143-46, 1987*

Esophageal Cancer:

Negative Observational Study: In a study of 178 pts., an intake >113,000 IU/mo. of retinol was associated with 3 times the risk of an intake of <41,000 IU (*Graham S et al. Nutritional epidemiology of cancer of the esophagus. Am J Epidemiol 131:454-67, 1990*).

Gastric Cancer: *Stehr PA et al. Am J Epidemiol 121:65-70, 1985*

Laryngeal Cancer: *Graham S et al. Dietary factors in the epidemiology of cancer of the larynx. Am J Epidemiol 113(6):675-80, 1981*

Lung Cancer: *Bond GG et al. Dietary vitamin A and lung cancer: Results of a case-control study among chemical workers. Nutr Cancer 9:109-21, 1987*

Prostate Cancer: *Kolonel LN et al. Vitamin A and prostate cancer in elderly men: Enhancement of risk. Cancer Res 47(11):2982-85, 1987*

Plasma/serum retinol levels may inversely correlate with cancer risk.

General:

Observational Study: Serum vitamin A concentrations and subsequent cancer development was monitored in a gp. of 36,265 subjects. 766 cases of cancer were eventually diagnosed. Serum retinol levels were 3.3% lower in men and 2.8% lower in women than in controls. Cancer risk was inversely associated with serum retinol levels (*Knekt P et al. Serum vitamin A and subsequent risk of cancer: Cancer incidence follow-up of the Finnish Mobile Clinic Health Examination Survey. Am J Epidemiol 132:857-70, 1990*).

Cervical Cancer: *Orr JW Jr et al. Nutritional status of patients with untreated cervical cancer. II. Vitamin assessment. Am J Obstet Gynecol 151(5):632-35, 1985*).

Esophageal Cancer: *Lipman T et al. Esophageal zinc content in human squamous esophageal cancer. J Am Coll Nutr 6:41-46, 1987*

Gastric Cancer: *Stähelin HB et al. Cancer, vitamins, and plasma lipids: Propective Basel study. J Natl Cancer Inst 73(6):1463-8, 1984*

Head and Neck Cancer: *de Vries N, Snow GB. Relationships of vitamins A and E and beta-carotene serum levels to head and neck cancer patients with and without second primary tumours. Eur Arch Otorhinolaryngol 247:368-70, 1990*

Lung Cancer: *Kune GA et al. Serum levels of β-carotene, vitamin A and zinc in male lung cancer cases and controls. Nutr Cancer 12:169-76, 1989*

Prostate Cancer: *Hsing A et al. Serologic precursors of cancer: retinol, carotenoids, tocopherol and risk of prostate cancer. J Natl Cancer Inst 82:941-46, 1990; Reichman M et al. Serum vitamin A and subsequent development of prostate cancer in the first National Health and Nutrition Examination Survey Epidemiologic Follow-up Study. Cancer Res 50:2311-15, 1990*

Serum levels of vitamin A and its transport proteins (prealbumin and retinal-binding protein) may be lower in cancer patients due to malnutrition as a consequence of the disease, rather than because of a feature of cancer *per se*.

Observational Study: Compared to 30 healthy subjects, mean serum vitamin A and prealbumin of 30 breast cancer pts. with distal metastases were lower, but the differences were not significant. In regard to retinal-binding protein, the differences between healthy subjects and pts. with either breast cancer or benign breast disease were significant (p<0.05). All differences were reduced by comparing the cancer pts. with the benign breast disease pts. rather than with the healthy controls; however, RBP remained significantly lower. Since RBP is highly sensitive to inadequate protein intake and closely correlated with degree of trauma, this finding may be due to secondary factors rather than to the cancer inself (*Basu TK et al. Serum vitamins A and E, β-carotene, and selenium in patients with breast cancer. J Am Coll Nutr 8(6):524-28,1989*).

Low serum retinol levels are associated with a diminished response to chemotherapy.

Observational Study: Serum alpha-tocopherol and retinol levels of 37 women with breast cancer who were to undergo initial chemotherapy and of 35 controls were analyzed. Among the pts. with serum retinol levels equal to or greater than the control mean, 83% responded to chemotherapy, 17% remained stable and none progressed. Among the pts. with serum retinol levels below the control mean, 36% responded, 24% remained stable and 40% progressed. There were no differences in tocopherol levels between gps., suggesting that differences in retinol are not the result of general nutritional debilitation and that specific nutritional or metabolic differences relating to vitamin A may exist (*Brown RR et al. Correlation of serum retinol levels with response to chemotherapy in breast cancer. Meeting Abstract. Proc Am Assoc Cancer Res 22:184, 1981*).

Administration of vitamin A may prevent and even reverse leukoplakia.

Experimental Double-blind Study: Fishermen in Kerala, India who chewed tobacco-containing betel quids were administered vitamin A 60 mg/wk for 6 mo. Leukoplakia remitted in 57% and micronucleated cells were reduced by 96%; formation of new leukoplakia was completely suppressed. The protective effect could be maintained for at least 8 additional mo. by lower doses (*Stich HF et al. Remission of precancerous lesions in the oral cavity of tobacco chewers and maintenance of the protective effect of β-carotene or vitamin A. Am J Clin Nutr 53:298S-304S, 1991*).

Experimental Study: Natives of Guam, Taiwan, the Philippines, India, Peru and Canada who chew tobacco mixtures were studied. Vitamin A 1-200,000 IU/wk produced a substantial reduction in frequency of micronucleated mucosal cells and remission of leukoplakias within 3-6 mo. of treatment; it also reduced the frequency of new leukoplakias. Micronucleated mucosal cells and leukoplakia returned when the supplements were discontinued. Vitamin A 50,000 IU/wk. maintained the protective effect for the 12-mo. post-treatment period (*Stich H et al. Remission of oral precancerous lesions of tobacco/areca nut chewers following administration of beta carotene or vitamin A, and maintenance of the protective effect. Cancer Det 15:93-8, 1991*).

Administration of vitamin A or of its synthetic analogs may improve the clinical course of certain cancers.

Review Article: A vast amt. of lab data have clearly demonstrated the potent antiproliferative and differentiation - inducing effects of vitamin A and its synthetic analogues. Since several interventional trials have clearly indicated that natural vitamin A at clinically tolerable doses has only limited activity against neoplastic processes, clinical work has focused on synthetic deriviatives. In human cancer prevention, retinoids have been most effective for skin diseases, while several noncutaneous premalignancies are currently receiving more attention. Definite anti-cancer activity has been documented in <u>oral leukoplakia</u>, <u>laryngeal papillomatosis</u>, <u>superficial bladder carcinoma</u>, <u>cervical dysplasia</u>, <u>bronchial metaplasia</u>, and <u>preleukemia</u>. Significant therapeutic advances are also occurring in drug-resistant and refractory malignancies including advanced <u>basal cell cancer</u>, <u>mycosis fungoides</u>, <u>melanoma</u>, <u>acute promyelocytic leukemia</u>, and <u>squamous cell carcinoma</u> (*Lippman SM, Meyskens ML Jr. Vitamin A derivatives in the prevention and treatment of human cancer. J Am Coll Nutr 7(4):269-84, 1988*).

Bladder Cancer:

Experimental Controlled Study: After transurethral resection of superficial bladder tumors, pts. randomly received either Etretinate once daily or no treatment. 85 pts. were in the treatment gp. and 72 pts. were controls. After 2 yrs., the recurrence rate was 18% in the treatment gp. and 38% in the controls (p<0.01).

Etretinate administration had a high recurrence inhibitory effect (p<0.05) in the cases of relapse, multiple tumors, and tumors less than 1 cm. 22.3% of pts. had side effects, primarily dry lips, cheilitis, stomatitis and dermal desquamation (Yoshida O et al. [*Prophylactic effect of etretinate on the recurrence of superficial bladder tumors: Results of a randomized control study.* *Hinyokika Kiyo* 32(9):1349-58, 1986).

Leukemia:

Experimental Study: 2/4 pts. with acute promyelocytic leukemia were treated with isotretinoin (13-*cis*-retinoic acid), and 2/4 were treated with all-*trans*-retinoic acid. All 4 received 45 mg/m^2 daily for 3 months. All 4 pts. were pancytopenic and had bone marrow infiltration with blastic promyelocytes. The 2 pts. treated with isotretinoin were well during treatment with no infection or hemorrhagic syndrome. Peripheral blood counts failed to improve; 1 died of cardiac ischemia on day 65, the other later went into complete remission with conventional chemotherapy. Of the 2 pts. treated with all-*trans*-retinoic acid, the neutrophil count returned to normal on day 9 and 18 and the platelet count returned to normal on day 42 and 24, respectively. Complete response (normal bone marrow maturation and karyotype) was observed on day 62 and 33, respectively. Hemoglobin was corrected by day 60 and 90, respectively. At 9 mo. follow-up, while on maintenance therapy with IM methotrexate and purinethol, both were still in complete remission. In 3 pts. toxicity was limited to dryness of skin and mucosa and minor increases in liver enzymes and triglycerides; the fourth pt. had bone pain from day 4 to day 30 (*Chomienne C et al. Retinoic acid therapy for promyelocytic leukaemia. Letter. Lancet 2:746-47, 1989*).

Experimental Study: 23/24 pts. with acute promyelocytic leukemia treated with the all-*trans*-isomer of retinoic acid 45 mg/m^2 daily obtained complete remission. Disseminated intravascular coagulation either disappeared rapidly or was not observed after treatment onset (*Huang ME et al. Use of all-trans-retinoic acid in the treatment of acute promyelocytic leukemia. Am J Hematol 28:124-27, 1988*).

Skin Cancer:

Experimental Double-blind Study: Following completion of surgery, radiotherapy or both, 103 pts. who were disease-free after primary treatment for squamous-cell cancers of the larynx, pharynx, or oral cavity randomly received either isotretinoin (13-*cis*-retinoic acid) 50-100 mg/m^2 of body-surface area per day or placebo. After 12 mo., there were no significant differences between the 2 gps. in the number of local, regional, or distant recurrences of the primary cancers. However, the isotretinoin gp. had significantly fewer second primary tumors. After a median follow-up of 32 mo., only 2 pts. in the isotretinoin gp. had second primary tumors compared to 12 in the placebo gp. (p=0.005). Multiple second primary tumors occurred in 4 pts., all of whom were in the placebo gp. (*Hong WK et al. Prevention of second primary tumors with isotretinoin in squamous-cell carcinoma of the head and neck. N Engl J Med 323:795-801, 1990*).

- and Beta-carotene:

Combined supplementation may reduce the risk of certain cancers.

Cervical Cancer:

Observational Study: The vitamin A and beta-carotene intake as well as cellular retinol-binding protein (CRBP) levels were assessed for 49 women with dysplastic changes or carcinoma in situ (CIS) and 49 matched controls. Women consuming less than ave. vitamin A and beta-carotene were 3 times as likely to develop severe dysplasia and 2 3/4 times as likely to develop CIS. CRBP levels in the cervical tissue samples were inversely correlated with the severity of the dysplasia (*Wylie-Rosett JA et al. Influence of vitamin A on cervical dysplasia and carcinoma in situ. Nutr Cancer 6(1):49-57, 1984*).

Oral Cancer:

Experimental Double-blind Study: Members of the Phillipine Ifugao tribe who chew betel quid, a tobacco-like plant mixture that promotes cellular damage, received weekly doses of vitamin A 150,000 IU, beta-carotene 180 mg, canthaxanthin 180 mg or placebo. Both at baseline and after 9 wks., 3-5% of the cells from inside the cheek had genetic damage in both the placebo and canthaxanthin groups, while the percentage of damaged cells decreased in the vitamin A gp. from 4% to 2% and in the beta-carotene group from 3.5% to 1%. The lack of protective activity of canthaxanthin, which is a good trapper of singlet oxygen but cannot be converted into vitamin A, suggests that vitamin A and beta-carotene exert their inhibitory effect on the formation of micronuclei by a mechanism not involving the scavenging of free radicals (*Stich HF et al. Use of the micronucleus test to monitor the effect of vitamin A, beta-carotene and canthaxanthin on the buccal mucosa of betel nut/tobacco chewers. Int J Cancer 34(6):745-50, 1984*).

Vitamin B6:

Theoretical Discussion: Since B6 is a co-enzyme in the biosynthesis of thymidine, a deficiency of which can increase mutagenesis, a B6 deficiency along with contact with carcinogens could lead to tumor initiation (*Prior F. Theoretical involvement of vitamin B6 in tumor initiation. Med Hypotheses 16:421-8, 1985*).

Blood levels may be reduced.

> **General Observational Study:** The vitamin B6 status of 12 non-medicated patients (ave. age 58) with newly diagnosed malignancies of the oral cavity, throat, lung, or prostate and bladder was determined by coenzyme stimulation of RBC alanine aminotransferase activity and plasma pyridoxal phosphate level. All subjects had smoked for over 25 years. Typical B6 intakes were close to 2 mg daily. All pts. and none of 3 controls had coenzyme stimulation values indicative of B6 deficiency. Low pyridoxal phosphate levels were observed in 67% of pts. and none of the controls (*Chrisley BM et al. Vitamin B6 status of a group of cancer patients. Nutr Res 6(9):1023-30, 1986*).

> **Cervical Cancer:** *Ramaswamy P, Natarajan R. Vitamin B6 status in patients with cancer of the uterine cervix. Nutr Cancer 6:176-80, 1984*

> **Liver Cancer:** *Zaman SN et al. Vitamin B6 concentrations in patients with chronic liver disease and hepatocellular caricnoma. Br Med J 293:175, 1986*).

Deficiency is associated with enhanced carcinogenesis.

> **Animal Experimental Study:** Mice deficient in vitamin B6 demonstrated enhanced tumor susceptibility, increased tumor size, and a lengthened regression time, probably due to defective cell-mediated processes (*Ha C et al. The effect of B-6 on host susceptibility to Moloney SarcomaVirus-induced tumor growth in mice. J Nutr 114:938-45, 1984*).

Vitamin B12:

A vitamin B12 deficiency may present a blood picture and bone marrow appearance which can be mistaken for leukemia (*Dokal IS et al. Vitamin B-12 and folate deficiency presenting as leukaemia. Br Med J 300:1263-64, 1990*).

- and Folic Acid:

Combined supplementation may reduce cell atypia in bronchial squamous metaplasia, a precancerous condition, in cigarette smokers.

> **Experimental Double-blind Study:** 73 men with metaplasia and a history of 20 or more pack-years of smoking randomly received either 10 mg folate plus 500 µg hydroxycobalamin daily or placebo. After 4 mo., direct cytological examination showed greater reduction of atypia in the treated gp. compared to controls (*Heimburger DC et al. Improvement in bronchial squamous metaplasia in smokers treated with folate and vitamin B12: Report of a preliminary randomized, double-blind intervention trial. JAMA 259(10):1525-30, 1988*).

Vitamin C:

Intake may inversely correlate with cancer risk.

General Review Article: "Approximately 90 epidemiologic studies have examined the role of vitamin C or vitamin C-rich foods in cancer prevention, and the vast majority have found statistically significant protective effects. Evidence is strong for cancers of the esophagus, oral cavity, stomach, and pancreas. There is also substantial evidence of a protective effect in cancers of the cervix, rectum, and breast. Even in lung cancer . . . there is recent evidence of a role for vitamin C" (*Block G. Epidemiologic evidence regarding vitamin C and cancer. Am J Clin Nutr 54:1310S-14S, 1991*).

Breast Cancer:

Review Article: In a review of data from 12 case-controlled studies, about 25% of postmenopausal breast cancers could be prevented with diet. In reviewing data from around the world, vitamin C (as a marker of vegetable and fruit intake) reduced cancer risk in postmenopausal women. Increasing vitamin C intake to 380 mg/d would lower breast cancer rates in the US alone by 16% (*Howe G et al. Dietary factors and risk of breast cancer: Combined analysis of 12 case-control studies. J Natl Cancer Inst 82:561-9, 1990*).

Cervical Cancer: *Verreault R et al. A case-control study of diet and invasive cervical cancer. Int J Cancer 43:1050-54, 1989*

Colorectal Cancer: *Kune S et al. Case-control study of dietary etiological factors: the melbourne colorectal cancer study. Nutr Cancer 9:21-42, 1987*

Esophageal Cancer: *Guo W et al. Correlations of dietary intake and blood nutrient levels with oesphageal cancer mortality in China. Nutr Cancer 13:121-27, 1990*

Gastric Cancer:

Review Article: "Epidemiological studies have consistently shown a strong negative association between ascorbic acid intake and the incidence of gastric cancer. The hypothesis that the endogenous formation of N-nitroso compounds may be an important etiological factor in the pathogenesis of this disease provides a useful model . . . . Ascorbic acid is an effective inhibitor of N-nitrosamine formation *in vitro*. It can also reduce significantly gastric nitrosation in man when taken at moderate doses ($\geq$100 mg). However, there exist a large number of important variables whose influence on the effectiveness of ascorbic acid remain unknown . . . " (*Kyrtopoulos SA. Ascorbic acid and the formation of N-nitroso compounds: possible role of ascorbic acid in cancer prevention. Am J Clin Nutr 45:1344-50, 1987*).

Laryngeal Cancer: *Graham S et al. Dietary factors in the epidemiology of cancer of the larynx. Am J Epidemiol 113(6):675-80, 1981*

Lung Cancer: *Fontham ETH et al. Dietary vitamins A and C and lung cancer risk in Louisiana. Cancer 62:2267-73, 1988*

Plasma/serum ascorbic acid levels may be lower in cancer patients than in normals.

General Observational Study: In a survey and 13-yr. follow-up of 4,224 men, plasma vitamin C was consistently significantly lower in cancer pts. than in controls; the lowest value was found for gastric cancer and corresponded to a below-ave. consumption of citrus fruits (*Stähelin HB et al. Cancer, vitamins, and plasma lipids: Prospective Basel study. J Natl Cancer Inst 73(6):1463-8, 1984*).

Cervical Cancer: *Orr JW Jr et al. Nutritional status of patients with untreated cervical cancer. II. Vitamin assessment. Am J Obstet Gynecol 151(5):632-35, 1985*

Plasma ascorbic acid may be inversely correlated with cancer risk.

General Observational Study: In a prospective study of 3000 males, baseline plasma vitamin C was significantly lower for subjects who later developed cancers (*Gey KF et al. Plasma levels of antioxidant vitamins in relation to ischemic heart disease and cancer. Am J Clin Nutr 45(5 Suppl):1368-77, 1987*).

Urinary ascorbic acid may be depressed in bladder cancer (*Schlegel JU et al. The role of ascorbic acid in the prevention of bladder tumor formation. J Urol 103(2):155-59, 1970*).

Leukocyte ascorbic acid may be low in <u>familial adenomatous polyposis</u> (*Spigelman A et al. Vitamin C levels in patients with familial adenomatous polyposis. Br J Surg 77:508-09, 1990*).

Supplementation may inhibit the development of <u>large bowel polyps</u> (which may become cancerous) in predisposed patients.

> **Experimental Double-blind Study:** In a 2-yr. randomized study, 19 pts. with polyposis coli received ascorbic acid 3g/d while 17 received placebo. At 9 mo. of follow-up, there was a reduction in polyp area in the treated gp. (p<0.03). There were also trends toward reduction in both number and area of rectal polyps during the middle of the trial. A labeling study of rectal epithelium with tritiated thymidine also hinted at a treatment effect (*Bussey HJ et al. A randomized trial of ascorbic acid in polyposis coli. Cancer 50(7):1434-39, 1982*).

- and <u>Vitamin E</u>:

> **Negative Experimental Double-blind Study:** In a 4-yr. study, 58 pts. with familial adenomatous polyposis randomly received ascorbic acid 4 g/d plus alpha-tocopherol 400 mg/d either with a low-fiber cereal or with a grain fiber supplement (Kellogg's All-Bran 22.5 g/d), or received placebo capsules and a low-fiber cereal. Vitamins C and E showed virtually no effect (*DeCosse JJ et al. Effect of wheat fiber and vitamins C and E on rectal polyps in patients with familial adenomatous polyposis. J Natl Cancer Inst 81(17):1290-97, 1989*).

> **Experimental Double-blind Study:** 129 pts. believed to be free of polyps after removal of at least one adenomatous colorectal polyp randomly received either ascorbic acid 400 mg and alpha-tocopherol 400 mg or placebo. After 2 yrs., polyps were observed during colonoscopy in 40.4% of 70 treated pts. and in 50.7% of 67 controls. After adjustment for differences between gps. in demographic and dietary factors before study entry, the relative risk of polyp occurrence was 0.86 (95% confidence limits 0.51-1.45). Results suggest that any reduction in the rate of polyp recurrence is small, and a larger study would be required to ensure that an effect of this size was not due to chance (*McKeown-Eyssen G et al. A randomized trial of vitamins C and E in the prevention of recurrence of colorectal polyps. Cancer Res 48(16):4701-05, 1988*).

Supplementation may be beneficial in cancer treatment.

> **Case Report:** A 70 year old white male had a radical nephrectomy for adenocarcinoma of the kidney. Three mo. later, he developed multiple lesions in the lungs and liver and perioartic lymphadenopathy and started on IV vitamin C 30 g twice weekly. A few weeks later his exam was totally normal with a dramatic improvement in pulmonary nodules and complete resolution of the periaortic lymphadenopathy on x-ray. On follow-ups extending 3 and 1/2 yrs., he has been free of all evidence of cancer (*Riordan HD et al. Case study: High-dose intravenous vitamin C in the treatment of a patient with adenocarcinoma of the kidney. J Orthomol Med 5(1):5-7, 1990*).

> **Negative Experimental Double-blind Study:** 100 advanced <u>large bowel cancer</u> pts. who had received no chemotherapy were treated with either vitamin C 10 gms daily for a median of 2.5 months or placebo. There were no differences in survival rates between the 2 gpts., although none of the pts. on vitamin C died while taking it (*Moertel CG et al. High-dose vitamin C versus placebo in the treatment of patients with advanced cancer who have had no prior chemotherapy: A randomized double-blind comparison. N Engl J Med 312:137-141, 1985*).

>> *Note: In rebuttal, Linus Pauling Ph.D. claims that the negative results were due to premature discontinuation of vitamin C after 2.5 months which, in addition to not providing sufficient time for vitamin C to demonstrate its effectiveness, caused a rebound effect which may have worsened the patients' status. He concludes that the Moertel study only shows that vitamin C should not be given to cancer patients for a short time and then withdrawn (Int Clin Nutr Rev 5(4):163-5, 1985).*

> **Review Article:** *In vitro* and *in vivo* results suggest that sodium ascorbate could be useful in the management of neoplasms. Vitamin C may kill certain tumor cells, may increase the cell killing effect of certain tumor therapeutic agents and may stimulate the host's immune system against the residual tumor cells. *In vitro* data also suggest that the irrational use of vitamin C may be harmful; thus further study of its effects using animal tumor models must be done before assaying its role in the treatment of cancer (*Prasad KN. Modulation of the effects of tumor therapeutic agents by vitamin C. Life Sci. 27(4):275-80, 1980*).

Negative Experimental Double-blind Study: 150 pts. with advanced cancer received ascorbic acid 10 gm or placebo. Sixty "evaluable" pts. received vitamin C and 63 similar randomized pts. received a lactose placebo, while 27 of the randomized pts. elected not to participate. All but 9 of the 123 pts. had previously received radiation, chemotherapy, or both. Neither vitamin C nor placebo improved survival times which averaged 51 days; however those who withdrew only survived 25 days, raising the question as to how the decision to withdraw may have influenced survival. The authors note that, in contrast to the earlier Pauling and Cameron study, a larger proportion of pts. in this study had received radiation and/or chemotherapy (*Creagan ET et al. N Engl J Med 301:687-90, 1979*).

Experimental Controlled Study: Vitamin C 10 gm daily in divided doses was given orally to "hopelessly ill" patients. Mean survival times were 300 days longer when they were compared to historical controls. Survival for longer than 1 yr. after the "date of untreatability" was observed in 22% of the experimental gp. but only 0.4% of historical controls. In addition, 370 non-random concurrent controls showed the same survival statistics (*Cameron E, Pauling L. Supplemental ascorbate in the supportive treatment of cancer: Reevaluation of prolongation of survival times in terminal human cancer. Proc Natl Acad Sci U S A 75:4538-42, 1978; Cameron E, Pauling L. Supplemental ascorbate in the supportive treatment of cancer: Prolongation of survival times in terminal human cancer. Proc Natl Acad Sci U S A 73:3685-9, 1976*).

> *Note: This study has been criticized on the following grounds:*
> *1. Lack of a prospective random double-blind study.*
> *2. Lack of rigidly-defined criteria for untreatability.*
> *3. Failure to match pts. by histological identification of type and origin of cancer cells.*
> *4. Failure to ensure that cases and controls adhere to their medication schedules.*
> *(Comroe J Jr. Proc Natl Acad Sci U S A 75:4543, 1978).*

Supplementation may reduce adriamycin toxicity.

Animal Experimental Study: Ascorbic acid had no effect on the anti-tumor activity of adriamycin (ADR) in mice inoculated with leukemia L1210 or Ehrlich ascites carcinoma, but it significantly prolonged the life of animals treated with ADR. Also, significant prevention of ADR-induced cardiomyopathy in guinea pigs by ascorbic acid was proven by electron microscopy (*Shimpo K et al. Ascorbic acid and adriamycin toxicity. Am J Clin Nutr 54:1298S-1301S, 1991*).

Supplementation may enhance the effect of radiation therapy.

Experimental Controlled Study: 50 previously untreated pts. randomly received radiation therapy either with or without vitamin C 5 g daily in divided doses. After 1 mo., 87% of the study gp. compared to 55% of the controls showed a complete response to treatment (disappearance of all known disease). After 4 mo., 63% of the study gp. compared to 45% of the controls continued to show a complete response. After 1 mo., progressive disease was seen in 3% of the study gp. and 5% of the controls; after 4 mo. progressive disease was seen in 20% of the study gp. compared to 7% of the controls. In the control gp., the 6-mo. survival rate was 45% in pts. without disease and 55% in those with disease; in the study gp. it was 67% in those without disease and 33% in those with disease. In addition subjective responses favored vitamin C including pain and anorexia. A comparison of other objective parameters such as weight loss and anemia also favored vitamin C (*Gupta S. Effect of radiotherapy on plasma ascorbic acid concentration in cancer patients. Unpublished thesis - summarized in Hanck AB. Vitamin C and Cancer. Prog Clin Biol Res 259:307-20, 1988*).

Supplementation may reduce the risk of stomach cancer.

Review Article: It has been repeatedly demonstrated that nitrites and nitrates can be converted to carcinogenic nitrosamines and nitrosamides and that vitamin C can block these conversions *in vitro* and *in vivo*. In addition, supplementation with vitamin C has been associated with decreased mutagenicity of gastric juice and several epidemiological studies have shown reduced risk of gastric cancer in populations consuming high levels of foods rich in vitamin C. Also, atrophic gastritis, while not a precancerous condition, may develop to metaplasia and dysplasia, and epidemiological studies have suggested that dietary vitamin C reduces the risk of its development (*Singh VN, Gaby SK. Premalignant lesion: role of antioxidant vitamins and β-carotene in risk reduction and prevention of malignant transformation. Am J Clin Nutr 53:386S-90S, 1991*).

- and <u>Vitamin B$_{12}$</u>:

Combined supplementation may inhibit carcinogenesis.

Animal Experimental Study: Inhibited the mitotic activity of transplantable mouse tumors and produced a 100% survival rate, while neither vitamin alone at the same dosage had any effect on mitosis or morphology of the cells studied. Microscopic exam of ascites fluid from treated mice showed a few tumor cells in various stages of disintegration which later disappeared (*Poydock ME et al. Inhibiting effect of vitamins C and B$_{12}$ on the mitotic activity of ascites tumors. <u>Exp Cell Biol</u> 47(3):210-17, 1979*).

- and <u>Vitamin K</u>:

Combined supplementation may have a synergistic effect in inhibiting cancer cell growth.

In vitro Experimental Study: When given separately, vitamin C or K$_3$ had a growth inhibiting action against cultured human breast cancer, oral epidermoid carcinoma, and endometrial cells only at high concentrations. When combined, however, they had a synergistic effect, with inhibition of cell growth occurring at 10-50 times lower concentrations. At these lower concentrations, they have no apparent toxicity (*Noto V et al. Effects of sodium ascorbate (vitamin C) and 2-methyl-1,4-naphthoquinone (vitamin K$_3$) treatment on human tumor cell growth in vitro. I. Synergism of combined vitamin C and K$_3$ action. <u>Cancer</u> 63:901-06, 1989*).

Vitamin D:

Intake may inversely correlate with the risk of <u>colon cancer</u> (*Garland CF, Garland FC, Gorham ED. Can colon cancer incidnece and death rates be reduced with calcium and vitamin D? <u>Am J Clin Nutr</u> 54:193S-201S, 1991*).

Serum level may inversely correlate with the risk of <u>colon cancer</u> (*Garland CF et al. Serum 25-hydroxyvitamin D and colon cancer: Eight-year prospective study. <u>Lancet</u> 1176-78, 1989*).

Patients whose <u>breast cancers</u> have vitamin D receptors survive longer than those with receptor-negative tumors, possibly because of the antiproliferative effect of vitamin D (*Colston KW et al. Possible role for vitamin D in controlling breast cancer cell proliferation. <u>Lancet</u> 1:188-91, 1989*).

1,25 dihydroxy vitamin D$_3$ inhibits cancer cell proliferation in melanoma, breast, bone and leukemia cells *in vitro* (*Editorial. Vitamin D: New perspectives. <u>Lancet</u> 1:1122-23, 1987*). However, it remains to be established whether vitamin D or its analogues can produce significant antitumor effects without unacceptable toxicity (*Colston KW et al. Possible role for vitamin D in controlling breast cancer cell proliferation. <u>Lancet</u> 1:188-91, 1989; Reichel H et al. The role of the vitamin D endocrine system in health and disease. <u>N Engl J Med</u> 320(15):980-91, 1989*).

Vitamin E:

Intake may inversely correlate with cancer risk.

Cervical Cancer: *Verreault R et al. A case-control study of diet and invasive cervical cancer. <u>Int J Cancer</u> 43:1050-54, 1989*

Gastric Cancer: *Buiatti E et al. A case-control study of gastric cancer and diet in Italy: association with nutrients. <u>Int J Cancer</u> 45:899-901, 1990*

Skin Cancer: *Stryker W et al. Diet, plasma levels of beta carotene and alpha tocopherol, and risk of malignant melanoma. <u>Am J Epidemiol</u> 13:597-611, 1990*

Serum levels may inversely correlate with cancer risk.

General:

Observational Study: Prediagnostic serum samples from 766 cases of cancer and 1419 matched controls were assayed. Individuals with a low level of α-tocopherol had about a 1.5-fold risk of cancer compared to those with a higher level. The strength of the association between serum α-tocopherol level and cancer risk varied for different cancer sites and was strongest for some GI tract cancers and for the combined gp. of cancers unrelated to smoking. The association was strongest among nonsmoking men and among women with low levels of serum selenium (*Knekt P et al. Vitamin E and cancer prevention. Am J Clin Nutr 53:283S-6S, 1991*).

Bowel Cancer: *Stahelin HB et al. J Natl Cancer Inst 73:1463-8, 1984.*

Breast Cancer: *Wald NJ et al. Plasma retinol, beta-carotene and vitamin E levels in relation to the future risk of breast cancer. Br J Cancer 49:321-4, 1984*

Cervical Cancer: *Palan PR et al. Plasma levels of antioxidant beta-carotene and alpha-tocopherol in uterine cervix dysplasias and cancer. Nutr Cancer 15:13-20, 1991*

Head and Neck Cancer: *de Vries N, Snow GB. Relationships of vitamins A and E and beta-carotene serum levels to head and neck cancer patients with and without second primary tumours. Eur Arch Otorhinolaryngol 247:368-70, 1990*

Lung Cancer: *LeGardeur BY et al. A case-control study of serum vitamins A, E, and C in lung cancer patients. Nutr Cancer 14:133-40, 1990*

Skin Cancer: *Stryker W et al. Diet, plasma levels of beta carotene and alpha tocopherol, and risk of malignant melanoma. Am J Epidemiol 13:597-611, 1990*

Supplementation may reduce cancer risk.

General:

Animal Experimental Study: Following topical DMBA application to the buccal pouch, numerous large tumors were observed in unsupplemented hamsters. In contrast, none of the DMBA-treated, vitamin E-supplemented animals had grossly visible tumors. There was evidence of dysplasia and carcinoma in situ undergoing degenerative changes. The gross, histologic and immunohistochemical results are persuasive evidence for a relationship between immunostimulation by vitamin E and the prevention of tumor development by the immune-mediated destruction of early foci of dysplasia and carcinoma in situ (*Shklar G et al. Prevention of experimental cancer and immunostimulation by vitamin E (immunosurveillance). J Oral Pathol Med 19:60-64, 1990*).

Breast Cancer:

Theoretical Discussion: Tocopherol can reduce the incidence of mammary tumors in experimental animal models and there is human data indicating that tocopherol supplementation may benefit benign breast disease and mammary dysplasia, both of which are associated with an increased risk of breast cancer. Clinical trials are needed to test the hypothesis that vitamin E will reduce breast cancer risk (*London RS et al. Breast cancer prevention by supplemental vitamin E. J Am Coll Nutr 4(5):559-64, 1985*).

Colon Cancer:

Experimental Study: Vitamin E supplements reduced stool mutagen levels by as much as 79% (*Bruce WR, Dion PW. Studies relating to a fecal mutagen. Am J Clin Nutr 33:2511-12, 1980*).

- and <u>Vitamins A and C</u>:

Experimental Controlled Study. 72 pts. who had recently had adenomatous polyps removed received vitamin A 30,000 IU, vitamin C 1 gm and vitamin E 70 mg for up to 2 yrs., while an additional 78 pts. did not receive treatment. Among pts. followed for 12-18 mo. who received vitamins, 7.6% experienced recurrence of polyps compared to 41% of controls (*Deleon M et al. Vitamin A, vitamin C, and vitamin E and lactulose in the prevention of recurrence of adenomatous polyps: Preliminary results of a controlled study. Meeting Abstract. Gut 30:1511-12, 1989*).

Liver Cancer:

Animal Experimental Study: Results of studies of experimental hepatocarcinogenesis in rats suggest that vitamin E could prevent the very early events (the induction of phenotypically-altered foci), but could no longer affect the later stages (the evolution of foci into persistent nodules) (*Ura H et al. Effect of vitamin E on the induction and evolution of enzyme-altered foci in the liver of rats treated with diethylnitrosamine. Carcinogenesis 8:1595-1600, 1987*).

Supplementation may reduce the risk of stomach cancer.

Review Article: Vitamin E is effective in preventing the nitrosation of amino substances under physiological conditions. Data strongly suggest that alpha-tocopherol, when ingested simultaneously with food, may reduce human exposure to carcinogenic N-Nitrosamine (*Lathia D, Blum A. Role of vitamin E as nitrite scavenger and N-nitrosamine inhibitor: a review. Int J Vitam Nutr Res 59(4):430-38, 1989*).

Supplementation by local injection may promote regression of experimental oral cancer.

Animal Experimental Study: Following the experimental induction of epidermoid carcinomas in the buccal pouch of hampsters, vitamin E was injected locally twice weekly in 20 of the animals. After 4 wks., microscopic examination of the buccal pouches of treated animals showed small epidermoid carcinomas with degeneration of tumor cells and a dense infiltrate of leukocytes, lymphocytes, and histiocytes. Buccal pouches of control animals showed large, well-differentiated or moderately differentiated epidermoid carcinomas (*Shklar G et al. Regression by vitamin E of experimental oral cancer. J Natl Cancer Inst 78(5):987-92, 1987*).

Supplementation may enhance the effect of chemotherapeutic drugs.

Adriamycin (Doxorubicin):

In vitro Experimental Study: The growth of human prostatic carcinoma cells in culture was inhibited by both adriamycin and vitamin E in a dose-related manner. The effect of vitamin E was additive or synergistic depending upon dosage. Vitamin E, even in higher concentrations, had minimal inhibitory effects on normal mouse fibroblasts, despite its marked toxicity for several malignant cell types (*Ripoll EAP et al. Vitamin E enhances the chemotherapeutic effects of adriamycin on human prostatic carcinoma cells in vitro. J Urol 136:529-31, 1986*).

Vincristine:

In vitro Experimental Study: Vitamin E enhanced the growth inhibitory effect of vincristine on mouse melanoma cells (*Prasad KN et al. Vitamin E increases the growth inhibitory and differentiating effects of tumor therapeutic agents on neuroblastoma and glioma cells in culture. Proc Soc Exp Biol Med 164(2):158-63, 1980*).

Supplementation may protect against the adverse side-effects of chemotherapeutic drugs.

Adriamycin (Doxorubicin):

Negative Experimental Double-blind Study: 25 pts. randomly received either vitamin E 1600 IU daily or placebo (vitamin C 400 IU daily) 0-3 days prior to treatment with doxorubicin. The results failed to support the efficacy of vitamin E as protection against doxorubicin-induced alopecia. However, hair retention was great enough in several pts. receiving vitamin E to perhaps warrant further study of vitamin E plus scalp hypothermia (*Ingle R, Johnson DH. Failure of high-dose vitamin E to prevent doxorubicin-induced alopecia. Abstract. Oncol Nurs Forum 15(2, Suppl):163, 1988*).

Note: This study failed to follow the recommendation of the authors of the earlier positive study (see directly below) that vitamin E must be started 5-7 days prior to chemotherapy.

Negative Experimental Controlled Study: D,L-alpha tocopherol acetate 1600 IU starting 7 days prior to chemotherapy was ineffective in preventing adriamycin-induced alopecia (*Martin-Jimenez M et al. Failure of high-dose tocopherol to prevent alopecia induced by doxorubicin. Letter. N Engl J Med 315(14):894-95, 1986*).

Negative Experimental Study: 20 pts. with different types of solid tumors began alpha-tocopherol acetate 400 IU every 6 hours. Seven days later, they began adriamycin 50-60 mg/m^2/cycle of treatment. The vitamin was administered until hair loss developed and then stopped. 18 pts. (90%) had hair loss requiring the use of a wig, and 2 (10%) had minor hair loss. It was concluded that vitamin E was ineffective in preventing hair loss under these conditions (*Perez JE et al. High-dose alpha-tocopherol as a preventative of doxorubicin-induced alopecia. Cancer Treat Rep 70:1213-14, 1986*).

Experimental Study: 69% of pts. on adriamycin 40 mg/m^2/treatment cycle receiving 1600 IU D,L-alpha tocopherol acetate daily did not develop alopecia. Those who did develop alopecia were believed to have received vitamin E too late before chemotherapy, as it should be started 5-7 days prior to commencement (*Wood L. Possible prevention of adriamycin-induced alopecia by tocopherol. Letter. N Engl J Med 312(16):1060, 1985*).

Bleomycin:

Animal Experimental Study: Vitamin E reduced bleomycin-induced lung fibrosis in mice (*Prasad KN et al. Vitamin E increases the growth inhibitory and differentiating effects of tumor therapeutic agents on neuroblastoma and glioma cells in culture. Proc Soc Exp Biol Med 164(2):158-63, 1980*).

- with Beta-carotene:

Supplementation may act synergistically to regress tumors.

Animal Experimental Study: A combination of vitamin E succinate and beta-carotene administered orally in vegetable oil was effective in regressing induced epidermoid cancers of the hamster buccal pouch. Tumors continued to increase in size in untreated animals and in hamsters supplemented orally with vitamin E or beta-carotene, although the tumors were not as extensive in the vitamin E or beta-carotene-treated animals (*Shklar G et al. Regression of experimental cancer by oral administration of combined alpha-tocopherol and beta-carotene. Nutr Cancer 12:321-25, 1989*).

- -

MINERALS

GENERAL:

Drink hard versus soft water.

Observational Study: Repeated negative correlations were found to occur, at both the national and provincial levels, between Canadian mortality from cancers of the digestive tract and calcium, magnesium and lithium levels in drinking water. As a consequence, water hardness is also inversely correlated with these diseases (*Norie IH, Foster HD. Water quality and cancer of the digestive tract: The Canadian experience. J Orthomol Med 4(2):59-69, 1989*).

Observational Studies: People drinking soft water have a higher incidence of colon cancer, while those eating high calcium diets have a lower incidence of colon cancer (*Science News 3/2/85 p. 141 and 9/21/85 p. 187*).

Note: Since absorption of elements in drinking water is usually twice that of foods (as there are no chelating agents present), they may have a greater influence than if in foods. Water hardness is usually caused by dissolved calcium and magnesium although, in a few areas, hardness may also result from iron or aluminum salts. The concentrations of these elements is usually small in relation to that in the food. The beneficial influence of water hardness may be from alkalinity or from competition between divalent ions. Toxic elements, such as lead and cadmium, may be leached from pipes in soft water areas because of low pH; also, the intestinal absorption of lead and cadmium may be retarded by the presence of competing ions in hard water, i.e. calcium and magnesium. (Borgman RF. Dietary factors in essential hypertension. Prog Food Nutr Sci 9:109-47, 1985).

Calcium:

Cancer may be associated with hypercalcemia.

> **Review Article:** 5% of hospital pts. with a malignancy have hypercalcemia. One of the current theories suggests that a protein-like parathyroid hormone is produced by the tumor; the other postulates the release of bone-resorbing cytokines from secondary tumors in the bone (*Heath DA. Hypercalcaemia in malignancy: Fluids and biphosphonate are best when life is threatened. Br Med J 298:1468-69, 1989*).

Administration may enhance the efficacy of radiation therapy.

> **Experimental Study:** Administration of calcium dihydromonophosphate enhanced the efficacy of radiotherapy in patients with tumors of the <u>bones</u> and <u>vulva</u> (*Iakovkeva SS. [Use of calcium salts in treatment of malignant tumors.] Arkh Patol 42(9):93-94, 1980*).

Colon Cancer

Calcium nutriture may inversely correlate with cancer risk (*Sorenson AW et al. Calcium and colon cancer: A review. Nutr Cancer 11:135-45, 1988*).

> **Review Article:** "Calcium likely reduces lipid damage in the colon by complexing with fat to form mineral-fat complexes or soaps. It has been shown in an increasing number of animal experiments that calcium has the ability to inhibit colon cancer. In limited studies in man, the colon hyperproliferation associated with increased risk for colon cancer has been reversed for short periods by administration of supplemental dietary calcium" (*Wargovich MJ, Lynch PM, Levin B. Modulating effects of calcium in animal models of colon carcinogenesis and short-term studies in subjects at increased risk for colon cancer. Am J Clin Nutr 54:202S-5S, 1991*).

Supplementation may reduce the adverse effects of bile acids and free ionized fatty acids in the colon, thus reducing their mutagenic effect and reducing the risk of colon cancer (*Appleton GV et al. Inhibition of intestinal carcinogenesis by dietary supplementation with calcium. Br J Surg 74(6):523-25, 1987; Buset M et al. Protection from toxicity of biliary and fatty acids on human colonic epithelial cells by calcium. Abstract. Proc Annu Meet Am Assoc Cancer Res 30:A1930, 1989; Newmark HL et al. Colon cancer and dietary fat, phosphate, and calcium: A hypothesis. J Natl Cancer Inst 72(6):1323-25, 1984*).

> **Negative Observational Study:** In a prospective study, subjects with sigmoid colon cancer had lower fat intakes than the other subjects; thus the protective effect of calcium appears unrelated to fat intake. Also, analysis of the interaction between total calcium and fat intake on colon cancer risk showed no significant effect (*Stemmermann G et al. The influence of dairy and nondairy calcium on subsite large-bowel cancer risk. Dis Colon Rectum 33:190-94, 1990*).

Supplementation may reduce the mucosal hyperproliferative state in high-risk patients.

> **Experimental Study:** Ornithine decarboxylase is an enzyme involved in polyamine synthesis which is related to mucosal hyperproliferation. 7 men with existing adenomatous polyps or a history of adenomas received calcium carbonate 1,250 mg daily. After 1 wk., mean ODC activity of colonic mucosa decreased by half in 4/7 pts. (*Dr. Freda Arlow, Henry Ford Hospital, Detroit - Presentation at the Am. Coll. of Gastroenterology meeting, 1989*).

> **Review Article:** Short term studies *in vitro* and *in vivo* of the proliferative behavior of human and animal colon mucosa indicate that calcium modulates proliferative response, and preliminary clinical studies suggest that the hyperproliferative mucosa of pts. at high risk for colon cancer may become decidedly less proliferative when subjects are given oral calcium (*Wargovich MJ. Calcium and colon cancer. J Am Coll Nutr 7(4):295-300, 1988*).

Experimental and In vitro Studies: 9 pts. at high risk for developing colon cancer received 1.5 gm calcium daily. After 4-8 wks., the colonic epithelial cells in 6/9 pts. showed a statistically significant decrease in their [3H]thymidine labeling indices in tissue culture so that they resembled those of pts. at low risk of developing colon cancer. Biopsies from each of the 9 pts. exhibited a decrease in proliferation when they were cultured *in vitro* with a high level of $CaCl_2$ (2.2 mM compared to 0.1 mM, the optimum value for proliferation). 2 adenomas and 2 carcinomas, in contrast to normal cells, exhibited no growth inhibition at this level, however, indicating that the growth inhibition induced by high extracellular calcium levels is lost at a stage in tumor development before cells become malignant (*Buset M et al. Inhibition of human colonic epithelial cell proliferation in vivo and in vitro by calcium. <u>Cancer Res</u> 46(10):5426-30, 1986*

Experimental Study: Patterns of proliferation of the epithelial cells lining colonic crypts in rectal mucosal biopsies of 10 pts. with family histories of colon cancer were examined and found to be characteristic of pts. with familial colon cancer. They were given 1.25 gm calcium daily and, after 2-3 mo., the number of rapidly proliferating cells in their colonic epithelium had significantly decreased and was almost the same as in people at low risk for colon cancer (*Lipkin M, Newmark H. Effect of added dietary calcium on colonic epithelial-cell proliferation in subjects at high risk for familial colonic cancer. <u>N Engl J Med</u> 313:1381-4, 1985*).

- and <u>Phosphorus</u>:

Low dietary calcium to phosphorus ratios are associated with an increased cancer risk (*Lipkin M, Newmark H. Effect of added dietary calcium on colonic epithelial-cell proliferation in subjects at high risk for familial colonic cancer. <u>N Engl J Med</u> 313:1381-4, 1985*).

- and <u>Vitamin D</u>:

Intake may inversely correlate with cancer risk.

Theoretical Discussion: "Epidemiological evidence now suggests that control of colon cancer with calcium and/or vitamin D may be possible. . . . With regard to efficacy, calcium intakes of 1800 mg/d in men and 1500 mg/d in women would appear to be suitable targets for reducing the incidence of colon cancer. . . . The epidemiologic data suggest that sufficient vitamin D from ultraviolet light or from the diet that would raise the serum 25-hydroxyvitamin D concentration to the 67-102 nmol/L range would the reduce the incidence of colon cancer markedly. . . . Large-scale trials are urgently needed" (*Garland CF, Garland FC, Gorham ED. Can colon cancer incidence and death rates be reduced with calcium and vitamin D? <u>Am J Clin Nutr</u> 54:193S-201S, 1991*).

Endometrial Cancer

Intake may inversely correlate with cancer risk.

Observational Study: In a study of the diets of 168 women with endometrial cancer and of 334 controls, calcium intake was inversely associated with endometrial cancer, as was consumption of yogurt or cheese at least once a month (*Barbone F et al. Diet and endometrial cancer. Abstract. <u>Am J Epidemiol</u> 132:783, 1990*).

- and <u>Vitamin D</u>:

Administration may increase the efficacy of chemotherapy.

Experimental Study: Administration of calcium gluconate and lactate in combination with vitamin D was found to enhance the efficacy of thioTEPA and other antineoplastic agents against <u>Hodgkin's disease</u> and <u>lung cancer</u> (*Iakovkeva SS. [Use of calcium salts in treatment of malignant tumors.] <u>Arkh Patol</u> 42(9):93-94, 1980*).

<u>Chlorine</u>:

WARNING: Consumption of chlorinated tap water is correlated with the risk of <u>bladder cancer</u>.

Observational Study: The relationship between chlorinated tap water intake and bladder cancer was assessed by comparing about 3000 cases among Caucasians living in 10 areas of the US with about 5500 controls. Risk of bladder cancer increased with intake level of beverages made with tap water. The odds ratio for the highest vs. lowest quintile of tap water consumption was 1.43 (95% confidence interval). The risk gradient with intake was restricted to persons with at least a 40-yr. exposure to chlorinated surface water and was not found among long-term users of nonchlorinated ground water. Duration of exposure to chlorinated surface water was associated with bladder cancer risk among women and nonsmokers of both sexes. Results are consistent with environmental chemistry and toxicologic data demonstrating the presence of genotoxic by-products of chlorine disinfection in treated surface waters (*Cantor KP et al. Bladder cancer, drinking water source, and tap water consumption: A case-control study. J Natl Cancer Inst 79(6):1269-79, 1987*).

Copper:

Depressed tissue copper levels are found in some types of malignancies, most of which are of the catabolic or highly metastatic type (*Watts DL. The nutritional relationships of copper. J Orthomol Med 4(2):99-108, 1989*).

Serum copper levels may rise during the growth of some malignancies and return to normal with remission (*Aspin N, Sass-Kortsak A. Copper, in F Bronner, J Coburn, Eds. Disorders of Mineral Metabolism Volume I. Trace Minerals. New York, Academic Press, 1981; Dickerson JWT. Nutrition of the cancer patient, in HH Draper, Ed. Advances in Nutritional Research, Volume 5. New York, Plenum Press, 1983*).

Observational Study: In a study of 100 pts., malignant tissue concentrations of copper averaged 46% higher than those of normal tissues (*Margalioth EJ et al. Copper and zinc levels in normal and malignant tissues. Cancer 52:868-72, 1983*).

Administration of copper salicylates may be beneficial.

Animal Experimental Study: The addition of copper salicylates decreased tumor growth, decreased metastases, and increased survival of animals with certain types of neoplasms (*Sorenson RJ et al. Antineoplastic activities of some copper salicylates, in DD Hemphill, Ed. Trace Substances in Environmental Health XVI. Columbia, Missouri, University of Missouri, 1982*).

Fluorine:

WARNING: Ingestion may be carcinogenic.

Review Article: Results of a National Toxicity Program (US) study suggest that fluoride may cause bone cancer in rodents; however these results are only very preliminary. This study was mandated by the US Congress in 1977 following a report of a 5% increase in cancer rates in cities having fluoridated water supplies. Subsequent studies by other investigators, however, have failed to confirm those findings (*Fluoride linked to bone cancer in federal study. Med Trib December 28, 1989*).

In vitro Experimental Study: 45-135 ppm fluoride (as NaF) caused a dose-dependent unscheduled DNA synthesis in human oral keratinocytes within 4 hours (*Tsutsui T et al. Induction of unscheduled DNA synthesis in cultured human oral keratinocytes by sodium fluoride. Mutation Res. 140:43-48, 1984*).

Note: The concentration of NaF in toothpaste and mouthwash is 23 times this high, suggesting that both may be carcinogenic (Sutton PRN. Letter. N Z Med J 98(775):207, 1985).

Germanium (Carboxyethyl germanium sesquioxide "Ge-132"):

An organic germanium compound formed by the hydrolysis of trihalogenopropionic acid, followed by the addition of trihalogenogermane to acrylic acid.

Administration may inhibit tumor growth.

Experimental Double-blind Study: Pts. with unresectable lung cancer received either chemotherapy plus Ge-132 or chemotherapy plus placebo. After 3 mo., the proportion of partial and complete responses in stage IV pts. was significantly higher in the Ge-132-treated patients. Although their survival also tended to be longer, the difference was not significant (*Mizushima M et al. Some pharmacological and clinical aspects of a novel organic germanium compound Ge-132, in Kelim & Samochowiec, Eds. 1st Int Conf on Germanium. Hanover, Germany, Oct. 1984. Semmelweis-Verlag, 1985*).

Experimental Study: Following oral administration of Ge-132 1000 mg/d for 10 days, natural killer cell activity in 18 cancer pts. was augmented at 3 days, but depressed at 10 days in all patients. In intermittent oral administration, however, more than half of the pts. with augmented NK activity at day 3 maintained the high activity level at day 10 (*Tanaka N et al. [Augmentation of NK activity in peripheral blood lymphocytes of cancer patients by intermittent Ge-132 administration.] Gan To Kagaku Ryoho 11(6):1303-6, 1984*).

Iodine:

Intake may be inversely correlate with the risk of breast, endometrial and ovarian cancer.

Review Article (breast cancer): Women with low iodine levels often have symptoms relating to severe hyperplasia and fibrocystic disease of the breast, precancerous lesions which have been corrected by iodine replacement in clinical trials (*Eskin BA. Biol. Trace Element Res. 5:399-412, 1983*).

Review Article (breast, endometrial and ovarian cancer): Geographic differences in the rates of breast, endometrial and ovarian cancer appear to be inversely correlated with iodine intake, suggesting that low iodine intake may produce increased gonadotrophin stimulation leading to a hyperestrogenic state characterized by relatively high production of estrone and estradiol and a relatively low estriol to estrone plus estradiol ratio which may increase the risk of these cancers (*Stadel VV. Dietary iodine and the risk of breast, endometrial, and ovarian cancer. Lancet 1: 890-91, 1976*).

Iron:

WARNING: Excessive iron intake may foster carcinogensis.

Iron can catalyze the production of oxygen radicals (*Hallivell B, Gutteridge JM. Oxygen free radicals and iron in relation to biology and medicine: Some problems and concepts. Arch Biochem Biophys 246:501-14, 1986*) which may be proximate carcinogens (*Ames BN. Dietary carcinogens and anticarcinogens: Oxygen radicals and degenerative diseases. Science 221:1256-64, 1983; Cerutti PA. Proxidant states and tumor promotion. Science 227:375-81, 1985*).

Iron may be a limiting nutrient for the growth and development of cancer cells; thus excess iron may increase the chances that cancer cells will survive and flourish (*Bergeron RJ et al. Influence of iron on in vivo proliferation and lethality of L1210 cells. J Nutr 115:369-74, 1985; Weinberg ED. Iron withholding: A defense against infection and neoplasia. Physiol Rev 64:65-102, 1984*).

Positive evidence:

General

Observational Study: In a survey of over 14,000 adults (the first US National Health and Nutrition Examination Survey), among the 242 men in whom cancer later developed, the mean total iron-binding capacity (inversely related to total iron body stores) was significantly lower (p<0.01) and transferrin saturation was significantly higher (p=0.002) than among 3113 who remained free of cancer at follow-up. Women did not have the same finding; however a *post hoc* examination yielded a relative risk of 1.3 associated with a very high transferrin saturation. In women with at least 6 yrs. of follow-up, the relative risk associated with a very high transferrin saturation was 1.5 (*Stevens RG et al. Body iron stores and the risk of cancer. N Engl J Med 319(16):1047-52, 1988*).

Observational Study: Higher available body iron stores in men, but not dietary intake of iron, was associated with a higher cancer risk. The estimate of iron intake based on a 24-hr. dietary-recall questionnaire was not associated with serum measures of iron status, possibly because the reporting period of

24 hrs. was too short to be a reliable index of dietary intake (*Stevens RG et al. Iron-binding proteins and risk of cancer in Taiwan. J Natl Cancer Inst 76:605-10, 1986*).

Breast Cancer

Animal Experimental Study: Rats were divided into 3 gps. and were fed a standard diet low, adequate, or high in iron. The animals were injected with the carcinogen 1-methyl-1-nitrosourea 3 wks. after initiation of the diet. The low-iron gp. showed few mammary tumors compared to the adequate and high-dose iron groups. Tumor incidence increased in the low-iron gp. when their low hematocrits and body wts. were restored to normal. Tumor incidence later plateaued in the adequate-iron gp.; however, tumor incidence continued to rise in the high-iron group. Results suggest that excess iron intake is a contributing factor to the development of breast cancer (*Thompson H et al. Effect of iron deficiency and excess on the induction of mammary carcinogenesis by l-methyl-l-nitrosourea. Carcinogenesis 12:1111-4, 1991*).

Hodgkin's Lymphoma

Observational Study: Tissue iron accumulation was found in the lymph nodes of 28 untreated pts. with Hodgkin's disease (*Dumont AE et al. Siderosis of lymph nodes in patients with Hodgkin's disease. Cancer 38(3):1247-52, 1976*).

Lung Cancer

Observational Study: The relationship between two indirect measures of tissue iron stores (anemia and total iron-binding capacity) as well as recent iron use and the subsequent risk of cancer was explored in a cohort of 174,507 persons. Women, but not men, who reported recent iron use (suggesting a history or iron deficiency) had a lower risk of lung cancer; anemia was also associated with lower lung cancer risk in women. TIBC, which is inversely related to body iron stores, was inversely related to the risk of lung cancer in women in a graded fashion (*Selby JV, Friedman GD. Epidemiologic evidence of an association between body iron stores and risk of cancer. Int J Cancer 41(5):677-82, 1988*).

Negative Evidence:

General

Observational Study: Because transferrin saturation is subject to the influence of disease status, and because the 1988 study of Stevens et al (*see above*) suggested increased cancer risk with increased body iron stores as assessed by TS but reported only a weak association, the same follow-up study was analyzed using a similar analytic design but a longer follow-up period and controlled more carefully for initial health status. An association between TS and the risk of cancer was not found. Because TS is not a satisfactory index of body iron stores, prospective studies using a better index, such as serum ferritin, are needed (*Yip R et al. Is there an association between iron nutrition status and the risk of cancer? Abstract. Am J Clin Nutr 53:P-31, 1991*).

Prostate Cancer

Observational Study: 25 pts. with moderately differentiated prostatic carcinoma stage D (Jewett) showed a significant decrease in serum iron (*Picurelli L et al. [Determination of serum Fe in prostatic pathology.] Actas Urol Esp 14(4):262-3, 1990*) (*in Spanish*).

Observational Study: Dietary records of 55 black pts. with prostate cancer were compared to those of matched controls. An inverse relationship was noted between dietary intake of iron and risk for developing prostate cancer for the 30 to 49-year-old group (p<0.05) (*Kaul L et al. The role of diet in prostate cancer. Nutr Cancer 9:123-28, 1987*).

Stomach Cancer

Observational Study: Stored serum samples were analyzed in a gp. of subjects who later developed stomach cancer (233 cases) or lung cancer (84 cases). An increased risk for developing stomach, but not lung, cancer was associated with low serum ferritin levels prior to the onset of the disease. The risk remained high for all subjects with low serum ferritin levels 5 yrs. or more prior to cancer diagnosis. Low serum ferritin combined with achlorhydria produced a 10-fold increase in subsequent risk (*Akiba S et al. Serum ferritin and stomach cancer risk among a Japanese population. Cancer 67:1707-12, 1991*).

Magnesium:

Intake may inversely correlate with cancer incidence and mortality.

Review Article: Animal studies report increased cancer in magnesium-deficient diets and a preventive effect in animals fed excess magnesium. Epidemiologic studies suggest that magnesium levels in water, soil, food and air are inversely related to cancer mortality (*Blondell JM. The anticarcinogenic effect of magnesium. Med Hypotheses 6:863-871, 1980*).

Nickel:

WARNING: Exposure may be correlated with the risk of nasopharyngeal and lung cancer (*Sunderman FW Jr. Mechanisms of nickel carcinogenesis. Scand J Work Environ Health 15(1):1-12, 1989*).

Selenium:

Intake may inversely correlate with cancer risk.

Review Article: Past epidemiological studies suggesting an association of selenium nutrition or blood levels and cancer incidence and mortality are reviewed. In a re-analysis of data indicating an inverse association between cancer incidence and selenium forage crop levels in the U.S., results confirmed an inverse association between selenium availability and total cancer mortality in both males and females (*Clark LC. The epidemiology of selenium and cancer. Fed Proc 44:2584, 1985*).

Deficiency may be associated with increased cancer risk.

Note: Ingestion of selenomethionine (which is plant-derived) will produce higher levels blood and tissue selenium levels than ingestion of selenocysteine (which is animal-derived) as animals treat selenomethionine as methionine. They thus incorporate it into proteins in place of methionine and, when catabolized, it becomes nutritionally available for incorporation into glutathione peroxidase. Selenocysteine, by contrast, is only incorporated into selenoproteins such as glutathione peroxidase and is excreted once the enzyme reaches control levels. Thus selenium levels merely reflect differences in the plant and animal components of the diet (Burk RF. Letter. JAMA 262(6):775, 1989).

Review Article: Recent research has failed to substantiate earlier claims that selenium was carcinogenic. A large proportion of animal studies showing a positive effect of selenium found at least a 35% reduction in tumor incidence, suggesting that a dietary deficiency of selenium may increase carcinogenesis in certain circumstances. Epidemiologic studies have confirmed that cancer pts. tend to have lower blood or plasma selenium levels than controls. Prospective studies suggest that it is unlikely that this correlation is due to an effect of cancer upon selenium metabolism (*Combs GF, Clark LC. Can dietary selenium modify cancer risk? Nutr Rev 43:325-31, 1985*).

Breast Cancer: *McConnell KP et al. The relationship between dietary selenium and breast cancer. J Surg Oncol 15(1):67-70, 1980*

Gastrointestinal Cancer: *Guo W et al. Correlations of dietary intake and blood nutrient levels with oesphageal cancer mortality in China. Nutr Cancer 13:121-27, 1990*

Pancreatic Cancer: *Burney PGJ et al. Serologic precursors of cancer: Serum micronutrients and the subsequent risk of pancreatic cancer. Am J Clin Nutr 49:895-900, 1989*

Skin Cancer: *Clark LC et al. Plasma selenium and skin neoplasms: A case control study. Nutr Cancer 6(1):13-21, 1984).*

Supplementation may inhibit carcinogenesis.

Experimental Placebo-controlled Study: 40 healthy Chinese miners found to have low selenium concentrations in plasma and hair randomly received either selenium 300 μg/d in high selenium malt cakes or placebo. After 1 yr., there was a 178% increase in serum and a 195% increase in hair selenium concentrations. Serum glutathione peroxidase activity increased by 156%, while lipid peroxidase levels decreased by almost 75% as compared to the placebo group. Also, lymphocyte DNA damage induced by both ultaviolet irradiation and carcinogens was reduced. Liver function was unaffected by selenium supplementation. Results suggest that selenium supplementation is safe and effective for the prevention of cancer in people with low selenium status (*Yu S et al. Intervention trial with selenium for the prevention of lung cancer among tin miners in Yunnan, China: A pilot study. Biol Trace Element Res 24:105-9, 1990).*

Review Article: For now, insufficient evidence exists to recommend that people, other than those living in areas of profound selenium deficiency in central China, supplement their diet with selenium (*Willett WC, Stampfer MJ. Selenium and cancer. Br Med J 297:573-74, 1988).*

In vitro and Animal Experimental Studies: The viability of human breast cancer cells was inhibited *in vitro* in a dose-dependent manner by selenium supplementation, while a normal diploid human cell line was relatively resistant. Parenteral administration of sodium selenite also significantly inhibited the growth of cancerous cell lines transplanted into mice without apparent ill effects (*Watrach AM et al. Inhibition of human breast cancer cells by selenium. Cancer Lett 25:41-47, 1984).*

Supplementation may reduce the tissue damage from chemotherapy.

Experimental Study: 23 pts. with ovarian cancer or metastatic endometrial cancer received cytotoxic chemotherapy with or without selenium supplementation (sodium selenate 200 μg/d). Sodium selenate significantly decreased the capacity of blood platelets to produce thromboxane A2 (which is increased in ovarian cancer) and prevented the chemotherapy-associated increase in creatine kinase activity (an indicator of the amt. of tissue damage) (*Sundstrom H et al. Supplementation with selenium, vitamin E and their combination in gynaecological cancer during cytotoxic chemotherapy. Carcinogenesis 10:273-78, 1989).*

- and Vitamin A:

Combined deficiencies may be associated with an increased risk of lung cancer.

Observational Study: In a 4 year case-control study of 51 cancer patients investigating the relationship between serum concentrations of selenium and vitamins A and E, inadequate vitamin A or beta-carotene intake was associated with an increased incidence of lung cancer among smoking men with low serum selenium (*Salonen J et al. Risk of cancer in relation to serum concentrations of selenium and vitamin A and E: Matched case-control analysis of prospective data. Br Med J 290:417-20, 1985).*

- and Vitamin E:

Vitamin E may potentiate the ability of selenium to inhibit cancer growth.

Observational Study: Blood samples of 36,365 subjects aged 15-99 who were free of cancer were stored. 6-10 yrs. later, the stored samples of 150 subjects who had developed gastrointestinal cancer were analyzed. Subjects with low serum vitamin E or selenium were more likely to develop upper GI cancer, but not cancer of the colon or rectum. The association with upper GI cancer was strongest in men (*Knekt P et al. Serum vitamin E, serum selenium, and the risk of gastrointestinal cancer. Int J Cancer 42:846-50, 1988).*

Observational Study: In a 4 year case-control study of 51 cancer patients investigating the relationship between serum concentrations of selenium and vitamins A and E, fatal cancer corresponded to selenium deficiency and vitamin E contributed to this effect (*Salonen J et al. Risk of cancer in relation to serum concentrations of selenium and vitamin A and E: Matched case-control analysis of prospective data. Br Med J 290:417, 1985*).

Animal Experimental Study: Mammary tumors were induced in rats maintained on a high polyunsaturated fat (20%) corn oil diet to increase oxidant stress. The addition of vitamin E facilitated the anticarcinogenic effect of selenium, but only when it was present during the proliferative phase (*Horvath PM, Ip C. Synergistic effect of vitamin E and selenium in the chemoprevention of mammary carcinogenesis in rats. Cancer Res 43(11):5335-41, 1983*).

Sodium:

High intake may be associated with an increased risk of colorectal cancer.

Observational Study: The sodium and potassium intakes of 715 pts. with colon cancer and 727 healthy controls were studied. High sodium intake in men was associated with an increased risk of colorectal cancer. The association was also seen in women, but to a much lesser degree. In women, a high potassium to sodium ratio was protective (*Kune G et al. Dietary sodium and potassium intake and colorectal cancer risk. Nutr Cancer 12:351-59, 1989*).

Zinc:

Both zinc deficiency and zinc excess may inhibit experimental tumor growth (*Song MK et al. Effect of different levels of dietary zinc on longevity of Balb/c mice inoculated with plasmacytoma MOPC 104E. J Natl Cancer Inst 72:647-52, 1984*).

Tumors may lower intestinal zinc absorption capacity while raising their zinc uptake rate; as a result, other tissues may become hypozincemic and hypercalcemic. In tumor-bearing mice, a zinc-excess diet is beneficial as they are generally zinc-deficient; the diet normalizes zinc organ concentrations resulting in increased survival time (*Song MK et al. Zinc, calcium, and magnesium metabolism: effects on plasmacytomas in Balb/c mice. Am J Clin Nutr 49:701-07, 1989*).

Esophageal Cancer

Dietary deficiency may contribute to the induction of esophageal cancer.

Review Article: While other trace elements may also alter the incidence of esophageal carcinoma, studies of these elements are not as conclusive as the epidemiological and experimental studies linking dietary zinc deficiency with an increased incidence of human esophageal carcinoma (*Barch DH. Esophageal cancer and microelements. J Am Coll Nutr 8(2):99-107, 1989*).

Plasma levels may be decreased in esophageal cancer (*Lipman T et al. Esophageal zinc content in human squamous esophageal cancer. J Am Coll Nutr 6:41-46, 1987*).

Lung Cancer

Experimental Controlled Study: Pts. with bronchogenic carcinoma often have low serum zinc and sometimes have markedly elevated renal zinc losses. Among a gp. of pts., low serum zinc and high urine zinc concentrations significantly correlated with depressed T cell phytohemagglutinin response. Oral zinc sulfate 220 mg 3 times daily was then given to some of the pts. with hyperzincuria. After 6 wks., treated pts. had normalization of T cell phytohemagglutinin response, while controls had no improvement. Results suggest that a mild subclinical zinc deficiency may exist in some lung cancer pts. which may cause abnormal T cell function, and that supplementation may normalize T cell function in those patients. The effect of supplementation on the course of the disease, however, is unknown (*Allen JI et al. Association between urinary zinc excretion and lymphocyte dysfunction in patients with lung cancer. Am J Med 79(2):209-15, 1985*).

Prostate Cancer

Serum levels may be low compared to patients with benign prostatic hypertrophy (*Whelen P et al. Zinc, vitamin A and prostatic cancer. Br J Urol 55(5):525-8, 1983*).

Prostatic tissue levels are low compared to normals (*Habib FK et al. Metal-androgen interrelationships in carcinoma and hyperplasia of the human prostate. J Endocrinol 71(1):133-41, 1976*).

Prostatic tissue levels may be low compared to patients with prostatic hyperplasia (*Romics I, Katchalova L. Spectrographic determination of zinc in the tissues of adenoma and carcinoma of the prostate. Int Urol Nephrol 15(2):171-76, 1983*).

Cadmium may stimulate the growth of prostatic epithelium by replacing zinc (*see also: "Cadmium" below*).

In vitro Experimental Study: Cadmium, a known antagonist of zinc, was found to have the ability to stimulate the growth of human prostatic epithelium at low concentrations, suggesting that cadmium may promote carcinogenesis by replacing zinc in the prostate (*Webber MM. Effects of zinc and cadmium on the growth of human prostatic epithelium in vitro. Nutr Res 6:35-40, 1986*).

Observational Study: As measured by atomic absorption spectrometry, there were distinct differences in zinc and cadmium content in the nuclear fractions of malignant tissues in comparison with BPH and normal tissues. The highest values of cadmium were obtained in the nuclear fractions of poorly-differentiated carcinomas, along with the lowest levels of zinc (*Feustel A, Wennrich R. Determination of the distribution of zinc and cadmium in cellular fractions of BPH, normal prostate and prostatic cancers of different histologies by atomic and laser absorption spectrometry in tissue slices. Urol Res 12(5):253-56, 1984*).

- -

OTHER NUTRITIONAL FACTORS

Alkoxyglycerols:

Shark liver oil has the highest concentration next to mother's milk and bone marrow.

Example: "Ecomer" (AB Astra) 250 mg capsules (each containing 50 mg alkoxyglycerols) 2 caps 2-3 times daily

Administration may reduce the cancer mortality rate (*Brohult A et al. Biochemical effects of alkoxyglycerols and their use in cancer therapy. Acta Chem Scand 24:730, 1970*).

Administration may produce tumor regression.

General

Review Article: "By combining multiple biological activities in one molecule, alkyl analogues of 2-PLC represent a unique new class of antitumor drugs. They modulate the adoptive immune system by suppressing antigen-specific effector cells and activating non-specific host defense cells. They change the invasive and differentiative behavior of tumor cells and they induce a selective destruction of neoplastic cells. Although proven to have potent tumor therapeutic activity in animal tumor models, their therapeutic efficacy in humans requires confirmation in the larger phase I/II trials now under way" (*Andreesen R. Ether lipids in the therapy of cancer. Prog Biochem Pharmacol 22:118-31, 1988*

Uterine Cancer

Experimental Study: When administered prior to radiation treatment, pts. with uterine cancer who received alkoxyglycerols in capsules containing 85% free alkylglycerols (AB Astra) 200 mg 3 times daily prior to radiation treatment demonstrated regression of tumor growth. This regression was remarkably higher for pts. <60 yrs. old compared to those >60 and was demonstrated by a change in the quotient between the incidence of early and advanced stages (*Brohult A et al. Reduced mortality in cancer patients after administration of alkoxyglycerols. Acta Obstet Gynecol Scand 65(7):779-85, 1986; Brohult A et al. Regression of tumour growth after administration of alkoxyglycerols. Acta Obstet Gynecol Scand 57(1):79-83, 1978*).

Administration may reduce injuries caused by radiation therapy.

Cervical Carcinoma

Experimental Study: The incidence of injuries following radiation therapy for carcinoma of the uterine cervix was markedly decreased by the administration of alkylglycerols, both in regard to more severe injuries such as fistulas and in regard to less harmful injuries. In this study, recto-vaginal and vesico-vaginal fistulas were reduced 47% by prior administration of alkylglycerols with capsules containing 85% free alkylglcerols (AB Astra) 200 mg 3 times daily (*Brohult A et al. Effect of alkoxyglycerols on the frequency of fistulas following radiation therapy for carcinoma of the uterine cervix. Acta Obstet Gynecol Scand 58(2):203-07, 1979*).

Experimental Study: Compared to controls, complex injuries due to the combination of radiation injury and tumor growth were reduced to about 1/3 in pts. receiving alkylglycerols before, during and after radiation treatment. When alkylglycerol capsules (AB Astra) 200 mg 3 times daily were only administered during and after radiation treatment, no effect was observed on complex injuries, although injuries due to radiation only were significantly decreased (*Brohult A et al. Effect of alkoxyglycerols on the frequency of injuries following radiation therapy for carcinoma of the uterine cervix. Acta Obstet Gynecol Scand 56(4):441-48, 1977*).

Amino Acids:

- Arginine:

Supplementation may retard tumor growth through immunomodulation.

Animal Experimental Study: Tumor-bearing mice were randomly assigned to a regular diet supplemented with either 1% arginine or glycine. The mean tumor latency period and ave. tumor incidence were not significantly different between groups. However, in the gp. inoculated with an immunogenic neuroblastoma, and the other with a minimally immunogenic clonal variant, arginine, but not glycine, markedly retarded tumor growth and significantly prolonged median survival (*Reynolds J et al. Arginine as an immunomodulator. Abstract. Surg Forum 38:415-18, 1987*).

May inhibit target cells in leukemia.

In vitro Animal Experimental Study: A K562 cell line isolated from a pt. with chronic leukemia was cocultivated with activated mice macrophages. Tumor target cells were not metabolically inhibited by the elimination of amino acids. However, with the addition of L-arginine to an otherwise amino acid-free culture, the activated macrophage cytotoxic effector mechanism was expressed, probably affecting mitochondrial respiration, aconitase activity, and DNA synthesis in the cancer cells (*Hibbs JB et al. L-arginine is required for the expression of the activated macrophage effector mechanism causing selective metabolic inhibition in target cells. J Immunol 138:550-65, 1987*).

- Cysteine:

N-acetylcysteine, some of which is converted to cysteine in the body, may be a natural intermediary in cysteine detoxification mechanisms. A precursor to intracellular glutathione, it is generally safe in doses up to 10 gm daily even during pregnancy; however it has a nauseating taste and smell and can cause vomiting (*Braverman ER, Pfeiffer CC. The Healing Nutrients Within. New Canaan, Conn., Keats Publishing, 1987*).

N-acetylcysteine administration may reduce the toxicity of chemotherapeutic agents.

Note: N-acetylcysteine prevents chemotherapy-induced liver and heart toxicity only to the extent that it is converted into cysteine in the body (Miller LF, Rumack BH. Clinical safety of high oral doses of acetylcysteine. Semin Oncol 10(1 Suppl 1):76-85, 1983); thus cysteine supplementation may be equally effective.

Adriamycin (Doxorubicin)

Animal Experimental Study: While N-acetylcysteine prevents adriamycin cardiotoxitiy in mice, it may interfere with its antitumor activity (*Schmitt-Gräff A, Scheulen ME. Prevention of adriamycin cardiotoxicity by niacin, isocitrate or N-acetyl-cysteine in mice. A morphological study. Pathol Res Pract 181(2):168-74, 1986*).

Negative Experimental Controlled Study: NAC failed to be clinically effective in blocking the cardiotoxicity of doxorubicin (*Myers C et al. A randomized controlled trial assessing the prevention of doxorubicin cardiomyopathy by N-acetylcysteine. Semin Oncol 10:53-5, 1983*).

Cyclophosphamide

Animal Experimental Study: Four times the dose of N-acetylcysteine as cyclophosphamide, given one-half hour before the dose of cyclophosphamide, prevented CPS-induced hemorrhagic cystitis and lengthened survival times (*Levy L, Vredevoe DL. The effect of N-acetyl cysteine on cyclophosphamide immunoregulation and antitumor activity. Semin Oncol 10(1 Suppl 1):7-16, 1983*).

> *Note: Metabolism of cyclophosphamide by liver enzymes results in cytostatic products and acrolein which is urotoxic. N-acetylcysteine reacts with acrolein to prevent its urotoxicity without interfering with the beneficial immunomodulatory effects of cycloposphamide (Palermo MS et al. Immunomodulation exerted by cyclophosphamide is not interfered by N-acetyl cysteine. Int J Immunopharmacol 8(6):651-55, 1986).*

Ifosfamide

Review Article: While ifosfamide is invaluable in treating resistant testis tumors and may even hold hope for treating renal cell carcinoma, its causes a severe, restrictive hemorrhagic cystitis which appears preventable with the oral administration of acetylcysteine (Mucomyst) (*Watson RA. Ifosfamide: Chemotherapy with new promise and new problems for the urologist. Urology 24(5):465-68, 1984*).

Topical application of N-acetylcysteine ointment may reduce skin reactions, prevent hair loss and protect the mucus membranes of the eyes from the adverse effects of radiation therapy (*Kim JA et al. Topical use of N-acetylcysteine for reduction of skin reaction to radiation therapy. Semin Oncol 10(1 Suppl 1):86-88, 1983*).

- D-Glucaric Acid:

Found in abundance in cruciferous vegetables, sweet cherries and citrus.

Supplementation may help to combat carcinogenesis.

Review Article: Glucuronidation is a principal conjugation pathway for disposing of carcinogens. Animal studies suggest that elevated levels of β-glucuronidase is linked with various disease states including cancer, and that carcinogenesis may be controlled by reducing the rate of de-glucuronidation by β-glucuronidase inhibitors such as D-glucaro-1,4-lactone and its precursors such as D-glucaric acid. Also, β-glucuronidase activity has been found to be positively correlated with estrogen levels in human mammary cancer and, in a study of chemically induced rat mammary cancers, dietary D-glucarate markedly reduced estradiol, as well as progesterone, levels (*Walaszek Z. Potential use of D-glucaric acid derivatives in cancer prevention. Cancer Lett 54:1-8, 1990*).

- Glutamine:

May protect against enteritis from radiation therapy.

Animal Experimental Study: When, following radiation, the diets of laboratory rats were supplemented with glutamine, there was improved healing of radiation enteritis (*Klimberg S. Prevention of radiogenic side effects using glutamine-enriched elemental diets. Recent Results Cancer Res 121:283-5, 1991*).

- Phenylalanine and
Tyrosine:

Dietary restriction may increase natural killer cell activity and decrease platelet aggregation, two indices associated with decreased tumor growth and metastasis.

Experimental Study: 9 healthy subjects consumed low-protein foods supplemented with formula diets free of tyrosine and phenylalanine to maintain total daily intake of tyrosine at 2.4 mg/kg and phenylalanine at 3.5 mg/kg. Plasma tyrosine but not plasma phenylalanine decreased (p<0.05). Platelet aggregation decreased. Natural killer, T-helper, and T-cytotoxic/supressor lymphocyte numbers proportionally increased relative to neutrophils (p<0.05). Natural killer cell activity increased in 6/9 subjects (*Norris JR et al. Tyrosine- and phenylalanine-restricted formula diet augments immunocompetence in healthy humans. Am J Clin Nutr 51:188-96, 1990*).

Dietary restriction may inhibit cancer growth in malignant melanoma.

Negative Experimental Study: Pts. with advanced malignant melanoma fed restricted diets limited to 8 mg/kg lean body wt. of total Phe and Tyr failed to respond (*Lawson DH et al. The effect of a phenylalanine and tyrosine restricted diet on elemental balance studies and plasma aminograms of patients with disseminated malignant melanoma. Am J Clin Nutr 41:73-84, 1985*).

Experimental Study: Restriction of Phe and Tyr resulted in tumor stabilization and/or remission in malignant melanoma pts. (*Lorincz AB et al. Tumor response to phenylalanine-tyrosine limited diets. J Am Diet Assoc 54:198-205, 1969*).

Experimental Study: 3/5 malignant melanoma pts. placed on a diet restricted in Phe and Tyr exhibited correlations between adherence to dietary protocol and regressive changes in the disease (*Demopoulos HB. Effects of reducing the phenylalamine-tyrosine intake of patients with advanced malignant melanoma. Cancer 19:657-64, 1966*).

Carotenoids:

Note: Only a small percentage of beta-carotene is converted into vitamin A, and this conversion is impaired in liver disease and hypothyroidism.

General Review Article: In reviewing the experimental evidence for carotenoid inhibition of mutagenicity, malignant transformation, tumor formation, and immunoenhancement, it is clear that, although a mechanism for its effects cannot yet be identified, the overwhelming evidence in these systems would indicate that carotenoids exert an important influence in modulating the actions of carcinogens (*Krinsky NI. Effects of carotenoids in cellular and animal systems. Am J Clin Nutr 53:238S-46S, 1991*).

Intake may be inversely correlated with the risk of certain cancers - independent of the effect of vitamin A (*see also "Vitamin A and Beta-Carotene" below*).

General

Observational Study: This case-control study compared estimated intakes of carotene and carotene-rich fruits and vegetables during the year before diagnosis in 96 men with lung cancer, 75 men with other epithelial cancers and 97 hospital controls. Compared to men in the lowest third of carotene intake, the smoking-adjusted odds ratios for men in the middle and upper thirds of carotene intake were 0.67 and 0.45, respectively, for lung cancer and 0.63 and 0.65, respectively, for other epithelial cancers. Ave. dietary carotene intakes were 24% lower in lung cancer pts. and 10% lower in pts. with other epithelial cancers than in controls. Ave. intakes of all 4 categories of carotene-rich fruits and vegetables were lower in both gps. of cancer pts. than in controls. For both lung and other epithelial cancers, estimated carotene intake was more strongly protective than was the total intake of carotene-rich vegetables and fruits (g/d) or of any of the 4 subgroups of vegetables and fruits, suggesting that the protective substance is carotene itself rather some other component of vegetables and fruits (*Harris RWC et al. A case-control study of dietary carotene in men with lung cancer and in men with other epithelial cancers. Nutr Cancer 15:63-8, 1991*).

Review Article: Low intake of vegetables and fruits and carotenoids is consistently associated with an increased risk of lung cancer in both prospective and retrospective studies, and low levels of serum or plasma β-carotene are consistently associated with the subsequent development of lung cancer. However, the importance of other carotenoids, other consitutents of vegetables and fruits, and other nutrients whose levels in the blood are partially correlated with those of β-carotene has not been adequately explored. Also, smoking is associated with reduced intake of carotenoids and lowered blood β-carotene levels and has not always been adequately controlled. While prospective and retrospective studies suggest that carotenoids may reduce the risk of certain other cancers, too few studies have looked at these sites to examine the consistency of the evidence (*Ziegler RG. A review of epidemiologic evidence that carotenoids reduce the risk of cancer. J Nutr 119:116-22, 1989*).

Breast Cancer

Negative Observational Study: The dietary histories of 133 Dutch women of Caucasian origin with newly diagnosed breast cancer and of 238 healthy controls were obtained. Beta-carotene intakes were similar in both gps. and no significant trend was seen for fruit or vegetable product consumption (*Van 'T Veer P et al. Dietary fiber, beta-carotene and breast cancer: Results from a case-control study. Int J Cancer 4:825-28, 1990*).

Cervical Cancer: *Verreault R et al. A case-control study of diet and invasive cervical cancer. Int J Cancer 43:1050-54, 1989*).

Colon Cancer: *West D et al. Dietary intake and colon cancer: Sex- and anatomic site-specific associations. Am J Epidemiol 130:883-94, 1989*).

Esophageal Cancer: *Decarli A et al. Vitamin A and other dietary factors in the etiology of esophageal cancer. Cancer 10:29-37, 1987*).

Gastric Cancer: *Buiatti E et al. A case-control study of gastric cancer and diet in Italy: association with nutrients. Int J Cancer 45:899-901, 1990*).

Laryngeal Cancer: *Mackerras D et al. Carotene intake and the risk of laryngeal cancer in coastal Texas. Am J Epidemiol 128:980-88, 1988*).

Lung Cancer

Review Article: "One of the most consistent epidemiological findings in nutrition research has been an association between β-carotene intake and status and reduced lung cancer risk, particularly risk of squamous cell cancer. . . . Large-scale NCI-sponsored in"ervention trials with subjects at high risk of developing lung cancer are currently underway using β-carotene" (*Singh VN, Gaby SK. Premalignant lesions: role of antioxidant vitamins and β-carotene in risk reduction and prevention of malignant transformation. Am J Clin Nutr 53:386S-90S, 1991*).

Skin Cancer: *Stryker W et al. Diet, plasma levels of beta carotene and alpha tocopherol, and risk of malignant melanoma. Am J Epidemiol 13:597-611, 1990*).

Vulvar Cancer

Observational Study: Diets of 201 cancer pts. and 342 controls were compared. There was a definite association between a decreased intake of alpha-carotene (but not with beta-carotene) and cancer risk (*Ziegler R et al. Diet and the risk of vulvar cancer. Am J Epidemiol 132:778, 1990*).

Plasma/serum levels may be lower in cancer patients than in controls.

General

Observational Study: Prediagnostic serum samples from 436 cases of cancer in 9 sites (colon, rectum, pancreas, lung, melanoma, basal cell of skin, breast, prostate, bladder) and 765 matched controls were assayed. Serum beta-carotene levels showed a strong protective association with lung cancer, suggestive protective associations with melanoma and bladder cancer, and a suggestive but nonprotective association with rectal cancer (*Comstock GW et al. Prediagnostic serum levels of carotenoids and vitamin E as related to subsequent cancer in Washington County, Maryland. Am J Clin Nutr 53:260S-4S, 1991*).

Observational Study: Prediagnostic plasma samples from 204 men who subsequently died of cancer and of 2421 controls were assayed. There were significantly lower mean carotene levels for all cancer, bronchus cancer, and stomach cancer (all p<0.01). The relative risk of subjects with low carotene (<0.23 μmol/L) was significantly elevated (p<0.05) for lung cancer. Higher risks were noted for all cancer (p<0.01) if both carotene and retinol were low (*Stähelin HB et al. β-carotene and cancer prevention: the Basel study. Am J Clin Nutr 53:265S-9S, 1991*).

Breast Cancer: *Potischman N et al. Breast cancer and dietary and plasma concentrations of carotenoids and vitamn A. Am J Clin Nutr 52:909-15, 1990*).

Cervical Cancer: *Palan PR et al. Plasma levels of antioxidant beta-carotene and alpha-tocopherol in uterine cervix dysplasias and cancer. Nutr Cancer 15:13-20, 1991*).

Gastric Cancer: *Stähelin HB et al. Cancer, vitamins, and plasma lipids: Prospective Basel study. J Natl Cancer Inst 73(6):1463-8, 1984*).

Lung Cancer: *Kune GA et al. Serum levels of β-carotene, vitamin A and zinc in male lung cancer cases and controls. Nutr Cancer 12:169-76, 1989*).

Skin Cancer

Observational Study: In a study of subjects 18 yrs. and older visiting a dermatology clinic for the first time due to pigmented skin lesions, plasma beta-carotene levels, but not alpha-carotene levels, were inversely associated with risk of malignant melanoma (*Stryker W et al. Diet, plasma levels of beta carotene and alpha tocopherol, and risk of malignant melanoma. Am J Epidemiol 13:597-611, 1990*).

The lower blood levels in cancer patients may be due to malnutrition rather than to the presence of cancer.

Observational Study: There were no differences in total plasma carotenoids and pro-vitamin A precursors between well-nourished normal volunteers and cancer pts., while malnourished cancer and non-cancer pts. had significantly lower values of both. In all gps., most of the circulating carotenoids were the non-pro-vitamin A precursors. Results suggest that differences in carotenoid levels between cancer pts. and normals are due to their nutritional state rather than to the presence of cancer (*Meguid M et al. Plasma carotenoid profiles in normals and patients with cancer. J Parenter Enteral Nutr 12(2):147-51, 1988*).

Tissue levels in cancerous tissue may be lower than in adjacent normal tissue.

Observational Study: Compared to adjacent normal tissues, levels of beta-carotene were lower in cancerous tissue from uterine tumors as well as from diseased tissue taken from the cervix, endometrium, ovary, breast, colon, lung, liver and rectum (*Palan P et al. Decreased B-carotene tissue levels in uterine leiomyomas and cancers of reproductive and nonreproductive organs. Am J Obstet Gynecol 161:1649-52, 1989*).

Supplementation with beta-carotene may inhibit carcinogenesis.

Non-melanoma Skin Cancer

Negative Experimental Double-blind Study: 1805 pts. who had had a recent nonmelanoma skin cancer randomly received either beta-carotene 50 mg or placebo daily. After 5 yrs. of follow-up, there was no difference between the gps. in the rate of occurrence of the first new nonmelanoma skin cancer. Active treatment showed no efficacy either in the pts. whose initial plasma beta-carotene level was in the lowest quartile or in those who currently smoked. The was also no significant difference between treated and control gps. in the mean number of new nonmelanoma skin cancers per patient-year (*Greenberg ER et al. A clinical trial of beta carotene to prevent basal-cell and squamous cell cancers of the skin. N Engl J Med 323:789-95, 1990*).

Oral Cancer

Review Article: Beta-carotene suppresses micronuclei in exfoliated oral mucosa cells from subjects at risk for oral cancer and is active in reversing leukop›akia; it is possible that it may prevent second primary tumors in pts. cured of their initial cancer who have an increased risk of developing new cancers of the upper aerodigestive tract (*Garewal HS. Potential role of β-carotene in prevention of oral cancer. Am J Clin Nutr 53:294S-7S, 1991*).

<u>Butyric Acid</u>:

A 4-carbon fatty acid which is produced by the anaerobic bacteria of the human colon and serves as the major energy source for colorectal epithelium.

The major metabolite when fiber is exposed to colonic flora (*Effects of short-chain fatty acids on a human colon carcinoma cell line. Nutr Rev 46(1):11-12, 1988*).

Promotes the differentiation of cultured malignant cells (*Jass JR. Diet, butyric acid and differentiation of gastrointestinal tract tumors. Med Hypotheses 18:133-18, 1985*).

In vitro Experimental Study: Butyrate enhanced cell differentiation for an antigen-producing human breast carcinoma cell line (*Prasad KN, Sinha PK. Effect of sodium butyrate on mammalian cells in culture: A review. In Vitro 12:125-32, 1976*).

May be a major cancer-inhibiting metabolite in the human colon (*Effects of short-chain fatty acids on a human colon carcinoma cell line. Nutr Rev 46(1):11-12, 1988*).

In vitro Experimental Study: Butyrate significantly suppressed the growth of malignant cells of a human colon carcinoma cell line (*Whitehead RH et al. Effects of short-chain fatty acids on a new human colon carcinoma cell line (LIM 1215). Gut 27:1457-63, 1986*).

Diminished stool butyric acid may suggest increased risk of colon cancer (*Wright JV. Butyrate determination and colon cancer. Int Clin Nutr Rev 9(2):66-67, 1989*).

<u>"Cartilage Anti-angiogenesis Factor"</u>:

Animal cartilage contains a protein which may inhibit tumor growth by inhibiting tumor angiogenesis (*Folkman J et al. Induction of angiogenesis during the transition from hyperplasia to neoplasia. Nature 339:58-61, 1989; Langer R et al. Isolations of a cartilage factor that inhibits tumor neovascularization. Science 193:70-72, 1976*).

Administration may be beneficial.

Experimental Study: Oral and subcutaneous administration of Catrix, a specific preparation of bovine tracheal cartilage rings, resulted in a high response rate in 31 cases of a variety of clinical malignancies (response rate 90%, 61% complete) following years of full dose therapy. The usual dosage was eight 375 mg capsules every 8 hours. Therapy was usually started by injection, and maintenance dosage was given orally. Responders included glioblastoma multiforme and cancers of the pancreas and lungs well as cancers of the ovary, rectum, prostate, cervix, thyroid, and an inoperable squamous cancer of the nose. There was no evidence of toxicity (*Prudden JF. The treatment of human cancer with agents prepared from bovine cartilage. J Biol Response Mod 4(6):551-584, 1985*).

In vitro Experimental Study: Catrix, an acidic mucopolysaccharide complex derived from bovine tracheal cartilage, was evaluated in the human tumor stem cell assay system using 3 human tumor cell lines and fresh biopsy specimens from 22 pts. with malignant tumors. *In vitro* efficacy was demonstrated against a human myeloma cell line as well as against ovarian, pancreatic, colon, testicular, and sarcoma biopsy specimens. The effective *in vitro* concentrations appear to be achievable *in vivo* (*Durie BG et al. Antitumor activity of bovine cartilage extract (Catrix-S) in the human tumor stem cell assay. J Biol Response Mod 4(6):590-95, 1985*).

Animal Experimental Study: An extract of shark cartilage was given to rabbits whose corneas had been implanted with a transplanted tumor. After 19 days, all controls had large tumors forming under the cornea while treated animals did not develop tumor masses despite continued growth of tumor cells. It took 500 gm of calf cartilage to produce 1 mg of a substance causing 70% inhibiton of vascular growth, slightly less inhibition than with 1/000th as much shark cartilage as starting material. The abundance of this factor in shark cartilage, in contrast to cartilage from mammalian sources, may help to explain the rarity of neoplasms in these animals (*Langer R, Lee A. Shark cartilage contains inhibitors of tumor angiogenesis. Science 221:1185-87, 1983*).

<u>Coenzyme Q$_{10}$</u>:   30 mg daily

May reduce cardiac toxicity from adriamycin therapy.

Experimental Controlled Study: Some of 80 pts. receiving chemotherapy with adriamycin also received CoQ$_{10}$. The QTc-duration was significantly prolonged and the QRS voltage was significantly decreased only in pts. who did not receive CoQ$_{10}$ (*Okuma K et al. [Protective effect of coenzyme Q$_{10}$ in cardiotoxicity induced by adriamycin.] Gan To Kagaku Ryoho 11(3):502-08, 1984*) (*in Japanese*).

Experimental Controlled Study: 9/15 pts. with adenocarcinoma of the lung who were treated with adriamycin also received CoQ$_{10}$. Using definitive impedence cardiography, all pts. on adriamycin alone showed depressed cardiac output, while only one pt. receiving adriamycin and CoQ$_{10}$ demonstrated an unsustained reduction in cardiac output by day 28 (*Folkers K et al. New progress on the biomedical and clinical research on Coenzyme Q, in K Folkers, Y Yamamura, Eds. Biomedical and Clinical Aspects of Coenzyme Q, Volume 3. Amsterdam, Elsevier/North Holland Biomedical Press, 1981:399-412*).

<u>Essential (polyunsaturated) Fatty Acids</u> (<u>PUFA</u>):

The relationship between dietary polyunsaturates and cancer has been controversial.

Reviews and Discussions

Review Article: While past studies have implied that high dietary PUFA levels can worsen cancer, recent evidence has shown that the degree of tumorigenicity correlates inversely with PUFA content. *In vitro* studies examining the effects of various PUFA supplements demonstrate that tumor cells are more sensitive to cytotoxic PUFA than non-tumor cells. GLA (gamma linolenic acid) and AA (arachidonic acid) have been shown to be the most effective in killing tumor cells. While sensitivity of cancer cells to PUFA varies, tests conclude that all cancer cell lines can be killed by one or more PUFA combinations (*Begin ME. Fatty acids, lipid peroxidation and diseases. Proc Nutr Soc 49:261-7, 1990*).

Review Article: "Studies in animals show that PUFA are required for the growth of cancers; the amt. required is considered to be greater than that which satisfies the EFA requirement of the host. At this time there is no indication from epidemiological studies that PUFA intake is associated with increased risk of breast or colon cancer, which have been suggested to be promoted by high-fat diets in humans" (*Dupont J et al. Food uses and health effects of corn oil. Am J Clin Nutr 9(5):438-70, 1990*).

Theoretical Discussion: Polyunsaturated fatty acids induce increases in the synthesis of series-2 postaglandins which, in turn, could result in depressing natural killer cell activity. As NK-cells are the first line of defense against tumor cells, this effect could increase cancer risk (*Barone J, Hebert JR. Dietary fat and natural killer cell activity. Med Hypotheses 25(4):223-26, 1988*).

Review Aricle: Epidemiological data suggest that polyunsaturates are associated with a higher incidence of tumors than are saturated fats (*Hopkins GJ, West CE. Possible roles of dietary fats in carcinogenesis. Life Sci. 19:1103-16, 1976*).

Review Article: The impression that polyunsaturated fatty acid diets might be implicated in colon cancer has no support either from clinical experience, epidemiological research or experimental studies (*Heyden S. Editorial: Polyunsaturated fatty acids and colon cancer. Nutr Metabol 17:321-28, 1974*).

Review Article: No convincing case has been made that polyunsaturated fatty acids cause cancer. Nevertheless, people consuming PUFA in quantity might consider taking supplements of vitamin E and should bear in mind the view that saturated, monounsaturated, and polyunsaturated fatty acids should be consumed in equal amounts (*Editorial: Are PUFA harmful? Br Med J October 6, 1973, pp. 1-2*).

Studies Suggesting A Harmful Effect

Observational Study: 230 cases of <u>colon</u> cancer were matched to 390 controls. Men, but not women, who consumed a high amt. of polyunsaturated fats had an almost 4-fold risk for developing colon cancer (*West D *et al. Dietary intake and colon cancer: Sex- and anatomic site-specific associations. Am J Epidemiol 130:883-94, 1989).*

Observational Study: 100 pts. with <u>malignant melanomas</u> had a significantly higher percentage of polyunsaturated fatty acids in the triglycerides of subcutaneous adipose tissue than did matched controls ($p < 0.01$) and there were significantly more controls than pts. who had a low percentage of linoleic acid in the triglycerides. Results suggest that increased consumption of dietary polyunsaturates may have a contributory effect in the etiology of melanoma (*Mackie BS et al. Melanoma and dietary lipids. Nutr Cancer 9(4):219-26, 1987*).

Observational Study: The total mortality of people ingesting a PUFA-enriched prudent diet high in polyunsaturated vegetable oils and low in saturated fat and cholesterol, even though they suffered less ischemic heart disease than those consuming an ordinary diet, was virtually equal to that of the control (ordinary diet) gp., largely due to an excess of deaths due to cancer. This difference in cancer mortality, however, is of borderline statistical significance (*Pearce ML, Dayton S. Incidence of cancer in men on a diet high in polyunsaturated fats. Lancet 1:464-67, 1971*).

Note: Of the 31 cases of fatal carcinomas in the experimental group, 12 were found in persons who adhered less than 20% of the time to the experimental diet, which leaves 19 cases who adhered to the diet greater than 20% of the time compared to 17 fatal cancer cases in the control group. Thus, if we exclude patients in the experimental group who adhered to their diet only very occasionally, there is no basis for finding an excess of deaths in the experimental group (Heyden S. Editorial: Polyunsaturated fatty acids and colon cancer. Nutr Metabol 17:321-28, 1974).

Studies Refuting a Harmful Effect

In vitro Experimental Study: Polyunsaturated fatty acids (especially those containing 3,4 or 5 double bonds) killed incubated human breast, lung and prostate cancer cells at concentrations which had no adverse effects on human fibroblasts or on normal animal cell lines. When human cancer cells and normal human fibroblasts were co-cultured in the absence of PUFAs, the malignant cells outgrew the normal ones. When eicosapentaenoic acid (EPA, 20:5n-3), gamma-linolenic acid (GLA, 18:3n-6) or arachidonic acid (AA, 20:4n-6) were added to the co-cultures, the normal cells outgrew the malignant ones (*Bëgin ME et al. Selective killing of human cancer cells by polyunsaturated fatty acids. Prostaglandins Leukotrienes Med 19(2):177-86, 1985*).

Obervational Study: In reviewing the 13-year experience of the Diet and Coronary Heart Disease Study of the New York City Health Department, there was no evidence of an association between excess cancer mortality and high polyunsaturated fatty acid diets (*Singman HS et al. Cancer mortality and polyunsaturated fatty acids. Mt Sinai J Med 40(5):677-80, 1973*).

- <u>Omega-3 Fatty Acids (Fish Oils)</u>:

Eicosapentaenoic acid (EPA) and docosahexaenoic acid (DHA).

Highest in cold water fish. Available in a refined form as "MaxEPA" (18% EPA).

Suggested MaxEPA dosage: 3 - 9 gm daily in divided doses (or 10 ml concentrate twice daily)

WARNING: Supplementation may require additional vitamin E intake to prevent increased membrane peroxidation and cellular damage (*Laganiere S, Fernandes G. High peroxidizability of subcellular membrane induced by high fish oil diet is reversed by vitamin E. Clin Res 35:A565, 1987*).

Animal Experimental Study: Mice were fed cod liver oil (rich in n-3 PUFA), corn oil or cottonseed oil as part of a nutritionally adequate diet. After 28 days, short- and long-term indicators of free-radical activity and lipid peroxidation were significantly increased in rats fed the PUFA-enriched diet. The n-3 fatty acids of fish oils are highly unstable, and therefore have an increased tendency to peroxidize *in vivo*. Increasing evidence indicates that tumorigenesis may occur via lipid peroxidation associated with the metabolism of the n-3 bonds of PUFA; thus increased intake of these fatty acids may comprise a cancer risk (*Odeleye OE, Watson RR. Health implications of the n-3 fatty acids. Letter. Am J Clin Nutr 53:177-81, 1991*).

Indomethacin, a chemical cyclooxygenase inhibitor, has been shown to inhibit carcinogenesis in animal models (*McCormick DL et al. Cancer Res 45:1803-8, 1985*). Since EPA is also a cyclooxygenase inhibitor, it may have a similar effect.

Omega-3 fatty acids may inhibit carcinogenesis.

In vitro Experimental Study: The longer malignant tumor cells were grown with EPA and the higher the dose, the less invasive the cells became (*Reich R et al. Eicosapentaenoic acid reduces the invasive and metastatic activities of malignant tumor cells. Biochem Biophys Res Commun 160:559-64, 1989*).

Observational Study: Breast cancer incidence and mortality rates were compared to estimates of the consumption of fish and other foods and nutrients. Of the dietary components considered, percent of calories from fish was the factor most strongly correlated with breast cancer rates after statistical adjustment for dietary fat intake (*Kaizer L et al. Fish consumption and breast cancer risk: An ecological study. Nutr Cancer 12:61-68, 1989*).

Animal Experimental Study: Mice bred to develop colorectal cancer were fed diets high in either ω-3 fatty acids, high in saturated fat, or high in both saturated and monounsaturated fat. After 4 wks., tumors were much smaller in mice fed the high ω-3 fatty acid diet compared to mice in the other 2 gps. (*Sakaguchi M et al. Relationship of tissue and tumor fatty acids to dietary fat in experimental colorectal cancer. Gut 30:1449, 1989*).

Animal Experimental Study: High levels of dietary fish oil inhibited the growth of human breast carcinoma xenografts in athymic mice as compared to the normal laboratory diet (p<0.001) (*Pritchard GA et al. Lipids in breast carcinogenesis. Br J Surg 76(10):1069-73, 1989*).

- Omega-6 Fatty Acids:

$$\text{Linoleic acid} \rightarrow \text{gammalinolenic acid (GLA)} \rightarrow \text{DGLA} \rightarrow \text{PGE}_1$$

Due to contradictory findings, the effect of linoleic acid upon human carcinogenesis is uncertain.

A. Studies suggesting an inhibitory effect upon carcinogenesis:

Animal Experimental Study: Oral administration of safflower oil (73% linoleate in triglyceride form) resulted in marked improvement in some of a gp. of animals with spontaneous tumors (*Iwamoto KS et al. Linoleate therapy for spontaneous cancer in animals. Abstract. FASEB J 3(3, Part I):A471, 1989*).

Animal Experimental Study: Cats and dogs with advanced cancer received injections of sodium linoleate, the water-soluble salt of linoleic acid. In 1 cat, the total tumor burden in the ascites dropped after 1 treatment to about 2% of its initial value, suggesting a direct action upon the tumor cells rather than on the pleural surfaces and, in one dog, sodium linoleate injected directly into a fibrosarcoma caused a significant shrinkage of the tumor (*Bennett LR et al. Cancer therapy with linoleate. Abstract. FASEB J 2(5):A1192, 1988*).

Animal and In vitro Experimental Studies: Linoleic acid was found to be the major component in a microsomal fraction from the small intestine of mice that was responsible for preventing the proliferation of Ehrlich ascites tumor cells, and an i.p. injection of sodium linoleate into mice 1 day after inoculation with Ehrlich ascites tumor cells increased the median survival from 18 to 48 days and completely prevented tumor growth in 40% of the mice. In addition, sodium linoleate was more effective *in vitro* in killing human chronic lymphocytic leukemia lymphocytes than in killing normal lymphocytes. Results suggest that linoleic acid plays a significant role in keeping the small intestine from developing primary cancers (*Norman A et al. Antitumor activity of sodium linoleate. Nutr Cancer 11(2):107-15, 1988*).

Observational Study: Dietary records of 55 black pts. with prostate cancer were compared to those of matched controls. An inverse relationship was noted between dietary intake of linoleic acid and risk for developing prostate cancer for the more-than-50-years-old group (p<0.04) (*Kaul L et al. The role of diet in prostate cancer. Nutr Cancer 9:123-28, 1987*).

Review Article: Linoleic acid has shown potent proliferation-suppressive effects on malignant cells in culture (*Booyens J et al. Dietary fats and cancer. Med Hypotheses 17(4):351-62, 1985*).

B. Studies suggesting a promotional effect upon carcinogenesis:

Review Article: The results of studies using animal experimental models of cancer have suggested that linoleic acid may promote mammary carcinogenesis, although most human diets contain more linoleic acid than the amt. required for maximum enhancement of tumor yields in animals (*Carroll KK. Lipid oxidation and carcinogenesis. Prog Clin Biol Res 206:237-44, 1986*).

C. Studies suggesting a mixed effect upon carcinogenesis:

Animal Experimental Study: Female rats received either high or low linoleic acid diets before and after inoculation with syngeneic tumor models. In most models, tumor growth was identical in both groups. In an adrenal cortical carcinoma, however, growth was significantly increased while, in a myeloid leukemia, growth was significantly decreased (*Kort WJ et al. Influence of the linoleic acid content of the diet on tumor growth in transplantable rat tumor models. Ann Nutr Metab 30(2):120-28, 1986*).

Animal Experimental Study: Female rats received either a high or a low linoleic acid diet during their whole lifespan. Spontaneous tumor incidence and median survival times were not significantly different. However, the numbers of reticulendothelial tumors and adrenocortical carcinomas were significantly higher in the animals on the low linoleic acid diet, while there were a greater number of mammary tumors in the high linoleic acid gp. due to a high incidence of tumor multiplicity (*Kort WJ et al. Spontaneous tumor incidence in female brown Norway rats after lifelong diets high and low in linoleic acid. J Natl Cancer Inst 74(2):529-36, 1985*).

It has been suggested that the production of gammalinolenic acid (GLA) from dietary linoleic acid is sometimes blocked due to a defect in the enzyme delta-6-desaturase, and that this blockage may promote carcinogenesis. If so, supplementation with a source of GLA such as evening primrose oil may theoretically inhibit carcinogenesis by restoring normal prostaglandin E series metabolism (*Booyens J, Katzeff IE. Cancer: A simple metabolic disease? Med Hypotheses 12(3):195-201, 1983; Horrobin DF. The reversibility of cancer: The relevance of cyclic AMP, calcium, essential fatty acids, and prostaglandin E1. Med Hypotheses 6:469-86, 1980*).

Animal Experimental Study: High levels of dietary evening primrose oil inhibited the growth of human breast carcinoma xenografts in athymic mice as compared to the normal laboratory diet (p<0.001) (*Pritchard GA et al. Lipids in breast carcinogenesis. Br J Surg 76(10):1069-73, 1989*).

Experimental Study: 21 pts. with untreatable cancers received 18-36 caps daily of evening primrose oil 500 mg (containing 45 mg each of GLA with vitamin E 10 mg). There was apparent clinical improvement in all cases. Most pts. noted marked subjective improvement; in many cases there were objective improvements such as weight gain and reduction of tumor mass. 4/21 pts. showed radiological evidence of improvement. In 11 pts. with primary hepatocellular carcinoma, most demonstrated a reduction in liver size; ave. survival time increased from 42 days in an unsupplemented gp. to 90 days. Of the remaining 10 cases, 3 are continuing to improve 32-41 mo. after commencing supplementation and 1 died in an accident after having been free of evidence of malignancy for 9 months. In regard to the 4/10 who died from their cancer, improvement lasted from 2 wks. to 4 months (*Van der Merwe et al. Oral gamma-linoleic acid in 21 patients with untreatable malignancy. An ongoing pilot open clinical trial. Br J Clin Pract 41(9):907-15, 1987*).

Animal Experimental Study: Breast-cancer-prone rats were fed a carcinogen. In addition, half were fed a high fat diet in which 20% of the fat was corn oil (high in linoleic acid), while the rest were fed the same high fat diet in which evening primrose oil was substituted for corn oil. In the rats fed corn oil nearly twice as many mammary tumors developed as in the rats fed primrose oil (*El-Ela SH et al.   Effects of dietary primrose on mammary tumorigenesis. Lipids 22(12):1041-44, 1987*).

In vitro Experimental Study: When human breast, lung and prostate cancer cells and normal human fibroblasts were co-cultured in the absence of PUFAs, the malignant cells outgrew the normal ones. When, however, gamma linolenic or arachidonic acid was added to the co-cultures, the normal cells outgrew the malignant ones at concentrations which had no adverse effects on human fibroblasts or on normal animal cell lines (*Bëgin ME et al.   Differential killing of human carcinoma cells supplemented with n-3 and n-6 polyunsaturated fatty acids.   J Natl Cancer Inst 77:1053-62, 1986; Bëgin ME et al.   Selective killing of human cancer cells by polyunsaturated fatty acids.   Prostaglandins Leukotrienes Med 19(2):177-86, 1985*).

Negative Animal Experimental Study: Mice bearing murine sarcoma allografts were fed either standard laboratory diets or diets supplemented with evening primrose oil. At the end of the treatment period, there was no significant difference in tumor volumes between the 2 gps. (*Ramchurren N et al.   Effects of gamma-linolenic acid on murine cells in vitro and in vivo. S Afr Med J 68(11):795-98, 1985*).

- with vitamin C:

   Experimental Controlled Study: In a study of pts. with primary hepatic carcinoma, supplementation with evening primrose oil and vitamin C was associated with a doubling of the mean survival time for 11 pts. with one surviving more than 300 days (*van der Merwe CF.   The reversibility of cancer.   S Afr Med J 65:712, 1984*).

- with vitamin C, pyridoxine and zinc:

   Negative Experimental Controlled Study: 54 pts. with Dukes's C colorectal cancer randomly received either 500 mg evening primrose oil (Efamol) capsules 6 daily in divided doses (each containing 45 mg GLA and 10 mg natural vitamin E) or placebo. In addition, all pts. received vitamin C 125 mg, pyridoxine 25 mg and zinc sulfate 5 mg daily. There was no significant difference in the pattern of disease progression between the 2 groups (*McIllmurray MB, Turkie W.   Controlled trial of gamma linolenic acid in Dukes's C colorectal cancer.   Br Med J 294:1260, 1987*).

- Omega-3 and
  Omega-6 fatty acids:

   Supplementation with both eicosapentaenoic acid (EPA), an omega-3 fatty acid, and gamma-linolenic acid (GLA), an omega-6 fatty acid, has been proposed as prophylaxis against the possible tumorigenic effect of dietary fats. Such supplementation would counteract a combination of inhibited desaturase enzymes and a concomitant free cellular supply of dietary arachidonic acid which may be causally related to carcinogenesis (*Booyens J et al.   Dietary fats and cancer.   Med Hypotheses 17(4):351-62, 1985*).

   Oils rich in omega-3 fatty acids may be superior to those rich in linoleic acid (an omega-6 fatty acid) in inhibiting the growth of malignant tumors (*Braden LM, Carroll KK.   Dietary polyunsaturated fat in relation to mammary carcinogenesis in rats.   Lipids 21(4):285-8, 1986; Cameron E et al.   Nutr Res Vol. 9, 1989; Nelson RL et al.   A comparison of dietary fish oil and corn oil in experimental colorectal carcinogenesis.   Nutr Cancer 11:215-20, 1988; Reddy B et al.   Effect of diets high in omega-3 and omega-6 fatty acids on initiation and postinitiation stages of colon carcinogenesis.   Cancer Res 51:487-91, 1991*).

   Increasing the ratio of omega-3 to omega-6 essential fatty acids may reduce cancer risk.

   Review Article: Data from the large MRFIT study showed that the 18:3 ω3/18:2 ω6 ratio and the ratio of total ω3/ω6 fatty acids in the diet are negatively correlated with the risk for cancer mortality (*Dolecek TA, Grandits G.   Dietary polyunsaturated fatty acids and mortality in the multiple risk factor intervention trial (MRFIT), in AP Simopoulos et al, Eds.   Health Effects of ω3 Polyunsaturated Fatty Acids in Seafoods.   World Rev Nutr Diet 66:205-17, 1991*).

   Review Article: In animal models of breast cancer, both a high level of dietary fat and a certain amt. of omega-6 fatty acid (linoleic acid) appear to be required to obtain the maximal carcinogenic effect of dietary fat. Although polyunsaturated fats are more effective than saturated fats in promoting mammary cancer in animals, human epidemiologial data has failed to find a correlation between dietary polyunsaturates and breast cancer mortality; however, this failure could be explained on the basis that the diets of most countries contain sufficient linoleic acid for maximum carcinogenic effect, so that the observed correlation between dietary fat and breast cancer mortality could be attributed to the amt. rather than the type of dietary fat. In regard to colon tumors, there is less indication of differences between saturated and polyunsaturated fats, and the requirement for omega-6 fatty acid seems to be less. In regard to pancreatic lesions, the level of omega-6 fatty acid required for maximal carcinogenic effect appears to be higher than for mammary tumors. For all 3 types of experimental cancer, high levels of fish oils (omega-3 fatty acids) appear to be inhibitory (*Carroll KK. Dietary fats and cancer. Am J Clin Nutr 53:1064S-7S, 1991*).

Review Article: There is compelling evidence that industrialized Western societies have been selectively depleting the dietary availability of omega-3 EFA's by hydrogenation, milling and selection of omega-3 poor foods (e.g. safflower oil, sunflower oil and corn oil). Currently, the daily intake of omega-6 EFA's may be 8-10 times higher than that recommended. The results of animal studies with experimental tumors suggest that diets should not only emphasize a greatly reduced intake of total fat, but also achieving more balance between the relative amts. of omega-3 and omega-6 EFA's (*Kearney R. Promotion and prevention of tumour growth: Effects of endotoxin, inflammation and dietary lipids. Int Clin Nutr Rev 7(4):157-68, 1987*).

Omega-9 fatty acids :

Oleic acid is a monounsaturate primarily found in olive oil.

Compared to the essential (omega-3 and omega-6) fatty acids, oleic acid may enhance (or more weakly inhibit) tumor growth.

Animal Experimental Study: High levels of dietary evening primrose oil or fish oil inhibited the growth of human breast carcinoma xenografts in athymic mice as compared to supplementation with olive oil or the normal lab diet (p<0.001) (*Pritchard GA et al. Lipids in breast carcinogenesis. Br J Surg 76(10):1069-73, 1989*).

Negative Animal Experimental Study: Rats were studied with experimentally-induced mammary tumors. Animals fed high-fat diets rich in linoleic acid (such as safflower or corn oil) exhibited an increased incidence and decreased latent period compared to those fed high-fat diets rich in oleic acid or coconut oil. Prostaglandin E_2 levels in the tumor lipid fatty acid content correlated with the incidence of tumors. In addition, dose-response studies indicated a threshold lying between 20% and 33% fat as calories which needed to be exceeded before tumor promotion was manifested. These results suggest that high fat intake is a necessary, but not a sufficient, condition for tumor promotion, and that the proportion of essential polyunsaturates *vis a vis* monounsaturates and saturates is a critical determinant of the fat effect (*Cohen LA. Fat and endocrine-responsive cancer in animals. Prev Med 16(4):468-74, 1987*).

In vitro Experimental Study: Gamma-linolenic acid (omega-6 series) and eicosapentaenoic (omega-3 series) suppressed the proliferation of human larynx carcinoma cells in culture, while oleic acid produced significant growth enhancement (*Booyens J, Katzeff IE. Suppression of proliferation of human larynx carcinoma cells in culture by gamma-linolenic and eicosapentaenoic acids with stimulation by oleic acid. IRCS J Med Sci 14:396, 1986*).

Review Article: Oleic acid, an omega-9 monounsaturated non-essential fatty acid present in vegetable oils and abundant in olive oil, has been shown to stimulate malignant cell proliferation *in vitro*, while the essential fatty acids of both the omega-3 and omega-6 series appear to have a protective effect. Findings that polyunsaturated fatty acids may be tumorigenic are most likely due to their oleic acid content (*Booyens J et al. Dietary fats and cancer. Med Hypotheses 17:351-62, 1985*).

Phytosterols:

Cholesterol analogs found in plants which may be protective against colon cancer.

Observational Study: 3-day composite diets of 4 study gps. of 18 Seventh-day Adventist (SDA) pure vegetarians, 50 SDA lacto-ovo-vegetarians, 50 SDA nonvegetarians, and 50 general population nonvegetarians were analyzed for their sterol composition and the plant sterol/cholesterol ratios were calculated. Results suggest that the absolute amts. of cholesterol consumed as a factor by itself might not be as significant in colon carcinogenesis as its relationship to total plant sterols in the diet (*Nair PP et al. Diet, nutrition intake, and metabolism in populations at high and low risk for colon cancer: Dietary cholesterol, beta-sitosterol, and stigmasterol. Am J Clin Nutr 40(4 suppl.):927-30, 1984*).

Superoxide Dismutase:

Provides a natural defense against the potentially damaging superoxide radical generated by aerobic metabolism.

May be diminished in tumors.

Observational Study: Diminished amts. of manganese-containing superoxide dismutase have been found in all tumors examined, and lowered amts. of copper/zinc-containing superoxide dismutase have been found in many tumors. At the same time, tumors have been shown to produce superoxide radicals. Diminished SOD along with superoxide radical production may lead to many of the observed properties of cancer cells (*Oberley LW, Buettner GR. Role of superoxide dismutase in cancer: A review. Cancer Res 39:1141-49, 1979*).

Supplementation may ameliorate radiation cystitis and colitis in patients receiving radiation therapy of pelvic tumors, such as bladder or prostate carcinomas.

Review Article: Double-blind trials have shown that SOD (Orgotein) 4-8 mg given sub-cutaneously 15-30 min. after completion of each fractional radiation dose, improved bowel and bladder function, and lessened the need for analgesics and anti-diarrheal medication (*Petkau A. Scientific basis for the clinical use of superoxide dismutase. Cancer Treat Rev 13:17-44, 1986*).

Supplementation may reverse the leukopenia induced in patients by radiation or chemotherapy (*Villasor RP. Superoxide dismutase treatment of myelosuppression resulting from cancer chemotherapy, in AP Autor, Ed. Pathology of Oxygen. New York, Academic Press, pp. 303-14*).

- -

COMBINED NUTRITIONAL SUPPLEMENTATION

General

Clinical Observations: Cancer pts. were treated with a regimen consisting of vitamin C 12 g/d along with large amts. of other nutrients and advice about food selection. Usually, the other nutrients consisted of niacin or niacinamide 1.5-3g/d, pyridoxine 250 mg/d, other B vitamins in variable amts., vitamin E 800 IU/d, beta-carotene 30,000 IU/d, selenium 2-500 μg/d, and other minerals. There were 3 cohorts: a cohort of 40 pts. with cancer of the breast, ovary, uterus, or cervix, a cohort of 61 pts. with other kinds of cancer, and a cohort of 31 similar pts. who did not follow the regimen. A Hardin Jones biostatistical analysis of mortality data for these cohorts was performed. Results indicated that mean survival time for the 31 pts. who did not follow the regimen was 5.7 months. 80% of the pts. in the other 2 cohorts were considered good responders, with a mean survival time of 122 mo. for 32 pts. with cancer of the breast, ovary, uterus or cervix, and 72 mo. for pts. with other kinds of cancer. 20% were poor responders, with a mean survival time of 10 months (*Hoffer A, Pauling L. Hardin Jones biostatistical analysis of mortality data for cohorts of cancer patients with a large fraction surviving at the termination of the study and a comparison of survival times of cancer patients receiving large regular oral doses of vitamin C and other nutrients with similar patients not receiving those doses. J Orthomol Med 5(3):143-54, 1990*).

Clinical Observations: 41 pts. were given dietary instructions (reduce red meats; increase green vegetables; avoid sugar, coffee, cocoa and milk products). They were also given daily supplements of vitamin B complex '50', niacin 1.5-3 g, vitamin A 25-50,000 IU, vitamin C to bowel tolerance (minimum 12 g), vitamin E 800 IU, magnesium 500 mg, selenium 4-500 μg, zinc 30-50 mg, and beta-carotene 30-60,000 IU. While the entire program appeared advantageous, unless pts. ingested high doses of vitamin C for at least 2 months, their prognosis was very poor. For example, at follow-up 5-7 yrs. later, all 5 pts. who failed to take vitamin C were dead with a mean survival of 7 months. The 1 pt. who took 3 gm of vitamin C survived 10 months, while 4/6 pts. who took 12 or more gm. of vitamin C were still alive and the mean survival of that group was 53 months. Results with subsequent pts. have been similar (*Hoffer A. Orthomolecular Medicine for Physicians. New Canaan, Conn., Keats Publishing, 1989*).

Pre-Leukemia

> **Case Report:** A 25-year-old male complained of a 2-3 yr. period of progressive malaise, fatigue and headache. Pre-leukemia was diagnosed on the basis of blood and bone marrow studies. He was placed on a regime which included large daily doses of antioxidants consisting of a multivitamin along with folic acid 1 mg, vitamin A 25 mg, vitamin C 1 gm, vitamin E 800 IU, selenium 400 µg, zinc 30 mg, β-carotene 50 mg, cysteine 2 gm and N-acetyl cysteine 3 gm. He was also given phenylalanine 3 gm and tyrosine 3 g for the treatment of depression. After 3 mo., his full blood count was entirely normal. 6 mo. after his bone marrow biopsy, a repeat biopsy was entirely normal (*Braverman ER. Reversal of pre-leukaemia with antioxidants: a case report. J Nutr Med 2:313-15, 1991*).

- -

MICROORGANISMS

Lactobacillus Acidophilus:

Administration may help to prevent colon cancer.

> **Experimental Crossover Study:** 21 healthy young subjects were fed viable lactobacillus acidophilus cultures with milk in concentrations similar to those in commercial acidophilus milk and LA yogurt cultures. The fecal concentrations of bacterial enzymes known to catalyze the conversion of procarcinogens to proximal carcinogens were significantly reduced by the end of one month, but not when milk was given without the LA, suggesting that LA in milk may help to prevent cancer of the colon (*Goldin BR, Gorbach SL. The effect of milk and lactobacillus feeding on human intestinal bacterial enzyme activity. Am J Clin Nutr 39:756-61, 1984*).

> **In vitro Experimental Study:** L. acidophilus and Bifidobacterium degraded nitrites *in vitro* (*Dodds KL, Collins-Thompson DL. Incidence of nitrite-depleting lactic acid bacteria in cured meats and in starter cultures. J Food Protection 47:7-10, 1984*).

> **Review article:** The link between diet and colon cancer can be explained, in part, by the alterations in fecal bacterial enzyme activity induced by the Western-style high beef, high fat, low fiber diet. These alterations can be normalized in experimental animals by the addition of Lactobacillus acidophilus to the diet (*Gorbach SL. The intestinal microflora and its colon cancer connection. Infection 10(6):379-84, 1982*).

> **Experimental Study:** The addition of viable Lactobacillus acidophilus supplements to the diet of omnivores significantly decreased fecal bacterial beta-glucuronidase and nitroreductase activities, both of which are known to catalyze reactions that may result in the formation of proximal carcinogens. Thirty days after supplements were curtailed, fecal enzyme levels returned to baseline (*Goldin BR et al. Effect of diet and Lactobacillus acidophilus supplements on human fecal bacterial enzymes. J Natl Cancer Inst 64(2):255-61, 1980*).

> **In vitro Experimental Study:** L. acidophilus and Bifidobacterium degrated nitrosamines *in vitro* (*Rowland IR, Grasso P. Degradation of N-nitrosamines by intestinal bacteria. Appl Microbiol 29:7-12, 1975*).

Administration may prevent radiotherapy-associated diarrhea.

> **Experimental Controlled Study:** Some of a gp. of 24 pts. with gynecologic malignancies and scheduled for internal and external pelvic irradiation received 150 ml of a fermented milk product daily supplying them with live L. acidophilus bacteria with 6.5% lactulose as the substrate. The ingestion of L. acidophilus successfully prevented radiotherapy-induced diarrhea (*Salminen E et al. Preservation of intestinal integrity during radiotherapy using live Lactobacillus acidophilus cultures. Clin Radiol 39:435-7, 1988*).

- -

TOXIC MINERALS

Arsenic:

WARNING: Exposure is associated with fatal internal organ cancers as well as non-lethal skin cancers (*Chen C-J et al. Arsenic and cancer. Letter. Lancet 1:414-15, 1988*).

Observational Study: In a study of copper smelter workers, whose increased incidence of respiratory cancer is believed to be due to airborne arsenic, there was a relative risk of 6.0 for men initially employed at 16.9 yrs. of age with heavy exposure as compared to those employed at 31.9 yrs. of age with only light exposure (*Lee-Feldstein A. A comparison of several measures of exposure to arsenic. Matched case-control study of copper smelter employees. Am J Epidemiol 129(1):112-124, 1989*).

Cadmium:

WARNING: Cadmium exposure is associated with increased cancer risk.

Review Article: A combination of all available data from the most recent follow up of causes of deaths among cadmium workers in 6 different cohorts suggests that long-term, high-level exposure to cadmium is associated with an increased risk of prostatic and lung cancer (*Elinder CG et al. Cancer mortality of cadmium workers. Br J Ind Med 42(10):651-55, 1985*).

Increased in prostatic tissue in prostatic cancer.

Observational Study: As measured by atomic absorption spectrometry, there were distinct differences in the cadmium content in the nuclear fractions of malignant tissues in comparison with BPH and normal prostatic tissue, with the highest cadmium levels being in the nuclear fractions of poorly-differentiated carcinomas (*Feustel A, Wennrich R. Zinc and cadmium in cell fractions of prostatic cancer tissues of different histological grading in comparison to BPH and normal prostate. Urol Res 12(2):147-50, 1984*).

Observational Study: As measured by atomic absorption spectroscopy, cadmium levels in carinomatous prostatic tissue were markedly increased compared to normal controls (129.79 ± 22.22 vs. 5.15 ± 0.62 nmol/g). Dihydrotestosterone levels in the malignant tissue were proportional to the cadmium concentrations (*Habib FK et al. Metal-androgen interrelationships in carcinoma and hyperplasia of the human prostate. J Endocrinol 71(1):133-41, 1976*).

CANDIDIASIS

See Also: IMMUNODEPRESSION
INFECTION

Overgrowth of candida albicans in mucous membranes, or hypersensitivity to the organism, is claimed by some authors to cause a poly-symptomatic syndrome (which may include mental symptoms, irritable bowel syndrome, premenstrual syndrome, etc.) even in the absence of infection.

At the present time, however, the American Academy of Allergy and Immunology considers the concept of a "candidiasis hypersensitivity syndrome" to be unproven. According to the Academy, "the diagnosis, the special laboratory tests, and the special aspects of treatment should be considered experimental and reserved for use with informed consent in appropriate controlled trials" (*Position statement: Candidiasis hypersensitivity syndrome. J Allergy Clin Immunol 78(2):271-73, 1986*).

- -

DIETARY FACTORS

Sugar-free diet.

In vitro Experimental Study: Candida albicans failed to grow in human saliva unless it was supplemented with glucose (*Samaranayake LP et al. The proteolytic potential of candida albicans in human saliva supplemented with glucose. J Med Microbiol 17(1):13-22, 1984*).

Experimental Study: The urinary sugar patterns of 100 women with recurrent candida vulvovaginitis were studied and elevated patterns of glucose, arabinose and ribose were found. These excretion patterns correlated well with the excessive oral ingestion of dairy products, artificial sweeteners and sucrose. Eliminating excessive use of these foods brought about a dramatic reduction in the incidence and severity of the illness (*Horowitz BJ et al. Sugar chromatography studies in recurrent Candida vulvovaginitis. J Reprod Med 29(7):441-43, 1984*).

Yeast- and mold-free diet.

Observational Study: Blood serum from 76 mold-allergic patients was studied using a RAST test. Cross reactivity between several genera of fungi was observed (*Hoffman DR, Kozak PP. Shared and specific allergens in mold extracts. J Allergy Clin Immunol 63:213, 1979*).

Experimental Double-blind Study: Pts. with chronic urticaria reacted to candida albicans antigens as well as to other types of yeast and fungi (*James J, Warren RP. An assessment of the role of candidia albicans and food yeast in chronic urticaria. Br J Dermatol 84:227-37, 1971*).

Experimental Study: 49/255 pts. with chronic urticaria reacted to candida albicans antigens. 55% of these pts. also reacted to brewer's yeast. After treatment with a low-yeast diet and anti-fungal therapy, 27/49 experienced a clinical cure. Similar results were obtained employing a yeast-free diet in the treatment of mucous colitis (*Holti G. Candida allergy, in Winner & Hurley, Eds. Symposium on Candida Infections. Edinburgh, Livingstone Publishers, 1966*).

- -

VITAMINS

Folic Acid:

May be deficient.

Observational Study: Deficient in serum in 15% of 101 pts. with candida allergy or toxicity (*Galland L. Nutrition and candidiasis. J Orthomol Psychiatry 14:50-60, 1985*).

Riboflavin:

May be deficient.

Observational Study: 29% of 17 pts. with candida allergy or toxicity showed evidence of riboflavin deficiency based on the RBC glutathione reductase activity coefficient, although none of 59 pts. were riboflavin-deficient based on microbiological assays (*Galland L. Nutrition and candidiasis. J Orthomol Psychiatry 14:50-60, 1985*).

Vitamin A:

May be deficient.

Observational Study: Deficient (< 25 mg/dl in serum) in 13% of 101 pts. with candida allergy or toxicity. None of these pts. was deficient in serum carotene, which was elevated in 4 patients. Since the vitamin A deficiency is most likely due to impairment of beta-carotene oxygenase, which is primarily found in the intestinal mucosa, these pts. most likely have intestinal candidiasis (*Galland L. Nutrition and candidiasis. J Orthomol Psychiatry 14:50-60, 1985*).

Observational Study: 13 pts. with mucocutaneous candidiasis were found to have vitamin A deficiency despite normal carotene levels (*Montes LF et al. Hypovitaminosis A in patients with mucocutaneous candidiasis. J Infect Dis 128:227-230, 1973*).

Supplementation may enhance resistance to candida infection (*Cohen BE, Elin RJ. Enhanced resistance to certain infections in vitamin A-treated mice. Plast Reconstr Surg 54(2):192-94, 1974*).

Vitamin B$_6$:

May be deficient.

Observational Study: 26/39 pts. with candida allergy or toxicity were found to be deficient in plasma pyridoxal-5-phosphate, while only 5/59 were deficient in pyridoxine. Results suggest impaired phosphorylation of pyridoxine (*Galland L. Nutrition and candidiasis. J Orthomol Psychiatry 14:50-60, 1985*).

Vitamin C:

May prevent the impairment of leukocyte function due to myeloperoxidase activation by Candida albicans.

Experimental Study: Ascorbic acid stimulated neutrophil motility and lymphocyte transformation by inhibition of the peroxidase/H_2O_2/halide system both *in vitro* and *in vivo* (*Anderson R. Ascorbate-mediated stimulation of neutrophil motility and lymphocyte transformation by inhibition of the peroxidase/H_2O_2/halide system in vitro and in vivo. Am J Clin Nutr 34:1906-11, 1981*).

May enhance the efficacy of amphotericin B.

In vitro Experimental Study: Ascorbic acid enhanced the lethal but not the permeabilizing effect of amphotericin B on Candida albicans cells. It is assumed that ascorbic acid acted as a pro-oxidant, augmenting the oxidation-dependent killing of fungal cells induced by amphotericin B (*Brajtburg J et al. Effects of ascorbic acid on the antifungal action of amphotericin B. J Antimicrob Chemother 24(3):333-7, 1989*).

- -

MINERALS

Copper:

Deficiency may impair the ability of neutrophils to kill candida.

In vitro Animal Experimental Study: Neutophils from cattle with copper deficiency induced by molybdenum or iron had an impaired ability to kill ingested candida albicans and were less viable than those from copper-supplemented cattle (*Boyne R, Arthur JR. Effects of molybdenum or iron induced copper deficiency on the viability and function of neutrophils from cattle. Res Vet Sci 41(3):417-19, 1986*).

High levels may increase candida virulence.

In vitro and Animal Experimental Study: Cultures of candida albicans in the yeast phase were found to be more virulent than cultures grown in the mycelial phase, and copper was found to suppress filamentation of candida in culture. When copper was injected into mice, the filamentous phase became as virulent as the yeast phase (*Vaughn VJ, Weinberg ED. Candida albicans dimorphism and virulence: Role of copper. Mycopathologia 64(1):39-42, 1978*).

Iron:

Deficiency may predispose to candida infections, and correction of the deficiency may be associated with healing.

Negative Clinical Observation: Iron replacement has produced neither benefit nor exacerbation of candidiasis in any pt., except those with sideropenic anemia (*Galland LD. Nutrition and Candida albicans, in J Bland, Ed. 1986: A Year in Nutritional Medicine. New Canaan, Connecticut, Keats Publishing, 1986*).

Observational Study: Serum ferritin was deficient in 10/101 pts. with candida allergy or toxicity (*Galland L. Nutrition and candidiasis. J Orthomol Psychiatry 14:50-60, 1985*).

Experimental Study: Among a gp. of pts. with hypochromic anemia and low serum iron (without concomitant deficiency of folate or vitamin B_{12}), C. albicans was isolated more often and in greater number from the saliva of malnourished pts. with mouth lesions. Therapy with oral ferrous sulfate was associated with a rapid clearing of the mouth lesions and a fall in salivary candida count (*Fletcher J et al. Mouth lesions in iron-deficient anemia: Relationship to candida albicans, saliva and to impairment of lymphocyte transformation. J Infect Dis 131:44-50, 1975*).

Experimental Study: Several pts. with chronic mucocutaneous candidiasis associated with reduced cellular immunity and iron deficiency demonstrated rapid improvement in clinical manifestations following iron administration (*Higgs JM, Wells RS. Mucocutaneous candidiasis. Br J Dermatol (Suppl) 86:88-102, 1972*).

While low levels of iron-binding proteins are associated with candida allergy, toxicity and infection, elevated levels of unbound serum iron <u>encourage</u> candida growth.

Animal Experimental Study: Mice received IV injections of candida albicans either with or without iron overload. Excessive iron clearly promoted the proliferation of inoculated candida (*Abe F et al. Experimental candidiasis in iron overload. Mycopathologica 89(1):59-63, 1985*).

Observational Study: Elevated serum iron and lowered serum transferrin were associated with predisposition to candidiasis in leukemic pts. (*Caroline L et al. Elevated serum iron, low unbound transferrin and candidiasis in acute leukemia. Blood 34(4):441-51, 1969*).

Magnesium: 6-12 mg/kg/day as an organic salt (ascorbate, citrate, lactate, orotate, etc.)

May be deficient.

Clinical Observation: Magnesium deficiency appears to be the commonest biochemical abnormality in chronic candidiasis patients. Many pts. fail to respond to magnesium oxide (including mixtures with amino acids); organic magnesium salts often produce a better response, especially when combined with pyridoxine 50-1000 mg/day and vitamin D 400-1000 IU/day (*Galland LD. Nutrition and Candida albicans, in J Bland, Ed. 1986: A Year in Nutritional Medicine. New Canaan, Connecticut, Keats Publishing, 1986*).

Experimental Study: Among 50 pts. with normocalcemic latent tetany, 34% suffered from recurrent or chronic candida infection by history, 24% showed evidence of active infection and 48% demonstrated type I hypersensitivity to C. albicans extract on intradermal testing. Treatment with oral antifungal drugs and allergy desensitization to Candida produced complete relief of symptoms in 44% of the pts., with remission occurring for symptoms of depression, irritable bowel syndrome, fatigue, premenstrual tension, headache, anxiety and back pain (*Galland L. Normocalcemic tetany and candidiasis. Magnesium 4(5-6):339-44, 1985*).

Experimental Study: 41 pts. with candida allergy or toxicity underwent a magnesium loading test. None had a normal result. In many cases, baseline magnesium excretion was elevated, suggesting impaired renal magnesium conservation. In addition, 10/10 pts. had a positive Chvostek's sign for latent tetany, consistent with neuromuscular excitability secondary to magnesium deficiency (*Galland L. Nutrition and candidiasis. J Orthomol Psychiatry 14:50-60, 1985*).

Selenium:

Deficiency may predispose to candida infection.

Animal Experimental Study: Following IV injections of candida albicans, deaths in selenium-deficient mice began several days earlier than deaths in selenium-supplemented animals. Similarly, 3 days after an injection, significantly more microorganisms were found in the organs of selenium-deficient mice than in selenium-supplemented ones. Selenium deficiency was also demonstrated to impair the ability of mouse neutrophils to kill candida in *in vitro* tests (*Boyne R, Arthur JR. The response of selenium-deficient mice to candida albicans infection. J Nutr 116(5):816-22, 1986*).

Zinc:

Reduced plasma (but not erythrocyte) zinc may be associated with candida infection.

Observational Study: Compared to controls, plasma zinc was significantly lower in 29 women with recurrent vaginal candidiasis (p=0.015). These differences were even greater when adjusted for dietary and supplemental zinc with the use of analyses of covariance. No differences in RBC zinc were found between the two gps. (*Edman J et al. Zinc status in women with vulvovaginal candidiasis. Am J Obstet Gynecol 155(5):1082-1085, 1986*).

Deficiency may facilitate candida infection.

In vitro Animal Experimental Study: Compared to controls, polymorphonuclear leukocytes from zinc-deficient rhesus monkey infants displayed impaired phagocytosis of candida albicans (*Haynes DC et al. Studies of marginal zinc deprivation in rhesus monkeys: VI. Influence on the immunohematology of infants in the first year. Am J Clin Nutr 42(2):252-62, 1985*).

Candida infection may cause zinc deficiency (*Parratt D. Nutrition and immunity. Proc Nutr Soc 39(2):133-40, 1980; Salvin SB, Rabin BS. Resistance and susceptability to infection. Effects of dietary zinc. Cell Immunol 87(2):546-52, 1984*)

Reduced plasma (but elevated erythrocyte) zinc may be associated with candida allergy or toxicity.

Observational Study: 14/83 (16.9%) pts. with candida allergy or toxicity had a plasma zinc level of <80 mg/dl, and 30/83 (36.1%) had a level <100 mg/dl. Based on the literature of experimental zinc deficiency in humans, the plasma levels suggested that 17.3% of pts. showed significant risk of zinc deficiency. Paradoxically, all pts. with low plasma zinc also had elevated levels of RBC zinc (*Galland L. Nutrition and candidiasis. J Orthomol Psychiatry 14:50-60, 1985*).

Supplementation may prevent candida infection.

Animal Experimental Study: When mice which are normally susceptible to candida albicans infections were fed a high-zinc diet, they became more resistant to infection. When mice which are normally resistant to candida albicans infections were fed a low-zinc diet, they became more susceptible to infection (*Salvin SB, Rabin BS. Resistance and susceptability to infection in inbred murine strains. IV. Effects of dietary zinc. Cell Immunol. 87(2):546-52, 1984*).

- -

OTHER NUTRITIONAL FACTORS

Biotin:

Required for the growth of C. albicans (*Burkholder PR. Vitamin deficiencies in yeasts. Am J Botany 30:206-11, 1943; Littman, ML, Miwatani T. Effect of water-soluble vitamins and their analogues on growth of Candida albicans. 1. Biotin, pyridoxamine, pyridoxine and fluorinated pyrimidines. Mycopathologia et Mycologia Applicata 21:81-108, 1963*).

Deficiency *in vitro* is associated with the conversion of candida to the more pathogenic fungal form.

> **In vitro Experimental Study:** Candida albicans in a chemically-defined basal medium supplemented with biotin at optimal and suboptimal concentrations for growth developed predominantly into yeast and mycelial phases, respectively (*Yamaguchi H. Mycelial development and chemical alteration of candida albicans from biotin insufficiency. Sabouraudia 12(3):320-28, 1974*).
>
>> *Note: Oral administration of biotin is not likely to have a significant effect on Candida growth patterns as the concentration achieved in the small intestine and colon is too low (T Iwata - personal communication - reported in Galland LD. Nutrition and Candida albicans, in J Bland, Ed. 1986: A Year in Nutritional Medicine. New Canaan, Connecticut, Keats Publishing, 1986*).

Caprylic Acid:

An aliphatic straight-chain fatty acid that occurs naturally in coconut oil.

Supplementation (when complexed to a resin) may be beneficial.

> **Experimental Study:** 16 pts. who exhibited +2 to +4 candida growth on stool cultures using BCG agar plates received 1800 mg daily of a commercial caprylic acid preparation (Capricin). After 16 days a second stool culture revealed 30-90% reduction. 3 pts. with +4 candida growth received 2700 mg daily leading to a 70-100% reduction in 2 pts. and complete elimination in one. 6 pts. with +4 candida growth received 3600 mg daily. After 2 wks., stool cultures for all 6 showed complete elimination. These results seemed to correlate with symptom scores on subjective questionnnaires, with the greatest subjective relief noted in pts. with the highest symptom scores (*Crinnion WJ. Clinical trial results on Neesby's Capricin. Unpublished manuscript . Probiologic, Inc., 1803 132nd Avenue, N.E., Bellevue, WA 98005, USA, September 10, 1985*).

> **Experimental Study:** 3 cases of severe intestinal candidiasis were treated successfully with a caprylic acid ion exchange complex, with complete disappearance of candida from stool specimens in all pts. within several days (*Neuhauser I., Gustus E. Successful treatment of intestinal moniliasis with fatty acid-resin complex. Arch Intern Med 93:53-60, 1954*).

> **Experimental Study:** Buffered caprylic acid produced a prompt and dramatic response in slowly progressing thrush infections which had been resistant to standard therapy (*Keeney E. Bull Johns Hopkins Hosp 78:333-39, 1946*).

Cysteine or
Cystine:

> WARNING: Like glucose, these amino acids are readily utilized carbon sources, and thus supplementation with them will enhance candida growth in the yeast form (*Griffin D. Fungal Physiology. Wiley-Interscience, 1981, pp.124-125*).

Omega-3 Fatty Acids:

May be deficient.

Observational Study: 104 pts. with candida allergy or toxicity were studied. In regard to essential fatty acid metabolism, the most common abnormality found in RBC and plasma phospholipid fatty acid studies was a general depression of all components of the omega-3 fatty acid family, and two or more physical findings of EFA deficiency (dry skin; flaky paint dermatitis; follicular keratoses; brittle nails; dry, straw-like hair) were present in 65% (*Galland L. Nutrition and candidiasis. J Orthomol Psychiatry 14:50-60, 1985*).

Observational Study: Ave. RBC membrane and plasma phospholipids for 24 pts. with chronic symptoms typical of mold sensitivity and yeast susceptibility were compared with those of controls. All measured components of the omega-3 fatty acid family were significantly reduced in the pts. (*Truss CO. Metabolic abnormalities in patients with chronic candidiasis: The acetaldehyde hypothesis. J Orthomol Psychiatry 13:66-93, 1984*).

Successful symptomatic treatment with nystatin may be accompanied by changes in omega-3 fatty acid levels.

Experimental Study: Ave. RBC membrane and plasma phospholipids (expressed as area percent of total phospholipids) for 5 pts. with chronic symptoms typical of mold sensitivity and yeast susceptibility both before and 2-9 mo. following successful symptomatic treatment with nystatin were compared. Levels of 20:5n3 (EPA), which were depressed prior to treatment, decreased still further in plasma but increased towards normal in RBC membranes. Levels of 22:5n3, which were normal, became sightly depressed only in plasma, and levels of 22:6n3, which were depressed, became normal (*Truss CO. Metabolic abnormalities in patients with chronic candidiasis: The acetaldehyde hypothesis. J Orthomol Psychiatry 13:66-93, 1984*).

Omega-6 Fatty Acids:

Levels may be abnormal.

Observational Study: 2/3 of 104 pts. with candida allergy or toxicity demonstrated abnormalities in RBC and plasma phospholipid omega-6 fatty acid concentrations. An elevated arachidonic acid (AA) concentration was the most common abnormality. In addition, there was evidence of a block in the the elongation and further desaturation of AA (*Galland L. Nutrition and candidiasis. J Orthomol Psychiatry 14:50-60, 1985*).

Observational Study: Ave. RBC membrane and plasma phospholipids (expressed as area percent of total phospholipids) for 24 pts. with chronic symptoms typical of mold sensitivity and yeast susceptibility were compared with those of controls. For the omega-6 family, levels of linoleic acid (18:2n6) were significantly elevated in pts., while levels of elongated members, adrenic acid (22:2n6) and 22:5n-6, were significantly depressed. Levels of DGLA (20:3n6) were elevated in pts. only in the RBC assay, and arachidonic acid (20:4n6) levels were not significantly different (*Truss CO. Metabolic abnormalities in patients with chronic candidiasis:The acetaldehyde hypothesis. J Orthomol Psychiatry 13:66-93, 1984*).

Successful symptomatic treatment with nystatin may be associated with a trend towards normalization.

Experimental Study: Ave. RBC membrane and plasma phospholipids (expressed as area percent of total phospholipids) for 5 pts. with chronic symptoms typical of mold sensitivity and yeast susceptibility both before and 2-9 mo. following successful symptomatic treatment with nystatin were compared. Levels of linoleic acid (18:2n6), which had been elevated, decreased into the normal range; levels of DGLA (20:3n6), which had been elevated only in RBC membranes, decreased in RBC membranes almost to the normal range and remained normal in plasma; levels of arachidonic acid (10:4n6) were normal both before and after; levels of adrenic acid (22:4n6), which had been slightly depressed, became normal; levels of 22:5n6, which had also been depressed, also became normal in plasma and increased towards normal in RBC membranes (*Truss CO. Metabolic abnormalities in patients with chronic candidiasis: The acetaldehyde hypothesis. J Orthomol Psychiatry 13:66-93, 1984*).

Pantethine:

A metabolic intermediate which is the stable disulfide form of pantetheine - a derivative of pantothenic acid and a precursor of Coenzyme A.

May theoretically reduce the adverse effects of aldehydes by increasing the activity of aldehyde dehydrogenase, the enzyme which metabolizes them. This could be beneficial to pts. believed to be reacting to overproduction of acetaldehyde by candidia albicans (*Truss CO. Metabolic abnormalities in patients with chronic candidiasis: The acetaldehyde hypothesis. J Orthomol Psychiatry 13:66-93, 1984*).

Experimental Study: Administration of pantethine prior to alcohol ingestion reduced acetaldehyde levels in the blood of human volunteers and in the liver of experimental animals. Since ethanol levels were unaffected, this reduction is believed to have been due to an increase in aldehyde dehydrogenase activity (*Watanabe A et al. Lowering of blood acetaldehyde but not ethanol concentrations by pantethine following alcohol ingestion: Different effects in flushing and non-flushing subjects. Alcohol Clin Exp Res 9:272, 1985*).

In vitro Experimental Study: Pantethine increased aldehyde dehydrogenase activity by as much as 71% (*Watanabe A et al. Lowering of blood acetaldehyde but not ethanol concentrations by pantethine following alcohol ingestion: Different effects in flushing and non-flushing subjects. Alcohol Clin Exp Res 9:272, 1985*).

> *Note: Pantethine is unlikely to be effective in patients who flush after alcohol ingestion, probably due to a weak aldehyde dehydrogenase enzyme (Watanabe A et al. Lowering of blood acetaldehyde but not ethanol concentrations by pantethine following alcohol ingestion: Different effects in flushing and non-flushing subjects. Alcohol Clin Exp Res 9:272, 1985).*

Propionic Acid:

A three-carbon fatty acid which occurs in small amounts in dairy products.

Selectively inhibits filamentous fungi such as the mycelial form of candida albicans.

In vitro Animal Experimental Study: Propionic acid was fed to broilers and its effect on intestinal flora was measured via the litter. Propionic acid reduced mycelial-producing fungi, but had no effect on budding yeast (*Arnfa RS et al. Relationship between yeast and mold population in litter of broilers fed dietary fungistatic compounds. Poultry Sci 59(7):1557, 1980*).

In vitro Experimental Study: Propionic acid inhibited several species of mycelial-forming fungi (*Bandelin FJ. The effect of pH on the efficiency of various inhibiting compounds. J Am Pharm Assoc Sci Ed 47:691-94, 1958*).

Sorbic Acid:

A straight chain 2,4-hexadienoic fatty acid derivative.

Widely used as a food preservative.

Review Article: *"Sorbate is an effective inhibitor of many microorganisms, including yeasts, molds and many bacteria. It is used in the preservation of a wide variety of products throughout the world"* (*Sofos JN, Busta FF. Antimicrobial activity of sorbate. J Food Protection 44(8):614-22, 1981*).

Local application of a 1-3% solution of potassium sorbate may relieve symptoms of vulvovaginal candidiasis.

Experimental Study: In 122 cases of vaginal fungal infections, local application gave prompt symptomatic relief with disappearance of the organisms (*McKennon DA, Rodgerson EB. Use of potassium sorbate for treatment of fungal infections. Obstet Gynecol 45:108-10, 1975*).

Undecylenic Acid:

An 11-carbon mono-unsaturated organic fatty acid with anti-fungal activity which naturally occurs in sweat.

Administration may be beneficial.

In vitro Experimental Study: Was effective against C. albicans, but less so than caprylic acid (*Neuhauser I. Successful treatment of intestinal moniliasis with fatty acid-resin complex. Arch Intern Med 93:53-60, 1954*).

> *Note: The accuracy of the comparison between the 2 fatty acids has been questioned as the author failed to control for pH, since Peck and Rosenfeld (see below) found that a pH of 5.8 or less is often sufficient to inhibit fungal growth.*

In vitro Experimental Study: Was about 6 times as effective an antifungal as caprylic acid (*Peck SM, Rosenfeld H. The effects of hydrogen ion concentration, fatty acids and vitamin C on the growth of fungi. J Invest Dermatol 1:237-65, 1938*).

- -

OTHER FACTORS

Rule out hydrochloric acid deficiency:

Candida albicans requires a pH of 7.4 for optimal growth and becomes completely inhibited at pH 4.5 (*Bolivar R, Bodey GP. Candidiasis of the gastrointestinal tract, in GP Bodey, V Fainstein, Eds. Candidiasis. New York, Raven Press, 1985*).

> *Note: H2-receptor antagonists, by decreasing gastric acidity, frequently encourage candida overgrowth in gastric juice, especially in women (Boero M et al. Candida overgrowth in gastric juice of peptic ulcer subjects on short- and long-term treatment with H2-receptor antagonists. Digestion 28(3):158-63, 1983).*

Lactobacillus Acidophilus:

Has a beneficial effect on the distribution of intestinal and vaginal microflora and on the metabolic activities of fecal enzymes in addition to having a direct anti-candida effect (*Lactobacillus feeding alters human colonic bacterial enzyme activities. Nutr Rev 42(11):374-76, 1984*).

> **Experimental Study:** 11 women with documented candidal vaginitis and a history of 5 or more infections annually ingested 1 cup daily of yogurt containing live LA cultures for 6 mo. after a 6 mo. baseline. There was a significant 3-fold decrease in the incidence of candidal vaginitis while ingesting LA compared to baseline. No significant colonization by the LA strains was observed (*Yogurt ingestion decreases candidal vaginitis infection threefold. Infect Dis News November, 1989, p.4*).

> **In vitro Experimental Study:** Candida albicans grew at pH 4.6 or above in nutrient broth containing 5% glucose but was retarded at pH 7.7 by filtrates of lactobacillus acidophilus (*Collins EB, Hardt P. Inhibition of candida albicans by lactobacillus acidophilus. J Dairy Sci 63:830-32, 1980*).

> **Experimental Study:** Vaginal implantation of non-fermented acidophilus milk, yogurt, or low-fat milk for preventing recurrence of candida vaginitis subsequent to treatment with nystatin was studied in 30 women following random assignment. Within 3 mo., there were 3 reinfections among pts. who received no milk product compared to 1 reinfection among those using yogurt, 1 among those using non-fermented acidophilus milk, and none among those using low-fat milk. Results suggest that lactose may selectively stimulate indigenous or applied lactobacilli with a concomitant increase in the production of inhibitors (*Collins EB, Hardt P. Inhibition of candida albicans by lactobacillus acidophilus. J Dairy Sci 63:830-32, 1980*).

Local application may be beneficial.

> **Clinical Report:** 20 pts. reported that they cured their candidia vulvovaginitis with preparations containing viable LA cultures (*Will TE. Lactobacillus overgrowth for treatment of moniliary vulvovaginitis. Letter. Lancet 2:482, 1979*).

CAPILLARY FRAGILITY

See Also: EDEMA

VITAMINS

Vitamin C:

Increased capillary fragility is a sign of scurvy.

Supplementation may be beneficial, especially if deficient.

> **Negative Experimental Study:** 7 pts. receiving continuous ambulatory peritoneal dialysis and 4 receiving hemodialysis, to whom ascorbate supplements had not been prescribed for at least 12 mo., received ascorbate 25 mg/d for the first mo., 50 mg/d for the second mo. and no supplementation for the third month. Whole blood ascorbate was below normal in 6/11 pts. at the start but was normal in 10/11 pts. while taking ascorbate 50 mg/d. Correction of ascorbate deficiency had no effect on capillary fragility tests (*Tomson CR et al. Correction of subclinical ascorbate deficiency in patients receiving dialysis: effects on plasma oxalate, serum cholesterol, and capillary fragility. Clin Chim Acta 180(3):255-64, 1989*).

> **Experimental Double-blind Study:** 94 institutionalized elderly received vitamin C 1 gm daily or placebo. After 3 mo., the experimental gp. had reduced petechial hemorrhages and purpura (*Schorah CJ et al. The effect of vitamin C supplements on body weight, serum proteins, and general health of an elderly population. Am J Clin Nutr 34(5):871-76, 1981*).

> **Experimental Study:** 10 pts. with hiatal hernia and esophageal reflux who developed vitamin C deficiency due to intolerance of "acid" foods were supplemented with vitamin C. Subsequently, scattered deficiency symptoms disappeared and both capillary fragility tests and serum ascorbic acid levels returned toward normal (*Hiebert CA. Gastroesophageal reflux and ascorbic acid deficiency. Ann Thorac Surg 24(2):108-12, 1977*).

> **Experimental Placebo-controlled Study:** 12 diabetics, 6 of whom had symptomatic retinopathy (aged 25-71) and 24 controls aged 21-61 were studied. Half of the diabetics and a quarter of the controls were found to have an intake of vitamin C which was less than the recommended 315 mg/wk. The diabetics randomly received either placebo for 1 mo. followed by vitamin C 1 g daily for 2 mo. (Gp. 1) or vitamin C for 2 mo. followed by placebo for 1 mo. (Gp. II). In all subjects during testing, by applying negative pressure to the anterior forearm surface, an increase of negative pressure led to a logarithmic increase in the number of petechiae observed. The diabetics showed petechiae at much lower negative pressures than the controls, and all diabetics with retinopathy had very fragile capillaries. In Gp. I, capillary fragility failed to change during placebo treatment. Capillary strength in all diabetics improved during vitamin C treatment. In Gp II capillary strength in 4/6 diabetics deteriorated on placebo treatment. No retinal changes were observed during vitamin C treatment (*Cox BD, Butterfield WJ. Vitamin C supplements and diabetic cutaneous capillary fragility. Br Med J 3:205, 1975*).

Vitamin E:

Supplementation may be beneficial.

> **Experimental Study:** 7 cases of purpura due to vascular changes caused by infection, drugs or unknown causes were treated with oral doses of α-tocopherol nicotinate 400-600 mg daily. 6/7 showed remarkable improvement of petechiae with their complete disappearance after 5-21 days along with improvements in other clinical symptoms (*Fujii T. The clinical effects of vitamin E on purpuras due to vascular defects. J Vitaminology 18:125-30, 1972*).

Experimental Study: 17 children with purpura received α-tocopherol acetate 2-400 mg daily. After 4-23 days (ave. 12 days), capillary resistance became normal or nearly so (*Cerloczy F, Bencze B. Ernährungsforschung 7:295, 1962; Cerloczy F et al. Acta Paediat Sci Huag (Hungary) 7:363, 1966*).

Experimental Study: 5 pts. with thrombocytopenic purpura received 2-400 mg α-tocopherol acetate daily. Within 7-14 days, platelet counts and capillary fragility returned to normal or near normal (*Skelton F et al. Science 163:762, 1946*).

- -

MINERALS

Zinc:

Deficiency may be associated with senile purpura.

Observational Study: 20 pts. with senile purpura aged 65-99 had lower serum zinc levels than 20 controls despite no significant differences in the mean serum concentration of albumin, the main binder of zinc (*Haboubi NY et al. Zinc deficiency in senile purpura. J Clin Pathol 38:1189-91, 1985*).

- -

OTHER NUTRITIONAL FACTORS

Bioflavonoids:

Administration may be beneficial (*Timberlake CF, Henry BS. Anthocyanins as natural food colorants. Prog Clin Biol Res 280:107-21, 1988*).

Experimental Study: Bioflavonoids minimized capillary bleeding during tonsillectomy and adenoid surgery as well as post-operative bleeding (*Ryan RE. A new aid to tonsil and adenoid surgery. Clin Med 5:327, 1958*).

- Anthocyanosides:

Bilberry (Vaccinium myrtillus) is a rich source.

Administration of an extract may be beneficial.

Experimental Study: Following oral administration of anthocyanosides, pts. with varicose veins and ulcerative dermatitis had a substantial drop in capillary leakage. Anthocyanosides were found to protect altered capillary walls by increasing the endothelium barrier-effect through stabilization of membrane phospholipids, and by increasing the biosynthetic processes of the acid mucopolysaccharides of the connective ground substance through restoration of the altered mucopolysaccharidic pericapillary sheath (*Mian E et al. [Anthocyanosides and the walls of microvessels: further aspects of the mechanism of action of their protective effect in syndromes due to abnormal capillary fragility.] Minerva Med 68(52):3565-81, 1977*).

- Hesperidin:

Deficiency is associated with altered capillary permeability and resistance, along with pain in the extremities marked by effort, debility and lassitude (*Scarborough H. Deficiency of vitamin C and vitamin P in man. Lancet 2:644, 1940*).

- with Vitamin C:

Combined administration may be beneficial.

Experimental Study: 40 menopausal women, mean age 51, were treated. 14 had nocturnal leg cramps, 15 easy bruising, and 11 spontaneous nosebleeds. In all cases, symptoms worsened during the time of the month in which their menses had formerly occurred. They received hesperidin 200 mg and vitamin C 200 mg after each meal and at bedtime for 2 wks. followed by 100 mg of each 4 times daily for 4 weeks. Once symptoms had disappeared, the dosage was reduced to 200 mg of each daily and then supplementation was discontinued. 4/14 with nocturnal leg cramps noted that symptoms were under control within 2 wks., and the rest within an ave. of 7 weeks. 11/15 pts. with easy bruising improved after 8 wks., while the other 4 responded by 16 weeks. Nosebleeds stopped in 6-11 wks. in the 8/11 cases which were moderate, and the dosage was successfully reduced to 400 mg/d of hesperidin and vitamin C for a year. Of the remaining 3/11 cases, 1 was under control in 3 mo., and remained so on 400 mg of each daily. The other 2 pts. improved but their nosebleeds were never completely controlled until they stopped spontaneously in the 4th year (*Horoschak A. Nocturnal leg cramps, easy bruisability and epistaxis in menopausal patients: Treated with hesperidin and ascorbic acid. Del State Med J January, 1959, pp. 19-22*).

Experimental Study: The combination of vitamin C 1.5 gm and bioflavonoids (hesperidine methyl-chalcone 150 mg and esculine 15 mg) given IV reduced the tendency towards capillary bleeding (microscopic hematuria) caused by anti-coagulants in 21 pts. without interfering with normal blood clotting. In 1 pt., a trial of vitamin C alone was unsuccessful (*Shapiro S, Spitzer JM. The use of Cepevit (ascorbic acid plus "p" factors) in drug-induced hypoprothrombinemia. Angiology 5:64-71, 1954*).

CARDIAC ARRHYTHMIAS

See Also: ATHEROSCLEROSIS

DIETARY FACTORS

Avoid <u>saturated fat</u>.

Animal Experimental Study: Long-term feeding of saturated animal fat to rats increased their susceptibility to develop cardiac arrhythmias under ischemic stress (*Charnock JS et al. Dietary fats and oils in cardiac arrhythmia in rats. <u>Am J Clin Nutr</u> 53:1047S-9S, 1991*).

Animal Experimental Study: In young rats, a diet that had been enriched with saturated fatty acids exacerbated arrhythmias induced by ischemia or by coronary artery reperfusion *in vivo* as well as those caused by catecholamine-stress *in vitro* (*McLennan PL et al. Reversal of the arrhythmogenic effects of long-term saturated fatty acid intake by dietary n-3 and n-6 polyunsaturated fatty acids. <u>Am J Clin Nutr</u> 51:53-58, 1990*).

Avoid heavy <u>alcohol</u> intake.

Review Article: Atrial fibrillation might be the first sign of heart damage due to alcohol abuse. It usually takes over 10 yrs. of chronic abuse before symptoms become overt (*Moushmoush B, Abi-Mansour P. Alcohol and the heart. The long-term effects of alcohol on the cardiovascular system. <u>Arch Intern Med</u> 151:36-42, 1991*).

Review Article: "In addition to supraventricular arrhythmias that often normalize spontaneously, there is an increased incidence of sudden death that peaks at about 50 years of age in the alcoholic population" (*Regan TJ. Alcohol and the cardiovascular system. <u>JAMA</u> 264(3):377-81, 1990*).

Animal Experimental Study: Since alcohol is known to produce magnesium deficits, and there is a demonstrated magnesium dietary deficiency in the West which is associated epidemiologically with cardiac disease and hypertension, the effect of acute magnesium deficiency on the response of canine coronary arteries was studied. Results suggest that alcohol may cause serious cardiac complications such as arrhythmias or sudden death if magnesium intake or metabolism is impaired (*Altura BM et al. Magnesium deficiency potentiates coronary arterial spasms induced by alcohol. Abstract. <u>J Am Coll Nutr</u> 8(5):456, 1989*).

Avoid <u>caffeine</u>.

Negative Experimental Double-blind Crossover Study: 70 cardiac pts. randomly received 300 mg caffeine (equivalent to 3 cups of coffee) or placebo. There were no significant differences in regard to cardiac arrhythmias. In a second study, 35 pts. with a history of MI received 300 mg caffeine followed by a second 150 mg dose after 4 hrs. without evidence of increased ventricular ectopic activity (*Myers MG. Caffeine and cardiac arrhythmias. <u>Ann Intern Med</u> 114:147-50, 1991*).

Review Article: "There are clearly people who have serious cardiac arrhythmias due to caffeine consumption" (*W. Gary Flamm, dierector of the Office of Toxicological Sciences, Center for Food Safety and Applied Nutrition, Federal Drug Administration, USA - quoted in <u>FDA Consumer</u> 12/87-1/88*).

Experimental Study: 7 normal volunteers and 12 pts. received oral coffee or IV caffeine citrate. 7 pts. had mitral valve prolapse, 1 had cardiomyopathy, 7 had symptoms of syncope or near syncope and 4 had palpitations. Cardioactive drugs were stopped 24 hrs. and caffeine 48 hrs. before the procedure. Atrial and ventricular pacing were accomplished with a digital stimulator. Although there was no significant change in conduction intervals, caffeine significantly shortened the effective refractory period of the high and low rt. atrium, the AV node and the rt. ventricle while increasing the effective refractory period of the left atrium. 2 pts. had unsustained ventricular tachycardia in response to programmed ventricular stimulation after caffeine; 3 controls had sustained atrial flutter-fibrillation in response to atrial extrastimuli only after caffeine; before caffeine, only 1 pt. had sustained tachycardia whereas 6 had sustained atrial flutter-fibrillation afterwards; 1 pt. had sustained atrioventricular nodal-reentry tachycardia only after caffeine (*Dobmeyer DJ et al. The arrhythmogenic effects of caffeine in human beings. N Engl J Med 308(14):814-16, 1983*).

VITAMINS

Vitamin D:

Supplementation may cure the sick sinus syndrome.

Case Report: A 77-year-old woman with systolic hypertension develped episodes of atrial fibrillation. Over the next yr., the episodes became more frequent and digoxin became increasingly ineffective in converting her to regular sinus rhythm, and quinidine was inconsistent in preventing the episodes. For the next 2 yrs., she was left in atrial fibrillation. Following a bout of neuralgia, she began taking vitamin D drops for the treatment of osteoporosis, which her rheumatologist had advised years earlier due to probable compression of the spinal nerve root secondary to that diagnosis. Vitamin D relieved the neuralgia and normal sinus rhythm reappeared. A review of her history revealed that the abnormal sinus rhythm started shortly after the pt. stopped taking the vitamin D drops for neuralgia a few years previously. Vitamin D appears to provide a role in the impulse formaton of the sinus node by facilitating transport of calcium during the action potential (*Kessel L. Sick sinus syndrome cured by vitamin D. Geriatrics 45:83-5, 1990*).

Vitamin E:

Supplementation may prevent ventricular fibrillation due to myocardial ischemia.

Animal Experimental Study: After occlusion of the coronary artery in rats to produce myocardial ischemia, there was a significant decrease in the ventricular fibrillation threshold in the placebo gp., while no decrease in threshold occurred in the vitamin E-treated rats (*Fuenmayor AJ et al. Vitamin E and ventricular fibrillation threshold in myocardial ischemia. Jpn Circ J 53:1229-32, 1989*).

MINERALS

Magnesium:

Supplementation may prevent and correct arrhythmias.

Review Article: "The association between marked hypomagnesemia and arrhythmias, particularly those associated with digitalis intoxication, has long been recognized. More recently, acute intervention with magnesium in patients who are not hypomagnesemic has demonstrated arrhythmia suppression in 3 settings: digitalis intoxication, long QT-related arrhythmias and arrhythmias after acute myocardial infarction. Although the electrophysiologic effects of magnesium are not clearly understood, magnesium treatment is emerging as an important adjunct in managing certain serious ventricular arrhythmias" (*Roden DM. Magnesium treatment of ventricular arrhythmias. Am J Cardiol 63(14):43G-46G, 1989*).

Arrhythmias may respond to supplementation whether or not serum magnesium is low; however, in the presence of hypomagnesemia, more magnesium may be required.

Experimental Blinded Study: 9 pts. with symptomatic atrial fibrillation and deficient serum magnesium levels required twice as much digoxin as did normomagnesemic patients (*DeCarli C et al. Serum magnesium levels in symptomatic atrial fibrillation and their relation to rhythm control by intravenous digoxin. Am J Cardiol 57:956, 1986*).

May prevent toxic arrhythmias caused by digitalis, perhaps because they tend to produce a loss of intracellular potassium (*Cohen L, Kitzes R. Magnesium deficiency and digitalis toxicity. JAMA 251:730, 1984; Cohen L, Kitzes R. Magnesium sulfate and digitalis-toxic arrhythmias. JAMA 249:2808-10, 1983*).

The antiarrhythmic activity of magnesium is more likely to be due to a metabolic, rather than to a pharmacologic, mechanism (*Frustaci A et al. Myocardial magnesium content, histology, and antiarrhythmic response to magnesium infusion. Letter. Lancet 2:1019, 1987*).

Potassium:

Deficiency (which may exist despite normal serum potassium levels) is associated with arrhythmias as well as decreased tolerance to cardiac medications and EKG alterations.

Observational Study: In a study of 590 pts. admitted to a coronary care unit, hypokalemia, often in the absence of diuretic use, occurred in 17% of the 211 pts. with acute MI. Pts. with acute MI and a potassium level of <4.0 mEq/L (4.0 mmol/L) had an increased risk of ventricular arrhythmias (59% vs. 42%) (*Kafka H et al. Serum magnesium and potassium in acute myocardial infarction. Influence on ventricular arrhythmias. Arch Intern Med 147(3):465-69, 1987*).

Observational Study: Serum potassium concentration was an inverse predictor of ventricular tachycardia and frequent unifocal PVC's early in acute myocardial infarction (*Nordrehaug J et al. Serum potassium concentration as a risk factor of ventricular arrhythmias early in acute myocardial infarction. Circulation 71(4):645-9, 1985*).

Supplementation to correct potassium deficits may be beneficial.

Experimental Controlled Study: 32 hypertensive pts. with previous diuretic-induced hypokalemia, normal 24-hr. ambulatory ECG monitoring, and normal exercise testing were treated with 100 mg hydrochlorothiazide (HCTZ) daily (Gp. 1) to induce hypokalemia or with a combination of HCTZ and amiloride (Gp. 2) to attempt to maintain plasma potassium levels in the normal range during diuretic therapy. Those Gp. 1 pts. with increased ventricular ectopic activity (VEA) during HCTZ therapy were subsequently potassium-repleted with amiloride and supplemental potassium chloride. One Gp. 1 pt. died suddenly after 12 days of HCTZ therapy; autopsy findings suggested an arrhythmic death. 6 Gp. 1 pts. who had increased VEA with HCTZ treatment had reductions in VEA following amiloride or supplemental potassium chloride. Gp. 2 pts. did not have a significant increase in VEA. Thus, diuretic therapy appears to cause VEA primarily by inducing electrolyte changes (*Holland OB et al. Ventricular ectopic activity with diuretic therapy. Am J Hypertens 1(4 Pt 1):380-85, 1988*).

Experimental and Observational Study: Serum and red blood cell potassium was measured in 17 pts. with EKG abnormalities. Although some of the abnormalities were typical of potassium deficiency, most were nonspecific T wave changes which are commonly attributed (without substantiation) to ischemia. Serum potassium levels were normal but RBC potassium levels were below normal in all cases and returned to normal (as did the EKG abnormalities) after treatment with potassium salts (*Sangiori GB et al. Serum potassium levels, red-blood-cell potassium and alterations of the repolarization phase of electrocardiography in old subjects. Age Ageing 13:309, 1984*).

Magnesium and
Potassium:

May be more effective when administered together when the level of either is deficient due to the inability of the heart muscle to hold on to potassium in the absence of magnesium (*Dychner T, Wester PO. Magnesium and potassium in serum and muscle in relation to disturbances of cardiac rhythm, in Magnesium in Health and Disease. Spectrum Publishing Company, 1980, pp. 551-7; Shils ME. Experimental human magnesium depletion. Medicine 48(1):61-85, 1969*).

Zinc to Copper Ratio:

An increased ratio may cause premature ventricular contractions.

Animal Experimental Study: Copper deficiency in mice was associated with bradycardia, coupled beats, ectopic ventricular foci, premature atrial beats and sudden death (*Klevay LM. Atrial thrombosis, abnormal electrocardiograms and sudden death in mice due to copper deficiency. Atherosclerosis 54(2):213-24, 1985*).

Case Reports: 3 pts. are described (*Spencer JC. Direct relationship between the body's copper/zinc ratio, ventricular premature beats and sudden cardiac death. Letter. Am J Clin Nutr June, 1979, pp. 1184-5*).

– –

OTHER NUTRITIONAL FACTORS

Aspartic Acid:

- with Magnesium and Potassium:

Administration of potassium and magnesium aspartate (1 gm of each twice daily) may be beneficial.

> **Review Article:** Potassium/magnesium aspartate is useful in the treatment of cardiac arrhythmias. Aspartates speed the onset of the therapeutic effects of digitalis while reducing both its maintenance dosage and potential cardiotoxic effects. Hyperkalemia is the only significant contraindication (*Grujic M, Perinovic M. [Treatment of acute myocardial infarction and chronic heart failure with K-Mg aspartate.] Med Welt 25 (50):2124-6, 1974*) (*in German*).

Carnitine:

Supplementation may be beneficial.

> **Animal Experimental Study:** The thresholds for electrically-induced atrial fibrillation were measured in experimental animals. Carnitine 100 mg/kg IV had much less of an antiarrhythmic effect than quinidine 5 mg/kg but, after atropinization, it was similar in effect to quinidine without causing the BP depression seen with quinidine (*DiPalma JR et al. Cardiovascular and antiarrhythmic effects of carnitine. Arch Int Pharmacdyn Ther 217(2):246-50, 1975*).

Coenzyme Q_{10}:

Supplementation may be beneficial.

> **Experimental Study:** 27 pts. with ventricular premature beats (VPBs) and no clinical findings of organic cardiopathies received coenzyme Q_{10}. Results were beneficial in 6/27 (22%), consisting of 1 pt. with hypertension and 5 pts. with diabetes mellitus. In the remaining 2 pts. with diabetes, the frequency of VPBs was reduced by 50% or more during treatment. The mean reduction of VPBs frequency in the 5 responders plus the additional 2 diabetic pts. was 85.7%, suggesting that CoQ_{10} exhibits an effective antiarrhythmic action not merely on organic heart disease but also on VPBs supervening in diabetes mellitus (*Fujioka T et al. Clinical study of cardiac arrhythmias using a 24-hour continuous electrocardiographic recorder (5th report): Antiarrhythmic action of conenzyme Q_{10} in diabetics. Tohoku J Exp Med 141(suppl):453-63, 1983*).

> **Experimental Study:** 4 pts. with intractable supraventricular tachyarrhythmias received CoQ_{10} 30 mg. After 1-2 wks., the arrhythmias were controlled either with CoQ_{10} alone or with the addition of another drug (*Imanishi S et al. Jpn J Clin Exp Med 58:216-19, 1981*) (*in Japanese*).

Essential Fatty Acids:

Supplementation may reduce the risk of arrhythmias.

> **Animal Experimental Study:** Long-term feeding of polyunsaturated fatty acids from sunflower seed oil (rich in omega-6 fatty acids) to rats reduced their susceptibility to develop cardiac arrhythmias under ischemic stress (*Charnock JS et al. Dietary fats and oils in cardiac arrhythmia in rats. Am J Clin Nutr 53:1047S-9S, 1991*).

> **Animal Experimental Study:** Dietary crossover to n-3 (tuna-fish oil) or n-6 (sunflower-seed oil) PUFA-supplemented diets to young rats at 9 mo. who had been raised on a commercial stock diet supplemented with saturated fatty acids reduced arrhythmias and mortality induced by ischemia or by coronary artery reperfusion *in vivo* as well as those caused by catecholamine-stress *in vitro*. The n-3 PUFAs were most effective (*McLennan PL et al.*

Reversal of the arrhythmogenic effects of long-term saturated fatty acid intake by dietary n-3 and n-6 polyunsaturated fatty acids. Am J Clin Nutr 51:53-58, 1990).

Taurine:

Arrhythmias characteristic of acute myocardial ischemia may be partly due to loss of intracellular taurine (*Crass MF, Lombardini JB. Release of tissue taurine from the oxygen-deficient perfused rat heart. Proc Soc Exp Biol Med 157:486-8, 1978; Lombardini JB, Cooper MW. Elevated blood taurine levels in acute and evolving myocardial infarction. J Lab Clin Med 98(6):849-59, 1981*).

Much like magnesium, taurine affects membrane excitability by normalizing potassium flux in and out of the heart muscle cell (*Chazov EL et al. Taurine and electrical activity of the heart. Circ Res 35 Suppl. 3:11-21, 1974; Shustova TI et al. [Effect of taurine on potassium, calcium and sodium levels in the blood and tissues of rats.] Vopr Med Khim 32(4):113-116, 1986*).

Supplementation may prevent digitalis-induced arrhythmias (*Sebring LA, Huxtable RJ. Cardiovascular actions of taurine, in Sulfur Amino Acids: Biochemical & Clinical Aspects, 1983*).

- -

OTHER FACTORS

Rule out food and chemical sensitivities.

Case Reports:
1. A 60 year-old male truck driver was resuscitated following ventricular fibrillation. When fed he immediately developed bloating, PVCs and hypotension on 3 occasions. He noted that milk or eggs usually precipitated these symptoms as well as gasoline fumes.
2. A 65 year-old female presented with an 8 yr. history of recurrent atrial fibrillation along with arthritis, blurring of vision, coughing spells and generalized muscle pain. Challenge with various chemicals would produce her symptoms.
(*Rea WJ, Suits CW. Cardiovascular disease triggered by foods and chemicals, in JW Gerrard, Ed. Food Allergy: New Perspectives. Springfield, Illinois, Charles C. Thomas, 1980*).

CARDIOMYOPATHY

See Also: ALCOHOLISM

DIETARY FACTORS

Avoid alcohol.

Excessive intake is known to be associated with the development of cardiomyopathy due to one or more of the following:
1. direct toxic injury by alcohol to the myocardium
2. nutritional disturbances (beri-beri)
3. toxic effects of substances contained in alcoholic beverages (e.g. cobalt)

(*Burch GE, Giles TD. Alcoholic cardiomyopathy, in B Kissin, H Begleiter, Eds. The Biology of Alcoholism: Vol. 3: Clinical Pathology. New York, Plenum Press, 1974*).

- -

VITAMINS

Vitamin E:

Supplementation may protect against the cardiotoxic effects of alcohol.

Animal Experimental Study: Mice pretreated with vitamin E by injection prior to injection of a large dose of alcohol exhibited much less evidence of myocardial cell damage than control mice (*Retzki J et al. J Toxicol Clin Toxicol 20:319-31, 1983*).

Supplementation may protect against cardiomyopathy caused by magnesium deficiency.

Animal Experimental Study: Hamsters receiving a magnesium-deficient diet had less myocardial damage if they were supplemented with vitamin E, with greater protection at higher doses. Results suggest that the cardiomyopathy of magnesium deficiency may be due to a reduction in the threshold antioxidant capacity of the cardiovascular system (*Freedman AM et al. Magnesium deficiency-induced cardiomyopathy: Protection by vitamin E. Biochem Biophys Res Commun 170:1102-6, 1990*).

- -

MINERALS

Magnesium:

Deficiency may be associated with the development of cardiomyopathy.

Review Article: Cardiac changes produced by experimental magnesium deficiency resemble those produced in mice fed large quantities of alcohol and are particularly prominent in myocardial mitochondriae. Also, chronic alcohol ingestion causes decreased muscle magnesium (*Burch BE, Giles TD. The importance of magnesium deficiency in cardiovascular disease. Am Heart J 94:649-56, 1977*).

Selenium:

Deficiency is associated with the development of cardiomyopathy.

Case Report: A 17 year-old girl who had been on total parenteral nutrition for 17 mo. following extensive bowel resection diet after a cardiac arrest secondary to septic shock. 7 mo. prior to her demise, severe selenium deficiency was diagnosed, selenium was added to the infusion, and plasma selenium concentrations increased. Autopsy showed evidence of cardiomyopathy due to prolonged selenium deficiency (*Lockitch G et al. Cardiomyopathy associated with nonendemic selenium deficiency in a Caucasian adolescent. Am J Clin Nutr 52:572-77, 1990*).

Review Article: The possibility of selenium deficiency should be thought of in cases of alcoholic cardiomyopathy (*Goldman IS, Kantrowitz NE. Cardiomyopathy associated with selenium deficiency. Letter. N Engl J Med 305:701, 1982*).

Case Report: A 2 year-old girl with dyspnea, cardiomegaly and CHF was found to have minimal selenium in her diet and a low serum selenium and improved with supplementation (*Collipp PJ, Chen SY. Cardiomyopathy and selenium deficiency in a two-year-old girl. Letter. N Engl J Med 304:1304-5, 1981*).

- -

OTHER NUTRITIONAL FACTORS

L-Carnitine:

Deficiency may cause cardiomyopathy.

Experimental Study: 5 pts. with endocardial fibroelastosis were found to have systemic carnitine deficiency which responded to supplementation (*Tripp ME et al. Systemic carnitine deficiency presenting as familial endocardial fibroelastosis: A treatable cardiomyopathy. N Engl J Med 305:385, 1982*).

Coenzyme Q: 100-150 mg daily in divided doses

WARNING: Caution should be used in withdrawing supplementation, as clinical and hemodynamic rebound events may occur within a few weeks.

May be deficient.

Observational Study: Blood CoQ_{10} levels were significantly lower in pts. with dilated cardiomyopathy (98% of whom were NY Heart Assoc. Class III or IV) than controls (*Langsjoen PH, Folkers K. Long-term efficacy and safety of coenzyme Q_{10} therapy for idiopathic dilated cardiomyopathy. Am J Cardiol 65:521-3, 1990*).

Observational Study: The tissue levels of CoQ_{10} in endomyocardial biopsy samples and blood from 43 pts. with cardiomyopathy were determined. Pts. of New York Heart Assoc. class IV had lower (p<0.01) levels of CoQ_{10} than those of class I. Pts. of classes III and IV had lower (p<0.0001) levels than those of classes I and II (*Folkers K et al. Biochemical rationale and myocardial tissue data on the effective therapy of cardiomyopathy with coenzyme Q_{10}. Proc Natl Acad Sci U S A 82(3):901-04, 1985*).

Supplementation may be beneficial.

Experimental Double-blind Study: 20 pts. with stable dilated cardiomyopathy of different etiologies (New York Heart Assoc. Class II or III) randomly received CoQ_{10} 100 mg or placebo for 60 days in either order with a 30 day washout period between treatments. After CoQ_{10} treatment, mean left ventricular ejection fraction increased from 45.7% to 49.2% (p<0.001 vs. placebo). Other parameters of cardiac function also improved. There were no side effects (*Pogessi L et al. Effect of coenzyme Q_{10} on left ventricular function in patients with dilative cardiomyopathy. Curr Ther Res 49:878-86, 1991*).

Negative Experimental Double-blind Study: 16 pts. mitochondrial myopathies who had responded to 6 mo. of supplementation to ubidecarenone (CoQ_{10}) 2 mg/kg/d in an open multicentric trial by showing at least a 25% decrease of post-exercise lactate levels were further treated with either CoQ_{10} or placebo. After 3 mo., no significant differences between the 2 gps. were observed (*Bresolin N et al. Ubidecarenone in the treatment of mitochondrial myopathies: a multi-center double-blind trial. J Neurol Sci 100(1-2):70-8, 1990; Scarlato G et al. Multicen-*

ter trial with ubidecarenone: treatment of 44 patients with mitochondrial myopathies. Rev Neurol (Paris) 147(6-7):542-8, 1991).

Negative Experimental Double-blind Crossover Study: 25 pts. with dilated cardiomyopathy (NY Heart Assoc. Class I, II and III) received CoQ$_{10}$ 100 mg/d and placebo in either order for 4 mo. each. Treatment with CoQ$_{10}$ failed to influence hemodynamic parameters, the EKG, the incidence of ventricular arrhythmias or exercise tolerance, and it was not possible to demonstrate any therapeutic effect (*Permanetter B et al. [Lack of effectiveness of coenzyme Q$_{10}$ (ubiquinone) in long-term treatment of dilated cardiomyopathy.] Z Kardiol 78(6):360-5, 1989).*

Experimental Double-blind Crossover Study: 19 pts. with chronic myocardial disease who were found to have low or borderline low blood levels of CoQ$_{10}$. All showed significant improvement following supplementation (*Langsjoen PH et al. Effective treatment with coenzyme Q$_{10}$ of patients with chronic myocardial disease. Drugs Exp Clin Res 11(8):577-79, 1985).*

Experimental Double-blind Crossover Study: 2 gps. of pts. with NY Heart Assoc. class III or IV cardiomyopathies received CoQ$_{10}$ and placebo in either order. These pts., who were steadily worsening and expected to diet within 2 yrs. with conventional therapy, generally showed an extraordinary clinical improvement (*Langsjoen PH et al. Response of patients in classes III and IV of cardiomyopathy to therapy in a blind and crossover trial with coenzyme Q$_{10}$. Proc Natl Acad Sci U S A 82(12):4240-44, 1985).*

Experimental Double-blind Study: Daily administration of CoQ$_{10}$ for 12 wks. increased cardiac ejection fraction significantly, reduced shortness of breath and increased muscle strength. These improvements lasted as long as 3 yrs. in pts. treated continuously, but cardiac function deteriorated when CoQ$_{10}$ was discontinued. Of the 80 pts. treated, 89% improved with supplementation (*Folkers K et al. Biochemical rationale and myocardial tissue data on the effective therapy of cardiomyopathy with coenzyme Q$_{10}$. Proc Natl Acad Sci U S A 82:901, 1985).*

CARPAL TUNNEL SYNDROME

See Also: MUSCLE CRAMPS
NEURALGIA AND NEUROPATHY

SIGNS AND SYMPTOMS

1. Pains in hands, elbows, shoulders or knees
2. Morning stiffness of fingers
3. Impaired finger flexion
4. Transitory nocturnal paralysis of arm and hand
5. Paresthesias of hands - possibly also of face
6. Painful adduction rotation of the thumb at metacarpophalangeal joint
7. Weakness of hand grip
8. Fluctuating edema in hands, feet or ankles
9. Impaired tactile sensations in fingers
10. Tenderness over carpal tunnel
11. Dropping of objects
12. Nocturnal muscle spasms in extremities

OFFICE EVALUATION

1. Hold the hands out with palms up.
2. Bend the fingers at the 2 outer joints only, leaving the metacarpophalangeal joints in a straight line with the wrists.
3. Bring the tips of the fingers down to the palms of the hands, right to the crease that separates fingers from hands.
4. If any of these 16 joints cannot be bent completely and without pain, carpal tunnel syndrome is suspected.

(Ellis JM, Presley J. Vitamin B6: The Doctor's Report. New York, Harper & Row, 1973).

VITAMINS

Vitamin B6: 100 mg. daily   (3 month trial)

>WARNING: Pyridoxine supplementation may <u>cause</u> a sensory neuropathy in doses as low as 200 mg daily over 3 years (usually 2-5 gm daily). The neurotoxicity is believed to due to exceeding the liver's ability to phosphorylate pyridoxine to the active coenzyme, pyridoxal phosphate. The resulting high pyridoxine blood level could be directly neurotoxic or may compete for binding sites with pyridoxal phosphate resulting in a relative deficiency of the active metabolite (*Parry GJ, Bredesen DE. Sensory neuropathy with low-dose pyridoxine. Neurology 35:1466-8, 1985*). Supplementation in the form of pyridoxal phosphate should thus avoid this danger.

May be deficient.

>**Observational Study:** Plasma pyridoxal phosphate levels were measured in 8 pts. with idiopathic carpal tunnel syndrome (3 of whom had had surgical decompensation at least 12 mo. earlier) and compared to those of 6 controls. The ave. level in the controls was almost 2.5-fold above the ave. level in CTS patients. The difference was statistically significant (p<0.01). Results strongly suggest that vitamin B6 deficiency may accompany CTS. "Part of the total work-up of pts. with CTS should include a nutritional evaluation, in particular, a determination of vitamin B6 status" (*Fuhr JE et al. Vitamin B6 levels in patients with carpal tunnel syndrome. Arch Surg 124:1329-30, 1989*).

Observational Study: The specific activities and % deficiencies of RBC glutamic oxaloacetic transaminase (EGOT) were found to suggest severe vitamin B6 deficiencies in 4 pts. evaluated at the time of surgery to relieve the compression of CTS (*Ellis J et al. Therapy with vitamin B6 with and without surgery for treatment of patients having the idiopathic carpal tunnel syndrome. Res Comm Chem Pathol Pharmacol 33(2):331, 1981*).

Improvement from supplementation is said to start in a few weeks with complete cure in 8-12 weeks for 85% of patients. Many of the others are said to benefit from pyridoxal-5[1]-phosphate or from the addition of magnesium.

Experimental Study: 22 pts. (39 hands) with CTS were studied to determine if thenar muscle weakness and atrophy, complications of sustained and unattended CTS, could be prevented and halted by treatment with 50-300 mg pyridoxine daily for a minimum of 12 weeks. All hands were relieved of paresthesia and pain of median nerve districtuion except one for a 97.4% cure rate. 9 pts. were followed-up for more than a decade. Function of abductor pollicis brevis and opponens pollicis muscles in the thenar eminence of thumbs was greater following many yrs. of treatment as were range of finger flexion of proximal interphalangeal joints of fingers and pounds pinch (*Ellis JM, Folkers K. Clinical aspects of treatment of carpal tunnel syndrome with vitamin B6. Ann N Y Acad Sci 585:302-20, 1990*).

Negative Experimental Double-blind Study: 15 pts. randomly received vitamin B6 or placebo. After 10 wks., 10 of the pts. improved; however, there was no advantage to vitamin B6 as compared to placebo (*Stransky M et al. Treatment of carpal tunnel syndrome with vitamin B6: a double-blind study. South Med J 82(7):841-2, 1989*).

Experimental Controlled Study: Pts. were placed on 50 mg pyridoxine 3 times daily which was later increased to 100 mg twice daily. While, retrospectively, 14.3% of a previous gp. of pts. treated conservatively experienced satisfactory relief of symptoms, 68% of pyridoxine-treated pts. experienced such relief, and there were no adverse effects (*Kasdan ML, Janes C. Carpal tunnel syndrome and vitamin B6. Plast Reconstruct Surg 79(3):156-62, 1987*).

Experimental Placebo-controlled Study: Based on the judgement of their physicians as well as on the results of distal motor latency and conduction measurements of the median nerve, 27/28 pts. treated with pyridoxine hydrochloride 100 mg daily for 5-18 wks. improved substantially, compared to only 1/4 pts. treated with placebo for 15-36 wks. (*Driskell JA et al. Effectiveness of pyridoxine hydrochloride treatment on carpal tunnel patients. Nutr Rep Int 34:1031-40, 1986*).

Experimental Single-blind Crossover Case Study: A pt. with severe CTS had markedly reduced basal specific activity of RBC glutamic-oxaloacetic transaminase and the enzyme was also deficient in pyridoxal phosphate. He received 2 mg daily of pyridoxine. After 11 wks., all but marginal symptoms were relieved, the EGOT activity deficiency was reduced from about 70% to 50% and pyridoxal phosphate remained deficient. Vitamin B6 was increased to 100 mg daily and, after 12 wks., he had nearly achieved a "ceiling" EGOT level and the pyridoxal phosphate deficiency was eliminated. Placebo administration for 9 wks. led to worsened clinical symptoms and laboratory values. After administration of vitamin B6 100 mg daily for 12 wks., the pt. became asymptomatic and laboratory values normalized again (*Ellis J et al. Clinical results of a cross-over treatment with pyridoxine and placebo of the carpal tunnel syndrome. Am J Clin Nutr 32:2040-6, 1979; Folkers K et al. Biochemical evidence for a deficiency of vitamin B6 in the carpal tunnel syndrome based on a crossover clinical study. Proc Natl Acad Sci U S A 75(7):3410-2, 1978*).

- and Riboflavin:

To become the coenzyme pyridoxal-5[1]-phosphate, dietary pyridoxine is converted by a kinase to pyridoxine 5[1]-phosphate and then a riboflavin-containing enzyme oxidizes it; thus a riboflavin deficiency may cause an identical syndrome.

Case Report: A pt. with a 3-yr. history of CTS was found to be deficient in both vitamin B6 and riboflavin as based on a reduction in the specific activities of RBC glutamic-oxaloacetic transaminase (vitamin B6) and RBC glutathione reductase (riboflavin) to the 30% levels. After 5 mo. of supplementation with riboflavin, there was nearly complete disappearance of the CTS without a change in the specific activity of RBC glutamic-oxaloacetic transaminase. Combined riboflavin and pyridoxine increased (p<0.001) the specific activities of both enzymes to normal levels with total disappearance of the CTS. Objectively, the strength of pinch of both hands increased (p<0.001) on treatment with riboflavin and further increased (p<0.001) on the combined treatment (*Folkers K et al. Enzymology of the response of the carpal tunnel syndrome to riboflavin and to combined riboflavin and pyridoxine.* Proc Natl Acad Sci U S A *81(22):7076-8, 1984*).

- -

MINERALS

Lithium:

WARNING: Carpal tunnel syndrome may develop as a side effect of high-dosage lithium administration (*Deahl MP. Lithium-induced carpal tunnel syndrome.* Br J Psychiatry *153:250-1, 1988; Wood KA, Jacoby RJ. Lithium induced hyperthyroidism presenting with carpal tunnel syndrome. Letter.* Br J Psychiatry *149:386-7, 1986*).

CATARACT

See Also: DIABETES MELLITUS

GENERAL

There are no clinical or epidemiological data which would support the conclusion that inadequate nutrition contributes directly to the deterioration of the mature human lens. The results of animal studies suggest that severe restrictions of certain nutrients, usually in young animals, initiates a chain of events which culminates in loss of transparency. This damage may reflect primarily an interference in growth and development of the lens rather than failure to meet daily needs (*Bunce GE. Nutrition and cataract. Nutr Rev 37(11):337-43, 1979*).

- -

DIETARY FACTORS

Moderate calorie restriction.

May delay cataract formation.

Animal Experimental Study: Feeding the Emory mouse, which is believed to be the best model for human senile cataracts, a diet which was restricted in calories by about 21% delayed the onset of cataracts in the first study to demonstrate *in vivo* the delay of senile-type cataracts. To the extent that cataract formation is due to lens protein oxidation and/or an inability to proteolytically remove damaged protein, it would appear that calorie restriction results in enhanced protection against lens oxidative stress or in prolonged proteolytic function (*Taylor A et al. Moderate caloric restriction delays cataract formation in the Emory mouse. FASEB J 3(6):1741-46, 1989*).

Eat fruits and vegetables.

Observational Study: In a study of plasma levels of vitamin C, vitamin E and carotenoids of 112 subjects aged 40-70 which included 77 cataract pts., persons who consumed fewer than 3.5 servings of fruit or vegetables daily had an increased risk of both cortical and posterior subcapsular cataract (OR=5.0, p<0.05; OR=12.9, p<0.01, respectively) (*Jacques PF, Chylack LT Jr. Epidemiologic evidence of a role for the antioxidant vitamins and carotenoids in cataract prevention. Am J Clin Nutr 53:352S-5S, 1991*).

Restrict sugar.

The monosaccharides D-glucose, D-galactose, D-xylose and L-arabinose enter the lens through diffusion from the aqueous humor and have provided an experimental animal model of caractogenesis. When, in animal studies, they are excessive in the diet, sugar alcohol products accumulate in the lens as they are not efficiently metabolized and have slower rates of diffusion out of the lens than the parent sugars. Accumulation causes hypertonicity and osmotic swelling which, if sustained, causes rupture of the fiber cells (*Kinoshita JH. Invest Ophthalmol 4:786-99, 1965*). In addition, an *in vitro* study has suggested that alteration of lens crystallins may occur leading to gradual deterioration of the structural order of the lens (*Stevens VJ et al. Proc Natl Acad Sci U S A 75:2918-22, 1978*).

Restrict dairy products:

Lactose intake may be directly associated with cataract risk, especially in people who have hereditary deficiencies which interfere with galactose metabolism.

Note: As many as 47% of patients with presenile cataracts have been found to have genetic abnormalities of galactose metabolism (Halbert M. Prevent cataracts in galactosemia carriers by diet? Med Tribune 24(12):14, 1983).

Review Article: Fragmentary data suggest that a risk of cataract secondary to lactose and galactose ingestion is present in certain subpopulations. In these gps., the lens could be exposed to intermittent episodes of hypergalactosemia due to the presence of a partial enzyme deficiency in the galactose metabolic pathway, and/or the presistence of a high adult jejunal lactase activity, and/or to a large and repeated consumption of either whole lactose or easily absorbed lactose (hydrolyzed forms and nonpausteurized yogurt) (*Couet C et al. Lactose and cataract in humans: A review. J Am Coll Nutr 10(1):79-86, 1991*).

Observational Study: 73 pts. aged 40-70 were compared to 33 similarly-aged controls. There was a non-significant 2-fold increase in cataract risk for subjects with a high lactose intake, while a statistically significant increase in cataract risk was found for subjects with both a high lactose intake and low levels of RBC galactokinase (p<0.05) (*Jacques PF et al. Lactose intake and senile cataract. Abstract. J Am Coll Nutr 7(5):424, 1988*).

Observational Study: 5/22 pts. under age 50 with presenile cataracts were heterozygous for galactokinase deficiency; 2/22 were heterozygous for galactose uridyl transferase deficiency (*Prchal JT et al. Association of presenile cataracts with heterozygosity for galactosaemic states and with riboflavin deficiency. Lancet 1:12-13, 1978*).

VITAMINS

Folic Acid:

Intake may be inversely correlated with the prevalence of cataracts (*Jacques PH et al. Vitamin intake and senile cataract. Abstract. J Am Coll Nutr 6(5):435, 1987*).

Riboflavin:

WARNING: Cataract patients should not receive more than 10 mg of riboflavin supplementation daily since the combination of light, ambient oxygen and riboflavin/FAD can generate free radicals and induce cataracts (*Varma S et al. Light-induced damage to ocular lens cation pump: Prevention by vitamin C. Proc Natl Acad Sci U S A 76:3504-06, 1979; Varma S et al. Protection against superoxide radicals in rat lens. Ophthalmic Res 9:421-31, 1977*).

Riboflavin is a precursor of flavin adenine dinucleotide which is required as a coenzyme for glutathione reductase. Since lenticular reduced glutathione is diminished in all forms of human cataract, an association between riboflavin deficiency and cataract formation has been postulated (*Skalka HW, Prchal JT. Cataracts and riboflavin deficiency. Am J Clin Nutr 34(5):861-63, 1981*).

Deficiency may increase the risk of cataracts.

Observational Study: In a Indian study, riboflavin deficiency (assessed by measuring glutathione reductase) was found in 81% of a gp. of 37 pts. aged 48-80 compared to 12.5% of 16 controls aged 48-60 with minor eye complaints. However, thiamine and pyridoxine deficiencies were more prevalent in the controls, suggesting that both gps. may have been malnourished (*Bhat KS. Nutritional status of thiamine, riboflavin and pyridoxine in cataract patients. Nutr Rep Int 36(3):685-92, 1987*).

Observational Study: In a study of 173 cataract pts., 20% of those under age 50 were deficient in riboflavin, as were 34% of those over age 50, while none of 16 normals over age 50 was riboflavin-deficient (*Skalka HW et al. Riboflavin deficiency and cataract formation. Metab Pediatr Ophthalmol 5(1):17-20, 1981*).

Negative Observational Study: In a study of the riboflavin status of healthy young adults, presenile and senile cataract pts., and young and older pts. with clear lenses, there was no evidence of an association between riboflavin deficiency and early cataract formation, either idiopathic or secondary. Older cataract pts. had more riboflavin deficiency, while older pts. with clear lenses did not have riboflavin deficiency. Results suggest that the degree of riboflavin deficiency encountered in the general population may not be cataractogenic (*Skalka HW, Prchal JT. Cataracts and riboflavin deficiency. Am J Clin Nutr 34(5):861-63, 1981*).

Animal Experimental Study: Kittens given a riboflavin-deficient diet developed cataracts (*Gershoff SN et al. J Nutr 68:75-88, 1959*).

- and <u>Galactose</u>:

> **Animal Experimental Study:** Riboflavin-deficient rats showed a higher incidence of galactose-induced cataracts than riboflavin-sufficient animals (*Review: Riboflavin deficiency, galactose metabolism and cataract. Nutr Rev 34:72-79, 1976*).

> **Review Article:** Excessive amts. of galactose increase the need for riboflavin (*Lerman S. Arch Ophthalmol 65:81, 1961*).

Supplementation may be beneficial.

Experimental Study: 18 pts. with lens opacities and 6 pts. with fully developed cataracts were supplemented with riboflavin 15 mg daily. Within 24-48 hrs., all pts. noted improvement. After 9 mo., all opacities and cataracts had disappeared (*Sydenstricker - U. of Georgia and U. of Georgia Hospital - reported in C Gerras et al, Eds. The Encyclopedia of Common Diseases. Emmaus, Penn., Rodale Press, 1976*).

<u>Vitamin C</u>:

Intake may be inversely correlated with cataract risk.

Observational Study: In a study of 112 subjects aged 40-70 which included 77 cataract pts., low vitamin C intake was associated with an increased risk of cortical cataract (OR=3.7; p<0.10) and posterior subcapsular cataract (OR=11.0, p<0.05) (*Jacques PF, Chylack LT Jr. Epidemiologic evidence of a role for the antioxidant vitamins and carotenoids in cataract prevention. Am J Clin Nutr 53:352S-5S, 1991*).

Observational Study: The self-reported consumption of supplementary vitamins by 175 cataract pts. was compared with that of 175 individually matched, cataract-free subjects. The latter gp. used significantly more supplementary vitamin C (p=0.01). Subjects taking vitamin C supplements alone had a 70% decrease in cataract risk compared to non-users of vitamin C supplements (*Robertson JM et al. Vitamin E intake and risk of cataracts in humans. Ann N Y Acad Sci 570:372-82, 1989*).

Ascorbate concentrations in the aqueous humor may be lower in patients with cortical cataracts than in patients with nuclear cataracts, despite similar levels in both the blood and in the lens (*Chandra DB et al. Vitamin C in the human aqueous humor and cataracts. Int J Vitam Nutr Res 56:165-9, 1986*).

Ascorbate concentrations may be lower in cataractous human lenses than in normal lenses (*Wilczek M. Zawartosc witaminy C w roznych typach zacm. Klin Oczna 38:477-80, 1968*).

Blood level may be inversely correlated with cataract risk.

Observational Study: In a study of plasma levels of vitamin C of 112 subjects aged 40-70 which included 77 cataract pts., the odds ratio of posterior subcapsular cataract for persons with low plasma vitamin C was 11.3 (p<0.10) (*Jacques PF, Chylack LT Jr. Epidemiologic evidence of a role for the antioxidant vitamins and carotenoids in cataract prevention. Am J Clin Nutr 53:352S-5S, 1991*).

Observational Study: While blood ascorbic acid concentrations were similar in pts. with cortical and nuclear cataracts, the level of ascorbic acid in the aqueous humor was lower in pts. with cortical cataracts, suggesting sluggish transport of ascorbate from the blood. The lower aqueous ascorbate in this gp. could not be accounted for by any dietary deficiency and thus appears to be metabolically related (*Chandra DB et al. Vitamin C in the human aqueous humor and cataracts. Int J Vitam Nutr Res 56(2):165-68, 1986*).

Total ascorbic acid concentration (both reduced and oxidized) in the human lens decreases with progressing cataract due to rapid oxidation of vitamin C (*Lohmann W. Exp Eye Res 43:859-62, 1986*).

Supplementation may be effective in preventing cataracts.

Animal Experimental Study: Cataracts were induced in a litter of rat pups by administering selenite, which is believed to induce cataracts as a result of oxidative stress to the lens. Pretreatment with vitamin C had a significant protective effect in preventing the development of selenite-induced cataracts (*Devamanoharan P et al. Prevention of selenite cataract by vitamin C. Exp Eye Res 52:563-8, 1991*).

In vitro Animal Experimental Study: Since excessive free radical oxidation is thought to be a cause of cataracts, rat lenses were maintained in a special solution that caused free radical damage. When vitamin C, an antioxidant, was added to the solution, the lenses were significantly protected (*Varma SD, Richards RD. Light-induced damage to ocular lens cation pump: Prevention by vitamin C. Proc Natl Acad Sci U S A 76:3504-06, 1979*).

Supplementation may reverse incipient cataracts.

Experimental Study: Pts. with incipient cataracts and low vitamin C status were supplemented with 350 mg ascorbic acid daily. Marked improvement usually occurred within the first 2 wks. and, after 4-8 wks., vision was improved in 60%. Cataracts which had already formed were not affected (*Bouton SM Jr. Vitamin C and the aging eye. Arch Intern Med 63:930-45, 1939*).

Experimental Study: 90% of 60 pts. with 113 incipient cataracts showed "good results" following 2 series of daily injections of 10 days each of 50-100 mg ascorbic acid. The earlier the treatment was given in the development of cataracts, the more effective it was (*Muhlmann V et al. Vitamin C therapy of incipient senile cataract. Arch Oftalmol B Aires 14:552-75, 1939*).

- and Vitamin A:

Combined supplementation may be beneficial.

Experimental Study: 450 pts. with incipient cataracts were placed in a nutritional program consisting of ascorbic acid 1 gm daily and vitamin A 20,000 IU daily. While similar pts. had previously required surgery after about 4 yrs., only a small gp. of supplemented pts. required surgery and, in some, cataracts did not progress in up to 11 yrs. (*Atkinson D. Malnutrition as an etiological factor in senile cataract. Eye Ear Nose Throat Mon 31:79-83, 1952*).

Vitamin D:

Blood level may be inversely correlated with cataract risk (*Jacques PF et al. Nutritional status in persons with and without senile cataract: Blood vitamin and mineral levels. Am J Clin Nutr 106(3):337-40, 1988*).

Vitamin E:

Dietary intake may be inversely associated with cataract risk.

Observational Study: The self-reported consumption of supplementary vitamins by 175 cataract pts. was compared with that of 175 individually matched, cataract-free subjects. The latter gp. used significantly more supplementary vitamin E (p=0.004). There was a 56% decrease in cataract risk in subjects who took only vitamin E supplements compared to subjects who did not take vitamin E (*Robertson JM et al. Vitamin E intake and risk of cataracts in humans. Ann N Y Acad Sci 570:372-82, 1989*).

Blood level may be inversely associated with cataract risk (*Jacques PF et al. Antioxidant status in persons with and without senile cataract. Arch Ophthalmol 106(3):337-40, 1988*).

Supplementation may be effective in preventing cataracts.

Animal Experimental Study: Pretreatment with vitamin E decreased the cataractogenic damage induced by irradiation from whole body exposure to single, acute doses of neutrons or gamma rays (*Ross WM, Creighton MO,*

Trevithick JR. Radiation cataractogenesis induced by neutron or gamma irradiation in the rat lens is reduced by vitamin E. Scan Micros *4:641-50, 1990).*

In vitro Animal Experimental Study: The addition of vitamin E to the perfusion solution of isolated rabbit corneal endothelium doubled its survival time, suggesting that vitamin E may be beneficial in restoring corneal function when it has undergone oxidative damage (*Neuwirth-Lux O, Billson F. Vitamin E and rabbit corneal endothelial cell survival.* Aust N Z J Ophthalmol *15(4):309-14, 1987).*

Animal Experimental Study: Adult rats, some pretreated for 2 wks. with daily injections of vitamin E, were made diabetic by an IV streptozotocin injection. In the animals that had not received vitamin E, changes appeared in the lenses as the hyperglycemia continued, while the lenses of the vitamin E-treated animals showed minimal changes (*Ross WM et al. Modelling cortical cataractogenesis: III. In vivo effects of vitamin E on cataractogenesis in diabetic rats.* Can J Ophthalmol *17(2):61-66, 1982).*

In vitro Animal Experimental Study: Since excessive free radical oxidation is thought to be a cause of cataracts, rat lenses were maintained in a special solution that caused free-radical damage when exposed to daylight. When vitamin E, an antioxidant, was added to the solution, the lenses suffered only 1/5 as much damage (*Varma SD et al. Photoperoxidation of lens lipids: prevention by vitamin E.* Photochem Photobiol *36(6):623-36, 1982).*

- -

MINERALS

Calcium:

The stability of the lens protein gel may depend upon maintaining a low internal level of calcium ions (*Duncan G, Jacob TJ. Calcium and the physiology of cataract.* Ciba Found Symp *106:132-52, 1984).*

May be elevated in the lens (*Ringvold A et al. The calcium and magnesium content of the human lens and aqueous humour. A study in patients with hypocalcemic and senile cataract.* Acta Ophthalmol (Copenh) *66(2):153-56, 1988; Stanojevïk-Paovïc A et al. Macro- and microelements in the cataractous eye lens.* Ophthalmic Res *19(4):230-34, 1987).*

> *Note: It appears that elevated lens calcium levels occur subsequent to cataract formation (McLaren DS.* Nutritional Opthalmology, *Second Edition. London, Academic Press, 1980).*

Copper:

Plasma levels may be reduced (*Bhat KS. Plasma calcium and trace minerals in human subjects with mature cataract.* Nutr Rep Int *37:157-63, 1988).*

Magnesium:

Metabolism may be abnormal.

Observational Study: While the magnesium content of the lens was found to be unaffected by cataract development in either senile or hypocalcemic cataract, the magnesium aqueous/serum ratio was elevated in cataract pts., suggesting a possible connection between magnesium metabolism and cataract development (*Ringvold A et al. The calcium and magnesium content of the human lens and aqueous humour. A study in patients with hypocalcemic and senile cataract.* Acta Ophthalmol (Copenh) *66(2):153-56, 1988).*

Selenium:

Required for the functioning of glutathione peroxidase, an important anti-oxidant in the lens (*Whanger P, Weswig P. Effects of selenium, chromium and antioxidants on growth, eye cataracts, plasma cholesterol and blood glucose in selenium deficient, vitamin E supplemented rats.* Nutr Rep Int *12:345-58, 1975).*

May be deficient in cataractous lenses (*Swanson A, Truesdale A. Elemental analysis in normal and cataractous human lens tissue.* Biochem Biophys Res Comm *45:1488-96, 1971).*

Blood levels may be elevated (*Jacques PF et al. Nutritional status in persons with and without senile cataract: Blood vitamin and mineral levels. Am J Clin Nutr 106(3):337-40, 1988*).

Excessive ingestion may cause cataracts.

> **Animal Experimental Study:** Excess selenium was found to cause cataracts in rats (*McLaren DS. Nutritional Opthalmology, Second Edition. London, Academic Press, 1980*).

Zinc:

Deficiency may cause cataracts.

> **Case Report:** A child with acrodermatitis enteropathica, a zinc-deficiency disease, developed bilateral cataracts, suggesting that zinc deficiency may have an etiologic role (*Racz P et al. Bilateral cataract in acrodermatitis enteropathica. J Pediatr Ophthalmol Strabismus 16(3):180-82, 1979*).

> **Animal Experimental Study:** Most trout fed a zinc-deficient diet developed cataracts, while no trout on the same diet supplemented with zinc developed them (*Ketola HG. J Nutr 109:965-69, 1979*).

Plasma levels may be reduced (*Bhat KS. Plasma calcium and trace minerals in human subjects with mature cataract. Nutr Rep Int 37:157-63, 1988*).

Levels in the lens of patients with mature senile cataract may be elevated (*Stanojevïk-Paovïc A et al. Macro- and microelements in the cataractous eye lens. Ophthalmic Res 19(4):230-34, 1987*).

Supplementation may be beneficial.

> **Animal Experimental Study:** Histologic examination of specimens of anterior lens capsules of rabbits have shown that small doses of zinc sulfate 0.1% stimulate mitotic activity of the lens epithelium, suggesting that this treatment may benefit pts. with early senile cataract (*Chuistova IP et al. [Experimental morphologic foundation for the usage of zinc in the treatment of cataract.] Oftalmol Zh 7:396, 1985*) (*in Russian*).

> **Review Article:** In senile cataract glucose utilization is disturbed due to loss of activity of some key zinc-dependent enzymes in the lens. Zinc supplementation improves the impaired glucose metabolism occurring in old age, and prolonged administration of zinc aspartate is indicated for the prophylaxis and therapy of senile cataract. In the presence of magnesium deficiency, magnesium salts should also be given. Also, cation eliminating exogenous or endogenous factors must be taken into consideration (*Heinitz M. [Clinical and biochemical aspects of the prophylaxis and therapy of senile cataract with zinc aspartate.] Klin Monatsbl Augenheilkd 172(5):778-83, 1978*) (*in German*).

- -

OTHER NUTRITIONAL FACTORS

Bioflavonoids:

Certain flavonoids such as quercetin and naringin (found in the flowers, fruit and rind of grapefruit) have been shown to inhibit aldose reductase, an enzyme involved in the synthesis of sorbitol from glucose.

> *Note: Sorbitol is not easily transported in or out of cells and thus accumulates intracellularly, drawing water in by osmosis while low molecular weight compounds are lost in an attempt to maintain osmotic equilibrium. Diabetic animals have been shown to be unusually prone to accumulate sorbitol leading, possibly, to the development of cataracts and other complications (Cogan DG et al. Aldose reductase and complications of diabetes. Ann Intern Med 101:82-91, 1984).*

Administration of certain bioflavonoids may be beneficial.

Animal Experimental Study: Oral quercitin given to diabetic rodents resulted in a significant decrease in sorbitol accumulation in lens tissue and, when given continuously, in a delay in the onset of cataracts (*Varma SD et al. Diabetic cataracts and flavonoids. Science 195:205-06, 1977*).

- and Vitamin E:

Experimental Study: 97% of 50 pts. with senile cortical cataracts demonstrated arrest in the progress of lens opacification following regular adminstration of bilberry (Vaccinium myrtillus) extract and vitamin E (*Bravetti G. Preventive medical treatment of senile cataract with vitamin E and anthocyanosides: Clinical evaluation. Ann Ottalmol Clin Ocul 115:109, 1989*).

Carotenoids:

Blood level may be inversely correlated with cataract risk (*Jacques PF, Chylack LT Jr. Epidemiologic evidence of a role for the antioxidant vitamins and carotenoids in cataract prevention. Am J Clin Nutr 53:352S-5S, 1991; Jacques PF et al. Nutritional status in persons with and without senile cataract:. Blood vitamin and mineral levels. Am J Clin Nutr 48:152-58, 1988; Jacques PF et al. Antioxidant status in persons with and without senile cataract. Arch Ophthalmol 106(3):337-40, 1988*).

May prevent photodamage to the lens by singlet oxygen (*Varma SD et al. Ocular damage by hematoporphyrin and light. In vitro studies with lens. Lens Res 3:319-33, 1986; Zigler JS, Goosey JD. Singlet oxygen as a possible factor in human senile cataract development. Curr Eye Res 3:59-65, 1984*).

Cysteine or Methionine:

Oxidation within the lens is associated with cataract formation (*Garner MH, Spector A. Selective oxidation of cysteine and methionine in normal and senile cataractous lenses. Proc Natl Acad Sci U S A 77(3):1274-77, 1980; Truscott RJ, Augusteyn RC. Oxidative changes in human lens proteins during senile nuclear cataract formation. Biochim Biophys Acta 492(1):43-52, 1977*).

Supplementation may retard cataract formation.

Theoretical Discussion: Glutathione protects the lens from the destructive effects of ultraviolet light but its concentration diminishes with age due to a decrease in the activity of the enzyme necessary for its synthesis. Perhaps a diet higher in cysteine or methionine, the rate-limiting amino acids in glutathione synthesis, would retard the age-related decline in glutathione levels and thus prevent cataract formation (*Cole H. Enzyme activity may hold the key to cataract activity. JAMA 254(8):1008, 1985*).

Dimethylglycine:

Administration may be beneficial.

Clinical Observation: DMG, which has been proven to prevent posterior subcapsular cataracts in experimental animals, frequently appears to reverse early posterior subcapsular cataracts in clinical practice when given at a dosage of 125 mg twice daily (*Todd GP. Nutrition, Health & Disease. Norfolk, Virginia, The Donning Company, 1985*).

Taurine:

One of the major free amino acids in the lens (*Kuck JFR Jr. Composition of the lens, in JB Bellows, Ed. Cataract and Abnormalities of the Lens. New York, Grune & Stratton, 1975:69-96, 1975*).

Local instillation may delay cataract formation in animals following ionizing radiation (*Fedorenko BS et al. Effect of taurine and vita-iodurol on the incidence of experimental radiation-induced cataracts. Bestn Oftalmol 6:67-69, 1978; Fedorenko BS et al. Der Einfluss von Taurin auf die Dynamik der Entwicklung experiementeller Katarakte bei Tieren. Radiobiol Radiother 19:452-58, 1978*).

Local instillation may reverse senile cataracts.

Experimental Controlled Study: 50 pts. received regular instillation of a 4% taurine solution into their eyes while another 50 pts. received regular instillation with a vitamin solution. After 6 mo., only the taurine-instilled pts. demonstrated increased visual acuity (*Vodovokov AM, Glotova NM. Results of treating senile cataracts with taurine. Vestn Oftalmol 2:44-45, 1981*).

- -

COMBINED NUTRIENTS

Intake may be inversely correlated with cataract risk.

Observational Study: Risk factors for age-related nuclear, cortical, posterior subcapsular, and mixed cataracts were evaluated for 1380 ophthalmology outpatients aged 40-79. Regular use of <u>multivitamin</u> supplements decreased risk (OR=0.63) for all cataract types. Dietary intake of <u>riboflavin</u>, <u>vitamin C</u>, <u>vitamin E</u> and <u>carotene</u>, which have anitoxidant potential, was protective for cortical, nuclear, and mixed cataract; intake of <u>niacin</u>, <u>thiamine</u>, and <u>iron</u> also decreased risk. Similar results were found in analyses that combined the antioxidant vitamins (OR=0.40) or considered the individual nutrients (OR=0.48-0.56) (*Leske MC et al. The Lens Opacities Case-Control Study: Risk factors for cataract. Arch Ophthalmol 109(2):244-51, 1991*).

Observational Study: The self-reported consumption of supplementary vitamins by 175 cataract pts. was compared to that of 175 controls. The latter gp. was found to use significantly more supplementary <u>vitamin C</u> (p=0.01) and <u>vitamin E</u> (p=0.004). The results suggested that supplementation was associated with at least a 50% reduction in the risk of cataracts (*Robertson J McD et al. A possible role for vitamins C and E in cataract prevention. Am J Clin Nutr 53:346S-51S, 1991*).

Animal Experimental Study: The frequency of advanced cataracts was much greater in mice maintained on a liquid anitoxidant-free diet (not containing any <u>vitamin C</u> or <u>vitamin E</u>) as compared to controls on the normal laboratory diet (*Mansour SA et al. Effect of antioxidant (vitamin E) on the progress of catracts in emory mice. Abstract. Invest Ophthalmol Vis Sci 25:138, 1984*).

Plasma levels may be reduced.

Observational Study: In a study of plasma levels of <u>vitamin C</u>, <u>vitamin E</u> and <u>carotenoids</u> of 112 subjects aged 40-70 which included 77 cataract pts., plasma levels in the pts. were lower in at least 2 of the 3 nutrients; however the differences were statistically significant only when the vitamins were analyzed as a combined index (*Jacques PF et al. Antioxidant status in persons with and without senile cataract. Arch Ophthalmol 106(3):337-40, 1988*).

CELIAC DISEASE

See Also: DERMATITIS HERPETIFORMIS

VITAMINS

Folic Acid:

Plasma levels usually indicate deficiency, and megaloblastic anemia is frequently present in adults, but uncommon in children. While correction occurs coincidentally with the improvement in absorption resulting from a gluten-free diet, folic acid should be given orally until recovery is complete (*Passmore R, Eastwood MA. Davidson and Passmore: Human Nutrition and Dietetics. Edinburgh, Churchill Livingstone, 1986, p. 440*).

Vitamin A:

May be deficient due to malabsorption of fats (*Passmore R, Eastwood MA. Davidson and Passmore: Human Nutrition and Dietetics. Edinburgh, Churchill Livingstone, 1986, p. 141*).

Vitamin B_6:

Absorption may be impaired (*Reinken L, Zieglauer H. Vitamin B6 absorption in children with acute celiac disease and in control subjects. J Nutr 108:1562, 1978*).

Depression, which is common in adult patients, may be treated successfully with pyridoxine.

Experimental Study: 12 depressed adult celiacs who had been on a gluten-free diet for years received supplementation with 80 mg pyridoxine daily. After 6 mo., depression had significantly improved in all patients (*Hallert C, Astrom J, Walan A. Reversal of psychopathology in adult celiac disease with the aid of pyridoxine (vitamin B6). Scand J Gastroenterol 18:299, 1983*).

Vitamin B_{12}:

May be deficient due to malabsorption (*Kokkonen J, Similä S. Gastric function and absorption of vitamin B12 in children with celiac disease. Eur J Pediatr 132(2):71-75, 1979*).

Vitamin D:

May be deficient due to malabsorption of fats (*Passmore R, Eastwood MA. Davidson and Passmore: Human Nutrition and Dietetics. Edinburgh, Churchill Livingstone, 1986, p. 141*).

Vitamin E:

May be deficient due to malabsorption of fats (*Passmore R, Eastwood MA. Davidson and Passmore: Human Nutrition and Dietetics. Edinburgh, Churchill Livingstone, 1986, p. 141*).

Vitamin K:

May be deficient due to malabsorption of fats (*Passmore R, Eastwood MA. Davidson and Passmore: Human Nutrition and Dietetics. Edinburgh, Churchill Livingstone, 1986, p. 141*).

- -

MINERALS

Copper:

May be deficient due to malabsorption (*Goyens P et al. Copper deficiency in infants with active celiac disease. J Pediatr Gastroenterol Nutr 4(4):677-80, 1985; Jameson S et al. Copper malabsorption in coeliac disease. Sci Total Environ 42(1-2):29-36, 1985*).

Iron:

Deficiency causes over 90% of the anemia which is usually present in patients. Correction of the anemia occurs coincidentally with the improvement in absorption which results from a gluten-free diet but, until recovery is complete, it is advisable to give iron to patients with hypochromic anemia (*Passmore R, Eastwood MA. Davidson and Passmore: Human Nutrition and Dietetics. Edinburgh, Churchill Livingstone, 1986, p. 440*).

Experimental Study: In a gp. of 54 pediatric pts., mild iron deficiency anemia or evidence of iron deficiency without anemia were common at the time of the diagnosis. Treatment with a gluten-free diet without iron supplementation eliminated all evidence of iron deficiency and completely normalized lab values. Subsequent challenge with gluten resulted in the rapid reappearance of suboptimal iron balance as evidenced by a decrease in serum ferritin (*Ståhlberg MR, Savilahti E, Siimes MA. Iron deficiency in coeliac disease is mild and it is detected and corrected by gluten-free diet. Acta Paediatr Scand 80(2):190-3, 1991*).

Experimental Study: 20 pediatric pts. aged 1.2-16.6 yrs. (mean 7.5 yrs.) were studied longitudinally during periods of gluten-free and gluten-containing diets. Their hemoglobin concentrations did not show any significant differences in relation to shifts in diet. A few had mild anemia. Their iron status, as judged from mean corpuscular volume, serum iron serum transferrin and saturation %, appeared to be generally insufficient. However, the only significant change related to shifts in diet was an increase of serum iron during the first period of the gluten-free diet. Dietary intakes of iron proved to be insufficient, regardless of the type of diet (*Hjelt K, Krasilnikoff PA. The impact of gluten on haematolgical status, dietary intakes of haemopoietic nutrients and vitamin B$_{12}$ and folic acid absorption in children with coeliac disease. Acta Paediatr Scand 79(10):911-19, 1990*).

Selenium:

May be deficient.

Observational Study: The selenium content of washed erythrocytes was determined in 24 celiac children on a gluten-containing diet and 25 on a gluten-free diet. In gluten loading, the selenium level was significantly lower than in the healthy control group. Selenium rose slightly in the erythrocytes of celiac children kept on a gluten-free diet but did not reach the lower limit of the physiological value. As celiac children were found to have increased sensitivity to oxidative stress and decreased activity of the selenium-containing antioxidant, glutathione peroxidase, the necessity of supplementing the trace element is raised (*Boda M, Nëmeth I. [Selenium levels in erythrocytes of children with celiac disease.] Orv Hetil 130(39):2087-90, 1989*) (*in Hungarian*).

Observational Study: Significantly lower levels of selenium (p<0.001) were found both in 37 celiac pts. on a gluten-containing diet and 36 on a gluten-free diet with respect to healthy controls. In pts. on the gluten-containing diet, the selenium deficit can be attributed to malabsorption, while in pts. on a gluten-free diet it may be due to the diet itself. As low serum selenium levels have been observed in several neoplasias, and celiac pts. show an increased incidence of GI tumors, long-term monitoring of the diet and selenium status is suggested in pts. with a persistent selenium deficit (*Cortigiani L et al. [Selenium in celiac disease.] Minerva Pediatr 41(11):539-42, 1989*) (*in Italian*).

Zinc:

Prior to gluten elimination, there is increased turnover and loss of endogenous zinc despite normal absorption at physiological intakes (*Crofton RW et al. Zinc metabolism in celiac disease. Am J Clin Nutr 52(2):379-82, 1990*).

- -

OTHER FACTORS

Avoid <u>gluten</u>.

Gluten is found in wheat, rye, oats, barley (including malt) and buckwheat.

Experimental Study: 314 infants and children were diagnosed on the basis of a flat proximal small bowel mucosa when untreated and an unequivocal response and remission on a gluten-free diet (GFD). In 91 pts., interruptions of the GFD were documented by repeated intestinal biopsies. 81% had a flat mucosa after 0.25-14.67 yrs. off the diet, while in 12% a successive deterioration of the mucosa occurred during 0.5-6.67 yrs. after interruption of the GFD without becoming flat. 6.6% had a normal intestinal mucosa after 2.24-6.92 yrs. off the diet, while 3 pts. were off the diet less than 2 yrs. and are thus still under study. A mucosal relapse within 2 yrs. after stopping the GFD was observed in 21/24 (87.5%) pts. studied longitudinally during planned challenges. It is concluded that only a minority (6.6%) will not relapse after an interruption of the GFD, while another small gp. (12%) will deteriorate very slowly; thus routine gluten challenges are not justifiable (*Shmerling DH, Franckx J. Childhood celiac disease: A long-term analysis of relapses in 91 pts.* <u>J Pediatr Gastroenterol Nutr</u> *5(4):565-69, 1986*).

Observational Study: Of 71 children suspected of having malabsorption, 16/17 diagnosed histologically as having childhood celiac disease had elevated antibodies to the alpha-gliadin fraction of wheat gluten (94% sensitivity). Of the 54 with normal biopsies, 48 had normal levels of alpha-gliadin antibodies (88% specificity) (*Kelly J et al. Alpha-gliadin antibodies in childhood celiac disease. Letter.* <u>Lancet</u> *September 7, 1985, p. 558*).

Rule out <u>lactase deficiency</u> causing intolerance to dairy products.

Many adult celiacs have low levels of intestinal lactase which is secondary to the disease process, probably due to reduced epithelial cells and alterations in the function of individual cells (*Plotkin GR, Isselbacher KJ. Secondary disaccharidase deficiency in adult celiac disease.* <u>N Engl J Med</u> *271:1033-7, 1964*).

CEREBROVASCULAR DISEASE

See Also: ATHEROSCLEROSIS
HYPERTENSION

DIETARY FACTORS

Eat fresh fruits and vegetables.

Observational Study: The relation between the 24 hr. dietary potassium intake (assessed by 24 hr. diet recall) at baseline and subsequent stroke-associated mortality was examined for 859 men and women (aged 50-79 yrs.). After 12 yrs., 24 stroke-associated deaths had occurred. The relative risks of stroke-associated mortality in the lowest tercile of potassium intake, as compared with that in the top two terciles combined, were 2.6 (p=0.16) in men and 4.8 (p=0.01) in women. In multivariate analyses, a 10 mmol increase in daily potassium intake (one extra helping of fruits or vegetables daily) was associated with a 40% reduction in the risk of stroke-associated mortality (p<0.001). This effect was independent of other dietary variables and of known cardiovascular risk factors. Results suggest that an increase in fruit and vegetable consumption may help to prevent cardiovascular disease (*Khaw KT, Barrett-Connor E. Dietary potassium and stroke-associated mortality. A 12-year prospective population study. N Engl J Med 316(5):235-40, 1987*).

Observational Study: A low incidence of cerebrovascular disease was associated with geographical regions where fresh fruit and vegetable consumption was high (*Acheson RM, Williams DRR. Does consumption of fruit and vegetables protect against stroke? Lancet 1:1191-93, 1983*).

Animal protein may be preferable to vegetable protein.

Observational Study: During 16 yrs. of follow-up among 7591 Japanese men, 409 stroke cases were identified. The intake of animal protein was significantly negatively associated with the incidence of both fatal and non-fatal thromboembolic strokes in multivariate models. Although the high intercorrelation of such dietary factors as protein, potassium and calcium makes it difficult to examine their separate effects, in this cohort calcium and animal protein had a stronger effect than potassium (*Lee CN et al. Dietary potassium and stroke. Letter. N Engl J Med 318(15):995-96, 1988*).

Theoretical Discussion: While coronary disease is correlated with consumption of foods of animal origin, cerebrovascular disease correlates with consumption of plant proteins. The author proposes that steroidal estrogens and plant metabolites which mimic estrogens (phyto-estrogens) are atherogenic and suggests that digestion products of phyto-estrogens pass through the blood/brain barrier while steroidal estrogens cannot. Rich sources of phyto-estrogens include soybeans and peanuts (*Seely S. Diet and cerebrovascular disease. Nutr Health 2:173-9, 1983*).

Limit alcohol consumption.

Excessive alcohol consumption (>300 g/wk) may increase the chance of hemorrhagic, but not thromboembolic, strokes, perhaps due to its inhibition of platelet aggregation, while moderate drinking (50-150 g/wk) may reduce stroke risk.

Observational Study: 177 male stroke pts. were compared with an equal number of matched controls. Daily or almost daily consumption equivalent to 1 or 2 drinks conferred the lowest relative risk of brain infarction (odds ratio 0.09). Risk rose substantially as drinking exceeded moderation, with consumption of >300 g/wk resulting in an odds ratio of 6.38. Among men who drank rarely or never, the risk of stroke was relatively low, but well above that for people who consumed 50-150 g of alcohol weekly. Regularity of consumption conbributed much to the benefit (*Markku Kaste, chairman of neurology, U. of Helskinki, Finland - reported at the Am. Heart Assoc. stroke meeting, 1991*).

Observational Study: For a large gp. of middle-aged female nurses, alcohol intake was associated with a decreased risk of ischemic stroke. For 5-14 gm alcohol daily (3-9 drinks/wk.) the relative risk was 0.3; for 15 gm daily it was 0.5. In contrast, alcohol intake tended to be associated with an increased risk of subarachnoid hemorrhage; for 5-14 gm daily the relative risk was 3.7 (*Stampfer MJ et al. A prospective study of moderate alcohol consumption and the risk of coronary disease and stroke in women. N Engl J Med 319:267-73, 1988*).

Observational Study: In a study of the 12-yr. incidence of stroke in 8000 males of Japanese ancestry, hemorrhagic stroke incidence increased steadily with the amt. of alcohol consumed. 2-3 drinks weekly was associated with more than double the risk, while heavy drinking was associated with almost triple the risk, independent of other risk factors. The differences in risk of thromboembolic stroke between abstainers and heavy drinkers, however, were insignificant (*Donahue RP et al. Alcohol and hemorrhagic stroke. The Honolulu Heart Program. JAMA 255(17):2311-14, 1986*).

Experimental Study: In a study using healthy volunteers, a 5-oz glass of wine did not inhibit platelet aggregation unless taken with a meal high in saturated fats, when it had a significant inhibitory effect compared to the meal alone (*Littleton JM. Interactions between ethanol and dietary fat in determining human platelet function. Thromb Haemost 51(1):50-53, 1984*).

Alcoholic binges may acutely cause stroke (*Wilkins MR, Kendall MJ. Stroke affecting young men after alcoholic binges. Br Med J 291:1342, 1985*).

Reduce serum cholesterol. (*see "ATHEROSCLEROSIS" for nutritional and dietary means.*)

There is an inverse relation between serum cholesterol level and the risk of death from hemorrhagic stroke in middle-aged American men, but its impact is overwhelmed by a positive association of higher serum cholesterol levels with death from nonhemorrhagic stroke as well as total cardiovascular disease (*Iso H et al. Serum cholesterol levels and six-year mortality from stroke in 350,977 men screened for the Multiple Risk Factor Invervention Trial. N Engl J Med 320-904-10, 1989*).

– –

VITAMINS

Vitamin B$_6$:

Promotes conversion of homocysteine (toxic) to cystathionine; thus B$_6$ deficiency is theorized (originally by Kilmer McCully, M.D., Professor of Pathology, Harvard Medical School) to cause arterial damage due to build-up of homocysteine. (The incidence of heterozygous homocystinuria due to cystathionine synthase deficiency is about 1 in 70.)

Note: See also "Folic acid" and "Betaine" in "ATHEROSCLEROSIS."

Observational Study: Hyperhomocysteinemia was detected in 16/38 pts. with cerebrovascular disease (42%), 7/25 pts. with peripheral vascular disease (28%), and 18/60 pts. with coronary vascular disease (30%) compared to none of 27 normal controls. After adjustment for the effects of conventional risk factors, the lower 95% confidence limit for the odds ratio for vascular disease among pts. with hyperhomocysteinemia as compared to normals was 3.2. The geometric-mean peak serum homocysteine level was 1.33 times higher in pts. with all vascular disease than in normals (p=0.002). The presence of cystathionine beta-synthase deficiency was confirmed n 18/23 pts. with vascular disease who had hyperhomocysteinemia. Results suggest that hyperhomocysteinemia is an independent risk factor for vascular disease which is probably due in most instances to cystathionine beta-synthase deficiency (*Clarke R et al. Hyperhomocysteinemia: an independent risk factor for vascular disease. N Engl J Med 324(17):1149-55, 1991*).

Note: The authors also found an inverse relation between both RBC folate and serum vitamin B$_{12}$ levels and hyperhomocysteinemia. They believe that there are probably multiple mechanisms involved in the pathogenesis of hyperhomocysteinemia and suggest that the relative contributions of genetic and nutritional factors require further study (Clarke R et al. Homocysteinemia: a risk factor for vascular disease. Letter. N Engl J Med 325(13):966-7, 1991).

Experimental Study: 25 pts. developing occlusive cerebrovascular disease before the age of 50 were studied. Heterozygous homocystinuria was diagnosed on the basis of excessive homocysteine accumulation after methionine loading and by the presence of cystathionine synthetase deficiency in skin fibroblasts. The disorder was found in 7 of the pts. (28%). Abnormal homocysteine metabolism improved in 10/11 pts. with ischemic vascular disease supplemented with B6 (*Boers GHJ et al. Heterozygosity for homocystinuria in premature peripheral and cerebral occlusive arterial disease. N Engl J Med 313:709-15, 1985*).

Observational Study: Compared to 17 controls, 19 pts. with arteriosclerotic cerebrovascular disease demonstrated significantly elevated plasma homocysteine concentrations measured as cysteine-homocysteine mixed disulfide, suggesting that moderate homocysteinuria might be a risk factor for arteriosclerotic cerebrovascular disease (*Brattstrom LE et al. Moderate homocysteinemia: A possible risk factor for arteriosclerotic cerebrovascular disease. Stroke 15(6):1012-16, 1984*).

Animal Experimental Study: Arteriosclerotic plaques were found in the aorta and arteries of rabbits given homocysteine thiolactone, methionine or homocysteic acid. Pyridoxine prevented thrombosis and pulmonary embolism but did not prevent arteriosclerotic plaques (*McCully KS, Wilson RB. Homocysteine theory of arteriosclerosis. Atherosclerosis 22(2):215-27, 1975*

- -

MINERALS

Calcium:

Intake may be negatively correlated with the incidence of thromboembolic strokes.

Observational Study: During 16 yrs. of follow-up among 7591 Japanese men, 409 stroke cases were identified. The intake of calcium was significantly negatively associated with the incidence of both fatal and non-fatal thromboembolic strokes in multivariate models. Although the high intercorrelation of such dietary factors as protein, potassium and calcium makes it difficult to examine their separate effects, in this cohort calcium and animal protein had a stronger effect than potassium (*Lee CN et al. Dietary potassium and stroke. Letter. N Engl J Med 318(15):995-96, 1988*).

Chromium:

Elevated hair chromium may be associated with damage to the cerebral arteries.

Observational Study: While the hair chromium levels of pts. with hyperlipemia and coronary heart disease were similar to those of healthy controls (p<0.02), significantly higher hair chromium values were observed in pts. with cerebral hemorrhage and cerebral thrombosis than in healthy subjects (p<0.001) (*Huang G et al. Hair chromium levels in patients with vascular diseases. Biol Trace Elem Res 29:133-7, 1991*).

Magnesium:

Supplementation may be beneficial in cerebral vasospasm and ischemia.

Theoretical Discussion: Recent evidence suggests that magnesium may act by opposing calcium-dependent cerebral arterial vasoconstriction; it may also antagonize the increase in intracellular calcium caused by ischemia and thus prevent cell damage and death. Magnesium may thus have a role in the treatment of cerebral vasospasm and ischemia, such as occurs in subarachnoid hemorrhage, ischemic stroke, and brain trauma (*Sadeh M. Action of magnesium sulfate in the treatment of preeclampsia-eclampsia. Stroke 20(9):1273-75, 1989*).

Potassium:

Intake may be negatively correlated with stroke-associated mortality.

Observational Study: During 16 yrs. of follow-up among 7591 Japanese men, 409 stroke cases were identified. The intake of potassium was significantly negatively associated only with the incidence of the small group of fatal thromboembolic strokes in multivariate models. Although the high intercorrelation of such dietary factors as protein, potassium and calcium makes it difficult to examine their separate effects, in this cohort calcium and animal protein had a stronger effect than potassium (*Lee CN et al. Dietary potassium and stroke. Letter. N Engl J Med 318(15):995-96, 1988*).

Observational Study: The relation between the 24 hr. dietary potassium intake (assessed by 24 hr. diet recall) at baseline and subsequent stroke-associated mortality was examined for 859 men and women (aged 50-79 yrs.). After 12 yrs., 24 stroke-associated deaths had occurred. The relative risks of stroke-associated mortality in the lowest tercile of potassium intake, as compared with that in the top two terciles combined, were 2.6 (p=0.16) in men and 4.8 (p=0.01) in women. In multivariate analyses, a 10 mmol increase in daily potassium intake (one extra helping of fruits or vegetables daily) was associated with a 40% reduction in the risk of stroke-associated mortality (p<0.001). This effect was independent of other dietary variables and of known cardiovascular risk factors. Results suggest that an increase in fruit and vegetable consumption may help to prevent cardiovascular disease (*Khaw KT, Barrett-Connor E. Dietary potassium and stroke-associated mortality. A 12-year prospective population study. N Engl J Med 316(5):235-40, 1987*).

Potassium iodide and
Niacin hydroiodide:

Combined supplementation may reduce anxiety and depression associated with cerebral atherosclerosis.

Experimental Double-blind Crossover Study: 17 female and 13 male domiciled ambulatory pts. aged 58-90 randomly received either the combination of potassium iodide 135 mg and niacinamide hydroiodide 25 mg (Iodo-Niacin, Cole) 2 tabs 3 times daily after meals or placebo after all medications previously administered for anxiety, depression and behavioral symptoms were stopped for 1 week. After 4 wks., supplements and placebos were withheld for 1 wk. and the gps. were crossed over for another 4 weeks. According to the ratings of the investigator and the charge nurse, supplementation resulted in moderate relief of depression in 10 pts. and of anxiety in 4 patients. 17 pts. experienced slight relief of anxiety, depression or behavioral symptoms (not the same 17 pts. in each case). Placebo resulted in moderate anxiety relief in 1 pt., behavioral improvement in 1 pts. and depression relief in 2 pts.; 5 pts. had slight relief of anxiety symptoms, 2 had slight relief of behavioral symptoms, and 13 had slight relief of depression. Pts. in both gps. had minor side-effects (*Stern FH. The management of cerebral atherosclerosis. Psychosomatics 9:229-34, 1968*).

- -

OTHER NUTRITIONAL FACTORS

Omega-3 Fatty Acids (Fish Oils):

Eicosapentaenoic acid (EPA) and docosahexaenoic acid (DHA).

Highest in cold water fish. Available in a refined form as "MaxEPA" (18% EPA).

Suggested MaxEPA dosage: 3 - 9 grams daily in divided doses (or 10 ml. concentrate twice daily)

WARNING: Supplementation may require additional vitamin E intake to prevent increased membrane peroxidation and cellular damage (*Laganiere S, Fernandes G. High peroxidizability of subcellular membrane induced by high fish oil diet is reversed by vitamin E. Clin Res 35:A565, 1987*).

Supplementation may protect against decreases in cerebral blood flow and cerebral edema in the presence of an acute carotid occlusion.

Animal Experimental Study: Gerbils were fed either a standard diet or a diet supplemented with menhaden fish oil (high in eicosapentaenoic acid) for 2 months. Ischemia was produced by bilateral carotid occlusion for 10 min., followed by reperfusion for 60 minutes. In control animals, cerebral blood flow was decreased 30 and 60 min. after reperfusion and brain water was increased, while in experimental animals cerebral blood flow did not fall during reperfusion and edema did not appear (*Black KL et al. Eicosapentaenoic acid: Effect on brain prostaglandins, cerebral blood flow and edema in ischemic gerbils. Stroke 15(1):65-69, 1984*).

CERVICAL DYSPLASIA

See Also: CANCER

VITAMINS

Folic Acid: 5 mg. twice daily (3 month trial)

Deficiency (best measured by RBC folate as serum folate may be normal) may be associated with the use of oral contraceptives (*Steiff R. Folate deficiency and oral contraceptives. JAMA 214:105-08, 1970*) and may be correlated with cervical dysplastic changes (*Lindenbaum J et al. Oral contraceptive hormones, folate metabolism, and the cervical epithelium. Am J Clin Nutr April, 1975, pp. 346-53*).

> *Note: The characteristic changes in cervicovaginal smears believed to be due to systemic B_{12} or folic acid deficiency include proportionate cellular and nuclear enlargement, multinucleation and absence of hyperchromasia. These changes were commonly found along with papilloma-virus cytopathic effects (30/57=52%) and carcinoma-in-situ (CIN) I or II (42/57=73%). Corresponding biopsies confirmed focal folic acid deficiency-like changes in 23/57=40% which were almost always observed in close proximity to papillomavirus cytopathic changes; CIN I-III was also present in 36/57=63%. These results suggest that changes in smears previously thought to be specific for folic acid deficiency may also be associated with papillomavirus infection and concomitant CIN (Fekete PS, Hammami A. Folic acid deficiency-like changes in cervicovaginal smears: A possible manifestation of papillomavirus infection? Abstract. Acta Cytologica 31(5):679, 1987*).

Observational Study: Red cell folate levels of a gp. of young women were lower in subjects on combination-type oral contraceptive agents (OCAs) for at least 6 mo. (189 ng/ml) than in those not on OCAs (269 ng/ml), and lowest in subjects on OCAs with cervical dysplasia (162 ng/ml) (*Butterworth CE et al. Improvement in cervical dysplasia associated with folic acid therapy in users of oral contraceptives. Am J Clin Nutr 35:73-82, 1982*).

Supplementation may be beneficial.

Experimental Double-blind Study: 47 young women with mild or moderate dysplasia who had been on combination-type oral contraceptive agents for at least 6 mo. received either 10 mg oral folate daily or placebo. After 3 mo., cervical biopsies showed significant improvement only in the women receiving folate. The dysplasia completely disappeared in 7 women receiving folate, while 4 women on placebo showed progression to carcinoma-in-situ (*Butterworth CE et al. Improvement in cervical dysplasia associated with folic acid therapy in users of oral contraceptives. Am J Clin Nutr 35:73-82, 1982*).

Experimental Study: Following treatment with folic acid 10 mg daily, 100% of cases reverted to normal as determined by colposcopy/biopsy examination (*Whitehead N et al. Megaloblastic changes in the cervical epithelium. Association with oral contraceptive therapy and reversal with folic acid. JAMA 226:1421-4, 1973*).

Vitamin A: 60,000 IU daily for 2 months; then 25,000 IU daily

Low intake may be associated with increased risk (*Romney SL et al. Retinoids and the prevention of cervical dysplasias. Am J Obstet Gynecol 141(8):890-4, 1981*).

Observational Study: From a gp. of 87 cases with abnormal uterocervical cytology and 82 controls, a subset of cases was matched to controls for age, ethnicity, socioeconomic status, and parity. Those cases with severe dysplasia or carcinoma in situ were more likely to have a total dietary vitamin A intake below the pooled median and/or a beta-carotene intake below the pooled median than were normal matched controls (p<0.05; p<0.025). Odds ratios revealed a 3 times greater risk for severe dysplasia and a 2 3/4 times greater risk for CIS in women with lowered vitamin A or beta-carotene intake (*Wylie-Rosett JA et al. Influence of vitamin A on cervical dysplasia and carcinoma in situ. Nutr Cancer 6(1):49-57, 1984*).

Retinol binding protein may be reduced both in the blood and in cervical tissue (*Romney SL et al. Retinoids and the prevention of cervical dysplasias. Am J Obstet Gynecol 141(8):890-4, 1981; Wylie-Rosett JA et al. Influence of vitamin A on cervical dysplasia and carcinoma in situ. Nutr Cancer 6(1):49-57, 1984*).

Topical application of retinyl acetate may increase plasma retinol and retinol binding protein.

Experimental Placebo-controlled Study: 41 women self-administered a retinyl acetate gel. After 7 days, there was an increase in both the concentrations of plasma retinol and retinol binding protein which receded after the gel was discontinued. No significant changes were noted in controls (*Palan PR et al. Vaginal hydrolysis of retinyl acetate: increase in plasma retinol and retinol binding protein in women with cervical dysplasias. Biochem Med Metab Biol 40(3):282-90, 1988*).

Topical application of synthetic retinoids may be beneficial.

Experimental Study: 36 pts. with cervical intraepithelial neoplasia were treated with 4 consecutive 24-hr. applications of retinoids via an inert collagen sponge in a cervical cap. Complete regression was seen in 2/14 (14%) pts. treated with lower concentrations and in 10/22 (45%) pts. treated with higher concentrations (*Weiner SA et al. A phase I trial of topically applied trans-retinoic acid in cervical dysplasia - clinical efficacy. Invest New Drugs 4(3):241-44, 1986*).

Vitamin C: 300 mg. daily

Low intake may be associated with increased risk (*Romney SL et al. Retinoids and the prevention of cervical dysplasias. Am J Obstet Gynecol 141(8):890-4, 1981*).

Observational Study: The dietary habits of 49 women with cervical abnormalities were compared to those of 49 matched negative controls. Mean daily vitamin C intake was 80 mg for cases compared to 107 mg for controls (p<0.01). Similarly, 29% of cases compared to 3% of controls had a vitamin C intake less than 50% of the RDA, yielding a 10-fold increase in risk of cervical dysplasia as estimated by odds ratio (p<0.05). Multiple logistic analysis indicated that low vitamin C intake is an independent contributor to risk of severe cervical dysplasia when age and sexual activity variables are controlled (*Wassertheil-Smoller S et al. Dietary vitamin C and uterine cervical dysplasia. Am J Epidemiol 114(5):714-24, 1981*).

Plasma levels may be low.

Observational Study: 46 pts. with 1 positive or 2 consecutive suspicious Pap smears for cervical dysplasia were found to have significantly lower vitamin C levels (0.36 mg/dl) than 34 controls with no gynecological dysfunction (0.75 mg/ml) (*Romney SL et al. Plasma vitamin C and uterine cervical dysplasia. Am J Obstet Gynecol 151(7):976-80, 1985*).

Vitamin E:

Plasma levels may be decreased (*Palan PR et al. Plasma levels of antioxidant beta-carotene and alpha-tocopherol in uterine cervix dysplasias and cancer. Nutr Cancer 15:13-20, 1991*).

- -

MINERALS

Selenium:

Deficiency is correlated with an increased risk of epithelial cancers (*Prasad K, Ed. Vitamins, Nutrition and Cancer. New York, Karger, 1984*).

Serum levels may be reduced (*Dawson E et al. Serum vitamin and selenium changes in cervical dysplasia. Fed Proc 43:612, 1984*).

OTHER NUTRITIONAL FACTORS

<u>Beta-carotene</u>:

Low intake may be associated with increased risk (*Romney SL et al. Retinoids and the prevention of cervical dysplasias. Am J Obstet Gynecol 141(8):890-4, 1981*).

Observational Study: From a gp. of 87 cases with abnormal uterocervical cytology and 82 controls, a subset of cases was matched to controls for age, ethnicity, socioeconomic status, and parity. Those cases with severe dysplasia or carcinoma in situ were more likely to have a total dietary vitamin A intake below the pooled median and/or a beta-carotene intake below the pooled median than were normal matched controls (p<0.05; p<0.025). Odds ratios revealed a 3 times greater risk for severe dysplasia and a 2 3/4 times greater risk for CIS in women with lowered vitamin A or beta-carotene intake (*Wylie-Rosett JA et al. Influence of vitamin A on cervical dysplasia and carcinoma in situ. Nutr Cancer 6(1):49-57, 1984*).

Plasma/serum levels may be low (*Brock K et al. Nutrients in diet and plasma and risk of in situ cervical cancer. J Natl Cancer Inst 80:580-5, 1988; Harris RWC et al. Cancer of the cervix uteri and vitamin A. Br J Cancer 53:653-9, 1986; Palan PR et al. Plasma levels of antioxidant beta-carotene and alpha-tocopherol in uterine cervix dysplasias and cancer. Nutr Cancer 15:13-20, 1991*).

CHRONIC FATIGUE SYNDROME

See Also: FATIGUE

VITAMINS

Vitamin B$_{12}$:

Supplementation may be beneficial.

Clinical Observation: Supplementation appears to give symptomatic improvement (*Lapp CW. Chronic fatigue syndrome is a real disease. North Carolina Family Physician 43(1):6-11, 1992*).

- with Folic acid and Liver extract:

Negative Experimental Double-blind Crossover Study: 15 pts. who met the Centers for Disease Control (US) criteria for chronic fatigue syndrome received IM a solution of bovine liver extract containing folic acid and cyanocobalamin (LEFAC). Although pts. responded to both LEFAC and placebo by several criteria of functional status, the placebo response appeared to be strong and no significant differences were found between LEFAC and placebo (*Kaslow JE, Rucker L, Onishi R. Liver extract-folic acid-cyanocobalamin vs placebo for chronic fatigue syndrome. Arch Intern Med 149(11):2501-3, 1989*).

- -

MINERALS

Germanium:

Bis-carboxyethyl germanium sesquioxide (Ge-132) may stimulate gamma-interferon production (*Kidd PM. Germanium-132 (Ge-132): Homeostatic normalizer and immunostimulant. A Review of its preventive and therapeutic efficacy. Int Clin Nutr Rev 7(1):11-20, 1987*).

Administration of bis-carboxyethyl germanium sesquioxide (Ge-132) may be beneficial.

Clinical Observations: Clinicians report that between 20% and over 50% of their pts. given Ge-132 150-500 mg/d note substantial to marked symptom relief (*Faloona GR, Levine SA. The use of organic germanium in chronic Epstein-Barr Virus Syndrome (CEBVS): An example of interferon modulation of herpes reactivation. J Orthomol Med 3(1):29-31, 1988*).

Magnesium:

Many of the symptoms of CFS are similar to those of magnesium deficiency: anorexia, nausea, learning disability, personality change, weakness, tiredness, and myalgia (*Cox IM, Campbell MJ, Dowson D. Red blood cell magnesium and chronic fatigue syndrome. Lancet 337:757-60, 1991*).

Red cell concentrations may be low.

Negative Observational Study: Compared to 18 controls matched for age, sex, and socioeconomic status, serum, whole blood and RBC magnesium levels did not differ from those of controls (*Deulofeu R et al. Magnesium and chronic fatigue syndrome. Letter. Lancet 338:641, 1991*).

Negative Observational Study: Compared to lab norms, RBC magnesium levels for 15/20 pts. with CFS for over 1 yr. meeting the Centers for Disease Control case definition for CFS were normal, while for 5 pts. they were raised (*Gantz NM. Magnesium and chronic fatigue. Letter. Lancet 338:66, 1991*).

Observational Study: 20 pts. had lower RBC magnesium than did 20 healthy controls matched for age, sex, and social class (*Cox IM, Campbell MJ, Dowson D. Red blood cell magnesium and chronic fatigue syndrome. Lancet 337:757-60, 1991*).

Supplementation may be beneficial.

Experimental Double-blind Study: 32 pts. randomly received either 50% magnesium sulfate (1 g in 2 ml) IM every wk. or placebo injections. After 6 wks., treated pts. claimed to have improved energy levels, better emotional state, and less pain, as judged by changes in the Nottingham health profile. 12/15 treated pts. said they had benefited from treatment, and in 7/15 pts. energy scores improved from the maximum to the minimum. By contrast, 3/17 controls felt better and 1/17 had a better energy score. RBC magnesium, which initially was low, returned to normal in all pts. on magnesium but in only 1 pt. on placebo (*Cox IM, Campbell MJ, Dowson D. Red blood cell magnesium and chronic fatigue syndrome. Lancet 337:757-60, 1991*).

Note: The supplementary dosage represents an additional magnesium intake of <1 mmol daily. Since the minimum UK recommended dietary intake of magnesium is 12 mmol, it is difficult to imagine how so small a dosage could be so effective in the absence of gross dietary magnesium deficiency or malabsorption (Young IS, Trimble ER. Magnesium and chronic fatigue syndrome. Letter. Lancet 337:1094-5, 1991).

See Also:

Experimental Double-blind Study: *Durlach J. Chronic fatigue syndrome and chronic primary magnesium deficiency (CFS and CPMD). Magnes Res 5(1):68, 1992*

- -

OTHER NUTRITIONAL FACTORS

Coenzyme Q10:

Supplementation may be beneficial.

Clinical Observation: Supplementation appears to give symptomatic improvement (*Lapp CW. Chronic fatigue syndrome is a real disease. North Carolina Family Physician 43(1):6-11, 1992*).

Clinical Observation: Several health care professionals have recommended that pts. take 2-4 30 mg caps daily (*Goldberg A. CFIDS Chronicle, Summer/Fall 1989*).

Essential Fatty Acids:

Metabolism may be abnormal.

Theoretical Discussion: Findings suggesting a relationship between essential fatty acid metabolism and the post-viral fatigue syndrome include the susceptibility of people with atopic eczema to viral infestions, the occasional precipitation of an atopic syndrome by viral infections, and the occurrence of a fatigue syndrome following viral infections. Key elements of the hypothesis that abnormal EFA metabolism is involved in the syndrome are the facts that interferon requires 6-desaturated EFAs in order to exert its anti-viral effects, that people with atopic eczema have low levels of 6-desaturated EFAs, and that viruses, as part of their attack strategy, may reduce the ability of cells to make 6-desaturated EFAs (*Horrobin DF. Post-viral fatigue syndrome, viral infections in atopic eczema, and essential fatty acids. Med Hypotheses 32(3):211-7, 1990*).

Administration may be beneficial.

Experimental Double-blind Study: 63 pts. with a good employment and mental health history who had post-viral fatigue syndrome for 1 yr. or longer randomly received Efamol Marine, a mixture of 80% of evening primrose oil and 20% of concentrated fish oil, or placebo. Baseline plasma EFA levels were low. After 3 mo., plasma EFA levels had risen to normal, and monounsaturated and saturated fatty acids had come down to normal in the treated group. After 1 mo., 74% of treated pts. and 23% of those on placebo rated themselves as better than at baseline. After 3 mo., 85% of treated pts. rated themselves as better than at baseline compared to only 17% of those on placebo, a highly significant difference (p<0.0001). Without exception, all the individual symptoms, including fatigue, aches and pains and depression, showed a highly significantly greater improvement on the fatty acid supplement than on placebo. There were no side effects (*Behan PO, Behan WM, Horrobin D. Effect of high doses of essential fatty acids on the postviral fatigue syndrome. Acta Neurol Scand 82(3):209-16, 1990; Behan PO, Behan WMH. Essential fatty acids in the treatment of post-viral fatigue syndrome, in DF Horrobin, Ed. Omega-6 Essential Fatty Acids: Pathophysiology and Roles in Clinical Medicine. New York, Alan R. Liss, 1990:275-82*).

CONGESTIVE HEART FAILURE

See Also: ATHEROSCLEROSIS
CARDIOMYOPATHY
HYPERTENSION

MINERALS

Calcium:

Increasing myocardial muscle cell calcium may be beneficial.

Review Article: Positive inotropic interventions aim to increase the cytosolic calcium ion concentration in the myocardium, including the use of digitalis glycosides, beta-agonists and amrinone (*Opie LH. Principles of therapy for congestive heart failure. Eur Heart J 4 Suppl. A:199-208, 1983*).

Reducing vascular smooth muscle calcium may be beneficial.

Experimental Study: Intercellular vascular smooth muscle calcium results in vasoconstriction and may thus potentially increase afterload in chronic CHF. In a study of the response to nifedipine, a calcium channel blocking agent, calcium antagonism resulted in significant afterload reduction and hemodynamic improvement in chronic CHF (*Prida XE et al. Evaluation of calcium-mediated vasoconstriction in chronic congestive heart failure. Am J Med 75(5):795-800, 1983*).

Magnesium:

Myocardial and serum magnesium may be abnormal.

Observational Study: In a gp. of 199 pts., the serum magnesium concentration was <1.6 mEq/L in 38 pts. (19%), within normal range in 134 (67%) and >2.1 mEq/L in 27 (14%) (*Gottlieb SS et al. Prognostic importance of the serum magnesium concentration in patients with congestive heart failure. J Am Coll Cardiol 1694):827-31, 1990*).

Review Article and Observational Study: In CHF there is a loss of magnesium (along with elevation of intracellular sodium and reduction of intracellular potassium) due to activation of the renin-angiotensin-aldosterone system. This deficiency may, in turn, add to the elevation of intracellular sodium and reduction of intracellular potassium since magnesium is necessary for the function of the Na-K pump. In 297 pts. with diuretic-treated CHF, 37% had hypomagnesemia and 43% had low muscle magnesium (*Wester PO, Dyckner T. Intracellular electrolytes in cardiac failure. Acta Med Scand [Suppl] 707:33-36, 1986*).

Review Article: CHF is often associated with hypomagnesemia as well as magnesium tissue deficits. Cardiac glycosides and diuretics (loop and distal types) often exacerbate, or result in, hypomagnesemia, which may lead to cardiac arrhythmias and sudden cardiac death. Deficits in extracellular and vascular tissue magnesium lead to peripheral vasoconstriction which may contribute to the increase in peripheral vascular resistance commonly noted. More attention must be paid to monitoring magnesium levels in tissues (possibly using lymphocytes) and in plasma, and deficits must be corrected. The nonspecific vasodilator properties of Mg^{++} together with its ability to unload the heart should be considered as an important adjunctive tool in CHF management (*Altura BM, Altura BT. Biochemistry and pathophysiology of congestive heart failure: Is there a role for magnesium? Magnesium 5(3-4):134-43, 1986*).

Abnormal serum magnesium levels may be associated with a poorer prognosis.

Observational Study: In a gp. of 199 pts., pts. with hypomagnesemia had more frequent ventricular premature complexes and episodes of ventricular tachycardia than did pts. with a normal serum magnesium concentrations (p<0.05). Even though the 2 gps. were similar with respect to severity of heart failure and neurohormonal variables, pts. with hypomagnesemia had a significantly worse prognosis during long-term follow-up (45% vs. 71% 1-yr. survival; p<0.05). Pts. with hypermagnesemia had more severe symptoms, greater neurohormonal activation and worse renal function than did pts. with a normal serum magnesium but tended to have fewer ventricular arrhythmias. Hypermagnesemic pts. also had a worse prognosis than did those with a normal serum magnesium (37% vs. 71% 1-yr. survival; p<0.05) (*Gottlieb SS et al. Prognostic importance of the serum magnesium concentration in patients with congestive heart failure. J Am Coll Cardiol 1694):827-31, 1990*).

Supplementation may assist in the correction of muscle potassium deficiencies as well as in correction of the disturbed relation between extra- and intracellular electrolytes.

Experimental Study: It was found that, for pts. with CHF, a deficiency of muscle potassium could not be corrected when there was also a concomitant magnesium deficiency. In addition, magnesium infusions changed the disturbed relation between extra- and intracellular electrolytes towards normal (*Wester PO, Dyckner T. Intracellular electrolytes in cardiac failure. Acta Med Scand [Suppl] 707:33-36, 1986*).

Potassium:

Myocardial and serum potassium may be deficient.

Review Article and Observational Study: In CHF the activation of the renin-angiotension-aldosterone system causes potassium losses, while the secondary hyperaldosteronism may give rise to low intracellular potassium through a direct permeability effect on the cell membrane. In addition, magnesium loss (which is also due to activation of the renin-angiotension-aldosterone system) leads to further loss of intracellular potassium as magnesium is necessary for the function of the Na-K pump. In 297 pts. with diuretic-treated CHF, 42% had hypokalemia and 52% had depletion of muscle potassium (*Wester PO, Dyckner T. Intracellular electrolytes in cardiac failure. Acta Med Scand [Suppl] 707:33-36, 1986*).

Review Article: CHF is often associated with hypokalemia as well as potassium tissue deficits. Cardiac glycosides and diuretics (loop and distal types) often exacerbate, or result in, hypokalemia, which may lead to cardiac arrhythmias and sudden cardiac death. Potassium deficits may contribute to the increase in peripheral vascular resistance commonly noted. More attention must be paid to monitoring potassium levels in tissues (possibly using lymphocytes) and in plasma, and deficits must be corrected (*Altura BM, Altura BT. Biochemistry and pathophysiology of congestive heart failure: Is there a role for magnesium? Magnesium 5(3-4):134-43, 1986*).

Supplementation may be beneficial.

Review Article: "Because hypokalemia is known to predispose patients to ventricular arrhythmias, it may be prudent to aggressively maintain serum potassium levels in patients with heart failure in the range of 4 to 5 mEq/liter" (*Francis GS. Interaction of the sympathetic nervous system and electrolytes in congestive heart failure. Am J Cardiol 65(10):24E-27E, 1990*).

Review Article: In pts. with CHF, "potassium can modify both the mechanical and electrical properties of the heart, it can exert diuretic effects, and it can reduce the frequency and complexity of potentially lethal ventricular tachyarrhythmias" (*Packer M. Potential role of potassium as determinant of morbidity and mortality in patients with systemic hypertension and congestive heart failure. Am J Cardiol 65(10):45E-51E, 1990*).

Sodium:

Myocardial sodium may be elevated, while serum sodium may be reduced.

Review Article and Observational Study: In CHF the activation of the renin-angiotension-aldosterone system causes sodium retention, while the secondary hyperaldosteronism may give rise to elevated intracellular sodium through a direct permeability effect on the cell membrane. In addition, magnesium loss (which is also due to activation of the renin-angiotension-aldosterone system) leads to further retention of intracellular sodium as magnesium is necessary for the function of the Na-K pump. In 297 pts. with diuretic-treated CHF, 12% had hyponatremia and 57% had excessive muscle sodium (*Wester PO, Dyckner T. Intracellular electrolytes in cardiac failure. Acta Med Scand [Suppl] 707:33-36, 1986*).

- -

OTHER NUTRITIONAL FACTORS

Coenzyme Q$_{10}$:   100 mg daily in divided doses

WARNING: Withdrawal of supplementation should be done cautiously as clinical and hemodynamic rebound effects may occur within a few weeks.

Deficiency in myocardial tissues is common (*Kitamura N et al. Myocardial tissue level of coenzyme Q$_{10}$ in patients with cardiac failure, in K Folkers, Y Yamamura, Eds., Biomed. & Clin. Aspects of Coenzyme Q. Vol. 4. Amsterdam, Elsevier/North Holland Biomedical Press, 1984:243-252*).

Observational Study: The levels of CoQ$_{10}$ in blood and endomyocardial biopsies were found to be significantly decreased in various gps. of pts. with myocardial failure (dilated and restrictive cardiomyopathy and alcoholic heart disease). The deficiency was more pronounced with increasing symptoms (*Mortensen SA et al. Coenzyme Q$_{10}$: clinical benefits with biochemical correlates suggesting a scientific breakthrough in the management of chronic heart failure. Int J Tissue React 12(3):155-62, 1990*).

Supplementation may be beneficial.

Experimental Study: Nearly 2/3 of a gp. of 40 pts. in severe heart failure (NY Heart Assoc. Classes III & IV) showed objective and subjective improvement following treatment with CoQ$_{10}$ 100 mg daily, including 69% of pts. with cardiomyopathy and 43% of pts. with ischemic heart disease (*Mortensen SA et al. Coenzyme Q$_{10}$: clinical benefits with biochemical correlates suggesting a scientific breakthrough in the management of chronic heart failure. Int J Tissue React 12(3):155-62, 1990*).

Experimental Study: 11 pts. with moderate to severe heart failure received ubidecarenone 60 mg/d in addition to conventional treatment with digitalis and diuretics. After 8 mo., most pts. showed a significant improvement in clinical symptoms and in quality of life. Furthermore, there was a statistically significant decrease in left atrium dimensions (p<0.01), end-diastolic (p<0.01) and end-systolic (p<0.05) left ventricular diameters and a significant reduction in the distance of the septum from the e point of the mitral valve (p<0.05), an expression of significant improvement in cardiac output (*Topi PL, Davini A, Squarcini G. [Efficacy of ubidecarenone in the treatment of patients with cardiac insufficiency.] Minerva Cardioangiol 37(5):255-8, 1989*) (*in Italian*).

Experimental Double-blind Crossover Study: 19 NY Heart Assoc. class III and IV heart failure pts. received CoQ$_{10}$ 100 mg daily and placebo for 3 mo. each. While receiving CoQ$_{10}$, 18/19 pts. significantly improved according to the results of impedance cardiography; while on placebo, heart function deteriorated. There were no adverse side-effects (*Langsjoen et al. Proc Natl Acad Sci U S A. 82:4240, 1985*).

Experimental Study: 20 pts. with CHF due either to ischemic or hypertensive heart disease were treated with coenzyme Q$_{10}$ 30 mg daily for 1-2 months. 55% reported subjective improvement, 50% showed a decrease in NY Heart Assoc. functional class, and 30% showed a "remarkable" decrease in chest congestion on chest x-ray. CoQ$_{10}$ also prevented the negative inotropic effect of beta-blocker therapy without apparently reducing the beneficial effect of beta-blockers on myocardial oxygen consumption. Its positive inotropic effect was not as potent as that of digitalis (*Tsuyusaki T et al. Mechanocardiography of ischemic or hypertensive heart failure, in Y Yamamura et al, Eds. Biomed. & Clin. Aspects of Coenzyme Q. Vol. 2. Amsterdam, Elsevier/North Holland Biomedical Press, 1980:273-88*).

Double-blind Experimental Study: 100/197 pts. with coronary arteriosclerosis, hypertensive heart failure or congestive heart failure resulting from valvular disease received either CoQ$_{10}$ 30 mg daily or placebo. After 2-4 wks., CoQ$_{10}$ increased the degree of overall improvement and reduced liver enlargement and anginal symptoms. The degree of improvement for anginal symptoms was significantly higher in the CoQ$_{10}$ gp. (p<0.025) and the degree of improvement in liver enlargement was also significantly higher (p<0.05) (*Hashiba K et al. Heart 4:1579-89, 1972*) (*in Japanese*).

<u>Taurine</u>:   2 gm two-three times daily

Supplementation may be beneficial.

> **Animal Experimental Study:** Congestive heart failure was produced in rabbits with surgically-induced aortic regurgitation. Mortality after 8 wks. in the untreated gp. was 53% compared to 10% in the taurine treated group. Taurine 100 mg/kg maintained cardiac function, while cardiac function deteriorated signficantly in untreated rabbits (*Takihara K et al. Beneficial effect of taurine in rabbits with chronic congestive heart failure. <u>Am Heart J</u> 112:1278, 1986*).

> **Experimental Double-blind Crossover Study:** Taurine 6 gm daily in divided doses or placebo was given to 14 pts. in addition to conventional treatment in a randomized crossover design for 4 wks. each with a 2-wk. wash-out period in between. 11/14 (79%) improved on taurine compared to 3/14 (21%) on placebo. Compared to placebo, taurine significantly improved NY Heart Assoc. functional class, pulmonary crackles, and chest film abnormalities. While heart-failure scores failed to change significantly on placebo, their decrease was highly significant on taurine ($p < 0.001$) during which pre-injection period (corrected for heart rate) and the quotient of pre-ejection period/left ventricular ejection time decreased. No pt. worsened during taurine administration, but 4 pts. did during placebo (*Azuma J et al. Therapeutic effect of taurine in congestive heart failure: A double-blind crossover trial. <u>Clin Cardiol</u> 8:276-82, 1985; Azuma J et al. Taurine and failing heart: Experimental and clinical aspects. <u>Prog Clin Biol Res</u> 179:195-213, 1985*).

> **Experimental Double-blind Crossover Study:** Taurine 2 gm 3 times daily or placebo was given to 62 pts. in a randomized crossover design for 4 wks. each. After 4 wks. of taurine, there was a highly significant improvement in dyspnea, palpitations, crackles, edema, cardiothoracic ratio on x-ray and NY Heart Assoc. functional class. Taurine was significantly more effective than placebo ($p < 0.05$), suggesting that it is clinically beneficial (*Azuma J et al. Double-blind randomized crossover trial of taurine in congestive heart failure. <u>Curr Ther Res</u> 34(4):543-57, 1983*).

<u>Coenzyme Q$_{10}$ versus</u>
<u>Taurine</u>:

> **Experimental Double-blind Study:** 17 pts. with CHF secondary to ischemic or idiopathic dilated cardiomyopathy (ejection fraction >50%) received either taurine 3 g/d or CoQ$_{10}$ 30 mg/d. After 6 wks., a significant treatment effect was observed on systolic left ventricular function in the taurine-treated gp. but not in the CoQ$_{10}$-treated gp. (*Azuma J, Sawamura A, Awata N. Usefulness of taurine in chronic congestive heart failure and its prospective application. <u>Jpn Circ J</u> 56(1):95-9, 1992*).

CONSTIPATION

See Also: **Irritable Bowel Syndrome**

DIETARY FACTORS

High <u>fiber</u> diet.

> Example: 1/2 cup of 100% wheat bran cereal (9 gm of dietary fiber) daily with increases by 1/2 cup increments as tolerated to 2 - 3 cups daily

A bulk-forming laxative.

Bran reduces the total emptying time of the GI tract in patients with a prolonged intestinal transit time (≥48 h), but not in those with shorter transit times (*Fantus B et al. Roentgen-ray study of intestinal motility as influenced by bran.* <u>*JAMA*</u> *114:404-08, 1940*).

"Change in dietary pattern is one of the main causes of the high prevalence of constipation in the Western world. . . . In the colon fibre increases stool bulk, holds water, and also acts as a substrate for colonic microflora, further increasing stool bulk by increasing bacterial, water and salt content and producing hydrogen, methane, and other gases that augment the bulking effect. It decreases transit time, reduces intracolonic pressure, and produces a softer stool" (*Taylor R. Management of constipation: High fiber diets work.* <u>*Br Med J*</u> *300:1063-64, 1990*).

> **Review Article:** In all studies reviewed, bran increased the stool weight and decreased the transit time. Statistical evaluation showed, however, that constipated pts. had lower stool outputs and slower transits whether or not they had taken bran, and they responded less well to bran than controls, suggesting that bran can be expected to be only partially effective in restoring normal stool weight and transit time in constipated pts. (*Müller-Lissner SA. Effect of wheat bran on weight of stool and gastrointestinal transit time: A meta analysis.* <u>*Br Med J*</u> *296:615-17, 1988*).

- -

VITAMINS

<u>Folic Acid:</u>   up to 60 mg daily as needed

If deficient, supplementation may be beneficial.

> **Experimental Study:** 3 women with folate deficiency presented with chronic constipation along with restless legs, depression, tiredness, depressed ankle jerks and impaired vibratory sensation and recovered with supplementation (*Botez MI et al. Neurologic disorders responsive to folic acid therapy.* <u>*Can Med Assoc J*</u> *15:217, 1976*).

<u>Pantothenic Acid:</u>   250 mg daily

Deficiency may cause constipation (*Bean WB, Hodges RE. Pantothenic acid deficiency induced in human subjects.* <u>*Proc Soc Exp Biol Med*</u> *86:693-98, 1954; Thornton GHM et al.* <u>*J Clin Invest*</u> *34:1073, 1955*).

Supplementation may be beneficial.

> **Review Article:** Dexpanthenol, the alcohol of pantothenic acid, is readily oxidized in the cells to pantothenic acid - which stimulates peristalsis at therapeutically efective doses. Several open and 2 double-blind studies have found oral dexpanthenol to be effective in the treatment of chronic functional constipation. As its physiologic

action is in favorable contrast to that of normal laxatives, dexpanthenol can be recommended for pregnant women, children and the elderly (*Hanck AB, Goffin H. Dexpanthenol (Ro 01-4709) in the treatment of constipation. Acta Vitaminol Enzymol 4(1-2):87-97, 1982*).

Clinical Observation and Theoretical Discussion: Individuals have reported the use and indispensibility of pantothenic acid over years for the treatment of constipation. It may work by strengthening and improving the metabolism of cells and tissues involved in peristalsis (*Williams RJ. The expanding horizon in nutrition. Texas Rep Biol Med 19(2):245-58, Summer, 1961*).

Clinical Observation: Paralytic ileus was treated successfully by supplementation with pantothenic acid (*Jacques JE. Pantothenic acid in paralytic ileus. Lancet 2:861-62, 1951*).

-- --

MINERALS

Magnesium Hydroxide: 30 ml daily   (onset in 3-6 hrs.)

An osmotic laxative.

Magnesium preparations may evacuate the bowel rapidly when taken in high doses, but they result in a watery stool, considerable urgency in defecation, and occasionally incontinence (*Taylor R. Management of constipation. Br Med J 300:1063-64, 1990*). In addition, they may cause hypermagnesemia, particularly in patients with poor renal function (*Mordeo JP et al. Extreme hypermagnesemia as a cause of refractory hypertension. Ann Intern Med 83:657-58, 1975*).

Supplementation may be preferable to administration of bulk laxatives in elderly long-term hospitalized patients.

Experimental Controlled Study: 64 geriatric long-stay pts. aged 65 or older and on laxatives received either magnesium hydroxide 25 ml daily or a bulk laxative 8.7 g daily. Magnesium hydroxide caused a more frequent bowel habit (12.2 vs. 10.4/4 wks., p<0.001) than the bulk laxative and bisacodyl for an additional laxative effect was not needed as often as with the bulk laxative (2.3 vs. 3.3/4 wks., p<0.01). Also the stool consistency was more normal during the magnesium hydroxide treatment. In 2 pts. serum magnesium was >1.25 mmol/L after magnesium hydroxide treatment, but there were no clinical signs of hypermangesiuma (*Kinnunen O, Salokannel J. Constipation in elderly long-stay patients: Its treatment by magnesium hydroxide and bulk-laxative. Ann Clin Res 19(5):321-23, 1987*).

-- --

OTHER FACTORS

Rule out food sensitivities.

Clinical Observation: Food allergy can be confused with the various symptoms of acute and chronic colitis. One pt. may develop constipation while another may develop diarrhea (*Rinkel HJ et al. Food Allergy. Springfield, Illinois, Charles C. Thomas, 1951*).

Observational Study: 40 pts. with G.I. "allergy." Constipation as well as gas, bloating and pain were the most common complaints. All showed physical evidence of hypothyroidism and had lowered basal metabolic rates. X-rays most frequently showed disharmonic or spastic colon (*Gay LP. Gastrointestinal Allergy. J Missouri Med Assoc 29:7-10, 1932*).

Lactobacillus Acidophilus: (may require weeks to months for beneficial effects)

Administration may be beneficial.

Experimental Study: Successful implantation of LA was followed by symptom relief in mucous colitis, irritable colon, idiopathic ulcerative colitis, and various other disorders causing constipation (*Rettger LF et al. Lactobacillus Acidophilus. Its Therapeutic Application. New Haven, Yale U. Press, 1935*).

CROHN'S DISEASE

See Also: ULCERATIVE COLITIS

DIETARY FACTORS

GENERAL:

There is a wide range of nutritional disturbances that may be found in Crohn's patients which need to be recognized early on and treated (*Harries AD, Heatley RV. Nutritional disturbances in Crohn's disease. Postgrad Med J 50:690-7, 1983*).

> **Experimental Crossover Study:** 28 malnourished pts. spent 2 mo. on an ordinary diet followed by 2 mo. on the same diet with the addition of a low-residue liquid nutritional supplement. All anthropometric measurements, serum proteins, creatinine height index and circulating T lymphocytes increased significantly, while serum orosomucoid levels dropped significantly - suggesting that disease activity was reduced. The benefits appeared to be due to the higher calorie intake with the oral supplement (*Harries AD et al. Controlled trial of supplemented oral nutrition in Crohn's disease. Lancet 1:8330, 1983*).

High fiber, low sugar diet.

> **Experimental Study:** Subjects were placed on a 2-wk. baseline diet followed by a test diet of the same composition, but with an added 120 gm sugar. With the addition of sugar, fecal bile acid concentrations increased and the oro-anal transit time decreased. Bacterial fermentation activity also increased, which was thought to partially explain the increase in total and secondary bile acids in the feces. Since these alterations in colonic activity are associated with elevated risk for Crohn's disease, sugar may increase the disease risk (*Kruis W et al. Influence of diets high and low in refined sugar on stool qualities, gastrointestinal transit time and fecal bile acid excretion. Gastroenterology 92:1483, 1987*).

> **Negative Observational Study:** Compared to 30 pts. with ulcerative colitis, 30 pts. with irritable bowel syndrome, and 30 pts. with minor orthopedic conditions, 30 Crohn's disease pts. consumed significantly more refined sugar. When interviewed within 6 mo. of diagnosis, however, 15 Crohn's pts. consumed similar amts. of sugar as compared to members of the other 3 groups. When interviewed 7-36 mo. after diagnosis, 15 other Crohn's pts. consumed significantly more refined sugar as compared to members of the other 3 groups. Results suggest that the high sugar consumption of Crohn's pts. is a secondary phenomenon without etiologic importance (*Järnerot G et al. Consumption of refined sugar by patients with Crohn's disease, ulcerative colitis, or irritable bowel syndrome. Scand J Gastroenterol 18(8):999-1002, 1983*).

> **Experimental Controlled Study:** 80% of pts. on a low carbohydrate diet which excluded all refined sugar had symptom relief within 18 mo., while 40% of pts. on a high carbohydrate diet which was high in refined sugar had to discontinue the diet due to flare-ups (*Brandes JW, Lorenz-Meyer H. [Sugar free diet: A new perspective in the treatment of Crohn disease? Randomized, control study.] Z Gastroenterol 19(1):1-12, 1981*).

> **Observational Study:** 120 pts. with Crohn's, 100 with ulcerative colitis and matched controls were interviewed by questionnaire. Crohn's pts. ate significantly more sugar than either controls or pts. with ulcerative colitis, and their use of sugar had changed little since symptom-onset (*Mayberry JF et al. Increased sugar consumption in Crohn's disease. Digestion 20:323-6, 1980*).

> **Experimental Controlled Study:** 32 Crohn's pts. were treated with a fiber-rich unrefined carbohydrate diet in addition to conventional management and followed for a mean of 4 years and 4 months. Their course was compared retrospectively with that of 32 matched pts. who had received no dietary instruction. Hospital admissions were significantly fewer and shorter in the diet-treated pts. (111 vs. 533 days). Whereas 5 of the controls required intestinal

surgery, only 1 diet-treated pt. required it. There were no cases of intestinal obstruction among the diet-treated pts. (*Heaton KW et al. Treatment of Crohn's disease with an unrefined-carbohydrate, fibre-rich diet. Br Med J 2:764-6, 1979*).

- -

VITAMINS

Folic Acid:

Serum folate may be low due to inadequate intake and/or poor absorption (*Elsborg L, Larsen L. Folate deficiency in chronic inflammatory bowel disease. Scand J Gastroenterol 14:1019-24, 1979; Hodges P et al. Vitamin and iron intake in patients with Crohn's disease. J Am Diet Assoc 84(1):52-8, 1984*).

Reduced folate may be due to the use of sulfasalazine (*Baum CL et al. Antifolate actions of sulfasalazine on intact lymphocytes. J Lab Clin Med 97(6):779-84, 1981*).

Folate supplementation may reduce diarrhea (*Carruthers LB. Chronic diarrhea treated with folic acid. Lancet 1:849, 1946*).

Riboflavin:

Intake may be inadequate (*Hodges P et al. Vitamin and iron intake in patients with Crohn's disease. J Am Diet Assoc 84(1):52-8, 1984*).

Thiamine:

Intake may be inadequate (*Hodges P et al. Vitamin and iron intake in patients with Crohn's disease. J Am Diet Assoc 84(1):52-8, 1984*).

Vitamin A:

Intake may be inadequate (*Hodges P et al. Vitamin and iron intake in patients with Crohn's disease. J Am Diet Assoc 84(1):52-8, 1984*).

May be deficient (*Main ANH et al. Vitamin A deficiency in Crohn's disease. Gut 24(12):1169-1175, 1983; Schoelmerich J et al. Zinc and vitamin A deficiency in patients with Crohn's disease is correlated with activity but not with localization or extent of the disease. Hepatogastroenterol 32(1):34-8, 1985*).

Supplementation has failed to be beneficial in long-term controlled trials.

> **Experimental Double-blind Study:** 86 pts. in remission failed to benefit from 50,000 IU twice daily (*Wright JP et al. Gastroenterology 88(2):512-14, 1985*).

Vitamin B6:

Intake may be inadequate (*Hodges P et al. Vitamin and iron intake in patients with Crohn's disease. J Am Diet Assoc 84(1):52-8, 1984*).

Vitamin B12:

Blood levels may be reduced (*Elsborg L. Vitamin B12 and folic acid in Crohn's disease. Dan Med Bull 29(7):362-5, 1982*).

Vitamin C:

Blood levels may be reduced (*Gerson CD, Fabry EM. Ascorbic acid deficiency and fistula formation in regional enteritis. Gastroenterology 67:428, 1974; Hughes RG, Williams N. Leukocyte ascorbic acid in Crohn's disease. Digestion 17:272, 1978*).

Localized deficiency may be associated with fistula formation.

Observational Study: 26 pts. without fistula formation had 47% more ascorbate concentrated at diseased when compared to undiseased intestine, while 26 pts. with fistulas had only 23% more ascorbate at diseased sites, suggesting that an inability to concentrate ascorbate may be related to fistula formation (*Pettit SH, Irving MH. Does local intestinal ascorbate deficiency predispose to fistula formation in Crohn's disease? Dis Colon Rectum 30(7):552-57, 1987*).

Vitamin D:

May be deficient.

Observational Study: Mild deficiency was common and severe deficiency (25-OHD levels less than 8 nmol/l) was encountered. Deficiency was more common in pts. with active vs. inactive disease. Plasma 25-OHD levels were significantly correlated with hemoglobin and ESR. Evidence of secondary hyperparathyroidism and osteomalacia was noted (*Dibble JB et al. A survey of vitamin D deficiency in gastrointestinal and liver disorders. Quart J Med 53:119-34, 1984*).

Vitamin K:

May be deficient, especially when the disease occurs in the terminal ileum.

Observational Study: 18/58 (31%) pts. with chronic GI disorders were found to have evidence of vitamin K deficiency; all pts. with deficiency had either Crohn's of the terminal ileum or ulcerative colitis treated with sulfasalazine or antibiotics (*Krasinski SD et al. The prevalence of vitamin K deficiency in chronic gastrointestinal disorders. Am J Clin Nutr 41(3):639-43, 1985*).

If deficient, supplementation may be beneficial.

Experimental Study: 18 pts. with either Crohn's of the terminal ileum or ulcerative colitis treated with sulfasalazine or antibiotics who were found to have vitamin K deficiency were supplemented with vitamin K. Abnormal prothrombin levels returned toward normal (*Krasinski SD et al. The prevalence of vitamin K deficiency in chronic gastrointestinal disorders. Am J Clin Nutr 41(3):639-43, 1985*).

- -

MINERALS

Calcium:

May be deficient due to loss of absorptive surfaces, steatorrhea, corticosteroid treatment, and vitamin D deficiency (*Rosenberg IH et al. Nutritional aspects of inflammatory bowel disease. Annu Rev Nutr 5:463-84, 1985*).

Iron:

Intake may be inadequate in women (*Hodges P et al. Vitamin and iron intake in patients with Crohn's disease. J Am Diet Assoc 84(1):52-8, 1984*).

May be deficient due to chronic blood loss through the gut (*Rosenberg IH et al. Nutritional aspects of inflammatory bowel disease. Annu Rev Nutr 5:463-84, 1985*).

Magnesium:

While serum levels are rarely decreased, intracellular levels are frequently low and may be associated with weakness, anorexia, hypotension, confusion, hyperirritability, tetany, convulsions, and EKG or EEG abnormalities (*Rosenberg IH et al. Nutritional aspects of inflammatory bowel disease. Annu Rev Nutr 5:463-84, 1985*).

Review Article: Magnesium deficiency is a frequent complication of inflammatory bowel disease which occurs in 13-88% of patients due primarily to decreased intake, malabsorption and increased intestinal losses. Parenteral magnesium requirements are at least 120 mg daily, and oral requirements may be as great as 700 mg daily (*Galland L. magnesium and inflammatory bowel disease. Magnesium 7(2):78-83, 1988*).

Selenium:

Blood levels may be low (*Penny WJ et al. Relationship between trace elements, sugar consumption, and taste in Crohn's disease. Gut 24(4):288-92, 1983*).

Zinc:

May be deficient.

Review Article: The prevalence of zinc deficiency ranges from 35-45% in stable outpatients with inflammatory bowel disease. Depressed serum zinc levels correlate with the degree of hypoalbuminemia and may be depressed in response to acute inflammation. Measurement of immune function, zinc-dependent proteins or enzymes and their response to a zinc supplement can help confirm zinc deficiency in borderline cases. Underlying mechanisms postulated as causing the deficiency include impaired intestinal absorption, increased endogenous losses, or low dietary intake due to anorexia (*Hendricks KM, Walker WA. Zinc deficiency in inflammatory bowel disease. Nutr Rev 46(12):401-08, 1988*).

If deficient, supplementation may reverse the signs and symptoms of zinc deficiency.

Review Article: Case reports of severe zinc deficiency in inflammatory bowel disease have shown pts. to be rapidly responsive to oral supplements of 210-750 mg zinc sulfate per day. Little information exists, however, on which to make recommendations for mild to moderate zinc deficiency (*Hendricks KM, Walker WA. Zinc deficiency in inflammatory bowel disease. Nutr Rev 46(12):401-08, 1988*).

- -

OTHER FACTORS

Rule out food sensitivities.

A. Specific food sensitivities:

Observational Study: 7/11 pts. showed skin test reactivity to milk, wheat and soy protein. Five of these had allergic symptoms and 4 had complaints of food allergy or cellular lymphocyte sensitivity to various food proteins reflected in an elevated Stimulation Index. 6 pts. demonstrated elevated sIgG4 to several food proteins despite negative sIgE reactions. The antigen most frequently associated with elevated sIgG4 levels was egg protein and the highest sIgG4 levels of egg and milk protein occurred in skin test negative patients (*Frieri M et al. Preliminary investigation on humoral and cellular immune responses to selected food proteins in patients with Crohn's disease. Ann Allergy 64:345-51, 1990*).

Observational Study: In a study of 71 pts., those without an ileostomy most consistently had exacerbations from nuts, raw fruit and tomatoes. Those with an ileostomy most consistently had exacerbations from nuts, raw fruit, corn, carbonated drinks, shellfish and pickles (*McDonald PJ, Fazio VW. What can Crohn's patients eat. Euro J Clin Nutr 42:703-08, 1988*).

Review Article: "No simple relationship between eating particular foods and disease activity . . . has emerged. . . . Patients with inflammatory bowel disease have enhanced immune responses against food antigens, but also against other antigens in the gut, particularly bacteria and bacterial products. . . . Expression of these immune responses may contribute to inflammation, and dietary alterations can induce remission. It seems just as likely that changes in faecal consistency and bacterial content are responsible for improvement, as that the withdrawal of a specific food antigen is responsible. Finally, however, there are striking geographical variations. . . . Epidemiological studies have shown that increasing westernisation leads to a higher incidence. . . . These emerging trends, as people of different races take up similar life-styles, point convincingly to environmental causes. While 'food allergy' remains the language of the enthusiast, a 'major influence of the constituents of the diet' seems likely to be an aetiological factor of greater significance" (*Hodgson HJF. Inflammatory bowel disease and food intolerance. J R Coll Physicians London 20(1):45-48, 1986*).

Observational Study: Compared to 100 controls, total serum IgE was not significantly different for 50 pts. matched for sex and age. However, in regard to RAST results with 10 selected foods, the percentage of positive reactions to specific IgE was significantly higher in Crohn's patients. In Crohn's disease with colic or ileocolic involvement, the percentage of pts. with a positive response to RAST was significantly greater than in Crohn's disease with ileal involvement. Results suggest a greater absorption of antigens through the diseased wall (*Brignola C et al. Dietary allergy evaluated by PRIST and RAST in inflammatory bowel disease. Hepatogastroenterology 33(3):128-30, 1986*).

Observational Study: Pts. with inflammatory bowel disease had significantly elevated serum levels of both IgG and IgM but normal levels of IgA. Serum IgE concentration, as well as the prevalence of pts. with "high IgE" were significantly increased. Among pts. with inflammatory bowel disease, those with Crohn's disease or those in relapse had the highest IgE levels (*Levo Y et al. Serum IgE levels in patients with inflammatory bowel disease. Ann Allergy 56(1):85-87, 1986*).

Observational Study: Lactose intolerance was found in 25-35% of pts. with inflammatory bowel disease compared to 5-10% of the normal population, suggesting that a low lactose diet may be beneficial (*Meryn S. [Role of nutrition in acute and long-term therapy of chronic inflammatory bowel diseases.] Wien Klin Wochenschr 98(22):774-79, 1986*).

Experimental Controlled Study: 20 pts. with active disease received either an unrefined carbohydrate fibre-rich diet or a diet which excluded specific foods to which a pt. was intolerant (as determined by a prior water fast followed by single food provocations). 7/10 pts. on the exclusion diet remained in remission for 6 mo. compared with 0/10 on the unrefined CH diet. In an uncontrolled study, an exclusion diet allowed 51/77 pts. to remain well on the diet alone for periods of up to 51 months, and with an annual relapse rate of <10% (*Jones VA et al. Crohn's disease: Maintenance of remission by diet. Lancet 2:177-80, 1985*).

B. Elemental (protein-free) and polymeric (protein-containing) liquid diets.

Experimental Study: 96/113 pts. with acute CD treated with an elemental diet between 1977 and 1988 went into remission. This remission rate was comparable to that achieved with steroids (*Teahon K et al. Ten years' experience with an elemental diet in the management of Crohn's disease. Gut 31:1133-7, 1990*).

Experimental Controlled Study: 30 pts. with active CD who would otherwise have been treated with steroids randomly received either an elemental diet (Vivonex) or a polymeric (protein-containing) diet (Fortison). Assessment after 10 and 28 days showed that clinical remission occurred in 12/16 (75%) pts. on the elemental diet compared with 5/14 (36%) pts. on the polymeric diet (p<0.03). Dietary treatment resulted in little change in the nutritional state or in various laboratory indices of activity over a 4-wk. period (*Giaffer MH et al. Controlled trial of polymeric versus elemental diet in treatment of active Crohn's disease. Lancet 1:816-19, 1990*).

Experimental Double-blind Study: 14 pts. with active CD received either an elemental or a polymeric diet via nasogastric tube. After 28 days, the clinical remission rate was significantly better for the polymeric than for the elemental group. However, long-term remission rates were disappointing for both gps. as only 2 pts., both in the polymeric gp., were well after 1 year (*Park RHR et al. Double blind trial comparing elemental and polymeric diet as primary therapy for active Crohn's disease. Gut 30:A1453-54, 1988*).

Experimental Controlled Study: 15 children with active CD of the small intestine randomly received either an elemental diet (Flexical) or IM ACTH followed by oral prednisolone with sulphasalazine. The elemental diet was equally effective in inducing an improvement in the Lloyd-Still disease activity index, erythrocyte sedimentation rate, C-reactive protein and albumin concentrations, and body weight as the high-dose steroid regimen. Linear growth, as assessed from height velocity over 6 mo., was significantly greater in the children receiving an elemental diet (*Sanderson IR et al. Remission induced by an elemental diet in small bowel Crohn's disease. Arch Dis Child 62(2):123-27, 1987*).

DERMATITIS HERPETIFORMIS

See Also: CELIAC DISEASE

MINERALS

Selenium:

Selenium-containing glutathione peroxidase may be reduced (*Juhlin L et al. Blood glutathione-peroxidase levels in skin diseases: Effect of selenium and vitamin E treatment. Acta Dermatovener (Stockholm) 62:211-14, 1982*).

Zinc:

Epidermal zinc levels may be reduced (*Michäelsson G, Ljunghall K. Patients with dermatitis herpetiformis, acne, psoriasis and Darier's disease have low epidermal zinc concentrations. Acta Derm Venereol (Stockh) 70(4):304-8, 1990*).

- -

OTHER NUTRITIONAL FACTORS

Para Amino Benzoic Acid: 200 mg. four to five times daily

Supplementation may be beneficial.

> **Experimental Study:** PABA was a successful treatment, even in pts. who were not controlling their intake of gluten (*Zarafonetis CJD et al. Paraaminobenzoic acid in dermatitis herpetiformis. Arch Dermatol Syphilol 63:115-132, 1951*).

- -

OTHER FACTORS

Rule out food sensitivities.

> **Gluten:**
>
> **Observational Study:** There was no correlation between dietary gluten intake and the degree of enteropathy in 51 pts. on a normal diet; however biopsy specimens were normal in 24/31 pts. on a gluten-free diet, all previously having been abnormal. 18 pts. on gluten-containing diets had normal jejunal histology and in 7 of these pts. all tests of small intestinal morphology and function were entirely normal. Intestinal permeability was abnormal and serum antigliadin antibodies were present in most pts. with enteropathy. Studies of acid secretion in 7 pts. showed that hypochlorhydria or achlorhydria did not lead to abnormal permeability in the absence of enteropathy. Results show that objective tests will detect abnormalities in most pts., including some with histologically normal jejunal biopsy specimens, although there is a small gp. in whom all conventional intestinal investigations are entirely normal (*Gwakrodger DJ et al. Small intestinal function and dietary status in dermatitis herpetiformis. Gut 32(4):377-82, 1991*).
>
> **Review Article:** A gluten-free diet is the therapy of choice. IgG, IgA and IgM antibodies against gliadin (the principal protein in gluten-containing grains) have been identified in DH pts., along with elevated serum gluten levels (*Int Clin Nutr Rev 4(2):100, 1984*).

Observational Study: In a study of 45 pts., morphological changes in the mucosa of the small intestine were associated with higher intakes of gluten, although gastric morphologic and functional changes also characteristic of DH (e.g. achlorhydric atrophic gastritis) did not appear to be associated with gluten intake (*Andersson H et al. Influence of the amount of dietary gluten on gastrointestinal morphology and function in dermatitis herpetiformis. Hum Nutr Clin Nutr 38C:279-85, 1984*).

Experimental Study: 12 pts. whose skin rashes had been effectively controlled for an ave. of over 7 yrs. without medication on a gluten-free diet were challenged with gluten. After an ave. of 12 wks., the rash returned in 11/12, suggesting that a life-long gluten-free diet is required (*Leonard J et al. Gluten challenge in dermatitis herpetiformis. N Engl J Med 308:816, 1983*).

Milk:

Observational Study: Using an ELISA assay, a significantly increased prevalence (p<0.001) of serum IgG antibodies reactive with wheat gliadin, bovine milk or ovalbumin was found in 75% (33/44) adult pts. compared to normals. IgA anti-milk antibodies were detected in pts. irrespective of whether they were on a gluten-free diet (*Barnes RM, Lewis-Jones MS. Isotype distribution and serial levels of antibodies reactive with dietary protein antigens in dermatitis herpetiformis. J Clin Lab Immunol 30(2):87-91, 1989*).

Case Report: 74 year-old man with characteristic lesions, upper abdominal pain and loose stools for 10 yrs. was treated with a milk-free diet which improved his dermatitis in less than a week but only slightly lessened his dyspepsia. Both the dermatitis and the dyspepsia were completely controlled with a gluten and milk-free diet, while reintroduction of milk and milk proteins caused recurrence of the dermatitis. After 4 mo. of a gluten-free diet, reintroduction of gluten no longer provoked recurrence of the dermatitis (*Engquist A, Pock-Steen OC. Dermatitis herpetiformis and milk-free diet. Lancet 2:438, 1971*).

Case Report: Pt. improved on a gluten and milk-free diet, although only milk provocation resulted in recurrence of the dermatitis (*Pock-Steen OC, Niordson AM. Milk sensitivity in dermatitis herpetiformis. Br J Dermatol 83:614-19, 1970*).

Rule out hydrochloric acid deficiency.

Note: While gastric anacidity had been reported in the past to be a relatively common condition which was associated with various dermatologic disorders and a number of other illnesses, the presence of achlorhydria is no longer accepted unless a potent parietal-cell stimulant (such as histamine) is employed in gastric analysis. More recent studies suggest that histamine-fast anacidity is uncommon before the fifth decade of life and, although it probably does not occur in a normal stomach, its presence is not necessarily associated with symptoms (Rappaport EM. Achlorhydria: Associated symptoms and response to hydrochloric acid. N Engl J Med 252(19):802-5, 1955).

Observational Study: 4 pts. underwent a fractional gastric analysis following a routine Ewald test meal. Hypoacidity was defined as values for total and free acids of 1/2 normal or less, while hyperacidity was defined as values 10-15 points above normal or values which were relatively high at the start of the test. 3/4 (75%) of the pts. were found to have hypoacidity, while 1/4 (25%) had hyperacidity. For 1 pt., the severity of the eruption correlated with both the presence of GI symptoms and abnormal gastric secretions while, for 2 pts., the severity of the eruption correlated with abnormal gastric secretions but there were no GI complaints (*Ayres S. Gastric secretion in psoriasis, eczema and dermatitis herpetiformis. Arch Dermatol Syphilol 20:854-57, 1929*).

DIABETES MELLITUS

See Also: ATHEROSCLEROSIS
CATARACTS
NEURALGIA and NEUROPATHY
ULCERS (SKIN)

OVERVIEW

1. To improve glucose tolerance.

Many studies have shown that high fiber, high complex carbohydrate diets are beneficial. A diet high in fat is deleterious, and saturated fats should be replaced by mono- and polyunsaturates. While sugar seems to have an adverse effect, recent studies comparing the glycemic response to both simple and complex carbohydrates have suggested that each food which is rich in carbohydrates needs to be separately evaluated.

In regard to specific nutrients, the evidence for manipulating them is considerably weaker. Increasing the intake of organic chromium either separately or by supplementing with high-chromium brewer's yeast is best documented. A marginal vitamin C deficiency is common and appears to contribute to disordered glycoregulation. Limited controlled studies also suggest that biotin and pyridoxine alpha-ketoglutarate may be beneficial. Many other nutrients have been found to be relevant, but the evidence for supplementation is generally weak.

Deficiencies of several minerals have been shown to have an adverse effect. A magnesium deficiency is the most common disturbance in mineral metabolism found in insulin-dependent (type II) diabetes. Deficiencies of chromium, copper, manganese and zinc are associated with glucose intolerance, while deficiencies of phosphorus and potassium are associated with insulin resistance.

2. To reduce diabetic complications.

a. Neuropathy

Supplementation with several members of the vitamin B complex has been reported to be beneficial. Vitamin B$_6$ is lower in patients with neuropathy and, in an open study, patients with both neuropathy and a B$_6$ deficiency improved following supplementation. Similarly, there appears to be a relationship between vitamin B$_{12}$ nutriture and neuropathy. In open studies, inositol supplementation was associated with improved sensory nerve function and evoked nerve action potential amplitudes (although a double-blind study failed to confirm these findings), and biotin supplementation has also been associated with objective improvement. The administration of evening primrose oil, a rich source of gamma-linolenic acid, has been shown under double-blind conditions to be beneficial.

b. Nephropathy

The development of nephropathy was retarded in diabetic rats when they were supplemented with nicotinamide, but evidence is lacking that human diabetics would also benefit.

c. Retinopathy

Magnesium is particularly low in diabetics with proliferative retinopathy, but it is not known if supplementation would be beneficial.

d. Microangiopathy

A marginal <u>vitamin C</u> deficiency may foster the development of microangiopathy as may deficiencies of <u>magnesium</u> and <u>phosphorus</u>. Diabetics appear have an increased requirement for <u>Vitamin E</u>, and supplementation may be preventative.

- -

> *KEY: A = may affect microangiopathy*
> *G = may affect glucose tolerance*
> *K = may affect nephropathy*
> *M = may affect mortality*
> *N = may affect neuropathy*
> *R = may affect retinopathy*

- -

DIETARY FACTORS

Avoid <u>obesity</u>.
(G)

> *Obesity is defined as a body weight 20-30% above the ideal.*

The exaggerated serum insulin levels observed after administration of glucose to maturity-onset diabetic patients correlate with the degree of obesity and do not differ quantitatively from the hyperresponse of insulin to glucose in obesity (*Karam JH et al. The relationship of obesity and growth hormone to serum insulin levels. Ann N Y Acad Sci 131(1):374-87, 1965; Karam JH et al. Excessive insulin response to glucose in obese subjects as measured by immunochemical assay. Diabetes 12(3):197-204, 1963*).

> **Review Article:** In the overweight pt., calorie restriction can improve tissue sensitivity to insulin (*DeFronzo RA, Ferrannini E. Insulin resistance. A multifaceted syndrome responsible for NIDDM, obesity, hypertension, dyslipidemia, and atherosclerotic cardiovascular disease. Diabetes Care 14(3):173-94, 1991*).

> **NIH Consensus Development Conference:** The risk of non-insulin-dependent (type II) diabetes accelerates with increased body weight and both the duration of obesity and specific distribution of excess body fat, with a higher risk associated with excess upper body fat ("beer bellies") than to excess fat in the hips and thighs. Nearly 80% of the 10 million Americans with type II diabetes were obese at disease onset. However, although type II diabetes is rare among thin people, the theory that weight control can prevent development of the disease is unproven (*National Institutes of Health Consensus Development Conference [USA], December 8-10, 1986*).

<u>Low fat</u> diet.   (<30% of calories)
(G,M)

A high fat diet causes glucose intolerance and insulin resistance due to tissue-specific alterations in transmembrane signaling (*Nagy K et al. High-fat feeding induces tissue-specific alteration in proportion of activated insulin receptors in rats. Acta Endocrinol (Coph) 122(3):361-68, 1990; Watarai T et al. Alteration of insulin-receptor kinase activity by high-fat feeding. Diabetes 37(10):1397-404, 1988*).

A high fat diet is more atherogenic for diabetics than it is for normals.

> **Review Article (M):** In 1927, Joslin wrote: "With an excess of fat diabetes begins and from an excess of fat diabetics die, formerly of coma, recently of arteriosclerosis." Atherosclerosis is the most common complication of diabetes. Currently, with prospective intervention trials in diabetics still lacking, the physician must rely on the reasonable assumption that the atherogenic effect of lipoproteins in the diabetic is the same as, but more pronounced than, that in the nondiabetic. There is strong evidence from primary prevention studies in nondiabetics that reduction in LDL level and elevation in HDL level each reduces the risk of coronary artery disease, and a secondary intervention study showed a similar benefit with the reduction of plasma triglyceride concentrations. It is essential that physicians pay attention to the control of plasma lipid disorders in their diabetic pts. (*Steiner G. Editorial: From an excess of fat, diabetics die. JAMA 262(3):398-99, 1989*).

Replace saturated fats with mono- and polyunsaturates.
(G)

> May reduce serum glucose levels (*Trevisan M et al. Consumption of olive oil, butter, and vegetable oils and coronary heart disease risk factors. JAMA 263:688-92, 1990*).

> Replacing saturated fat with poly- and monounsaturates may be preferable to replacing it with complex carbohydrates as this substitution avoids inducing the deleterious effects on carbohydrate and lipoprotein metabolism caused by a low-fat, complex carbohydrate diet (*Garg A et al. Comparison of a high-carbohydrate diet with a high-monounsaturated-fat diet in patients with non-insulin-dependent diabetes mellitus. N Engl J Med 319(13):829-34, 1988; Reaven GM. Dietary therapy for non-insulin-dependent diabetes mellitus. Editorial. N Engl J Med 319(13):862-64, 1988*).

High complex carbohydrate diet.   (55-60% of calories with 12-20% of calories as protein)
(G)

> WARNING: A low-fat, complex carbohydrate diet may increase plasma VLDL triglyceride, lower HDL cholesterol and cause deterioration in glycemic control in patients with non-insulin-dependent DM in some studies; thus its routine acceptance must be questioned (*Reaven GM. Dietary therapy for non-insulin-dependent diabetes mellitus. Editorial. N Engl J Med 319(13):862-64, 1988*).

> > **Experimental Crossover Study (G):** 3 women and 5 men with type II diabetes (mean age 66) received either 40% or 60% of total calories in carbohydrates while fat intake in both diets varied from 20-40% of total calories. After completion of 2 diet periods of 6-wks. each, evidence indicated that glycemic control deteriorated during the high-carbohydrate diet: Plasma glucose concentrations were significantly higher throughout the day and both insulin response and 24h urinary glucose excretion were significantly greater as were total and very-low-density-lipoprotein (VLDL) triglyceride concentrations. Although total plasma cholesterol was similar, plasma VLDL cholesterol concentration increased and plasma low-density-lipoprotein cholesterol concentrations decreased on the 60% carbohydrate diet (*Coulston AM. Persistence of hypertriglyceridemic effect of low-fat high-carbohydrate diets in NIDDM patients. Diabetes Care 12:94-101, 1989*).

> **Review Article:** On the basis of clinical investigations, the American, British and Canadian Diabetes Associations currently recommend that diabetics use generous amts. of complex carbohydrate and fiber and restrict their use of saturated fat and cholesterol. For example, the American Diabetes Association now recommends a diet providing about 55-60% of calories as carbohydrate (*Anderson JW. Recent advances in carbohydrate nutrition and metabolism in diabetes mellitus. J Am Coll Nutr 8(Suppl):61S-67S, 1989*).

> **Review Article (G):** The rate of the small intestine amylolytic digestion appears to be a major determinant of the glycemic response. Studies of diabetes using high fiber, high legume diets have almost uniformly noted improvements in glycemic control and blood lipid profile; similar improvements have also been noted when foods were selected on the basis of their slow rates of digestion and flatter glycemic response despite relatively small changes in fiber content. Reasons for altered rates of digestion include fiber, food form, the nature of the starch, antinutrients, etc. Through reducing the rate of digestion of starchy food post prandially, "slow release" starchy foods blunt many gut hormone responses, and prolong free fatty acid and ketone body suppression. Also, increased starch losses to the colon may enhance small chain fatty acid production. All these events may modify carbohydrate and lipid metabolism (*Jenkins DJ et al. Starchy foods and fiber: Reduced rate of digestion and improved carbohydrate metabolism. Scand J Gastroenterol Suppl 129:132-41, 1987*).

High soluble fiber diet.   (up to 40 g/d or 15-25 g/1,000 kcal)
(G)

> Soluble or viscous fibers are found in legumes (guar gum), fruit (pectins), cereals (such as oats) and green vegetables (such as okra).

> > WARNING: High fiber diets may worsen diabetic control in non-insulin-dependent patients who are poorly controlled with oral hypoglycemic agents and who may require the addition of insulin 4 times daily to achieve maximum improvements in diabetic control (*Scott AR et al. Comparison of high fibre diets, basal insulin supplements, and flexible insulin treatment for non-insulin dependent (type II) diabetics poorly controlled with sulphonylureas. Br Med J 297:707-10, 1988*).

Improves glucose tolerance by slowing gastric emptying and intestinal absorption of glucose due to its physical viscosity (*Meyer JH et al. Intragastric vs intraintestinal viscous polymers and glucose tolerance after liquid meals of glucose. Am J Clin Nutr 48:260-66, 1988*).

Review Article (G): "The benefits from high fibre intake are not massive but may improve diabetic control that is otherwise only fairly good. . . . The advantages of eating natural fibre reside in the simultaneous avoidance of possibly injurious diet - for example, saturated fats or quickly digested carbohydrates in excess - and the fact that, almost inevitably, such fibre will be eaten with slow release carbohydrate" (*Hockaday TDR. Fibre in the management of diabetes: Natural fibre useful as part of total dietary prescription. Br Med J 300:1334-36, 1990*).

NIH Consensus Development Conference (G): The benefit of high fiber intake is controversial. Though some studies have suggested that fiber helps to control blood glucose levels and to reduce plasma cholesterol concentrations, fiber-rich diets are often "unpalatable" and may be contraindicated in pts. with autonomic neuropathy (*National Institutes of Health Consensus Development Conference [USA], December 8-10, 1986*).

Observational Study (G): Diabetes is rare in African villagers who eat large amts. of fiber but is common in Western countries where people eat fiber-depleted diets (*Trowell HC. Dietary-fiber hypothesis of the etiology of diabetes mellitus. Diabetes 24(8):762-65, 1975*).

Specific Fibers

Cereal Fibers:

   Experimental Controlled Study (G): Gps. of 6 drawn from a pool of 16 diabetics received test meals containing varying ratios of whole cereal grains (barley or cracked wheat) to milled flour. There was a significant trend to a lower glycemic index with increasing proportion of whole cereal grains in the test bread (p<0.05) and with lower *in vitro* digestibility (p<0.001), suggesting that breads containing a high proportion of whole cereal grains may reduce the postprandial blood glucose profile in diabetics as they are more slowly digested (*Jenkins DJA et al. Wholemeal versus wholegrain breads: Proportion of whole or cracked grain and the glycaemic response. Br Med J 297:958-63, 1988*).

Glucomannan:

   Experimental Double-blind Study (G): 27 white pts. (17 on insulin; 10 on oral medication) were placed on a high-fiber, high carbohydrate, low fat diet; in addition they randomly received either 4.2 gm konjac-glucomannan (Mannan Life Dietary Fibre®, Tsuruta Shokuhin Co., Japan) or placebo. After 12 wks., the gel fiber had significant beneficial effects on glycemic control, insulin requirement and HDL cholesterol levels in the insulin-treated subjects while, in all subjects, increased intakes of dietary fiber were associated with significant decreases in total serum protein and increases in serum albumin. Results suggest that supplementation of the recommended diabetic diet with glucomannan may be beneficial to insulin-dependent diabetics (*Vorster HH et al. Benefits from supplementation of the current recommended diabetic diet with gel fibre. Int Clin Nutr Rev 8(3):140-46, 1988*).

Guar Gum:

Soluble gums are the most effective fibers in reducing glucose levels (*Hallfrisch J. Dietary sugars and carbohydrate metabolism in type II diabetes. J Am Coll Nutr 6(5):385-96, 1987*).

   Experimental Double-blind Study (G): Type II diabetic pts. received either guar granules or wheat bran (placebo) in 5 gm sachets to sprinkle on food with a 2-wk. separation between trial and placebo periods. After 4 wks., mean fasting plasma glucose concentration and glycosylated hemoglobin were significantly lower after guar than after placebo and total plasma cholesterol decreased due to decreased LDL cholesterol. Postprandial insulin was reduced as was enteroglucagon concentration. In addition, when guar was eaten with a standardized test meal, there was a 50% reduction in the incremental area under the postprandial glycemic curve. Side effects were increased stool frequency and looseness during the first week (*Fuessel HS et al. Guar sprinkled on food: Effect on glycaemic control, plasma lipids and gut hormones in non-insulin dependent diabetic patients. Diabetic Med 4(5):463-68, 1987*).

Leguminous Fiber:

Observational Study (G): The association between the intake of carbohydrates, body mass index (BMI), and the 4-y incidence of impaired glucose tolerance and diabetes mellitus was investigated in 175 elderly men and women aged 64-87 who were normoglycemic at baseline. The habitual intake of legumes was inversely related to the incidence of glucose intolerance (*Feskens EJM, Bowles CH, Kromhout D. Carbohydrate intake and body mass index in relation to the risk of glucose intolerance in an elderly population. Am J Clin Nutr 54:136-40, 1991*).

Experimental Crossover Study (G): 18 non-insulin-dependent and 9 insulin-dependent diabetics were put on a high carbohydrate diet containing leguminous fiber (HL) for 6 wks. and a standard low carbohydrate diet (LC) for 6 wks. in random order. Preprandial and mean 2 hr. postprandial blood glucoses were significantly lower on the HL diet in both gps., as were several measures of diabetic control. In addition, total cholesterol was significantly reduced in both gps. and the HDL/LDL cholesterol ratio increased significantly in the NIDDM gp., suggesting that use of a LC diet is no longer justified (*Simpson HCR et al. A high-carbohydrate leguminous fiber diet improves all aspects of diabetic control. Lancet 1:1-5, 1981*).

Oat Gum:

Experimental Controlled Study (G): 9 healthy, fasting subjects consumed 50 mg glucose in a drink, 50 g glucose with 14.5 g of specifically prepared oat gum, and 50 g glucose with 14.5 mg guar gum. Each test meal was scheduled at least 3 days apart. Plasma glucose and insulin increases after the glucose drink were greater than after both gum meals between 20 and 60 min ($p<0.01$). The responses to the two gum meals were nearly identical (*Braaten JT et al. Oat gum lowers glucose and insulin after an oral glucose load. Am J Clin Nutr 53:1425-30, 1991*).

Pea Fiber:

Experimental Controlled Study (G): 8 healthy subjects received 4 different meals. The control meal consisted of boiled ground beef mixed with glucose and lactulose. To this was added either wheat bran, sugar beet fiber or pea fiber in randomized order at least 3 days apart. Only the addition of pea fiber (15 g pure fiber) significantly reduced the area under the incremental blood glucose curve ($p<0.05$). None of the fibers significantly affected the area under the insulin-response curve, although all of them reduced it. Mouth-to-cecum transit time was not decreased by pea fiber, but was decreased by the other 2 fibers ($p<0.05$) (*Hamberg O et al. Blood glucose response to pea fiber: Comparisons with sugar beet fiber and wheat bran. Am J Clin Nutr 50:324-28, 1989*).

Pectin:

Experimental Study (G): Insulin-dependent diabetics were given a milk shake of skim milk, vanilla and 7 gms of apple pectin (equivalent to 2 apples) 10 min. before a meal of meat, rice, cheese and bread. Following the meal 35% less insulin was required to return blood sugar levels to baseline (*Poynard T et al. Reduction of post-prandial insulin needs by pectin as assessed by the artificial pancreas in insulin-dependent diabetics. Diabete Metab 8(3):187-89, 1982*).

Psyllium:

Experimental Placebo-controlled Crossover Study (G): 18 non-insulin-dependent pts. randomly received psyllium (two 3.4 g packets, each mixed in water) and placebo in either order immediately before both breakfast and dinner. For meals eaten immediately after psyllium ingestion, maximum postprandial glucose elevation was reduced by 14% at breakfast and 20% at dinner relative to placebo. Postprandial serum insulin concentrations after breakfast were reduced by 12%. Second-meal effects after lunch showed a 31% reduction in postprandial glucose elevation (*Pastors JG et al. Psyllium fiber reduces rise in postprandial glucose and insulin concentrations in patients with non-insulin-dependent diabetes. Am J Clin Nutr 53:1431-5, 1991*).

<u>Vegetarian</u> diet.
(G,M)

Diabetes mellitus is positively associated with the level of animal fat consumption (*West KM, Kalbfleisch JM. Influence of nutritional factors on prevalence of diabetes. <u>Diabetes</u> 20:99-108, 1971*), and is more common in beef eating populations than in vegetarian populations (*Snowdon DA, Phillips RL. Does a vegetarian diet reduce the occurrence of diabetes? <u>Am J Public Health</u> 75:507-12, 1985; West KM. <u>Epidemiology of Diabetes and Its Vascular Lesions</u>. New York, Elsevier North-Holland, 1978*).

Associated with reduced risk of death from diabetes.

> **Observational Study (G):** During 21 yrs. of follow-up, the risk of diabetes as an underlying cause of death among 25,600 caucasian Seventh-day Adventists was 1/2 of the risk for all American caucasians. Within this population, the male vegetarians (those who consumed fish rarely and meat/poultry less than once weekly) had a substantially lower risk than non-vegetarians of diabetes as an underlying or contributing cause of death. The prevalence of reported diabetes was lower for both vegetarian males and females compared to non-vegetarians. These associations were not due to differences in weight, other dietary factors or physical activity and were stronger in males than in females (*Snowdon DA, Phillips RL. Does a vegetarian diet reduce the occurrence of diabetes? <u>Am J Public Health</u> 75(5):507-12, 1985*).

Eat <u>whole-food snacks</u> instead of sugary, manufactured snacks ("junk foods").
(G)

> **Experimental Study (G):** 10 healthy subjects consumed 4 different snack meals, similar in fat and total energy content. Two snacks were based on sugary, manufactured products (chocolate-coated candy bar; cola drink with potato chips) and two on whole foods (raisins and peanuts; bananas and peanuts). After the processed food snacks, plasma glucose levels tended to rise higher and to fall lower than after the whole-food snacks. One subject had pathologic insulinemia after both manufactured snacks but normal responses after both whole-food snacks (*Oettle GJ et al. Glucose and insulin responses to manufactured and whole-food snacks. <u>Am J Clin Nutr</u> 45:86-91, 1987*).

Restrict <u>sucrose</u>:
(G,K,R)

Intake may be related to the risk of diabetes.

> **Observational Study:** Yemenites who have lived in Israel for over 25 yrs. have a significantly greater prevalence of diabetes mellitus. While no sugar was eaten in Yemen, about 20% of carbohydrates ingested by Yemenites in Israel is in the form of sucrose. Fat consumption in Yemen was mainly of animal origin and its quantity was much the same as the total of animal fat and margarine consumed by Jews living in Israel, although Yemenites in Israel also consume about 16 g of soya, olive, and sesame oil. There is no significant difference in the amt. of protein consumption, nor in the total amt. of carbohydrate consumption or in the proportion of calories derived from carbohydrates (*Cohen AM et al. Change of diet of Yemenite Jews in relation to diabetes and ischaemic heart-disease. <u>Lancet</u> 2:1399-401, 1961*).

Results of studies investigating the effect of sucrose upon glucose tolerance, hyperlipidemia and diabetic complications have been mixed due to differences in the background diet, the degree of diabetic control and individual variations in sucrose sensitivity.

> **Negative Observational Study (G):** The association between the intake of carbohydrates, body mass index (BMI), and the 4-y incidence of impaired glucose tolerance and diabetes mellitus was investigated in 175 elderly men and women aged 64-87 who were normoglycemic at baseline. There was no relationship between the intake of sugar products and the development of glucose intolerance; however, there was a significant association (p<0.01) between the intake of pastries and the development of glucose intolerance (*Feskens EJM, Bowles CH, Kromhout D. Carbohydrate intake and body mass index in relation to the risk of glucose intolerance in an elderly population. <u>Am J Clin Nutr</u> 54:136-40, 1991*).

> *Note: These results suggest that the fat content, rather than the sugar content, of sweet deserts may contribute to glucose intolerance.*

Negative Review Article (G): The vast majority of data show no untoward effects from sucrose, and diabetics could have up to a teaspoon of sugar, honey, or molasses, or other sweetener in a food serving (*Bankhead CD. Diabetics do fine on sugar snacks in short-term trial. Med World News, August 14, 1989*).

Negative Double-blind Crossover Study (G): 9 well-controlled type II diabetics had sucrose 45 g or aspartame 162 mg added to their usual diet for 6 wks. in either order. Neither addition adversely affected glycemic control, lipids, glucose tolerance, or insulin action (*Colagiuri S et al. Metabolic effects of adding sucrose and aspartame to the diet of subjects with noninsulin-dependent diabetes mellitus. Am J Clin Nutr 50:474-78, 1989*).

Animal Experimental Study (G): Rats were fed equal amts. of high-sucrose or high-starch diets. Whole-body glucose disposal was impaired by sucrose feedings because of a major impairment of insulin action at the liver with a smaller contribution from peripheral tissues (*Storlien LH et al. Effects of sucrose vs starch diets on in vivo insulin action, thermogenesis, and obesity in rats. Am J Clin Nutr 47:420-27, 1988*).

Review Article (G,K,R): In about 30% of subjects, a high sugar diet can result in an increase in insulin in fasting blood. Other studies have reported a decreased response to insulin; the development of retinopathy; an increase in size and change in structure in the glomeruli with deposition of calcium salts in, and disease of, the kidney; and liver enlargement, enzyme changes and an increase in its proportions of fat and collagen (*Yudkin J. Metabolic changes induced by sugar in relation to coronary heart disease and diabetes. Nutr Health 5(1/2):5-8, 1987*).

Review Article (G): Sucrose alone may be a very important etiologic factor in diabetes in the 10% of the population which is carbohydrate sensitive. In the rest of the population, sucrose still must be considered an important risk factor due to its synergistic interaction with dietary cholesterol and triglycerides (*Reiser S, Szepesi B. SCOGS report on the health aspects of sucrose consumption. Letter. Am J Clin Nutr 31:9-11, 1978*).

Sucrose increases urinary chromium excretion, and glucose intolerance is a sign of chromium deficiency (*see "Chromium" below*).

Experimental Controlled Study: 37 pts. consumed sequentially for 6 wks. each a diet containing 35% of calories from complex carbohydrates and 15% from sucrose, and a diet containing 15% of calories from complex carbohydrates and 35% from sucrose. Chromium content of each diet was 16 μg/1000 calories. 27/37 had an increase in urinary chromium excretion during the high sucrose diet compared to the low sucrose diet ranging from 10-300%, while 10/37 had no change. Absorption of chromium did not differ between the 2 diet periods (*Kozlovsky AS et al. Effects of diets high in simple sugars on urinary chromium losses. Metabolism 35(6):515-18, 1986*).

Substitute fructose for sucrose.

WARNINGS:

1. Fructose, when used as a major source of dietary carbohydrate, may induce copper deficiency which, in turn, may adversely affect glucose tolerance (*see "Copper"*).

Experimental Study: Subjects fed fructose as 20% of their diet developed biochemical evidence of decreased copper status and cardiac rhythm disturbances occurred with unexpected frequency - either due to the high-fructose diet or to the copper deficiency (*Reiser S et al. Indices of copper status in humans consuming a typical American diet containing either fructose or starch. Am J Clin Nutr 42:242-51, 1985*).

2. The fructose moiety of the sucrose molecule may be responsible for adverse changes in serum lipids similar to those noted after sucrose consumption.

Experimental Crossover Study: 10 hyperinsulinemic and 11 nonhyperinsulinemic men consumed a diet similar to one currently consumed in the US with 20% of the kcal from either fructose or high-amylose cornstarch for 5 wks. each in a crossover design. In the hyperinsulinemic men the intake of fructose significantly increased the total triglycerides and their lipoprotein distribution; total and VLDL lipoprotein cholesterol; apoproteins B-100, C-II, C-III; and uric acid. In the nonhyperinsulinemic men total triglycerides, total and LDL cholesterol and uric acid were significantly greater after the consumption of fructose than after cornstarch. Results indicate that, in a diet high in saturated fatty acids and cholesterol, fructose increases the levels of risk factors associated with heart disease, especially in hyperinsulinemic men (*Reiser S et al. Blood lipids, lipoproteins, apoproteins, and uric acid in men fed diets containing fructose or high-amylose cornstarch. Am J Clin Nutr 49:832-39, 1989*).

3. The addition of fructose to the diet may increase insulin resistance (*Beck-Nielsen H et al. Impaired cellular insulin binding and insulin sensitivity induced by a high-fructose feeding in normal subjects. Am J Clin Nutr 33:273-78, 1980; Hallfrisch J et al. Effects of dietary fructose on plasma glucose and hormone responses in normal and hyperinsulinemic men. J Nutr 113:1819-26, 1983*).

Fructose, when used as a short-term replacement of other carbohydrate sources in the diabetic diet, may improve glycemic control.

Note: Glycemic responses in insulin-dependent diabetics appear to be largely determined by the glucose component of food (*Hughes TA et al. Glycemic responses in insulin-dependent diabetic patients: effect of food composition. Am J Clin Nutr 49:658-66, 1989*).

Review Article (G): Acute human feeding trials have shown that the blood glucose response after fructose is similar to raw corn starch and about 2/3 the size of the response after sucrose (*Thorburn AW et al. Fructose-induced in vivo insulin resistance and elevated plasma triglyceride levels in rats. Am J Clin Nutr 49:1155-63, 1989*).

Avoid alcohol.
(G)

If the diabetes is well-controlled, the blood glucose level will not ordinarily be affected by the moderate use of alochol (*Franz MJ. Diabetes mellitus: Considerations in the development of guidelines for the occasional use of alcohol. J Am Diet Assoc 83:147-52, 1983*).

May decrease insulin sensitivity (*Avogaro A et al. Alcohol impairs insulin sensitivity in normal subjects. Diabetes Res 5:23-27, 1987*).

Avoid nitrosamines in children's diets.

Streptozocin, a chemical related to the nitrosamines, is used to induce diabetes in experimental animals.

Observational Study: 339 children with juvenile diabetes aged 0-14 were compared to 528 non-diabetic controls. Compared to controls, the diabetic children had a high frequency of nitrosamine consumption, as well as a high frequency of foods rich in protein or carbohydrate (*Dahlquist GG et al. Dietary factors and the risk of developing insulin dependent diabetes in children. Br Med J 300:1302-6, 1990*).

— —

COMBINED DIET

High complex carbohydrate and plant fiber (HCF) diet.
(G, R)

The HCF diet is high in cereal grains, legumes and root vegetables and restricts simple sugar and fat. 70-75% of calories come from complex carbohydrates, 15-20% from protein and 5-10% from fat, with a total fiber content of almost 100 gm daily. (More information and dietary guidelines are available from: *HCF Nutrition Research Foundation, 1872 Blairmore Rd., Lexington, Ky. 40502, USA*).

The HCF diet has led to discontinuation of insulin therapy in approx. 60% of type I diabetics, and has significantly reduced doses in the other 40% (*Vahouny G, Kritchevsky D. Dietary Fiber in Health and Disease. New York, Plenum Press, 1982; Anderson JW, Ward K. High-carbohydrate, high-fiber diets for insulin-treated men with diabetes mellitus. Am J Clin Nutr 32:2312-21, 1979; Anderson JW. High polysaccharide diet studies in patients with diabetes and vascular disease. Cereal Foods World 22:12-22, 1977*).

Experimental Controlled Crossover Study (G): After 1 wk. baseline. 10 type I diabetics randomly received either a high-carbohydrate (70%), high-fiber (70 g) (HCHF) diet or a low-carbohydrate (39%), low-fiber (10 g) (LFLC) diet. After a 6-wk. washout period, the gps. were switched over. Compared with the LCLF diet, the HCHF diet reduced basal insulin requirements (p<0.025), increased carbohydrate disposed of per unit insulin (p<0.0008), and lowered total (p<0.0004) and HDL (p<0.0013) cholesterol. Glycemic control and other lipid fractions did not differ significantly (*Anderson JW et al. Metabolic effects of high-carbohydrate, high-fiber diets for insulin-dependent diabetic individuals. Am J Clin Nutr 54:936-43, 1991*).

May be associated with decreased risk of developing retinopathy.

Observational Study (R): On the basis of 3-day food diaries, diabetics without retinopathy had significantly higher daily intakes of total carbohydrate, water-soluble dietary fibers, insoluble dietary fibers, and glucose and a significantly lower proportion of total daily calories as protein than did pts. with retinopathy (*Roy MS et al. Nutritional factors in diabetics with and without retinopathy. Am J Clin Nutr 50:728-30, 1989*).

Restrict cow's milk.
(G)

May decrease the risk of type I diabetes.

Review Article: Various cow-milk preparations have been reported to be diabetogenic in 2 animal models of insulin-dependent diabetes mellitus. While the suggestion of an inverse relationship between breast-feeding and IDDDM remains controversial, a possible negative relationship is observed between breast-feeding at age 3 mo. and IDDM risk. Also, there is a significant positive correlation between consumption of unfermented cow's milk protein and the incidence of IDDM in various countries (*Scott FW. Hypothesis. Cow milk and insulin-dependent diabetes mellitus: is there a relationship? Am J Clin Nutr 51:489-91, 1990*).

Eat a wide variety of foods.

Associated with less macrovascular disease in type II diabetics.

Observational Study: Arterial wall indices (compliance over the aorto-iliac segment and pulse wave damping at the common femoral and post. tibial arteries) were measured by Doppler ultrasound in type II diabetics and normal controls. Significant correlations were found between total food variety (p<0.01), and plant food variety (p<0.05), and each arterial wall index when the diabetics and controls were grouped together. 13-19% of the variance was explained by food variety (*Wahlqvist ML et al. Food variety is associated with less macrovascular disease in those with type II diabetes and their healthy controls. J Am Coll Nutr 8(6):515-23, 1989*).

– –

VITAMINS

Niacin:
(G,K)

A component of glucose tolerance factor (GTF); thus a deficiency will interfere with GTF synthesis (*Mertz W. Effects and metabolism of glucose tolerance factor. Nutr Rev 33(5):129-35, 1975*).

In type I diabetics, supplementation with nicotinamide may slow down beta-cell destruction and/or enhance their regeneration.

Experimental Double-blind Study (G): One wk. after starting intensive insulin therapy, 9/16 newly-diagnosed insulin-dependent diabetics aged 10-35 ingested nicotinamide (Nicobion 500, Astra) 3 gm daily while 7/16 ingested a placebo. Pts. then gradually reduced their insulin dose. Nicotinamide was discontinued if insulin was still required after 6 months. Insulin was discontinued successfully in 6/9 pts. in the nicotinamide gp. for 3, 6, 8, 27, 32, and 36 mo., and in 5 pts. in the placebo gp. for 1, 1, 1, 8 and 9 months. After 12 mo., none of the placebo gp. and 3 pts. in the nicotinamide gp. remained in remission. One of these pts. relapsed at 27 mo.; the other 2 remain in remission (*Vague PH et al. Nicotinamide may extend remission phase in insulin-dependent diabetes. Lancet 1:619-20, 1987*).

In type II diabetics, supplementation with niacin may improve glycemic control.

> WARNING: In type II diabetics, niacin supplementation may result in deterioration of glycemic control and an increase in plasma uric acid (*Garg A, Grundy SM. Nicotinic acid as therapy for dyslipidemia in non-insulin-dependent diabetes mellitus. JAMA 264(6):723-26, 1990*).

> **Case Reports:** 4 pts. with type II diabetes were supplemented with nicotinic acid 500 mg/d for 1 mo. followed by 250 mg/d. Blood sugar levels fell to normal and the 2 pts. on oral hypoglycemic agents were able to discontinue them. All experienced a water diuresis over a period of several mo. that resulted in a loss of 20-30 lbs. (*Cleary JP. Vitamin B3 in the treatment of diabetes mellitus: Case reports and review of the literature. J Nutr Med 1:217-25, 1990*).

Supplementation may retard the development of nephropathy (*Wahlberg G et al. Protective effect of nicotinamide against nephropathy in diabetic rats. Diabetes Res. 2:307, 1985*).

Thiamine: 100 mg. daily (2 week trial)
(N)

Required in glucose metabolism to form thiamine diphosphate which acts in the direct oxidative pathway.

May be marginally deficient (*Saito N et al. Blood thiamine levels in outpatients with diabetes mellitus. J Nutr Sci Vitaminol (Tokyo) 33(6):421-30, 1987*).

Thiamine deficiency is known to be associated with a neuropathy which responds to supplementation.

> **Review Article (N):** Treatment of acute thiamine deficiency neuropathy consists of thiamine 50 mg IM daily for several days followed by 2.5-5 mg orally (*Skelton WP III, Skelton NK. Thiamine deficiency neuropathy: It's still common today. Postgrad Med 85(8):301-06, 1989*).

Supplementation may decrease the symptoms of sensory neuropathy in diabetics.

> **Clinical Observation (N):** About 80% of diabetic pts. with sensory neuropathy were found to improve with thiamine supplementation (*Mirsky, Stanley, M.D., pres. of N.Y. affiliate of Am. Diabetes Assoc. & author of Diabetes: Controlling It the Easy Way, Random House, 1981.*)

Vitamin A:

Plasma/serum levels may be reduced, probably due to reduced mobilization from the liver (*Basu TK et al. Serum vitamin A and retionol-binding protein in patients with insulin-dependent diabetes mellitus. Am J Clin Nutr 50:329-31, 1989; Wako Y et al. Vitamin A transport in plasma of diabetic patients. Tohoku J Exp Med 149:133-43, 1986*).

Vitamin B6:
(G,N)

May be deficient (*Hollenbeck CB et al. The composition and nutritional adequacy of subject-selected high carbohydrate, low fat diets in insulin-dependent diabetes mellitus. Am J Clin Nutr 38(1):41-51, 1983; Rao RH et al. Failure of pyridoxine to improve glucose tolerance in diabetics. J Clin Endocrinol Metab 50(1):198-200, 1980*).

May be particularly low in diabetics with diabetic neuropathy (*McCann VJ, Davis RE. Serum pyridoxal concentrations in patients with diabetic neuropathy. Aust N Z J Med 8:259-61, 1978*).

Supplementation may reduce symptoms of diabetic neuropathy.

> **Negative Experimental Double-blind Study (N):** After 6 wks., pyridoxine 150 mg daily did not produce greater benefit than placebo on neuropathic symptoms or motor nerve conduction velocity in pts. with neuropathy (*Levin ER et al. The influence of pyridoxine in diabetic peripheral neuropathy. Diabetes Care 4:606, 1981*).

Experimental Study (N):   10 insulin-dependent diabetics with neuropathy and signs of pyridoxine deficiency were supplemented with 50 mg pyridoxine 3 times daily. Most noted some initial relief of pain and paresthesias in about 10 days. Improvement continued throughout the experimental period with amelioration or resolution of symptoms. Each pt. noted that the eyes "felt better." After the experimental period 7/10 pts. requested to be maintained on the supplementation. Within 3 wks., those who stopped noted a recurrence of symptoms which abated when supplementation was resumed (*Jones CL, Gonzales V. Pyridoxine deficiency: A new factor in diabetic neuropathy. J Am Podiatry Assoc 68(9):646-53, 1978*).

Supplementation may cure gestational diabetes.

Experimental and Observational Study (G):   13/14 pregnant women shown by the oral glucose tolerance test to have gestational diabetes had an increased urinary xanthurenic acid excretion after an oral tryptophan load, indicating a relative pyridoxine deficiency. All were treated with pyridoxine 100 mg daily for 14 days after which the deficiency was corrected and glucose tolerance improved considerably. Only 2/14 then had sufficiently impaired glucose tolerance to justify the diagnosis of gestational diabetes (*Coelingh Bennink HJT, Schreurs WHP. Improvement of oral glucose tolerance in gestational diabetes by pyridoxine. Br Med J 3:13-15, 1975*).

Supplementation does **not** improve glucose tolerance in type II diabetics, even if they are B6-deficient.

Experimental Study (G):   13 adult maturity-onset diabetics, including 7 who were vitamin B6-deficient, as assessed by the stimulation of RBC glutamic oxaloacetic transaminase *in vitro* by pyridoxal phosphate, failed to demonstrate significant alterations in either oral glucose tolerance or insulin response to glucose following supplementation with pyridoxine hydrochloride 40 mg twice daily for 3 wks. (*Rao RH et al. Failure of pyridoxine to improve glucose tolerance in diabetics. J Clin Endocrinol Metab 50(1):198-200, 1980*).

Supplementation may inhibit nonenzymatic glycosylation of hemoglobin and improve oxygen delivery in type II diabetics.

Experimental Double-blind Crossover Study: 15 type II diabetics randomly received pyridoxine 50 mg 3 times daily and placebo for 6 wk.s in either order. Prior to supplementation, tests of vitamin B6 nutriture (RBC aspartate aminotransferase activity; alanine aminotransferase activity) were normal. Supplementation failed to produce a consistent change in fasting blood glucose. However, HbAlc levels decreased in 6/9 pts. and rose again in 5/6 pts. after B6 was discontinued. The mean reduction in HbAlc level was about 6%. These changes were greater than expected, based on changes in fasting blood glucose. Supplementation also decreased hemoglobin oxygen affinity (*Solomon LR, Cohen K. Erythrocyte O2 transport and metabolism and effects of vitamin B6 therapy in type II diabetes mellitus. Diabetes 38:881-86, 1989*).

In normals, subclinical vitamin B6 deficiency may be associated with insulin resistance.

Experimental Study (G):   Elderly subjects ate self-selected diets followed by a vitamin B6-deficiency period of up to 30 days and a repletion period. Insulin levels increased 131% in men as a result of vitamin B6 deficiency and increased with repletion; however, post-study values remained above baselines. In women, insulin levels increased 30% and returned to baseline with B6 repletion. Plasma glucose levels rose 13% in men during the deficiency period, but returned to normal with repletion. No changes were noted in glucose tolerance tests. Results suggest that vitamin B6 deficiency provokes insulin resistance, especially in men (*Ribaya-Mercado J et al. Vitamin B6 deficiency elevates serum insulin in elderly subjects. Ann N Y Acad Sci 585:531-3, 1990*).

Negative Observational Study (G):   16 clinically normal subjects with pyridoxine deficiency (diagnosed by RBC transaminase activity and the 6 hr. tryptophan loading test) were compared to 16 controls. The deficient subjects had fasting normoglycemia with hypoinsulinemia (p<0.01) and a normal postglucose increment to insulin, but peak blood glucose and incremental glucose were significantly lower than in the controls (p<0.01), suggesting enhanced sensitivity to the hypoglycemic action of insulin. Supplementation resulted in a tendency for insulin levels to rise (results not significant) and a significant increase in growth hormone levels. It is suggested that impairment in growth hormone reserve may be the basis for the increased insulin sensitivity (*Rao RH. Glucose tolerance in subclinical pyridoxine deficiency in man. Am J Clin Nutr 38(3):440-44, 1983*).

Vitamin B$_{12}$:
(N)

Absorption in diabetics, both with and without intrinsic factor, is normal (*Fossati P et al.   Etude de l'absorption de la vitamine B$_{12}$ marquée isolée et associée au facteur intrinsèque chez le diabétique.   Diabete 20(1):23-31, 1972*).

Serum levels may be low in patients with <u>diabetic neuropathy</u> (*Bedi T et al.   A study of serum vitamin B$_{12}$ in various peripheral neuropathies.   J Assoc Physicians India 21(6):473-79, 1973; Khan MA et al.   Vitamin B$_{12}$ deficiency and diabetic neuropathy.   Lancet 2:768, 1969*).

Reduced tissue cobalamins as a result of diabetes may cause <u>diabetic neuropathy</u>.

Animal Experimental Study (N):   24 rats made diabetic showed muscle wasting and severe growth retardation and were found to have excessive urinary methylmalonic acid excretion but no abnormalities in the excretion of pyruvic or other ketoacids.   The serum total cobalamin was almost double that of controls.   Following an injection of methylcobalamin, an active form of B$_{12}$, the methylmalonic aciduria was abolished within 24 hours.   Since it is known that impaired tissue availability or utilization of cobalamins may rapidly produce neurological disorders, results suggest that a disturbance in tissue cobalamin enzymes are an important factor in the development of diabetic neuropathy (*Bhatt HR et al.   Can faulty vitamin B$_{12}$ (cobalamin) metabolism produce diabetic neuropathy? Letter.   Lancet 2:572, 1983*).

Parenteral supplementation may benefit <u>peripheral neuropathy</u>.

Experimental Study (N):   7 men and 4 women with diabetic neuropathy received methylcobalamin 2,500 μg intrathecally which was repeated several times with a 1-mo. interval between injections.   Symptoms in the legs, such as paresthesia, burning pains, and haviness, dramatically improved.   The effect appeared within a few hours to 1 wk. and lasted from several mo. to 4 years.   There were no side effects (*Ide H et al.   Clinical usefulness of intrathecal injection of methylcobalamin in patients with diabetic neuropathy.   Clin Ther 9(2):183-92, 1987*).

Animal Experimental Study (N):   For rats made diabetic, continuous treatment with methylcobalamin had an ameliorative effect on the peripheral nerve lesions in experimental diabetic neuropathy (*Yagihashi S et al.   In vivo effect of methylcobalamin on the peripheral nerve structure in streptozotocin diabetic rats.   Horm Metab Res 14(1):10-13, 1982*).

Experimental Study (N):   5 pts. with known diabetic neuropathy, 3 of whom were in good diabetic control, received 30 μg vitamin B$_{12}$ parenterally 3 times weekly.   All pts. had a marked subjective improvement; however, none showed objective evidence of improvement (*Davidson S.   The use of vitamin B$_{12}$ in the treatment of diabetic neuropathy.   J Fla Med Assoc 15:717-20, 1954*).

Experimental Study (N):   12 pts. with objective neurologic disturbances for which no other cause beside diabetes could be found were treated with crystalline vitamin B$_{12}$ IM for 3-13 months.   Generally 15-30 y were given daily for 7-14 days, followed by a maintenance dosage of 15-30 y once or twice weekly.   3/12 showed complete neurologic remission, 1/12 showed a complete remission after a partial relapse, 3/12 showed almost complete remission, 3/12 were improved and 2/12 were questionably improved (*Sancetta SM et al.   The use of vitamin B$_{12}$ in the management of the neurological manifestations of diabetes mellitus, with notes on the administration of massive doses.   Ann Intern Med 35:1028-48, 1951*).

Vitamin C: 500 mg - 2 grams daily
(A,G,K,N,R)

Frequently depressed in both the plasma and leukocytes of diabetics even despite adequate dietary vitamin C (*Cunningham J et al.   Reduced mononuclear leukocyte ascorbic-acid content in adults with insulin-dependent diabetes mellitus consuming adequate dietary vitamin C.   Metabolism 40:146-9, 1991; Jennings PE et al.   Vitamin C metabolites and microangiopathy in diabetes mellitus.   Diabetes Res 6(3):151-54, 1987; Som S et al.   Ascorbic acid metabolism in diabetes mellitus.   Metabolism 30:572-77, 1981*).

Note: Animal studies suggest that this is due to increased urinary excretion (Zebrowski EJ, Bhatnagar PK.   Urinary excretion pattern of ascorbic acid in streptozotocin diabetic and insulin treated rats.   Pharm Res Commun 11(2):95-103, 1979), disrupted vitamin C transport across cell membranes (Cunningham JJ.   Altered vitamin C transport in diabetes mellitus. Med Hypotheses. 26:263-65, 1988; Mann GV. Hypothesis: The role of vitamin C in diabetic angiopathy. Persp Biol Med 17:210-17, 1974), and increased oxidation to dehydroascorbic acid (Som S et al. Ascorbic acid metabolism in diabetes mellitus. Metabolism 30(6):572-7, 1981).

A deficiency of vitamin C provokes disorders in glycoregulation reminiscent of diabetes, while diabetes brings about disorders in ascorbic acid metabolism which may lead to a vitamin C deficiency in some tissues. This vicious circle can be cut by an increased supply of ascorbic acid (*Ginter EM, Chorvathova V. Vitamin C and diabetes mellitus. Nutr Health 2:3-11, 1983*).

Dehydroascorbic acid (DHAA), whose structure is closely related to alloxan, causes diabetes mellitus in rats (*Patterson JW. The diabetogenic effect of dehydroascorbic acid and dehydroisoascorbic acids. J Bio Chem 183:81, 1950*).

Findings suggesting that diabetics have elevated DHAA levels (*Banerjee A. Blood dehydroascorbic acid and diabetes mellitus in human beings. Ann Clin Biochem 19(Pt 2):65-70, 1982; Som S et al. Ascorbic acid metabolism in diabetes mellitus. Metabolism 30(6):572-77, 1981*) have not been confrimed in more recent studies (*Jennings PE et al. Vitamin C metabolites and microangiopathy in diabetes mellitus. Diabetes Res 6(3):151-54, 1987; Newill A et al. Plasma levels of vitamin C components in normal and diabetic subjects. Ann Clin Biochem 21(Pt 6):488-90, 1984*). However, even if plasma DHAA levels in diabetics are normal, decreased ascorbic acid levels result in an elevated DHAA/AA ratio which may be a reflection of increased oxidative stress, suggesting that diabetics may be less able to prevent oxidative damage (*Jennings PE et al. Vitamin C metabolites and microangiopathy in diabetes mellitus. Diabetes Res 6(3):151-54, 1987*).

Although large doses of ascorbic acid can cause a rise in DHAA levels with an associated elevation in blood sugar (*Chatterjee IB et al. Synthesis and some major functions of vitamin C in animals. Ann N Y Acad Sci 258:24, 1975*), DHAA disappears after continued administration of ascorbic acid and the accumulation of DHAA seems to be an indication of ascorbic acid deficiency (*Banerjee S. Physiological role of dehydroascorbic acid. Indian J Physiol Pharmacol 21(2):85-93, 1977*).

> *Note: The addition of "capillary active" bioflavonoids or of glutathione may prevent ascorbic acid supplementation from raising DHAA levels (Clemetson AB. Ascorbic acid and diabetes mellitus. Med Hypotheses 2:193-4, 1976) (see "Bioflavonoids" and "Glutathione" below).*

Experimental Controlled Study: 22 diabetics with and without microangiopathy were compared to 22 age-matched controls. At baseline, the pts. had low vitamin C concentrations and elevated DHAA/AA ratios. Three wks. after initiating supplementation with ascorbic acid 1 gm daily, ascorbate levels had increased in both diabetic gps. and were maintained in the controls. However, these levels fell by 6 wks. in both diabetic groups. The ratio of DHAA to AA fell in all gps. by 3 wks., but increased again in the diabetic gps. by 6 weeks. Results show that vitamin C supplementation only partially and temporarily corrects disturbances in vitamin C metabolism in diabetes (*Sinclair A et al. Disturbed handling of ascorbic acid in diabetic patients with and without microangiopathy during high dose ascorbate supplementation. Diabetol 34:171-5, 1991*).

A marginal vitamin C deficiency may contribute to the development of angiopathy, since low insulin levels and hyperglycemia accelerate the cellular changes leading to atherosclerosis by impairing ascorbic acid uptake into the vascular epithelium, and studies have correlated experimental ascorbic acid deficiencies with atherogenic processes, presumably by altering glycosaminoglycan metabolism (*Kapeghian JC, Verlangieri AJ. The effects of glucose on ascorbic acid uptake in heart endothelial cells: Possible pathogenesis of diabetic angiopathies. Life Sci 34(6):577-84, 1984*).

Supplementation may improve glucose tolerance.

WARNING: ascorbic acid supplementation may skew the results of urine tests for glucose

Observational Study (G): Plasma vitamin C levels were inversely correlated with fasting blood sugar levels for a group of 241 subjects (*Esk C et al. Correlation of plasma ascorbic acid with cardiovascular risk factors. Clin Res 38:A747, 1990*).

Experimental Study (G): Pts. were given 500 mg vitamin C twice daily. After 10 days, glucose tolerance was improved in all pts. (*Sandhya P, Das UN. Vitamin C therapy for maturity onset diabetes mellitus: Relevance to prostaglandin involvement. IRCS J Med. Sci 9(7):618, 1981*).

Supplementation may significantly depress <u>cutaneous capillary fragility</u> .

> **Experimental Placebo-controlled Study:**   12 diabetics, 6 of whom had symptomatic retinopathy (aged 25-71) and 24 controls aged 21-61 were studied. Half of the diabetics and a quarter of the controls were found to have an intake of vitamin C which was less than the recommended 315 mg/wk. The diabetics randomly received either placebo for 1 mo. followed by vitamin C 1 g daily for 2 mo. (Gp. 1) or vitamin C for 2 mo. followed by placebo for 1 month (Gp. II). In all subjects during testing by applying negative pressure to the anterior forearm surface, an increase of negative pressure led to a logarithmic increase in the number of petechiae observed. The diabetics showed petechiae at much lower negative pressures than the controls, and all diabetics with retinopathy had very fragile capillaries. In Gp. I, capillary fragility failed to change during placebo treatment. Capillary strength in all diabetics improved during vitamin C treatment. In Gp II capillary strength in 4/6 diabetics deteriorated on placebo treatment. No retinal changes were observed during vitamin C treatment (*Cox BD, Butterfield WJ. Vitamin C supplements and diabetic cutaneous capillary fragility. <u>Br Med J</u> 3:205, 1975*).

Supplementation may lower <u>cholesterol</u> and <u>triglycerides</u> in type II diabetics.

> **Experimental Study:**   60% of maturity-onset diabetic pts. with hypercholesterolemia given 500 mg ascorbic acid daily for 1 yr. experienced at least a 40% reduction in cholesterol levels along with a moderate decline of triglyceridemia. Since significantly lower vitamin C concentrations have been found in the blood and particularly in the leukocytes of these pts., these results suggest that the long-term administration removed the tissue ascorbate deficiency and improved the liver's ability to compensate for the increased endogenous synthesis of cholesterol by enhanced transformation to bile acids (*Ginter E et al. Hypocholesterolemic effect of ascorbic acid in maturity-onset diabetes mellitus. <u>Int J Vitam Nutr Res</u> 48(4):368-73, 1978*).

Supplementation may reduce RBC sorbitol levels (*Vinson JA et al. In vitro and in vivo reduction of erythrocyte sorbitol by ascorbic acid. <u>Diabetes</u> 38:1036-41, 1989*).

> *Note (A,K,N,R): Sorbitol accumulation in tissues is associated with the development of cataracts, retinopathy, neuropathy and other complications of diabetes (Cogan DG et al. Aldose reductase and complications of diabetes. <u>Ann Intern Med</u> 101:82-91, 1984*).

<u>Vitamin E:</u>
(A,G)

> WARNING: As vitamin E may reduce the insulin requirement, diabetics on insulin should be started on 100 IU or less daily and the dosage raised slowly with adjustment of the insulin dose (*Vogelsang A. Vitamin E in the treatment of diabetes mellitus. <u>Ann N Y Acad Sci</u> 52:406, 1949*).

Diabetics appear to have an increased requirement for vitamin E (*Lubin B, Machlin L. Biological aspects of vitamin E. <u>Ann N Y Acad Sci</u> 1982, p. 393*).

Deficiency may promote cellular damage due to free radical oxidation (*Galli C, Socin A. Biological actions and possible uses of vitamin E. <u>Acta Vitaminol Enzymol</u> 4:245-52, 1984*).

Supplementation may reduce the risk of developing diabetes.

> **Animal Experimental Study (G):**   90 diabetes-prone rats were fed either a high- or low-vitamin E diet for 6 mo. or until they became diabetic. 5/45 animals on the high E diet vs. 11/45 on the low E diet became diabetic. Thymus vitamin E levels were significantly higher (p<0.005) in the high E asymptomatic rats compared to the high E diabetic rats, suggesting that high dietary vitamin E may decrease the incidence of diabetes in animals which are able to accumulate sufficient amounts of the vitamin in the thymus (*Behrens WA et al. Effect of dietary vitamin E on the vitamin E status in the BB rat during devlopment and after the onset of diabetes. <u>Ann Nutr Metab</u> 30:157-65, 1986*).

Supplementation may reduce platelet hyperaggregability which may contribute to microvascular disease and premature atherosclerosis.

> **Review Article (A):**   Vitamin E might be a favorable adjunct to treatment. It is effective in reversing abnormal platelet aggregation and is relatively non-toxic. In studies on diabetic pts. and animals, vitamin E supplementation

normalizes TXA$_2$ production by inhibiting platelet thromboxane release and restores aortic PGI$_2$ production. For example, thromboxane levels of pts. receiving dl-alpha tocopherol acetate 400 mg/d for 4 wks. returned to levels observed in healthy controls. In addition, vitamin E might influence plasma cholesterol levels, reduce the risk for angina, alleviate the symptoms of intermittent claudication, and reduce LDL peroxide formation. Thus, supplementation might prevent or delay the development of diabetic vascular complications (*Gisinger C et al. Vitamin E and platelet eicosanoids in diabetes mellitus.* <u>*Prostaglandins Leukot Essent Fatty Acids*</u> *40:169-76, 1990*).

Experimental Double-blind Study (A): 22 type I pts. without significant vascular disease received 400 IU vitamin E daily. After 4 wks., there was a significant reduction of induced platelet thromboxane A$_2$ production at each ADP concentration and at 2 or 3 collagen concentrations. Metabolic control was unchanged, suggesting that the effect of vitamin E is not dependent on the quality of diabetic control. Platelet aggregation, which was not significantly increased in pts. compared to healthy controls, was significantly reduced only at one collagen concentration. Results suggest that vitamin E treatment might be promising for the prevention of diabetic angiopathy (*Gisinger C et al. Effect of vitamin E supplementation on platelet thromboxane A$_2$ production in type I diabetic patients.* <u>*Diabetes*</u> *37:1260-64, 1988*).

> *Note: previous research has shown that inhibition of thromboxane A$_2$ production may be a more sensitive index of inhibition of platelet function than aggregation itself (Gisinger C et al. Effect of vitamin E supplementation on platelet thromboxane A$_2$ production in type I diabetic patients.* <u>*Diabetes*</u> *37:1260-64, 1988).*

Experimental Double-blind CrossoverStudy (A): 9 type I diabetics received either 1 gm vitamin E daily or placebo. After 35 days, supplementation resulted in decreased platelet aggregation (*Colette C et al. Platelet function in type I diabetes: Effects of supplementation with large doses of vitamin E.* <u>*Am J Clin Nutr*</u> *47:256-61, 1988*).

Supplementation may assist healing of lesions of <u>necrobiosis lipoidica diabeticorum</u>.

Case Report: "Moderately good success" following vitamin E 400 IU daily (*Ayres S Jr., Mihan R. Vitamin E and dermatology.* <u>*Cutis*</u> *16:1017-1021, 1975*).

Case Reports: A diabetic woman with a large, yellow ulcerating lesion on the right leg received 150 mg. of vitamin E twice weekly plus 100 mg. orally 3 times daily after meals. After 2 wks., the ulcers closed and normal skin formation began. Another woman with 3 lesions which had been present for a yr. received the same treatment with clearing of the lesions in 3 wks. (*Block MT. Vitamin E in the treatment of diseases of the skin.* <u>*Clin Med*</u> *60:31, 1953*).

Supplementation may assist healing of <u>gangrene</u>.

Case Reports: 3/3 pts. with gangrene of the toes had excellent results from treatment with 100-150 mg. of vitamin E orally 3 times daily and 150 mg. IM 2-3 times weekly. Strongly recommended by the author (in conjunction with antibiotics) even in advanced cases to prevent debridement and amputation (*Block MT. Vitamin E in the treatment of diseases of the skin.* <u>*Clin Med*</u> *60:31, 1953*).

Supplementation may reduce nonenzymatic protein glycosylation, one of the mechanisms of cellular ageing and perhaps a cause of end-organ damage.

Experimental Conrolled Study: 2 gps. of 10 type I diabetics received 600 and 1,200 mg, respectively, of vitamin E daily, while a third gp. served as a control. After 2 mo., glycemic indices did not change significantly; however, fasting concentrations of labile HbA1 and glycosylated proteins decreased significantly only in pts. receiving vitamin E (*Ceriello A et al. Vitamin E reduction of protein glycosylation in diabetes.* <u>*Diabetes Care*</u> *14:68-72, 1991*).

_ _

MINERALS

<u>Calcium:</u>
(G)

Diabetes appears to enhance the deposition of calcium in arterial walls which may contribute to the development of hypertension and atherosclerosis (*Neubauer B. A quantitative study of peripheral arterial calcification and glucose tolerance in elderly diabetics and non-diabetics. <u>Diabetologia</u> 7:409-13, 1971; Turlapaty PD et al. Ca^{2+} uptake and distribution in alloxan-diabetic rat arterial and venous smooth muscle. <u>Experientia</u> 36(11):1298-99, 1980*).

Increased serum calcium concentrations may be associated with impaired glucose tolerance as well as with hyperlipidemia and hypertension (*Lind L et al. Relation of serum calcium concentration to metabolic risk factors for cardiovascular disease. <u>Br Med J</u> 297:960-63, 1988*).

Serum ionized calcium may be depressed (*Fogh-Andersen N et al. Lowered serum ionized calcium in insulin treated diabetic subjects. <u>Scand J Clin Lab Invest Suppl</u> 165:93-97, 1983*).

Hair calcium levels may be elevated.

> *Note: Elevated hair calcium levels are sometimes suggestive of a calcium deficiency.*

> **Observational Study (G):** 60% of 118 ambulatory pts. with a wide range of clinical problems were found to have an abnormal glucose tolerance test, including all pts. with elevated hair calcium levels (*Tamari GM, Roma, Z. Hair mineral levels and their correlation with abnormal glucose tolerance. <u>Cytobiol Rev</u> 9(4):191-6, 1985*).

Calcium deficiency may be a cause of diabetes.

> **Theoretical Discussion:** In old age, low calcium and vitamin D intake, short solar exposure, decreased intestinal absorption, and falling renal function with insufficient 1,25-dihydroxyvitamin D synthesis all contribute to calcium deficiency, secondary hyperparathyroidism, bone loss and possibly calcium shift from the bone to soft tissue, and from the extracellular to the intracellular compartment, blunting the sharp concentration gap between these compartments. Consequences may include a decrease in cellular function due to blunting of the difference in extracellular-intracellular calcium, leading to diabetes mellitus (*Fujita T. Aging and calcium as an environmental factor. <u>J Nutr Sci Vitaminol (Tokyo)</u> 31 Suppl S15-9, 1985*).

<u>Chromium:</u>
(G,N)

A necessary component of glucose tolerance factor (GTF) - a substance present in brewer's yeast known to improve glucose tolerance in laboratory animals by potentiating the effect of insulin on carbohydrate metabolism (*Haylock SJ et al. Separation of biologically active chromium-containing complexes from yeast extracts and other sources of glucose tolerance factor (GTF) activity. <u>J Inorg Biochem</u> 18(3):195-211, 1983; Mertz W, Schwarz K. Chromium (III) and the glucose tolerance factor. <u>Arch Biochem Biophys</u> 85:292-5, 1959*).

Glucose intolerance is one of the signs of chromium deficiency (*Freund H et al. Chromium deficiency during total parenteral nutrition. <u>JAMA</u> 241(5):496-8, 1979*), and chromium nutriture may affect glucose uptake in insulin-sensitive tissues (*Mertz W. Chromium occurrence and function in a biological system. <u>Physiol Rev</u> 49:163-230, 1969*).

> **Experimental Double-blind Crossover Study (G):** 11 females and 6 males without diabetes mellitus were studied. Those with glucose concentrations >5.56 mmol/L but <11.1 mmol/L 90 min after an oral glucose challenge were designated as hyperglycemic; the rest of the gp. served as controls. All subjects were placed on a low-chromium diet containing chromium in the lowest quartile of normal intake. After a 4-wk. baseline, subjects randomly received either chromium 200 µg/d or placebo for 4 wks.; then, after a 1 wk. washout period, the gps. were switched over. The low-chromium diet was associated with detrimental effects on glucose toelrance, insulin and glucagon in the hyperglycemic subjects. Glucose tolerance, circulating insulin and glucagon all improved in the hyperglycemic gp. during chromium vs. placebo supplementation, while these measures were unchanged in the

control gp. throughout the study (*Supplemental-chromium effects on glucose, insulin, glucagon, and urinary chromium losses in subjects consuming controlled low-chromium diets. Am J Clin Nutr 54:909-16, 1991*).

Serum chromium levels may be positively correlated with serum insulin levels (*Liu VJ, Abernathy RP. Chromium and insulin in young subjects with normal glucose tolerance. Am J Clin Nutr 25(4):661-67, 1982*).

Supplementation (in its trivalent form) may improve glucose tolerance.

Experimental Double-blind Crossover Study (G):   11 type II diabetics on stable doses of oral hypoglycemic agents randomly received chromium 200 µg/d as chromium tripicolinate 1.6 mg and placebo in either order with a 2 wk. wash-out period between trials. After 6 wks. of treatment, fasting blood sugar decreased an ave. of 18% (32 mg/dl) and glycosylated hemoglobin decreased 10%. Both changes were statistically significant. There were no changes after placebo administration (*Evans GW. The effect of chromium picolinate on insulin controlled parameters in humans. Int J Biosoc Med Res 11(2):163-80, 1989*).

Experimental Double-blind Study (G):   85 elderly women (ages 59-82), 62% of whom were on medications that could affect glucose metabolism, were divided into "high risk" and "low risk" categories on the basis of a 2 hr. GTT and received either chromium (CrCl3 200 µg) or placebo. After 10 wks. there were no significant differences between experimental subjects and controls except for a small but significant improvement after a GTT in the high risk, non-medicated group. This sub-group was found to have a significantly lower median chromium intake compared to the experimental low risk non-medicated group, suggesting that suboptimal chromium status may account for the difference. Because it appears that medications may have obscured this effect in the medicated subjects, the researchers suggest that future studies omit medicated subjects (*Martinez OB et al. Dietary chromium and effect of chromium supplementation on glucose tolerance of elderly Canadian women. Nutr Res 5:609-20, 1985*).

Negative Experimental Double-blind Study (G):   2 gps. of diabetic and non-diabetic subjects received either 68 µg chromium daily in the form of brewer's yeast or tortula yeast placebo. While hair chromium increased about 25% for both gps. supplemented with chromium, the decrease in fasting blood sugar among chromium-supplemented diabetics (from 204 to 194 mg/dl) was not significant compared to placebo (*Hunt AE et al. Effect of chromium supplementation on hair chromium concentration and diabetic status. Nutr Res 5:131-140, 1985*).

If deficient, supplementation may improve diabetic neuropathy:

Case Report (N):   A female diabetic on long-term total parenteral nutrition developed peripheral neuropathy along with glucose intolerance, weight loss, and other metabolic disturbances that failed to respond to increased insulin. Chromium balance was negative and blood and hair chromium levels were below normal. After chromium supplementation with chromium 250 microng daily to her infusate, her nerve conduction studies became normal and insulin could be discontinued (*Jeejeebhoy KN et al. Chromium deficiency, glucose intolerance, and neuropathy reversed by chromium supplementation, in a patient receiving long-term total parenteral nutrition. Am J Clin Nutr 30(4):531-38, 1977*).

- with Niacin:

Supplementation may improve glucose tolerance.

Experimental Study (G):   16 healthy elderly volunteers received either chomium 200 µg, nicotinic acid 100 mg, or both, daily. After 28 days, fasting glucose and glucose tolerance were unaffected by either nutrient alone; however, the combination reduced the glucose area integrated total (indicative of improved glucose tolerance) by 15% (p<0.025) and decreased fasting blood glucose by 7% (*Urberg M et al. Evidence for synergism between chromium and nicotinic acid in the control of glucose tolerance in elderly humans. Metabolism 36:896-99, 1987*).

Copper:
(A,G,K,N,R)

Deficiency may impair glucose intolerance

Negative Animal Experimental Study (G):   Copper deficiency in rats was associated with impaired glucose tolerance only when fed fructose or glucose, but not when fed starch. Of the 2 monosaccharides, fructose was more diabetogenic. The data indicate that copper deficiency *per se* does not impair glucose tolerance (*Fields M et al. Impairment of glucose tolerance in copper-deficient rats: Dependency on the type of dietary carbohydrate. J Nutr 114(2):393-97, 1984*).

Case Reports (G):   2 healthy men, aged 21 and 30 yrs., were fed a low-copper diet (0.7-0.8 mg/d) for 6 or 5 months. The diet was supplemented daily with 0.5, 0 and 3.5 mg of copper as sulfate during the respective dietary periods. Control of energy intake and physical activity prevented change in body weight. Glucose tolerance tests were done at the end of the control (30 days), depletion 120 or 90 days and repletion (30 days) periods. For the GTT, 1/2 g/kg as a 25% solution was infused IV in 3-5 min. and 7 samples were collected between 2.5 and 60 min. Ave. glucose concentration at each point after glucose infusion increased by 38 mg/dl during depletion and decreased by 24 mg/dl during repletion. Ave. insulin concentration declined by 10 µU/ml during depletion and further by 25 µU/ml during repletion. During repletion, although insulin concentration was lower, glucose clearance was more rapid (*Klevay LM et al. Diminished glucose tolerance in two men due to a diet low in copper. Abstract. Am J Clin Nutr 37:717, 1983*).

Animal Experimental Study (G):   Copper-deficient rats have significantly higher blood glucose levels after an oral glucose load compared with copper-supplemented rats (*Reiser S et al. Role of dietary fructose in the enhancement of mortality and biochemical changes associated with copper deficiency in rats. Am J Clin Nutr 38:214-22, 1983*).

Copper deficiency in animals is associated with increased tissue concentrations of sorbitol when fructose or sucrose rather than starch is the source of dietary carbohydrate (*Fields M et al. Accumulation of sorbitol in copper deficiency: Dependency on gender and type of dietary carbohydrate. Metabolism 38(4):371-75, 1989*).

> *Note (A,K,N,R): Sorbitol accumulation in tissues is associated with the development of cataracts, retinopathy, neuropathy and other complications of diabetes (Cogan DG et al. Aldose reductase and complications of diabetes. Ann Intern Med 101:82-91, 1984).*

Iron:
(G)

Reduction of elevated serum ferritin levels (ferritin is a major iron storage protein) may be beneficial.

Experimental Study (G):   9/18 poorly-controlled type II diabetics had elevated serum ferritin levels, while serum iron and total iron-binding capacity were normal in all cases. None had a disorder known to cause iron storage. All 9 pts. with elevated ferritin were treated with the iron chelating agent desferrioxamine 10 mg/kg IV twice weekly for 9-26 treatments, depending upon response. 8/9 had an improvement in blood sugar which was frequently dramatic and permitted discontinuation of insulin injections and oral hypoglycemic agents for all of them. Serum cholesterol, triglycerides and hemoglobin A1c levels also improved considerably. In 1 pt. with high serum ferritin and in all 7 pts. with normal serum ferritin, treatment with desferrioxamine failed to improve diabetic control (*Cutler P. Desferrioxamine therapy in high-ferritin diabetes. Diabetes 38:1207-10, 1989*).

Magnesium:
(A,G,K,M,N,R)

General Review Article (A,G,K,M,N,R):
1. Not only is magnesium deficiency the most common disturbance in mineral metabolism observed in insulin-dependent diabetes, but low blood magnesium levels are associated with both the acute metabolic and late chronic complications.
2. Essential for glucose homeostasis, magnesium is a co-factor in glucose transport and regulates energy production in liver mitochrondria.
3. Magnesium also functions in the release of insulin and the maintenance of the pancreatic beta cells associated with insulin production and release, and increases the affinity and number of insulin receptors.
4. Magnesium deficiency is associated with beta cell atrophy, and insulin deficiency is associated with magnesium depletion.
5. Other than acute ketoacidosis, the most frequent cause of secondary hypomagnesemia is diabetes.

6. The etiology of hypomagnesemia in diabetics includes increased urinary excretion with glucosuria, an inverse association between plasma magnesium and blood glucose, hyposecretion of insulin and adrenalin, modification of vitamin D metabolism, and lack of pyridoxine.

7. Magnesium depletion is also associated with several diabetic complications including cardiovascular, ocular, neurological, renal, osteoarticular, and metabolic, and magnesium losses during ketoacidosis can have life-threatening effects on the myocardium and skeletal muscles. Hypomagnesemia is also linked to microvascular disorders including hypertension and retinopathy.

8. Magnesium supplementation restores low blood and tissue levels, produces a protective effect against cardiovascular disease, and might aid in the prevention of vascular complcations associated with diabetes and possibly in the pathophysiology of the disease.

(*Elamin A, Tuvemo T. Magnesium and insulin-dependent diabetes mellitus. Diabetes Res Clin Pract 10:203-9, 1990*).

Frequently low in diabetics, especially those with coronary heart disease or proliferative retinopathy.

> **Review Article:** Diabetes mellitus is the most common pathological state in which secondary magnesium deficiency occurs. Plasma magnesium levels, which are more often decreased than RBC magnesium, are correlated mainly with the severity of the diabetic state, glucose disposal and endogenous insulin secretion. Mechanisms involved relate to insulin and epinephrine secretion, modifications of vitamin D metabolism, decrease of blood phosphorus, vitamin B6 and taurine levels, increase of vitamin B5, vitamin C and glutathione turnover, and treatment with high levels of insulin and biguanides. Retinopathy and microangiopathy are correlated with the drop of plasma and RBC magnesium (*Durlach J, Collery P. Magnesium and potassium in diabetes and carbohydrate metabolism. Review of the present status and recent results. Magnesium 3(4-6):315-23, 1984*).

Insulin enhances magnesium uptake; it has been proposed that this effect is an important component of insulin's effect on ion translocation, with intracellular magnesium serving as second messenger for insulin (*Lostroh AJ, Krahl. Magnesium, a second messenger for insulin: Ion translocation coupled to transport activity. Adv Enz Regul 12:73-81, 1974*).

During diabetic ketosis, both hypo- and hypermagnesemia can develop (*Martin HE. Clinical magnesium deficiency. Ann N Y Acad Sci 156:891-900, 1969*).

The similarity of small coronary arteriopathy of experimental magnesium deficiency to that of diabetes suggests that chronic magnesium loss may contribute to the cardiovascular complications, including the arrhythmias of diabetes (which have been attributed to small coronary arterial disease) (*Ditzel J. Morphologic hemodynamic changes in the small blood vessels in diabetes mellitus. N Engl J Med 250:541-46, 1954; James TN. Pathology of small coronary arteries. Am J Cardiol 20:679-91, 1967*).

Supplementation may improve insulin response and action.

> **Experimental Blinded Crossover Study (G):** 8 elderly, moderately obese pts. with non-insulin-dependent DM received a weight-maintenance diet containing at least 250 g carbohydrate and an ave. of 317 mg magnesium per day. In addition, they randomly received 2 g magnesium daily or placebo in random order for 4 wks. with a 2-wk. washout period in between. Glucose metabolism was unchanged on placebo; however, both acute insulin response and glucose disappearance constant increased significantly with magnesium supplementation. At the end of the supplementation period, these values were positively and significantly correlated with increased RBC magnesium content. In addition, during euglycemic-hyperinsulinemic testing, the glucose infusion rate was significantly higher during the final hour of the experiment in supplemented pts., and the net increase in glucose infusion rate was significantly correlated with increased RBC magnesium (*Paolisso G et al. Improved insulin response and action by chronic magnesium administration in aged NIDDM subjects. Diabetes Care 12:265-69, 1989*).

Manganese:
(G)

Levels in diabetics are one-half those of normals (*Kosenko LG. Klin Med 42:113, 1964*).

An important cofactor in the key enzymes of glycolysis (*Wimhurst JM, Manchester KL. Comparison of ability of Mg and Mn to activate the key enzymes of glycolysis. FEBS Letters 27:321-6, 1972*).

Deficiency can lead to glucose intolerance which can be reversed by supplementation (*Baly D et al. Effect of manganese deficiency on insulin binding, glucose transport and metabolism in rat adipocytes. J Nutr 120:1075-9, 1990*).

Case Reports (G): A 21 year-old insulin-dependent diabetic received oral manganese chloride 3-5 mg daily which resulted in a consistent fall in blood glucose, often to severely hypoglycemic levels, with modification of the GTT. On the other hand, oral manganese failed to affect the blood sugar level in 3 middle-aged diabetics, 3 juvenile diabetics and 1 case of diabetes resulting from chronic pancreatitis (*Rubenstein AH et al. Hypoglycemia induced by manganese. Nature 194:188-9, 1962*).

Phosphorus:
(A,G,R)

Hypophosphatemia, which is common in diabetics, is associated with an impaired response to insulin (*DeFronzo RA, Lang R. Hypophosphatemia and glucose intolerance: Evidence for tissue insensitivity to insulin. N Engl J Med 303(22):1259-63, 1980*).

Insulin-dependent diabetics appear to have a fluctuating disorder in the oxygen-releasing capacity of their erythrocytes. Transient decreases in red cell oxygen delivery appears to lead to dilatation of the venous part of the microcirculation associated with increased transcapillary plasma permeation. Combined with microrheologic alterations (increased RBC aggregation, increased blood viscosity, and decreased red cell deformability), these changes may play a role in the pathogenesis of diabetic angiopathy. The position of the oxyhemoglobin dissociation curve is positively correlated with levels of RBC 2,3-diphosphoglycerate (2,3-DPG) which, in turn, varies in response to the plasma concentration of inorganic phosphate (*Ditzel J. Changes in red cell oxygen release capacity in diabetes mellitus. Fed Proc 38(11):2484-88, 1979; Ditzel J. Oxygen transport impairment in diabetes. Diabetes 25:832-8, 1976*).

Dietary enrichment with phosphates may thus improve RBC oxygen-releasing capacity (and thereby help to prevent the development of angiopathy) by preventing the inhibitory effect of a low concentration of inorganic phosphorus on red cell oxygen delivery (*Freyler H. [Modern trends in the treatment of diabetic retinopathy.] Wien Klin Wochenschr 89(4):101-06, 1977*).

Experimental Study (G): When evaluated after 2 yrs. of supplementation with dibasic calcium phosphate 2 gm 3 times daily with meals, type I diabetic pts. felt less tired and diabetic control was improved. They showed no evidence of adverse effects including soft tissue calcification, urinary calculus formation, hyper- or hypocalcemia (*Ditzel J. Oxygen transport impairment in diabetes. Diabetes 25:832-8, 1976*).

Potassium:
(G)

WARNING: Diabetics commonly have decreased plasma aldosterone levels, making them liable to severe hyperkalemia from potassium supplementation (*Perez GO et al. Potassium homeostasis in chronic diabetes mellitus. Arch Intern Med 137(8):1018-22, 1977*). Even diabetics without aldosterone deficiency may have a reduced capacity to excrete an oral potassium load coupled with an enhanced capacity to transfer potassium intracellularly (*Smoller S et al. Blunted kaliuresis after an acute oral potassium load in diabetes mellitus. Am J Med Sci 295(2):114-21, 1988*).

Tissue levels may be reduced (*Sjogren A et al. Magnesium, potassium and zinc deficiency in subjects with type II diabetes mellitus. Acta Med Scand 224:461-63, 1988*).

Review Article: Potassium depletion in diabetes is well known and increases the noxious cardiorenal effects of magnesium deficiency (*Durlach J, Collery P. Magnesium and potassium in diabetes and carbohydrate metabolism. Review of the present status and recent results. Magnesium 3(4-6):315-23, 1984*).

Potassium deficiency may cause a reversible decrease in peripheral insulin levels and insulin resistance at the postreceptor sites.

Experimental Study (G): Caloric deprivation in 20 obese non-diabetic subjects (15 mmol K in a protein-modified fast) was followed by a negative potassium balance, decreased serum potassium, decreased peripheral insulin levels, increased insulin receptors and a striking reduction of peripheral glucose utilization. The addition of oral potassium chloride supplementation (64 mmol daily) was associated with significantly higher peripheral insulin levels and improvement of peripheral glucose utilization (*Norbiato G et al. Effects of potassium supplementation* *on insulin binding and insulin action in human obesity: Protein-modified fast and refeeding. Europ J Clin Invest 44:414-9, 1984).*

Glucose administration may provoke hyperkalemia.

Experimental Study: 7/13 diabetics had a history of spontaneous hyperkalemia which could be provoked by oral glucose administration, and plasma aldosterone concentration was decreased in all 13. Abnormalities of potassium homeostasis are probably related to insulin and mineralocorticoid deficiency. Diabetic pts. with hypoaldosteronism have the potential for severe hyperkalemia should renal or extrarenal mechanisms for potassium homeostasis be challenged by severe acidosis, diminished renal function, marked hyperglycemia, or administration of potassium salts or potassium-sparing diuretics (*Perez GO et al. Potassium homeostasis in chronic diabetes mellitus. Arch Intern Med 137(8):1018-22, 1977).*

Zinc:
(G)

May be malabsorbed from the gut (*Kinlaw WB et al. Abnormal zinc metabolism in type II diabetes mellitus. Am J Med 75(2):273-77, 1983).*

Tissue levels may be depressed (*Sjogren A et al. Magnesium, potassium and zinc deficiency in subjects with type II diabetes mellitus. Acta Med Scand 224:461-63, 1988).*

Plasma, lymphocyte, granulocyte and platelet zinc may be depressed (*Pai LH, Prasad A. Cellular zinc in patients with diabetes mellitus. Nutr Res 8(8):889-98, 1988).*

Serum zinc may be elevated and may correlate with insulin levels, possibly reflecting a deficient storage or a chronic hypersecretion of insulin in hyperglycemic patients (*Mateo MC et al. Serum zinc, copper and insulin in diabetes mellitus. Biomedicine 29(2):56-58, 1978).*

Urinary zinc may be elevated (*Kinlaw WB et al. Abnormal zinc metabolism in type II diabetes mellitus. Am J Med 75(2):273-77, 1983; Sjogren A et al. Magnesium, potassium and zinc deficiency in subjects with type II diabetes mellitus. Acta Med Scand 224:461-63, 1988).*

Deficiency may adversely affect carbohydrate and fat metabolism even when serum levels are normal.

Experimental Study (G): 6 non-diabetic young men were alternately fed diets containing either 16.5 or 5.5 mg zinc. While serum zinc was unchanged, the low zinc diet was associated with a significant increase in fasting blood glucose and a significant increase in the percent of total fatty acids as arachidonic acid. Results suggest that a low zinc intake mildly alters carbohydrate and fat metabolism before a change in serum zinc is evident (*Solomon SJ, King JC. Effect of low zinc intake on carbohydate and fat metabolism in men. Fed Proc 42:391, 1983).*

– –

OTHER NUTRITIONAL FACTORS

Bioflavonoids:
(A,G,N,R)

Administration may enhance insulin secretion (*Hii CST, Howell SL. Effect of flavonoids on insulin secretion and $^{45}Ca^{2+}$ handling in rat islets of Langerhans. J Endocrinol 107(1):1-8, 1985).*

Administration of certain "capillary active" bioflavonoids such as rutin or quercetin will prevent vitamin C from being oxidized in the jejunum to dehydroascorbic acid which is damaging to capillary endothelial cells (*see "Vitamin C" above*) (*Clemetson AB. Ascorbic acid and diabetes mellitus. Med Hypotheses 2:193-4, 1976; Clemetson AB, Anderson L. Plant polyphenols as antioxidants for ascorbic acid. Ann N Y Acad Sci 136:339, 1966).*

Administration may strengthen capillary basement membranes (*see "VASCULAR FRAGILITY"*).

Administration may decrease blood flow resistance and reduce stasis and resulting ischemia.

Experimental Study (A): 18 pts. received Daflon 500 mg 6 tablets daily. After 28 days, there was a decrease of blood viscosity and a better RBC disaggregability process under shear (*Lacombe C et al. Hemorheological improvement after Daflon 500 mg treatment in diabetes. Int Angiol 7(2 Suppl):21-24, 1988*).

Certain flavonoids such as quercetin and naringin (found in the flowers, fruit and rind of grapefruit) have been shown to inhibit aldose reductase, an enzyme involved in the synthesis of sorbitol from glucose (*Humber LG. The medicinal chemistry of aldose reductase inhibitors. Prog Med Chem 24:299-343, 1987; Varma SD. Inhibition of aldose reductase by flavonoids: Possible attenuation of diabetic complications. Prog Clin Biol Res 213:343-58, 1986*).

> *Note: Sorbitol is not easily transported in or out of cells and thus accumulates intracellularly, drawing water in by osmosis while low molecular weight compounds are lost in an attempt to maintain osmotic equilibrium. Diabetic animals have been shown to be unusually prone to accumulate sorbitol leading, possibly, to the development of cataracts, retinopathy, neuropathy and other complications (Cogan DG et al. Aldose reductase and complications of diabetes. Ann Intern Med 101:82-91, 1984).*

> *Note: The potential for aldose reductase inhibitors is illustrated by Sorbinil, a drug known to be a potent aldose reductase inhibitor. When Sorbinil was given to 11 diabetics with neuropathy unresponsive to numerous drugs in a placebo-controlled study, 8/11 pts. noted moderate to marked relief, usually starting the 3rd or 4th day. Each of the 4 who also had amyotrophy had improvement in pain and mild to moderate improvement in muscle strength which was confirmed by tests of autonomic nerve function and nerve conduction velocity (Jaspan J et al. Treatment of severely painful diabetic neuropathy with an aldose reductase inhibitor: Relief of pain and improved somatic and autonomic nerve function. Lancet 2:758-62, 1983).*

Animal Experimental Study: Oral quercitin given to diabetic rodents resulted in a significant decrease in sorbitol accumulation in lens tissue and, when given continuously, in a delay in the onset of cataracts (*Varma SD et al. Diabetic cataracts and flavonoids. Science 195:205-06, 1977*).

Biotin:
(G,N)

May work both synergistically with insulin and independently in lowering blood glucose levels.

Experimental Placebo-controlled Study (G): Pts. with insulin-dependent DM were removed from insulin therapy and treated with biotin 16 mg daily or placebo for 1 week. Fasting blood sugar levels fell significantly in pts. on biotin, while they rose as expected in pts. on placebo. Since biotin levels are typically elevated in diabetics, the authors speculate that it may be abnormally bound and/or biologically unavailable (*Coggeshall JC et al. Biotin status and plasma glucose in diabetics. Ann N Y Acad Sci 447:389-92, 1985*).

Supplementation may be beneficial in diabetic peripheral neuropathy.

Experimental Study (N): High doses of biotin by injection were given for 1-2 yrs. to 3 pts. with severe peripheral neuropathy. Within 4-8 wks. there was a marked improvement in clinical and lab findings. The authors speculate that, in diabetes, biotin may be deficient, inactive or unavailable causing disordered activity of pyruvate carboxylase which is biotin-dependent. This would lead to accumulation of pyruvate and/or depletion of aspartate, both of which play an important role in nervous system metabolism (*Koutsikos D, Agroyannis B, Tzanatos-Exarchou H. Biotin for diabetic peripheral neuropathy. Biomed Pharmacother 44(10):511-14, 1990*).

Coenzyme Q_{10}: (ubiquinone)
(G)

Blood levels may be reduced (*Kishi T et al. Bioenergetics in clinical medicine. XI. Studies on coenzyme Q and diabetes mellitus. J Med 7:307, 1976*).

Supplementation may be beneficial.

Experimental Study (G): 15 diabetics received CoQ10 60 mg daily. After 3 mo., insulin synthesis and secretion was promoted and blood sugar control was facilitated (*Shimura Y, Hogimoto S. Jpn J Clin Exp Med 58:1349-532, 1981*) (*in Japanese*).

Experimental Study (G): For 20 pts. undergoing initial treatment, CoQ10 administration stimulated insulin synthesis and peripheral glucose utilization (*Kihara A et al. Diagnosis Treatm 66:2327-32, 1978*) (*in Japanese*).

Experimental Study (G): 39 stable diabetics received 120 mg CoQ7 [interchangeable in the body for CoQ10] daily for 2-18 weeks. Fasting blood sugar was reduced by at least 20% in 12/39 pts (36%) and by at least 30% in 12/39 pts. (31%), while ketone bodies fell by at least 30% in 13/22 pts. (59%) (*Shigeta Y et al. Effect of coenzyme Q7 treatment on blood sugar and ketone bodies of diabetics. J Vitaminol 12:293, 1966*).

Glutathione:

A tripeptide composed of the amino acids cysteine, glutamic acid and glycine.

Reduces dehydroascorbic acid to vitamin C in red blood cells. Frequently low in diabetics which may be a cause of increased levels of dehydroascorbic acid (*Banerjee S. Physiological role of dehydroascorbic acid. Indian J Physiol Pharmacol 21(2):85-93, 1977*) which is thought to have destructive effects (*See "Vitamin C" above*).

Inositol:
(N)

May be decreased in peripheral nerves (*Greene DA et al. Correction of myo-inositol depletion in diabetic human sural nerve by treatment with an aldose reductase inhibitor. Abstract. Diabetes 36(Suppl 1):86A, 1987; Mayhew JA et al. Free and lipid inositol, sorbitol and sugars in sciatic nerve obtained post-mortem from diabetic and control subjects. Diabetologia 24:13-15, 1983*).

> **Negative Observational Study (N):** Compared to controls, mean sural nerve levels of *myo*-inositol were not decreased in diabetics, with or without neuropathy, and were not associated with any of the neuropathological end-points of diabetes (*Dyck PJ et al. Nerve glucose, fructose, sorbitol, myo-inositol, and fiber degeneration and regeneration in diabetic neuropathy. N Engl J Med 319(9):542-48, 1988*).

Supplementation has been associated with improvement in neuropathy, perhaps because sorbitol accumulation (and the resulting adverse effects upon peripheral nerves) may be a direct effect of *myo*-inositol loss (*Greene DA et al. Are disturbances of sorbitol, phosphoinositide, and Na$^+$-K$^+$-ATPase regulation involved in pathogenesis of diabetic neuropathy? Diabetes 37(6):688-93, 1988; Wuarin-Bierman L, Zahnd GR. Current aspects of research on the pathogenesis of diabetic neuropathy. Diabete Metab 12(6):319-24, 1986*).

> *Note: Inositol content of foods is analyzed in: Clements RS Jr, Darnell B. Myo-inositol content of common foods: Development of a high-myo-inositol diet. Am J Clin Nutr 33:1954-1967, 1980*

Negative Experimental Study (N): 5 pts. and 3 non-diabetics received *myo*-inositol 20 g/d (40x the normal dietary amt.). After 14 days, peripheral nerve function as measured by motor conduction velocity and resistance to ischemia was unchanged (*Arendrup K et al. High-dose dietary myo-inositol supplementation does not alter the ischaemia phenomenon in human diabetics. Acta Neurol Scand 80(2):99-102, 1989*).

Negative Experimental Double-blind Study (N): 28 young diabetics (whose neurophysiological parameters most frequently showed values in the lower normal range or just below) received either inositol 6 gm daily or placebo. After 2 mo., there were no differences in vibratory perception threshold, motor and sensory conduction velocity or amplitude of nerve potential, and muscle tissue *myo*-inositol levels were unchanged (*Gregersen G et al. Oral supplementation of myoinositol: Effects on peripheral nerve function in human diabetics and on the concentration in plasma, erythrocytes, urine and muscle tissue in human diabetics and normals. Acta Neurol Scand 67:164-72, 1983*).

Experimental Study (N): 20 pts. with diabetic neuropathy demonstrated significant improvement in sensory nerve function after the total mean daily *myo*-inositol intake was increased from 772 to 1648 mg (*Clements RS Jr et al. Dietary myo-inositol intake and peripheral nerve function in diabetic neuropathy. Metabolism 28:477, 1979*).

Experimental Study (N): 7 pts. supplemented with *myo*-inositol 500 mg twice daily for 2 wks. demonstrated substantial increases in the amplitude of evoked nerve action potentials but no significant changes in the conduction velocities (*Salway JG et al. Effect of myo-inositol on peripheral-nerve function in diabetes. Lancet 2:1282-84, 1978*).

Omega-3 Fatty Acids:
(G)

Most important member: Eicosapentaenoic acid (EPA) which is particularly high in cold water fish. Available in a refined form as "MaxEPA" (18% EPA).

Suggested MaxEPA dosage: 3 - 9 grams daily in divided doses (or 10 ml. concentrate twice daily)

WARNINGS:

1. In type I diabetes, supplementation with MaxEPA may increase total cholesterol (*Haines AP et al. Effects of a fish oil supplement on platelet function, heamostatic variables and albuminuria in insulin-dependent diabetics. Thromb Res 43:643-55, 1986; Vandongen R et al. Hypercholesterolaemic effect of fish oil in insulin-dependent diabetic patients. Med J Aust 148:141-43, 1988*).

> *Note: MaxEPA contains 30% saturated fats compared to cod liver oil, which is also rich in omega-3 fatty acids, which only contains 15% saturated fats and may lower LDL cholesterol in type I diabetics (Jensen T et al. Partial normalization by dietary cod-liver oil of increased microvascular albumin leakage in patients with insulin-dependent diabetes and albuminuria. N Engl J Med 321:1572-77, 1989*).

2. In type II diabetes, supplementation may impair insulin secretion and elevate basal hepatic glucose output (*Friday KE et al. Omega-3 fatty acid supplementation has discordant effects on plasma glucose and lipoporteins in type II diabetes. Abstract. Diabetes 36(Suppl 1):12A, 1987; Glauber H et al. Adverse metabolic effect of omega-3 fatty acids in non-insulin-dependent diabetes mellitus. Ann Intern Med 108(5):663-68, 1988; Hendra T et al. Effects of fish oil supplements in NIDDM subjects. Diab Care 13:821-29, 1990*).

3. Supplementation may require additional vitamin E intake to prevent increased membrane peroxidation and cellular damage (*Laganiere S, Fernandes G. High peroxidizability of subcellular membrane induced by high fish oil diet is reversed by vitamin E. Clin Res 35:A565, 1987*).

Supplementation may decrease insulin resistance in type II diabetics (*Popp-Snijders C et al. Dietary supplementation of omega-3 polyunsaturated fatty acids improves insulin sensitivity in non-insulin-dependent diabetics. Diabetes Res 4:141-47, 1987; Popp-Snijders C et al. Dietary supplementation of omega-3 fatty acids improve insulin sensitivity in non-insulin dependent diabetes. Neth J Med 28:531-32, 1985*).

Supplementation may improve the lipoprotein profile.

Experimental Double-blind Crossover Study: 18 type I diabetics received cod-liver-oil (rich in omega-3 fatty acids) or olive-oil (rich in oleic acid) supplementation. After 8 wks. on cod liver oil, the plasma concentration of HDL cholesterol increased and the concentrations of VLDL cholesterol and triglycerides decreased (p<0.05 for all comparisons), but the level of LDL cholesterol did not change. In contrast, during supplementation with olive oil, the concentration of LDL cholesterol decreased and the levels of VLDL cholesterol and triglyceride increased (p<0.05 for all comparisons), but there was no change in the level of HDL cholesterol (*Jensen T et al. Partial normalization by dietary cod-liver oil of increased microvascular albumin leakage in patients with insulin-dependent diabetes and albuminuria. N Engl J Med 321:1572-77, 1989*).

Experimental Study: Type II diabetics received 8 gm ω-3 fatty acids daily. After 8 wks., total cholesterol decreased by 11%, VLDL decreased by 51%, and triglycerides decreased by 33% (*Friday KE et al. Omega-3 fatty acid supplementation has discordant effects on plasma glucose and lipoproteins in type II diabetes. Abstract. Diabetes 36(Suppl 1):12A, 1987*).

Supplementation may increase RBC membrane fluidity, thus potentially reducing symptoms due to impaired red cell deformability (such as intermittent claudication).

Experimental Controlled Study: Dietary sardine oil 2.7 gm daily was given to diabetic and control subjects. Compared to controls, RBC membrane fluidity was lower in the diabetics prior to supplementation. After 4 wks., membrane fluidity was increased in both diabetics and controls, and remained elevated for the entire 8 wk. study, with disappearance of the difference in RBC membrane fluidity between diabetics and controls (*Kamada T et al. Dietary sardine oil increases erythrocyte membrane fluidity in diabetic patients. Diabetes 35:604-11, 1986*).

Supplementation may partially normalize increased microvascular albumin leakage and reduce blood pressure in type I diabetics with albuminuria.

Experimental Double-blind Crossover Study: 18 type I diabetics received cod-liver-oil (rich in omega-3 fatty acids) or olive-oil (rich in oleic acid) supplementation. After 8 wks., the mean transcapillary escape rate of albumin significantly decreased (P<0.01), and the BP significantly decreased (p<0.05) when pts. received cod liver oil but not when they received olive oil. There was no correlation, however, between cod liver oil's effect on the trans-capillary escape rate of albumin and its effect on BP (*Jensen T et al. Partial normalization by dietary cod-liver oil of increased microvascular albumin leakage in patients with insulin-dependent diabetes and albuminuria. N Engl J Med 321:1572-77, 1989*).

Omega-6 Fatty Acids:
(A,G,M,N)

linoleic acid → gammalinolenic acid → DGLA → PGE_1

High linoleic acid diet is associated with decreased progression of microangiopathy and cardiac ischemia.

Experimental Controlled Study (A,M): Half of a gp. of 102 newly diagnosed diabetics were placed on a normal Western diet while the rest were placed on a linoleic acid enriched diet. After 5 yrs., 3 males in the normal diet gp. but none in the linoleic acid gp. had died of MI. Of the survivors, 6% of males and 4% of females in the linoleic acid gp. had cardiac ischemia vs. 22% of males and 16% of females in the control group. The incidence of microangiopathy was also significantly lower in the linoleic acid gp. (27% of males and 32% of females vs. 62% of males and 55% of females) (*Houtsmuller AJ et al. Favourable influences of linoleic acid on the progression of diabetic micro and macroangiopathy. Nutr Metab 24 (Supp. 1):105-18, 1980*).

High linoleic acid diet is associated with a less atherogenic lipoprotein profile.

Experimental Crossover Study: 14 pts. with noninsulin-dependent DM alternately received a diet with a low polyunsaturated to saturated fat ratio (P:S 0.3) and one with a P:S of 1.0. After 30 wks. on the high P:S diet, total and LDL-cholesterol declined by 7.6% (p<0.01) and 9.8% (p<0.01), respectively. VLDL- HDL2-, and HDL3-cholesterol were not affected (*Heine RJ et al. Linoleic-acid-enriched diet: long-term effects on serum lipoprotein and apolipoprotein concentrations and insulin sensitivity in noninsulin-dependent diabetic patients. Am J Clin Nutr 49:448-56, 1989*).

Prostaglandin E_1 (PGE_1), which is derived from linoleic acid, has insulin-like actions and potentiates insulin effects (*Haessler HA, Crawford JD. Insulin-like inhibition of lipolysis and stimulation of lipo-genesis by prostaglandin E1. J Clin Invest 46:1065-70, 1967*).

The first step in the conversion of linoleic acid to PGE_1 requires delta-6-desaturase, an enzyme whose activity may be inhibited in diabetes, as suggested by animal models (*Mercuri O et al. Depression of microsomal desaturation of linoleic to gamma-linolenic acid in the alloxan-diabetic rat. Biochim Biophys Acta 116:409-11, 1966*).

Administration of evening primrose oil, which is high in the PGE_1 precursor gamma linolenic acid (the compound formed by the action of delta-6-desaturase on linoleic acid), may benefit diabetic neuropathy.

Experimental Double-blind Study (N): 22 pts. whose neuropathy was demonstrated both clinically and by nerve function tests received either evening primrose oil 4 gm daily or placebo. After 6 mo., all 8 neurophysiologic variables tested (including motor and sensory nerve function, and cutaneous sensitivity to cold and hot stimuli) improved in the EPO gp., but worsened in the placebo gp. (p<0.001) (*Jamal GA et al. Treatment of diabetic neuropathy with gamma-linolenic acid (GLA) as everning primrose oil (Efamol). J Am Coll Nutr 6:86, 1987; Jamal GA et al. Gamma-linolenic acid in diabetic neuropathy. Lancet 1:1098, 1986*).

<u>Pyridoxine Alpha-ketoglutarate (PAK)</u>:
(G)

Administration may improve glycoregulation.

Experimental Double-blind Study (G): A gp. of 30 insulin-treated type I diabetics and a gp. of 30 phenformin-treated type II diabetics were each randomly divided into 2 sub-groups. Half of each gp. received PAK 600 mg 3 times daily, while half received placebo. After 4 wks., both gps. receiving PAK showed significant decreases in fasting glucose, glycosylated hemoglobin, lactate and pyruvate compared to pre-treatment levels. All values returned to pre-treatment levels within 3 wks. of discontinuing PAK. There were no side-effects or abnormalities in CBC, liver enzymes or BUN. Results suggested that PAK "potentiated the effects of insulin and phenformin" (*Passariello N et al. Effects of pyridoxine alpha-ketoglutarate on blood glucose and lactate in type I and type II diabetics. <u>Int J Clin Pharmacol Ther Toxicol</u> 21:252-56, 1983*).

_ _

COMBINED NUTRITIONAL SUPPLEMENTATION

<u>Vitamin A</u>,
<u>Vitamin C</u>,
<u>Vitamin E</u>, and
<u>Selenium</u>:
(R)

Combined supplementation may benefit <u>retinopathy</u>.

Experimental Study (R): 19/20 pts. with diabetic retinal changes had improvement or no progression of retinopathy for several yrs. while receiving a high-dose antioxidant regimen providing 500 μg selenium, 800 IU vitamin E, 1 gm vitamin C, and 10,000 IU vitamin A daily (*Crary EJ, Mc Carty MF. Potential clinical applications for high-dose nutritional antioxidants. <u>Med Hypotheses</u> 13:77-98, 1984*).

_ _

OTHER FACTORS

Rule out <u>hydrochloric acid deficiency</u>.

Note: While gastric anacidity had been reported in the past to be a relatively common condition which was associated with a number of illnesses, the presence of achlorhydria is no longer accepted unless a potent parietal-cell stimulant (such as histamine) is employed in gastric analysis. More recent studies suggest that histamine-fast anacidity is uncommon before the fifth decade of life and, although it probably does not occur in a normal stomach, its presence is not necessarily associated with symptoms (Rappaport EM. Achlorhydria: Associated symptoms and response to hydrochloric acid. <u>N Engl J Med</u> 252(19):802-5, 1955).

Experimental Controlled Study: Vagal response to feeding was evaluated in 17 insulin-dependent diabetics, 24 post-vagotomy pts. and 10 normals. Compared to normals, diabetics both with and without neuropathy had a decreased acid secretion and delayed gastric emptying following sham feeding similar to vagotomized patients. This was not due to hyperglycemia, since 3 pts. given IV insulin during sham feeding showed the same abnormality. (*Richardson CT et al. Diabetics have reduced acid secretion and delayed digestion. <u>Am Family Physician</u> June, 1978, p. 143*).

Observational Study: Gastric acid output in response to insulin-produced hypoglycemia and pentagastrin was measured in 18 diabetic pts. with autonomic neuropathy. 2/18 were achlorhydric while the rest responded normally to pentagastrin. 10/16 of these pts., however, had low acid output evoked by insulin-induced hypoglycemia. Results suggest that vagal impairment is common in diabetics with autonomic symptoms (*Hosking DJ et al. Vagal impairment of gastric secretion in diabetic autonomic neuropathy. <u>Br Med J</u> June 14, 1975, pp. 588-90*).

Observational Study: 50 pts. under age 40 and 50 pts. ages 40 and older were randomly selected from a gp. in whom gastric analysis had been performed. 18% of the younger gp. and 64% of the older gp. were achlorhydric, an incidence considerably higher than that reported for normals. Of the 41/100 with achlorhydria, 11 (27%) were anemic compared to 3 (5.1%) of the 59 non-achlorhydric patients. Similarly, 7/41 with achlorhydria (17%) had neuritis vs. 2/59 (3%) of the non-achlorhydric patients. These differences suggest a causal association (*Rabinowich IM. Achlorhydria and its clinical significance in diabetes mellitus. Am J Dig Dis 16:322-32, 1949*).

Review Article: Based on a review of 8 studies, the ave. incidence of achlorhydria was 32.8% (*Joslin EP et al. The Treatment of Diabetes Mellitus, 8th Edition. Lea & Febiger, 1946*).

If deficient, supplementation with hydrochloric acid may benefit neuritis due to inadequate thiamine absorption.

Case Reports (N): 3 pts. with severe neuritis are described whose diabetes was under good control and who had failed to benefit from thiamine supplementation. After receiving hydrochloric acid supplementation, all showed marked improvement. An additional large gp. of cases showed similar results (*Rabinowich IM. Achlorhydria and its clinical significance in diabetes mellitus. Am J Dig Dis 16:322-32, 1949*).

Brewer's Yeast:
(G)

The richest known source of glucose tolerance factor (GTF) (*Mertz W. Effects and metabolism of glucose tolerance factor. Nutr Rev 33(5):129-35, 1975*).

Administration may improve glucose tolerance and lipid metabolism.

Experimental Single-blind Study (G): 24 elderly subjects (including 8 non-insulin-dependent diabetics) randomly received either chromium-rich brewer's yeast 9 gm daily or chromium-poor tortula yeast. After 8 wks., glucose tolerance, insulin sensitivity and total lipids improved only in the gp. receiving brewers' yeast (*Offenbacher E, Stunyer F. Beneficial effect of chromium-rich yeast on glucose tolerance and blood lipids in elderly patients. Diabetes 29:919-25, 1980*).

Chromium may not be essential to glucose tolerance factor.

In vitro Experimental Study: Fractions of extracts of brewer's yeast were purified. Although addition of chromium to the growth medium increased the yield of glucose tolerance factor, the purified substance contained no chromium and GTF activity was isolated in cationic and anionic small amino-acid or peptide-like molecules (*Davies DM et al. The isolation of glucose tolerance factors from brewer's yeast and their relationship to chromium. Biochem Med 33(3):297-311, 1985*).

In vitro Experimental Study: An insulin-enhancing factor was isolated from brewer's yeast grown on a chromium-containing medium. The active fraction was found to have little more than a background level of chromium, while the major chromium-containing fraction was found not to have insulin-enhancing activity (*Held DD et al. Isolation of a non-chromium insulin-enhancing factor from brewer's yeast. Fed Proc 43:472, 1984*).

DIARRHEA

See Also: CELIAC DISEASE
CONSTIPATION
IRRITABLE BOWEL SYNDROME

Diarrhea can be sub-divided into osmotic and secretory forms:

Osmotic diarrhea: The result of the accumulation of non-absorbale solutes in the gut lumen.

1. Ingestion of poorly absorbable solutes

> Examples: Magnesium sulfate, sodium sulfate, citrate-containing laxatives, some laxatives (such as $Mg(OH)_2$), mannitol, sorbitol

2. Maldigestion

3. Mucosal transport defects

Secretory diarrhea: The result of the effect of a secretory stimulus on the intestinal mucosa.

1. Inhibition of absorption

2. Secretion of water and electrolytes resulting in a net luminal gain.

Generally, osmotic diarrhea stops upon fasting or upon discontinuation of ingestion of the poorly absorbable solute, while secretory diarrhea persists despite fasting and the stools are larger in volume and more watery. For acute diarrhea, traveler's diarrhea, and some cases of chronic diarrhea, the most imporant aspect of therapy is prevention or correction of salt and water depletion (*Krejs GJ. Diarrhea, in JB Wyngaarden & LH Smith Jr., Eds. Cecil. Textbook of Medicine, 18th edition. Philadelphia, W. B. Saunders, 1988*).

- -

DIETARY FACTORS

Treat malnutrition to prevent persistent diarrhea.

> **Observational Study:** 756 Indian children were followed prospectively. Children who developed persistent diarrhea were compared with population controls and controls with acute diarrhea. The mean weight for age in the children with persistent diarrhea was significantly lower than that in the population controls and the diarrheal controls. Weight for age of $\leq 70\%$ was associated with persistent diarrhea in both case-control analyses, suggesting that prevention of malnutrition and intensive management of acute diarrhea in malnourished children should help reduce the risk of persistent diarrhea (*Bhandari N et al. Association of antecedent malnutrition with persistent diarrhoea: A case-control study. Br Med J 298:1284-87, 1989*).

Treat malnutrition to prevent growth retardation due to diarrhea.

> **Observational Study:** In a study of Colombian children, nutritional supplementation was shown to completely offset the negative effect of diarrheal disease on length (*Lutter CK et al. Nutritional supplementation: Effects on child stunting because of diarrhea. Am J Clin Nutr 50:1-8, 1989*).

High protein diet.

Chronic diarrhea may result in significant protein loss (*Gardner FH. Nutritional management of chronic diarrhea in adults. JAMA 180:147-52, 1962*).

Avoid caffeine.

Experimental Study: The administration of caffeine 75-300 mg (amts. contained in many beverages) resulted in striking net secretion in the jejunum which lasted at least 15 min. as well as net secretion in the ileum 35 min later. These patterns correlated best with the passage of the intestinal bolus of caffeine rather than plasma caffeine levels. Small intestinal transit times were unchanged, however. Results suggest that methylxanthine-induced small intestinal secretion may play a role in the symptoms experienced by some pts. with functional diarrhea (*Wald A et al. Effect of caffeine on the human small intestine. Gastroenterology 71(5):738-42, 1976*).

Avoid excess fiber.

May induce diarrhea (mushy to pasty stools) along with increased stool frequency, a sense of incomplete evacuation, and excess rectal gas (*Saibil F. Diarrhea due to fiber overload. Letter. N Engl J Med 320(9):599, 1989*).

Eat honey.

Consumption may be beneficial in treating acute bacterial diarrhea in children.

Experimental Controlled Study: 159 children with acute gastroenteritis were given electrolyte solutions containing sodium, potassium and chloride to drink, to which either glucose or honey was added. The time taken to recover from bacterial, but not non-bacterial, diarrhea was significantly shortened (p=0.026) when oral rehydration solutions containing honey were compared to solutions containing only glucose (*Haffejee IE, Moosa A. Honey in the treatment of infantile gastroenteritis. Br Med J 290:1866-67, 1985*).

- -

VITAMINS

Folic Acid:

Preferentially absorbed in the jejunum; thus any diarrheal problem associated with jejunal disorders will eventually need supplemental folic acid 5 mg daily (*Gardner FH. Nutritional management of chronic diarrhea in adults. JAMA 180:147-52, 1962*).

Supplementation may be beneficial.

Experimental Controlled Study: Half of 76 children aged 1-44 mo. admitted with acute diarrhea lasting <7 days were randomly given oral folate 5 mg every 8 hrs. until normal, formed stools were passed in addition to standard treatment. The mean recovery time in the folate gp. was significantly lower than in the controls (p<0.0001) (*Haffejee IE. Effect of oral folate on duration of acute infantile diarrhoea. Letter. Lancet 2:334-35, 1988*).

Experimental Study: 8 pts. with chronic diarrhea from diverse etiologies were treated with folic acid 40-60 mg daily with restoration of normal or almost normal stools in 2-5 days which reversed when folate was discontinued, suggesting that long-standing diarrhea is associated with the development of folate deficiency (*Carruthers LB. Chronic diarrhea treated with folic acid. Lancet 1:849-50, 1946*).

Niacin:

Diarrhea is common in pellagra.

Observational Study: 20/45 (44%) pts. with cutaneous pellagra had diarrhea. 42/45 showed inflammation on sigmoidoscopy, and rectal biopsies showed inflammation in all cases. Diarrhea stopped within one wk. of starting vitamin therapy in all cases (*Segal I et al. Rectal manifestations of pellagra. Int J Color Dis 1(4):238-43, 1986*).

Vitamin A:

May become deficient in children with persistent diarrhea (*Usha N et al. Early detection of vitamin A deficiency in children with persistent diarrhoea. Letter. Lancet 1:422, 1990*).

Vitamin B$_{12}$:

Chronic diarrhea associated with ileal lesions (blind loops, ileal resection, regional ileitis, etc.) may inhibit vitamin B$_{12}$ absorption due to bacterial interference. In addition, in the presence of steatorrhea, insoluble calcium soaps are formed, which prevents calcium from coupling with the vitamin for the purposes of transport across the mucosa (*Gardner FH. Nutritional management of chronic diarrhea in adults. JAMA 180:147-52, 1962*).

Vitamin C:

Chronic diarrhea depletes the body stores of ascorbic acid and may result in low plasma levels (*Gardner FH. Nutritional management of chronic diarrhea in adults. JAMA 180:147-52, 1962*).

Vitamin K:

Chronic diarrhea can cause a vitamin K deficiency which can be prevented by oral administration of vitamin K 2-10 mg daily (*Krejs GJ. Diarrhea, in JB Wyngaarden & LH Smith Jr., Eds. Cecil, Textbook of Medicine, 18th edition. Philadelphia, W. B. Saunders, 1988*).

- -

MINERALS

Bismuth:

Administration may be effective.

Review Article: Bismuth subsalicylate is effective prophylactically for traveler's diarrhea, and has shown modest efficacy in treating traveler's diarrhea and acute and chronic diarrhea in children. Neurological toxicity has been rare with bismuth subsalicylate and colloidal bismuth subcitrate. However, recent studies have demonstrated intestinal absorption of bismuth and sequestration in multiple tissue sites even over a 6-wk. period, suggesting that treatment periods with any bismuth-containing compound should last no longer than 6-8 wks. followed by 8-wk. bismuth-free intervals (*Gorbach SL. Bismuth therapy in gastrointestinal diseases. Gastroenterology 99(3):863-75, 1990*).

Copper:

Chronic diarrhea in children, especially when accompanied by malabsorption, is associated with lower copper levels. Hair determinations appear to be more sensitive than plasma values to changes in copper status (*Rodríguez A et al. Zinc and copper in hair and plasma of children with chronic diarrhea. Acta Paediatr Scand 74(5):770-74, 1985*).

Iron:

Chronic diarrhea associated with malabsorption will, over a period of years, deplete the body stores of iron, and treatment of anemia related to vitamin deficiencies will be incomplete unless iron stores are replaced (*Gardner FH. Nutritional management of chronic diarrhea in adults. JAMA 180:147-52, 1962*).

Magnesium:

Magnesium ingestion may induce diarrhea (*Fine KD, Santa Ana CA, Fordtran JS. Diagnosis of magnesium-induced diarrhea. N Engl J Med 324:1012-7, 1991*).

Diarrhea even for a few days in young children may cause magnesium deficiency. In adults it may arise in pts. with prolonged diarrhea from any cause. As oral magnesium salts are poorly absorbed and can cause diarrhea, a daily addition of 20-30 mmol magnesium (10 mmol/kg for children) to an IV infusion prevents deficiency (*Passmore R,*

Eastwood MA. Davidson and Passmore: Human Nutrition and Dietetics. Eighth Edition. Ediburgh, Churchill Livingstone, 1986).

Potassium:

Electrolyte losses often account for the listnessness, fatigue, and abdominal distension noted in chronic diarrhea. Potassium is probably the most important loss, reflecting tissue depletion rather than specific changes in the circulating plasma levels. The loss of potassium alters bowel motility, promotes anorexia, and thus introduces a cycle of further bowel distress. Supplemental potassium salts (ex.: KCl 3-6 gm daily) should be given (*Gardner FH. Nutritional management of chronic diarrhea in adults. JAMA 180:147-52, 1962*).

Sodium:

Sodium depletion, while not usually as serious as that of potassium, can occur with even moderate chronic diarrhea (*Gardner FH. Nutritional management of chronic diarrhea in adults. JAMA 180:147-52, 1962*).

Zinc:

Chronic diarrhea in children, especially when accompanied by malabsorption, is associated with lower zinc levels. Hair determinations appear to be more sensitive than plasma values to changes in their zinc status (*Rodríguez A et al. Zinc and copper in hair and plasma of children with chronic diarrhea. Acta Paediatr Scand 74(5):770-74, 1985*).

Supplementation may be beneficial in acute infantile diarrhea, especially if deficient.

Experimental Double-blind Study: 64 Bangladesh children aged 3-24 mo. with acute diarrhea randomly received zinc acetate 15mg/kg/d or placebo for 14 days. Compared to controls, the addition of zinc enabled a 25% increase in linear growth predominantly over the 4th to 9th wk. after presentation with acute diarrhea (*Behrens RH et al. Zinc supplementation during diarrhoea, a fortification against malnutrition? Letter. Lancet 336:442-43, 1990*).

Experimental Placebo-controlled Study: In a randomized trial, 50 infants with acute dehydrating diarrhea received oral zinc sulfate 20 mg twice daily or placebo following rehydration. While the diarrheal duration and frequency of the zinc-supplemented gp. were lower, the differences were not significant. However, when only pts. with relatively severe initial zinc depletion were considered, the diarrheal duration and frequency were significantly lower in the zinc-supplemented infants (*Sachdev HP et al. A controlled trial on utility of oral zinc supplementation in acute dehydrating diarrhea in infants. J Pediatr Gastroenterol Nutr 7(6):877-81, 1988*).

- -

OTHER NUTRITIONAL FACTORS

Omega-6 fatty acids:

In an *in vitro* study, linoleic acid inhibited adhesion of enteropathogenic E. coli (EPEC) to HEp-2 cells. As adhesion to these cells correlates with the attachment of EPEC to the intestinal mucosa, linoleic acid deficiency, primarily a condition of children, could increase susceptibility to EPEC diarrhea. Therefore supplementation of inadequate diets by a source of linoleic acid may prevent diarrhea due to colonization of the intestinal mucosa by EPEC (*Chart H, Said B, Rowe B. Linoleic acid adhesion of enteropathogenic Escherichia coli to HEp-2 cells. Letter. Lancet 338:126-7, 1991*).

- -

OTHER FACTORS

Rule out hydrochloric acid deficiency.

Experimental Study: Hydrochloric acid suplementation was effective in "gastrogenous" (i.e. achlorhydric) chronic diarrhea (*Bulletin Gen. de Therapeutique, Paris - abstracted in JAMA 39:55, 1902*).

Rule out <u>food sensitivities</u>.

General

Observational Study: Endoscopy of infants with colitis revealed patchy erythema with loss of visible vascularity and very occasional, mild, superficial ulceration. Histology revealed an excess of both mucosal eosinophils and IgE-containing cells, compatible with an IgE-mediated process. The main foods implicated were milk, soy and beef (*Jenkins HR et al. Food allergy: the major cause of infantile colitis. <u>Arch Dis Child</u> 59(4):326-9, 1984*).

Clinical Observations: Food allergy can be confused with the various symptoms of acute and chronic colitis. One pt. may develop constipation while another may develop diarrhea. Some of the most violent reactions are associated with acute diarrhea. For example, the eating of 2 Brazil nut meats produced a continuous diarrhea in one person for 4 days which was associated with a 15 lb. weight loss. As the intestinal irritability produced by the allergic reaction was such as to make the presence of any food particles irritating enough to flare the diarrhea, it was necessary to stop all food by mouth for 2 days to achieve remission. In another case, a similar reaction was induced by 2 bites of solid maple sugar (*Rinkel HJ et al. <u>Food Allergy</u>. Springfield, Illinois, Charles C. Thomas, 1951*).

Fruit Juice

Experimental Study: Diarrhea in 3/7 children aged 14-27 mo. with a 3-mo. history of chronic non-specific diarrhea remitted when fruit juice was eliminated (*Hyams JS et al. Carbohydrate malabsorption following fruit juice ingestion in young children. <u>Pediatrics</u> 82(1):64-68, 1988*).

Milk

Bahna SL, Heiner DC. <u>Allergies to Milk</u>. New York, Grune and Stratton, 1980

Gryboski JD. Gastrointestinal milk allergy in infants. <u>Pediatrics</u> 40:354, 1967

<u>Bacterial Cultures</u>:

<u>General</u>:

Review Article: Numerous studies both *in vivo* and *in vitro* indicate that Lactobacilli can compete with pathogenic species and displace them. Other bacterial species which may have a protective role include Lactobacillus casei, Streptococcus faecium and Bifidobacterium bifidum. These bacteria are thought to produce antimicrobial substances which inhibit the growth of pathogenic bacterial species and may ultimately be useful for both prevention and therapy of diarrhea (*Fernandes CF et al. Control of diarrhoea by Lactobacilli. <u>J Appl Nutr</u> 40(1):32-41, 1988*).

<u>Bifidobacterium</u>:

Administration may be beneficial for the treatment of pediatric diarrhea (*Hotta M et al. Clinical effects of Bifidobacterium preparations on pediatric intractable diarrhea. <u>Keio J Med</u> 36(3):298-314, 1987*

Administration of Bifidobacterium longum-containing yogurt may protect against erythromycin-induced diarrhea.

Experimental Single-blind Study: 10 healthy volunteers took erythromycin 1 gm orally twice daily for two 3-day study periods with a 3-wk. interval between them. Over each 3-day study period they took, together with erythromycin, 3 B. longum (BA) or 3 placebo yogurts daily in random order. Fecal weight, stool frequency, and abdominal complaints were significantly increased when erythromycin was given with placebo yogurt but not when BA yogurt was being taken (*Colombel JF et al. Yoghurt with bifidobacterium longum reduces erythromycin-induced gastrointestinal effects. Letter. <u>Lancet</u> 2:43, 1987*).

<u>Lactobacillus acidophilus</u>

Administration may be beneficial (*Speck ML. Lactobacilli as dietary supplements and manifestations of their functions in the intestines, in B Hallgren, Ed. <u>Nutrition and the Intestinal Flora</u>. Stockholm, Almqvist & Wiksell International, 1983:93-98*).

Experimental Study: Humans ingesting low-fat milk containing L. acidophilus demonstrated a significant reduction in the levels of intestinal E. coli which increased to presupplemental levels within 4 wks. after discontinuation (*Ayebo AD et al. Effect of feeding Lactobacillus acidophilus milk upon fecal flora and enzyme activity in humans. J Dairy Sci 62(Suppl 1):44, 1979*).

Experimental Controlled Study: The effects of L. acidophilus-containing yogurt and Neomycin-kaopectate as treatment of infantile diarrhea were compared using 45 infants aged 1-27 months. Those treated with yogurt recovered more rapidly (*Niv M et al. Yogurt in the treatment of infantile diarrhea. Clin Ped 2:407-11, 1963*)

Experimental Study: L. acidophilus was effective in treating both viral and antibiotic-produced diarrheas (*Beck C, Necheles H. Beneficial effects of administration of lactobacillus acidophilus in diarrhea and other intestinal disorders. Am J Gastroenterol 35:522-27, 1961*).

Experimental Study: L. acidophilus milk was more effective than antibiotics in treating infantile diarrhea (*Tomic-Karovic K et al. Der Lactobacillus Acidophilus in der Therapie bei Säuglingsdiarrhoen. Neue Oest Z Kinderheilk 6:1-7, 1961*).

- with Lactobacillus bulgaricus:

Administration may prevent ampicillin-related diarrhea.

Experimental Double-blind Study: 79 adult in-pts. randomly received 1 pkt. of L. acidophilus and L. bulgaricus (Lactinex) or placebo 4 times daily during the first 5 days of ampicillin therapy. Diarrhea occurred in 9/43 (21%) receiving placebo and in 3 (8.3%) pts. receiving Lactinex. This difference was not statistically significant (p=0.21). When the pts. with diarrhea unrelated to ampicillin were excluded (50%), the incidence of ampicillin-related diarrhea in the placebo gp. (14%) was significantly greater (p=0.03) than in the Lactinex gp. (0%) (*Gotz V et al. Prophylaxis against ampicillin-associated diarrhea with a lactobacillus preparation. Am J Hosp Pharm 36:754-57, 1979*).

Lactobacillus GG:

Administration may be beneficial.

Experimental Study: 5 pts. with relapsing C. difficile colitis received L. GG as a concentrate in 5 ml of skim milk (10^{10} viable bacteria). After 7-10 days, 4 pts. had a total remission and no further relapses, while the fifth relapsed after a 3-day remission, received metronidazole for 10 days followed by L. GG, and then had no further relapses (*Gorbach SL et al. Successful treatment of relapsing Clostridium difficile colitis with Lactobacillus GG. Letter. Lancet 2:1519, 1987*).

Streptococcus faecium:

Administration may be beneficial for enteritis and acute diarrhea (*Camarri E et al. A double-blind comparison of two different treatments for acute enteritis in adults. Chemotherapy 27:466-70, 1981; D'Appuzzo V, Salzberg R. Die behandlung der akuten diarrhoe in der padiatrie mit Streptococcus faecium: resultate einer doppelblindstudie. Ther Umsch 39:1033-35, 1982*

Streptococcus faecium SF68:

Administration may be beneficial, especially when diarrhea is due to pathogenic microorganisms (*Bruno F, Frigerio G. Eine neuartige moglichkeit zur behandlung der enteritis - Kontrollierte doppel-blindversuche mit dem stam SF68. Schweiz Rundsch Med/Prax 70:1717-20, 1981; Lewenstein A et al. Effect of Streptococcus faecium C-68, a new approach for the treatments of diarrheal diseases. Curr Ther Res 26:967-81, 1979*).

DUMPING SYNDROME

DIETARY FACTORS

Macronutrients:

Experimental Study: For 62 pts. with dumping syndrome after gastric resection, breakfast meals of carbohydrate and foods containing a mixture of carbohydrate and fat were more quickly evacuated from the gastric stump than protein meals. Doubling the amt. of fat in the mixture of carbohydrate and fat (up to 40 g) induced no significant deceleration in gastric stump evacuation; moreover, in some cases evacuation was accelerated. Mineral water ingested before breakfast significantly decelerated gastric stump evacuation after the protein breakfast but failed to affect evacuation after the other breakfasts (*Saakian AG et al. [Effect of different types of food loads on the rate of emptying of the gastric stump in patients with the dumping syndrome after gastric resection.] Vopr Pitan (5):18-21, 1988*).

High fiber diet.

- Guar Gum:

Experimental Double-blind Study: Guar gum 5 gm/meal prevented dumping syndrome and increased tolerance to foods not previously tolerated in 9/11 pts. (*Harju E, Larmi TKI. Efficacy of guar gum in preventing the dumping syndrome. J Parenter Enteral Nutr 7(5): 470-2, 1983*).

- Pectin:

Experimental Study: 12 pts. recovering from abdominal surgery developed characteristic G.I. distress and hypoglycemia after drinking a glucose solution. When 1/3 oz. pectin was added to the solution, gastric emptying time was prolonged to near normal in 6 pts., while in 5 the emptying time was slowed but not normalized. In all 11, blood glucose levels were more stable and symptoms were minimized (*Leeds AR et al. Pectin in the dumping syndrome: Reduction of symptoms and plasma volume changes. Lancet 1:1075-8, 1981*).

-Wheat Bran:

Experimental Study: 65 pts. with dumping syndrome after gastric resection were studied. The addition of 10-20 g of wheat bran to semolina porridge significantly (p<0.05) inhibited the rate of gastric stump and small intestine evacuation, and in 1/3 of pts. it reduced manifestations and duration of the syndrome (*Saakian AG et al. [Effects of wheat bran on the rate of gastric stump and small intestine evacuation in patients with dumping syndrome after stomach resection.] Vopr Pitan (5):18-21, 1990*).

- -

VITAMINS

Folic Acid:

Supplementation may be beneficial.

Case Report: 51 year-old male post-partial gastrectomy for pyloric stenosis resulting from duodenal ulcer presented with severe diarrhea and abdominal pain which failed to respond to standard treatments. X-rays showed that the stoma was functioning perfectly, although precipitately. Folic acid 5 mg orally twice daily was given. By the next day his stools were reduced from 8-14 daily to 4 and since the second day stools have been reduced to 2 formed stools daily although all medication has been discontinued (*Young C. Folic acid in dumping syndrome. Letter. Can Med Assoc J 65:72, 1951*).

DYSMENORRHEA

VITAMINS

Niacin:

Supplementation may be beneficial.

Experimental Study: About 90% of 80 pts. treated with niacin 100 mg twice daily and, during cramps, every 2-3 hrs. were relieved of menstrual cramps which had been severe enough to require bed rest, time-loss or heavy sedation. The effectiveness of niacin seemed to be enhanced by the addition of ascorbic acid 300 mg and rutin 60 mg daily, probably because, by improving capillary permeability, they enhanced the vasodilating effect of the niacin. Supplementation had to start at least 7-10 days prior to menses to be effective, and its benefits often remained for several months after discontinuation. The niacin dosage may be increased 50-100 mg or more, to maintain flushing with each dose, for maximum effect. A preliminary trial suggests that niacinamide may be as effective. Pts. were warned to expect flushing and/or itching and occasional slight dizziness 15 min. after taking niacin (*Hudgins AP. Vitamins P, C and niacin for dysmenorrhea therapy. West J Surg Gynecol 62:610-11, 1954*).

Experimental Study: 87.5% of 40 pts. were were relieved of menstrual cramps after starting supplementation with niacin 100 mg every morning and evening, and 100 mg every 2-3 hrs. during cramps. These pts. had no other procedures or conditions (pregnancy, conization of the cervix or other surgery) which could account for their relief (*Hudgins AP. Am Pract Digest Treat 3:892-3, 1952*).

Vitamin E:

Supplementation may be beneficial.

Experimental Study: Pts. with algomenorrhea studied while in pain were supplemented with vitamin E until an analgesic effect was reached; 9 pts. had resumption of pain following naloxone administration. Compared to baseline, beta-endorphin-like immunoreactivity was increased in 7 pts. studied 15 min. after vitamin E administration. There was evidence that the efficacy of vitamin E depended upon the pathogenesis of the algomenorrhea. In some pts. for whom vitamin E had a strong analgesic effect, naloxone failed to cause the pain to return (*Kryzhanovskiï GN et al. [Endogenous opioid system in the realization of the analgesic effect of alpha-tocopherol.] Biull Eksp Biol Med 105(2):148-50, 1988*).

Experimental Placebo-controlled Study: 100 young women (ages 18-21) with spasmotic dysmenorrhea received either alpha-tocopherol tablets 50 mg 3 times daily or placebo for 10 days premenstrually and for the next 4 days. After 2 cycles, 34/50 (68%) in the experimental gp. improved compared to 9/50 (18%) of the controls (*Butler EB, McKnight E. Vitamin E in the treatment of primary dysmenorrhoea. Lancet 1:844-7, 1955*).

- -

MINERALS

Iron:

Supplementation may be beneficial.

Experimental Single-blind Study: 12 pts. with primary dysmenorrhea, most of whom had iron-deficiency anemia, reported diminution or complete disappearance of menstrual pain following iron supplementation for the treatment of iron deficiency. They were not told in advance that iron supplementation might affect their menstrual pain (*Shafer N. Iron in the treatment of dysmenorrhea: A preliminary report. Curr Ther Res 7:365-6, 1965*).

Magnesium:

May be reduced (*Henrotte JG et al. Les variations de la magnesemie liee au sexe, leurs relations avec l'excitabilite et la fatigue. CR Soc Biol 167:843-47, 1973*).

Supplementation may be beneficial.

Experimental Double-blind Study: 21 pts. aged 16-42 with primary dysmenorrhea randomly received magnesium (Magnesiocard 3x5 mmol granulate) or placebo on the day preceding menstruation and on the first and second days of the menstrual cycle. After 6 cycles, compared to placebo, magnesium had only a slight effect on the first day of the cycle; on the second and third days it had a therapeutic effect on both back and lower abdominal pain. Pts. on magnesium also demonstrated a marked reduction in absences from work due to dysmenorrhea (*Fontana-Klaiber H, Hogg B. [Therapeutic effects of magnesium in dysmenorrhea.] Schweiz Rundsch Med Prax 79(16):491-4, 1990*).

Experimental Double-blind Study: 50 pts. with primary dysmenorrhea received magnesium (Mg 5-longoral, Artesan GmbH) or placebo. After 6 mo., 21/25 women in the experimental gp. improved. Magnesium treatment was associated with a reduction of prostaglandin F_2 alpha in menstrual blood to 45% of its baseline value, as compared to 90% of baseline in women treated with placebo; therefore, in addition to its direct muscle relaxant and vasodilatory effect, magnesium appears to inhibit the biosynthesis of PGF_2 alpha (*Seifert B et al. [Magnesium — a new therapeutic alternative in primary dysmenorrhea.] Zentralbl Gynakol 111(11):755-60, 1989*).

- with Vitamin B6:

Increases the influx of Mg^{++}, which has an antispasmotic effect, into the myometrial cell (*Abraham GE. Primary dysmenorrhea. Clin Obstet Gynecol 21(1):139-45, 1978*).

Combined supplementation may be beneficial.

Experimental Study: Pts. received aminoacid-chelated magnesium and pyridoxine 100 mg of each every 2 hrs. as needed during menses and 4 times daily throughout the cycle until RBC magnesium returned to normal (4.7-7 mg/100 ml). There was a progressive decrease in intensity and duration of menstrual cramps over 4-6 months (*Abraham GE. Primary dysmenorrhea. Clin Obstet Gynecol 21(1):139-45, 1978*).

OTHER NUTRITIONAL FACTORS

Essential fatty acids:

Administration of the E series prostaglanins may promote uterine relaxation (*Abraham GE. Primary dysmenorrhea. Clin Obstet Gynecol 21(1):139-45, 1978*).

Administration of natural sources of gamma-linolenic acid, precursor of prostaglandin E_1, such as evening primrose oil, may theoretically be beneficial; however, their efficacy has yet to be proven (*Rees MC. Human menstruation and eicosanoids. Reprod Fertil Dev 2(5):467-76, 1990*).

ECZEMA
(ATOPIC DERMATITIS)

VITAMINS

<u>Vitamin A</u>:

Supplementation may be beneficial.

      WARNING: High doses may be toxic and thus must be given under close medical supervision.

    Experimental Study: 10 children with chronic eczema received oral vitamin A palmitate 25,000-200,000 IU daily for 3-21 months. 3/9 who tolerated it showed some improvement and 6 had marked improvement with a decrease in skin dryness. There was no evidence of vitamin A toxicity (*Strosser AV, Nelson LS. Synthetic vitamin A in the treatment of eczema in children. <u>Ann Allergy</u> 10:703-4, 1952*).

<u>Vitamin C</u>:

Supplementation may be beneficial.

    Experimental Double-blind Crossover Study: 10 pts. with severe atopic dermatitis aged 3-21 randomly received 50-75 mg/kg of slow-release vitamin C and placebo in either order with a 2 wk. washout period in between. By 3 mo., treated pts. noted significant decreases in symptom scores. Treated pts. required half as many antibiotic courses for skin infections as those given placebo. Improvements in lymphocyte transformation and neutrophil chemotaxis were also seen, suggesting that vitamin C may act by boosting the immune response (*Kline, Glen, U. of California at San Francisco - reported in <u>Med World News</u>, April 24, 1989*).

- -

MINERALS

<u>Copper</u>:

Serum copper concentration may be elevated (*David TJ et al. Serum levels of trace metals in children with atopic eczma. <u>Br J Dermatol</u> 122(4):485-89, 1990*).

    Negative Observational Study: Compared to 19 controls, mean serum copper was not significantly different for 21 eczematous children aged 2-14 (*Di Toro R et al. Zinc and copper status of allergic children. <u>Acta Paediatr Scand</u> 76(4):612-17, 1987*).

Hair copper concentration may be elevated (*Di Toro R et al. Zinc and copper status of allergic children. <u>Acta Paediatr Scand</u> 76(4):612-17, 1987*).

<u>Iron</u>:

Serum ferritin (major iron storage protein), but not serum iron or iron-binding capacity, may be depressed (*David TJ et al. Serum levels of trace metals in children with atopic eczema. <u>Br J Dermatol</u> 122(4):485-89, 1990*).

<u>Selenium</u>:

The blood level of glutathione peroxidase, a sensitive indicator of its selenium content, may be reduced (*Juhlin L et al. Blood glutathione-peroxidase levels in skin diseases: Effect of selenium and vitamin E treatment. <u>Acta Derm Venereol (Stockh)</u> 62:211-14, 1982*).

Supplementation may be beneficial.

- with <u>vitamin E</u>:

Negative Experimental Double-blind Study: 60 pts. with atopic dermatitis were supplemented with selenium-enriched yeast. Gp. 1 took 600 µg of selenium alone, Gp. 2 took 600 µg selenium plus 600 IU of vitamin E and Gp. 3 took a placebo. After 12 wks., there was a significant increase in whole blood selenium and the activity of selenium-dependent glutathione peroxidase in platelets in Gps. 1 and 2 and the concentration of vitamin E in plasma in Gp. 2. However, there was no significant difference in the 3 gps. in the severity of the eczema or the concentration of selenium either before or after the 12 wks. of supplementation, suggesting that, although the supplement was absorbed and bioavailable, it did not enter the skin or produce a worthwhile improvement (*Fairris GM et al. The effect on atopic dermatitis of supplementation with selenium and vitamin E. <u>Acta Derm Venereol (Stockh)</u> 69(4):359-62, 1989*).

Experimental Study: 50/506 pts. with various skin disorders (including eczema and atopic dermatitis) and low glutathione peroxidase levels were treated with tablets containing 0.2 mg selenium as Na_2SeO_3 and 10 mg tocopheryl succinate. The clinical effect was encouraging and the glutathione peroxidase levels increased slowly over 6-8 weeks (*Juhlin L et al. Blood glutathione-peroxidase levels in skin diseases: Effect of selenium and vitamin E treatment. <u>Acta Derm Venereol (Stockh)</u> 62:211-14, 1982*).

<u>Zinc</u>:

Serum levels may be reduced (*David TJ et al. Low serum zinc in children with atopic eczema. <u>Br J Dermatol</u> 111(5):597-601, 1984; Endre L et al. [Incidence of food allergy and zinc deficiency in children treated for atopic dermatitis.] <u>Orv Hetil</u> 130(46):2465-69, 1989*).

Negative Observational Study: Compared to 112 controls, 134 children with atopic eczema showed no significant difference in serum zinc concentrations (*David TJ et al. Serum levels of trace metals in children with atopic ecezma. <u>Br J Dermatol</u> 122(4):485-89, 1990*).

Supplementation may be beneficial.

Clinical Observation: Out of 40 cases, supplementation with chelated zinc 50 mg 3 times daily [along with any other indicated nutritional treatments] was followed by full remission in all except one severe case which showed a partial response. Improvement may take up to 6 wks. and full remission from 3-8 mo. (*Wright JV. <u>Dr. Wright's Book of Nutritional Therapy</u>. Emmaus, Penn, Rodale Press, 1979*).

- -

OTHER NUTRITIONAL FACTORS

<u>Omega-3 Fatty Acids</u>:

Eicosapentaenoic acid (EPA) and docosahexaenoic acid (DHA).

Highest in cold water fish. Available in a refined form as "MaxEPA" (18% EPA).

Suggested MaxEPA dosage: 3 - 9 grams daily in divided doses (or 10 ml. concentrate twice daily)

WARNING: Supplementation may require additional vitamin E intake to prevent increased membrane peroxidation and cellular damage (*Laganiere S, Fernandes G. High peroxidizability of subcellular membrane induced by high fish oil diet is reversed by vitamin E. <u>Clin Res</u> 35:A565, 1987*).

Supplementation may be beneficial.

Experimental Double-blind Study: The diets of pts. were supplemented with 10 gm fish oil (1.8 gm EPA) or placebo. After 12 wks., the experimental gp. had reduced scaling, itching, and overall subjective severity of skin leions compared to controls. Improvement corresponded with changes in serum phospholipids indicative of an increased EPA intake (*Bjorneboe A et al. Effect of dietary supplementation with eicosapentaenoic acid in the treatment of atopic dermatitis. Br J Dermatol 117(4):463-69, 1987*).

Omega-6 Fatty Acids:

$$\text{linoleic acid} \rightarrow \text{GLA} \rightarrow \text{DGLA} \rightarrow \text{prostaglandin } E_1$$

Evening primrose oil is rich in GLA, the conversion of which from linoleic acid may be reduced in atopic eczema. (Suggested adult dosage: 2 gm twice daily.)

Observational Study: Compared to 22 controls, 25 mothers of children with atopic eczema had a significantly greater proportion of linoleic acid, and a smaller proportion of DGLA (derived from GLA), in their breast milk than the controls (*Wright S et al. Breast milk fatty acids in mothers of children with atopic eczema. Br J Nutr 62(3):693-98, 1989*).

Experimental Double-blind Study: 50 young adult pts. had variable but higher levels of linoleic acid and lower levels of LA metabolites than did healthy controls.   During administration of EPO, they showed no significant change in LA, a slight elevation in GLA, significant increases in DGLA and PGE₁ in the higher dose gps., and a significant increase in arachidonic acid when all gps. were considered together (*Manku MS et al. Reduced levels of prostaglandin precursors in the blood of atopic patients: Defective delta-6-desaturase function as a biochemical basis for atopy. Prostaglandins Leukotrienes Med. 9(6):615-28, 1982*).

Supplementation of omega-6 fatty acids may be beneficial.

Experimental Study: 179 pts. with moderate to severe atopic dermatitis which had required treatment with steroids more potent than 1% hydrocortisone for least 2 yrs. were treated with evening primrose oil (Epogram®, Scotia, England) 2 gm twice daily after meals while continuing on their regular medications. After a median of 11 mo., 111/179 (62%) were rated as improved. Most pts. began to respond within 12 wks. but a few required longer treatment. Many pts. were able to reduce or stop their medications and there were minimal side effects (*Stewart JCM et al. Treatment of severe and moderately severe atopic dermatitis with evening primrose oil (Epogram): A multi-centre study. J Nutr Med 2:9-15, 1991*).

Meta-analytic Study: The results of 9 placebo-controlled clinical studies, 4 of which were crossover studies, on the effects of EPO (Epogram) were reviewed.   In the parallel studies, both pt. and doctor scores showed a highly significant improvement over baseline (p<0.0001) due to EPO; for both scores the effect of EPO was significantly better than placebo.   Similar results were found in the crossover trials, although the difference between EPO and placebo in the doctors' global score failed to reach significance.   The effects on itch were particularly striking, as there was no placebo response, while there was a substantial and highly significant response to EPO (p<0.0001) (*Morse PF et al. Meta-analysis of placebo-controlled studies of the efficacy of Epogram in the treatment of atopic eczema: relationship between plasma essential fatty changes and treatment response. Br J Dermatol 121:75-90, 1989*).

Negative Experimental Double-blind Study: 123 pts. with moderately severe eczema randomly received either evening primrose oil 6-8 gm daily (adults) or 2-4 gm daily (children) or placebo. No significant benefits of EPO, as compared to placebo, were found, and plasma EFA levels failed to rise during treatment (*Bamford JT et al. Atopic eczema unresponsive to evening primrose oil (linoleic and gamma-linolenic acids). J Am Acad Dermatol 13:959-65, 1985*).

Note: This study has been criticized as, in both gps., plasma concentrations of DGLA, a marker for EPO treatment, increased, suggesting that somehow members of the placebo gp. may have received EPO (Horrobin DF, Stewart C. Evening primrose oil in atopic eczema. Letter. Lancet 1:864-65, 1990). In any event, patient compliance was extremely poor (Wright S. Essential fatty acids in clinical dermatology. J Nutr Med 1:301-13, 1990).

- -

OTHER FACTORS

Rule out food sensitivities.

Review Article: "Although the case remains unproved, when conventional management has not succeeded a place for dietary manipulation seems reasonable, but under careful supervision" (*Rubin P. Role of diet in treating atopic eczema. Editorial Comment. Br Med J 297:1459, 1988*).

Experimental Double-blind Study: 132 children with severe atopic dermatitis were evaluated for food hypersensitivity using double-blind placebo-controlled oral food challenges. 59% experienced at least one immediate hypersensitivity response. Definite diagnosis of food allergy and initiation of an appropriate elimination diet resulted in significant improvement in the majority of pts. with atopic dermatitis and food hypersensitivity (*Sampson HA. Food hypersensitivity as a pathogenic factor in atopic dermatitis. N Engl Reg Allergy Proc 7(6):511-19, 1986*).

Observational Study: GI permeability was investigated by measuring the relative urinary excretion rates of the inert di- and monosaccharides lactulose and rhamnose following their oral administration. 26 children with atopic eczema had a higher median lactulose/rhamnose ratio than a control gp. of 29 children who were either healthy or who had various noneczematous dermatoses. This increased permeability may be a primary abnormality of the gut or may reflect intestinal mucosal damage caused by local hypersensitivity reactions to food antigens (*Pike MG et al. Increased intestinal permeability in atopic eczema. Int J Dermatol 25(5):301-04, 1986*).

Observational Study: 35.7% of 56 adult pts. had serum antibodies against wheat gliadin and/or milk using ELISA, compared with 9.2% of the controls (p<0.0005), and 30.4% had IgG antibodies reactive with gliadin compared with 6.5% of the controls (p<0.0005), suggesting that antigen absorption from the gut may play a role in the pathogenesis of the disease (*Finn RA et al. Serum IgG antibodies to gliadin and other dietary antigens in adults with atopic eczema. Clin Exp Dermatol 10(3):222-28, 1985*).

Experimental Double-blind Study: 33 afflicted children underwent a 10 day elimination of allergic foods followed by food challenges. 35 challenges elicited symptoms, 31 of which involved the skin, 17 the gastrointestinal tract, 8 the nasal passages and 6 the respiratory tract within 10 - 90 minutes. All 60 placebo challenges were negative (*Sampson HA, Jolie PL. Increased plasma histamine concentrations after food challenges in children with atopic dermatitis. N Engl J Med 311:371-6, 1984*).

Experimental Double-blind Study: Over 50% of 26 afflicted children with high serum IgE levels developed cutaneous signs after food challenges (*Sampson HA. Role of immediate food sensitivity in the pathogenesis of atopic dermatitis. J Allergy Clin Immunol 71:473-80, 1983*).

Observational Study: Polyethylene glycol was used as a probe molecule to measure GI absorption which was found to be greater in pts. with known food allergy and/or eczema than in normals, suggesting either that abnormal food absorption precedes and causes eczema or that eczema also affects the GI tract causing increased absorption secondarily (*Jackson P et al. Intestinal permeability in patients with eczema and food allergy. Lancet 1:1285, 1981*).

Experimental Double-blind Crossover Study: 20/36 afflicted children completed a 12 wk. double-blind, crossover trial of an egg and cow's milk exclusion diet. 14 responded more favorably to the antigen-avoidance diet versus only 1 to the control diet. There was no correlation between positive prick test to egg and cow's milk antigen and response to the trial diet (*Atherton DJ et al. A double-blind crossover trial of an antigen-avoidance diet in atopic eczema. Lancet February 25, 1978 pp. 401-3*).

Rule out hydrochloric acid deficiency.

Note: While gastric anacidity had been reported in the past to be a relatively common condition which was associated with a number of illnesses, the presence of achlorhydria is no longer accepted unless a potent parietal-cell stimulant (such as histamine) is employed in gastric analysis. More recent studies suggest that histamine-fast anacidity is uncommon before the fifth decade of life and, although it probably does not occur in a normal stomach, its presence is not necessarily associated with symptoms (Rappaport EM. Achlorhydria: Associated symptoms and response to hydrochloric acid. N Engl J Med 252(19):802-5, 1955).

Experimental and Observational Study: Of 106 cases of subacute or chronic eczema which had resisted all forms of local treatment, 26 (25%) had no HCl and only 27 (26%) had normal HCl levels. The severity of the condition seemed to correlate with the extent of the HCl deficiency and also seemed to be associated with signs of B complex deficiency. Supplementation of HCl and vitamin B complex was followed by improvement in the HCl deficient patients (*Allison JR. The relation of deficiency of hydrochloric acid and vitamin B complex in certain skin diseases. South Med J 38:235-241, 1945*).

Observational Study: 11 pts. underwent a fractional gastric analysis following a routine Ewald test meal. Hypoacidity was defined as values for total and free acids of 1/2 normal or less, while hyperacidity was defined as values 10-15 points above normal or values which were relatively high at the start of the test. 8/11 (72%) of the pts. were found to have hypoacidity, while 2/11 (18%) had normal acid and 1/11 (9%) had hyperacidity. For 7/11 (63%) of the pts., the severity of the eruption correlated with both the presence of GI symptoms and abnormal gastric acid levels (*Ayers S. Gastric secretion in psoriasis, eczema and dermatitis herpetiformis. Arch Dermatol Syph 20:854-57, 1929*).

Case Report: A 52 year-old pt. with a 46 yr. history of eczema as well as a history of gas in the stomach and bowels for at least the past year presented with a red, lichenified face and a less severe eruption on the hand and thigh. The pt. was found to be deficient in hydrochloric acid and was treated with dilute HCl. For nearly 1 yr. the patient's skin condition has been practically normal (*Ayers S. Gastric secretion in psoriasis, eczema and dermatitis herpetiformis. Arch Dermatol Syph 20:854-57, 1929*).

EDEMA

(including CAPILLARY HYPERPERMEABILITY)

See Also: CARPAL TUNNEL SYNDROME
PREGNANCY AND ILLNESS
PREMENSTRUAL SYNDROME

DIETARY FACTORS

Eat adequate protein.

Protein deficiency is a known cause of edema.

In the presence of protein deficiency, excessive sodium or potassium intake is more likely to result in gross edema (*McGuire EA, Young VR. Nutritional edema in a rat model of protein deficiency. J Nutr 116(7):1209-24, 1986*).

Low salt diet. (70-90 meq of sodium daily)

Standard treatment for idiopathic edema (*Ponce P, Pello-Gomes E. [Idiopathic edema, tubular metabolism of water and sodium.] Acta Med Port 4(5):236-41, 1991*) (*in Portuguese*).

Fails to correct the physiologic defect in idiopathic edema of excessive sodium resorption in the proximal renal tubule (*Ponce P, Pello-Gomes E. [Idiopathic edema, tubular metabolism of water and sodium.] Acta Med Port 4(5):236-41, 1991*) (*in Portuguese*).

- -

VITAMINS

Vitamin B6:

May block the effect of estrogen upon sodium retention (*Edelstein B. The Woman Doctor's Medical Guide for Women. William Morrow and Co., 1982*).

Supplementation may be beneficial.

Case Report: A woman with a history of marked fluid retention during pregnancy continued to have moderate fluid retention following her last pregnancy despite sodium restriction and diuretics which was exacerbated by eating ham. She started supplementation with pyridoxine 25 mg daily and noted loss of ankle edema by the next day and a 10-pound weight loss after one week. She subsequently continued the B6 and the edema did not return (*Peterson M. Winning the water retention battle. Let's Live June, 1981, pp. 48-51*).

Vitamin E:

Supplementation may be beneficial.

Experimental Study: Capillary permeability was increased in human skin by using chemicals such as histamine, acetylcholine and α-chymotrypsin which was then reduced by the administration of α-tocopherol acetate 450 IU for 5-7 days (*Kamimura M. et al. Vitamins 28:129, 1961*).

- -

OTHER NUTRITIONAL FACTORS

Bioflavonoids :

Administration may reduce capillary permeability.

> **Review Article:** Edematous syndromes, both generalized and localized, due to capillary hyperpermeability, may be corrected by administration of vitamin "P" (bioflavonoids) (*Lagrue E, Behar A, Maurel A. [Edematous syndromes caused by capillary hyperpermeability. J Mal Vasc 1493):231-5, 1989) (in French).*

> **Experimental Study:** 13 diabetics with microcirculatory disorders received Daflon (micronized flavonoid fraction) 500 mg daily in addition to their regular treatments while 15 controls made no changes. At baseline, labelled albumin retention (a measure of capillary permeability) was abnormal in both groups. After 1 mo., it became normal in all but 1 of the treated pts., and that pt. improved, but remained abnormal in the controls. Treatment was withdrawn and, after 5.5 ± 1.0 mo., the test was again abnormal in both gps. (*Behar A et al. Capillary filtration and lymphatic resorption in diabetes. Int Angiol 8(4 Suppl):27-9, 1989*).

> **Book:** The benzopyrones (which include the flavonoids) control edema, reducing the swelling and pain associated with many diseases (*Casley-Smith JR & Casley-Smith JR. High-Protein Oedemas and the Benzo-Pyrones. Hagerstown, MD, J. B. Lippincott, 1986*).

> **Animal Experimental Study:** Various flavonoids were found to reduce capillary permeability in rabbits (*Paris R, Moury J. [Effects of diverse flavonoids upon capillary permeability.] Ann Pharm Franc 22:489-93, 1964*).

- Anthocyanosides:

Bilberry (Vaccinium myrtillus) is a rich source.

Administration of an extract may reduce capillary permeability.

> **Experimental Study:** Following oral administration of anthocyanosides, pts. with varicose veins and ulcerative dermatitis had a substantial drop in capillary leakage. Anthocyanosides were found to protect altered capillary walls by increasing the endothelium barrier-effect through stabilization of membrane phospholipids, and by increasing the biosynthetic processes of the acid mucopolysaccharides of the connective ground substance through restoration of the altered mucopolysaccharidic pericapillary sheath (*Mian E et al. [Anthocyanosides and the walls of microvessels: further aspects of the mechanism of action of their protective effect in syndromes due to abnormal capillary fragility.] Minerva Med 68(52):3565-81, 1977*).

> **Animal Experimental Study:** In rabbits and rats, a bilberry anthocyanosides preparation exhibited a vasoprotective effect by preventing chemically-induced increases in capillary permeability (*Lietti A. Studies on Vaccinium myrtillus anthocyanosides. I. Vasoprotective and anti-inflammatory activity. Arzneimittelforschung 26(5):829-32, 1976*).

- Hesperidin:

Deficiency is associated with altered capillary permeability and resistance, along with pain in the extremities marked by effort, debility and lassitude (*Scarborough H. Deficiency of vitamin C and vitamin P in man. Lancet 2:644, 1940*).

- with Vitamin C:

> Combined administration may be beneficial (*Beiler JM. Biochemistry of the synergists. Ascorbic acid and hesperidin. Exp Med Surg 12:563-69, 1955; Horoschak S. Clinical application of the synergists: ascorbic acid and hesperidin. Exp Med Surg 12:570, 1954; Martin GJ. Hesperidin and ascorbic acid: conclusions. Exp Med Surg 12:597, 1954*).

OTHER FACTORS

Rule out <u>food sensitivities</u>.

Clinical Observations: "I often recommend an empirical elimination diet from which common allergens (wheat, milk, eggs, corn, coffee, tea, alcohol, yeast, citrus, and sugar) are removed for several weeks. Although edema is usually not their primary complaint, many patients report a pronounced diuresis and loss of edema fluid during the first several days of the diet. Foods that cause a return of a patient's presenting symptoms often cause fluid retention as well" (*Gaby AR. Idiopathic edema: 'Overlooked' causes. Letter. <u>Hospital Pract</u> Feb. 15, 1986, p. 21*).

Clinical Observations: Edema is a very reliable and accurate index in detecting a food reaction which may cause the body to suddenly retain as much as 4 percent of its body weight as edema fluid. This weight is gained within 6-8 hrs. after ingesting the guilty food is ingested, and lost within 18-24 hrs. after the food is removed from the diet (*Brenerman JC. <u>Basics of Food Allergy</u>. Springfield, IL, Charles C. Thomas, 1978*).

EPILEPSY

DIETARY FACTORS

GENERAL

Review Article: Epileptic pts. should have normal, well-balanced meals at regular intervals, and children should not be allowed to take very large meals as these may predispose them to seizures (*Passmore R, Eastwood MA. Davidson and Passmore: Human Nutrition and Dietetics. Edinburgh, Churchill Livingstone, 1986:471*).

Avoid alcohol.

Review Article: Regular alcohol consumption can cause recurring seizures in otherwise normal people. They are usually only once or twice yearly. The degree of risk is directly related to the amt. of alcohol consumption and returns to normal once a person gives up alcohol. Alcohol withdrawal can also trigger seizures. These seizures are often multiple and occur 10-48 hrs. after discontinuing or reducing alcohol intake. Alcohol-provoked seizures are usually tonic-clonic seizures with a normal EEG and CT-scan. Pts. who have partial seizures usually have a history of brain damage, head trauma or stroke (*Baulac M, Laplane D. [Alcohol and epilepsy.] Rev Prat 40(4):307-11, 1990*) (in French).

Avoid caffeine.

Caffeine, a methylxanthine, is a stimulant and is proconvulsant (*Marangos PJ et al. The benzodiazepines and inosine antagonize caffeine-induced seizures. Psychopharmacology (Berlin) 72(3):269-73, 1981*).

Ketogenic (low-carbohydrate, high fat) diet:

WARNING: Introduction of this diet should be done during hospitalization.

WARNING: May cause hyperlipidemia, hypoglycemia, protein deficiency and kidney stones (*Herzberg GZ et al. Urolithiasis associated with the ketogenic diet. J Pediatr 117(5):743-5, 1990*).

Found to be particularly useful in the treatment of intractable absence-type epilepsy in children (*De Vivo DC. How to use other drugs (steroids) and the ketogenic diet, in PL Morselli, CE Pippenger, and JK Penry, Eds. Antiepileptic Drug Therapy in Pediatrics. New York, Raven Press, 1983:283-92*).

The diet is initiated by fasting the patient for 24-36 hours. A maximum of 1000 ml/24 h of fluid intake is allowed by water or low calorie drinks. The child is then placed on a high fat diet with a ratio of lipids to carbohydrates and proteins combined 4:1 by weight. In the medium chain triglyceride modification, a 50% MCT emulsion is prepared by liquidizing equal quantities of MCT oil and cold boiled water. When this diet is well tolerated, and if ketosis is being maintained, slow introduction of solid food can be initiated and gradually increased in amount over 4-6 days. Fluids should be restricted only if ketosis is unstable. If ketosis is inadequate and seizures are recorded, the diet needs further adjustments. Vomiting, diarrhea and abdominal pain are possible side effects (*Yutsis PI. Nutritional management of epilepsy in children, in P Yanick Jr, R Jaffe, Eds. Clinical Chemistry & Nutrition Guidebook: A Physician's Desk Reference. Volume One. T&H Publishing, 1988*).

Review Article: While ketogenic diets may be effective for the rare child whose seizures cannot be controlled by drugs, they are unhealthy for growing children (*R Passmore, MA Eastwood. Davidson and Passmore: Human Nutrition and Dietetics. Edinburgh, Churchill Livingstone, 1986:471*).

- -

VITAMINS

<u>Folic Acid</u>:

Total brain folate apparently is depleted following experimentally induced seizures, suggesting that folic acid metabolism is intimately involved in the epileptogenic process (*Smith DB, Obbens EAMT. Antifolate-antiepileptic relationships, in MI Botez, EH Reynolds, Eds. <u>Folic Acid in Neurology, Psychiatry, and Internal Medicine</u>. New York, Raven Press, 1979*).

Blood and cerebrospinal fluid folate levels are frequently reduced by certain anticonvulsants such as phenytoin, primidone and phenobarbital (*Smith DB, Obbens EAMT. Antifolate-antiepileptic relationships, in MI Botez, EH Reynolds, Eds. <u>Folic Acid in Neurology, Psychiatry, and Internal Medicine</u>. New York, Raven Press, 1979*). Low cerebrospinal fluid folate levels may be due to interference with the conversion of folate into a form which can pass the blood-brain barrier.

Experimental Study: While, with folate supplementation, low serum folate concentrations rose in pts. on anticonvulsants, low cerebrospinal fluid folate levels failed to rise (*Mattson R et al. Folate therapy in epilepsy. <u>Arch Neurol</u> 29:78, 1973*).

Supplementation may be beneficial.

WARNING: A number of uncontrolled studies suggest that folate supplementation may have an epileptogenic effect. Several controlled studies, however, have failed to confirm this observation, suggesting that such an effect is very rare (*Smith DB, Obbens EAMT. Antifolate-antiepileptic relationships, in MI Botez, EH Reynolds, Eds. <u>Folic Acid in Neurology, Psychiatry, and Internal Medicine</u>. New York, Raven Press, 1979*).

WARNING: Administration of folic acid supplements to pts. on anticonvulsants can result in a marked fall in serum vitamin B_{12} levels (*Hunter R et al. Effect of folic-acid supplement on serum-vitamin-B_{12} levels in patients on anticonvulsants. <u>Lancet</u> September 27, 1969*).

WARNING: Administration of folic acid supplements may lower serum barbiturate and anticonvulsant levels (*Mattson R et al. Folate therapy in epilepsy. <u>Arch Neurol</u> 29:78, 1973*).

Experimental Double-blind Study: Pts. on phenytoin supplemented with oral folate for a minimum of 1 yr. had a significant improvement in seizure frequency, although those given placebo also showed some improvement (*Givverd FB et al. The influence of folic acid on the frequency of epileptic attacks. <u>Eur J Clin Pharmacol</u> 19(1):57-60, 1981*).

Negative Experimental Study: Correction of serum folate deficiencies in epileptics on anticonvulsants failed to significantly alter seizure frequency or severity or psychological test performance (*Mattson R et al. Folate therapy in epilepsy. <u>Arch Neurol</u> 29:78, 1973*).

If blood levels are reduced, oral supplementation may prevent gingival hyperplasia from phenytoin.

Experimental Controlled Study: 23 children with DPH-treatment for >1 yr., and 8 children with short-term DPH treatment, were randomly assigned to gps. with and without daily supplementation of folic acid (folacin 5 mg). Despite DPH levels in many cases below the lower reference value, seizure control was good. Plasma and RBC folate levels were within or above the given reference values in all but 1 child. After 1 yr., there were no significant changes in the size of the gingival hyperplasias. However, 9 severely retarded DPH-treated adults whose serum DPH levels were above the higher reference values, and whose plasma and RBC folate levels were below the reference value, showed a significant reduction in the size of gingival hyperplasia following 1 yr. of folate supplementation. Seizure control was unchanged (*Bäckman N et al. Folate treatment of diphenylhydantoin-induced gingival hyperplasia. <u>Scand J Dent Res</u> 97(3):222-32, 1989*).

Topical application as a mouthwash may prevent gingival hyperplasia from phenytoin.

Experimental Blinded Study: 15 pts. with gingival hyperplasia received either folic acid 2 mg twice daily and a placebo mouthwash for 2 min. twice daily, placebo tablets and a folic acid mouth wash (5 ml with 1 mg folic acid/ml), or placebo tablets and placebo mouth wash. Over a 6-mo. period, the topical folic acid significantly inhibited gingival hyperplasia, while neither the oral folic acid or placebo gps. improved (*Drew HJ et al. Effect of folate on phenytoin hyperplasia. J Clin Periodontol 14:350, 1987*).

Niacin:

Supplementation may potentiate the effect of anticonvulsants.

Animal Experimental Study: Nicotinamide had an anticonvulsant effect in mice but was ineffective against maximal electroshock. At doses that were ineffective by themselves, it potentiated the anticonvulsant activity of phenobarbital without potentiating its toxicity (*Bourgeois BFD et al. Potentiation of the antiepileptic activity of phenobarbital by nicotinamide. Epilepsia 24:238-44, 1983*).

Clinical Observation: Several pts. were unable to achieve good control with anticonvulsants as the required dosages made them so drowsy and sluggish that they were unable to function normally. They were supplemented with vitamin B3 1 gram 3 times daily. After they were on the supplement for several mo., the anticonvulsant dose could be slowly reduced while monitoring carefully for an increase in seizure frequency (*Hoffer A. Niacin Therapy in Psychiatry. Springfield, Ill., Charles C. Thomas, 1962*).

Thiamine:

Deficiency may be associated with seizures.

Observational Study: 16 neurological pts. with diagnosed thiamine deficiency exhibited epileptic or epileptiform manifestations and produced irritative activity on EEG recordings which was attributable to the deficiency state. Results suggest that thiamine deficiency may provoke epileptic manifestations in pts. who have a subclinical predisposition to seizures (*Keyser A. Epileptic manifestations and vitamin B1 deficiency. Eur Neurol 31:121-5, 1991*).

Blood levels may be low - perhaps due to anticonvulsants (*Krause KH et al. B vitamins in epileptics. Biblthca Nutr Dieta 38:154-67, 1986*).

Vitamin B6:

Blood levels may be low - perhaps due to anticonvulsants (*Krause KH et al. B vitamins in epileptics. Bibl Nutr Dieta 38:154-67, 1986*).

Pyridoxine binds to glutamate decarboxylase which converts glutamic acid to the inhibitory neurotransmitter gamma-aminobutyric acid (GABA). Defective binding of pyridoxine may reduce GABA levels which reduces the seizure threshold. Large doses of pyridoxine compensate for the binding defect and should be considered in any infant with hard to control seizures (*Crowell GF, Roach ES. Pyridoxine-dependent seizures. Am Fam Physician 27(3):183-87, 1983*).

Deficiency is known to cause seizures in humans and experimental animals (*Coursin DB. Vitamin B6 and brain function in animals and man. Ann N Y Acad Sci 166:7-15, 1969*).

Experimental Study: 8 healthy young women were fed a defined formula diet almost devoid of vitamin B6. Within 12 days, 2 women exhibited abnormal EEG tracings which were rapidly reversed by repletion of vitamin B6 at the 0.5 mg/d level (*Kretsch MJ et al. Electroencephalographic changes and periodontal status during short-term vitamin B-6 depletion of young, nonpregnant women. Am J Clin Nutr 53:1266-74, 1991*).

If deficient, supplementation may be beneficial.

Case Report: Following supplementation with 200 mg pyridoxine daily which was raised to 300 mg daily after 1 mo., a female patient's RBC glutamic oxaloacetic transaminase (EGOT) rose from 34 units (deficient) to 68 units (normal) and seizure activity decreased from an ave. of 2.1 seizures per mo. to 0.5 seizures per month. During this time manganese rose from 2.6 to 5.8 ppb. After 7 mo. the pt. stopped pyridoxine and, 2 mo. later, she was averaging 6 seizures per month (*Sholer A, Pfeiffer CC. Vitamin B6 and the treatment of mental disease. Int Clin Nutr Rev 8(3), 1988*).

Vitamin D:

Anticonvulsant drugs interfere with vitamin D and calcium metabolism in some manner not well understood; serum calcitriol levels are normal, while calcifediol levels are depressed (*Flodin NW. Pharmacology of Micronutrients. New York, Alan R. Liss, Inc., 1988*).

Vitamin E:

Blood levels may be low - perhaps due to anticonvulsants (*Higashi A et al. Serum vitamin E concentration in patients with severe multiple handicaps treated with anticonvulsants. Paed Pharmacol 1:129-34, 1980; Ogunmekan AO. Plasma vitamin E levels in normal children and in epileptic children with and without anticonvulsant therapy. Trop Geog Med 37:175-77, 1985; Ogunmekan AO. Vitamin E deficiency in animals and man. Can J Neurol Sci 6:43-45, 1979*).

Patients may have increased lipid peroxidation products in the plasma which may be reduced with supplementation (*Kovalenko VM et al. [Alpha-tocopherol in the complex treatment of several forms of epilepsy.] Zh Neuropathol Psikhitv 6:892-97, 1984*).

Supplementation may reduce seizures.

Experimental Double-blind Study: Compared to age-matched controls, serum vitamin E levels were markedly reduced in epileptics on anticonvulsant medications. Pts. randomly received either 250 IU alpha tocopherol daily or placebo. After 9 mo., 2/3 of the adult pts. receiving vitamin E showed an 11% to a >50% reduction in seizures, while 2/6 children taking vitamin E improved (*Sullivan C et al. Seizures and natural vitamin E. Letter. Med J Aust 152:613-14, 1990*).

Experimental Double-blind Study: 24 epileptic children refractory to anticonvulsants received either D-alpha-tocopherol acetate (vitamin E 400 IU/d) or placebo in addition to their anticonvulsant medication. After 3 mo., there was a statistically significant improvement in seizure control in 10/12 (83.3%) of the experimental subjects (for whom seizure frequency was reduced by >60%) compared to none of the 12 controls. In 6 of the experimental pts., seizures were reduced 90-100% When pts. on placebo were switched to vitamin E, seizure frequency was reduced 70-100% in all of them. There were no side effects (*Ogunmekan AO, Hwang PA. A randomised double blind, placebo-controlled, clinical trial of D-alpha-tocopherol acetate (vitamin E) as add-on therapy for epilepsy in children. Epilepsia 30(1):84-89, 1989*).

Experimental Study: 18 children aged 5-12 with tonic-clonic generalized seizures (at least 6 per mo.) received vitamin E 400 mg daily in addition to their anti-epileptic drugs, the dosages of which were kept fixed. After 2 mo., 16/18 pts. had improved seizure control with a 50-75% reduction of seizures. The 16 who responded were on 1-2 anti-epileptic medications, had normal or mildly abnormal EEG changes, and normal mentation. The 2 non-responders were on 3 anti-epileptic drugs, had diffusely abnormal EEGs, and subnormal mentation. There were no side effects (*Ogunmekan AO. Is there a role for vitamin E therapy in epilepsy? Int Clin Nutr Rev 8(1):50-52, 1988*).

- -

MINERALS

Calcium:

Serum calcium levels are rarely of value in the work-up of an adult patient. Seizures as the presenting symptom of hypocalcemia occur primarily in neonates and rarely in pts. with hypoparthyroidism, in whom other clinical signs (such as tetany) are usually present (*Bohr T. Evaluation and treatment of seizures. Letter. N Engl J Med 324(17):1213-14, 1991*).

Anticonvulsant drugs interfere with calcium and vitamin D metabolism in some manner not well understood. Calcium levels are depressed and rickets or osteomalacia may result (*Flodin NW. Pharmacology of Micronutrients. New York, Alan R. Liss, Inc., 1988*).

Intracellular calcium (Ca^{++}) influx is essential for neuronal excitability independent from synaptic function. In fact, abnormal Ca^{++} metabolism may play a dominant role in both the initiation and propagation of seizure discharge, and calcium channel blockers may represent a new therapeutic modality (*Meyer FB. Calcium, neuronal hyperexcitability and ischemic injury. Brain Res Bran Res Rev 14(3):227-43, 1989*).

Copper:

Deficiency may cause seizures (*Sorenson JRJ. Therapeutic uses of copper, in JO Nriagu, Ed. Copper in the Environment. Part II: Health Effects. New York, John Wiley & Sons, 1979:83-162*).

Case Report: A 21-month-old boy was admitted to the hospital because of repeated seizures and failure to thrive. He had blonde, curly hair, spurring of the femora and tibiae, and mild anemia. The mother and maternal uncle had copper deficiency with mild symptoms. Oral copper supplementation was followed by general improvement, but as soon as it was reduced or stopped hypocupremia and seizures resumed (*Mëhes K, Petrovicz E. Familial benign copper deficiency. Arch Dis Child 57(9):716-18, 1982*).

Serum levels may be elevated, at least partly due to anticonvulsants (*Palm R, Hallmans G. Zinc and copper metabolism in phenytoin therapy. Epilepsia 23(5):453-61, 1982; Tutor JC et al. Serum copper concentration and hepatic enzyme induction during long-term therapy with anticonvulsants. Clin Chem 28(6):1367-70, 1982*).

It has been hypothesized that anticonvulsant drugs are activated *in vivo* by forming copper complexes (*Sorenson JRJ. The anti-inflammatory activities of copper complexes, in H Sigel, Ed. Metal Ions in Biological Systems. New York, Marcel Dekker, Inc., 1982, vol. 14, pp. 77-124*).

Magnesium:

Hypomagnesemia may be associated with either grand mal or multifocal seizures (*Hall RCW, Joffe JR. Hypomagnesemia: physical and psychiatric symptoms. JAMA 224(13):1749-51, 1973*).

Blood levels of epileptics may be reduced (*Benga I et al. Plasma and cerebrospinal fluid concentrations of magnesium in epileptic children. J Neurol Sci 67(1):29-34, 1985; Shoji Y. Serum magnesium and zinc in epileptic children. Brain Dev 5(2):200, 1983*).

Cerebrospinal magnesium levels may be increased (*Benga I et al. Plasma and cerebrospinal fluid concentrations of magnesium in epileptic children. J Neurol Sci 67(1):29-34, 1985*).

Negative Observational Study: 7/8 pts. had total CSF magnesium levels in the normal range. In one pt. who had been in status epilepticus for one mo., during which the plasma magnesium was low, the total CSF magnesium level was low (*Hirschfelder AD, Haury VG. Variations in magnesium and potassium associated with essential epilepsy. Arch Neurol Psychiatry 40:66-78, 1938*).

If deficient, supplementation may be beneficial.

Experimental and Observational Study: 75% of 21 children (age 9 - 14) were deficient and most of these improved after administration of magnesium chloride solution (5 mg/kg daily) (*Pediatria Romania 31(4):343-347, 1982*).

Case Report: Immediately following 4 hrs. of continuous exercise in heat, a 23-year-old man displayed epileptic-type convulsions while, 1 wk. earlier, he completed an identical exercise program without convulsions at normal room temperature. Upon assessment, the only abnormality found was that, during the exercise in heat, an abnormally low serum magnesium prevailed for most of the test. Treatment with phenobarb and magnesium chloride enteric tablets reversed the biochemical abnormality. He subsequently heat acclimatized and repeated similar exercise tests as before without any ill effects (*Jooste PL et al. Epileptic-type convulsions and magnesium deficiency. Aviat Space Environ Med 50(7):734-35, 1979*).

Supplementation may be beneficial despite lack of evidence of deficiency.

Animal Experimental Study: Parenteral magnesium sulfate was able to directly suppress neuronal burst firing and interictal EEG spike generation at serum levels below those producing paralysis, corroborating the clinical observation that magnesium can produce an anticonvulsant effect in pts. apart from neuromuscular blockade and suggesting that it may have clinical applicability in treating a wider range of acute convulsions (*Gorges LF, Gücer G. Effect of magnesium on epileptic foci. Epilepsia 19(1):81-91, 1978*).

Experimental Study: 30 epileptic children with grand mal or petit mal seizures were given magnesium 450 mg daily and their anticonvulsants were discontinued. 29/30 showed marked improvement. One child, age 13, had a 10-yr. history of epilepsy which could not be controlled by drugs, was severely depressed and showed signs of mental retardation. After receiving magnesium, his seizures stopped and he became mentally alert (*Barnet LB. J Clin Physiol 1:25, 1959*).

Experimental Study: 10 pts. failed to benefit from 2 gms 4 times daily of oral magnesium chloride in enteric stearic acid-coated tablets. However, a retained rectal enema of 30 gm magnesium sulfate in 90 cc water usually aborted a series of convulsions temporarily, magnesium sulfate 1 gm IM almost, but not quite, always caused convulsions to cease. Magnesium sulfate 1 gm IV usually stopped the convulsions with the exception of one pt. (*Hirschfelder AD, Haury VG. Variations in magnesium and potassium associated with essential epilepsy. Arch Neurol Psychiatry 40:66-78, 1938*).

Manganese:

Blood levels may be low (*Carl GF et al. Association of low blood manganese concentration with epilepsy. Neurology 36:1584-87, 1986; Dupont CL, Tanaka Y. Blood manganese levels in children with convulsive disorder. Biochem Med 33(2):246-55, 1985; Papavasiliou PS et al. Seizure disorders and trace metals: Manganese tissue levels in treated epileptics. Neurology 29:1466, 1979*).

Supplementation may be beneficial.

Clinical Observation: Manganese supplementation may be helpful in controlling both major and minor motor seizures (*Pfeiffer CC, LaMola S. Zinc and manganese in the schizophrenias. J Orthomol Psychiatry 12:215-234, 1983*).

Experimental Study: A boy with seizures which were unresponsive to medications was found to have a blood manganese level which was half the normal value; when supplemented, he had fewer seizures and improvement in gait, speech and learning. (*Tanaka Y. Low manganese level may trigger epilepsy. JAMA 238:1805, 1977*).

Potassium:

Serum levels are increased during seizures, while the cerebrospinal fluid level usually remains normal (*Hirschfelder AD, Haury VG. Variations in magnesium and potassium associated with essential epilepsy. Arch Neurol Psychiatry 40:66-78, 1938; McQuarrie I. Ann Intern Med 6:497, 1932*).

Selenium:

Supplementation may be beneficial for early childhood seizures.

Experimental Study: 4 children with intractable seizures during the first 6 mo. of life, intolerance to anticonvulsants and repeated infections were found to be deficient in glutathione peroxidase. This deficiency may increase the risk of recurrent seizures in children due to peroxidation stress. Two of the children had low intracellular enzyme activity but normal whole blood selenium and high plasma glutathione peroxidase concentrations. The other 2 had low intracellular glutathione peroxidase activity along with low circulating glutathione peroxidase and low whole blood selenium.. Anticonvulsants were discontinued and selenium (the metal in the active site of glutathione peroxidase) was supplemented. All 4 children showed clinical improvement (*Weber GF et al. Glutathione peroxidase deficiency and childhood seizures. Lancet 337:1443-4, 1991*).

Zinc:

Serum levels may be reduced (*Barbeau A, Donaldson J. Zinc, taurine, and epilepsy. Arch Neurol 30:52-58, 1974; Shoji Y. Serum magnesium and zinc in epileptic children. Brain Dev 5(2):200, 1983*).

The availability of excess zinc, delivered either by dietary supplementation or by injection, has been found to protect against the development of seizures in at least 3 different animal models of epilepsy (*Sterman MB et al. Zinc and seizure mechanisms, in J Morley, MB Sterman, J Walsh, Eds. Nutritional Modulation of Neural Function. New York, Academic Press, 1988:307-19*).

Anticonvulsants may cause zinc deficiency either by reducing zinc absorption in the gut by chelation or by causing diarrhea.

Experimental and Observational Study: 2 pts. presented with diarrhea and brownish-red scaly eruptions which followed substitution of high dose sodium valproate for phenytoin. Serum zinc concentrations were abnormally low. The diarrhea and rashes responded to zinc supplementation (*Lewis-Jones MS et al. Cutaneous manifestations of zinc deficiency during treatment with anticonvulsants. Br Med J 290:603-4, 1985*).

Deficiency may cause seizures.

Convulsions in chronic alcoholics may be associated with dietary zinc deficiency (accompanied by reduced blood and liver zinc and increased urine zinc) and may respond to zinc supplementation (*Prasad AS et al. Determination of zinc in biological fluids by atomic absorption spectrophotometry in normal and cirrhotic subjects. J Lab Clin Med 66:508-16, 1965; Sullivan JF, Lankford HG. Zinc metabolism and chronic alcoholism. Am J Clin Nutr 17:57-72, 1965*).

Zinc to Copper Ratio:

Since serum zinc is low and copper high in epileptics, seizures are theorized to occur when the zinc/copper ratio falls suddenly in the absence of adequate taurine (*Barbeau A, Donaldson J. Zinc, taurine, and epilepsy. Arch Neurol 30:52-58, 1974*).

_ _

OTHER NUTRITIONAL FACTORS

Biotin:

Blood levels may be low - perhaps due to anticonvulsants (*Krause KH et al. B vitamins in epileptics. Biblthca Nutr Dieta 38:154-67, 1986*).

Choline: Start with 4 gm daily.
                Increase to 12 - 16 gm daily by the third month.

Supplementation may be beneficial in treating complex partial seizures.

Negative Animal Experimental Study: The results of rat experiments suggest that sustained complex partial seizure activity eventually results in cellular damage; thus it may be a goal in the management of human epilepsy to control such seizure activity. The cholinergic system may play a role in generating or maintaining this type of seizure activity, and anticholinergics may protect against it provided they are given prior to commencement of the seizures (*Olney JW et al. Excitotoxic mechanisms of epileptic brain damage. Adv Neurol 44:857-77, 1986*).

Experimental Study: Following 4 mo. of supplementation with oral choline 12-16 g/d, 3 pts. with intractable complex partial seizures had shorter seizure duration and less post-seizure fatigue (but a slight increase in seizure frequency) and considered themselves much improved. A 4th pt. whose plasma choline only increased 21%, compared to 75-300% increases in the other 3 pts., failed to improve (*McNamara JO et al. Effects of oral choline on human complex partial seizures. Neurology 30(12):1334-36, 1980*).

<u>Dimethyl Glycine</u>:   100 mg. twice daily

DMG is formed from betaine in the metabolism of homocysteine to methionine and is a precursor of glycine, a neuroinhibitory amino acid.

Supplementation may be beneficial.

>   **Animal Experimental Study:** Mice were given various dosages of N,N-dimethylglycine followed by pentylenetetrazol after 10 minutes. N,N-dimethylglycine produced a significant dose-dependent decrease in seizure incidence (p<0.001) and a significant increase in the latency to the first seizure (*Freed WJ. N,N-dimethylglycine, betaine, and seizures. Letter. <u>Arch Neurol</u> 41(11):1129-30, 1984*).

>   **Negative Experimental Study:** 5 epileptics who were refractory to standard treatment failed to respond to DMG 90 mg 3 times daily (*Roach ES, Gibson P. Failure of N,N-dimethylglycine in epilepsy. Letter. <u>Ann Neurol</u> 14(3):347, 1983*).

>   **Case Report:** A 22 year-old man with long-standing mental retardation and mixed complex, partial and grand mal seizures had been having 16-18 generalized seizures per week despite phenobarbitol and carbamazepine for the previous 6 months. Within 1 wk. of starting DMG 90 mg twice daily, his seizure frequency dropped to 3 per week. Two attempts to withdraw the DMG caused dramatic increases in seizure frequency (*Roach ES, Carlin L. N,N-dimethylglycine for epilepsy. Letter. <u>N Engl J Med</u> 307:1081-82, 1982*).

<u>D,L-Glutamic Acid</u>:

Brain tissue contains an enzyme which synthesizes glutamine from L-glutamic acid and ammonia.

Administration of D,L-glutamic acid may reduce <u>petit mal</u> and <u>psychomotor</u> seizures.

>   **Case Reports:** 8 pts. with seizures usually associated with slow wave activity received D,L-glutamic acid hydrochloride at the dosage required to maintain a urinary pH of 5.0 (approx. 4 g 3 times daily). Petit mal and psychomotor, but not grand mal, seizures were reduced in frequency, and both mental and physical alertness were increased. Usually pts. were more energetic and happier, mood swings were less pronounced, behavior mannerisms were ameliorated, and they were more social. Side effects, including GI symptoms, were minimal, and taste objections were alleviated by administering the drug in capsules (*Price JC et al. dl-Glutamic acid hydrochloride in treatment of petit mal and psychomotor seizures. <u>JAMA</u> 122(17):1153-56, 1943*).

<u>Omega-6 Fatty Acids</u>:

>   WARNING: Supplementation may exacerbate <u>temporal lobe epilepsy</u> (*Holman CP, Bell AFJ. A trial of evening primrose oil in the treatment of chronic schizophrenia. <u>J Orthomol Psychiatry</u> 12:302-04, 1983; Vaddadi KS. The use of gamma-linolenic acid and linoleic acid to differentiate between temporal lobe epilepsy and schizophrenia. <u>Prostaglandins Med</u> 6:375-79, 1981*).

<u>Taurine</u>: 500 mg 3 times daily

Taurine is a neuroinhibitory amino acid.

Low brain taurine concentrations have been found at the site of maximal seizure activity (*Sturman J. Taurine in nutrition. <u>Compr Ther</u> 3:64, 1977; Van Gelder NM et al. Amino acid content of epileptogenic human brain: Focal versus surrounding regions. <u>Brain Res</u> 40:385-93, 1972*).

Urinary taurine excretion is decreased (*Hartley SG et al. Urinary excretion of taurine in epilepsy. <u>Neurochem Res</u> 14(2):149-52, 1989*).

>   *Note: Rao et al (Rao A et al. Urinary excretion of taurine in epilepsy. <u>Acta Neurol Scand</u> 68:421-23, 1983) reported increased taurine excretion using an older method. It is now known that those results were due to additional substances which are co-eluted with taurine using that method, yielding spuriously high values (Hartley SG et al. Urinary excretion of taurine in epilepsy. <u>Neurochem Res</u> 14(2):149-52, 1989).*

Platelet taurine may be reduced.

> **Observational Study:** Compared to 99 controls, platelet taurine concentrations were significantly lower in 114 pts. and there was no significant association between platelet taurine concentrations and serum drug concentrations (*Goodman HO et al. Antiepileptic drugs and plasma and platelet taurine in epilepsy. Epilepsia 30(2):201-07, 1989*).

Supplementation may be reduce seizures.

> **Review Article:** Taurine's "antiepileptic action, confirmed in several models of experimental epilepsy and in short-term clinical studies, does not seem to possess major clinical relevance since trials with a longer follow-up gave unsatisfactory results. Taurine's limited diffusibility across the blood-brain barrier may be the main factor restricting the anitepileptic effect of this compound" (*Durelli L, Tutani R. The current status of taurine in epilepsy. Clin Neuropharmacol 6(1):37-48, 1983*).

> **Experimental Study:** 25 children aged 4 mo. to 12 yrs. with daily frequent seizures despite vigorous anticonvulsant medication received 0.05-0.3 g/kg taurine daily. In addition, 12 of them received probenecid 0.5-1.0 g/d. Complete seizure control was achieved in a case of Lennox syndrome, >50% decrease in seizures was achieved in 1 case, <50% decrease in 4 cases, and no effects in 18 cases. The effects of taurine often manifest only temporarily. EEG abnormalities were not improved by taurine in the 21 cases examined except for one in which the EEG markedly improved along with seizure control. 4 pts. had side effects of drowsiness and ataxia (*Fukuyama Y, Ochiai Y. Therapeutic trial by taurine for intractable childhood epilepsies. Brain Dev 4(1):63-69, 1982*).

> **Experimental Double-blind Crossover Study:** 7 institutionalized adults and 2 ambulatory children with drug-resistant epilepsy received taurine 100 mg/kg/d or placebo in 3 divided doses for 2 mo. each in either order. During taurine treatment, 1/9 pts. had a practically 100% decrease in the number of convulsions, and 2/9 had about a 50% decrease. Placebo had no effect and there were no adverse side effects from taurine (*Airaksinen EM et al. Effects of taurine treatment on epileptic patients. Prog Clin Biol Res 39:157-66, 1980*).

> **Negative Experimental Study:** Oral taurine at doses of 375 - 8000 mg/d (16 -150 mg/kg/d) failed to improve seizure control for 6 pts. with mixed seizure disorders which had been refractory to standard anticonvulsant treatment (*Mantovani J et al. Effects of taurine on seizures and growth hormone release in epileptic patients. Arch Neurol 35:672, 1979*).

> **Experimental Study:** Pts. with focal epilepsy who had at least 3 daily convulsions despite maximal anticonvulsant therapy were supplemented with slowly increasing taurine dosages. Only when clinical suppression of seizures had been maintained for 5 days were the other anticonvulsant drugs slowly withdrawn. Antiseizure activity was evident at ranges between 200 mg and 1.5 g per day. At higher levels, worsening of the EEG was seen in some patients (*Barbeau A, Donaldson J. Zinc, taurine, and epilepsy. Arch Neurol 30:52-58, 1974*).

- -

OTHER FACTORS

Rule out food sensitivities.

General:

> **Experimental Study:** Based on their urinary glycoprotein-peptide-complex patterns, 4 epileptic children with autistic syndromes who were receiving anticonvulsants were treated with either a gluten-free and milk-reduced, or a milk-free and gluten-reduced diet. 3/4 had a reduction in seizure frequency. In addition, urinary peptide secretion was reduced, and some behaviors improved (*Reichelt KL et al. Gluten, milk proteins and autism: Dietary intervention effects on behavior and peptide secretion. J Appl Nutr 42(1):1-11, 1990*).

> **Experimental Double-blind Study:** 63 epileptic children were studied, 45 with recurrent headaches, abdominal symptoms, or hyperkinetic behavior, and 18 with epilepsy alone. Foods that provoked symptoms were first identified by a systematic reintroduction of foods singly into a limited control diet. 42 different foods caused seizures and symptoms in the 45 epileptic children with symptoms of migraines or hyperkinetic behavior, while the 18 children with epilepsy alone did not experience seizures or other symptoms following food reintroduction. When inciting foods were removed

from the diet of the children with combined symptoms, 36/45 recovered or improved. The problem foods were then reintroduced to 16 of the children in a double-blind manner, and seizures or other symptoms recurred in 15/16, while no symptoms recurred when placebo was given (*Egger J et al. Oligoantigenic diet treatment of children with epilepsy and migraine. J Pediatr 114:51-58, 1989*).

Double-blind Case Report: Epilepsy was precipitated by ingestion of specific foods and carefully controlled, double-blind confirmation of the food-epilepsy relationship was demonstrated (*Crayton JW et al. Epilepsy precipitated by food sensitivity: Report of a case with double-blind placebo-controlled assessment. Clin Electroencephalography 12(4):192-8, 1981*).

Double-blind Case Report: 29 year-old male had a 4 year history of syncope and grand mal epilepsy as well as double vision, tachycardia, dizziness, edema, and spontaneous bruising. EEG was entirely normal. Phenytoin and other anti-convulsants only partly controlled his seizures. Following a 6 1/2 day fast, his symptoms cleared. Challenge with foods and chemicals precipitated seizures. A double-blind challenge with peanuts using a Levine tube confirmed that he was reacting to the food (*Rea WJ, Suits CW. Cardiovascular disease triggered by foods and chemicals, in JW Gerrard, Ed. Food Allergy: New Perspectives. Springfield, Illinois, Charles C. Thomas, 1980*).

Aspartame:

Case Report: A 54-year-old female on maintenance imipramine 150 mg/day for 5 yrs. suddenly experienced a grand mal seizure followed by her first manic episode several wks. after switching from sugar to aspartame to sweeten as much as 1 gal iced tea daily. She did well after switching back to sugar (*Walton RG. Seizure and mania after high intake of aspartame. Psychosomatics 27(3):21820, 1986*).

Finegold Diet (salicylates and additives):

Case Report: A 3 1/2 year old male with tuberous sclerosis, mental retardation and uncontrolled seizures was studied. Using a reversal design, the Feingold (salicylate and food additive elimination) diet was presented and withdrawn 3 times, and each presentation resulted in substantial reductions in seizure frequency. During a 21-week follow-up, seizure frequency remained low despite the phasing out of 1 drug, and seizures were reportedly eliminated 1 yr. later, while hyperactive behavior was unchanged (*Haavik S et al. Effects of the Feingold diet on seizures and hyperactivity: A single-subject analysis. J Behav Med 2(4):365-74, 1979*).

FATIGUE

See Also: ANEMIA
CHRONIC FATIGUE SYNDROME
"HYPOGLYCEMIA" (FUNCTIONAL)

OVERVIEW

1. High-carbohydrate meals or the consumption of refined sugar may cause fatigue, possibly by increasing the transport of tryptophan across the blood/brain barrier.

2. A chronic high intake of caffeine may cause fatigue, as may caffeine withdrawal.

3. Marginal deficiencies of a number of essential nutrients, including folic acid, pantothenic acid, vitamin C, iron, magnesium, potassium, and zinc, may cause fatigue, and repletion of these deficiencies will restore normal energy levels.

4. Supplementation with potassium/magnesium aspartate may reduce fatigue and/or increase endurance.

5. Food sensitivities have been suggested as a cause of an "allergic tension-fatigue syndrome" characterized sometimes by sensory and motor fatigue.

- -

DIETARY FACTORS

Avoid high carbohydrate meals.

> **Experimental Study:** On different occasions, in counterbalanced order, 7 normal women fasted overnight, ate a standard breakfast, and at lunch either continued to fast or ate a high-carbohydrate, low-protein meal; a hedonically similar meal containing both carbohydrate and protein; or a high-protein, low-carbohydrate meal. Meals were isocaloric and equated for fat content. Only the carbohydrate meal significantly increased fatigue, which could not be attributed to hypoglycemia because plasma glucose remained elevated. Fatigue began approximately when the carbohydrate meal elevated the plasma tryptophan ratio but ended even though the ratio remained elevated (*Spring B et al. Psychobiological effects of carbohydrates. J Clin Psychiatry 50 Suppl:27-33, 1989*).

Avoid chronic use of caffeine and sugar.

> **Experimental Double-blind Study:** 22 coffee drinkers (3-7 cups/d) underwent a double-blind trial to test for caffeine withdrawal effects which consisted of a randomized crossover period of 1 d of decaffeinated coffee and 1 d of caffeinated coffee (100 mg). Withdrawal symptoms were headaches, drowsiness and fatigue (*Hughes JR et al. Caffeine self-administration, withdrawal, and adverse effects among coffee drinkers. Arch Gen Psychiatry 48:611-17, 1991*).

> **Experimental Double-blind Study:** 16 pts. complaining of symptoms such as depression, headaches, moodiness and fatigue consumed a caffeine- and refined-sucrose-free diet for up to 2 weeks. Those who improved were sequentially challenged double-blind with caffeine, cellulose placebo, sucrose-sweetened Kool-Aid, and aspartame-sweetened Kool-Aid for 6 days each. 7/16 pts. (44%) demonstrated a return of symptoms and mood disturbance when challenged with caffeine or refined sucrose, but not with cellulose or aspartame. Responders and non-responders could not be differentiated by the Profile of Mood States, the Beck Depression Inventory, or the MMPI, and both gps. showed similar symptoms of sleep disturbances, depression, fatigue, moodiness and irritability (*Christensen L. Psychological distress and diet - effects of sucrose and caffeine. J Appl Nutr 40(1):44-50, 1988*).

Observational Study: 22% of 83 hospitalized adult psychiatric pts. reported being high caffeine consumers (750 mg or more daily). 61% of the high consumers reported feeling tired easily on the State-Trait Anxiety Index, compared to 54% of the the moderate consumers (250-749 mg daily), and 24% of those consuming <250 mg caffeine daily. High caffeine consumers scored significantly higher on the State-Trait Anxiety Index and the Beck Depression Scale than moderate or low consumers and described significantly more clinical symptoms, felt that their physical health was not as good, and reported greater use of sedative-hypnotics and minor tranquilizers (*Greden JF et al. Anxiety and depression associated with caffeinism among psychiatric inpatients. Am J Psychiatry 135(8):963-6, 1978*).

Animal Experimental Study: In contrast to a single dose of caffeine, 6 weeks' treatment with caffeine greatly reduced the swimming capacity of mice. This detrimental effect was not due to an accumulation of toxic levels of caffeine, and motor coordination was unaffected. There was no deficiency of metabolic substrates, since glycogen, fat stores, blood glucose and fatty acid levels were not lower than in controls. It is proposed that caffeine may interfere with the ability to mobilize and spend metabolic substrates for energy requirements of skeletal muscle (*Estler CJ, Ammon HP, Herzog C. Swimming capacity of mice after prolonged treatment with psychostimulants. I. Effects of caffeine on swimming performance and cold stress. Psychopharmacology (Berlin) 58(2):161-6, 1978*).

- -

VITAMINS

General:

Combined marginal deficiencies can seriously reduce work performance.

Review Article: Combined marginal deficiencies of iron, vitamin C and B-group vitamins are widespread in developing countries. It is becoming clear that combined deficiencies of certain vitamins, or of iron and vitamins, although less severe than those causing the lesions of classic clinical deficiency, can seriously reduce work performance (*Bates CJ et al. Vitamins, iron, and physical work. Lancet 2:313-14, 1989*).

Vitamin B Complex:

- Folic Acid:

Deficiency may be associated with easy fatigability which may respond to supplementation.

Experimental Study: A gp. of 38 pts. is described with minor neurological signs but with depression, fatigue, lassitude, and burning feet and restless legs syndromes are the main subjective complaints. Supplementation with folic acid, starting with 10 mg/d, resulted in regression of the lasstitude, easy fatigability and depression in about 2-3 months. The burning feet and restless legs syndromes improved during the first 3 wks. (*Botez MI et al. Neuropsychological correlates of folic acid deficiency: facts and hypotheses, in MI Botez, EH Reynolds, Eds. Folic Acid in Neurology, Psychiatry, and Internal Medicine. New York, Raven Press, 1979:435-61*).

Experimental Study: 4 pts. with easy fatigability along with other symptoms were found to have low folate levels. As folate levels rose with supplementation, fatigue disappeared (*Clin Psychiatry News, April, 1976*).

- Pantothenic Acid: 250 mg. daily (calcium pantothenate)

Fatigue is the most prominent deficiency symptom - associated with insomnia, sullenness and depression.

Experimental Controlled Study: 10 healthy male volunteers received a low pantothenic acid diet, and 5 of them with supplemented with 10 mg pantothenic acid daily. After 63 days, the deprived men appeared listless and complained of fatigue (*Fry PC et al. Metabolic response to a pantothenic acid deficient diet in humans. J Nutr Sci Vitaminol 22:339-46, 1976*).

Experimental Study: Male volunteers from Iowa State Prison were given a formula diet adequate except for pantothenic acid. The men developed low blood pressure, dizziness, extreme fatigue, muscle weakness, sleepiness, stomach distress, constipation, rapid pulse on exertion, and continuous upper respiratory infections. Urine analyses quickly showed a decrease in adrenal hormones which fell progressively as the experiment continued. Digestive enzymes and gastric acid were markedly reduced, and both gastric and intestinal motility decreased (*Thornton GHM et al. J Clin Invest 34:1073, 1955*).

- Vitamin B₁₂:

Supplementation may be reduce tiredness.

Experimental Double-blind Crossover Study: 28 men and women who complained of tiredness but had normal serum B₁₂ levels and no physical findings were randomly given intramuscular injections of hydroxy-cobalamin 5 mg or placebo twice daily for 2 wks. followed by a 2-wk. rest period and the crossover treatment. Based on the sum of daily subjective scores, those who received placebo first felt significantly better in regard to "general well-being" (p=0.006) in the second period when they received B₁₂. However, those who initially received B₁₂ noted no differences between the B₁₂ and placebo periods, which suggests that the effects of B₁₂ may persist for a period of at least 4 weeks (*Ellis FR, Nasser S. A pilot study of vitamin B₁₂ in the treatment of tiredness. Br J Nutr 30:277-83,1973*).

Vitamin C:

If marginally deficient, supplementation may be beneficial.

Review Article: The results of many studies of the effect of vitamin C on physical performance have been equivocal, and most studies could not demonstrate an effect. However, a sub-optimal vitamin status results in an impaired working capacity which can be normalized by restoring vitamin C body pools (*Gerster H. The role of vitamin C in athletic performance. J Am Coll Nutr 8(6):636-43, 1989*).

Observational Study: In a survey of vitamin C intake among 411 dentists and their wives, there was a significant inverse relationship between vitamin C intake and fatigue, with the mean number of fatigue symptoms among the low vitamin C users being double that among the relatively high users of vitamin C (*Cheraskin E et al. Daily vitamin C consumption and fatigability. J Am Geriatr Soc 24(3):136-37, 1976*).

- -

MINERALS

Iron:

WARNING: only supplement if deficient - otherwise can be toxic.

Deficiency syndrome may be associated with fatigue and a diminished work capacity.

Note: Iron may be deficient despite the lack of anemia and a normal serum iron (Finch CA. Editorial: Evaluation of iron status. JAMA 251(15):2004, 1984).

Experimental Study: During intellectual activity, iron-deficient women demonstrated reduction in efficiency, more noticeable fatigue in the course of a working day and week, and deterioration of body functions. Repletion with iron supplements raised the work volume and improved its quality. It also improved the state of health, activity and mood (*Kuleschova EA, Riabova NV. [Effect of iron deficiency of the body on the work capacity of women engaged in mental work.] Ter Arkh 61(1):92-95, 1989) (in Russian*).

Review Article: Normal iron levels are necessary for normal work capacity. Independent of the anemia, an iron deficiency results in reduced exercise capacity. Elderly pts. complaining of increased fatigue should be screened for iron deficiency which, in their case, almost always results from blood loss (*Schultz BM, Freedman ML. Iron deficiency in the elderly. Baillieres Clin Haematol 1(2):291-313, 1987*).

Experimental Double-blind Study: About 2/3 of a gp. of chronically fatigued non-anemic women improved following iron supplementation (*Buetler E et al. Iron therapy in chronically fatigued non-anemic women: A double blind study. Ann Intern Med 52:378, 1960*).

Iron overload may be associated with disabling fatigue.

Observational Study: Among pts. with hereditary hemochromatosis, disabling fatigue, reported in over 80% of pts. at the time of diagnosis, is the most common symptom (*Niederau C et al. Survival and causes of death in cirrhotic and noncirrhotic patients with primary hemochromatosis. N Engl J Med 313:1256-62, 1985*). .

Magnesium:

Required for ATP synthesis.

Enhances transport of potassium into cells (*see "Potassium" below*).

Potassium:

Malaise is probably the most common deficiency symptom when potassium deficits are chronic, and muscular weakness is almost always noted (*Snively WD, Westerman RL. The clinician views potassium deficit. Minn Med June, 1965, pp. 713-19*).

Observational Study: In a study of older people (ave. age of men, 74.7 yrs.; ave. age of women, 73.7 yrs.), 60% of men and 40% of women were found to have an inadequate potassium intake, and low potassium intake was associated with weaker grip strength than normal for people matched by age, sex and weight (*Judge TG, Cowan NR. Dietary potassium intake and grip strength in older people. Gerontologia Clinica 13:221-26, 1971*).

Hyperkalemia during brief periods of intensive exercise may contribute to the development of fatigue (*Friedland J, Paterson D. Potassium and fatigue. Letter. Lancet 2:961-62, 1988; Kössler F et al. [Problems of muscular fatigue: relationship to stimulation conduction velocity and K(+) concentration.] Z Gesante Hyg 36(7):354-56, 1990; Vollestad NK, Sejersted OM. Biochemical correlates with fatigue. Eur J Appl Physiol 57:336-47, 1988*).

Zinc:

Leukonychia (white spots on fingernails), believed to be associated with marginal zinc deficiency, may be associated with lethargy.

Observational Study: 65% of 459 college students reported leukonychia. Sleep time and drowsiness were used as indicators of lethargy. Subjects with leukonychia typically reported longer sleep times (p<0.02) and were more likely to report drowsiness (p=0.10). 21/28 (75%) who reported themselves as "very often drowsy" had leukonychia in contrast to 5/11 (45.5%) who reported themselves as "never drowsy" (*Bakan P. Confusion, lethargy and leukonychia. J Orthomol Med 5(4):198-202, 1990*).

If marginally deficient, supplementation may improve muscle strength and endurance.

Experimental Study: After 15 days of supplementation with 135 mg zinc daily, isokinetic strength and isometric endurance of leg muscles were significantly improved. Results suggest that zinc supplementation may be of practical importance in many clinical situations where malabsorption or lower intake may induce zinc depletion and thereby influence muscle strength and fatigue (*Krotkiewski M et al. Zinc and muscle strength and endurance. Acta Physiol Scand 116(3):309-11, 1982*).

- -

OTHER NUTRITIONAL FACTORS

Aspartic Acid:

Aspartic acid is converted intracellularly into oxaloacetate, an important substrate in the energy-producing Krebs cycle, and is also a carrier molecule for the transport of potassium and magnesium into the cell.

- with potassium and magnesium:

Example: potassium/magnesium aspartate 1 gm twice daily

Supplementation may relieve chronic fatigue.

Review Article: Both uncontrolled and double-blind studies (totaling nearly 3000 subjects) have found that 75-91% of treated pts. experienced pronounced relief of fatigue during treatment with K^{++} and Mg^{++} aspartates in daily doses of 1 gm of each salt, compared to 5-25% of controls. A beneficial effect was usually noted after 4-5 days, but sometimes 10 days were required. Pts. usually continued treatment for 4-6 wks.; afterwards fatigue frequently did not return. Side effects, which were mild and uncommon, included mild GI distress and dryness of the mouth (*Gaby AR. Aspartic acid salts and fatigue. Curr Nutr Therapeut November, 1982*).

Experimental Double-blind Study: 46% of 145 pts. were placed on tablets containing 250 mg each of magnesium and potassium aspartates and told to take 2 tabs 4 times daily after meals and at bedtime, while 54% received placebo. 56/66 (85%) pts. receiving aspartates reported an increase in strength or physical activity over the 18 mo. of the study compared to only 9% of pts. on placebo. Of the pts. receiving aspartates, in 20/66 the fatigue was without a somatic basis, in 20/66 it was associated with anxiety neuroses, in 10/66 with GI disturbances, in 4/66 with menopause, in 5/66 the postpartum period and in 7/66 fatigue was a sequel of influenza. No side effects were noted (*Hicks J. Treatment of fatigue in general practice: A double-blind study. Clin Med January, 1964, pp. 85-90*).

Negative Review Article: The efficacy of aspartates for fatigue is considered unproven as the theoretical basis is questionable and estimation of the relief of fatigue is so subjective that it is extremely difficult to substantiate their effectiveness (*Council on drugs, new, drugs and developments in therapeutics. JAMA 183:362, 1963*).

Experimental Placebo-controlled Study: In a study of 71 pts., 91% of pts. given potassium/magnesium aspartates noted improvement compared to 5% of pts. given placebo (*Friedlander HS. Fatigue as a presenting symptom: Management in general practice. Curr Ther Res 4:441-9, 1962*).

Experimental Placebo-controlled Study: 84 women and 16 men with persistent tiredness believed to be unrelated to depression, some of whom had been symptomatic for >2 yrs., were placed on potassium and magnesium aspartates 4 tabs daily in divided doses. Aspartates were administered to 6% of the series for 2 wks., and to 68% for 4-6 weeks. The remaining 26% received placebos as well as the active medication in crossover studies. There was a positive therapeutic response, which developed gradually over 4-10 days, in 87% of the active treatment periods. After 4-6 wks. most improved pts. stopped the supplements and continued to do well (*Formica PE. The housewife syndrome: treatment with the potassium and magnesium salts of aspartic acid. Curr Ther Res March, 1962, pp. 98-106*).

Experimental Double-blind Study: 80% of over 2000 pts. treated with potassium and magnesium salts of aspartic acid experienced adequate subjective relief of fatigue compared to 20-26% who responded to placebo (*Agersborg HPK, Shaw DL Jr. Physiologic approach to the problem of fatigue - summarized in Shaw DL Jr et al. Management of fatigue: A physiologic approach. Am J Med Sci 243:758-69, 1962*).

Experimental Double-blind Studies:
1. 57 pts. without demonstrable organic disease received tablets containing 250 mg each of potassium and magnesium aspartates and were told to take 2 tabs after the morning and evening meals, while 28 similar pts. received placebo. After 4 wks., 49/57 (86%) in the experimental gp. felt better, were more able to cope with daily activities, and were not fatigued beyond normal tiredness after a full day's schedule compared to 7/28 (25%) controls. Onset of reponse in the experimental gp. took about 4 days for full benefit, and there was no evidence of central stimulation.
2. 32 pts. who complained primarily of fatigue but who had an organic disease whose treatment had been stable for at least 1 mo. received aspartates in the standard dose and placebo in a crossover trial for 4 wks. each. 21/32 were relieved of fatigue, 9/32 had a questionable response (i.e. they responded to the first medication received, whether aspartates or placebo, and continued to respond after the crossover) and 2/32 were unimproved. After placebo substitution for 4 wks., 3/32 were relieved, 4/32 were questionable and 25/32 were unimproved. Results correlated with objective data obtained with the electronic rheotome.
(*Shaw DL et al. Management of fatigue: A physiologic approach. Am J Med Sci 243:758-69, 1962*).

Experimental Double-blind Study: In a study 92 pts., 80% responded to potassium/magnesium aspartates compared to 9% of pts. given placebo (*Taylor BB. The fatigued worker: A double blind study of treatment with the potassium and magnesium salts of aspartic acid. West Med 2:535-8, 1961*).

- with <u>arginine</u>:

Supplementation with arginine aspartate may reduce both psychophysical and sexual asthenia (*Duruy A, Baujat JP. Traitment de l'asthénie physique, psychique et sexuelle par le Sargénor. Vie Méd 9:1589-90, 1965; Salomon C et al. Etude clinique de Sargénor dans les impuissances sexuelles secondaires. Psychol Méd 4:541-59, 1972*).

<u>L-Glutamine</u>: 500 mg. twice daily for 1 week, then
500 mg. 3 times daily for 1 week, then
1 gm. twice daily for 1 week as a trial

WARNING: Contraindicated in hyperammonemia.

Able to pass through the blood-brain barrier to increase brain levels of glutamate, an excitatory neurotransmitter (*Butterworth et al. Effect of asparagine, glutamine and insulin on cerebral amino acid neurotransmitters. J Can Sci Neurol 7(4):447-50, 1980*).

<u>Inosine</u>:

Supplementation may reduce fatigue by increasing the oxygen-carrying capacity of the blood (*DeVerdier CH, Westman M. Intravenous infusion of inosine in man: Effect on erythrocyte 2,3-diphosphoglycerate concentration and on blood oxygen affinity. Scand J Clin Lab Invest 32(3):205-10, 1973*).

- -

OTHER FACTORS

Rule out <u>food sensitivities</u>.

Said to sometimes cause an "allergic tension-fatigue syndrome" characterized by sensory and motor hyperactivity and/or sensory and motor fatigue.

Experimental Study: 42/44 pts. with a history of allergic tension-fatigue syndrome showed lymphocyte stimulation to a series of food extracts and additivies. There was a positive response to food in 40.9%, a positive response to additives in 18.1%, and a positive response to both in 36.6% Elimination diets prescribed in accordance with the *in vitro* results produced remissions in 38/42 pts. (86.3%), partial remissions in 2/42 (4.5%) and no change in 4/42 (9.0%) (*Valverde E et al. In vitro response of lymphocytes in patients with allergic tension-fatigue syndrome. Ann Allergy 45(3):185-88, 1980*).

Clinical Observations: 75% of a gp. of 50 pts. with tension-fatigue syndrome were found to have a history of nasal, ocular, respiratory, or skin allergy. Over half the pts. treated by an elimination diet had superior to excellent results, while an additional 16/50 had a good response (*Crook WG. Can Your Child Read? Is He Hyperactive? Jackson, Tenn., Professional Books, 1977*).

Experimental Double-blind Case Report: A child presenting with fatigue, irritability, headache and stomach ache had the symptoms reproduced by milk in capsules but not by placebo (*Crook WG. Can Your Child Read? Is He Hyperactive? Jackson, Tenn., Professional Books, 1977*).

Case Report: A 13 year-old boy with severe bronchial asthma was strikingly pale with dark circles under his eyes. He was morose, listless and lethargic and complained of musculoskeletal pains, headache and abdominal pain. He drank two pints of milk daily and ate chocolate or drank a cola-type beverage daily. Within 48 hrs. of starting milk and chocolate elimination, the facial pallor and the dark circles under his eyes almost completely disappeared. Most remarkable was the improvement in his mood and behavior. He became alert, cheerful, and interested in his surroundings. His physical complaints ceased and his asthma was easily controlled. After 3 wks., milk was added to his diet. Within 1 wk. his pallor and the dark circumorbital circles returned and he became morose. He was returned to the therapeutic diet with the same satisfactory result as before (*Weinberg EG, Tuchinda M. Allergic tension-fatigue syndrome. Ann Allergy 31:209-11, 1973*).

Clinical Observations and Case Reports: The fatigue related to chronic food allergy usually starts as intermittent episodes in association with some other allergic manifestation, especially GI symptoms, headaches or nasal allergy. It is usually more pronounced in the early morning, often decreases as the day progresses, and occurs despite a full night of sound sleep. Unlike exercise-related fatigue, there is a basal or pre-exertion fatigue or weakness which often requires a distinct effort or "push" to start the daily work. There are often cognitive difficulties, with memory impairment, mental sluggishness, and inability to concentrate or maintain attention. Various degress of depression may exist as well as muscle aching and soreness or drawing sensations in gps. of muscles. Sometimes there is edema, especially puffiness of the eyelids and fullness and discoloration of the infraorbital areas. Although sensitivity to wheat, corn, milk and eggs is most common, any food eaten regularly may be an offender. 5 case reports are presented as illustrations (*Randolph TG. Fatigue and weakness of allergic origin to be differentiated from "nervous fatigue" or neurasthenia. Ann Allergy 3:418-30,460, 1945*).

GALLBLADDER DISEASE
(CHOLECYSTITIS AND CHOLELITHIASIS)

DIETARY FACTORS

General:

Review Article: For pts. with cholelithiasis, the total calorie intake should be calculated based on each individual's energy requirement and should be restricted on overweight patients. The diet should contain approx. 15-20% of the daily calories from proteins, 30-35% from fat (mainly vegetable fat) and 40-55% from carbohydrates, especially complex carbohydrates. There should be adequate vitamins and minerals in the diet, and fiber consumption should be increased to 30-40 g/d. Finally, meals should be small and frequent (*Magnati G et al. [The dietary problem in cholelithiasis and patients at risk.] Acta Biomed Ateneo Parmense 57(5-6):169-77, 1986*).

Observational Study: 300 pts. (200 females; 100 males) and 200 controls (100 females; 100 males) were studied to ascertain the effects of 31 factors of irrational nutrition on the development and progress of cholecystitis. The most important factors were found to be <u>frequent consumption of fatty and fried foods and smoked foods</u>, <u>abundant meals</u>, and <u>decreased vegetable consumption</u> (*Koliado VB. [Effects of unbalanced diet on the etiology and course of cholecystitis.] Vopr Pitan (6):23-27, 1983*).

Negative Observational Study: 214 women aged 20-61 with no known history of gallstones had oral cholecystography. 11 cases of stone (5.1%) were discovered and these patients' diets were compared to those of 202 women without gallstones. No significant differences in calories, protein, fat or carbohydrate intake were found. In a second study, the diet of 50 pts. with known gallstones and that of 50 matched controls was compared. No significant differences were found once again (*Sarles H et al. Diet and cholesterol gallstones: A further study. Digestion 17(2):128-134, 1978*).

Observational Study: The incidence of gallstones in autopsy statistics was compared to diets in France, India, Japan, Portugal, South Africa, Sweden and Uganda. Low calorie diets, low lipid intakes and vegetable diets were associated with a low incidence of gallstones. When total calories were below 3,000 kcal, there was a positive correlation between calorie intake and gallstone incidence; in France, for example, in the 20 yrs. following the starvation caused by World War II, changes in the incidence of gallstones paralleled the changes in total calories, lipids and animal proteins. When calorie intakes were 3,000 kcal/d or higher, however, these correlations no longer existed. These results suggest that <u>a hypocaloric diet associated with a low fat intake and a low protein intake of mostly vegetable origin</u> is protective against cholelithiasis (*Sarles H et al. Diet and cholesterol gallstones: A multicenter study. Digestion 17(2):121-127, 1978*).

Increase <u>dietary fiber</u>.

Experimental Controlled Study: 13 pts. with radiolucent gallstones ate refined or unrefined carbohydrate diets for 6 wks. each, in random order. While the unrefined carbohydrate diet averaged 27 gms of fiber daily, the refined carbohydrate diet averaged only 13 gms of fiber daily. The bile saturation index was higher in 12/13 during the refined carbohydrate period (*Thornton JR et al. Diet and gallstones: Effects of refined carbohydrates on bile cholesterol saturation and bile acid metabolism. Gut 24:2-6, 1983*).

Experimental Study: 11 healthy individuals added 30 grams of wheat bran to their diet for 2 months. There was a decrease in bile saturation index in all 5 subjects whose initial index was 1 or higher but no change in those whose initial index was less than 1 (*Watts JM et al. The effect of added bran to the diet on the saturation of bile in people without gallstones. Am J Surg 135:321, 1978*).

Observational Study: The consumption of vegetables and fruits was lower in 101 gallstone pts. than in 101 matched controls, suggesting that the consumption of fiber may be protective (*Sarles H et al. Diet and cholesterol gallstones. A study of 101 patients with cholelithiasis compared to 101 matched controls. Am J Dig Dis 14:531-34, 1969*).

Avoid overconsumption of carbohydrates.

Animal Experimental Study: Since epidemiologic studies suggest that diets rich in carbohydrates may, in part, be responsible for the increasing incidence of pigment gallstone disease, two gps. of 8 prairie dogs were maintained on either a control, nonlithogenic chow, or a high carbohydrate (35% sucrose, 32% rich starch) diet for 2 months. The results indicate that, in the prairie dog, carbohydrate feeding results in increased biliary concentrations of phospholipids, calcium, and bilirubin, and the formation of calcium bilirubinate crystals, sludge and microscopic gallstones (*Conter RL et al. Carbohydrate diet-induced calcium bilirubinate sludge and pigment gallstones in the prairie dog. J Surg Res 40(6):580-87, 1986*).

Avoid sugar.

Negative Observational Study: In a study of 88,837 women aged 34-59, no significant association was found between the energy-adjusted intake of sucrose and the relative risk of symptomatic gallstones (*Maclure KM et al. Dietary predictors of symptom-associated gallstones in middle-aged women. Am J Clin Nutr 52:916-22, 1990*).

Observational Study: Gallstone formation in young people was correlated with an increased sugar intake (soft drinks and sweets) as well as an increased energy or fat intake, suggesting that sugar may increase cholesterol synthesis by stimulating insulin secretion (*Report: How sugar can get you stoned. New Scientist vol. 14, March 21, 1985*).

Observational Study: Dietary habits were reviewed for 267 hospitalized pts. with newly diagnosed gallstones and compared to 214 matched controls in the community and 359 hospital patient controls. Refined sugar intake in drinks and sweets was found to be a risk factor independent of obesity (*Scragg RK et al. Diet, alcohol, and relative weight in gall stone disease: A case-control study. Br Med J 288:1113-19, 1984*).

Vegetarian diet.

Observational Study: In a study of 88,837 women aged 34-59, compared to the lowest quintile of vegetable fat intake, the relative risk of symptomatic gallstones was 0.6 (95% confidence interval, 0.4-0.9), and the corresponding relative risk for vegetable protein intake was 0.7 (95% confidence interval, 0.6-0.) (*Maclure KM et al. Dietary predictors of symptom-associated gallstones in middle-aged women. Am J Clin Nutr 52:916-22, 1990*).

Observational Study: In a study of over 700 women aged 40-69 lasting several years, 632 omnivorous women had about twice the incidence of gallstones as 130 vegetarian women, perhaps because they ate more fat and less fiber (*Pixley F et al. Effect of vegetarianism on development of gall stones in women. Br Med J 291:11-12, 1985*).

Animal Experimental Study: Substitution of soy for casein (milk protein) significantly inhibited gallstone formation, and had a solubilizing effect when gallstones were preestablished (*Kritchevsky D, Klurfeld DM. Influence of vegetable protein on gallstone formation in hamsters. Am J Clin Nutr 32:2174, 1979*).

Observational Study: The incidence of gallstones in autopsy statistics was compared to diets in France, India, Japan, Portugal, South Africa, Sweden and Uganda. A vegetable (vegan) diet was associated with a low incidence of gallstones, while the consumption of both animal proteins and animal fats was each directly and strikingly correlated with the incidence of gallstones. For people consuming at least 3,000 kcal/d, however, this correlation no longer held (*Sarles H et al. Diet and cholesterol gallstones: A multicenter study. Digestion 17(2):121-127, 1978*).

Avoid legumes.

Experimental Controlled Study: Chileans and N. Am. Indians have one of the highest prevalence rates of cholesterol gallstones in the world, and legumes are common foods consumed by both populations. To test the hypothesis that legume intake may favor the production of biliary cholesterol supersaturation, 20 young males received 120 g of dry legumes/d and a control diet without legumes for a period of 1 mo. each. After the legume diet, LDL cholesterol decreased by 16% (p<0.001), while bile cholesterol saturation increased from a mean of 110% to 169% (p<0.001) (*Nervi F et al. Influence of legume intake on biliary lipids and cholesterol saturation in young Chilean men. Gastroenterology 96(3):825-30, 1989*).

Eat a regular breakfast.

Observational Study: Women who skipped breakfast or had only coffee experienced a much greater incidence of gallstones than those who ate a morning meal (*Capron JP et al. Meal frequency and duration of overnight fast: A role in gall-stone formation? Br Med J 283:1435, 1981*).

Avoid high animal fat intake.

Negative Observational Study: In a study of 88,837 women aged 34-59, no significant association was found between the energy-adjusted intake of animal fat or animal protein and the relative risk of symptomatic gallstones (*Maclure KM et al. Dietary predictors of symptom-associated gallstones in middle-aged women. Am J Clin Nutr 52:916-22, 1990*).

Observational Study: 267 hospital pts. with newly-diagnosed gallstones were compared to 241 matched controls from the community and 359 hospital controls. High fat intake in the young was found to be a risk factor (*Scragg RK et al. Diet, alcohol, and relative weight in gall stone disease: A case-control study. Br Med J 288:1113-19, 1984*).

Observational Study: The incidence of gallstones in autopsy statistics was compared to diets in France, India, Japan, Portugal, South Africa, Sweden and Uganda. There was a strking correlation between the intake of animal fats and the incidence of gallstones and a slight correlation between the intake of vegetable fats and the gallstone incidence. However, when the total calorie intake was at least 3,000 kcal/d, these correlations no longer held (*Sarles H et al. Diet and cholesterol gallstones: A multicenter study. Digestion 17(2):121-127, 1978*).

Fats which are solid at room temperature are less likely to provoke biliary colic than fats which are liquid (*Sarles H. Gallbladder contraction and type of fat. Letter. Lancet 2:1399, 1989*).

Experimental Study: Six normal volunteers ate 5 test meals containing various fats. Plasma CCK levels were measured and the gallbladder volume was calculated from ultasound measurements. The sodium salt of oleic acid (a monounsaturate) produced a significantly greater integrated CCK response than that of stearic acid (a saturated fatty acid). The gallbladder contracted to 3% of its initial volume after oleate but remained at 8% of its initial volume after stearate. Also, unsaturated triglycerides were found to be stonger stimulants than saturated ones (*Beardshall K et al. Saturation of fat and cholecystokinin release: implications for pancreatic carcinogenesis. Lancet 2:1008-10, 1989*).

> *Note: Long-chain fatty acids are solid if they are saturated and liquid if they are not (Sarles H. Gallbladder contraction and type of fat. Letter. Lancet 2:1399, 1989).*

Experimental Study: Gallbladder contraction in healthy volunteers was studied after a meal comprising of 20 g of various fats (trielaidin, trilaurin, triolein, soya lecithin, egg yolk, butter, corn oil, sunflower oil, cacao fat, hydrogenated coconut oil, olive oil). The action of saturated and unsaturated fats was not significantly different; fats liquid at room temperature resulted in a significantly greater contraction of the gallbladder (45%) than solid fats (25%) (*Sarles H et al. Etude de l'action des corps gras sur la contraction vésiculaire. I: Comparaison de l'action de divers corps gras. Nutritio Dieta 2:219-22, 1960*).

Moderate alcohol consumption.

Observational Study: 88,837 women aged 34-59 were followed for 4 yrs. after completing a detailed questionnaire about food and alcohol intake. An ave. alcohol intake of 5 g or more per day was associated with a 40% reduction in the risk of gallstones in nonobese women (*Maclure KM et al. Weight, diet, and the risk of symptomatic gallstones in middle-aged women. N Engl J Med 321(9):563-69, 1989*).

Observational Study: In a study of 267 hospital pts. with newly-diagnosed gallstone disease, 241 individually matched community controls and 359 controls who were pts. in the hospital, in both sexes increased intake of alcohol was associated with a decreased risk of developing gallstones (*Scragg RK et al. Diet, alcohol, and relative weight in gall stone disease: A case-control study. Br Med J 288:1113-19, 1984*).

Coffee consumption may inhibit cholesterol gallstone formation, but may cause acute gallbladder pain.

May inhibit the formation of cholesterol gallstones.

Animal Experimental Study: In dogs fed a control diet, administration of caffeine significantly increased hepatic bile flow and decreased the gallbladder/hepatic bile ratio for both bile acids and sodium. In dogs fed a high-cholesterol diet, caffeine significantly decreased the ratios for both bile acids and sodium, lowered gallbladder bile protein levels, normalized gallbladder stasis, and lowered serum cholesterol levels. In summary, caffeine prevented formation of cholesterol gallstones in this experimental model, perhaps due to alterations of multiple biliary parameters including inhibition of gallbladder absorption (*Lillemoe KD et al. Caffeine prevents cholesterol gallstone formation. Surgery 106(2):400-07, 1989*).

May cause pain in gallstone patients due to stimulation of gallbladder contractions.

Experimental Study: 6 healthy regular coffee drinkers ingested 165 ml each of regular and decaffeinated coffee and 400 ml of regular coffee. Both regular and decaffeinated coffee were found to give rise to increments in plasma cholecystokinin and contractions of the gallbladder (*Douglas BR et al. Coffee stimulation of cholecystokinin release and gallbladder contraction in humans. Am J Clin Nutr 52:553-56, 1990*).

VITAMINS

Vitamin C:

Deficiency may be associated with cholesterol gallstones (*Bergman F et al. Gallstone formation in guinea pigs under different dietary conditions. Effect of vitamin C on bile acid pattern. Med Biol 5992):92-8, 1981;Jenkins SA. Vitamin C status, serum cholesterol levels and bile composition in the pregnant guinea-pig. Br J Nutr 43(1):95-100, 1980*).

Supplementation may be beneficial (*Ginter E, Milu:s L. Reduction of gallstone formation by ascorbic acid in hamsters. Experientia 33(6):716-7, 1977; Peraza M et al. [Prevention of cholelithiasis with ascorbic acid. Experimental study in hamsters.] Rev Gestroenterol Mex 44(4):159-62, 1979*).

Negative Experimental Study: The biliary lipid composition was examined in 10 healthy persons before and after 7-15 days' treatment with large doses of ascorbic acid. No significant differences were found, suggesting that vitamin C most likely has no place in the medical treatment of cholesterol gallstones (*Pedersen L. Biliary lipids during vitamin C feeding in healthy persons. Scand J Gastroenterol 10(3):311-14, 1975*).

Vitamin E:

Deficiency may be associated with cholesterol gallstones (*Saito T. The preventive effect of vitamin E on gallstone formation. (1). A study of biliary cholesterol and bile acids in vitamin E-deficient hamsters. Arch Jpn Chir 56(3):247-61, 1987; Saito T. The preventive effect of vitamin E on gallstone formation. (2). A study of the prevention of gallstone formation and protection from liver disorder in hamsters. Arch Jpn Chir 56(3):262-75, 1987*).

Supplementation may reduce gallstone formation in patients with cholesterol stones.

Experimental Study: 10 pts. received 200 mg 3 times daily of d-α-tocopherol, and 2 received 100 mg 3 times daily. 5 pts. with cholesterol gallstones on the higher dosage showed reduced biliary cholesterol levels and increased glycine-conjugated bile acids, and all 5 had a corresponding improvement of the lithogenic index. These changes were not observed in the other patients. 2 of these pts. had bilirubin stones. In the other 5 pts., serum α-tocopherol levels were not raised adequately; 2 of these pts. received the lower dosage, while the T-tube had not been clamped before and throughout the study in the remaining 3 pts. which reduced the rise in α-tocopherol (*Saito T, Tanimura H. The preventive effect of vitamin E on gallstone formation. (3). A study of the biliary lipids in patients with gallstones. Arch Jpn Chir 56(3):276-88, 1987*).

OTHER NUTRITIONAL FACTORS

Choline:

Lecithin, a dietary source of choline, may increase the capacity of the bile to solubilize cholesterol (*Duff GL et al. Am J Med 11:92, 1951*).

Negative Placebo-controlled Study: 25 pts. with gallstones and radiologically functioning gallbladders received either lecithin 8 gm daily or placebo. Lecithin failed to affect the solubility of bile cholesterol (*Mamianetti A et al. [Biliary lipids and the cholesterol saturation rate in relation to lecithin administration by oral route.] Acta Gastroenterol Latinoam 9(2):89-94, 1979*) (*in Spanish*).

Supplementation may be beneficial.

Negative Experimental Study: 6 pts. with radiolucent cholelithiasis underwent randomized successive 3-wk. trials with beta-glycerophosphate, linoleic acid, or purified soybean lecithin. Soybean lecithin feeding effected a qualitative change in biliary lecithin with increased fatty acid unsaturation, but no significant improvement in biliary cholesterol saturation or lipid composition changes including a proportionate increase in biliary phospholipids resulted from any treatment program (*Holon KR et al. Effect of oral administration of 'essential' phospholipid, beta-glycerophosphate, and linoleic acid on biliary lipids in patients with cholelithiasis. Digestion 19(4):251-8, 1979*).

Experimental Study: 8 pts. aged 38-58 with gallstones were treated with "lecithin" 100 mg 3 times daily for 18-34 mo. and demonstrated significant increases in bile phospholipid content and cholate/cholesterol ratio as well as a significant decrease in bile cholesterol. In 1 pt., gallstones decreased in size and changed in shape (*Tuzhilin SA et al. The treatment of patients with gallstones by lecithin. Am J Gastroenterol 65(3):231-5, 1976*).

Experimental Study: Pts. with gallstones have an abnormally low phospholipid-cholesterol ratio in their bile (2:1 in pts. vs. 6:1 in normals). 6 of these pts. were given lecithin 10 gm daily which resulted in a doubling of the bile concentration of phospholipids (*Tompkins RK et al. Relationship of biliary phospholipid and cholesterol concentrations to the occurrence and dissolution of human gallstones. Ann Surg 172(6):936-45, 1970*).

- with <u>Cholic Acid</u>:

Negative Experimental Study: 6 pts. with radiolucent cholelithiasis received soybean lecithin plus cholic acid. After 6 mo., there was no therapeutic response indicative of gallstone dissolution in any of the pts. (*Holon KR et al. Effect of oral administration of 'essential' phospholipid, beta-glycerophosphate, and linoleic acid on biliary lipids in patients with cholelithiasis. Digestion 19(4):251-8, 1979*).

Experimental Study: 7 pts. with radiolucent gallstones and 2 pts. with radiolucent biliary tree stones were treated with purified soybean lecithin 2,250 mg daily and cholic acid 750 mg daily for 6 months. In 2 pts. the stones disappeared and in 1, the stones decreased in size. In all 5 pts. whose fasting bile samples were obtained before and during treatment, the lithogenic index of bile was reduced during treatment. Also during treatment, the biliary deoxycholic acid concentration increased and chenodeoxycholic acid concentration decreased (*Toouli J et al. Gallstone dissolution in man using cholic acid and lecithin. Lancet 2:1124-6, 1975*).

<u>Essential Fatty Acids</u>:

Rowachol (Rowa, Ltd., Eire), a proprietary "essential oil" preparation, lowers the bile lithogenic index (*Doran J et al. Gut 18:A977, 1977*).

Supplementation with Rowachol may be beneficial.

Note: The incidence of gallstones may be <u>higher</u> when fats come from polyunsaturates rather than from saturated fats and cholesterol.

Observational Study: The incidence of gallstones found at autopsy of 424 male pts. who had been on the standard American diet was compared to that of 422 male pts. who had been on a diet high in polyunsaturates and low in saturated fats and cholesterol. 14% of those on the standard diet had gallstones versus 34% of the others (*Sturdevant RA et al. Increased prevalence of cholelithiasis in men ingesting a serum-cholesterol-lowering diet. N Engl J Med 288(1):24-27, 1973*).

Experimental Study: 23 pts. took Rowachol 1 cap/10 kg/d for 6-12 months. 3 pts. had complete and 4 had partial dissolution of gallstones (*Bell GD, Doran J. Gall stone dissolution in man using an essential oil preparation. Br Med J 1:24, 1979*).

Taurine:

Hepatic conjugation of bile acids in humans proceeds with taurine if it is available (*Vessey DA. The biochemical basis for the conjugation of bile acids with either glycine or taurine. Biochem J 174:621-26, 1978*).

Supplementation may be beneficial.

Experimental Controlled Crossover Study: 18 hepatobiliary pts. with choledochostomies and a specific T-tube insertion randomly received an ordinary post-op soft diet for the first 5 post-op days followed by a taurine-supplemented soft diet (40 mumol/kg/d) for another 5 days or the same diets in reverse order. The taurine-supplemented diet increased the secretion and conjugation of bile acids in both gps. (*Wang WY, Liaw KY. Effect of a taurine-supplemented diet on conjugated bile acids in biliary surgical patients. JPEN J Parenter Enteral Nutr 15(3):294-7, 1991*).

Experimental Study: 4 healthy males received taurine 3.2 g/d for 2 wks., while another 5 healthy males were administered cholesterol 1 g/d for 2 wks. followed by taurine and cholesterol simultaneously for 2 weeks. Taurine administration alone increased taurine-conjugated bile acids, but did not alter either serum or biliary lipid composition. When taurine and cholesterol were administered together, both LDL cholesterol and the bile lithogenic index were increased (*Tanno N et al. Effect of taurine administration on serum lipid and biliary lipid composition in man. Tohoku J Exp Med 159(2):91-100, 1989*).

Animal Experimental Study: Mice were fed either a lithogenic diet either with or without taurine supplementation or a control diet. Results suggest that the inhibitory effect of dietary taurine on cholesterol gallstone formation is related to increased bile acid synthesis (*Nakamura-Yamanaka Y et al. Effect of dietary taurine on cholesterol 7 alpha-hydroxylase activity in the liver of mice fed a lithogenic diet. J Nutr Sci Vitaminol (Tokyo) 33(3):239-43, 1987*).

- -

OTHER FACTORS

Avoid obesity.

Observational Study: 88,837 women aged 34-59 were followed for 4 yrs. after completing a detailed questionnaire about food and alcohol intake. The age-adjusted relative risk for very obese women was 6.0 (95% confidence interval, 4.0 - 9.0), compared to normals. For slightly overweight women, the relative risk was 1.7 (95% confidence interval, 1.1 - 2.7). Overall, there was a linear relation between relative weight and the risk of gallstones (*Maclure KM et al. Weight, diet, and the risk of symptomatic gallstones in middle-aged women. N Engl J Med 321(9):563-69, 1989*).

Case Report: A 41-year-old woman with a large gallstone who was also 55 lbs overweight went on a 1000 calorie diet. Ater 15 mo., she had lost 42 lbs and her gallstone had disappeared. After 19 mo., she was down to her ideal weight and her gallbladder was functioning normally (*Thornton JR. Gallstone disappearance associated with weight loss. Letter. Lancet 2:478, 1979*).

Rule out food sensitivities.

Experimental Study: 69 pts. with gallstones or post-cholecystectomy syndrome were placed on an elimination diet consisting of beef, rye, soy, rice, cherry, peach, apricot, beet, and spinach. After 1 week, additional foods were added systematically and each symptom-provoking food was retested several times. All pts. were relieved of their symptoms, with improvements usually occurring in 3-5 days. Egg was by far the most frequent offender (93%), followed by pork (64%) and onion (52%) (*Breneman JC. Allergy elimination diet as the most effective gallbladder diet. Ann Allergy 26:83, 1968*).

Experimental Study: Ingestion of offending foods caused disturbances in emptying of the gallbladder, as evidenced by measurements of its size. Some differences between control and experimental measurements were seen at 1 hr., but the major differences were usually seen at the end of 2 hrs. and were associated with typical symptoms of a gallbladder attack along with such allergic symptoms as shortness of breath, sneezing, headaches and hives (*Necheles H et al. Allergy of the gallbladder: A study using the Graham-Cole test and the leukopenic index. Am J Dig Dis 7:238, 1940*).

Experimental Study: Pts. with bronchial asthma developed gallbladder distress after ingesting wheat which ceased after wheat elimination (*Graham EA et al. Diseases of the Gall Bladder and Bile Ducts. Philadelphia, Lea & Febiger, 1928*).

Rule out hydrochloric acid deficiency.

Experimental Study: 26/50 (52%) pts. with cholelithiasis showed evidence of gastric hyposecretion with the augmented histamine test, and 16/18 showed persistent reflux of duodenal fluid by the pyloric regurgitation test. Results suggest that, when gallstones form, duodenal reflux may be an associated factor that produces dysfunction and destruction of oxyntic cells. These changes may cause hyposecretion, while the presence of bile and pancreatic juices in the stomach may cause flatulent dyspepsia (*Capper WM et al. Gallstones, gastric secretion, and flatulent dyspepsia. Lancet 1:413-15, 1967*).

Clinical Observation: Gastric hyposecretion was usual when the gallbladder was non-functioning or atonic (*Twiss JR, Oppenheim E. Practical Management of Disorders of the Liver, Pancreas and Bile Ducts. London, 1955*).

Experimental Study: 49/110 (45%) pts. were found to have impaired acid output (*Wichels P, Brink J. Z klin Med 123:303, 1933*).

Experimental Study: 57/192 pts. with documented gallstones had gastric anacidity following an Ewald meal of bread and water, while another 29/192 had gastric hypoacidity, a total of 45% (*Gatewood. JAMA 81:904, 1923*).

GLAUCOMA

DIETARY FACTORS

Moderate protein diet.

> **Observational Study:** Based on a case-control study of 400 eye pts. including 52 with ocular hypertension and/or glaucoma, the pigmentary-disperson glaucomas, and likely also pseudoexfoliative glaucoma, are strongly associated with excessive protein intake (>3x US RDA) (*Lane BC. Diet and the glaucomas. Abstract. J Am Coll Nutr 10(5):536, 1991*).

Minimize dietary *trans fatty acids*.

> **Observational Study:** Based on a case-control study of 400 eye pts. including 52 with ocular hypertension and/or glaucoma, the pigmentary-disperson glaucomas, and likely also pseudoexfoliative glaucoma, are strongly associated with the intake of *trans* fatty acids (*Lane BC. Diet and the glaucomas. Abstract. J Am Coll Nutr 10(5):536, 1991*).

Avoid caffeine:

> **Case Reports:** 2 pts. with open-angle glaucoma responded to caffeinated, but not to decaffeinated, expresso with clinically significant increases in intraocular pressure 1 hr. later (*Davis RH. Does caffeine ingestion affect intraocular pressure? Letter. Ophthalmology 96(11):1680-81, 1989*).

> **Experimental Single-blind Crossover Study:** 13 pts. randomly received either coffee or herbal tea in either order. There was a statistically significant difference in the change in intraocular pressure between the 2 gps. at 90 min. after ingestion (p=0.003) which, however, was not clinically significant. There were no significant differences at 30 and 60 min. (*Higginbotham EJ et al. The effect of caffeine on intraocular pressure in glaucoma patients. Ophthalmology 96(5):624-26, 1989*).

- -

VITAMINS

Thiamine:

May be reduced due to decreased absorption (*Asregadoo ER. Blood levels of thiamine and ascorbic acid in chronic open-angle glaucoma. Ann Ophthalmol 11(7):1095-1100, 1979*).

In glaucoma, thiamine deficiency may be associated with optic nerve atrophy whose symptoms may be at least partly reversible.

> **Theoretical Discussion:** As thiamine is so vital in the metabolism of nervous and vascular tissues, there may be a connection between thiamine deficiency and atrophy of the optic nerve in glaucoma. Corticosteroids are well known to increase intraocular pressure. Beriberi, the classical thiamine deficiency disease, may cause atrophy of the endocrine glands and hypertrophy of the adrenals with increased corticosteroid secretion. In experimental animals, beriberi is associated with degeneration of the myelin sheaths and ganglion cells of the brain and spinal cord. It would seem that the ganglion cells of the eye would also be affected. In Guyana from 1952-56, the author failed to find glaucoma in East Indians, who were mainly vegetarians and fisheaters, and found a preponderance of chronic open angle glaucoma in blacks, whose diet was different and who were more likely to have hypovitaminosis B. Most cases of moderate optic atrophy associated with hypovitaminosis B could be cured with 100 mg thiamine and vitamin B complex given IM for 10 days and followed by oral supplements. Pts. with early or moderate cupping improved visually, and their fields remained static or improved slightly. Glaucomatous eyes

also improved, although not as much (*Asregadoo ER. Blood levels of thiamine and ascorbic acid in chronic open-angle glaucoma. Ann Ophthalmol 11(7):1095-1100, 1979*).

Vitamin A:

If deficient, supplementation may be beneficial.

Clinical Observation: Following supplementation with vitamin A, the intraocular pressures of several pts. with evidence of vitamin A deficiency dropped to normal, and they were able to discontinue their medications after a few months (*Todd GP. Nutrition, Health & Disease. Norfolk, Virginia, The Donning Company, 1985*).

Vitamin C:

Intake may be inversely correlated with intraocular pressure.

Observational Study: Ave. intraocular pressure of 31 subjects (ages 26-74) with a mean daily intake of 75 mg vitamin C was 22.33 mm Hg which was significantly higher (p<0.001) than that of a matched gp. with a mean daily intake of 1200 mg (15.15 mm Hg) (*Lane BC. Evaluation of intraocular pressure with daily, sustained closework stimulus to accommodation, lowered tissue chromium and dietary deficiency of ascorbic acid. 3rd International Conference on Myopia, Copenhagen & The Hague. Doc Ophthalmol 28:149-55, 1981*).

Intake may be inadequate.

Observational Study: Based on a case-control study of 400 eye pts. including 52 with ocular hypertension and/or glaucoma, primary open-angle glaucoma appears strongly associated with a deficiency of habitual daily ascorbic acid intake (*Lane BC. Diet and the glaucomas. Abstract. J Am Coll Nutr 10(5):536, 1991*).

Negative Observational Study: There was no significant difference in dietary intake between 38 pts. with chronic open-angle glaucoma (mean age 63 yrs.) and 12 normals (mean age 53 yrs.) (*Asregadoo ER. Blood levels of thiamine and ascorbic acid in chronic open-angle glaucoma. Ann Ophthalmol 11(7):1095-1100, 1979*).

May be deficient.

Negative Observational Study: There was no significant difference in blood ascorbic acid levels between 38 pts. with chronic open-angle glaucoma (mean age 63 yrs.) and 12 normals (mean age 53 yrs.) (*Asregadoo ER. Blood levels of thiamine and ascorbic acid in chronic open-angle glaucoma. Ann Ophthalmol 11(7):1095-1100, 1979*).

Observational Study: In a study of aqueous humor ascorbate concentration in 35 pts. with open-angle glaucoma, the results indicate that the majority of open-angle glaucomatous eyes do not involve a deficiency of ascorbate (*Lee P et al. Aqueous humor ascorbate concentration and open-angle glaucoma. Arch Ophthalmol 95(2):308-10, 1977*).

A glucose-uptake insulin-receptor potentiator, ascorbic acid putatively enables strong ciliary muscle eye-focusing activity, and a deficiency is associated with elevated intraocular pressure which tends to stretch the eye to reduce the need for focusing power (*Lane BC. Diet and the glaucomas. Abstract. J Am Coll Nutr 10(5):536, 1991*).

Supplementation may increase aqueous humor drainage by reducing the viscosity of hyaluronic acid (*Liu KM et al. Inhibition of oxidative degradation of hyaluronic acid by uric acid. Curr Eye Res 3(8):1049-53, 1984*).

Supplementation may reduce intraocular pressure.

Negative Experimental Study: 20 pts. failed to show changes in intraocular tension after 1 wk. of supplementation with vitamin C 3.5 g/kg/d in 4 divided doses (*Mehra KS. Relationship of pH of blood and aqueous with vitamin C. Ann Ophthalmol 10(1):83-92, 1978*).

Negative Experimental Study: 6 pts. with open angle glaucoma failed to benefit from the addition of 1.5 gm ascorbic acid 3 times daily for 3-12 wks. to their usual medications (*Fishbein SL, Goldstein S. The pressure lowering effect of ascorbic acid. Ann Ophthalmol 4:498-91, 1972*).

Experimental Controlled Study: 25 subjects (ave. age 63 yrs.) with moderate ocular hypertension received 0.5 gm ascorbic acid orally 4 times daily. After 6 days mean intraocular pressure fell significantly (*Linner E. The pressure lowering effect of ascorbic acid in ocular hypertension. Acta Ophthalmol (Copen) 47:685-9, 1969*).

Experimental Study: A single dose of 500 mg/kg ascorbic acid reduced intraocular pressure in 39/39 pts. by an ave. of 16 mm Hg but usually caused GI symptoms. Ascorbic acid 100-150 mg/kg 3-5 times daily resulted in almost normal intraocular pressures in 15/16 pts. by 45 days, some of whom were uncontrollable with acetazolamide and 2% pilocarpine, with only 3-4 days of GI symptoms (*Virno M et al. Oral treatment of glaucoma with vitamin C. Eye, Ear, Nose, Throat Monthly 46:1502-8, 1967*).

Experimental Study: Sodium ascorbate 0.4-1 g/kg IV or oral ascorbic acid 500 mg/kg successfully produced a significant lowering of intraocular pressure in patients. Oral ascorbic acid was most effective in chronic open-angle glaucoma and lasted for the length of the study (7 mo.) when given at a maintenance dosage of 125 mg/kg 3-5 times daily. Normal intraocular tension was achieved with ascorbic acid alone or in association with miotics. In some cases, ascorbic acid supplementation achieved normal intraocular tension when miotics alone were unable to control it (*Bietti GB. Further contributions on the value of osmotic substances as means to reduce intraocular pressure. Trans Ophthalmol Soc Aust 26:61-71, 1967; Trans Ophthamol Soc U K 86:247-54, 1966*).

Experimental Controlled Study: 22 normal subjects received 500 mg ascorbic acid orally twice daily. After 1 wk., intraocular pressure was significantly lower and returned to baseline by 1 wk. after ascorbic acid was discontinued (*Linner E. Intraocular pressure regulation and ascorbic acid. Acta Soc Med Upsal 69:225-32, 1964*).

- with <u>glycerin</u>:

> **Experimental Study:** 18 pts. with different types of glaucoma received an IV drip containing 0.5 g/kg glycerin and 0.28 g/kg sodium ascorbate (pH 7.7-7.4) for 7-60 minutes. Intraocular pressure was reduced in all but one pt. It began to fall in most cases within 15-20 min. and dropped to minimal levels within 30-60 minutes. The precentage intraocular pressure reduction varied from 20.6%-84.2% in the glaucomatous eyes and from 30.1%-64.9% in the normal eyes (*Shen T-M, Yu M-C. Clinical evaluation of glycerin-sodium ascorbate solution in lowering intraocular pressure. Chin Med J 1:64-68, 1975*).

Topical application may be beneficial.

Experimental Controlled Study: 10% aqueous solution of ascorbic acid was applied topically in one eye of 19 subjects (ave. age 63 yrs.) 3 times daily for 3 days resulting in a significant drop in mean intraocular pressure in the treated eye only (*Linner E. Intraocular pressure regulation and ascorbic acid. Acta Soc Med Upsal 69:225-32, 1964*).

- -

MINERALS

<u>Chromium</u>:

Erythrocyte levels may be reduced in primary open-angle glaucoma.

Observational Study: Based on a case-control study of 400 eye pts. including 52 with ocular hypertension and/or glaucoma, primary open-angle glaucoma appears strongly associated with RBC chromium deficiency and elevation of RBC vanadium, chromium's principle antagonist. Chromium is a glucose-uptake insulin-receptor potentiator which putatively enables sustained strong ciliary-muscle eye-focusing activity, and a deficiency is associated with elevated intraocular pressure which tends to stretch the eye to reduce the need for focusing power. The most significant biochemical differentiator between normals and persons with primary open-angle glaucoma is RBC chromium. Persons with diet-responsive RBC chromium ≤150 ng/ml are more likely to have undrugged intraocular pressures >20 mm Hg (odds ratio 95% confidence interval=1.4-16.4) (*Lane BC. Diet and the glaucomas. Abstract. J Am Coll Nutr 10(5):536, 1991*).

<u>Zinc to Copper ratio</u>:

May be decreased in the aqueous humor.

Observational Study: 44 pts. with glaucoma and cataract were found to have normal serum zinc and copper concentrations, with the highest mean copper concentration found in the glaucoma group. There was a significant negative correlation between the aqueous humor levels of zinc and copper in glaucoma patients. It was concluded that reduced zinc together with increased copper might be of importance in pts. with glaucoma (*Akyol N et al. Aqueous humour and serum zinc and copper concentrations of patients with glaucoma and cataract. Br J Ophthalmol 74(11):661-2, 1990*).

OTHER NUTRITIONAL FACTORS

Rutin:

A common plant constituent.

Administration may be beneficial.

Experimental Study: After 4 or more wks. of administration of rutin 20 mg 3 times daily, 17/26 eyes with uncomplicated primary glaucoma demonstrated a 15% or greater reduction in intraocular pressure and responded better to miotics (*Stocker FW. New ways of influencing the intraocular pressure. N Y State J Med 49:58-63, 1949*).

COMBINED NUTRITIONAL TREATMENT

Vitamin A, Vitamin C, Vitamin E and Protein:

Combined supplementation may be beneficial.

Clinical Observation: In West Africa, hundreds of pts. with primary glaucoma were successfully treated with vitamin C 3 g, vitamin A 180,000 IU and vitamin E 200 IU daily. Since many pts. were protein-deficient, a 20 gm protein supplement was also given daily. In most cases, ocular tension was reduced to normal within 1 wk., while earlier trials with 1/2 the dosages reduced tension to normal in 2-4 weeks (*Evans SC. Ophthalmic nutrition and prevention of eye disorder and blindness. Nutr Metab 21(suppl 1):268-72, 1977*).

OTHER FACTORS

Rule out food sensitivities in chronic simple glaucoma.

Case Reports: 113 pts. with chronic simple glaucoma were successfully treated by diagnosing atopic allergies and treating them with avoidance and immunotherapy. Some demonstrated an immediate rise in intraocular pressure of up to 20 mm upon antigen challenge (*Raymond LF. Allergy and chronic simple glaucoma. Ann Allergy 22:146-50, 1964*).

Case Reports: In 3 cases of chronic simple glaucoma, treatment with miotics and attempted desensitization with autogenous bacterial antigens was supplemented by the removal of food antigens (as determined from the pulse testing method of Coca) from their diets. In 1 case, ocular tension was brought under control only after the institution of an allergen-free diet. In the other 2 cases, surgery and medical treatment controlled the tension but failed to check the progressive visual field loss which showed marked improvement after the institution of an allergen-free diet (*Berens C et al. Allergy in glaucoma. Manifestations of allergy in three glaucoma patients as determined by the pulse-diet method of Coca. Ann Allergy 5:526-35, 1947*).

GOUT

DIETARY FACTORS

Low _purine_ diet (avoid meats, esp. organ meats, seafood, lentils, beans and peas).

May decrease uric acid by up to 1 milligram.

Restrict _alcohol_, especially _beer_ (which has a higher purine content than wine or spirits).

Beer consumption may be higher in patients with gout.

Observational Study: The major dietary difference of 61 men with gout versus controls was that 41% (25/41) of the afflicted men drank more than seven 12 ounce cans of beer daily compared to 17% of the healthy men which was associated with a significantly higher intake of purine nitrogen, half of which was derived from beer (_Gibson T et al. A controlled study of diet in patients with gout. Ann Rheum Dis 42(2):123-27, 1983_).

Increases lactate production which competes with uric acid for renal clearance (_Emmerson BT. Therapeutics of hyperuricaemia and gout. Med J Aust 141:31-6, 1984_).

Increases purine nucleotide degradation in the liver increasing oxypurine and thus uric acid production (_Emmerson BT. Therapeutics of hyperuricaemia and gout. Med J Aust 141:31-6, 1984_).

Avoid _fructose_.

Increases urate production, possibly leading to hyperuricemia (_Emmerson BT. Effect of oral fructose on urate production. Ann Rheum Dis 33:276, 1974; Henry RR, Crapo PA, Thorburn AW. Current issues in fructose metabolism. Annu Rev Nutr 11:21-39, 1991; Perheentupa J, Raivio K. Fructose-induced hyperuricaemia. Lancet 2:528, 1967_).

- -

VITAMINS

Folic Acid:

Inhibits xanthine oxidase which is required for uric acid production (_Kalckar HM, Klenow H. Milk xanthopterin oxidase and pteroylglutamic acid. J BiolChem 172:349-350, 1948_).

Note: Folic acid is only a weak inhibitor of human liver xanthine oxidase in vitro, and much of its inhibitory effect is secondary to trace contamination by pterin-6-aldehyde, a potent inhibitor of the enzyme (Boss GR et al. Failure of folic acid (pteroylglutamic acid) to affect hyperuricemia. J Lab Clin Med 96:783, 1980).

High dosage supplementation is said to reduce uric acid with greater safety than drugs (_Oster KA. Evaluation of serum cholesterol reduction and xanthine oxidase inhibition in the treatment of atherosclerosis, in Recent Advances in Studies on Cardiac Structure 3:73-80, 1973_).

Negative Experimental Study: Folic acid in oral doses of up to 1000 mg/d did not significantly lower the serum urate concentration nor decrease the urinary urate or total oxypurine excretion in 5 hyperuricemic subjects. The folate was well absorbed, as reflected by marked increases in serum and RBC folate concentrations, and up to 50% could be recovered in the urine. There was no evidence of clinical or laboratory toxicity (_Boss GR et al. Failure of folic acid (pteroylglutamic acid) to affect hyperuricemia. J Lab Clin Med 96:783, 1980_).

Niacin:

WARNING: Supplementation may be harmful.

May precipitate an attack of gout as nicotinic acid competes with uric acid for renal excretion (*Pfeiffer CC. Mental and Elemental Nutrients. New Canaan, Conn. Keats Publishing, 1975, p. 121*).

Vitamin A:

WARNING: Supplementation may be harmful.

Review Article: "Several lines of indirect evidence implicate vitamin A intoxication, associated mainly with impaired renal function, in the etiopathogensis of gouty arthritis. The enzyme xanthine oxidase is involved not only in the conversion of xanthine to uric acid but also in that of retinol to its more toxic metabolite, retinoic acid" (*Mawson AR, Onor GI. Gout and vitamin A intoxication: is there a connection? Semin Arthritis Rheum 20(5):297-304, 1991*).

Vitamin C:

May lower serum uric acid levels by increasing renal excretion.

Experimental Study: Supplementation with 4 gm or more vitamin C daily increased renal excretion of uric acid. While supplementation with < 8 gm/d of vitamin C did not affect serum uric acid levels, 8 gm daily decreased serum uric acid levels by 1.2 to 3.1 mg% (*Stein HB et al. Ascorbic acid-induced uricosuria: A consequence of megavitamin therapy. Ann Intern Med 84(4):385-8, 1976*).

- -

MINERALS

Zinc:

Plasma levels may be decreased during periods of disease activity (*Mataràn Pérez L et al. [Zinc in arthrosis and microcrystalline arthritis.] Rev Clin Esp 189(2):60-2, 1991*).

HEADACHE

See Also: "HYPOGLYCEMIA" (FUNCTIONAL)
PAIN
PREMENSTRUAL SYNDROME

DIETARY FACTORS

See Also: "Rule out food sensitivities" below

Low tryptophan diet

Serotonin is derived from tryptophan in the diet. Blood serotonin (which is at least 90% concentrated in platelets) may help provoke migraine (*Crook M. Migraine: A biochemical headache?* Biochem Soc Trans *9(4):351-57, 1981*); thus a low tryptophan diet may be beneficial.

Experimental Study: 10 women with recurrent migraine-like headache, flush, urticaria and itching excoriations were put on a diet in which the intake of foods with a high tryptophan to protein ratio was strongly restricted (which made the diet low in protein); serotonin-rich foods were excluded. On the diet, their migraine-like symptoms and skin manifestations were reduced and, in parallel, their severely disturbed 5-HT uptake kinetics in platelets were normalized, suggesting that impairment of 5-HT uptake in platelets contributes to the pathogenesis of some migraine-like headaches (*Unge G et al. Effects of dietary protein-tryptophan restriction upon 5-HT uptake by platelets and clinical symptoms in migraine-like headache.* Cephalalgia *3(4):213-18, 1983*).

High carbohydrate diet

A high carbohydrate diet may increase the availability of tryptophan to the brain, and thus promote brain serotonin synthesis, through provoking insulin secretion (*Curzon G. Influence of plasma tryptophan on brain 5-HT synthesis and serotonergic activity, in B Haber et al, Eds.* Serotonin: Current Aspects of Neurochemistry and Function. *New York, Plenum Press, 1981:207-19; Fernstrom JD. Dietary precursors and brain transmitter formation.* Annu Rev Med *32:413-25, 1981*).

Due to the involvement of brain serotonin in the anti-nociceptive system, a high carbohydrate diet may help to alleviate migraine headaches (*Sicuteri F. Endorphins, opiate receptors and migraine headache.* Headache *17:253-56, 1978*).

- with a low tryptophan diet:

Experimental Study: 7 migraine pts. (4 with classic, 3 with common migraine) were placed on a carbohydrate-rich diet in which the intake of foods with a high tryptophan to protein ratio was strongly restricted and serotonin-rich foods were excluded. After 50 days, 3/4 pts. with classic migraine noted a marked improvement in migraine frequency which began within 4 weeks. None of the 3 pts. with common migraine improved (*Hasselmark L et al. Effect of a carbohydrate-rich diet, low in protein-tryptophan, in classic and common migraine.* Cephalalgia *7:87-92, 1987*).

Low carbohydrate diet

Some migraine patients may develop headaches when hypoglycemic.

Experimental Study: Only 1/20 migraine pts. had a migraine identical with their usual symptoms during an insulin-produced hypoglycemia in the range of 20 mg% glucose (*Pierce J. Insulin-induced hypoglycemia in migraine.* JNNP *34:154-56, 1971*).

Observational Study: 5/36 pts. with both migraine and non-insulin-dependent diabetes mellitus had a marked reduction of migraines with the onset of diabetic control. For 4/36 pts. nocturnal-type hypoglycemia precipitated migraines, and 6/36 pts. had migraines precipitated by missing a meal (*Blau JN, Pike DA. Effect of diabetes on migraine. Lancet 2:241-43, 1970*).

A low sucrose diet may reduce migraine headaches in patients with reactive hypoglycemia.

Experimental Study: 74 migraine pts. who associated their attacks with fasting or with the mid-morning or mid-afternoon fasting state underwent a 5-hr., 100 gm glucose tolerance test. The curves of 6 pts. were classified as diabetic and 56 pts. exhibited a curve consistent with degrees of reactive hypoglycemia (serum glucose of <65 mg% or a drop of 75 mg% with 1 hr.). Following dietary therapy with a low sucrose, 6 meal regimen (protein:fat:carbohydrate ratio = 20:45:35), all pts. with a diabetic glucose tolerance curve showed an improvement of >75%, and 3 have been headache-free. 43/56 pts. with reactive hypoglycemic curves returned for follow-up. 27/43 (63%) showed >75% improvement, 17/43 (40%) showed 50-75% improvement, and 4/43 (9%) showed 25-50% improvement (*Dexter JD et al. The five hour glucose tolerance test and effect of low sucrose diet in migraine. Headache 18:91-94, 1978*).

A low carbohydrate diet may reduce migraine headaches in patients with reactive hypoglycemia.

Experimental Study: 11/92 pts. seen in more than a 17-month period had migraines that seemed to be associated with spontaneous hyperinsulinism. All improved or had complete symptom relief when placed on a low carbohydrate, high fat diet (150 gm protein, 190 gm fat, 75 gm carbohydrate) [sucrose content was unspecified] (*Wilkinson CF. Return of migrinoid headaches associated with spontaneous hypoglycemia. Am J Med Sci 218:209-12, 1949*).

- -

VITAMINS

Vitamin B6:

Supplementation may be beneficial in chronic headache induced by medications.

Review Article: Chronic use of ergotamine, opiate analgesics, and other medications used for pain relief, such as aspirin, may lead to medication-induced chronic headaches due to depletion of CNS endorphins with downregulating of receptor sites. The most successful treatments include an extremely gradual detoxification from the offending agents and concurrent use of pyridoxine to increase serotonin levels via pyridoxine-mediated pathways in order to raise pain thresholds (*Bernstein AL. Vitamin B6 in clinical neurology. Ann N Y Acad Sci 585:250-60, 1990*).

- -

MINERALS

Copper:

Dietary copper may trigger migraine headaches.

Review Article: The migraine-inducing effect of copper is associated with its role in the metabolism of vasoneuroactive amines, such as serotonin, tyramine, and catecholamines. Foods which contain high amounts of copper (such as chocolate, nuts, wheat germ and shellfish) or which increase the intestinal absorption of copper (such as citrus) or which bind and transport copper between blood and tissues (monosodium glutamate) are therefore potential headache triggering agents, especially when copper metabolism is abnormal (*Harrison DP. Copper as a factor in the dietary precipitation of migraine. Headache 26(5):248-50, 1986*).

Lithium:

Administration may reduce cluster headaches and the cyclic form of migraines (*Solomon SS, Lipton RB, Newman LC. Prophylactic therapy of cluster headaches. Clin Neuropharmacol 1492):116-30, 1991; Yung CY. A review of clinical trails of lithium in neurology. Pharmacol Biochem Behav 21 Suppl 1:57-64, 1984*).

Magnesium:

Premenstrual migraine headaches may be associated with low red blood cell magnesium levels.

> **Observational Study:** 26 female pts. with premenstrual tension had significantly lower RBC magnesium than 9 normals (p<0.01) despite no significant differences in serum magnesium levels (*Abraham GE, Lubran MM. Serum and red cell magnesium levels in patients with premenstrual tension. Am J Clin Nutr 34:(11)2364-66, 1981*).

May be deficient in pre-eclampsia which is strongly associated with a history of migraine headaches.

> **Observational Study:** 24 women with severe pre-eclampsia diagnosed before 34 wks.' gestation were compared to 48 matched controls. A history of headaches, particularly migraine, was identified as a significant risk factor in the pre-eclamptic women (*Moore MP, Redman CW. Case-control study of severe pre-eclampsia of early onset. Br Med J 287:580-83, 1983*).

> **Observational Study:** Women with pre-eclampsia were low in serum magnesium prior to therapy (*Weaver K. Magnesium in Health and Disease. Jamaica, N.Y., Spectrum Publications, 1980, p. 833*).

Supplementation may be beneficial in migraine headaches.

> **Experimental Study:** 3000 female pts. both pregnant and non-pregnant received 100-200 mg elemental magnesium as an amino acid chelate. 80% had a "good" response (*Weaver K. Magnesium and its role in vascular reactivity and coagulation. Contemp Nutr 12(3), 1987*).

> - with Vitamin B6 and dilute Adrenal Steroids:

>> **Clinical Observation:** 1500-2000 mg magnesium sulfate combined with 300-400 mg vitamin B6 and 5-10 cc's of a very dilute solution of mixed adrenal steroids given IV as a slow push over several min. (with the speed determined by the patient's tolerance of the "intense heat" felt with the injection) will substantially diminish or end acute migraine in most cases. Repetition of the dose if necessary usually removes any residual symptoms. Follow-up with IM magnesium sulfate 1 g twice weekly for several wks., tapering to once weekly and then less often as acute attacks diminish, along with 250-300 mg elemental magnesium as aspartate or citrate orally will substantially diminish or eliminate allergy/hypersensitivity-induced migraine. Unless extremely important, supplemental calcium should be avoided until migraine relief is achieved (*Wright JV. Magnesium can relieve migraine (and other magnesium-related matters). AAEM Newsletter, Winter, 1989, p. 14*).

- -

OTHER NUTRITIONAL FACTORS

Choline:

Red blood cell choline levels may be deficient in patients with cluster headache.

> **Experimental and Observational Study (cluster headache):** Compared to age-related controls, RBC choline concentrations were low in pts. both during and between cluster periods. During lithium treatment, choline levels rose 78 times (*de Belleroche J et al. Erythrocyte choline concentrations and cluster headache. Br Med J 288:268-70, 1984*).

<u>Omega-3 Fatty Acids (Fish Oils)</u>:

Eicosapentaenoic acid (EPA) and docosahexaenoic acid (DHA).

Highest in cold water fish. Available in a refined form as "MaxEPA" (18% EPA).

Suggested MaxEPA dosage: 3 - 9 gm daily in divided doses (or 10 ml concentrate twice daily)

WARNING: Supplementation may require additional vitamin E intake to prevent increased membrane peroxidation and cellular damage (*Laganiere S, Fernandes G. High peroxidizability of subcellular membrane induced by high fish oil diet is reversed by vitamin E.* <u>*Clin Res*</u> *35:A565, 1987*).

Supplementation may be beneficial.

Experimental Double-blind Study (<u>migraine headache</u>): 15 pts. with severe migraine unresponsive to medications experienced a significant reduction in headache frequency and intensity following supplementation with EPA 2.7 gm and DHA 1.8 gm daily (*Glueck CJ et al. Amelioration of severe migraine with omega-3 fatty acids: A double-blind, placebo-controlled clinical trial. Abstract.* <u>*Am J Clin Nutr*</u> *43:710, 1986*).

Experimental Double-blind Crossover Study (<u>migraine headache</u>): 6 chronic sufferers with severe, very frequent migraine were given 20 gm. fish oil or placebo daily in two 6-wk. treatment phases with a 3-wk. placebo crossover. Significant headache relief was found in 5/6 pts. in regard to both headache frequency and intensity (*Mc Carren T et al. Amelioration of severe migraine by fish oil (ω-3) fatty acids. Abstract.* <u>*Am J Clin Nutr*</u> *41:874a, 1985*).

<u>Tryptophan</u>: *See "<u>Low tryptophan</u> diet" above*

- -

OTHER FACTORS

Rule out <u>food sensitivities</u>.

General

Review Article: Early studies have suggested that about 30-40% of migraineurs benefit markedly by avoiding certain foods, and results of 4 recent double-blind studies support the role of food in causing migraine. Most foods that provoke migraine are commonly eaten but often not recognized as causative. A 1-mo. trial of eliminating foods which may be implicated is suggested (*Mansfield LE. Food allergy and migraine: Whom to evaluate and how to treat.* <u>*Postgrad Med*</u> *83(7):46-55, 1988*).

Experimental Double-blind Study (<u>migraine headache</u>): 6/43 adults with recurrent migraines became headache-free following an elimination diet and 13/43 experienced 66% or greater headache reduction. 11/16 skin test-positive pts. responded to the diet, while only 2/27 skin test-negatives did. Double-blind challenges provoked migraines in 5/7, while placebo challenges failed to provoke them (*Mansfield LE et al. Food allergy and adult migraine: Double-blind and mediator confirmation of an allergic etiology.* <u>*Ann Allergy*</u> *55:126, 1985*).

Experimental Double-blind Study (<u>migraine headache</u>): Foods which provoked migraine in 9 pts. with severe migraine refractory to medications were identified. The pts. were then given either sodium cromoglycate or placebo in a double-blind manner along with provoking foods. Sodium cromoglycate exerted a protective effect on the symptoms and immune complexes were not produced in the protected patients (*Monro J et al. Migraine is a food-allergic disease.* <u>*Lancet*</u> *2:719-21, 1984*).

Experimental Double-blind Study (<u>migraine headache</u>): 93% of 88 children with severe frequent migraine recovered on oligoantigenic diets; the causative foods were identified by sequential reintroduction, and the role of the foods provoking mgraine was established by a double-blind controlled trial in 40 of the children (*Egger J et al. Is migraine food allergy?: A double-blind controlled trial of oligoantigenic diet treatment.* <u>*Lancet*</u> *2:865-9, 1983*).

Experimental Study (migraine headache): Certain flavonoid phenolic compounds in foods and alcoholic beverages inhibit phenolsulfotransferase P (PST-P), an important enzyme which deactivates phenols. Pts. with a history of diet-induced migraine have lower platelet levels of PST-P, while both healthy controls and migraine pts. whose headaches are not food-induced have normal levels. Many red wines cause 100% inhibition of PST-P, while white wines, whiskey and brandy cause less inhibition, and vodka and gin least of all (*APA Psychiatric News June 7, 1985; Littlewood J et al. Platelet phenolsulfotransferase deficiency in dietary migraine. Lancet 1:983-6, 1982*).

Review Article: At least 25 syndromes have been described in which foods or food and drug combinations cause head and neck pain, including coloring and flavoring agents, alcoholic products, chocolate, coffee and tea, foods containing tyramine, vitamins, minerals, pesticides, and several others (*Seltzer S. Foods, and food and drug combinations, responsible for head and neck pain. Cephalalgia 2(2):111-24, 1982*).

Alcoholic Beverages (general)

Observational Study: 171 pts. aged 9-81 with different types of headache were surveyed. Nearly 50% reported alcohol was a precipitating factor. Alcohol was cited more often as a factor in migraine pts. (57.6%) than others (34.5%) (*Lipton R et al. Aspartame as a dietary trigger of headache. Headache 29:90-92, 1989*).

Aspartame

Observational Study: 171 pts. aged 9-81 with different types of headache were surveyed. 8.2% reported aspartame as a trigger. Three times more migraine pts. (10.6%) than pts. with other types of headache (3.4%) reported aspartame as a precipitating factor (*Lipton R et al. Aspartame as a dietary trigger of headache. Headache 29:90-92, 1989*).

Experimental Double-blind Study: Compared to placebo, 11 pts. who ingested aspartame experienced a significant increase in the frequency of migraines which also lasted longer (*Koehler SM, Glaros A. The effect of aspartame on migraine headaches. Headache 28(1):10-14, 1988*).

Negative Experimental Double-blind Study: Headache incidence among 40 pts. after aspartame ingestion was not significantly different than the incidence after placebo (*Schiffman, SS et al. Aspartame and susceptibility to headache. N Engl J Med 317:1181-15, 1987*).

Caffeine

Caffeine intake is correlated with headache prevalence.

Observational Study: In a cross-sectional study of 4558 Australians, the proportion of subjects reporting headache increased significantly with mean caffeine intake. A multiple logistic regression model showed that the association between headache prevalence and usual daily caffeine consumption remained significant in both males and females after controlling for age, adiposity, smoking, alcohol intake and occupation. The relative risk of headache for people consuming 240 mg of caffeine (4-5 cups of coffee or tea) daily is 1.3 for males and 1.2 for females. Coffee consumption had no significant effect over and above that attributable to its caffeine content (*Shirlow MJ, Mathers CD. A study of caffeine consumption and symptoms: Indigestion, palpitations, tremor, headache and insomnia. Int J Epidemiol 14(2):239-48, 1985*).

Withdrawal from regular caffeine consumption may cause headache.

Experimental Double-blind Study: 22 coffee drinkers (3-7 cups/d) underwent repeated double-blind trials to test for caffeine self-adminstration, withdrawal and adverse effects. Each trial consisted first of a randomized cross-over period of 1 d of decaffeinated coffee and 1 d of caffeinated coffee (100 mg). Next, subjects were given 2 d of concurrent access to the 2 coffees. The relative use of the 2 coffees was used to assess caffeine self-administration. Reliable caffeine self-administration occurred in 3/10 subjects in study 1 and 7/12 subjects in study 2. Withdrawal symptoms were headaches, drowsiness and fatigue. The major adverse effect from self-administration was tremulousness. The occurrence of headaches on substitution of decaffeinated coffee prospectively predicted subsequent self-administration of caffeine (*Hughes JR et al. Caffeine self-administration, withdrawal, and adverse effects among coffee drinkers. Arch Gen Psychiatry 48:611-17, 1991*).

Experimental Double-blind Study: 45 healthy subjects who habitually consumed 4-6 cups coffee/d were matched for sex, age and BP and randomly received either 5 cups (84 mg caffeine/cup) coffee/d for 6 wks. followed by 5 cups of decaffeinated coffee/d for the next 6 wks., or the reverse treatment. The mean caffeine intake for coffee drinkers was 435 mg/d, and for the decaffeinated gp., 30 mg/d. Even though 38/45 did not realize that they had changed from caffeinated to decaffeinated coffee, 19 recorded more complaints about headache during the first wk. of taking decaffeinated coffee, compared with the mean number of complaints they recorded during the other 11 weeks. Headaches started on the first or second day without caffeine and lasted from 1-6 days (*van Dusseldorp M, Katan MB. Headache caused by caffeine withdrawal among moderate coffee drinkers switched from ordinary to decaffeinated coffee: a 12 week double blind trial. Br Med J 300:1558-9, 1990*).

Review Article: Caffeine withdrawal headache begins with a feeling of "cerebral fullness" about 18 h after caffeine ingestion and quickly develops into a diffuse, throbbing, painful headache that is exacerbated by exercise. Discomfort peaks from 3-6 h after onset (*Greden JF et al. Caffeine-withdrawal headache: A clinical profile. Psychosomatics 21:411-18, 1980*).

Cheese

Reactions are believed to be due to its phenylethylamine content (*Sandler M et al. A phenylethylamine oxidising defect in migraine. Nature 250:335, 1974*).

Chocolate

Reactions have been blamed on its phenylethylamine content (at least 3 mg/2 oz bar) (*Sandler M et al. A phenylethylamine oxidising defect in migraine. Nature 250:335, 1974*).

Experimental Controlled Study (migraine headache): 36 pts. who attributed their migraines to chocolate received either phenylethylamine or placebo (lactose). 18/18 reported attacks 12 hrs. following phenylethylamine ingestion vs. 6/18 reported attacks following placebo (*Schweitzer JW et al. Chocolate, beta-phenylethylamine and migraine re-examined. Nature 257:256, 1975*).

Experimental Double-blind Study (migraine headache): 13/80 pts. developed attacks after chocolate but in only 2 could these reactions be reproduced with consistency (*Moffett AM et al. Effect of chocolate in migraine: A double-blind study. J Neurol Neurosurg Psychiatry 37:445, 1974*).

Negative Double-blind Study (migraine headache): 100 pts. showed no evidence of an increase in frequency of headaches following ingestion of tyramine, phenylethylamine or chocolate, despite their conviction that chocolate would cause them to develop headaches (*Moffett AM et al. Migraine and diet. Letter. Lancet 2:7885, 1974*).

Milk

Lactase deficiency may be associated with migraine headaches (*Ratner D et al. Milk protein-free diet for nonseasonal asthma and migraine in lactase-deficient patients. Isr J Med Sci 19:806-09, 1983*

Case Report: A 13 year-old boy was hospitalized because of headache, musculoskeletal and abdominal pains and bronchial asthma. Examination revealed pallor and dark circles under his eyes. Milk and chocolate were removed from his diet. There was marked improvement within 48 hrs., and reappearance of signs and symptoms with milk reintroduction (*Weinberg EG, Tuchinda M. Ann Allergy 31:209, 1973*).

Nitrates and Nitrites

(including hot dogs and other cured meats)

May precipitate migraine headaches (*Graham JR. Headache related to a variety of medical disorders, in O Appenzeller, Ed. Pathogenesis and Treatment of Headache. New York, Spectrum Publications, 1976*).

Red Wine

May precipitate migraine headaches due either to its tyramine content or to other factors.

Experimental Single-blind Study (migraine headache): 9/11 pts. who believed that their headaches could be provoked by red wine with a negligible tyramine content but not by gin or vodka developed migraines after challenge with red wine which was disguised to hide both color and flavor, while 0/8 similar pts. developed migraines after vodka which was similarly disguised. Neither challenge provoked migraines in other migrainous subjects or in healthy controls (*Littlewood JT et al. Red wine as a cause of migraine. Lancet 1:558-59, 1988*).

Tyramine

(found in aged cheeses, certain red wines, fermented sausages, sour cream, etc.)

A pharmacologically active substance which has been implicated in triggering migraines (*Hanington E. Preliminary report on tyramine headache. Br Med J 2:550-51, 1967*).

Releases serotonin from mast cells and norepinephrine from norepinephrine stores (*Zaimis E, in E Zaimis, Ed. Nerve Growth Factor and its Antiserum. London, Athlone Press, 1972*).

Tyramine ingestion may be of minor importance for the majority of migraineurs.

Experimental Study (migraine headache): 24 migraineurs were placed on a diet containing tyramine (aged cheeses, alcoholic drinks, fermented sausages and sour cream), phenylethylamine (chocolate), nitrates (hot dogs) and levodopa (broad bean pods), excluding these foods, or unregulated. In evaluating headaches occurring within 12 hrs. after ingestion, there were no significant differences in migraine severity in any group, although some headaches were time-locked to alcohol, chocolate and less so to citrus and nuts, suggesting that these substances may either have produced headaches or may merely have triggered impending attacks (*Medina JL, Diamond S. The role of diet in migraine. Headache 18:31-34, 1978*).

Experimental Double-blind Study (migraine headache): Administration of tyramine to pts. who benefited from a low-tyramine diet failed to provoke migraine attacks (*Moffett A et al. Effect of tyramine in migraine: A double-blind study. J Neurol Neurosurg Psychiatry 35:496-99, 1972*).

HEARTBURN
(REFLUX ESOPHAGITIS)

See Also: ULCERS (DUODENAL AND GASTRIC)

DIETARY FACTORS

Eat an early dinner.

May be associated with reduced gastric acidity.

Experimental Study: 23 healthy volunteers ate standarized meals at 7 am and 12 noon. They ate dinner at either 6 or 9 pm in random order, and the time of going to bed was standardized. With early dinner nocturnal pH was higher than with late dinner (p<0.001) (*Duroux P et al. Early dinner reduces nocturnal gastric acidity. Gut 30(8):106367, 1989*).

Avoid alcohol.

Relaxes the lower esophageal sphincter (LES) and decreases the peristaltic force (*Hogan WJ et al. Ethanol induced acute esophageal sphincter motor dysfunction. J Appl Physiol 32:755-60, 1972*).

Experimental Study: In a study of healthy volunteers, after only moderate amts. of alcohol (4 oz of scotch whiskey), there was a significant exposure of the distal esophagus to acid and the normal acid clearance of the esophagus in the supine position was impaired (*Vitale GC et al. The effect of alcohol on nocturnal gastroesophageal reflux. JAMA 258(15):2077-79, 1987*).

Stimulates gastric acid secretion (*Lenz HJ et al. Wine and five percent ethanol are potent stimulants of gastric acid secretion in humans. Gastroenterology 85(5):1082-87, 1983*).

Avoid carminatives (such as peppermint and spearmint).

These volatile oils have been shown to decrease LES pressure (*Sigmund CJ, McNally EF. The action of a carminative on the lower esophageal sphincter. Gastroenterology 56:13-18, 1969*).

Avoid chocolate.

May relax the lower esophageal sphincter.

Experimental Study: Ingestion of chocolate produced striking, immediate and sustained lowering of the pressure of the lower esophageal sphincter (*Babka JC, Castell DO. On the genesis of heartburn. The effects of specific foods on the lower esophageal sphincter. Am J Dig Dis 18(5):391-97, 1973*).

Effect on the LES may be due to its methylxanthine content, as chocolate syrup with a low fat content (1%) still lowers LES pressure (*Castell DO. Diet and the lower esophageal sphincter. Am J Clin Nutr 28:1296-98, 1975*).

May increase gastric acid secretion more than sugar.

Experimental Study: Symptomatic pts. with endoscopic demonstration of esophageal erosions and normal controls were given identical meals on two consecutive days and given the same activities. They could not lie flat, take medications or smoke cigarettes. On day one, they were given a chocolate drink after each meal. On day two, they were given a test solution of sugar of about the same volume, calories, and osmolality. In the pts., one hour after eating, there was a statistically significant increase in the amt. of acid exposure after the chocolate, as compared to the sugar, solution. In the controls, there was some increase in the amt. of acid after the meal, but it was not statistically significant (*Daniel Murphy, Bowman Gray School of Medicine, Winston-Salem, North Carolina - reported in Med Tribune October 7, 1987*).

Avoid coffee.

May both relax the lower esophageal sphincter and stimulate gastric acid secretion.

Experimental Study: 150 ml of caffeinated instant coffee at either pH 4.5 or 7.0 caused a decrease in fasting and postcibal LES pressure in 20 normal volunteers and 16 pts. with reflux esophagitis from 30 min. to at least 60 min. after ingestion. The magnitude and the duration of effect were greater after coffee at the lower pH (*Thomas FB et al. Inhibitory effect of coffee on lower esophageal sphincter pressure. Gastroenterology 79(6):1262-66, 1980*).

Experimental Study: 66 pts. with pain of possible esophageal origin received acid infusion (Berstein) tests. Compared to Berstein-negative pts., acid-sensitive pts. were sensitive to coffee infusion (p<0.01), even when adjusted to pH 7 (p<0.001) (*Price SF et al. Food sensitivity in reflux esophagitis. Gastroenterology 75(2):240-43, 1978*).

Experimental Study: Caffeine slightly relaxed the LES even in the dose range commonly encountered in 1-2 cups of coffee during the first 30-45 min. after ingestion, at the same time that it produced maximal stimulation of gastric acid (*Dennish GW, Castell DO. Caffeine and the lower esophageal sphincter. Am J Dig Dis 17:993-96, 1972*).

Avoid fatty meals.

Dramatically decreases lower esophageal sphincter pressure, even in normal subjects (*Nebel OT, Castell DO. Kinetics of fat inhibition of the lower esophageal sphincter. J Appl Physiol 35:6, 1973*)

Avoid milk.

Milk has only a transient neutralizing effect on gastric acidity followed by a rise in acid secretion (*Ippoliti AF et al. The effect of various forms of milk on gastric-acid secretion. Ann Intern Med 84:286-89, 1976*).

Experimental Study: In 6 healthy subjects, milk increased gastric acid secretion to >95% of the pentagastrin response (*McArthur K et al. Relative stimulatory effects of commonly ingested beverages on gastric acid secretion in humans. Gastroenterology 83:199-203, 1982*).

Avoid orange juice.

Causes disordered motility in the lower esophageal segment, suggesting that it may irritate the inflamed esophageal mucosa (*Babka JC, Castell DO. On the genesis of heartburn. The effects of specific foods on the lower esophageal sphincter. Am J Dig Dis 18(5):391-97, 1973*).

Experimental Study: 66 pts. with pain of possible esophageal origin received acid infusion (Berstein) tests. Compared to Berstein-negative pts., acid-sensitive pts. were sensitive to an orange juice infusion (p<0.01), even when adjusted to pH 7 (p<0.001) (*Price SF et al. Food sensitivity in reflux esophagitis. Gastroenterology 75(2):240-43, 1978*).

Avoid spicy foods.

Spicy foods most likely produce symptoms due to a direct irritant effect on the inflamed esophageal mucosa (*Castell DO. Diet and the lower esophageal sphincter. Am J Clin Nutr 28:1296-98, 1975*).

Avoid sugar.

May increase gastric acidity.

Experimental Study: The gastric juice of 7 healthy young volunteers was examined following 2 wks. on a high-sugar diet in which dietary starch was reduced by the same amt. that dietary sugar was increased. A test meal before breakfast revealed a 20% increase in peak gastric activity and a 250% increase in peak pepsin activity (*Yudkin J. Eating and ulcers. Letter. Br Med J February 16, 1980, pp. 483-4*).

Avoid tea.

May increase gastric acid secretion.

Experimental Study: 36 pts. with duodenal ulcer and 56 normal controls drank a 200 ml cup of tea which resulted in an acid secretory response which was almost equal to that after a maximal dose (0.04 mg/kg) of histamine. This effect was mainly due to its local chemical action upon the gastric mucosa (*Dubey P et al. Effect of tea on gastric acid secretion. Dig Dis Sci 29(3):202-06, 1984*).

Avoid tomato products.

Tomato juice, which has a somewhat acidic pH, causes disordered motility in the distal portion of the esophagus, suggesting that its effect may be due to direct irritation of an inflammed esophageal mucosa rather than a decrease of LES pressure (*Castell DO. Diet and the lower esophageal sphincter. Am J Clin Nutr 28:1296-98, 1975*).

Experimental Study: 66 pts. with pain of possible esophageal origin received acid infusion (Berstein) tests. Compared to Berstein-negative pts., acid-sensitive pts. were sensitive to a spicy tomato drink infusion (p<0.01), even when adjusted to pH 7 (p<0.001) (*Price SF et al. Food sensitivity in reflux esophagitis. Gastroenterology 75(2):240-43, 1978*).

HEPATITIS

See Also: ALCOHOLISM
INFECTION

DIETARY FACTORS

Low sugar diet.

Experimenal Study: 21 normal subjects received a typical American diet containing 25-30% sucrose for 18 days, and a "calorically diluted" diet containing less than 10% sucrose for 12 days. Serum GOT and GPT levels rose significantly when subjects consumed the high sucrose diet and returned to baseline levels on the low sucrose diet, with the rise apparently due both to surplus calories and excess sucrose consumption. In 2 subjects, the rise in enzyme levels on the high sucrose diet was so great that they had to be withdrawn from the study. Serum triglycerides were also significantly greater on the high sucrose diet. (*Porikos KP, van Itallie TB. Diet-induced changes in serum transaminase and triglyceride levels in healthy adult men. Role of sucrose and excess calories. Am J Med 75:624, 1983*).

Avoid alcohol ingestion.

Animal Experimental Study: 9 pairs of baboons were pair-fed an alcohol-containing or a control liquid diet. After 8-22 mo., alcohol consumption was associated with the development of a fatty liver along with mild inflammation, cellular degeneration and some fibrosis. In 3 animals, alcoholic hepatitis developed as defined by inflammation and "central hyaline sclerosis" (*Lieber CS, DeCarli LM. An experimental model of alcohol feeding and liver injury in the baboon. J Med Primatol 3:153-63, 1974*).

- -

VITAMINS

Vitamin A:

WARNING: Excessive vitamin A supplementation may cause hepatitis starting at dosages of 25-50,000 IU for at least several months (*Geubel AP et al. Liver damage caused by therapeutic vitamin A administration: estimate of dose-related toxicity in 41 cases. Gastroenterology 100(6):1701-9, 1991; Hathcock JN et al. Evaluation of vitamin A toxicity. Am J Clin Nutr 52(2):183-202, 1990*).

In alcoholic liver disease, enhanced microsomal degradation of retinoids, together with hepatic mobilization, promotes depletion. However, treatment is complicated by the fact that ethanol also enhances the toxicity of excess vitamin A (*Lieber CS. Interaction of alcohol with other drugs and nutrients. Drugs 40 Suppl 3:23-44, 1990*).

Vitamin B_{12}:

May be deficient despite normal or elevated serum levels since the diseased liver is unable to absorb B_{12} normally from the serum.

Observational Study: Compared to normals, liver content of cobalamin in 27 alcoholics was low while serum cobalamin and RBC cobalamin analogues were high, confirming earlier work which suggested that, in alcoholism and liver disease, cobalamin depletion in tissues may be masked by normal to high serum cobalamin and analogue levels. The failure of damaged liver to take up from the serum cobalamin and analogues, compounded by the release of these compounds and their binders from damaged liver into the serum, can account for these findings (*Kanazawa S, Herbert V. Total corrinoid, cobalamin (viamin B12), and cobalamin analogue levels may be normal in serum despite cobalamin in liver depletion in patients with alcoholism. Lab Invest 53(1):108-10, 1985*).

Observational Study: Blood levels of vitamin B_{12} were normal in a gp. of 41 pts. with alcoholic liver disease except for those with cirrhosis where it was raised (*Majumdar SK et al. Blood vitamin status (B_1, B_2, B_6, folic acid and B_{12}) in patients with alcoholic liver disease. <u>Int J Vitam Nutr Res</u> 52(3):266-71, 1982*).

Observational Study: Alcoholism was the most common disease correlate of vitamin B_{12} elevations in female general hospital patients. 61% of them had a serum B_{12} concentration greater or equal to 1000 ng/l compared to 17% of non-alcoholics. B_{12} elevations paralleled high SGOT, GGT and MCV values. In contrast, males far less often exhibited B_{12} elevations (*Goldman PA et al. A sex difference in the serum vitamin B_{12} levels of hospitalized alcoholics. <u>Curr Alcohol</u> 5:237-49, 1979*).

Plasma vitamin B_{12} levels may serve as an indicator of the severity of hepatitis and a predictor of mortality.

Observational Study: Elevated blood serum levels of free vitamin B_{12}, conforming to the disease severity and stage, were found in 168 pts. with viral hepatitis A, 13 with chronic active hepatitis, and 8 with mechanical jaundice of neoplastic origin with liver involvement. Correlations between cobalaminemia and other functional liver tests were observed (*Komar VI. [The blood level of cobalamin as an indicator of the functional status of the liver in jaundice of different etiologies.] <u>Lab Delo</u> (9):11-2, 1991*).

Observational Study: 320 pts. and 212 controls were tested for plasma B_{12} levels along with liver function studies. There was a positive corrrelation between high plasma B_{12} levels and liver function tests consistent with liver damage, and plasma B_{12} levels rose as death from alcoholic hepatitis approached (*Baker H et al. Plasma vitamin B_{12} titres as indicators of disease severity and mortality of patients with alcoholic hepatitis. <u>Alcohol Alcoholism</u> 22(1):15, 1987*).

Supplementation by injection may be beneficial in <u>viral hepatitis</u>.

Experimental Controlled Study: 13/26 pts. with viral hepatitis selected alternately received B_{12} 100 mcg IV daily in addition to standard treatment. While liver function tests were unmodified, the experimental gp. had less anorexia and jaundice and the mean duration of illness was 34.8 days compared to 45.8 days in the controls (*Jain ASC, Mukerji DP. Observations on the therapeutic value of intravenous B_{12} in infective hepatitis. <u>J Indian Med Assoc</u> 35:502-5, 1960*).

Experimental Controlled Study: IV B_{12} brought about rapid return of appetite and liver size to normal in pts. with viral hepatitis. In addition, the serum bilirubin returned to normal earlier (in 10 wks. compared to 18 wks. in the control gp.) and the mean duration of illness was reduced brom 54 to 48 days (*Campbell RE, Pruitt FW. Vitamin B_{12} in the treatment of viral hepatitis. <u>Am J Med Sci</u> 224:252, 1952*).

<u>Vitamin B_{12} and
Folic Acid</u>:

Combined supplementation may be beneficial in <u>viral hepatitis</u>.

Experimental Controlled Study: Two matched gps. of 44 pts. with acute viral hepatitis received a high protein, high carbohydrate, moderate fat diet. In addition, the experimental gp. received 30 μg vitamin B_{12} IM every other day and 5 mg of folic acid orally 3 times daily for the first 10 days of hospitalization. The mean duration of illness of the experimental gp. was 47.5 days as compared to 57.2 days for controls. The difference was most marked when total serum bilirubin was >15 mg/100 cc (17.2 days) but was appreciable (about 10 days) in those gps. where total serum bilirubin was 5-10 mg. While the total serum bilirubins of the entire experimental gp. were normal after the eleventh wk., 18 wks. were required by the control group. The bromsulfalein values of the experimental gp. all became normal by the eleventh wk. compared to 17 wks. in the controls. Finally, the pts. in the experimental gp. had a more rapid return of normal appetite (*Campbell RE, Pruitt FW. The effect of vitamin B_{12} and folic acid in the treatment of viral hepatitis. <u>Am J Med Sci</u> 229:8-15, 1955*).

<u>Vitamin C</u>:

Supplementation may be beneficial.

Experimental Controlled Study: Indicators of humoral and cellular immunity were studied for pts. with hepatitis A who received ascorbic acid 300 mg/d for 2-3 wks. and compared to those of pts. who did not receive the vitamin. Results established that vitamin C exerts a remarkable immunomodulating action in this illness and should be included in the treatment of all patients (*Vasil'ev VS, Komar VI, Kisel' NI. [Humoral and cellular indices of nonspecific resistance in viral hepatitis A and ascorbic acid.] Ter Arkh 61(11):44-6, 1989*).

Clinical Observation: 40-100 gm orally or IV. Said to be "one of the easiest diseases for ascorbic acid to cure" with paradoxical cessation of diarrhea despite oral supplementation within 1-2 days. Stools and urine return to normal color within 2-3 days in acute cases and patients feel fairly well in 2-4 days with clearing of jaundice in about 6 days (*Cathcart, RF III. The method of determining proper doses of vitamin C for the treatment of disease by titrating to bowel tolerance. J Orthomol Psychiatry 10:125-32, 1981*).

Clinical Observation: Pts. treated with 400-600 mg/kg were well and back to work in 3-7 days (*Klenner FR. Observations on the dose of administration of ascorbic acid when employed beyond the range of a vitamin in human pathology. J Appl Nutr 23(3&4):61-88, Winter, 1971*).

Experimental Study: 245 infected children received 10 gm ascorbic acid daily with rapid recovery (*Baetgen D. Results of the treatment of epidemic hepatitis in children with high doses of ascorbic acid in the years 1957 - 1958. Medizinische Monatschrift 15:30-36, 1961*).

Experimental Controlled Study: 10 gms. ascorbic acid was infused on several different occasions and compared with results of the previous year in patients who were not given the infusions. The infusions were associated with about a 50% reduction in the duration of the illness (*Baur H, Staub H. Treatment of hepatitis with infusions of ascorbic acid: Comparison with other therapies. Abstract. JAMA 156(5):565, 1954*).

May prevent serum hepatitis in surgical patients.

Negative Experimental Double-blind Study: For 2 days before surgery and 2 wks. afterwards, cardiac surgery pts. randomly received either 800 mg of vitamin C 4 times daily or a lactose placebo. 175 pts. completed the study. There was no significant difference in the incidence of posttransfusion hepatitis (p<0.50) or the clinical course of hepatitis between the 2 treatment gps. (*Knodell RG et al. Vitamin C prophylaxis for posttransfusion hepatitis: Lack of an effect in a controlled trial. Am J Clin Nutr 34:20 1981*).

> *Note: This study has been criticized by Linus Pauling who claims that the data demonstrate a reduction in the incidence of illness with vitamin C. Also pts. receiving vitamin C had more transfusions than the control group; thus if the ratio of cases of post-transfusion hepatitis per transfusion is calculated, there is a 40-50% reduction in those who received 3.2 gm. vitamin C daily (Pauling L. Vitamin C prophylaxis for posttransfusion hepatitis. Letter. Am J Clin Nutr 34(9):1978-80, 1981).*

Experimental Controlled Study: While 12/170 (7%) transfused pts. who received little or no vitamin C developed post-transfusion hepatitis, only 3/1,367 pts. (0.2%) who received ≥2 g vitamin C /d developed it (all non-B) (*Morishige F, Murata A. Vitamin C for prophylaxis of viral hepatitis B in transfused patients. J Int Coll Prev Med 5(1):54-58, 1978; Morishige F, Murata A. Vitamin C for prophylaxis of viral hepatitis B in transfused patients. J Int Acad Prev Med 5(1):54, 1978*).

Experimental Controlled Study: None of 1095 surgical pts. given 2 gm or more vitamin C daily developed serum hepatitis, while 7% (11/150) pts. given < 1.5 gm vitamin C developed the disease (*Murata A. Virucidal activity of vitamin C: Vitamin C for prevention and treatment of viral diseases, in T Hasegawa, Ed. Proc First Intersectional Congress Int Assoc Microbiol Soc, Volume 3. Tokyo U. Press, 1975:432-42*).

Vitamin E:

Hepatitis is often associated with low blood levels of vitamin E. A vitamin E deficiency can be manifested by accelerated RBC destruction and neuromuscular deficits, and thus should be treated by supplementation (*Machlin LJ. Use and safe of elevated dosages of vitamin E in adults. Int J Vitam Nutr Res Suppl 30:56-68, 1989*).

Observational Study: Low RBC alpha tocopherol was found in 3/27 (11.1%) pts. with chronic hepatitis, but their ratio of plasma alpha-tocopherol to plasma lipids was not necessarily reduced (*Suzuki T, Kawase T, Harada T. [Clinical study of vitamin E status in patients with chronic liver diseases.] Nippon Shokakibyo Gakkai Zasshi 88(4):1066-73, 1991*).

- -

MINERALS

<u>Calcium:</u>

Blood levels may be elevated in <u>viral hepatitis</u> (*Ford DJ, Reid IR. Hypercalcaemia associated with viral hepatitis. Letter.* <u>*Lancet*</u> *336:181, 1990*).

<u>Selenium:</u>

A low selenium content in grains is correlated with a high incidence of hepatitis B infections (*Yu SY et al. Chemoprevention trial of human hepatitis with selenium supplementation in China.* <u>*Biol Trace Elem Res*</u> *21(1-2):15-22, 1989*).

If the intake is low, supplementation may reduce the risk of <u>viral hepatitis</u>.

Experimental Controlled Study: 20,847 residents of a town in China received supplementation with selenium in the form of table salt fortification with 15 ppm anhydrous sodium selenite. After 3 yrs., the incidence of viral hepatitis in the town was significantly lower than that of controls provided with normal table salt (*Yu SY et al. Chemoprevention trial of human hepatitis with selenium supplementation in China.* <u>*Biol Trace Elem Res*</u> *21(1-2):15-22, 1989*).

- -

OTHER NUTRITIONAL FACTORS

<u>Amino Acids:</u>

Supplementation with mixed freeform amino acids may be beneficial in <u>alcoholic hepatitis</u>.

Experimental Controlled Study: 17/35 pts. with alcoholic hepatitis randomly received amino acids 70-85 gm IV daily. All 35 had similar clinical and biochemical features and received a 3000 kcal 100 gm protein diet. After 28 days, ascites and encephalopathy tended to improve more in the study group. Serum bilirubin and albumin improved only in the study group. 4 pts. died in the control gp., but none in the study gp. (*Nasrallah SM, Galambos JT. Aminoacid therapy of alcoholic hepatitis.* <u>*Lancet*</u> *2:1276-7, 1980*).

- <u>Methionine:</u>

Supplementation may be beneficial in <u>halothane hepatitis</u>.

Case Report: A 40 year-old female developed hepatitis due to halothane poisoning after gastric surgery for morbid obesity. After 5 wks., there was no sign of resolution of the hepatitis and methionine therapy was begun. 6 days after administration of 250 mg methionine orally 4 times daily, there was a 50% reduction of her serum bilirubin concentration (from 300 to 150 μmol/L). Significant reductions in the alkaline phosphatase and aspartate transaminase levels were also noted. She was discharged 3 wk.s after the start of methionine therapy; normal liver function tests have been found at follow-up (*Windsor JA, Wynne-Jones G. Halothane hepatitis and prompt resolution with methionine therapy: Case report.* <u>*N Z Med J*</u> *101:502-03, 1988*).

- <u>Taurine:</u>

Supplementation may be beneficial in <u>acute hepatitis</u>.

Experimental Double-blind Study: 63 pts. with acute hepatitis and serum bilirubin of >3 mg/dl randomly received either taurine 4 gm 3 times daily after meals or placebo. Compared to controls, there was a significant drop of bilirubin level soon afterwards and a remarkable drop in total bile acid levels within 1 week (*Matsuyama Y et al. The effect of taurine administration on patients with acute hepatitis, in K Kuriyama, RJ Huxtable, H Iwata, Eds.* <u>*Sulfur Amino Acids: Biochemical and Clinical Aspects*</u>. *New York, Alan R. Liss, Inc., 1983:461-68*).

Supplementation may <u>not</u> be beneficial in <u>chronic hepatitis</u>.

Experimental Double-blind Study: In a randomized study, taurine failed to improve enzymatic indices of liver injury in chronic hepatitis (*Podda M et al. Effects of ursodeoxycholic acid and taurine on serum liver enzymes and bile acids in chronic hepatitis. <u>Gastroenterology</u> 98(4):1044-50, 1990*).

<u>Catechin</u>:

Supplementation may be beneficial.

Experimental Double-blind Study: 338 pts. with HBs-Ag-positive chronic hepatitis received either cianidanol (catechin) 1.5 gm daily for 2 wks. followed by 2.25 gm daily for 14 wks. or placebo. The HBsAg titer decreased by at least 50% in 44/144 (31%) of treated pts. compared to 21/140 (15%) of controls (p<0.01). Liver function tests also tended to improve in those whose antibody titers fell. The only side effect was a transient febrile reaction in 13 pts. (*Suzuki H et al. Cianidanol therapy for HBs-antigen-positive chronic hepatitis: A multicentre, double-blind study. <u>Liver</u> 6:35, 1986*).

Experimental Double-blind Study: 160 pts. with acute viral hepatitis randomly received either (+)-cyanidanol-3 3 gm daily or placebo. The mean time for serum bilirubin to decrease to 1.3 mg/dl was 30.8 ± 3.5 days in the treated gp. and 52.2 ± 9.8 days in the controls (p<0.025). The time for SGOT to decrease to 100 IU/l was 17.98 ± 1.82 in the treated gp. and 26.53 ± 3.7 in the controls (p<0.025). The incidence of chronicity was unaltered by treatment and the elimination rate of HBsAg was identical in both groups (*Schomerus H et al. (+)-Cyanidanol-3 in the treatment of acute viral hepatitis: A randomized controlled trial. <u>Hepatology</u> 4(2):331-35, 1984*).

<u>Phosphatidyl choline</u>:

Supplementation may be beneficial.

Experimental Double-blind Study: 15 pts. with HBsAg negative chronic active hepatitis received polyunsaturated phosphatidyl choline (Essential Phospholipid, Nattermann, Germany) 3 g daily in addition to normal maintenance immunosuppressive therapy. Histological evidence of disease activity was significantly reduced in the treatment group (*Jenkins PJ et al. Use of polyunsaturated phosphatidyl choline in HBsAg negative chronic active hepatitis: Results of prospective double-blind controlled trial. <u>Liver</u> 2:77-81, 1982*).

HERPES SIMPLEX

See Also: INFECTION

VITAMINS

Vitamin C:

Supplementation may be beneficial.

> **Experimental Study:** 30/38 pts. with recurrent cold sores remained free of recurrences 4 yrs. after starting supplementation with vitamin C 1-2 gm daily. The other 8 pts. were able to inhibit the infection with several gms. of vitamin C at the first appearance of symptoms (*Lewin S. Vitamin C: Its Molecular Biology and Medical Potential. New York, Van Nostrand Reinhold Co., 1973*).

- and Bioflavonoids:

Supplementation may be beneficial.

> **Experimental Double-blind Study:** 14/38 herpes labialis pts. on vitamin C 200 mg and bioflavonoids 200 mg 3 or 5 times daily starting within 48 hrs. after the onset of symptoms and maintained for 3 days developed blisters versus 10/10 on placebo. Only 10/38 treated pts. demonstrated disruption of the vesicular membrane during the course of the infection compared to all 10 of the controls. The tendency toward vesicular formation was even further inhibited when treatment was determined to have been initiated within the first 12 hrs. after recognition of the initial symptoms. While the interval from initial onset to complete remission was 9.7 ± 2.8 days in the placebo gp., it was 4.2 ± 1.7 days in the 600 mg gp. and 4.4 ± 3.9 days in the 1000 mg group. The difference between the combined treatment gps. and controls was significant ($p<0.01$) (*Terezhalmy GT et al. The use of water-soluble bioflavonoid-ascorbic acid complex in the treatment of recurrent herpes labialis. Oral Surg 45:56-62, 1978*).

Vitamin E: Squeeze capsule onto cotton roll

Topical application may be beneficial.

> **Case Report:** Topical application of vitamin E gave a pt. complete relief of the pain of gingivostomatitis in 15 min. followed by complete recovery after 10 days (*Starasoler S, Haber GS. Use of vitamin E oil in primary herpes gingivostomatitis in an adult. N Y State Dent J 44(9):382-83, 1978*).

- -

MINERALS

Iron:

People with a history of recurrent herpes simplex labialis are more often iron-deficient than are controls matched for age and sex (*Chandra RK. 1990 McCollum Award Lecture: Nutrition and immunity: lessons from the past and new insights into the future. Am J Clin Nutr 53:1087-1101, 1991*).

Lithium:

Administration may reduce the recurrence of labial infections.

WARNING: As oral lithium has potentially serious adverse effects, it is generally not recommended as a treatment for herpes simplex.

Observational Study: In a retrospective study, the mean rate of recurrent labial herpes infections in 177 subjects receiving lithium prophylaxis for psychiatric illness was significantly reduced compared to the pretreatment period (p<0.001). In contrast, the mean rate of herpes infections of 59 subjects receiving other antidepressants was unchanged (p=0.53). Although the overall reduction in herpes infections was not significantly different between gps., the proportion of subjects reporting a reduction in infection rate was greater in the lithium gp. (71%) compared to the control gp. (52%) (p=0.07). These data compliment prior *in vitro* and clinical studies demonstrating a potential antiviral activity for lithium carbonate (*Amsterdam JD et al. A possible antiviral action of lithium carbonate in herpes simplex virus infections. Biol Psychiatry 27(4):447-53, 1990*).

Zinc:

Supplementation may be beneficial.

In vitro Experimental Study: Zinc sulfate 0.1 mM inhibited the synthesis of herpes simplex virus progeny, while 0.2 mM resulted in almost complete inhibition of replication (*Gordon YJ et al. Irreversible inhibition of herpes simplex virus replication in BSC-1 cells by zinc ions. Antimicrob Agents Chemother 8(3):377-80, 1975*).

- with Vitamin C:

Supplementation may be beneficial.

Experimental Study: Following an eruption, pts. with recurrent herpes simplex type I received zinc sulfate 100 mg and vitamin C 250 mg twice daily for 6 weeks. There was either (1) complete suppression of the eruption for an indefinite period; (2) a local tingling sensation but without an eruption or with local swelling and a very limited area of vesiculation which receded within 24 hrs.; or (3) a violent eruption which was not followed by any further eruption providing supplementation was continued (*Fitzherbert J. Genital herpes and zinc. Letter. Med J Aust 1:399, 1979*).

Topical application may be beneficial.

Experimental Study: 200 pts. with Type I or Type II herpes applied 0.25% zinc sulfate in a saturated solution of camphor water 8-10 times daily starting within 24 hrs. of the appearance of lesions. The lesions usually cleared within 3-6 days. With applications every 30-60 min., the itching, burning, stinging and pain usually disappeared within 2-3 hours. For women with vaginal herpes, a 0.25% zinc sulfate solution used as a douche also had excellent results (*Finnerty EF. Topical zinc in the treatment of herpes simplex. Cutis 37(2):130-31, 1986*).

Review Article: Long-term topical application of zinc appears to greatly reduce or eliminate recurrences of orolabial and genital herpetic infections (*Eby G. Use of topical zinc to prevent recurrent herpes simplex infection: Review of literature and suggested protocols. Med Hypotheses 17:157-65, 1985*).

OTHER NUTRITIONAL FACTORS

Adenosine 5[1]-monophosphate:

A naturally occurring purine nucleotide that is an intermediate in cellular metabolism and nucleic acid synthesis.

Available in aqueous and gel form for IM injection. Aqueous AMP is administered 25 mg IM every other day until significant remission occurs; then injections are reduced to twice and then to once a week. If complete remission occurs, treatment is stopped. The gel form, which is not available in the US, is administered at 100 mg IM 3 times a week. Again, treatment is reduced as remission occurs (*S. Harvey Sklar, M.D. - reported in CFS Forum 2(3), April 15, 1989*).

Low levels of AMP may be associated with herpetic infections.

Experimental Study: Blood samples of 65 pts. with either herpes zoster or herpes simplex consistently had abnormally low AMP levels and abnormally high levels of adenosine triphosphate (*Sklar SH. Herpesvirus infection. Letter. JAMA 237(9):871-72, 1977*).

Administration by IM injection may reduce pain and promote healing.

> WARNING: Readily converted into adenosine which can inhibit immune system functions. Although the dosages recommended appear to be too small to significantly affect systemic AMP levels, little is known about its toxic effects (*AMP for herpes infections. Med Sci Bull 7(12), August 1985*). Over 75 mg of aqueous AMP at once can cause transient cardiac symptoms (*S. Harvey Sklar, M.D. - reported in CFS Forum 2(3), April 15, 1989*).

Supplementation may be beneficial.

Experimental Study: 36 pts. with recurrent herpes labialis were treated with adenosine 5^1-monophosphate in 9-12 doses of 1.5-2 mg/kg on alternate days. The lesions dried up in 24-36 hrs., and pain disappeared within 48 hours. 23/36 pts. were free of recurrences for varying intervals extending over 2 yrs., while the remainder had a single recurrence (*Scklar SH, Buimovici-Klein E. Adensoine in the treatment of recurrent herpes labialis. Oral Surg 48(5):416-17, 1979*).

L-Lysine: 1 - 6 gm. daily between meals until healed (take with carbohydrate);
        then 500 mg. daily to prevent recurrence.

WARNING: follow cholesterol levels as lysine may stimulate the liver to increase its manufacture (*Schmeisser DD et al. Effect of excess dietary lysine on plasma lipids of the chick. J Nutr 113(9):1777-83, 1983*).

Supplementation, along with arginine restriction, may be beneficial.

lysine/arginine ratios of foods

good	bad
meat	chocolate (1:2)
potatoes	peanuts (1:3)
milk	other nuts
brewer's yeast	seeds
fish	cereal grains
chicken	gelatin
beans	carob
eggs	raisins

Experimental Placebo-controlled Study: 52 pts. with recurrent infections (oral, genital, or both) received L-lysine 1 gm 3 times daily or placebo. All pts. were instructed to avoid nuts, chocolate, and gelatin. After 6 mo., the treatment was rated as effective or very effective by 74% of those receiving lysine, compared to 28% of those receiving placebo (p<0.01). Mean number of herpes outbreaks were 3.1 in the lysine gp. compared to 4.2 in the placebo group, and lysine-treated pts. reported milder symptoms. There were no significant side effects (*Griffith RS et al. Success of L-lysine therapy in frequently recurrent herpes simplex infection. Dermatologica 175:183-90, 1987*).

Experimental Double-blind Crossover Study: 41 pts. taking an ave. daily dose of 1248 mg of L-lysine monohydrochloride showed evidence of a decreased recurrence rate and of decreased severity of symptoms during recurrences, but not of reduced healing time. A dose of 624 mg daily was ineffective (*McCune MA et al. Treatment of recurrent herpes simplex infections with L-lysine monohydrochloride. Cutis 34(4):366-73, 1984*).

Negative Experimental Double-blind Study: 21 pts. with recurring infections randomly received oral lysine HCl 400 mg 3 times daily or placebo at the start of an episode and were told to continue it for 4-5 months. In addition, all pts. avoided excessive ingestion of seeds, nuts or chocolate. Measures of episode frequency, duration and severity failed to detect substantial benefits from lysine either as prophylaxis or as treatment for episodes in progress (*DiGiovanna J, Blank H.   Failure of lysine in frequently recurrent herpes simplex infection.   Arch Dermatol 120:48-51, 1984*).

In vitro Experimental Study: Arginine deficiency suppressed herpes simplex virus replication in tissue culture while lysine, an analog of arginine, as an antimetabolite, antagonized the viral growth-promoting action of arginine (*Griffith RS et al.   Relation of arginine-lysine antagonism to Herpes simplex growth in tissue culture.   Chemotherapy 27:209-13, 1981*).

Experimental Double-blind Crossover Study: 65 pts. with recurrent herpes simplex labialis received either L-lysine monohydrochloride daily or placebo. After 12 wks., the gps. were crossed-over. On the whole, lysine prophylaxis had no effect on recurrence rates; however, significantly more pts. were recurrence-free during lysine than during placebo, suggesting that certain pts. may benefit (*Milman N et al.   Lysine prophylaxis in recurrent herpes simplex labialis: A double-blind crossover study.   Acta Dermatovener 60:85-87, 1980*

- -

COMBINED TOPICAL TREATMENTS

Lithium Succinate (8%),
Zinc Sulfate (0.05%) and
D.L Alpha Tocopherol (0.1%) ointment:

   Topical application may be beneficial.

   Experimental Double-blind Study: In a randomized study, 73 patients with recurrent genital herpes were treated within 48 hrs. of lesion onset with lithium ointment applied 4 times daily for 1 wk. or placebo. The ointment significantly reduced mean pain duration from 7 to 4 days. Time to complete healing was 7 days in the treatment gp. and 8 days in controls. 55% of the control gp. was excreting virus by the fourth or fifth day compared to 14% of treated patients. Moreover, in those still excreting virus, mean virus excretion was 30 times greater in the controls that in the treatment group. No side effects were noted; however, the long-term safety of topical lithium is unknown (*Skinner GR. Lithium ointment for genital herpes. Letter. Lancet 2:288, 1983*).

- -

OTHER FACTORS

Lactobacillus Acidophilus:

   Administration may be beneficial.

   Negative Experimental Double-blind Study: 80 mental retardates with oral ulcerations received Bacid, a viable human strain of L. acidophilus in 100 mg of carboxymethylcellulose base, 2 caps 4 times daily for 10 days or placebo during a 12-mo. study. The contents were mixed with 2 oz milk, held in the mouth for a few min., and then swallowed. About 90% of the lesions were clinically judged to be canker sores; the balance were cold sores (herpes simplex). 18/80 pts. had repeat episodes of oral ulcerations during the study; they were then switched to the alternative treatment. Bacid failed to affect the duration of healing of the lesions; its effect on pain could not be studied as the majority of the pts. were unable to communicate responsibly with respect to the degree of pain experienced (*Gertenrich RL, Hart RW. Treatment of oral ulcerations with Bacid (Lactobacillus acidophilus). Oral Surg 30(2):196-200, 1970*).

   Experimental Study: 38/40 patients given L. acidophilus tablets reported relief within 48 hours (*Rapoport L, Levine WI. Treatment of oral ulceration with lactobacillus tablets. Report of forty cases. Oral Surg. 20(5):591-93, 1965*).

HERPES ZOSTER

including POST-HERPETIC NEURALGIA

See Also: INFECTION

VITAMINS

<u>Vitamin B₁₂</u>: 500 μgm IM daily

Supplementation by injection may be beneficial.

Experimental Study: 21 pts. showed "dramatic response . . . as judged by relief of pain and the speed of disappearance of vesicles" with improvement starting the second or third day of treatment. None developed post-herpetic neuralgia (*Gupta AK, Mital HS. Cyanocobalamin (vitamin B₁₂) in the management of herpes zoster. Indian Pract 20(7):457-59, 1967*).

Clinical Observation: In cases of post-herpetic neuralgia, "my own routine is to inject 1 mg of cyanocobalamin daily for six days and weekly for six weeks" (*Hope-Simpson RE. Herpes zoster in the elderly. Geriatrics 22(9):151-59, 1967*).

<u>Vitamin C:</u>   10 grams daily (1 gm./hr.) until lesions dry up

Supplementation may be beneficial.

Experimental Study: 327 pts. were all cured following 3 days of IV vitamin C injections (*Zureick M. Treatment of shingles and herpes with vitamin C intravenously. J des Praticiens 64:586, 1950*).

Experimental Study: 8 pts. received injections of vitamin C. 7 reported cessation of pain within 2 hrs. after the first injection. 7 also showed drying of the blisters within 1 day and complete clearing in 3 days (*Klenner F. The treatment of poliomyelitis and other virus diseases with vitamin C. South Med Surg 111:209-14, 1949*).

- with <u>Bioflavonoids</u>:

Supplementation may be beneficial.

Experimental Controlled Study: 20 episodes of recurrent herpes labialis were treated with a complex of 600 mg of water-soluble bioflavonoids and 600 mg of ascorbic acid, admnistered in equal increments 3 times daily. 20 episodes were treated with dosages of 1000 mg of each administered 5 times daily, and 10 episodes were treated with a lactose placebo. Treatment was maintained for 3 days after initial symptom recognition. The water-soluble bioflavonoid-ascorbic acid complex reduced vesiculation and prevented disruption of the vesicular membrane; it was most effective when initiated during the prodromal stage. Optimum symptom remission was observed in 4.2 ± 1.7 days with the 600 mg dosage of the complex. No adverse reactions were reported (*Terezhalmy GT et al. The use of water-soluble bioflavonoid-ascorbic acid complex in the treatment of recurrent herpes labialis. Oral Surg 45(1):56-62, 1978*).

<u>Vitamin E:</u>   1200-1600 IU daily (6 month trial) (for <u>post-herpetic neuralgia</u>)

Supplementation may be beneficial.

Experimental Study: 13 pts. with chronic post-herpes zoster neuralgia received 400-1,600 IU vitamin E daily before meals. 9/13 experienced complete or almost complete control of pain, two were moderately improved, and two were slightly improved. Two of those who experienced complete or almost complete pain relief had had neuralgia for 13 and 19 yrs., respectively (*Ayres S, Mihan R. Post-herpes zoster neuralgia: Response to vitamin E therapy. Arch Dermatol 108:855-56, 1973*).

Negative Experimental Study: 6 female (ages 56-72) and 2 male (ages 60-64) pts. were given D-alpha tocopheryl acetate 400 IU daily before meals. After 2 wks. the dose was increased to 800 IU daily for 2 wks. and then to 1600 IU daily for 6 weeks. In addition, 2 women used vitamin E cream (50 IU/gm) topically. After 10 wks., 7/8 pts. noted no change in either severity or frequency of the neuralgia (*Cochrane T. Post-herpes zoster neuralgia: Response to vitamin E therapy. Letter. Arch Dermatol 111:396, 1975*).

Note: Ayres and Mihan have emphasized that 1200-1600 IU of D-alpha tocopheryl acetate or succinate for at least 6 months is necessary as well as avoiding any medication or foods (including mixed vitamins containing inorganic iron, white flour, vitamin-enriched cereals, and conjugated estrogens) which may inactivate vitamin E (Ayres S, Mihan R. Letter. Arch Dermatol 111:396, 1975).

— —

OTHER NUTRITIONAL FACTORS

<u>Adenosine Monophosphate</u>:

A naturally occurring purine nucleotide that is an intermediate in cellular metabolism and nucleic acid synthesis.

Available in aqueous and gel form for IM injection. Aqueous AMP is administered 25 mg IM every other day until significant remission occurs; then injections are reduced to twice and then to once a week. If complete remission occurs, treatment is stopped. The gel form, which is not available in the US, is administered at 100 mg IM 3 times a week. Again, treatment is reduced as remission occurs (*S. Harvey Sklar, M.D. - reported in CFS Forum 2(3), April 15, 1989*).

Low levels of AMP may be associated with herpetic infections.

Experimental Study: Blood samples of 65 pts. with either herpes zoster or herpes simplex consistently had abnormally low AMP levels and abnormally high levels of adenosine triphosphate (*Sklar SH. Herpesvirus infection. Letter. JAMA 237(9):871-72, 1977*).

Administration by IM injection may reduce pain and promote healing.

WARNING: Readily converted into adenosine which can inhibit immune system functions. Although the dosages recommended appear to be too small to significantly affect systemic AMP levels, little is known about its toxic effects (*AMP for herpes infections. Med Sci Bull 7(12), August 1985*). Over 75 mg of aqueous AMP at once can cause transient cardiac symptoms (*S. Harvey Sklar M.D. - reported in CFS Forum 2(3), April 15, 1989*).

Experimental Double-blind Study: 32 adult pts. with a vesicular rash of not >72 hrs. randomly received IM injections of either gel-sustained AMP 100 mg in 1 mg gelatin base or placebo 3 times/wk. for up to 4 wks. in acute herpes zoster. AMP moderately reduced the pain soon after the start of treatment, decreased desquamation time, and promoted faster healing of the skin than placebo. It also reduced virus shedding and cleared the virus faster than in placebo-treated subjects. Following 4 wks., 88% of AMP-treated pts. were pain-free, compared to 43% of placebo patients. All pts. who had not recovered from pain then started receiving AMP without breaking the code. All these pts. recovered from pain within 3 wks. after initiation of treatment. No recurrence of pain or lesions was experienced from 3-18 mo. following termination of treatment. There were no adverse side-effects during and after treatment (*Sklar SH et al. Herpes zoster. The treatment and prevention of neuralgia with adenosine monophosphate. JAMA 253(10):1427-30, 1985*).

Note: As the number of patients is small, and the groups were not comparable at the onset of therapy with respect to factors known to influence the natural history of varicella zoster infections (such as severity of disease at initiation of therapy), these results must be considered preliminary (Sherlock CH, Corey L. Adenosine monophosphate for the treatment of varicella zoster infections: A large dose of caution. Editorial. JAMA 253(10):1444-5, 1985).

"HYPERESTROGENISM"
(IMPAIRED ESTROGEN METABOLISM)

See Also: **BENIGN BREAST DISEASE**
CANCER
MENORRHAGIA
PREMENSTRUAL SYNDROME

Through hydroxylation in the liver, estrogen is metabolized as follows:

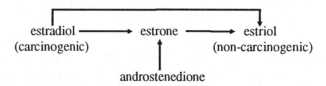

estradiol ⟶ estrone ⟶ estriol
(carcinogenic)   (non-carcinogenic)

androstenedione

Estradiol is secreted by the ovary. Estrone is converted from estradiol or from androstenedione which is secreted by the adrenal cortex. Except for a small amount from the ovary, estriol is converted in the liver from estrone as well as from estradiol by a circuitous route.

Estradiol and estrone are extremely active stimulants of breast and uterine tissue, while estriol is less stimulating and may even be anticarcinogenic (*Follingstad AH. Commentary: Estriol, the forgotten estrogen? JAMA 239(1):29-30, 1978; Cole P, MacMahon B. Oestrogen fractions during early reproductive life in the aetiology of breast cancer. Lancet 1:604-6, 1969*).

> **Observational Study:** Urine was collected from women in their reproductive years in areas of the world of high and low breast cancer risk. Results were strikingly consistent with the hypothesis that women who metabolize a high proportion of their estrogens to estriol are at low risk for breast cancer (*MacMahon B et al. Urine oestrogen profiles of Asian and North American women. Int J Cancer 14:161-67, 1974; Dickinson LE et al. Estrogen profiles of Oriental and Caucasian women in Hawaii. N Engl J Med 291:1211-13, 1974*).

In the presence of sub-optimal liver function and/or nutritional deficiencies, the conversion of estradiol and estrone to estriol is blocked, causing <u>PMT-A</u>, one of the types of <u>premenstrual syndrome</u>. PMT-A is associated with symptoms of anxiety, irritability and nervous tension, occurring as early as the mid cycle, becoming progressively worse during the luteal phase and sometimes followed by mild to moderate depression and improvement with menses. Patients have elevated blood estrogens (which are CNS stimulants) and decreased progesterone (a CNS depressant) during the luteal phase (*Abraham GE. Premenstrual tension syndromes: A nutritional approach. Anabolism 5(2):5-6, 1986*).

Also associated with increased estrogen levels is <u>prolonged menses</u> (over 4 days versus 3 days), <u>heavy bleeding</u> and an increased risk of <u>uterine fibroids, endometriosis</u> and <u>fibrocystic breast disease</u>.

> **Observational Study:** Women with periods of menstrual flow ≥ 1 wk. as well as cycles of 27 days or less had more than double the risk for endometriosis compared to women with shorter flow and longer cycles. Women with greater menstrual pain were also at higher risk for endometriosis, while both smoking and regular exercise, which lower endogenous estrogen levels, were associated with decreased risk (*Cramer DW et al. The relation of endometriosis to menstrual characteristics, smoking, and exercise. JAMA 255(14):1904-08, 1986*).

The metabolism of estrogen can be evaluated by calculating the <u>estrogen quotient</u>. A 24-hour urine is obtained for fractionated estrogens. If the sum of the estrone and the estradiol is greater than the estriol, women may be at greater risk for illnesses related to estrogen excess:

$$Eq = \frac{\text{Estriol } (\mu g/24 \text{ hrs})}{\text{Estrone } + \text{Estradiol } (\mu g/24 \text{ hrs})}$$

High Risk: below 0.7
Low Risk: above 1.0

Observational Study: 26 breast cancer pts. without endocrine treatment or recent surgery had an ave. estrogen quotient of 0.5 if premenopausal and 0.8 if postmenopausal. 62% had a quotient of <1.34. Controls had an ave. estrogen quotient of 1.2 if premenopausal and 1.3 if postmenopausal, and only 21% had a quotient of <1 (*Lemon HM et al. Reduced estriol excretion in patients with breast cancer prior to endocrine therapy. JAMA 196(13):1128-36, 1966*).

Elevated estrogen suppresses progesterone (*Abraham GE. Nutritional factors in the etiology of the premenstrual tension syndromes. J Reprod Med 28:446-64, 1983*), and reduced progesterone in the luteal phase is associated with an increased risk of breast cancer.

Observational Study: A prospective study of 1,083 infertile pts. revealed that the risk of breast cancer was 5.4 times greater in pts. with luteal (progesterone) deficiency than in pts. with a normal luteal phase and normal progesterone levels (*Cowan LD et al. Breast cancer incidence in women with a history of progesterone deficiency. Am J Epidemiol 114:209-17, 1981*).

- -

DIETARY FACTORS

High protein (about 1/2 gm protein/ lb. of body weight) diet.

Increases the cytochrome P-450-dependent hydroxylation of estradiol (*Kappas A et al. Nutrition - endocrine interactions: Induction of reciprocal changes in the delta-4-5-alpha-reduction of testosterone and the cytochrome p-450-dependent oxidation of estradiol by dietary macronutrients in man. Proc Natl Acad Sci U S A 80:7646-49, 1983*).

Low fat diet.

Dietary fat may increase estrogenic stimulation.

Experimental Study: Switching women from a high fat (40% of calories from fat) to a low fat (25% of calories from fat) diet resulted in a significant decrease in urinary excretion of 16-alpha-hydroxylated estrogens (which are associated with prolonged estrogenic stimulation and increased cancer risk) and a significant increase in catechol estrogens (which are associated with reduced bioactivity of estrogen) (*Longcope C et al. The effect of a low fat diet on oestrogen metabolism. J Clin Endocrinol Metab 64:1246-50, 1987*).

The effect of dietary fat on estrogen metabolism may be due to:

1. the stimulation of animal fats upon the growth of colonic bacteria which are capable of synthesizing estrogen as well as of breaking the estrogen-glucuronide linkages (*Goldin BR, Gorbach SL. The relationship between diet and rat fecal bacterial enzymes implicated in colon cancer. J Natl Cancer Inst 57:371-75, 1976*).

Observational Study: High fat diets were associated with metabolically very active anaerobic bacterial flora which were found to be able to produce estrone, estradiol and 17-methoxyestradiol from bacterial metabolites of cholesterol, suggesting that this is a mechanism by which dietary fat may influence estrogen patterns and breast cancer risk (*Hill MJ et al. Gut bacteria and aetiology of cancer of the breast. Lancet 2:472-73, 1971*).

2. increased arachidonic acid derived from animal fats. Arachidonic acid is the precursor of prostaglandin F_2 alpha which is luteolytic (*Dennefors BL et al. Progesterone and adenosine 3',5'-monophosphate formation by isolated human corpora lutea of different ages: Influence of human chorionic gonadotrophin and prostaglandins. J Clin Endocrinol Metab 3:227-34, 1943*) and thus could contribute to the increased estrogen/progesterone ratio seen in premenstrual syndrome (PMT-A).

<u>High fiber</u> diet.

May increase estrogen clearance and excretion.

> **Review Article:** For Western women, dietary fiber may be important in the prevention of breast cancer, and both the early onset of menarche and a high fat diet are risk factors in breast cancer. Breast cancer may be estrogen-dependent and dietary fiber may increase the fecal excretion of estrogen (*Hughes RE. Hypothesis: A new look at dietary fiber. <u>Hum Nutr Clin Nutr</u> 40C:81-86, 1986*).

> **Observational Study:** Peripheral and fecal estrogens were compared in 10 vegetarian and 10 omnivorous women who were menstruating regularly. The omnivorous women consumed 11-13 g/d of fiber compared to 25-33 g/d for vegetarian women. A significant negative correlation between fiber intake and fecal estrogens suggests that food fiber increases the clearance and fecal excretion of estrogens. Blood estrogen levels were significantly lower in the vegetarian women than in the omnivorous women (*Goldin BR et al. Estrogen excretion patterns and plasma levels in vegetarian and omnivorous women. <u>N Engl J Med</u> 307:1542-47, 1982*).

> - with a <u>low fat</u> diet.

>> **Experimental Study:** 17 healthy premenopausal women consumed a typical Western diet (40% of calories from fat, a polyunsaturate to saturate ratio (P:S) of 0.5, 400 mg cholesterol/d, and 12 g dietary fiber/d. After 4 wks., they were switched to a low-fat, high-fiber diet consisting of 25% of calories from fat, a P:S ratio of 1.0, 200 mg cholesterol/d, and 40 g dietary fiber/d. After 8-10 wks., 16/17 women had lower serum estrone sulfate levels on the low-fat, high-fiber diet. There was an ave. decrease of 36% with mean levels decreasing from 2.11 ± 0.25 nmol/L on the control diet to 1.29 ± 0.19 nmol/L on the experimental diet (p<0.001) (*Woods MN et al. Low-fat, high-fiber diet and serum estrone sulfate in premenopausal women. <u>Am J Clin Nutr</u> 49:1179-83, 1989*).

<u>Vegetarian</u> diet.

Benefits may be due to its low fat and high fiber content.

Vegetarians excrete 2-3 times more estrogen in their feces and have 50% lower mean plasma levels of unconjugated estrogens than do omnivores (*Goldin BR et al. Estrogen excretion patterns and plasma levels in vegetarian and omnivorous women. <u>N Engl J Med</u> 307:1542-47, 1982; Goldin BR et al. Effect of diet on excretion of estrogens in pre- and post-menopausal women. <u>Cancer Res</u> 41:3771-73, 1981*).

> **Experimental Controlled Study:** 39 women aged 21-52 were randomly assigned to continue their usual meat-eating diet, to change to a vegetarian diet, or to change to a predominantly vegetarian diet where fish was consumed 3 times a week. Change to the vegetarian or fish diet had little effect on total hormone concentrations; however, the amt. of estradiol was significantly decreased in the vegetarian gp. (*Bennett FC, Ingram DM. Diet and female sex hormone concentrations: an intervention study for the type of fat consumed. <u>Am J Clin Nutr</u> 52:808-12, 1990*).

> **Observational Study:** When premenopausal US women eating a Western high fat (40% of calories), low fiber diet were compared with age-matched vegetarians eating a moderate fat (30%), high fiber diet, the vegetarians were found to excrete 3 times as much estrogen in their feces and less estrogen excretion in their urine; plasma estrogen levels were 15-20% lower. Plasma estrogen was found to be positively associated with fat and negatively associated with fiber (*Gorbach SL, Goldin BR. Diet and the excretion and enterohepatic cycling of estrogens. <u>Prev Med</u> 16:525-31, 1987*).

Eat <u>broccoli</u>, <u>cauliflower</u>, and <u>cabbage</u>.

Vegetables from the Brassica genus, whether raw or lightly cooked, contain a chemical that promotes the inactivation of estrogen (*Jon Michnovicz & H. Leon Bradlow, Institute for Hormone Research, New York City - reported in <u>Science News</u>, June 16, 1990*).

Restrict <u>sugar</u> intake to below 10% of calories.

Sugar may impair estrogen metabolism in the liver.

Experimental Study: 15 normal young adult males reduced their usual sugar intake from about 150 gm/d to about 55 gm/d. After 3 wks., plasma estradiol concentrations fell 25% and returned to previous values after they resumed their higher level of sugar intake for 2 weeks (*Yudkin J, Eisa O. Dietary sucrose and oestradiol concentration in young men. Ann Nutr Metabol 32:53-55, 1988*).

Experimental Study: 21 normal adult males received a typical Western diet containing 25-30% sucrose for 18 days and a "calorically diluted" diet containing < 10% sucrose for 12 days. Serum GOT and GPT levels rose significantly on the high sucrose diet and returned to baseline levels on the low sucrose diet. The extent of the enzyme elevation was so great in 2 subjects that they had to be withdrawn from the study. Data analysis suggested that both surplus calories and excess sucrose consumption contributed to the rise in enzyme levels which, the authors suggest, may be indicative of hepatic injury (*Porikos KP, van Itallie TB. Diet-induced changes in serum transaminase and triglyceride levels in healthy adult men. Role of sucrose and excess calories. Am J Med 75:624, 1983*).

- -

VITAMINS

<u>Vitamin B Complex</u>:

If deficient, hepatic inactivation of estrogen may be impaired, and supplementation may be beneficial.

Experimental Study: In order to determine whether female pts. with signs and symptoms of nutritional deficiency also suffered from symptoms of estrogen excess, the nutritional status of pts. presenting with menorrhagia, metrorrhagia, cystic mastitis and/or premenstrual tension was investigated, as was the presence of these conditions among pts. presenting with signs and symptoms of nutritional deficiency. 104 pts. were studied. 37/39 pts. observed primarily because of the presence of lesions of nutritional deficiency presented with conditions suggestive of estrogen excess, while 52/52 pts. who presented with one or more of these conditions had signs or symptoms of vitamin B complex deficiency. Treatment of these conditions with vitamin B complex (containing thiamin 3-9 mg, riboflavin 4.5-9 mg and up to 60 mg of niacin and niacinamide along with the rest of the complex) was instituted with good results, suggesting that syndromes related to estrogen excess are caused by failure of the liver to inactivate estrogen because of deficiency of vitamin B complex (*Biskind MS. Nutritional deficiency in the etiology of menorrhagia, cystic mastitis and premenstrual tension, treatment with vitamin B complex. J Clin Endocrinol Metabol 3:227-34, 1943; Biskind MS et al. Nutritional deficiency in the etiology of menorrhagia, cystic mastitis and premenstrual tension, treatment with vitamin B complex. II. Further observations of treatment with the vitamin B complex. Surg Gynecol Obstet 78:49-57, 1944*).

Animal Experimental Study: Estrone pellets were implanted in the spleens of adult castrate female rats so that the absorbed estrogen passed through the liver before reaching the systemic circulation. On a normal diet the animals remained anestrous, but when they were placed on a vitamin B complex-free diet, protracted estrus occurred. The addition of brewer's yeast caused them to become anestrous, while subsequent dietary depletion again led to estrus, suggesting that the liver may have an important part in maintaining the body's estrogen level within the normal range and that a vitamin B deficiency may impair the hepatic estrogen-inactivating function (*Biskind MS, Biskind GR. Effect of vitamin B complex deficiency on inactivation of estrone in the liver. Endocrinology 31:109-114, 1942*).

- <u>Vitamin B6</u>: 100 mg. daily

If deficient, choline is unable to function properly as a lipotropic agent (*Engel RW. The relation of B-vitamins and dietary fat to the lipotropic action of choline. J Biol Chem 37:140, 1941*).

Deficiency lowers the hepatic clearance rate of estrogens resulting in hyperestrogenemia (*Abraham GE. Nutritional factors in the etiology of the premenstrual tension syndrome. J Reprod Med 28(7):446-464, 1983*).

<u>Vitamin E</u>:   800 IU daily (mixed tocopherols)

An anti-oxidant which may be effective in the treatment of both premenstrual syndrome and fibrocystic breast disease, illnesses which may be due to impaired estrogen metabolism (*London RS et al. The effect of alpha-tocopherol on premenstrual symptomatology: A double-blind trial.   J Am Coll Nutr 2:115-22, 1983; London RS et al.   Nutr Res 2:243-47, 1982).*

MINERALS

Iodine:

Low iodine intake may produce a state of increased effective gonadotrophin stimulation, which in turn may produce a hyperestrogenic state characterized by an increased estrogen quotient and an increased risk of estrogen-dependent tumors of the breast, uterus and ovary (*Stadel BV.   Dietary iodine and risk of breast, endometrial, and ovarian cancer.   Lancet 1:890-1, 1976*).

Supplementation may reduce the estrogen quotient.

Experimental Study: The estrogen quotient was significantly raised in 6/7 women presenting with a low estrogen quotient following treatment with sodium or potassium iodide 100-300 mg daily. In the seventh case, improvement was slight. Sustained treatment at a lower dose was associated with persistent improvement (*Wright JV. The oestrogen quotient. Int Clin Nutr Rev 11(3):144-5, 1991*).

OTHER NUTRITIONAL FACTORS

Bioflavonoids:

Examples: quercitin, apigenin

Inhibit human estrogen synthesis *in vitro* and may have a similar effect *in vivo* by competing with estrogen as a substrate (*Kellis Jr JT, Vickery LE.   Inhibition of human estrogen synthetase (aromatase) by flavones.   Science 255:1032-4, 1984*).

Methionine:

Precursor of S-adenosylmethionine which has been shown to be beneficial in treating cholestasis due to estrogen excess (*Padova C et al.   S-adenosyl-L-methionine antagonizes oral contraceptive-induced bile cholesterol supersaturation in healthy women: Preliminary report of a controlled randomized trial.   Am J Gastroenterol 79:941-44, 1984; Frezza M et al. Reversal of intrahepatic cholestasis of pregnancy in women after high dose S-adenosyl-L-methionine (SAMe) administration.   Hepatology 4:274-78, 1984*).

COMBINED NUTRITIONAL TREATMENT

Experimental Study: 160 healthy female students rated themselves on the following scale:

Endometriosis	2 points
Excessive menstrual hemorrhaging	2 points
Fibrocystic breast disease	2 points
Menses lasting 4 days	1 point
Menses lasting 5 or more days	2 points
Premenstrual symptoms:	
Water retention; weight gain	1 point
Anxiety; depression; hysteria	1 point
Craving for sweets	1/2 point
Irritability	1/2 point
Feeling depersonalized	1/2 point
Fainting; dizziness	1 point
Breast sensitivity	1 point

Increase in breast cysts	2 points
Backache; cramps; headache	1 point
Uterine fibroids	2 points

Students scoring 6 or more points were placed on a high protein, low fat, low sugar diet and were supplemented with pyridoxine, vitamin E, selenium, choline and inositol. After 6 mo., all noted at least some benefits including shorter menstrual periods, reduced menstrual hemorrhaging and premenstrual symptoms, reduced symptoms of fibrocystic breast disease, decreased size of uterine fibroids, etcetera. The author suggests a 2 mo. trial and notes that the first menses after starting the program (2-4 wks.) may be more disturbed as estrogen production increases before liver function, and thus estrogen metabolism, improves. 60-70% of symptomatic women are said to experience subjective improvement which will be reflected by an increase in the ratio of estriol to total estrogen (*Fredericks C. Female dysfunctions, hormones, cancer and nutrition. Let's Live January, 1984, pp. 14-17*).

_ _

OTHER FACTORS

Lactobacillus acidophilus:

Inhibits beta-glucuronidase, the fecal bacterial enzyme responsible for deconjugating liver-conjugated estrogen (*Goldin B, Gorsbach S. The effect of milk and lactobacillus feeding on human intestinal bacterial enzyme activity. Am J Clin Nutr 39:756-61, 1984*).

HYPERTENSION

See Also: ATHEROSCLEROSIS
DIABETES MELLITUS
PREGNANCY-RELATED ILLNESS

OVERVIEW

1. Dietary manipulation has been proven to be an effective treatment method. A high fiber, low fat (with a high percentage of polyunsaturates), low salt, low sugar diet is suggested.

2. Relatively higher intakes of calcium, magnesium and potassium, and a relatively lower intake of sodium, appear to be beneficial.

3. Early studies suggest that supplementation with vitamin C, coenzyme Q_{10}, omega-3 fatty acids from fish oils, taurine or tryptophan may be beneficial.

4. Elevated blood cadmium levels appear to be positively correlated to the risk of hypertension; zinc may counteract these effects. Lead and mercury exposures also increase the risk of hypertension.

- -

DIETARY FACTORS

Avoid obesity.

> **Review Article:** Insulin resistance and hyperinsulinemia are associated with hypertension. Much evidence indicates that the link between diabetes and essential hypertension is hyperinsulinemia. In the overweight pt., calorie restriction can improve tissue sensitivity to insulin (*DeFronzo RA, Ferrannini E. Insulin resistance. A multifaceted syndrome responsible for NIDDM, obesity, hypertension, dyslipidemia, and atherosclerotic cardiovascular disease. Diabetes Care 14(3):173-94, 1991*).

> **Review Article:** Weight reduction was found to reduce the risk of elevated arterial pressure as well as overall cardio-vascular morbidity and mortality. Weight control is 1 of only 3 nonpharmacological modalities with sufficient support to warrant a recommendation for inclusion in hypertension treatment programs (*Nonpharmacological approaches to the control of high blood pressure. Final report of the Subcommittee on Nonpharmacological Therapy of the 1984 Joint National Committee on Detection, Evaluation, and Treatment of High Blood Pressure. Hypertension 8(5):444-467, 1986*).

Low salt diet.

> See "*Sodium*" under "*MINERALS*" below.

High fiber diet.

> **Experimental Double-blind Study:** 46 lean pts. with BP between 140/95 and 195/110 mm Hg randomly received either 7 gm fiber from grains, citrus and vegetables ("Fibre Trim Plus" tablets, Farma Food) or placebo. After 3 mo., the fiber gp. showed a significant reduction in systolic BP from a mean of 157 to 147 mm Hg (p=0.004) and of diastolic BP from 97 to 92 mm Hg (p<0.001), while BP in the placebo gp. remained constant. Weights remained stable (*Schlamowitz P et al. Treatment of mild to moderate hypertension with dietary fibre. Letter. Lancet 2:622-23, 1987*).

Review Article: "Dietary fiber is one of the many dietary factors possibly affecting blood pressure. Populations with high-fiber intakes do not have the age-associated increase in blood pressure seen in Western people with low fiber intakes. Vegetarians and others with high fiber intakes have lower blood pressures than matched control subjects. Finally, addition of fiber to the diet lowers blood pressure of normotensive and hypertensive individuals. All of this evidence suggests fiber may have an important influence on blood pressure, but the independent effects of dietary fiber on blood pressure are not established" (*Anderson JW, Tietyen-Clark J. Dietary fiber: Hyperlipidemia, hypertension, and coronary heart disease. Am J Gastroenterol 81(10):907-19, 1986*).

Experimental and Observational Studies: 1.) 94 volunteers aged 18-60 were classified as to fiber intake on the basis of a 3-day dietary survey. Subjects with a high-fiber intake were found to have lower mean BPs than those with a low-fiber intake. 2.) 11 of those eating a high-fiber diet decreased their dietary fiber. After 4 wks., they showed increased mean BPs. 31 of those eating a low-fiber diet increased their dietary fiber. After 4 wks., they showed decreased mean BPs. 3.) 12 hypertensive volunteers were all found to have low-fiber diets and were placed on a high-fiber diet. After 6 wks., their mean BPs did not decrease significantly; however individual recordings varied substantially (*Wright A et al. Dietary fibre and blood pressure. Br Med J 2:1541-43, 1979*).

- Guar Gum:

   Experimental Study: 20 moderately overweight hypertensive men received guar gum 7 gm in water 3 times daily before meals. After 2 wks., systolic BP declined 9.8%, while diastolic BP declined 9%. BP values returned to baseline by the end of a 3-wk. washout period. The only side-effect was a transitory flatulence (*Krotkiewski M. Effect of guar gum on the arterial blood pressure. Acta Med Scand 222(1):43-49, 1987*).

Vegetarian diet.

Associated with lower systolic and diastolic BP.

   Experimental Crossover Controlled Study: 58 pts. aged 30-64 with mild untreated hypertension were allocated either to a control gp. eating a typical omnivorous diet or to 1 of 2 gps. eating an ovolactovegetarian diet for 1 of 2 six-wk. periods. A fall in systolic BP of the order of 5 mm Hg occurred during the vegetarian diet periods, with a corresponding rise on resuming a meat diet (*Margetts RM et al. Vegetarian diet in mild hypertension: A randomized controlled trial. Br Med J 293:1468-71, 1986*).

   Observational and Experimental Study: Systolic BP of 97 Seventh-day Adventist vegetarians was almost 5 mm Hg lower than that of 113 Morman omnivores and the diastolic BP was 4-5 mm Hg lower when adjusted for age, height and weight despite similar strengths of religious affiliations, consumption of alcohol, tea and coffee and use of alcohol. In a controlled intervention study, mean systolic and diastolic BP and serum cholesterol fell significantly during feeding with a vegetarian diet. Dietary analysis indicated that a vegetarian diet provided more polyunsaturated fat, fiber, vitamin C, vitamin E, magnesium, calcium and potassium and significantly less total fat, saturated fat and cholesterol than an omnivore diet (*Rouse IL et al. Vegetarian diet, blood pressure and cardiovascular risk. Aust N Z J Med 14(4):439-43, 1984*).

Benefits may be due to its high content of fiber, polyunsaturates, vegetable protein, potassium and/or magnesium (*Rouse IL et al. Blood pressure lowering effects of a vegetarian diet: Controlled trial in normotensive subjects. Lancet 1:5-9, 1983*).

   Experimental Study: Two of the notably largest dietary changes that occur on introduction of a vegetarian diet are increases in the dietary polysaturate to saturate ratio and fiber intake. When intakes of these nutrients were increased (in isolation from other dietary changes) to levels seen in vegetarians, no effects on BP attributable to the change were seen, suggesting that either a combination of these factors or some other aspect of the diet is responsible for the BP reduction (*Margetts BM et al. Vegetarian diet in mild hypertension: Effects of fat and fiber. Am J Clin Nutr 48:801-05, 1988*).

   Observational Study: 98 vegetarians were compared to a matched gp. of nonvegetarians. The ave. BP was 126/77 for the vegetarians and 147/88 for the control gp., a significant difference. Only 2% of the vegetarians had hypertension (BP above 160/95) compared to 26% of the non-vegetarians. Both gps. had a similar sodium intake and excreted the same amounts of sodium, while potassium intake and excretion was significantly higher in the vegetarians; thus it appears that the high potassium intake of vegetarians could account for the diet's anti-hypertensive effect (*Ophir O et al. Low blood pressure in vegetarians: The possible role of potassium. Am J Clin Nutr 37:755-762, 1983*).

Increase consumption of <u>raw foods</u>.

Experimental Study: For an mean duration of 6.7 mo., 32 pts. ingested an ave. of 62% of their calories in the form of uncooked food. Mean diastolic BP was significantly reduced by 17.8 mm Hg. In addition, there was a significant mean weight loss of 3.8 kg and 80% of those who smoked or drank alcohol abstained spontaneously (*Douglass J et al. Effects of a raw food diet on hypertension and obesity. South Med J 78(7):841, 1985*).

<u>Low fat</u> diet with a high ratio of polyunsaturates to saturates.

> *See Also: "Fatty Acids" below.*

Observational Study: In a study of 4903 Italian men and women aged 20-59, increased butter consumption was associated with significantly higher BP for men, while consumption of olive oil and vegetable oil was inversely associated with systolic BP in both sexes. This finding was adjusted for confounding effects of other risk factors for cardiovascular disease (*Trevisan M et al. Consumption of olive oil, butter, and vegetable oils and coronary heart disease risk factors. JAMA 263:688-92, 1990*).

Review Article: A significant reduction in BP has been observed during low-fat, high polyunsaturated fatty acid/saturated fatty acid ratio diets in a series of studies. Results suggest the active role of linoleic acid but the effects of decreased intake of saturated fats and the concomitant changes in the intake of other dietary components cannot be ruled out (*Iacono JM et al. Dietary polyunsaturated fat and hypertension. Ann Med 21(3):251-54, 1989*).

Animal Experimental Study: Wistar rats were placed on diets containing animal fat, partially-hydrogenated marine oil, cod-liver oil or sunflowerseed oil. After 5 wks., hypertension was induced by administration of sodium chloride in the drinking water. The rise in BP was greatest in the animals receiving animal fat. The hypotensive effect was greatest with cod-liver oil and least with sunflowerseed oil; the effect on rats fed partially hydrogenated marine oil was in-between (*Ziemlänski S et al. Effect of dietary fats on experimental hypertension. Ann Nutr Metab 29(4):223-31, 1985*).

Experimental Study: 84 middle-aged Finns were randomly allocated into 2 groups. In both gps., the proportion of energy from fats was reduced from 38-24%. In gp. I, the polyunsaturated/saturated fat ratio was increased from 0.2 to 0.9 while, in gp. II, it was only increased to 0.4. After 12 wks., mean systolic BP decreased 4 mm Hg in gp. I ($p<0.01$) and 3 mm Hg in gp. II ($p<0.01$). Mean diastolic BP decreased 5 mm Hg in Gp. I ($p<0.001$) and 4 mm Hg in gp. II ($p<0.01$). These reductions were reversed during a subsequent switch-back period. Results show no significant further BP reduction with more than a moderately increased P/S ratio when the saturated fat intake is markedly reduced (*Puska P et al. Dietary fat and blood pressure: An intervention study on the effects of a low-fat diet with two levels of polyunsaturated fat. Prev Med 14(5):573-84, 1985*).

<u>Low sugar</u> diet.

Animal Experimental Study: 75 spontaneously hypertensive rats were placed on a baseline diet which derived equal calories from sucrose, proteins and fats, one of two diets which derived the majority of calories from sucrose with decreases in calories from proteins or fats, or one of two diet which were relatively low in sucrose with a higher percentage of total calories from proteins or fats. After 1 yr., only 20% and 26% respectively, of the rats consuming the high-sucrose diets survived in contrast to 42% on the baseline diet, and 65% and 50%, respectively, on the low-sucrose diets. By 16.5 mo., all rats on the high-sucrose diets were dead, while 29% of rats on the baseline diet, and 43% and 35% of the rats on the low-sucrose diets were still alive. Postmortems suggested death from congestive heart failure. The BP of the rats consuming the high-sucrose diets were consistently significantly higher than those on the low-sucrose diets (*Zein M et al. Effects of excess sucrose ingestion on the lifespan of SHR. Abstract. J Am Coll Nutr 8(5):435, 1989*).

Experimental Study: Untreated, mild diabetic males were placed for 2 wks. on a baseline, intermediate sucrose, diet (35% fat, 15% protein, 120 gm sugar) and then randomized to one of five diets. BP levels dropped during the low and intermediate sucrose diets, and systolic BP rose on the high sucrose diet. Subjects on the high sucrose diet had reduced urinary potassium excretion which reflected a low dietary intake of this mineral due to the high sugar concentration of the diet. Results suggest that a high dietary sugar intake may raise systolic BP, and that this effect is partially modulated by a low-fat, high-carbohydrate diet, possibly because of changes in potassium intake (*Abraira C et al. Systolic blood pressure (B.P.) enhancing effect of dietary sucrose (S) in humans. J Am Coll Nutr 5:79, 1987*).

Experimental Study: The BP of 20 healthy normotensive men was examined after they had ingested various sugar solutions following an overnight fast. Ingestion of water, lactose or galactose produced no change in BP, while systolic BP 1 hr. after glucose ingestion rose significantly (10 mg Hg) for 2 hours and ingestion of sucrose produced a significant increase (9 mm Hg) that lasted for 1 hour (*Rebello T et al. Short-term effects of various sugars on antinatriuresis and blood pressure changes on normotensive young men. Am J Clin Nutr 38(1):84-94, 1983*).

Experimental Controlled Study: Ave. diastolic BPs of 26 normal subjects fed 200 gms sucrose daily over 5 wks. were significantly higher than those who avoided sucrose (78 mm Hg compared to 73 mm Hg) ($p < 0.01$). 8 of the 26 subjects showed sucrose sensitivity (*Ahrens RA, Natl. Acad. Sci., 1975 - summarized in Preuss HG, Fournier RD. Minireview: Effects of sucrose ingestion on blood pressure. Life Sci 30:879-86, 1982*).

Restrict alcohol.

Observational Study: Over 7000 men of Japanese descent were assessed. Alcohol, above a threshold of approx. 20 ml/d, was found to be positively, strongly, and independently correlated with systolic and diastolic BP, and this effect was independent of the effects of calcium and potassium. The effect of alcohol on BP was stronger than was either the separate or combined effects of calcium and potassium (*Criqui MH et al. Dietary alcohol, calcium, and potassium. Independent and combined effects on blood pressure. Circulation 80(3):609-14, 1989*).

Review Article: Epidemiological studies have pointed to alcohol consumption as a cause of hypertension, while clinical studies have demonstrated that, by reducing alcohol intake, hypertensive pts. can lower their BP. Still unresolved, however, is whether the alcohol-induced rise in BP is genuine hypertension, with its adverse pathological consequences, or not. The reduction in BP in response to decreased alcohol consumption is remarkably rapid (between 24 hr to 1 wk after cessation of alcohol intake) (*Beevers DG, Maheswaran R. Does alcohol cause hypertension or pseudo-hypertension? Proc Nutr Soc 47(2):111-14, 1988*).

Avoid caffeine.

Individuals who do not regularly consume caffeine may experience a slight increase in BP when exposed, but tolerance develops rapidly and BP returns to baseline (*Myers MG. Effects of caffeine upon blood pressure. Arch Intern Med 148(5):1189-93, 1988; Smits P et al. Circulatory effects of coffee in relation to the pharmacokinetics of caffeine. Am J Cardiol 56(15):958-63, 1985*).

Experimental Double-blind Study: 69 young, healthy subjects who regularly consumed caffeine randomly received 4-6 140 mL cups of filtered decaffeinated coffee per day and either an equal number of pills containing 75 mg caffeine or an equal number of placebo pills. No other source of caffeine was allowed. After 9 wks., BP was unaffected by the ingestion of caffeine (*Bak AAA, Grobbbee DE. Caffeine, blood pressure, and serum lipids. Am J Clin Nutr 53:971-5, 1991*).

Caffeine consumption may potentiate the stress-related rise in blood pressure in hypertension-prone men (*Lovallo WR et al. Caffeine may potentiate adrenocortical stress responses in hypertension-prone men. Hypertension 14(2):170-76, 1989*).

- -

COMBINED DIETARY INTERVENTIONS

Experimental Controlled Study: 199 pts. randomly received either a cardiovasoprotective diet or a usual diet along with drug therapy. The study diet included a significantly higher content of polyunsaturated fat, complex carbohydrates, calcium, magnesium and potassium. At entry, risk factors, drug therapy, mean BPs, and mean serum calcium, magnesium, potassium and sodium were comparable in both groups. After 8 wks., there were significantly lower mean systolic (140 ± 10.8 mm Hg) and diastolic (87.5 ± 7.80 mm Hg) pressures in the treatment gp. compared with mean systolic (150.0 ± 11.0 mm Hg) and diastolic (96.0 ± 6.8 mm Hg) pressures in the control gp. as well as when compared to initial mean systolic (152.2 ± 12.8 mm Hg) and diastolic (99.8 ± 7.2 mm Hg) pressures (*Singh RB et al. Can dietary changes modulate blood pressure and blood lipids in hypertension? J Nutr Med 2:17-24, 1991*).

Experimental Controlled Study: 91 middle-aged men and women with mild essential hypertension were divided into treatment and control groups. Pts. in the treatment gp. were instructed to reduce their daily salt intake to <70 mmol, to increase their potassium intake, reduce saturated fat, increase the polyunsaturated:saturated fatty acid ratio of the diet and, if necessary, to lose weight. Net decreases in BP were greatest in the first 3 mo. of the 1 yr. study. In men, the mean decrease was 11.3 mm Hg in systolic and 8.3 mm Hg in diastolic BP; in women, the decreases were 10.8 and 6.4 mm Hg, respectively (*Jula A et al. Long-term nonpharmacoloigcal treatment for mild to moderate hypertension. J Intern Med 227:413-21, 1990*).

Experimental Controlled Study: 189 pts. who were 10-49% overweight or whose sodium intake was >2800 mg/d were randomized into 3 groups: Gp. 1 - discontinue drug therapy and reduce overweight, excess salt, and alcohol; Gp. 2 - discontinue drug therapy; Gp. 3 - continue drug therapy. Drug therapy was resumed in Gps. 1 and 2 if BP rose to hypertensive levels. At 4 yrs., 30% of Gp. 1 pts. maintained at least a 4.5 kg weight loss (mean loss 1.8 kg); sodium intake fell 36% and a modest alcohol intake reduction was reported. 39% of pts. in Gp. 1 remained normotensive without drug therapy, compared to 5% in Gp. 2, suggesting that nutritional therapy may substitute for drugs in a sizable proportion of hypertensives (*Stamler R et al. Nutritional therapy for high blood pressure: Final report of a four-year randomized controlled trial - The hypertension control program. JAMA 257(11):1484-91, 1987*).

- -

VITAMINS

Vitamin A:

Lower intake may be associated with hypertension (*McCarron DA et al. Blood pressure and nutrient intake in the United States. Science 224(4656):1392-98, 1984*).

Vitamin C:

Lower intake may be associated with hypertension (*McCarron DA et al. Blood pressure and nutrient intake in the United States. Science 224(4656):1392-98, 1984*).

Lower blood levels may be associated with higher blood pressures.

Observational Study: In a study of 170 healthy men and women aged 19-70, plasma levels of vitamin C decreased as both systolic and diastolic BP increased (*Moran J et al. Dietary antioxidants and blood pressure - extended study. Clin Res 39:A419, 1991*).

Review Article: In 5 populations of essentially healthy people, BP has been found to correlate negatively with vitamin C status (*Trout DL. Vitamin C and cardiovascular risk factors. Am J Clin Nutr 53:322S-5S, 1991*).

Supplementation may reduce blood pressure.

Experimental Placebo-controlled Crossover Study: 20 adults, 12 of whom had borderline hypertension, took ascorbic acid 1 g/d or placebo in random order for 6 wks. each. Systolic BP decreased 6.3 mm Hg and pulse pressure decreased 6.9 mm Hg in the supplemented group, both in the normotensive and in the hypertensive subjects (*Osilesi O et al. Blood pressure and plasma lipids during ascorbic acid supplementation in borderline hypertensive and normotensive adults. Nutr Res 11:405-12, 1991*).

Experimental Double-blind Study: 23 borderline hypertensive women (systolic BP 140-160 mm Hg or diastolic BP 90-100 mg Hg) received ascorbic acid 1 g/d. After 3 mo., there was a 7 mm lowering of systolic pressure ($0.05<p<0.1$) and a 4 mm lowering of diastolic pressure ($0.05<p<0.1$) (*Kuo ET. Effect of vitamin C on blood parameters of hypertensive subjects. J Okla State Med Assoc 77:177-82, 1984*).

Vitamin D:

Higher intake may be associated with lower systolic blood pressure (*Sowers MF et al. The association of intakes of vitamin D and calcium with blood pressure among women. Am J Clin Nutr 42:135-42, 1985*).

- -

MINERALS

GENERAL:

Drink <u>hard</u> rather than soft <u>water</u>.

> **Review Article:** While the results of studies are mixed, most show that hard water is associated with lower BP levels than soft water. Since absorption of elements in drinking water is usually twice that of foods (as there are no chelating agents present), they may have a greater influence than if in foods. Water hardness is usually caused by dissolved calcium and magnesium although, in a few areas, hardness may also result from iron or aluminum salts. The concentrations of these elements is usually small in relation to that in the food. In areas where drinking water is hard, the incidences of hypertension, cardiovascular disease and stroke are often less than in soft water areas. The beneficial influence of water hardness may be from alkalinity or from competition between divalent ions. Toxic elements, such as lead and cadmium, may be leached from pipes in soft water areas because of low pH; also, the intestinal absorption of lead and cadmium may be retarded by the presence of competing ions in hard water, i.e. calcium and magnesium (*Borgman RF. Dietary factors in essential hypertension. <u>Prog Food Nutr Sci</u> 9:109-47, 1985*).

<u>Calcium</u>:   1000 - 2000 mg. daily   (2 month trial)

> **General Review Article:** "Epidemiologic findings . . . indicate that there is a threshold of the potential protective effect of adequate calcium intake, below which the risk of hypertension increases at a greater rate. The set point of this threshold, estimated at 700-800 mg/d, may be modified by a variety of factors including dietary patterns and components, lifestyle, and genetics. . . . In animal models of hypertension . . . greater amounts of calcium must be give to cause a blood pressure change comparable with that in normal animals, suggesting that in high-risk human populations in which calcium metabolism may be disordered, calcium intake may have to be increased to amounts >700-800 mg/d to demonstrate the blood-pressure-lowering effect. Calcium intake at or above the currently recommended daily allowance of 800 mg could be of potential benefit to certain racial groups, individuals ingesting excessive alcohol, and pregnant women, all of whom generally consume low amounts of calcium and who are at higher risk of developing hypertension" (*McCarron DA et al. Dietary calcium and blood pressure: modifying factors in specific populations. <u>Am J Clin Nutr</u> 54:215S-19S, 1991*).

Dietary calcium may be negatively correlated with blood pressure.

> **Observational Study:** Over 7000 men of Japanese descent were assessed. Calcium and potassium intake were inversely related to BP, were highly correlated (r=0.59), and their combined effect was greater than the effect of either alone (*Criqui MH et al. Dietary alcohol, calcium, and potassium. Independent and combined effects on blood pressure. <u>Circulation</u> 80(3):609-14, 1989*).

> **Review Article:** 10 published reports have identified an association between greater dietary calcium consumption and lower BP in humans (*McCarron DA, Morris CD. Metabolic consideratons and cellular mechanism related to calcium's antihypertensive effects. <u>Fed Proc</u> 45:2734-38, 1986*).

> **Review Article:** Reduced dietary calcium is the most consistent nutritional correlate of hypertension in the U.S. (*McCarron DA. Is calcium more important than sodium in the pathogenesis of essential hypertension? <u>Hypertension</u> 7(4):607-27, 1985*).

> **Review Articles:** Results from the evaluation of the First National Health and Nutrition Examination Survey (NHANES I) suggest that the correlation between low calcium intake and hypertension may be stronger than either high sodium or low potassium intakes and hypertension. Hypertensives were found to consume 18% less dietary calcium than normals. Of 10,372 adults who denied a history of hypertension and intentional dietary modification, dietary calcium was the only one of 17 nutrients examined which had a significant, consistent and independent association with BP among previously undiagnosed hypertensives (*Harlan WK et al. Blood pressure and nutrition in adults. The National Health and Nutrition Examination Survey. <u>Am J Epidemiol</u> 120:17-27, 1984; McCarron DA et al. Blood pressure and nutrient intake in the United States. <u>Science</u> 224(4656):1392-98, 1984*).

The relationship between dietary sodium and potassium and blood pressure may only be relevant when dietary calcium is low.

Observational Study: Using First National Health and Nutrition Examination Survey (NHANES I) data, at low calcium intakes (<400 mg/d for men and <800 mg/d for women), the sodium to potassium ratio was significantly related to BP (p<0.01) after controlling for age, body mass index, race, and gender. At higher calcium intakes neither the sodium to potassium ratio nor any other nutrient was related to either systolic or diastolic pressures. (The sodium to potassium ratio was more strongly related to blood pressure than either nutrient alone.) This interaction between these 3 minerals was evident in all race and gender groups (*Gruchow HW et al. Calcium intake and the relationship of dietary sodium and potassium to blood pressure. Am J Clin Nutr 48:1463-70, 1988*).

Alterations in calcium metabolism may be a primary factor in the development of hypertension.

Review Article: While certain studies suggest that increased calcium availability may be associated with increased BP, others suggest that a calcium deficiency may contribute to the pathogenesis of hypertensive disease. Calcium metabolic indices may predict and even determine dietary sodium sensitivity in hypertension, as well as the BP responsiveness to antihypertensive drug therapy. Moreover, oral calcium supplementation may posesss antihypertensive actions in specifically targeted renin subgroups of essential hypertensive subjects. It may ultimately be the calcium-regulating hormones, rather than circulating calcium levels, that mediate BP and possibly even the renin deviations observed among differing hypertensives (*Resnick LM et al. Calcium metabolism and the renin-aldosterone system in essential hypertension. J Cardiovasc Pharmacol 7 Suppl. 6:S187-93, 1985*).

Review Article: Epidemiological surveys, animal experiments, and clinical trials support an inverse relationship between calcium and BP. Current basic research "suggests that when adequate levels of available calcium are present in cells, calcium acts as a calcium channel blocker, controlling its own influx across the cell membrane" (*Henry HJ et al. Increasing calcium lowers blood pressure: The literature reviewed. J Am Diet Assoc 85:182-5, 1985*).

The hypotensive effects of calcium may be due to increased urinary sodium excretion.

Experimental Study: Pts. with mild to moderate hypertension were placed on a sodium-controlled diet (120-130 meq sodium/day) with either normal or high calcium (1000 mg ionic calcium) intake. On the fifth day, they were given a 2-liter isotonic saline load and urine was collected for 4 hours. The high calcium intake resulted in increases in urinary volume, urinary sodium excretion, and the urinary sodium to total urinary volume ratio. These changes were associated with a slight BP reduction (*Lasaridis A, Sofos A. Calcium diet supplementation increases sodium excretion in essential hypertension. Nephron 45:250, 1987*).

Experimental Study: 24 female pts. over age 40 received 800 mg calcium daily. After 12 wks., ave. systolic BP fell from 141.5 to 136.3 mm Hg and ave. diastolic BP fell from 84.5 to 81.1 mm Hg. Urinary sodium excretion was markedly elevated during calcium supplementation, suggesting that calcium supplementation may provide for the special needs of the hypertension pt. through an indirect, natriuretic mechanism (*Gilliland M et al. Preliminary report: Natriuretic effect of calcium supplementation in hypertensive women over forty. J Am Coll Nutr 6:139-43, 1987*).

Calcium excretion may be directly correlated with blood pressure.

Observational Study: In a study of 194 young males and 174 young females (ages 19-35), males with elevated BP had greater calcium excretion than normotensives despite adequate calcium status and an equivalent calcium intake (*Medeiros DM et al. Blood pressure in young adults as influenced by diet, anthropometrics, calcium status and serum lipids. Nutr Res 6:359-68, 1986*).

Serum calcium concentration may be directly correlated with blood pressure.

Observational Study: In a survey of 18,000 adults, serum calcium concentration (adjusted for albumin) was positively related to systolic and diastolic blood pressures (*Lind L et al. Relation of serum calcium concentration to metabolic risk factors for cardiovascular disease. Br Med J 297:960-63, 1988*).

Plasma ionized calcium may be <u>inversely</u> correlated with blood pressure.

> **Observational Study:** Indices of mineral metabolism in blood and urine were analyzed in relation to BP in 97 healthy subjects aged 18-82. In a multivariate analysis, after allowing for the effects of sex, body mass index and age, there was an inverse relationship between plasma ionized calcium and mean BP (p=0.0005); this was the only significant relationship found (*Hvarfner A et al. Indices of mineral metabolism in relation to blood pressure in a sample of a healthy population. <u>Acta Med Scand</u> 219(5):461-68, 1986*).

Supplementation may lower blood pressure.

> *Note: In an animal study in which dietary calcium intake was inversely correlated with systolic BP, signs of magnesium deficiency, calcium deposits in the kidneys, and histological lesions were noted in the high-calcium, low to normal magnesium group, suggesting that calcium supplementation without magnesium supplementation may upset the calcium-magnesium balance and result in kidney damage (Evans G et al. Association of magnesium deficiency with the blood pressure-lowering effects of calcium. <u>J Hypertens</u> 8:327-37, 1990).*

> **Review Article:** "Several clinical trials have tested the hypotensive effect of calcium supplementation. In some cases, no significant hypotensive effect of calcium up to 2.5 g/day was noted. In other trials, all placebo-controlled, an increase in dietary calcium intake showed a significant blood pressure lowering effect both in normotensive and hypertensive subjects. In both normals and hypertensives, the distribution of blood pressure responses is unimodal, and the effect may take 6-8 weeks to be evident. The magnitude of blood pressure reduction is modest" (*Moore TJ. The role of dietary electrolytes in hypertension. <u>J Am Coll Nutr</u> 8 Suppl S:68S-80S, 1989*).

> **Review Article:** Calcium supplementation, like that of sodium, has a heterogenous effect on BP in normal and hypertensive subjects. The magnitude of BP response to sodium supplementation seems to be less than that of calcium and to exert an effect in a smaller number of individuals. However, in comparison to the voluminous data regarding sodium, the evidence concerning calcium is quite scanty and requires further confirmation and study (*Weinberger MH. Salt intake and blood pressure in humans. <u>Contemp Nutr</u> 13(8), 1988*).

Copper:

Excessive dietary copper may be associated with primary pulmonary hypertension due to increased pulmonary vascular resistance.

> **Animal Experimental Study:** Rats placed on high copper diets had significantly higher systolic blood pressures than those with low copper intakes (*Lui CF, Medeiros D. Excess diet copper increases systolic blood pressure in rats. <u>Biol Trace Element Res.</u> 9:15, 1986*).

> **Animal Experimental Study:** IV infusion of copper sulfate in sheep produced a marked increase in pulmonary vascular resistance (*Ahmed I, Sackner M. Increased serum copper in primary pulmonary hypertension: A possible pathogenic link? <u>Respiration</u> 47:243-46, 1985*).

Serum copper levels may be elevated in primary pulmonary hypertension.

> **Observational Study:** Compared to 6 normal women, the mean serum copper level was significantly higher in 7 pts. with primary pulmonary hypertension, indicating that serum copper may be a cause or a marker of this entity (*Ahmed I, Sackner M. Increased serum copper in primary pulmonary hypertension: A possible pathogenic link? <u>Respiration</u> 47:243-46, 1985*).

In hypertensives, blood pressure may be directly correlated with urinary copper excretion.

> **Observational Study:** In a study of 63 early hypertensives and 63 matched controls, both systolic and diastolic blood pressures were significantly and positively correlated with urinary copper excretion (*Vivoli G et al. Zinc and copper levels in serum, urine and hair of humans in relation to blood pressure. <u>Sci Total Environ</u> 66:55-64, 1987*).

<u>Magnesium</u>:

Magnesium is a potent vasodilator because of its ability to displace calcium from the same smooth muscle cell surfaces as well as its interference with the metabolism of acetylcholine at the myoneural junction. With magnesium deficiency there is an increased flow of calcium into vascular muscle cells which increases contractility and potentiates the constrictor effects of humoral pressor substances. Reversible hypertension is a clinical finding in hypomagnesemia and magnesium depletion; 50% of magnesium-depleted patients are hypertensive and their blood pressure returns to normal with supplementation (*Anabolism 2(6):1, 1983; Altura BM, Altura BT. Magnesium ions and contraction of vascular smooth muscles: Relationship to some vascular diseases. Fed Proc 40(12):2672-9, 1981*).

Observational Study: In reviewing 61 dietary variables in 615 men of Japanese ancestry with no history of cardiovascular disease or hypertension living in Hawaii, magnesium intake had the strongest association with blood pressure in both univariate and multivariate analyses (*Joffres MR et al. Relationship of magnesium intake and other dietary factors to blood pressure: the Honolulu heart study. Am J Clin Nutr 45(2):469-75, 1987*).

Review Article: Pts. with low magnesium levels require a greater number of anti-hypertensive medications to control BP than pts. with normal magnesium levels (*Wester PO, Dyckner T. Magnesium and hypertension. J Am Coll Nutr 6(4):321-28, 1987*).

Observational Study: 1000 stable, treated essential hypertensives were studied. 4.5% had definite hypomagnesemia and, regardless of their potassium levels, required a greater number of anti-hypertensive drugs for the same degree of BP control as hypertensives with normal magnesium levels. Since normal serum magnesium may still be associated with cellular magnesium depletion, the prevalence of magnesium depletion may have been greater (*Whang R et al. Hypomagnesemia and hypokalemia in 1,000 treated ambulatory hypertensive patients. J Am Coll Nutr 1:317-322, 1982*).

Supplementation may reduce blood pressure in hypertensives.

Review Article: In 3 trials, magnesium supplementation administered to pts. on diuretics (diuretics are known to cause magnesium depletion) significantly lowered BP (6-12 mm Hg) while placebo had no effect. By contrast, in a single study, administration of magnesium or placebo to untreated pts. failed to affect BP. These studies suggest that magnesium supplementation may lower BP in magnesium-depleted patients (*Moore TJ. The role of dietary electrolytes in hypertension. J Am Coll Nutr 8 Suppl S:68S-80S, 1989*).

Review Article: While observational and clinical trial experience suggest a role for magnesium in hypertension, the evidence from epidemiologic studies is inconsistent and many of the clinical trails are small and methodologically imperfect. Large, rigorously controlled observational and interventional studies are needed to dispell the uncertainty (*Whelton PK, Klag MJ. Magnesium and blood pressure: Review of the epidemiologic and clinical trial experience. Am J Cardiol 63(14):26G-30G, 1989*).

- and <u>Potassium</u>:

Magnesium deficiency is associated with loss of cellular potassium (*Altura BM, Altura BT. Interactions of Mg and K on blood vessels: Aspects in view of hypertension. Magnesium 3(4-6):175-94, 1984*).

Review Article: Magnesium supplementation in association with potassium is more effective than potassium alone in restoring the anti-hypertensive efficacy of diuretics (*Wester PO, Dyckner T. Magnesium and hypertension. J Am Coll Nutr 6(4):321-28, 1987*).

<u>Phosphorus</u>:

- and <u>Calcium</u>:

Low dietary calcium to phosphorus ratios are associated with hypertension (*Parrot-Garcia M, McCarron DA. Nutr Rev 42:205-13, 1984; Nutr Rev 42:223-25, 1984*).

<u>Potassium:</u>

Dietary potassium may be inversely associated with blood pressure (*Khaw KT, Barrett-Connor E. The association between blood pressure, age, and dietary sodium and potassium: A population study. <u>Circulation</u> 77(1):53-61, 1988; McCarron DA et al. Blood pressure and nutrient intake in the United States. <u>Science</u> 224(4656):1392-98, 1984).*

Observational Study: In a study of 233 children aged 5-17 drawn at random who were followed for an ave. of 7 yrs., the mean systolic BP slopes were lower when potassium intake was higher. A rise in BP was on ave. 1 mm Hg lower in children in the upper part of the intake distribution compared with those in the lower part (*Gelijnse JM et al. Sodium and potassium intake and blood pressure change in childhood. <u>Br Med J</u> 300:899-902, 1990).*

Experimental Crossover Study: 10 healthy, normotensive men randomly received isocaloric diets (each lasting 9 days) providing either low (10 mmol/d) or normal (90 mmol/d) amts. of potassium, while sodium intake was maintained at the subjects' usual levels (120-200 mmol/d). The mean arterial pressure increased over the 9 days of the low-potassium diet from 90.9 ± 2.2 to 95.0 ± 2.2 mm Hg (p<0.05). Both mean arterial (p<0.01) and diastolic (p<0.005) pressures were significantly higher after the low-potassium diet than after the normal-potassium diet. In addition, a saline infusion further increased the mean arterial pressure in the potassium-depleted subjects but had no effect in the control gp. (p<0.05). Potassium depletion suppressed plasma aldosterone levels but had no effect on plsma renin activity or on arginine vasopressin or catecholamine levels (*Krishna GG et al. Increased blood pressure during potassium depletion in normotensive men. <u>N Engl J Med</u> 320:1177-82, 1989).*

Observational Study: 98 vegetarians were compared to a matched gp. of nonvegetarians. The ave. BP was 126/77 for the vegetarians and 147/88 for the control gp., a significant difference. Only 2% of the vegetarians had hypertension (BP above 160/95) compared to 26% of the non-vegetarians. Both gps. had a similar sodium intake and excreted the same amounts of sodium, while potassium intake and excretion was significantly higher in the vegetarians; thus it appears that the high potassium intake of vegetarians could account for the diet's anti-hypertensive effect (*Ophir O et al. Low blood pressure in vegetarians: The possible role of potassium. <u>Am J Clin Nutr</u> 37:755-762, 1983).*

Supplementation may reduce blood pressure in hypertensives.

Experimental Double-blind Study: 37 pts. with mildly increased BP and normal sodium intake randomly received either 48 mmol potassium daily or placebo. By the third wk., BP in the actively treated gp. had decreased significantly compared to the placebo gp. and, at 15 wks., the decrease reached its maximum. 13 pts. then underwent a further 9 wks. of treatment with 1/2 the dose of potassium. At the end of the second study period, their BP was still significantly lower compared with their baseline values but not with that of the placebo group (*Siani A et al. Controlled trial of long term oral potassium supplements in patients with mild hypertension. <u>Br Med J</u> 294:1453-56, 1987).*

Experimental Double-blind Crossover Study: 16 hypertensive pts. who had diuretic-induced hypokalemia randomly received either potassium chloride 60 mmol/day or placebo while continuing on diuretics. In 9/16, the mean BP fell by an ave. of 5.5 mm Hg (p=0.004) which correlated with a fall in plasma renin activity (*Kaplan NM et al. Potassium supplementation in hypertensive patients with diuretic-induced hypokalemia. <u>N Engl J Med</u> 312(12):746-49, 1985).*

- and a <u>low sodium diet</u>:

Negative Experimental Double-blind Study: 287 men aged 45-68 on long-term drug treatment for hypertension randomly received either 96 mmol potassium chloride (4 caps 3 times daily) daily or placebo. In addition, both gps. were advised to follow a low-sodium diet. After 12 wks., antihypertensive drugs were withdrawn and pts. were followed an ave. of 2.2 years. 79 pts. in each gp. required reinstitution of antihypertensive medications, and no significant differences in BP were observed between the 2 groups (*Grimm RH Jr et al. The influence of oral potassium chloride on blood pressure in hypertensive men on a low-sodium diet. <u>N Engl J Med</u> 322(9):569-74, 1990).*

Note: This study involved white men almost exclusively, while most positive studies have involved black men. In at least 2 studies that included both black and white subjects, only the blacks had a significant decrease in BP. Second, these results, while they affirm that potassium supplements will not prevent the return of an elevated pressure previously suppressed by medications, do not preclude the possibility that potassium could lower an elevated BP. Finally, the sodium restriction was associated with a significant decline in BPs in both groups. If increased BP after medication withdrawal could be prevented in some subjects by either a low-sodium diet or potassium supplementation, and both therapies operated by a similar mechanism but the effect of a low-sodium diet took precedence, the potential benefit of potassium supplementation could have been realized instead by sodium restriction (Kaplan NM, Ram CVS. Editorial. Potassium supplements for hypertension. N Engl J Med 322(9):623-24, 1990).

- and Calcium:

Both individual and combined intake may be inversely related to blood pressure.

Observational Study: Over 7000 men of Japanese descent were assessed. Calcium and potassium intake were inversely related to BP, were highly correlated (r=0.59), and their combined effect was greater than the effect of either alone (*Criqui MH et al. Dietary alcohol, calcium, and potassium. Independent and combined effects on blood pressure. Circulation 80(3):609-14, 1989*).

Selenium:

Low serum levels may be associated with elevated blood pressure.

Observational Study: In a study of 722 Finnish men, higher serum selenium levels were associated with lower BP, both systolic and diastolic, with a marked elevation of BP at the lowest levels of serum selenium concentration (*Salonen JT et al. Blood pressure, dietary fats, and antioxidants. Am J Clin Nutr 48:1226-32, 1988*).

Sodium:

Review Article: "It is no longer acceptable to recommend that simply lowering sodium chloride is an adequate intervention to prevent or treat high blood pressure. Correcting deficiencies in calcium, potassium, and magnesium intake should be our first step. The current data suggest that sodium chloride would not be a factor if these other cations are consumed in sufficient quantities" (*Mc Carron DA, Reusser ME. The integrated effects of electrolytes on blood pressure. The Nutr Rep 9(8), August, 1991*).

Epidemiologic studies of the correlation between salt consumption and blood pressure have had mixed results.

Positive Studies:

Meta-analyses of Observational Studies:
1. In an analysis of studies of 47,000 people in different communities throughout the world, a difference in sodium intake of 100 mmol/24 hr was associated with an ave. difference in systolic BP that ranged from 5 mm Hg at age 15-19 yrs. to 10 mm Hg at age 60-69. The differences in diastolic BP were half as great (*Law MR, Frost CD, Wald NJ. By how much does dietary salt reduction lower blood pressure? I - Analysis of observational data among populations. Br Med J 302:811-5, 1991*).
2. In an examination of data from 14 published studies that correlated BP in individuals against measurements of their 24 hr. sodium intake, the relationship was found to confirm the authors' estimates of the magnitude of the association based on comparisons between different populations (*Frost CD, Law MR, Wald NJ. II - Analysis of observational data within populations. Br Med J 302:815-8, 1991*).

Observational Study: The relationship between BP and 24 hr. urinary sodium was examined for over 10,000 men and women in 52 centers around the world. In individual subjects within centers, sodium excretion was significantly related to BP. 4 centers found very low sodium excretion, low BP, and little or no upward slope of BP with age. Across the other 48 centers sodium was significantly related to the slope of BP with age but not to median BP or prevalence of high BP. Overall, it was concluded that a drop of 2.2 mm Hg systolic and 0.1 mm Hg diastolic BP could be attained with a reduction of 100 mmol/day of sodium (*Intersalt co-operative research group. Intersalt: An international study of electrolyte excretion and blood pressure: Results for 24 hour urinary sodium and potassium excretion. Br Med J 297:319-28, 1988*).

Observational Study: In a study of 7354 Scottish men and women aged 40-59 yrs., results suggest that, although there was a weak correlation between sodium excretion and BP in both men and women, alcohol and potassium intakes appear to have a greater influence upon BP than does sodium intake (*Smith WCS et al. Urinary electrolyte excretion, alcohol consumption, and blood pressure in the Scottish heart study. Br Med J 297:329-30, 1988*).

Book: Essential hypertension is virtually unknown in various populations that consume a diet which is very low in salt (<1 g/d sodium) and high in potassium throughout their lifetime (*Denton D. Hunger For Salt: An Anthropological, Physiological and Medical Analysis. New York, Springer-Verlag, 1982:573*).

Negative Studies:

Negative Observational Study: Because of apparently elevated rates of hypertension in Gila Bend Papago indians and a high sodium level (440 mg/L) in the water supply, 342 indians and 375 non-indians living in the area 25 yrs. of age or older were interviewed. No consistent associations were found between any of the sodium values (dietary sodium intake and urinary sodium) and systolic or diastolic BP. Mean BP for the Gila Bend whites were lower in most age gps. than in comparison US white populations, and the prevalence of hypertension was not significantly higher than national rates (*Welty TK et al. Effects of exposure to salty drinking water in an Arizona community: Cardiovascular mortality, hypertension prevalence, and relationships between blood pressure and sodium intake. JAMA 255(5):622, 1986*).

Negative Observational Study: Among normotensive young adults, the less table salt reportedly consumed, the higher the systolic and diastolic BP measured (*Phillips K et al. Am J Public Health 75:405-6, 1985*).

Negative Observational Study: The intake of 17 nutrients was surveyed in over 10,000 adult Americans who denied a history of hypertension. Not only did a significant increase in sodium intake fail to distinguish hypertensive from normotensive subjects, but higher intakes of sodium were associated with lower mean systolic BP and lower absolute risk of hypertension (*McCarron DA et al. Blood pressure and nutrient intake in the United States. Science 224(4656):1392-98, 1984*).

Negative Observational Study: BP and salt intake was measured in 3566 men and women who had never been diagnosed as hypertensive. No significant difference in BP was found between those with the lowest and highest 10% of salt use, suggesting that moderate reduction of salt consumption by the general population to prevent hypertension is unjustified (*Holden RA et al. Dietary salt intake and blood pressure. JAMA 250:365-9, 1983*).

Roughly half of the hypertensive population, and a smaller percentage of normal population, is salt-sensitive.

Review Article: Salt-sensitive subjects are estimated to be 40-50% of the hypertensive population and about 30% of the general public (*Mc Carron DA, Reusser ME. The integrated effects of electrolytes on blood pressure. The Nutr Rep 9(8), August, 1991*).

Review Article: Half of the 30% of the population which is hypertensive is salt-sensitive; thus about 85% of the population can eat salt with impunity (*Michael J Horan, associate director for cardiology at the National Heart, Lung and Blood Institute, USA - reported in the Los Angeles Times March 19, 1990*).

Review Article: Recent evidence suggests that essential hypertension is a syndrome with elevated BP the common symptom. Approx. 60% of the hypertensive population has an increased BP sensitivity to salt intake; this gp. consists of at least 6 major entities: renal parenchymal disease, bilateral renal artery stenosis, primary aldosteronism, acromegaly, low renin essential hypertension, and nonmodulating essential hypertension (*Williams GH, Hollenberg NK. Sodium-sensitive essential hypertension: Emerging insights into an old entity. J Am Coll Nutr 8(6):490-94, 1989*).

Reducing dietary salt may increase blood pressure.

Experimental Study: Salt intake was varied in 27 white men in their mid-30's, some of whom were mildly hypertensive. On a high-salt diet, 10/27 (37%) had blood pressures which were at least 5 mm Hg higher than on a low-salt diet while, 13/27 (48%) had higher blood pressures when they ate less salt. In these men, lowering salt also raised serum cholesterol levels (*Brent M Egan, director of the hypertension program, Medical College of Wisconsin in Milwaukee - reported in the Los Angeles Times March 19, 1990*).

Increased dietary sodium may not account for the higher incidence of salt-sensitive hypertension in blacks.

Observational Study: White hypertensives were found to have a greater sodium intake that black hypertensives, and white normotensives a greater sodium intake than black normotensives. High sodium foods were significantly lower in diets of blacks than in whites. Intake of potassium was also significantly lower for blacks than for whites, as were intakes of grains, candy and soft drinks, alcohol and seafood (*Zemel P et al. Dietary mineral intake in normotensive and hypertensive blacks and whites. Abstract. J Am Coll Nutr 6(5):454, 1987*).

In rats, once hypertension has developed due to chronic excess salt ingestion, blood pressure remains elevated when the animals are placed on a low-salt diet (*Dahl LK et al. Effects of chronic excess salt ingestion. Modification of experimental hypertension in the rat by variations in the diet. Circ Res 22(1):11-18, 1968*).

Moderate sodium restriction may possibly delay or prevent the development of hypertension (*Kaplan NM. Non-drug treatment of hypertension. Ann Intern Med 102:359-73, 1985*).

Moderate sodium restriction may be associated with perhaps as much as a 5-10 mm Hg decrease in hypertensives who are salt-sensitive (*Falkner B. Sodium sensitivity: A determinant of essential hypertension. J Am Coll Nutr 7(1):35-41, 1988; Kawasaki T et al. The effect of high-sodium and low-sodium intakes on blood pressure and other related variables in human subjects with idiopathic hypertension. Am J Med 64:193-98, 1978; Weinberger MH et al. Definitions and characteristics of sodium sensitivity and blood pressure resistance. Hypertension 8(6 Pt 2):II127-34, 1986*).

Meta-analysis of Experimental Studies: In analyzing the results of 68 crossover trials and 10 randomized controlled trials of dietary salt reduction, in the trials in which salt reduction lasted 4 wks. or less the observed reductions in BP were less than those predicted while, in the trials in which salt reduction lasted 5 wks. or longer, the predicted reductions in individual trials closely matched a wide range of observed reductions (*Law MR, Frost CD, Wald NJ. III - Analysis of data from trials of salt reduction. Br Med J 302:819-24, 1991*).

Review Article: Advice on dietary salt intake is controversial. Diets with an extremely low salt content undoubtedly lower BP but are unacceptable to the healthy population. As to moderate salt restriction, it has not lowered BP in normotensive subjects and pts. with borderline BPs, and the effect has been small in mild hypertension. The suggestion that a moderate reduction would lower the whole population BP distribution curve is based on associations in intercultural studies between sodium intake and BP. It has been assumed in public health campaigns that the relation between salt intake and BP reported in some studies is causal. Recently, two sophisticated major epidemiological studies have failed to find a strong association between sodium intake and BP. Clearly, large-scale intervention trials are needed (*Editorial: Salt and blood pressure: the next chapter. Lancet 1:1301-02, 1989*).

Meta-analysis of Experimental Studies: A meta-analysis was performed of 5 randomized trials investigating the effect of salt restriction on hypertensive populations, of which none receive antihypertensive medications. Results indicate that any hypotensive effect of salt restriction is clinically irrelevant (*Graudal N, Galløe A. Effect of salt restriction on hypertension. Letter. Lancet 2:41-42, 1989*).

Review Article: While wide variations in salt intake have little effect on BP in normotensives, hypertensive subjects on average display a more pronounced pressor response to a high-salt inake and, conversely, tend to reduce BP with sodium restriction. However, many hypertensives have no appreciable change in BP with high vs. low sodium intake. Salt sensitivity is higher in blacks, pts. with low-renin essential hypertension, the elderly, and subjects with renal impairment. Plamsa renin activity is lower in salt-sensitive subjects, and those with low renin levels have a higher prevalence of salt sensitivity. Since renin levels tend to fall with aging and tend to be lower in blacks, the plasma renin activity level either reflects an expanded plasma/intravascular volume or may in some way be responsible for salt sensitivity (*Moore TJ. The role of dietary electrolytes in hypertension. J Am Coll Nutr 8 Suppl S:68S-80S, 1989*).

The degree of myocardial hypertrophy in essential hypertension due to dietary salt intake may be independent of blood pressure.

Observational Study: 60 white middle-aged men with previously untreated mild essential hypertension stage I or II were studied. Left ventricular mass was calculated and related to sodium excretion during the 24 hours prior to evaluation. Significant correlations of sodium excretion with diastolic diamteter to the left chamber (p<0.01) and with left ventricular mass (p<0.006) were observed, and 24 hr. sodium excretion was shown to be an independent determinant of left ventricular mass (p<0.05) (*Schmieder RE. Salt intake is related to the process of myocardial hypertrophy in essential hypertension. Letter. JAMA 262(9):1187-88, 1989*).

The effect of dietary sodium chloride upon blood pressure may be due, not solely to the presence of sodium in the salt, but to the effect of that specific salt.

> **Experimental Study:** 5 hypertensive men had normal BP when dietary sodium chloride was restricted to 0.23 gm of sodium daily. After 7 days of increasing sodium chloride intake to 5.52 gm daily, both systolic and diastolic BP increased (16 ± 2 and 8 ± 2 respectively). Replacing sodium chloride with the equivalent amt. of sodium in the form of sodium citrate abolished the BP increase. Both salts induced comparable sodium retention, and suppression of plasma renin activity and plasma aldosterone. However, supplemental sodium chloride increased plasma volume and urinary calcium excretion, wheras sodium citrate did not (*Kurtz TW et al. "Salt sensitive" essential hypertension in men. N Engl J Med 317(17):1043-48, 1987*).

Essential hypertension may result from an interaction between the response to environmental stress and sodium intake (*Poulter NR et al. Pulse rate and twenty-four hour urinary sodium content interact to determine blood pressure levels of male London civil servants. J Hypertens Suppl 6(4):S611-13, 1988; Sever PS, Poulter NR. A hypothesis for the pathogenesis of essential hypertension: the initiating factors. J Hypertens Suppl 7(1):S9-12, 1989; Staessen J et al. Sympathetic tone and relation between sodium intake and blood pressure in the general population. Br Med J 299:1502-03, 1989*).

Sodium/Potassium Ratio:

May be inversely correlated with blood pressure and have a greater impact on blood pressure than either nutrient alone (*Gruchow HW et al. Threshold effect of dietary calcium on blood pressure. J Hypertension 4(suppl 5):S355-57, 1986; Khaw KT, Barrett-Connor E. The association between blood pressure, age, and dietary sodium and potassium: A population study. Circulation 77(1):53-61, 1988; Smith WCS et al. Urinary electrolyte excretion, alcohol consumption, and blood pressure in the Scottish heart study. Br Med J 297:329-30, 1988*).

Decreases may be beneficial.

> **Review Article:** A therapeutic program based on dietary sodium alone or in combination with a diuretic will be more anti-hypertensive if the dietary intake of potassium is increased (*Haddy F. Dietary sodium and potassium in the genesis, therapy, and prevention of hypertension. J Am Coll Nutr 6:261-70, 1987*).

> **Review Article:** "Although the addition of potassium may reduce the hypertensive effect of a high-sodium intake, the potential hazards and considerable cost of large amounts of potassium supplements make this practice unacceptable. A more sensible approach is to reduce the intake of high-sodium, low-potassium processed foods and increase the intake of low-sodium, high-potassium natural foods. In addition, potassium chloride should be partially substituted for sodium chloride in cooking and at the table" (*Kaplan NM. Non-drug treatment of hypertension. Ann Intern Med 102:359-73, 1985*).

- and Calcium:

> **Observational Study:** In the First National Health and Nutrition Examination Survey (NHANES I), low calcium intake increased the impact of a high sodium/potassium ratio. The gp. at greatest risk for elevated systolic and diastolic BP ingested a Na/K ratio >1.36 and <400 mg calcium daily. When the Na/K ratio was <0.65, dietary calcium apparently had no effect (*Gruchow HW et al. Threshold effect of dietary calcium on blood pressure. J Hypertension 4(suppl 5):S355-57, 1986*).

Zinc:

Erythrocyte zinc levels may be elevated in hypertension (*Frithz G Ronquist G. Increased red cell content of zinc in essential hypertension. Acta Med Scand 205:647-49, 1979; Henrotte JG et al. Blood and tissue zinc levels in spontaneously hypertensive rats. J Am Coll Nutr 9(4):340-43, 1990*).

Supplementation may counteract the deleterious effects of cadmium on blood pressure (*see "Cadmium" below*).

– –

OTHER NUTRITIONAL FACTORS

Amino Acids:

- Taurine:

A sulfur amino acid.

Dietary intake of sulfur amino acids may be inversely correlated with systolic blood pressure.

Observational Study: In a Japanese farming village where the stroke incidence is nearly twice as high as the ave. stroke incidence in Japan, systolic BP was inversely correlated with urinary sulfate to nitrogen ratio - corresponding to the ratio of the dietary intake of sulfur amino acids derived from animal protein to the total protein intake (*Yamori Y et al. Studies on stroke prevention in animal models, and their supportable epidemiological evidence, in H Barnett et al, Eds. Cerebrovascular Diseases: New Trends in Surgical and Medical Aspects. Amsterdam: Elsevier/North Holland, 1981:47-62*).

Supplementation may reduce elevated blood pressure.

Experimental Blinded Study: 19 young pts. with borderline hypertension received either 6 gm daily of taurine or placebo. After 7 days, systolic and diastolic BP fell significantly in pts. receiving taurine (9.0 and 4.1 mm Hg), while no significant changes occurred in the placebo group. In addition, the rise in plasma epinephrine was blunted by taurine, suggesting that its anti-hypertensive effect may be mediated by a reduction in sympathetic tone (*Fujita T et al. Effects of increased adrenomedullary activity and taurine in young patients with borderline hypertension. Circulation 75:525, 1987*).

- L-Tryptophan:

May reduce blood pressure in essential hypertension.

Experimental Double-blind Study: 38 essential hypertensives randomly received either L-tryptophan 3 gm daily or placebo. In addition, after 1 wk., they also received either a protein- or a carbohydrate-enriched diet following a crossover design. While BP values of the 2 gps. were not significantly different at the start, after 3 wks. BP levels in the tryptophan gp. were significantly lower (p=0.05). Diet changes failed to affect the placebo gp.; however, those pts. in the tryptophan gp. who first received a carbohydrate-rich diet demonstrated larger BP decreases (*Lehnert H et al. Effects of L-tryptophan on blood pressure levels in essential hypertensives. Abstract. Clin Exp Theory Pract A9(1):208, 1987*).

Coenzyme Q10:   60 mg daily
                  (BP reduction takes 4-12 weeks)

Often deficient in hypertensives.

Observational Study: Enzymatic assays revealed that 39% of 59 pts. were deficient in CoQ10 compared to 6% of 65 controls (*Yamagami T et al. Bioenergetics in clinical medicine. Studies on coenzyme Q10 and essential hypertension. Res Commun Chem Pathol Pharmacol 11:273, 1975*).

Supplementation may reduce blood pressure in hypertensives.

Experimental Double-blind Crossover Study: 18 essential hypertensives received CoQ10 100 mg/d and placebo in either order for 10 wks. each with a 2-wk. washout period. Mean systolic and diastolic pressures fell significantly by 10.6 and 7.7 mm Hg, respectively, during CoQ10 treatment and failed to change during placebo treatment (*Digiesi V, Cantini F, Brodbeck B. Effect of coenzyme Q10 on essential arterial hypertension. Curr Ther Res 47:841-5, 1990*).

Experimental Study: 25 essential hypertensives received CoQ$_{10}$ 60 mg daily. After 8 wks., there was a highly significant decrease in mean BP and 54% had a mean BP reduction of >10% (*Yamagami T et al. Correlation between serum coenzyme Q levels and succinate dehydrogenase coenzyme Q reductase activity in cardiovascular disease and the influence of coenzyme Q administration, in K Folkers, Y Yamamura, Eds., Biomed & Clin Aspects of Coenzyme Q. Amsterdam, Elsevier Science Publishers, 1984:253-62*).

Fatty Acids:

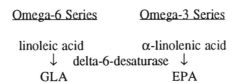

Supplementation with polyunsaturates, especially while reducing total and saturated fat intake, may be beneficial.

Experimental Double-blind Crossover Study: 46 elderly (≥60 yrs.) hypertensives with entry systolic BP ≥160 or diastolic BP ≥90 mm Hg randomly received 9 g/d of fish oil (omega-3 fatty acids) or 9g/d of corn oil (omega-6 fatty acids) in either order. Following a 4 wk. baseline period, each regimen was given for 8 wks. with a 3 wk. washout period in between. An isocaloric, low cholesterol diet was used throughout. Within gps., during the first treatment period, both fish oil and corn oil lowered all 4 BP measures (p<0.05); BPs were not furthered lowered during the second treatment period, compared to washout (*Margolin G et al. Blood pressure lowering in elderly subjects: A double-blind crossover study of ω-3 and ω-6 fatty acids. Am J Clin Nutr 53:562-72, 1991*).

Review Article: A significant reduction in BP has been observed during low-fat, high polyunsaturated fatty acid/saturated fatty acid ratio diets in a series of studies. Results suggest the active role of linoleic acid but the effects of decreased intake of saturated fats and the concomitant changes in the intake of other dietary components cannot be ruled out (*Iacono JM et al. Dietary polyunsaturated fat and hypertension. Ann Med 21(3):251-54, 1989*).

Negative Animal Experimental Study: After a control period on a low fat diet, rabbits were given diets enriched with oils containing different proportions of linoleic, gamma-linolenic and alpha-linolenic acids for 8 wks., and returned to the low fat control diet for 3 weeks. BP increased from the 4th wk. of fat feeding. At 8 wks., the BP increase was 10%, 13%, 15% and 14% respectively for primrose, starflower, safflower and olive oils (all p<0.001). Return to the low fat control diet for 3 wks. restored BPs to near control values (*Bursztyn PG, King MH. Fat induced hypertension in rabbits: The effects of dietary linoleic and linolenic acid. J Hypertens 4(6):699-702, 1986*).

- Oleic Acid:

Intake may be inversely correlated with blood pressure.

Observational Study: In a study of 76 sedentary middle-aged American men (aged 30-55) with resting BP's below 160/100 mm Hg, both systolic and diastolic BP's correlated significantly and inversely with monounsaturated fat consumption. Although polyunsaturated fat consumption also correlated inversely with diastolic BP, this relationship became nonsignificant when adjusted for an index of male adiposity. The correlations with monounsaturates were specific to oleic acid, while the correlation with polyunsaturates was specific to linoleic acid (*Williams PT et al. Associations of dietary fat, regional adiposity, and blood pressure in men. JAMA 257(23):3251-56, 1987*).

- Omega-3 Fatty Acids (Fish Oils):

Eicosapentaenoic acid (EPA) and docosahexaenoic acid (DHA).

Highest in cold water fish such as herring, mackerel, salmon, bluefish and tuna (or EPA and DHA can be derived in the body from α-linolenic acid).

Suggested dosage: 5-15 g/d in divided doses

WARNING: Supplementation may require additional vitamin E intake to prevent increased membrane per-oxidation and cellular damage (*Laganiere S, Fernandes G. High peroxidizability of subcellular membrane induced by high fish oil diet is reversed by vitamin E. Clin Res 35:A565, 1987*).

Intake may be inversely associated with blood pressure.

Observational Study: In a study of 722 Finnish men aged 54, estimated dietary intake of linolenic acid had an inverse association (p=0.048) with the mean resting BP (*Salonen JT et al. Blood pressure, dietary fats, and antioxidants. Am J Clin Nutr 48:1226-32, 1988*).

Tissue levels may be inversely associated with blood pressure.

Observational Study: Adipose tissue fatty acid composition was analyzed in 399 males (ave. age 47). An absolute 1% increase in linolenic acid was associated with a decrease of 5 mm Hg in the systolic, diastolic and composite mean arterial BP. While linolenic acid comprised only 1/8 the amt. of linoleic acid, it had a disproportionate association with BP, suggesting that omega-3 fatty acids may be helpful in the treatment and prevention of hypertension (*Berry EM, Hirsch J. Does dietary linolenic acid influence blood pressure? Am J Clin Nutr 44(3):336-49, 1986*).

Supplementation with fish oils (EPA and DHA) may reduce blood pressure.

Review Article: 8 studies, most conducted on pts. with mild hypertension, were reviewed. 6/8 reported significant declines in both systolic and diastolic BP, one reported a significant decline in only systolic BP, and one had negative findings. Overall, other studies suggest that a low-dose long-term ingestion of fatty fish can likewise be effective to reduce mildly elevated BP; however, no epidemiologic data on BP and ω3 fatty acid intake are available and, because of the confounding effect of other nutrients, no clear case can, so far, be made for a beneficial effect of fish consumption (*Singer P. Blood pressure-lowering effect of ω3 polyun-saturated fatty acids in clinical studies, in AP Simopoulos et al, Eds. Health Effects of ω3 Polyunsaturated Fatty Acids In Seafoods. World Rev Nutr Diet 66:329-48, 1991*).

Review Article: In the majority of 8 studies on normotensive subjects, only a weak and insignificant BP-lowering effect in response to ω3 polyunsaturated fatty acids was found. However, 6/7 studies of pts. with several risk factors for coronary heart disease other than hypertension revealed a significant fall of systolic anc diastolic BP with fish oil supplementation, suggesting that these pts. are appropriate candidates for sup-plementation (*Singer P. Blood pressure-lowering effect of ω3 polyunsaturated fatty acids in clinical studies, in AP Simopoulos et al, Eds. Health Effects of ω3 Polyunsaturated Fatty Acids In Seafoods. World Rev Nutr Diet 66:329-48, 1991*).

- Omega-6 Fatty Acids:

linoleic acid $\rightarrow$ GLA $\rightarrow$ DGLA $\rightarrow$ prostaglandin E$_1$

Evening primrose oil is a rich source of GLA.

Tissue levels may be inversely associated with blood pressure.

Negative Observational Study: Adipose tissue fatty acid composition was analyzed in 399 males (ave. age 47). Linoleic acid was unassociated with BP (*Berry EM, Hirsch J. Does dietary linolenic acid influence blood pressure? Am J Clin Nutr 44(3):336-49, 1986*).

Observational Study: BP was negatively correlated with linoleate concentration in adipose tissue of males (*Oster P et al. Blood pressure and adipose tissue linoleic acid. Res Exp Med (Berl) 175:287, 1979*).

Supplementation with linoleic acid or its metabolites may reduce blood pressure in hypertensives.

Experimental Study: Increasing dietary linoleate was associated with decreases in both systolic and diastolic BP in hypertensives (*Iacono JM et al. Effect of dietary fat on blood pressure in a rural Finnish population. Am J Clin Nutr 38:860, 1983*).

Experimental Study: Increasing linoleate in the diet of pts. was associated with BP reduction (*Rao RH et al. Effect of polyunsaturate-rich vegetables oils on blood pressure in essential hypertension. Clin Exp Hyperten 3:27, 1981*).

Experimental Study: A moderate increase in dietary linoleic acid significantly decreased diastolic BP in 8 borderline hypertensives within 4 weeks. The change was not due to reduced dietary sodium. A significant increase in creatinine excretion and clearance was noted, indicating improved kidney function (*Vergroesen AJ et al. The influence of increased dietary linoleate on essential hypertension in man. Acta Biol Med Ger 37(5-6):879-83, 1978*).

- omega-3 vs. omega-6 fatty acids:

Fish oil (high in eiscosapentaenoic and docosahexaenoic acids of the omega-3 family) may be more beneficial than vegetable oil (high in linoleic acid of the omega-6 family).

Experimental Double-blind Crossover Study: 33 pts. with mild hypertension randomly received omega-3 fatty acids 2.04 g/d from fish oil and linoleic acid (omega-6 fatty acid) 4.8 g/d from safflower oil for 12 wks. each with a 4 wk. washout period. All antihypertensive medication was discontinued. There were significant reductions in supine diastolic and sitting systolic BPs in the fish oil gp. with no significant changes in the safflower oil group. Fish oil supplementation was associated with a significant reduction in supine diastolic BP of 3.7 mm Hg. There was a significant decrease from pretreatment values for sitting diastolic, mean arterial and systolic BPs after fish oil supplementation. No adverse changes were noted on lipid profiles (*Radack K et al. The effects of low doses of N-3 fatty acid supplementation on blood pressure in hypertensive subjects: a randomized controlled trial. Arch Intern Med 151:1173-80, 1991*).

Experimental Double-blind Study: 33 normotensive, mildly hypercholesterolemic men randomly received 1 of 3 diets supplemented with linoleic acid 14.3 g/d, α-linolenic acid 9.2 g/d, or eicosapentaenoic acid plus docosahexaenoic acid (fish oils) 3.4 g/d following 3 wks. on the linoleic acid-supplemented diet. Diets were matched to provide similar amts. of the major classes of fatty acids and cholesterol. After 6 wks., systolic BP fell 5.1 mm ($p=0.01$) in the gp. receiving the EPA and DHA supplement as compared to the linoleic acid-supplement, while the α-linolenic acid supplement failed to affect BP (*Kestin M et al. n-3 fatty acids of marine origin lower systolic blood pressure and triglycerides but raise LDL cholesterol compared with n-3 and n-6 fatty acids from plants. Am J Clin Nutr 51:1028-34, 1990*).

Experimental Double-blind Study: 156 men and women with previously untreated, stable, mild essential hypertension randomly received either 6 g/d of 85% eicosapentaenoic and docosahexaenoic acids or 6 g/d of corn oil. In the fish oil gp., the mean systolic BP fell by 4.6 mm Hg ($p=0.002$), and diastolic BP fell by 3.0 mm Hg ($p=0.0002$); there was no significant change in the control group. The differences between gps. remained significant for both systolic ($p=0.0025$) and diastolic ($p=0.029$) BP after controlling for anthropometric, lifestyle, and dietary variables. The decreases in BP were larger as concentrations of plasma phospholipid n-3 fatty acids increased ($p=0.027$). Dietary supplementation with fish oil did not change mean BP in the subjects who ate fish 3 or more times/wk. as part of their usual diet, or in those who had a baseline concentration of plasma phospholipid n-3 fatty acids above 175.1 mg/L (*Bønaa KH et al. Effect of eicosapentaenoic and docosahexaenoic acids on blood pressure in hypertension. N Engl J Med 322:795-801, 1990*).

Experimental Study: 32 men with mild essential hypertension received either 10 ml or 50 ml of fish oil (3 or 15 g of ω-3 fatty acids) daily, 50 ml of safflower oil (39 g of ω-6 fatty acids), or 50 ml of a mixture of oils that approximated the types of fat present in the American diet. BP decreased in the men who received the high dose of fish oil (systolic BP by a mean of 6.5 mm Hg ($p<0.03$) and diastolic BP by 4.4 mm Hg ($p<0.015$), but not in the other gps. (*Knapp HR, FitzGerald GA. The antihypertensive effects of fish oil. N Engl J Med 320(16):1037-43, 1989*).

The combination of fish oil (high in the omega-3 fatty acids EPA and DHA) and evening primrose oil (high in the omega-6 fatty acid GLA) may be more beneficial than the combination of sunflower seed oil (high in the omega-3 fatty acid linoleic acid) and linseed oil (high in the omega-6 fatty acid α-linolenic acid).

Experimental Double-blind Crossover Study: Following 4 wks. on placebo capsules, 25 non-obese black pts. with mild-moderate uncomplicated essential hypertension randomly received either a combination of evening primrose (high in GLA) and marine oils (high in EPA) (Efamol-Marine), or sunflower seed (high in linoleic acid) and linseed oil (high in α-linolenic acid) capsules. After 12 wks., both gps. were placed again on placebo for 4 wks. and then crossed over for another 12 weeks. The mean systolic BP of pts. receiving Efamol-Marine was significantly lowered after 8 and 12 wks., while those receiving sunflower/linseed oil supplementation had no significant BP reduction (*Venter CP et al. Effects of essential fatty acids on mild to moderate hypertension. Prostaglandins Leukot Essent Fatty Acids 33(1):49-51, 1988*).

- -

OTHER FACTORS

Rule out <u>food sensitivities</u>.

Experimental Study: 15 migraineurs with diastolic BP of 100 mm Hg or greater followed a 5-day elimination diet consisting usually of lamb and pears. The exclusion diet and avoidance of other precipitants resulted in reduction of diastolic BP to 90 mm Hg or below in every patient. BP rose when foods causing reactions were tested and fell to normal when these foods were avoided (*Grant ECG. Food allergies and migraine. Lancet 1:966-9, 1979*).

Case Reports: 6 cases of hypertension are described with "definite and positive" evidence of a relationship between familial non-reaginic food allergy and hypertension. Food eliminations produced excellent clinical results in 2, good results in 2 and unfavorable results in 2 (*Price AS. The role of food allergy in hypertension: An experimental study. Rev Gastroenterol 10:233-45, 1943*).

Rule out <u>cadmium</u> toxicity.

Observational Study: 32 black female hypertensives aged 50-75 were compared with 30 normotensives. BP status, body mass and smoking status were the only variables significantly related ($p<0.05$) to blood cadmium level (*Fontana SA, Boulos BM. Blood cadmium level as affected by hypertension, smoking, occupation, and body mass. Am J Hypertens 1(3 Pt 3):158S-160S, 1988*).

Review Article: Occupational exposure to cadmium causes tubular and interstitial nephropathy, chemical pneumonitis and eventually pulmonary emphysema, and bone metabolism disturbances leading to osteomalacia. The effects on the kidneys may cause renal hypertension. In kidney specimens obtained from autopsies of pts. suffering from hypertension, cadmium and lead have been found in higher concentrations, but the role of cadmium in the pathogenesis of hypertension is still not well proven (*Petronio L. Chemical and physical agents of work-related cardiovascular diseases. Eur Heart J (Suppl 1):26-34, 1988*).

Observational Study: A statistically significant relationship between the height of diastolic BP and serum cadmium levels was observed in 100 pts. with essential hypertension (*Arora RB et al. Role of elements in pathophysiology of hypertension and antihypertensive drug development. Acta Pharmacol Toxicol (Copenh) 59 Suppl 7:344-47, 1986*).

Observational Study: Untreated hypertensives showed blood cadmium levels 3-4 times those of matched normotensives (*Glauser SC et al. Blood cadmium levels in normotensive and untreated hypertensive humans. Lancet 1:717-18, 1976*).

In hypertensives, elevated cadmium levels may be associated with reduced plasma zinc levels (*Arora RB et al. Role of elements in pathophysiology of hypertension and antihypertensive drug development. Acta Pharmacol Toxicol (Copenh) 59 Suppl 7:344-47, 1986; Bartolin R et al. [Blood cadmium and plasma zinc in hypertensive patients. Apropos of 76 cases.] Rev Med Interne 6(3):280-84, 1985*).

Cadmium-induced hypertension may be associated with increased renal copper and zinc excretion, possibly due to the cadmium-induced synthesis of metallothionein, a protein able to bind different metals (*Carmignani M, Boscolo P. Cardiovascular responsiveness to physiological agonists of male rats made hypertensive by long-term exposure to cadmium. Sci Total Environ 34(1-2):19-33, 1984*).

Zinc supplementation may counteract the adverse effect of cadmium on blood pressure.

Animal Experimental Study: Supplementation with a zinc chelate was able to reverse cadmium-induced experimental hypertension in rats (*Schroeder HA, Buckman J. Cadmium hypertension: Its reversal in rats by a zinc chelate. Arch Environ Health 14:693, 1967*).

Rule out <u>lead</u> toxicity.

Review Article: "Acute lead poisoning is characterized by saturnine colic and blood hypertension, secondary to diffuse arteriolar vasoconstriction . . . . Chronic lead poisoning causes nephroangiosclerosis complicated by hypertension." It is unknown whether low-dose chronic exposure causes vascular damage. Undecided is whether soft water may transport more suspended lead than hard water which may be responsible for hypertension (*Petronio L. Chemical and physical agents of work-related cardiovascular diseases. Eur Heart J (Suppl 1):26-34, 1988*).

Observational Study: Lead levels previously considered safe were found to be associated with increased BP (*Harlan WR et al. Blood lead and blood pressure. Relationship in the adolescent and adult US population. JAMA 253(4):530-34, 1985*).

Observational Study: The Second National Health and Nutrition Survey (NHANES II, 1976-1980) substantially supports the growing evidence from both animal and epidemiologic studies that a causal association exists between serum lead and hypertension (*Peirkle JL et al. The relationship between blood lead levels and blood pressure and its cardiovascular risk implications. Am J Epidemiol 121:246-58, 1985*).

Rule out <u>mercury</u> toxicity:

Review Article: "Occupational exposure to mercury (Hg) is involved in causing hypertension with a prevalence rate which is double that of the general population" (*Petronio L. Chemical and physical agents of work-related cardiovascular diseases. Eur Heart J (Suppl 1):26-34, 1988*).

"HYPOGLYCEMIA" (FUNCTIONAL)

See Also: ALCOHOLISM
HEADACHE
INNER EAR DYSFUNCTION
MUSCLE CRAMPS
RESTLESS LEGS SYNDROME

DIETARY FACTORS

High carbohydrate, high fiber diet.

Experimental Study: 8 pts. with postprandial hypoglycemia and previous gastric surgery received glucomannan, a potent gel-forming dietary fiber, in addition to a carbohydrate-rich breakfast. Addition of glucomannan improved reactive hypoglycemia from 2.3 mmol/L to 3.3 mmol/L after 2.6 gm and to 4.2 mmol/L after 5.2 gm, and decreased the postprandial rise in plasma insulin. Expiratory breath hydrogen excretion tended to decrease, reflecting improvement of carbohydrate metabolism. Also, addition of glucomannan to an intraduodenal sucrose solution significantly raised plasma glucose nadirs, indicating that it was effective during the intestinal phase (*Hopman WPM et al. Glucomannan prevents postprandial hypoglycemia in patients with previous gastric surgery. Gut 29(7):930-34, 1988*).

Clinical Observation: In our extensive experience, almost all individuals with reactive hypoglycemia respond favorably to high-carbohydrate, high-fiber diets restricted in simple sugars and providing 50-55% of energy as carbohydrate, 15-20% protein, 30-35% fat, 50 g plant fiber and <50 g simple carbohydrate daily. To accomplish this, individuals must usually limit milk and fruit intake, and severely limit or avoid fruit juices. This diet increases insulin sensitivity and facilitates glucose uptake. In addition, soluble fiber delays gastric emptying, slows glucose absorption, and minimizes blood glucose swings (*Anderson JW, Gustafson NJ. Dietary fiber in disease prevention and treatment. Compr Ther 13(1):43-53, 1987*).

Experimental Study: Of the different fibers, apple pectin and oat bran have the most pronounced effects on the hypoglycemic index (the fall in blood glucose in the 90 min. before reaching the nadir divided by the value of the nadir) (*Langseth L et al. Fd Cosmet Toxicol 16:129-38, 1978*).

High protein, low carbohydrate diet.

Said to be beneficial as the blood sugar response to protein ingestion in both normals and functional hypoglycemics is flatter than for glucose, suggesting that there may be a smaller subsequent hypoglycemic swing (*Conn JW. The glycemic response to isoglucogenic quantitites of protein and carbohydrate. J Clin Invest 15:665-71, 1936; Conn JW, Newburgh LH. The advantage of a high protein diet in the treatment of spontaneous hypoglycemia. J Clin Invest 15:673-78, 1936*).

Negative Clinical Observation: "In our experience, high protein diets are rarely effective in treating reactive hypoglycemia" (*Anderson JW, Gustafson NJ. Dietary fiber in disease prevention and treatment. Compr Ther 13(1):43-53, 1987*).

Experimental Study: Flat GTT curve pts. with hypoglycemic symptoms responded well to a high protein, low carbohydrate diet (*Shah S et al. Flat G.T.T.: The significance of the flat glucose tolerance test. J Kansas Med Soc November, 1975, pp. 263-67*).

Negative Experimental Study: 7 pts. with impaired glucose tolerance (3 with diabetes mellitus and 4 with post-prandial hypoglycemia) had a significant deterioration in glucose tolerance when they changed from a low protein, high carbohydrate diet to a high protein, low carbohydrate diet (*Anderson JW, Herman RH. Effects of* *carbohydrate restriction on glucose tolerance of normal men and reactive hypoglycemic patients. Am J Clin Nutr 28:748, 1975).*

Clinical Observations: In a gp. of over 350 pts. who presented with either spontaneous leg cramps (SLC) or restless legs (RL), approx. 2/3 pts. had SLC alone, while 1/3 experienced both SLC and RL. Although the calf and foot musculature usually was involved, occasionally pts. suffered cyclic cramps primarily in the upper thighs, low back or hands. There were also several cases of severe nocturnal carpal spasm and the "stiff man syndrome." With few exceptions, these pts. also experienced typical features of recurrent hypoglycemia which was confirmed by afternoon glucose tolerance testing and an attack of muscle cramps occasionally was precipitated concomitantly with a hypoglycemic episode during testing. Institution of a sugar-free, high protein diet with frequent nibbling and at least one night feeding was followed by prompt and persistent remission or striking alleviation of longstanding symptoms in the vast majority of pts., while symptom recurrence could usually be attributed to some dietary indiscretion within the preceeding 12 hours (*Roberts HJ. Spontaneous leg cramps and "restless legs" due to diabetogenic (functional) hyperinsulinism: A basis for rational therapy. J Fla Med Assoc 60(5):29-31, 1973*).

Experimental Study: 11/92 pts. seen in more than a 17-month period had migraines that seemed to be associated with spontaneous hyperinsulinism. All improved or had complete symptom relief when placed on a low carbohydrate, high fat diet (150 gm protein, 190 gm fat, 75 gm carbohydrate) [sucrose content was unspecified] (*Wilkinson CF. Return of migrinoid headaches associated with spontaneous hypoglycemia. Am J Med Sci 218:209-12, 1949*).

Experimental Study: As compared to high carbohydrate meals, high protein meals resulted in greater blood sugar stability with avoidance of hypoglycemic symptoms and higher metabolic rates (*Thorn GW et al. A comparison of the metabolic effects of isocaloric meals of varying compositions with special reference to the prevention of post-prandial hypoglycemic symptoms. Ann Intern Med 18(6):913-19, 1943*).

Avoid <u>refined carbohydrates</u>.

Case Report: A 56-year-old woman had attacks of faintness after meals containing sugar. Postprandial hypoglycemia was found and she was diagnosed as idiopathic reactive hypoglycemia. After sugar was eliminated from her diet, she had no further attacks (*Weiss M, Pilpel N, Dossoretz C. [Metabolic studies in reactive hypoglycemia.] Harefuah 118(12):691-2, 1990*) (*in Hebrew*).

Review Article: "Patients with bona fide meal-related reactive hypoglycemia should be treated primarily with dietary restriction of refined carbohydrates" (*Hofeldt FD. Reactive hypoglycemia. Endocrinol Metab Clin North Am 18(1):185-201, 1989*).

Experimental Study: "10 healthy subjects consumed 4 different snack meals, similar in fat and total energy content. Two snacks were based on sugary, manufactured products (chocolate-coated candy bar; cola drink with crisps) and two on whole foods (raisins and peanuts; bananas and peanuts). After the processed food snacks, plasma-glucose levels tended to rise higher and to fall lower than after the whole-food snacks. The area under the plasma insulin curve was 70% greater after the manufactured snacks than after the raisin-peanut snack. The banana-peanut snack evoked an intermediate insulin response. One subject had pathological insulinemia after both manufactured snacks but normal responses after both whole-food snacks. These findings suggest that foods and drinks containing added fiber-depleted sugars stress and sometimes overwhelm homeostatic mechanisms, but also suggest that the insulin response is influenced by the physical state of the food" (*Oettle GJ et al. Glucose and insulin responses to manufactured and whole-food snacks. Am J Clin Nutr 45:86-91, 1987*).

Experimental Study: 8 pts. (ages 19-52) with glucose nadirs <55 mg/dL accompanied by symptoms of reactive hypoglycemia, peak plasma cortisol of more than 18 μg/ml, and at least a 5 μg/ml rise in plasma cortisol from its value at the glucose nadir were placed on a low refined carbohydrate diet. Mean daily consumption of refined carbohydrates decreased from 147 gm to 20 gm, mean total carbohydrate consumption decreased from 307 to 221 gm, mean daily protein consumption increased from 89 to 99 gm, and mean fat consumption decreased from 107 to 95 grams. 7/8 became asymptomatic and the other was substantially improved. When total grams of refined carbohydrate increased, symptoms returned (*Sanders LR et al. Refined carbohydrate as a contributing factor in reactive hypoglycemia. South Med J 75:1072, 1982*).

Substitute fructose for glucose or sucrose as a sugar source.

Review Article: The ingestion of fructose, as compared to glucose, causes substantially less stimulation of plasma glucose and insulin responses. The disadvantage of large excursions of plasma glucose and insulin after high glucose and sucrose meals is well known in glucose intolerant and normotolerant individuals in whom subsequent reactive hypoglycemia may be observed (*Schwarz J-M et al. Thermogenesis in men and women induced by fructose vs glucose added to a meal. Am J Clin Nutr 49:667-74, 1989*).

Note: Unlike glucose, fructose is metabolized quickly to lactate under anerobic conditions so that tissue anoxia will enhance lactate formation from fructose and inhibit lactate clearance (Cook GC, Jacobson J. Individual variation in fructose metabolism in man. Br J Nutr 26(2):187-95, 1971). Since patients with panic attacks are prone to suffer an attack following a lactate infusion, fructose should probably be avoided as should sorbitol and xylitol which are converted into fructose.

Avoid alcohol.

Inhibits gluconeogenesis and promotes a fall in plasma glucose (*Rabin D. Hypoglycemia: Physiologic and diagnostic considerations, in GE Abraham, Ed. Radioassay Systems in Clinical Endocrinology. New York, Marcel Dekker, 1981:609-24*).

The increase in gastric acidity that follows alcohol ingestion might cause excessive release of gut secretagogues which augment beta-cell responsiveness to glucose fluctuations, leading to excessive insulin release (*Freinkel N, Getzger BE. Oral glucose tolerance curve and hypoglycemias in the fed state. N Engl J Med 280:820-8, 1969*).

- and Sucrose:

The combination of alcohol and a sucrose mixer (ex. gin and tonic) is more likely to provoke reactive hypoglycemia than alcohol alone.

Experimental Study: 14 men (9 normal wt. and 5 obese) aged 20-50 consumed a 50 g glucose load together with 50 g ethanol over an hr., their early plasma insulin response was significantly higher and their later fall in plasma glucose significantly lower than after drinking the same amt. of a starch solution (maize meal) and alcohol. In 4 subjects (3 of them normal wt.) plasma glucose concentrations dropped below 2.8 mmol/L after drinking the glucose-alcohol solution (*Baker SG et al. Alcohol-potentiated reactive hypoglycaemia depends on the nature of the carbohydrate ingested at the same time. Alcohol Alcohol 19(1):45-9, 1984*).

VITAMINS

Niacin:

Supplementation may be beneficial.

Theoretical Discussion: As both schizophrenia and alcoholism have the symptomatological state of hypoglycemia as a normal accompaniment to the disease, and niacin has been of value in both of these conditions, it appears that niacin may work by alleviating hypoglycemia (*Shansky A. Vitamin B3 in the alleviation of hypoglycemia. Drug Cosmetic Industry 129(4):68, 1981*

MINERALS

Chromium:

Supplementation may be beneficial.

Experimental Double-blind Crossover Study: 8 female pts. were supplemented with 200 μg chromium (as chromic chloride) daily. By 3 mo., hypoglycemic symptoms were alleviated and the glucose nadir following a glucose load was raised at 2-4 hours. In addition, insulin binding to red blood cells and insulin receptor number improved significantly. Results suggest that impaired chromium nutrition and/or metabolism may be a factor in the etiology of hypoglycemia (*Anderson RA et al. Effects of supplemental chromium on patients with symptoms of reactive hypoglycemia. Metabolism 36(4):351-55, 1987; Anderson RA et al. Chromium supplementation of humans with hypoglycemia. Fed Proc 43:471, 1984*).

<u>Magnesium</u>:   400 mg daily (6 week trial)

May reduce glucose-induced insulin secretion (*Curry DL et al. Magnesium modulation of glucose-induced insulin secretion by the perfused rat pancreas. Endocrinology 101:203, 1977*); thus deficiency may contribute to reactive hypoglycemia by enhancing glucose-induced insulin secretion.

May be reduced in women.

Observational Study: Compared to controls, 14 women with reactive hypoglycemia had low RBC, plasma and hair magnesium levels while, for 8 men with reactive hypoglycemia, these levels did not differ from those of controls (*Stebbing JB et al. Reactive hypoglycaemia and magnesium. Magnesium Bull 4(2):131-34, 1982*).

Supplementation may be beneficial.

Experimental Placebo-controlled Study: 14 women with reactive hypoglycemia and lower RBC, plasma and hair magnesium levels than normal controls were given magnesium 340 mg daily as magnesium sulfate. After 6 wks., blood glucose no longer dropped below fasting levels during glucose tolerance testing and in 3/14 pts., glucose tolerance was much improved. 7/14 (50%) supplemented women felt better vs. only 25% of the women on placebo. Non-responders tended to have either an elevated hair calcium to magnesium ratio or failure of urinary excretion of magnesium to increase with supplementation (*Stebbing JB et al. Reactive hypoglycaemia and magnesium. Magnesium Bull 4(2):131-34, 1982*).

— —

OTHER NUTRITIONAL FACTORS

<u>Omega-6 Fatty Acids</u>:

$$\text{linoleic acid} \rightarrow \text{GLA} \rightarrow \text{DGLA} \rightarrow \text{prostaglandin E}_1$$

Prostaglandin E_1 inhibits glucose-induced insulin secretion (*Gugliano D, Torella R. Prostaglandin E₁ inhibits glucose-induced insulin secretion in man. Prostaglandins Med 48:302, 1979*).

<u>L-Tryptophan</u>:

Dietary precursor to the neurotransmitter serotonin.

Serotonergic deficits may predispose individuals to hypoglycemia during a glucose tolerance test (*Roy A et al. Monamines, glucose metabolism, aggression towards self and others. Int J Neurosci 41(3-4):261-4, 1988*).

— —

OTHER FACTORS

Rule out <u>food sensitivities</u>.

Clinical Observation: Said to cause 75% of cases of functional hypoglycemia (*Breneman JC. Basics of Food Allergy. Springfield, Illinois, Charles C. Thomas, 1978*).

IMMUNODEPRESSION

See Also: AIDS
CANCER
CANDIDIASIS
INFECTION

GENERAL REVIEW ARTICLES

DIET

"The importance of diet in multiple aspects of the immune response is inescapable. Although only a few trials have attempted to apply knowledge derived from *in vitro* and animal data to humans, the ability to modulate or 'reset' the immune response by manipulating dietary intake will surely continue to be studied in the future" (*Corman LC. Effects of specific nutrients on the immune response. Selected clinical applications. Med Clin North Am 69(4):759-91, 1985*).

NUTRIENTS

Isolated deficiencies of micronutrients as a cause of immune dysfunction are rare with the exception of iron, vitamin A and zinc. However, micronutrient deficiencies frequently complicate protein-energy malnutrition and many systemic diseases. A slight excess intake of certain nutrients may be associated with enhanced immune responses, but all nutrients given in quantities beyond a certain threshold will reduce immune responses (*Chandra RK. 1990 McCollum Award Lecture. Nutrition and immunity: lessons from the past and new insights into the future. Am J Clin Nutr 53:1087-1101, 1991*).

- -

DIETARY FACTORS

Adequate dietary protein.

Deficiency is immunosuppressive (*Levy JA. Nutrition and the immune system, in DP Stites et al. Basic and Clinical Immunology. 4th Edition. Los Altos, Ca., Lange Medical Publications, 1982:297-305*).

Low fat diet.

Excessive lipid intake (particularly of cholesterol and of polyunsaturated fatty acids) is associated with immunodepression (*Chandra RK. Nutrition and immunity - Basic considerations. Part 1. Contemp Nutr 11(11), 1986; Levy JA. Nutrition and the immune system, in DP Stites et al, Eds. Basic and Clinical Immunology. 4th Edition. Los Altos, Ca., Lange Medical Publications, 1982:297-305*).

Low fat intake may enhance natural killer-cell activity (*Barone J et al. Dietary fat and natural-killer-cell activity. Am J Clin Nutr 50:861-67, 1989*).

Avoid sugar.

May impair cell-mediated immunity.

Experimental Study: 7 healthy adults ingested 75 gm glucose. *In vitro* lymphocyte transformation in response to PHA at 30 and 60 min. was significantly depressed to 79.4% and 83.3% of fasting levels, respectively. At 2 hrs., lymphocyte transformation had returned to fasting levels. Addition of physiologic doses of insulin decreased *in vitro* lymphocyte transformation by 40%. Results suggest that glucose ingestion may affect *in vitro* measures of cellular immunity by increasing serum insulin, which competes with mitogens for binding sites on lymphocytes. In addition, glucose may impair cell-mediated immunity *in vivo* (*Bernstein J et al. Depression of lymphocyte transformation following oral glucose ingestion. Am J Clin Nutr 30:613, 1977*).

May impair antibody production.

Experimental Animal Study: "As the nutritional quality of the diet was reduced by progressively diluting the diet with sucrose in 10 percent increments, the production of antibodies was decreased proportionately" (*Nalder BN et al. Sensitivity of the immunological response to the nutritional status of rats. J Nutr 102(4):535-41, 1972*).

May impair phagocytosis.

Experimental Study: Healthy volunteers ingested 100 gm portions of carbohydrate from glucose, fructose, sucrose, honey or orange juice. Each significantly decreased the phagocytic index (the capacity of neutrophils to engulf bacteria). Starch ingestion did not have this effect. The maximal decrease in phagocytic activity occurred between 1-2 hrs. after ingestion, but the values remained below control levels 5 hrs. after feeding (*Sanchez A et al. Role of sugars in human neutrophilic phagocytosis. Am J Clin Nutr 26:180, 1973*).

Avoid coffee.

May suppress lymphocyte response to mitogens (while increasing both suppressor T-cells and natural killer cells and the chemotactic activity of mononuclear cells).

Experimental Crossover Study: 15 men and women aged 19-49 who were regular coffee drinkers drank 5 cups of coffee daily (225 mg caffeine) for 5 wks. followed by 5 wks. of abstinence. At the end of the coffee period, lympohcyte responses to PHA and Con A mitogens were about one-third lower than during abstinence. While total T-lymphocytes, B-cells and helper T-cells were unaffected, the proportion of suppressor T-cells increased by >30% during coffee consumption and the proportion of natural killer cells increased by 50%, and chemotaxis activity of mononuclear cells was significantly higher (*Melamed I et al. Coffee and the immune system. Int J Immunol 12:129-34, 1990*).

Consumption may be associated with lower immunoglobulin levels.

Observational Study: In a study comparing 10 smokers to 10 non-smokers, it was found that the 5 high coffee consumers (4 or more cups daily) among the smokers had lower immunoglobulin levels than the 5 low or modest coffee consumers (<4 cups daily). This difference was significant for IgM ($p < 0.05$) (*Kraal JH. Immunoglobulin levels in relation to smoking and coffee consumption. Am J Clin Nutr 31(2):198-200, 1972*).

- -

VITAMINS

Vitamin A:

Deficiency reduces the response of both T and B lymphocytes to mitogens and antigens, while modest doses stimulate immune responses (*Chandra RK. Nutrition and immunity - Basic considerations. Part 1. Contemp Nutr 11(11), 1986*).

Deficiency may impair phagocytosis (*Ongsakul M et al. Impaired blood clearance of bacteria and phagocytic activity in vitamin A deficient rats. Proc Soc Exp Biol Med 178(2):204-8, 1985*).

Deficiency may be associated with decreased antibody responses to antigens (*Pasatiempo AMG et al. Vitamin A depletion and repletion: effects on antibody response to the capsular polysaccharide of Streptococcus pneumoniae, type III (SSS-III). Am J Clin Nutr 49:501-10, 1989; Smith SM et al. Impaired immunity in vitamin A deficient mice. J Nutr 117:857-65, 1987; Smith SM et al. Contrasting impairment in IgM and IgG responses of vitamin A deficient mice. Proc Natl Acad Sci U S A 84:5878-82, 1987*).

Plasma levels may be directly correlated with the frequency of antibody responses to antigens.

Observational Study: In 100 healthy people over age 60, those with higher plasma concentrations of vitamin A exhibited delayed hypersensitivity reactions to significantly more antigens than people with lower concentrations (p<0.01) (*Chavance M et al. Nutritional support improves antibody response to influenza virus in the elderly. Letter. Br Med J November 9, 1985, pp. 1348-49*).

Deficiency may impair secretory IgA production (*Dreizen S. Nutrition and the immune response - A review. Int J Vitam Nutr Res 49:220-28, 1978*).

Severe deficiency leads to atrophy of the thymus and spleen and a marked decrease in circulating leukocytes and lymphocytes (*Levy JA. Nutrition and the immune system, in DP Stites et al, Eds. Basic and Clinical Immunology. 4th Edition. Los Altos, Ca., Lange Medical Publications, 1982:297-305*).

Supplementation may reverse post-operative immunosuppression.

Experimental Controlled Study: Lymphocytes were counted on the first and seventh days post-surgery. The experimental gp., which received 300,000-450,000 units of vitamin A acetate for 7 days, showed no change, while the lymphocyte counts fell in the control gp. (*Cohen B et al. Reversal of postoperative immunosuppresion in man by vitamin A. Surg Gynecol Obstet 149:658-62, 1979*).

Supplementation may enhance responses to weak immunogens and reverse immunosuppression (*Nuwayri-Salti N, Murad T. Immunologic and anti-immunosuppressive effects of vitamin A. Pharmacology 30(4):181-87, 1985*).

While essentially nothing is known about the effects of high intakes of vitamin A on IgE production or immediate hypersensitivity, it can both increase and suppress cellular immune function depending upon the system tested and the concentration used (*Watson RR. Regulation of immunological resistance to cancer by beta carotene and retinoids, in Nutrition, Disease Resistance, and Immune Function. New York, Marcel Dekker, Inc., 1984:345-55*).

Vitamin B Complex:

Deficiencies are associated with decreased antibody responses and impaired cellular immunity (*Anderson R, Theron A. Effects of B-complex vitamins on cellular and humoral immune functions in vitro and in vivo. Int J Vitam Nutr Res 24:77-84, 1983; Chandra RK. Nutrition and immunity - Basic considerations. Part 1. Contemp Nutr 11(11), 1986*).

Supplementation may reduce postoperative immunosuppression.

Experimental Controlled Study: 31 pts. with gastric cancer received IV thiamine 107 mg, vitamin B_6 100 mg and vitamin B_{12} 1,000 µg daily for 14 days starting on the day of surgery. Compared to untreated pts., vitamin treatment reduced the postoperative suppression of blastogenic responses to PHA and PWM and enhanced the recovery of lymphocyte responsiveness at 4 wks. postoperatively (*Kurashige S et al. Effect of vitamin B complex on the immunodeficiency produced by surgery of gastric cancer patients. Jpn J Exp Med 58(4):197-202, 1988*).

- Folic Acid:

Deficiency is associated with impaired responses to mitogens *in vitro* and delayed hypersensitivity responses in both animals and man (*Levy JA. Nutrition and the immune system, in DP Stites et al, Eds. Basic and Clinical Immunology, 4th Edition. Los Altos, Ca., Lange Medical Publications, 1982:297-305; Beisel WR. Single nutrients and immunity. Am J Clin Nutr 35:417-68 [Suppl], 1982*).

- Pantothenic Acid:

Deficiency depresses humoral antibody responses to various antigens in experimental animals and man (*Beisel WR. Single nutrients and immunity. Am J Clin Nutr 35:417-68 [Suppl.], 1982*).

- Riboflavin:

Deficiency in animals is associated with a diminished ability to generate humoral antibodies in response to test antigens (*Beisel WR. Single nutrients and immunity. Am J Clin Nutr 35:417-68 [Suppl], 1982*).

- Vitamin B$_6$:

Since pyridoxine is required for normal nucleic acid and protein synthesis and for cellular multiplication, isolated pyridoxine deficiencies cause more profound effects on immune system functions than deficiencies of any other B gp. vitamin. Also, unlike any other B vitamin, deficiencies appear to inhibit cell-mediated immune functions as well as humoral responsiveness to a variety of test antigens (*Axelrod AE, Traketellis AC. Relationship of pyridoxine to immunological phenomena. Vitam Horm 22:591-607, 1964*).

Deficiency is associated with a reduction in number and function of both T and B lymphocytes, reduced delayed hypersensitivity responses, greatly diminished response to antigenic challenge, decreased secretion of immunoglobulins, reduced thymic epithelial cell function and reduced phagocytic activity of neutrophils (*Levy JA. Nutrition and the immune system, in DP Stites et al, Eds. Basic and Clinical Immunology. 4th Edition. Los Altos, Ca., Lange Medical Publications, 1982, pp. 297-305*).

Deficiency impairs interleukin 2 production and lymphocyte proliferation in the elderly which is reversible with repletion (*Meydani SN et al. Vitamin B-6 deficiency impairs interleukin 2 production and lympocyte proliferation in elderly adults. Am J Clin Nutr 53:1275-80, 1991*).

If deficient, supplementation may improve lymphocyte responses.

> **Experimental Single-blind Study:** 15 elderly persons aged 65-81. some of whom had low pre-supplement levels of pyridoxal-5-phosphate, received pyridoxine HCl 50 mg daily or placebo. After 1-2 mo., treated subjects showed significant increases in lymphocyte responses to mitogens and antigens, and percentages of T3$^+$ and T4$^+$ but not T8$^+$ cells increased significantly (*Talbott MC et al. Pyridoxine supplementation: Effect on lymphocyte responses in elderly persons. Am J Clin Nutr 46(4):659-64, 1987*).

> **Experimental Study:** 5/8 male hemodialysis pts. had B$_6$ deficiency (abnormal *in vitro* RBC glutamic-pyruvic transaminase activity), 3/8 had abnormal nitroblue tetrazolium tests (a measure of oxygen-dependent bactericidal neutrophil activity) and, in 5/8, the generation of chemotactic factors was abnormal. Following supplementation with pyridoxine 50 mg/day, the first two tests normalized and the third was significantly improved. In addition, while the absolute number of lymphocytes did not change, certain pts. showed functional enhancements of lymphocyte function, including a marked increase in lymphocyte transformation in response to mitogens (*Casciato DA et al. Nephron 38:9-16, 1984*).

- Vitamin B$_{12}$:

Deficiency is associated with impaired lymphocyte response to mitogens and a modest reduction in the phagocytic and bacteriocidal capacity of polymorphonuclear leukocytes (*Levy JA. Nutrition and the immune system, in DP Stites et al, Eds. Basic and Clinical Immunology. 4th Edition. Los Altos, Ca., Lange Medical Publications, 1982:297-305*).

In untreated primary pernicious anemia:

> 1. neutrophil phagocytosis is impaired (*Kaplan SS, Basford RE. Effect of vitamin B$_{12}$ and folic acid deficiencies on neutrophil function. Blood 47:801-5, 1976*).

> 2. lymphocyte function is impaired (*Das KC, Herbert V. The lymphocyte as a marker of past nutritional status: Persistence of abnormal lymphocyte deoxyuridine (uD) suppression test and chromosomes in patients with past deficiency of folate and vitamin B$_{12}$. Br J Haematol 38:219-33, 1978*).

Vitamin C: 1-3 gm daily to achieve immune enhancement (*Anderson R. The immunostimulatory, anti-inflammatory and anti-allergic properties of ascorbate. Adv Nutr Res 6:19-45, 1984*).

WARNING: In the presence of high levels of stress, large supplementary doses may impair the immune response.

> **Animal Study:** Large daily doses of vitamin C resulted in severe lymphopenia in stressed mice. Since stress abruptly increases adrenal corticosteroids in plasma following the release of vitamin C by the adrenals, it is hypothesized that large doses of vitamin C may maintain high levels of plasma corticosteroids which, in turn, may

reduce the organism's immune response when stress is present (*Richardson J. Vitamin C and immunosuppression. Med Hypotheses 21(4):383-85, 1986*).

Extreme deficiency impairs phagocyte function and cellular immunity (*Chandra RK. Nutrition and immunity - Basic considerations. Part 1. Contemp Nutr 11(11), 1986*).

Deficiency is associated with a reduced delayed hypersensitivity response that appears to be due to an inability to develop a local inflammatory response rather than to an immunologic defect in lymphocytes (*Levy JA. Nutrition and the immune system, in DP Stites et al, Eds. Basic and Clinical Immunology. 4th Edition. Los Altos, Ca., Lange Medical Publications, 1982:297-305*). This is true for a moderate deficiency (5-20 mg/d) despite the lack of scorbutic symptoms (*Jacob RA et al. Immunocompetence and oxidant defense during ascorbate depletion of healthy men. Am J Clin Nutr 54:1302S-9S, 1991*).

Deficiency is associated with inhibition of neutrophil mobility which, in turn, inhibits the formation of inflammatory reactions (*Beisel WR. Role of nutrition in immune system diseases. Compr Ther 13(1):13-19, 1987*).

Supplementation may enhance neutrophil motility and chemotaxis.

Experimental Study: 6 normal volunteers showed increased neutrophil motility 1 h after a single IV dose of 1 g ascorbate (*Anderson R. Ascorbate-mediated stimulation of neutrophil motility and lymphocyte transformation by inhibition of the peroxidase/H₂O₂/halide system in vitro and in vivo. Am J Clin Nutr 34(9):1906-11, 1981*).

Experimental Study: Healthy adults supplemented with a minimum of 2-3 gm ascorbate daily showed enhanced neutrophil chemotaxis (*Anderson R et al. The effects of increasing weekly doses of ascorbate on certain cellular and humoral immune functions in normal volunteers. Am J Clin Nutr 33(1):71-76, 1980*).

Supplementation may increase neutrophil phagocytosis.

Review Article: "Vitamin C represents the specific therapy for primary defects of phagocytic function in persons with recurrent infections" (*Patrone F, Dallegri F. Vitamin C and the phagocytic system. Acta Vitaminol Enzymol 1:5-10, 1979*).

Supplementation may increase immunoglobulin levels.

Negative Experimental Controlled Study: Elderly volunteers received either vitamin C 500 mg IM daily or placebo. After 1 mo., there was no change in serum concentrations of IgA, IgG or IgM (*Kennes B et al. Effect of vitamin C supplements on cell-mediated immunity in old people. Gerontology 29:305-10, 1983*).

Experimental Controlled Study: Healthy students received vitamin C 1 gm daily. After 77 days, their serum IgA and IgM levels showed a statistically significant increase compared to controls (*Prinz W et al. The effect of ascorbic acid supplementation on some parameters of the human immunological defense system. Int J Vitam Nutr Res 47(3):248-57, 1977*).

Experimental Study: Supplementation of normal subjects with 1 gm/d of vitamin C was associated with increases in serum levels of non-specific IgG and IgM. There were significant positive correlations between leukocyte ascorbic acid levels and both IgG and IgM levels (*Vallance S. Relationships between ascorbic acid and serum proteins of the immune system. Br Med J 2:437-38, 1977*).

Supplementation may increase complement concentrations (*Johnston CS et al. The effect of vitamin nutriture on complement component C1q concentrations in guinea pig plasma. J Nutr 117:764-68, 1987; Prinz W et al. The effect of ascorbic acid supplementation on some parameters of the human immunological defense system. Int J Vitam Nutr Res 47(3):248-57, 1977*).

Supplementation may increase lymphocyte blastogenesis in response to mitogens (*Anderson R et al. The effects of increasing weekly doses of ascorbate on certain cellular and humoral immune functions in normal volunteers. Am J Clin Nutr 33(1):71-76, 1980; Kennes B et al. Effect of vitamin C supplements on cell-mediated immunity in old people. Gerontology 29:305-10, 1983*).

Supplementation may improve delayed hypersensitivity skin reactions (*Kennes B et al. Effect of vitamin C supplements on cell-mediated immunity in old people. Gerontology 29(5):305-10, 1983*).

Vitamin D:

In its active form (1,25-dihydroxyvitamin D₃), it is an autoregulatory hormone which maintains a constant T-cell population after the T-cells are activated (*Nunn JD et al. Regulation of human tonsillar T-cell proliferation by the active metabolite of vitamin D₃. Immunology 59:479-84, 1986*).

Deficiency may depress cellular immune responses (*Toss G, Symreng T. Delayed hypersensitivity response and vitamin D deficiency. Int J Vitam Nutr Res 53(1):27-31, 1983*).

Vitamin E:

WARNING: Megadoses may impair cellular immunity and the bactericidal function of polymorphonuclear leukocytes.

Experimental Study: 18 healthy male volunteers received d,l-alpha-tocopheryl acetate 300 mg daily. After 21 days, there was diminished *in vitro* bactericidal activity of neutrophils and responsiveness of lymphocytes to PHA; however, when PHA was used for skin testing, DDH reactions were unchanged (*Prasad JS. Effect of vitamin E supplementation on leukocyte function. Am J Clin Nutr 33:606-8, 1980*).

Deficiency depresses immunoglobulin response to antigens, lymphocytic proliferative responses to mitogens and antigens, delayed dermal hypersensitivity reactions, and general host resistance (*Beisel WR et al. Single-nutrient effects on immunologic functions. JAMA 245(1):53-58, 1981*).

Supplementation may enhance immune responses (*Chandra RK. Nutrition and immunity - Basic considerations. Part 1. Contemp. Nutr. 11(11), 1986*). In addition to probably increasing the number of antibody-forming cells, supplementation enhances cell-mediated responses, including the delayed hypersensitivity reaction, and the clearance function of reticuloendothelial cells (*Levy JA. Nutrition and the immune system, in DP Stites et al, Eds. Basic and Clinical Immunology. 4th Edition. Los Altos, Ca., Lange Medical Publications, 1982:297-305*).

Experimental Double-blind Study: 32 healthy men and women ≥age 60 received dl-alpha-tocopheryl acetate 800 mg or placebo. After 30 days, in the supplemented gp., cumulative diameter and number of positive antigen responses in delayed-type hypersensitivity skin test response were elevated (p<0.05), IL-2 production and mitogenic response to optimal doses of concanavalin A were increased (p<0.05), and PGE₂ synthesis by peripheral blood mononuclear cells (p<0.005) and plasma lipid peroxides (p<0.001) were reduced. Results suggest that enhanced cell-mediated immunity may be mediated by a decrease in PGE₂ and/or other lipid-peroxidation products (*Meydani SN et al. Vitamin supplementation enhances cell-mediated immunity in healthy elderly subjects. Am J Clin Nutr 52:557-63, 1990*).

The elderly may require a higher intake to maintain immune function.

Animal Experimental Study: Vitamin E administered in high doses to aging animals caused several indices of immune function to be equal to those of younger animals, suggesting that they have higher vitamin E requirements than young animals in terms of immune system responsiveness (*Blumberg J. - reported in Med Tribune January 8, 1986*).

Observational Study: In a retrospective study of 100 healthy persons over age 60, there was a statistically significant correlation between serum vitamin E levels and the number of infections during the previous 3 years (*Chavance M et al. Immunologic and nutritional status among the elderly, in AL deWeck, Ed. Lymphoid Cell Function in Aging. Evrage, Rijswijk, 1984*).

- -

MINERALS

<u>Copper:</u>

Deficiency is associated with an increased incidence of infection and impairment of cell-mediated immunity. The function of the reticuloendothelial system is depressed and the microbicidal activity of granulocytes is reduced. Impaired antibody response to heterologous red blood cells and low levels of thymic hormone activity have been reported (*Chandra RK. Nutrition and immunity - Basic considerations. Part 1. <u>Contemp Nutr</u> 11(11), 1986; Chandra RK. Trace element regulation of immunity and infection. <u>J Am Coll Nutr</u> 4(1):5-16, 1985*).

Excess copper may suppress immune responses (*Pocino M et al. Influence of the oral administration of excess copper on the immune response. <u>Fund Appl Toxicol</u> 16:249-56, 1991*).

<u>Germanium Sesquioxide:</u>

Supplementation may induce gamma-interferon production leading to augmented natural killer cell activity and macrophage activation (*Aso H et al. Induction of interferon and activation of NK cells and macrophages in mice by oral administration of Ge-132, an organic germanium compound. <u>Microbiol Immunol</u> 29(1):65-74, 1985*).

Supplementation may improve impaired immune responses due to aging (*Mizushima Y et al. Restoration of impaired immunoresponse by germanium in mice. <u>Int Arch Allergy Appl Immunol</u> 63:338-39, 1980*).

<u>Iodine:</u>

Deficiency is associated with reduced microbicidal activity of polymorphonuclear leukocytes (*Chandra RK. Nutrition and immunity - Basic considerations. Part 1. <u>Contemp Nutr</u> 11(11), 1986*).

<u>Iron:</u>

Deficiency may result in impaired immunity due to impairment of bacteriocidal capacity of neutrophils and impairment of the lymphocyte proliferation response (*Chandra RK. Nutrition and immunity - Basic considerations. Part 1. <u>Contemp Nutr</u> 11(11), 1986; Chandra RK. Trace element regulation of immunity and infection. <u>J Am Coll Nutr</u> 4(1):5-16, 1985*).

> **Experimental and Observational Study:** In 21 pts. with iron deficiency anemia, the mean number of total lymphocytes, CD3 and CD4 subsets, and B lymphocytes were decreased, as was killer cell activity. After iron treatment, some of these parameters returned to normal (*Santos PC, Falcado RP. Decreased lymphocyte subsets and K-cell activity in iron-deficiency anemia. <u>Acta Haematol</u> 84:118-21, 1990*).

> **Review Article:** Data on the influence of iron deficiency on immune function are often confusing and contradictory. Abnormalities in cell-mediated immunity and ability of neutrophils to kill several types of bacteria are well established under experimental conditions in iron-deficient patients, although it remains uncertain whether these abnormalities result in an increased incidence and duration of infections (*Dallman P et al. Iron deficiency and the immune response. <u>Am J Clin Nutr</u> 46(2):329-34, 1987*).

Immunodepression can occur with as little as a 10% decrease in dietary iron (*Levy JA. Nutrition and the immune system, in DP Stites et al, Eds. <u>Basic and Clinical Immunology</u>. 4th Edition. Los Altos, Ca., Lange Medical Publications, 1982:297-305*).

<u>Magnesium:</u>

While magnesium deficiency has not been shown to cause deficient immune responses in humans, deficient immune responses have been found in mice and rats fed diets moderately deficient in magnesium for extended periods (*Beisel WR. Single nutrients and immunity. <u>Am J Clin Nutr</u> 35:417-68 (suppl), 1982*).

Magnesium-deficient animals have primarily a reduction in antibody-forming cells. Immunoglobulin levels are decreased, the humoral response to particular antigens is diminished, and thymic atrophy can take place (*Levy JA. Nutrition and the immune system, in DP Stites et al, Eds. Basic and Clinical Immunology. 4th Edition. Los Altos, Ca., Lange Medical Publications, 1982:297-305*).

Manganese:

Supplementation may enhance natural killer cell and macrophage activity (*Smialowicz RJ et al. Manganese chloride enhances natural cell-mediated immune effector cell function: Effects on macrophages. Immunopharmacol 9:1-11, 1985*).

Selenium: 50-200 µg total intake daily (70 kg adult)

> WARNING: Excessive intake may be immunosuppressive (*Diplock AT. Trace elements in human health with special reference to selenium. Am J Clin Nutr 45:1313-22, 1987*).

> **In vitro Experimental Study:** Neutrophil and natural killer cytotoxic function was affected by *in vitro* supplementation with sodium selenite of blood samples obtained from healthy volunteers. Effects included augmentation and suppression of neutrophil chemiluminescence and NK-mediated cytotoxicity, with augmentation at lower supplemental doses and suppression at higher doses. Results suggest that no benefit and potential harm may occur when supplementation is given to individuals whose selenium levels are already optimal; thus intracellular selenium assays should be performed or, better yet, functional assays for phagocytes and NK cells to determine if selenium supplementation is warranted (*LaBue M et al. Dosage window of selenium on phagocytic and natural killer cytotoxic responses. Int Clin Nutr Rev 8(4):198-203, 1988*).

When deficient:
1. cell-mediated immunity is impaired, especially when the deficiency is associated with a vitamin E deficiency (*Chandra RK. Trace element regulation of immunity and infection. J Am Coll Nutr 4(1):5-16, 1985*).
2. phagocytosis is decreased, and T cells appear to be coated by factors that suppress their response to mitogens and antigens (*Levy JA. Nutrition and the immune system, in DP Stites et al, Eds. Basic and Clinical Immunology. 4th Edition. Los Altos, Ca., Lange Medical Publications, 1982:297-305*).
3. Helper T cell numbers are diminished, and increase in response to supplementation (*Shils M et al. Selenium deficiency and immune functions in home TPN patients. Presentation at the American Society of Clinical Nutrition, 1983*).
4. humoral immunity may be impaired (*Mulhern SA et al. Deficient levels of dietary selenium suppress the antibody response to first and second generation mice. Nutr Res 5:201-10, 1985*).

Supplementation may enhance lymphocyte responses.

> **Experimental Double-blind Study:** 22 elderly institutionalized pts. received either selenium 100 µg/d as selenium-enriched yeast or placebo. At baseline, the mean response of lymphocytes to mitogens tended to be lower than responses in healthy adults, but remained within the 5-95% confidence interval limit for healthy adults. Baseline selenium concentrations were in the usual range for free-living adults aged >80 y from the same area. During supplementation the proliferative response to pokeweed mitogen significantly increased after 4 mo. (p<0.01) and reached the upper limit of the usual range for adults after 6 mo. (p<0.001) (*Peretz A et al. Lymphocyte response is enhanced by supplementation of elderly subjects with selenium-enriched yeast. Am J Clin Nutr 53:1323-8, 1991*).

Zinc:

> WARNING: Excessive intake (300 mg daily) may impair lymphocyte and neutrophil responses (*Bogden JD et al. Zinc and immunocompetence in the elderly: Baseline data on zinc nutriture and immunity in unsupplemented subjects. Am J Clin Nutr 46:101-09, 1987; Chandra RK. Excessive intake of zinc impairs immune responses. JAMA 252:1443-46, 1984*).

Deficiency may be associated with impaired humoral and cellular immune responses including T cell response and neutrophil chemotaxis. Thymic hormone activity is very low (*Chandra RK. Nutrition and immunity - Basic considerations. Part 1. Contemp Nutr 11(11), 1986; Chandra RK. Trace element regulation of immunity and infection. J Am Coll Nutr 4(1):5-16, 1985; Golden MHN et al. Effect of zinc on thymus of recently malnourished children. Lancet*

2:1057-9, 1977; Pekarek RS et al. Humoral and cellular immune responses in zinc deficient rats. Nutr Rep Int 16(3):267-76, 1977).

May regulate suppressor T-cell counts.

Experimental Study: 42 pts. with AIDS-related complex or cancer in remission and with severe, stable helper-T cell deficiency received 125 mg zinc gluconate twice daily. After 3 wks., while there was no significant change in helper-T cells, suppressor T-cells increased significantly in those with initially low suppppressor T-cell counts, and decreased significantly in those with initially normal or high suppressor T-cell counts (*Mathe G et al. A phase II trial of immunorestoration with zinc gluconate in immunodepressed cancer patients. Biomed Pharmacother 40(10):383-85, 1986*).

Supplementation may be beneficial.

Experimental Double-blind Partial Crossover Study: 63 elderly subjects aged 60-89 randomly received 15 mg zinc daily, 100 mg zinc daily or placebo in addition to a multivitamin/mineral supplement without zinc for 16 months. Natural killer cell activity was transiently enhanced by the 100 mg dose of zinc. However, there was a progressive improvement in delayed dermal hypersensitivity and in lymphocyte response to two mitogens which was significantly greater in the placebo gp., suggesting that it was due to components of the multivitamin/mineral supplement and was adversely affected by zinc supplementation (*Bogden JD et al. Effects of one year of supplementation with zinc and other micronutrients on cellular immunity in the elderly. J Am Coll Nutr 9(3):214-25, 1990*).

Experimental Study: Individuals over age 50 and most young Down's Syndrome children were found to have reduced concentrations of thymic hormone. This reduction could be completely prevented by the addition of zinc sulfate to plasma samples taken from these individuals and, in fact, induced concentrations of thymic hormone comparable to those of healthy young people (*Fabris N et al. Thymic hormone deficiency in normal ageing and Down's Syndrome. Is there a primary failure of the thymus? Lancet 1:983-86, 1984*).

Experimental and Observational Study: 22% of 203 elderly men and women (ages 60-97) were anergic; the same subjects were those with the lowest zinc intakes and serum zinc levels. 5 of these anergic subjects were supplemented with 55 mg zinc daily. After 4 wks., their immune responses had normalized (*Wagner PA et al. Zinc nutriture and cell-mediated immunity in the aged. Int J Vitam Nutr Res 53(1):94-101, 1983*).

Experimental Study: 83 normal volunteers received zinc sulfate 660 mg daily (150 mg elemental zinc). After 1 mo., the response of lymphocytes to mitogens *in vitro* was significantly improved. This effect was not correlated with initial serum zinc concentrations, suggesting that the effect of supplementation was not due to a pre-existing, latent zinc deficiency (*Duchateau J et al. Influence of oral zinc supplementation on the lymphocyte response to mitogens of normal subjects. Am J Clin Nutr 34:88-93, 1981*).

> *Note: The proposition that the immunoregulation of cell-mediated immunity is a pharmacological or medicinal effect of zinc is unsettled (Oral zinc and immunoregulation: A nutritional or pharmacological effect of zinc supplementation? Nutr Rev 40(3):72-4, 1982).*

- -

OTHER NUTRITIONAL FACTORS

Arginine:

May be deficient, especially during illness.

Review Article: Calculations based on creatinine excretion show that 0.8 gm of protein/kg body weight of the quality supplied by the usual American diet barely provides sufficient arginine for synthesizing the quantity of creatinine excreted daily in the urine of 70 kg adults. Human pts. who often consume less than this amt. of protein show a decline in creatinine excretion during illness, which suggests that their arginine intake is less than optimal (*Visek WJ. Arinine needs, physiological state and usual diets. A reevaluation. J Nutr 116(1):36-46, 1986*).

Augments T-lymphocyte activation in response to mitogens in clinical and experimental studies and enhances specific T cell antitumor immunity in experimental studies. It appears to mediate a direct effect on components of the immune system which results in enhanced production or use of lymphokines (*Reynolds JV et al. Immunomodulary mechanisms of arginine. Surgery 104(2):142-51, 1988*).

> **Experimental Study:** Arginine 30 g/d for 3 days increased the number of circulating CD56+ cells by a median of 32% (p<0.01) in 8 volunteers. This increase was associated with a mean rise of 91% in natural killer (NK) cell activity (p=0.003) and of 58% in the cell activity of their activated counterparts, lymphokine-activated-killer (LAK) cells, (p=0.001) in 13 volunteers. The substantial enhancement of human NK and LAK cell activity by arginine could be useful in many immunosuppressed states, including malignant disease, AIDS, and HIV infection, in which depressed NK cell activity is an important component of the disease process (*Park KGM et al. Stimulation of lymphocyte natural cytotoxicity by L-arginine. Lancet 337:645-6, 1991*).

> **Experimental Controlled Study:** In a randomized, prospective study, 30 cancer pts. undergoing major surgery received either L-arginine 25 g/d or isonitrogenous L-glycine 43 g/d for 7 days after surgery as a supplement to a graduated enteral diet. Supplemental arginine significantly enhanced the mean T-lymphocyte response (stimulation index) to a mitogen compared to glycine and increased mean CD4 phenotype (% T-cells) on post-op. days 1 and 7 (p<0.05) (*Daly JM et al. Immune and metabolic effects of arginine in the surgical patient. Ann Surg 208(4):512, 1988*).

Beta-carotene:

Modest doses stimulate immune responses (*Chandra RK. Nutrition and immunity - Basic considerations. Part 1. Contemp Nutr 11(11), 1986*).

> **Review Article:** "There is growing evidence from *in vitro* and *in vivo* laboratory animal studies that β-carotene can protect phagocytic cells from autooxidative damage, enhance T and B lymphocyte proliferative responses, stimulate effector T cell functions, and enhance macrophage, cytotoxic T cell and natural killer cell tumoricidal capacities, as well as increase the production of certain interleukins" (*Bendich A. Carotenoids and the immune response. J Nutr 119:112-115, 1989*).

Supplementation may enhance both T- and B-lymphocyte responses to mitogens (*Bendich A, Shapiro SS. Effect of β-carotene and canthaxanthin on the immune responses of the rat. J Nutr 2254-62, 1986*).

Supplementation may increase the precentage of lymphoid cells with surface markers for T-helper and natural killer cells.

> **Experimental Study:** 10 healthy men and 10 healthy women, mean age 56 yrs., randomly received various doses of supplementary beta-carotene. After 2 mo., the percentage of lymphoid cells with surface markers for T-helper and natural killer cells and cells with interleukin 2 and transferrrin receptors were significantly and substantially increased in peripheral blood mononuclear cells. While the plasma concentrations of beta-carotene were significantly elevated, there was no increase in the amt. of retinol, suggesting that the immunomodulation may be due to the carotenoid rather than to vitamin A (*Watson RR et al. Effect of β-carotene on lymphocyte subpopulations in elderly humans: evidence for a dose-response relationship. Am J Clin Nutr 53:90-4, 1991*).

> **Experimental Controlled Study:** After 1 wk., beta-carotene (Solatene[R] - Roche) 180 mg daily significantly increased the frequency of OKT4[+] cells (helper/inducer T cells) in normal volunteers; after 2 wks., it significantly increased the frequency of OKT3[+] cells (all T cells). The frequency of OKT8[+] cells (suppressor T cells) was unaffected compared to controls (*Alexander M et al. Oral beta-carotene can increase the number of OKT4[+] cells in human blood. Immunol Lett 9:221-24, 1985*).

L-Carnitine:

Supplementation may be beneficial.

> **In vitro Experimental Study:** L-carnitine increased the proliferative response of both murine and human lymphocytes following mitogenic stimulation, increased polymorphonuclear chemotaxis and, even at minimal concentrations, neutralized lipid-induced immunosuppression (*De Simone C et al. Vitamins and immunity: II. Influence of L-carnitine on the immune system. Acta Vitaminol Enzymol 4(1-2):135-40, 1982*).

Coenzyme Q10:

Supplementation may activate macrophages (*Saiki I et al. Macrophage activation with ubiquinones and their related compounds in mice. Int J Vitam Nutr Res 53:312-20, 1983*).

Dimethylglycine:

Supplementation may enhance both humoral and cell-mediated immunity.

Animal Experimental Study: Rabbits pretreated with DMG inoculated with either killed influenza virus or Salmonella typhi vaccine showed 3- to 5-fold higher antibody titers than controls. Lymphocyte transformation assays following inoculation with influenza virus showed a tenfold increase in mean proliferative response. Lymphocytes from animals immunized with typhoid vaccine showed a 4-fold increase in thymidine uptake. No toxicity or adverse effects were observed (*Reap EA, Lawson JW. Stimulation of the immune response by dimethylglycine, a nontoxic metabolite. J Lab Clin Med 115(4):481-86, 1990*).

Experimental Double-blind Study: Compared to age-matched controls who received calcium gluconate 300 mg daily, 10 healthy volunteers receiving DMG 120 mg daily along with calcium gluconate 180 mg daily showed a fourfold increase in antibody response to pneumococcal vaccine after 10 wks. (p<0.01). While production of leukocyte inhibitory factor in response to concanavalin A was similar in the 2 gps., those taking DMG had a significantly higher mean response of leukocyte inhibition factor to streptokinase-streptodornase (p<0.01) and to pneumococcal antigens after immunization with vaccine (p<0.001) (*Graber CD et al. Immunomodulating properties of dimethylglycine in humans. J Infect Dis 143(1):101-5, 1981*).

Experimental Double-blind Study: 20 subjects showed a fourfold increase in antibody response to pneumococcal vaccine compared to controls (p<0.01) as well as a significantly higher response of leukocyte inhibitory factor to streptokinase-streptodornase (p<0.01) and to pneumococcal antigens after immunization with vaccine (p<0.001). The *in vitro* responses to lymphocytes from pts. with diabetes and sickle cell disease to mitogens were increased almost three fold after addition of DMG. These results suggest that DMG enhances both humoral and cell-mediated immune reponses (*Graber CD et al. Immunomodulating properties of dimethylglycine in humans. J Infect Dis 143(1):101-5, 1981*).

Essential Amino Acids:

Deficiencies or imbalances interfere with protein synthesis, and thus with the production of immunoglobulins, interferons, and all other proteins necessary for host defenses (*Beisel WR. Single nutrients and immunity. Am J Clin Nutr 35(suppl):417-68, 1982*).

Essential Fatty Acids:

Deficiency may result in lymphoid atrophy and depressed immune responses (*Chandra RK. Nutrition and immunity - Basic considerations. Part 1. Contemp Nutr 11(11), 1986; DeWille JW et al. Effects of essential fatty acid deficiency, and various levels of dietary polyunsaturated fatty acids, on humoral immunity in mice. J Nutr 109(6):1018-27, 1979*).

Excess (for example, of arachidonic or linoleic acids) may induce atrophy of lymphoid tissue and diminish T cell immune responsiveness to antigenic stimulation (*Chandra RK. Nutrition and immunity - Basic considerations. Part 1. Contemp Nutr 11(11), 1986*).

Supplementation may improve immune responses.

Animal Experimental Study: Guinea pigs were fed diets supplemented with olive oil, fish oil (high in omega-3 fatty acids), or borage oil high in gamma-linolenic acid (an omega-6 fatty acid). The fish oil- and GLA-supplemented animals showed marked changes in polymorphonuclear leukocyte membrane structure and function associated with improved immune response. Long-term supplementation with fish oils (12 wks. or longer) also produced an inhibitory effect on oxidative processes otherwise associated with tissue damage and reduced immunological response (*Fletcher M, Ziboh V. Effects of dietary supplementation with eicosapentaenoic acid or gamma-linoleic acid on neutrophil phospholipid fatty acid composition and activation responses. Inflammation 14:585-97, 1990*).

- Omega-3 Fatty Acids:

WARNING: Fish oils, a rich source of omega-3 fatty acids, may decrease several indices of cell-mediated immunity.

Experimental Study: Subjects consumed a typical American diet (15% saturated, 15% monounsaturated, 5% omega-6 fatty acids, 1% omega-3 fatty acids, and 180 mg cholesterol/1000 calories) for 6 wks. and were then switched to a low-fat, low-cholesterol diet containing 5% saturated, 12% monounsaturated, 7.5% omega-6 fatty acids, 2.5% omega-3 fatty acids from fish oils, and 60 mg cholesterol/1000 calories. On the latter diet, omega-3 fatty acid plasma levels rose and prostaglandin E_2 levels decreased. Helper and suppressor T cell activity and numerous other indices of immune function also decreased, suggesting that an omega-3-enriched, low-fat diet may increase susceptibility to infection and disease (*Meydani S et al. Effect of low-fat, low cholesterol (LF-FCHL) diet enriched in N-3 fatty acids (FA) on the immune response of humans. FASEB J 5:1449A, 1991*).

Eicosapentaenoic acid (EPA) (a major component of fish oils) may affect the functions of several types of leukocytes critical to inflammation and immunity.

Experimental Study: 2 gps. of 6 adults with persistent asthma received either 0.1 or 4 gm of purified EPA ethyl ester daily. After 8 wks., both doses significantly increased the generation of leukotriene B_5 from EPA by polymorphonuclear and mononuclear leukocytes, while only the high dose decreased leukocyte arachidonic acid and the generation of leukotriene B_4 and prostaglandin E_2 from arachidonic acid. Only the high dose led to inhibition of polymorphonuclear leukocyte chemotaxis to multiple stimuli by a mean of 57-70%. Both doses increased the responses of T lymphocytes to a mitogen by a mean of at least 73% without modifying the numbers of helper and suppressor T lymphocytes (*Payan DG et al. Alterations in human leukocyte function induced by ingestion of eicosapentaenoic acid. J Clin Chem 6(5):402-10, 1986*).

- Omega-6 Fatty Acids:

linoleic acid $\rightarrow$ GLA $\rightarrow$ DGLA $\rightarrow$ Prostaglandin E_1

WARNING: Linoleic acid, linolenic acid and arachidonic acid may reduce T-cell responsiveness.

Animal Experimental Study: When tested several months after being injected with a potent carcinogen or after being infected with Mycoplasma pulmonis, mice on a diet enriched with linoleic acid, when compared to mice on diets enriched with oleic acid (a monounsaturate), palmitic acid (a saturated fatty acid) or eicosapentaenoic acid (an omega-3 fatty acid), were predisposed to suppression of T-cell-mediated cutaneous responses (*Bennett M et al. Dietary fatty acid effects on T-cell-mediated immunity in mice infected with mycoplasma pulmonis or given carcinogens by injection. Am J Pathol 126(1):103-13, 1987*).

Prostaglandin E_1 plays an important role in the regulation of T lymphocyte function; either a deficiency or an excess can have a deleterious effect (*Horrobin DF et al. The nutritional regulation of T lymphocyte function. Med Hypotheses 5:969-85, 1979*).

PGE_1 precursors such as linoleic acid and gammalinolenic acid (in addition to vitamin B_6, vitamin C and zinc) may theoretically be utilized to promote T cell activation, and supplementation with GLA could perhaps be beneficial (*Horrobin DF et al. The nutritional regulation of T lymphocyte function. Med Hypotheses 5:969-85, 1979*).

Glutamine:

After sepsis, surgery, trauma, and burns, both immune function (*Green DR, Faist E. Trauma and the immune response. Immunol Today 9:253-55, 1988*) and plasma glutamine concentrations (*Parry-Billings M et al. Does glutamine contribute to immunosuppression after major burns? Lancet 336:523-25, 1990; Stinnert JD et al. Plasma and skeletal muscle amino acids following severe burn injury in patients and experimental animals. Ann Surg 195:75-89, 1982*) are depressed.

Deficiency is immunosuppressive (*Kafkewitz D, Bendich A. Am J Clin Nutr 37:1025-30, 1983*), and falls in glutamine concentration affect T lymphocyte proliferation and macrophage function (*Parry-Billings M et al. Does glutamine contribute to immunosuppression after major burns? Lancet 336:523-25, 1990*).

Glycosaminoglycans:

May enhance antibody responses.

> **Animal and In vitro Experimental Study:** Catrix-S is a soluble derivative of bovine tracheal cartilage rings. It enhanced T-dependent and T-independent antibody responses *in vivo* in nude as well as in normal mice in a dose-dependent manner. *In vitro*, its enhancing activity on proliferative response was additive with that of dextran sulfate and lipopolysaccharide but not with chondroitin sulfate C; it appears to be related to the chondroitin sulfate component because both have similar effects on *in vivo* and *in vitro* antibody responses and because chondroitinase ABC inactivites it. Results indicate that its activity is due in part to a direct effect on B cells and/or to an indirect effect mediated by macrophages (*Rosen J et al. Immunoregulatory effects of Catrix. J Biol Response Mod 7(5):498-512, 1988*).

L-Ornithine:

WARNING: May suppress cytotoxic T lymphocyte activation, both *in vivo* and *in vitro* (*Dröge W et al. Suppression of cytotoxic T lymphocyte activation by L-ornithine. J Immunol 134(5):3379-83, 1985*).

Picolinic Acid:

May activate macrophages (*Ruffmann R et al. In vivo activation of macrophages but not natural killer cells by picolinic acid (PLA). J Immunopharmacol 6(4):291-304, 1984*).

Taurine:

Supplementation may increase both the phagocytic and bactericidal capacities of neutrophils (*Masuda M et al. Influences of taurine on functions of rat neutrophils. Jpn J Pharmacol 34(1):116-18, 1984*).

-- --

OTHER FACTORS

Rule out aluminum toxicity.

May be immunosuppressive (*Nordal KP et al. Aluminum accumulation and immunosuppressive effect in recipients of kidney transplants. Br Med J 297:1581-82, 1099*).

Rule out cadmium toxicity.

Cadmium adversely affects both humoral and cell-mediated immune response in animals (*Nath R et al. Molecular basis of cadmium toxicity. Prog Food Nutr Sci 8(1-2):109-63, 1984*).

Cadmium may inhibit natural killer cell function (*Stacey NH et al. Effects of cadmium on natural killer and killer cell functions in vivo. Environ Res 45:71-77, 1988*).

Rule out mercury toxicity.

In laboratory animals, mercuric chloride is able to trigger immune dysregulation in different species depending upon the genetic background of the strain tested (*Nordlind K. Toxic metals and immune function. Int Clin Nutr Rev 9(4):175-81, 1989*).

Rule out nickel toxicity.

May be immunosuppressive (*Nordlind K. Toxic metals and immune function. Int Clin Nutr Rev 9(4):175-81, 1989*).

INFECTION

See Also: CANDIDIASIS
HERPES SIMPLEX
HERPES ZOSTER
IMMUNODEPRESSION

OVERVIEW

1. A low fat, low cholesterol, low sugar diet may be beneficial.

2. Deficiencies of the following nutrients will increase susceptibility to infection and thus should be corrected: pantothenic acid, vitamin A, vitamin C, vitamin E, copper, iron, magnesium, phosphorus, selenium, zinc.

3. Excesses of the following nutrients will increase susceptibility to infection and thus should be corrected: vitamin A, copper, iron, zinc.

4. Supplementation with the following nutrients may reduce susceptibility to infection: vitamin A, vitamin C, vitamin E, zinc, essential fatty acids, quercetin.

5. Lactobacillus acidophilus has significant antibacterial activity *in vitro*. It may be beneficial intravaginally in bacterial vaginitis, and may have some efficacy aganst candida vaginitis when given orally.

6. Cadmium and lead toxicity will increase susceptibility to infection.

- -

DIETARY FACTORS

Avoid protein-calorie malnutrition.

> **Review Article:** Protein-calorie malnutrition is associated with increased susceptibility to infection (*Chandra RK. Trace element regulation of immunity and infection. J Am Coll Nutr 4(1):5-16, 1985*).

Low fat diet.

> **Review Article:** Excessive omega-6 PUFA metabolism due to high levels of dietary fat intake can encourage infection via prolonged inflammation, enhanced Gram negative survival, reticuloendothelial blockage, immunosuppression, and monokine depression (*Wan JM et al. Invited comment: lipids and the development of immune dysfunction and infection. JPEN J Parenter Enteral Nutr 12(6 Suppl):43S-52S, 1988*).

Low cholesterol diet.

> **Review Article:** Cholesterol excess increases susceptibility to infection with possible suppression of antibody production (*Beisel WR. Single nutrients and immunity. Am J Clin Nutr 35:417-68 (suppl), 1982*).

> **Review Article:** While cholesterol is a potent modulator of T lymphocyte and phagocyte functions in laboratory animals and in leukocyte cultures, its effect in humans is still uncertain (*Edelman R. Obesity: does it modulate infectious disease and immunity? Prog Clin Biol Res 67:327-37, 1981*).

367

Avoid <u>sugar</u>.

Sugar may weaken immune defenses against infection.

> **Experimental Study:** Ingestion of 100 gm of carbohydrate from glucose, fructose, sucrose, honey or orange juice but not starch significantly decreased the phagocytic index as measured by the capacity of neutrophils to engulf bacteria. Values were still below control values 5 hrs. after ingestion (*Sanchez A et al. Role of sugars in human neutrophilic phagocytosis. <u>Am J Clin Nutr</u> 26:180, 1973*).

- -

VITAMINS

<u>Pantothenic Acid:</u>

Deficiency may cause frequent upper respiratory infections (*Thornton GHM et al. <u>J Clin Invest</u> 34:1073, 1955*).

<u>Vitamin A:</u>

Deficiency is associated with increased susceptibility to infection (*Sommer A et al. Increased risk of respiratory disease and diarrhoea in children with pre-existing mild vitamin A deficiency. <u>Am J Clin Nutr</u> 40:1090-95, 1984*).

Supplementation causing vitamin A excess enhances lymphocytic response to antigens and antibody responses, and may diminish host susceptibility to infection (*Beisel WR. Single nutrients and immunity. <u>Am J Clin Nutr</u> 35:417-68 (suppl), 1982*).

> **Review Article:** Regarding children in developing countries, "the data on vitamin A suggest that strategies to improve micronutrient status may be extremely beneficial in terms of survival from infection" (*Editorial: Vitamin A and malnutrition/infection complex in developing countries. <u>Lancet</u> 336:1349-51, 1990*).

> **Review Article:** As mounting scientific evidence suggests that vitamin A status at the time of measles infection may be critical to its outcome, WHO and UNICEF recommend that, in countries where the fatality rate of measles is 1% or higher, vitamin A supplements should be provided to all infected children (*Editorial. Vitamin A for measles. <u>Lancet</u> 1:1067-68, 1987*).

> **Experimental Placebo-controlled Study:** 147 preschool-age children with a history of frequent respiratory illness randomly received either vitamin A 450 μg (1500 IU) daily or placebo. After 11 mo., supplemented children experienced 19% fewer episodes of respiratory symptomatology (p<0.05) compared to controls, even though their plasma retinol levels did not change. Children with prior histories of lower respiratory illness or of allergy benefited most (*Pinnock CB et al. Vitamin A status in children who are prone to respiratory tract infections. <u>Aust Paediatr J</u> 22(2):95-99, 1986*).

> **Observational Study:** In 100 healthy people over age 60, those with higher plasma concentrations of vitamin A reported less infections over the past 3 yrs., but the difference was not quite significant (p<0.07) (*Chavance M et al. Nutritional support improves antibody response to influenza virus in the elderly. Letter. <u>Br Med J</u> November 9, 1985, pp. 1348-49*).

<u>Vitamin C:</u>

Bacterial infections may reduce the cellular uptake of ascorbic acid (*Aleo JJ, Padh H. Inhibition of ascorbic acid uptake by endotoxin: Evidence of mediation by serum factor(s). <u>Proc Soc Exp Biol Med</u> 179(1):128-31, 1985*).

Infection in mammals is followed by an abrupt and often sustained fall in the blood, tissue and urine levels of ascorbic acid and by localization of the vitamin at the infected site (*Stacpoole PW. Role of vitamin C in infectious disease and allergic reactions. <u>Med Hypotheses</u> 1:42-46, 1975*).

Serum level may be negatively associated with the risk of <u>bronchitis</u>.

Observational Study: In a study of 9,074 white and black adult Americans aged 30 yrs. and older, after controlling for age, race, sex, calories, and pack-years of cigarette smoking, the serum vitamin C level was negatively associated with bronchitis (*Schwartz J, Weiss ST. Dietary factors and their relation to respiratory symptoms. The Second National Health and Nutrition Examination Survey. Am J Epidemiol 132(1):67-76, 1990*).

Supplementation may stimulate neutrophil motility and enhance phagocyte antimicrobial activity (*Anderson R. The immunostimulatory, anti-inflammatory and anti-allergic properties of ascorbate. Adv Nutr Res 6:19-45, 1984*).

Supplementation may reduce the severity and duration of the common cold.

Experimental Blinded Study: 16 college men with normal serum vitamin C levels who were free of antibodies of rhinovirus 16 received either vitamin C 500 mg 4 times daily or placebo. During the following wk., they spent many hours playing poker with 8 donors already infected with rhinovirus 16 colds. 6/8 treated men and 7/8 controls caught colds - suggesting that vitamin C failed to prevent colds. However, symptoms (number of coughs, sneezes and nose blows) were significantly milder in the vitamin C group (*Dick EC, chief of the respiratory virus research lab, U. of Wisconsin at Madison - reported in Med World News 12/28/87*).

Review Article: "It is now fairly clear that for preventing common colds, vitamin C has no worthwhile effect . . . . There is . . . a little more evidence for a small therapeutic effect . . . , but it is not clear which symptom it relieves or how" (*Truswell AS. Ascorbic acid. N Engl J Med 315(11):709, 1986*).

Review Article: "The present consensus of scientific opinion fails to support the view that ascorbic acid supplementation using 1 to 2 g/day doses is effective in reducing susceptibility to common colds. At best, such doses may lessen the severity and/or duration of symptoms" (*Beisel WR. Single nutrients and immunity. Am J Clin Nutr 35:417-68 (suppl), 1982*).

Negative Observational Study: Plasma ascorbic acid levels were studied for 28 submarine crewmen before, during and after a 68-day patrol. There were no significant health differences between those with the highest and those with the lowest levels (*Biersner RJ et al. Relationship of plasma vitamin C to the health and performance of submariners. J Appl Nutr 34(1):29-37, 1982*).

Experimental Double-blind Study: One twin from each of 95 pairs of identical twins ingested 1 g of ascorbic acid per day for 100 days while the other received a placebo. Vitamin C cut the duration of cold symptoms by 19% but did not prevent the occurrence of colds (*Carr AB et al. Vitamin C and the common cold: Using identical twins as controls. Med J Aust 2:411-12, 1981*).

Supplementation may increase serum interferon level in response to viral infections (*Geber WF et al. Effect of ascorbic acid, sodium salicylate, and caffeine on the serum interferon level in response to viral infection. Pharmacology 13(3):228-33, 1975*).

Supplementation may be beneficial in treating certain bacterial infections (*Rawal BD et al. Inhibition of Pseudomonas aeruginosa by ascorbic acid acting singly and in combination with antimicrobials: in-vitro and in-vivo studies. Med J Aust 1(6):169-74, 1974; Rawal BD. Ascorbic acid: Preferential lysis and catalase induction in antibiotic-resistant strains of Staphlococcus aureus. J Pharm Sci 62(5):837-38, 1973*

Supplementation may be beneficial in treating toxoplasmosis (*Seah SK. Letter. Vitamin C and experimental toxoplasmosis. Trans R Soc Trop Med Hyg 68(1):76-77, 1974*

Vitamin E:

Deficiency is associated with increased infections due to diminished membrane-related chemotaxis and ingestion (*Baehner RL, Boxer LA. Role of membrane vitamin E and cytoplasmic glutathione in the regulation of phagocytic functions of neutrophils and monocytes. Am J Pediatr Hematol Oncol 1(1):71-76, 1979*).

Observational Study: In 100 healthy people over age 60, the plasma alpha tocopherol concentration was negatively correlated (p<0.001) with the number of infections in the past 3 years (*Chavance M et al. Nutritional support improves antibody response to influenza virus in the elderly. Letter. Br Med J November 9, 1985, pp. 1348-49*).

Supplementation may enhance both humoral and cellular immune responses and increase phagocytic functions to stimulate body defenses against infectious agents (*Tengerdy RP. Vitamin E, immune response, and disease resistance. Ann N Y Acad Sci 570:335-44, 1989*).

_____

MINERALS

Copper:

WARNING: Excess copper may increase susceptibility to infection (*Beisel WR. Single nutrients and immunity. Am J Clin Nutr 35:417-68 (suppl.), 1982*).

During a bacterial infection, serum copper rises due to its removal from storage tissues in order to fight the infection which results in a reduction in tissue levels (*Watts DL. The nutritional relationships of copper. J Orthomol Med 4(2):99-108, 1989*).

Observational Study: In a study of 53 pts. with acute bacterial and viral infections, plasma copper increased in bacterial infections causing septicemia, pneumonia and meningitis, but was unchanged in pts. with erysipelas. The onset of change in copper occurred within a few days and persisted for several weeks. The changes appeared to be non-specific and independent of the agent causing infection (*Srinivas U et al. Trace element alterations in infectious diseases. Scand J Clin Lab Invest 48(6):495-500, 1988*).

Deficiency may be associated with increased susceptibility to infection due to impairment of cell-mediated immunity (*Chandra RK. Trace element regulation of immunity and infection. J Am Coll Nutr 4(1):5-16, 1985*).

Iron:

WARNING: Excess supplementation can increase bacterial growth and replication and the release of certain exotoxins (*Beisel WR. Single nutrients and immunity. Am J Clin Nutr 35:417-68 (suppl.), 1982*).

Deficiency may be associated with increased susceptibility to infection (*Beisel WR. Single nutrients and immunity. Am J Clin Nutr 35:417-68 (suppl), 1982*) as there is a slight decrease in the number of rosette-forming T cells and a significant impairment of lymphocyte response to mitogens and antigens. Polymorphonuclear leukocytes are unable to kill ingested bacteria and fungi in an efficient manner (*Chandra RK. Trace element regulation of immunity and infection. J Am Coll Nutr 4(1):5-16, 1985*).

Experimental Study: 16 pts. with recurrent staphylococcal furunculosis but without anemia had significantly lower serum iron concentrations than normal lab reference values, 8 controls with single furuncles, or 10 controls with acne conglobata. There were no significant differences in serum glucose or iron-binding capacity between the groups studied. After 3-4 weeks' treatment with iron supplements, furunculosis resolved in all but one patient (*Weijmer MC et al. Preliminary report: furunculosis and hypoferraemia. Lancet 336:464-66, 1990*).

Observational Study: 28 children (ages 10 mo.-10 yrs.) with undue susceptibility to middle ear and respiratory infections were found to have significantly lower serum iron (p<0.05) than 13 controls. Serum zinc was also significantly lower, but copper, magnesium, transferrin and ceruloplasmin did not differ between gps. (*Bondestam M et al. Subclinical trace element deficiency in children with undue susceptibility to infections. Acta Paediatr Scand 74(4):515-20, 1985*).

The effect of iron deprivation in limiting bacterial multiplication has considerable *in vitro* evidence; however, clinical data do not support the suggestion that iron deficiency protects against infection or that correction of iron deficiency, particularly if it is achieved gradually by oral iron therapy, increeases the incidence or severity of infectious disease in man (*Chandra RK. 1990 McCollum Award Lecture. Nutrition and immunity: lessons from the past and new insights into the future. Am J Clin Nutr 53:1087-1101, 1991*).

The hypoferremia of inflammation is not identical to iron deficiency; rather it is a redistribution of iron in the face of normal or increased iron stores, and thus may have the advantages of reducing the iron supply to pathogens without adverse effects on host resistance. Since hypoferremia is one of the most constant features of infectious disease, and since iron deprivation in bacterial cultures is regularly associated with inhibition of growth, it has been suggested that it may be an important host defence mechanism; however few clinical data support the importance of iron deficiency or overload in determining the severity or prevalence of infectious disease in man. Whether correcting the hypoferremia of inflammation may deleteriously affect existing infections has not been directly studied, although there are reports from developing countries of an increased incidence or severity of infectious disease after iron treatment (*Hershko C et al. Iron and infection. Br Med J 296:660-64, 1988*).

Magnesium:

The ability of animals to cope with infection may be influenced by magnesium nutriture (*Miller ER. Mineral X disease interactions. J Anim Sci 60(6):1500-7, 1985*).

Phosphorus:

The ability of animals to cope with infection may be influenced by phosphorus nutriture (*Miller ER. Mineral X disease interactions. J Anim Sci 60(6):1500-7, 1985*).

Selenium:

Deficiency may be associated with increased susceptibility to infection (*Boyne K et al. The response of selenium-deficient mice to Candida albicans infections. J Nutr 116?816-22, 1986*).

Plasma selenium levels may decrease during infections (*Srinivas U et al. Trace element alterations in infectious diseases. Scand J Clin Lab Invest 48(6):495-500, 1988*).

Zinc:

WARNING: Higher levels of supplementation may increase susceptibility to infection.

Experimental Study: 11 healthy adult men ingested 150 mg of elemental zinc twice daily. After 6 wks., there was a reduction in chemotaxis and phagocytosis of bacteria by polymorphonuclear leukocytes (*Chandra RK. Excessive intake of zinc impairs immune responses. JAMA 252(11):1443-46, 1984*).

General Review Article: Serum zinc levels decrease sharply in many infections. Levels slightly below normal are associated with optimal phagocytic function, and low zinc concentrations may decrease microbial virulence. Brief decreases in serum levels appear to have no detrimental effect on host immunity and may act as a protective measure by decreasing the ability of indigenous or infecting microbes to thrive. However, prolonged zinc deficiency in mammals is associated with depressed T-cell function (with near normal B-cell function) (*Sugarman B. Zinc and infection. Rev Infect Dis 5(1):137-47, 1983*).

Reduced hair and serum levels, and elevated urinary levels, are associated with increased susceptibility to infection.

Observational Study: In a study of 474 children aged 3-7, children with frequent upper respiratory tract infections (>6/yr) showed significantly lower hair zinc values, independent of their age (*Lombeck I et al. Hair zinc of young children from rural and urban areas in North Rhine-Westphalia, Federal Republic of Germany. Eur J Pediatr 147(2):179-83, 1988*).

Observational Study: Compared to age- and sex-matched controls, 20 pediatric pts. with recurrent upper respiratory tract infection had lower hair zinc (p=0.004) and higher urinary zinc (p=0.05), but similar levels of serum zinc. While they had lower-normal height for age, there was no difference in weight for height. No correlation was found between zinc levels and the duration of their complaints (*van Wouwe JP et al. Subacute zinc deficiency in children with recurrent upper respiratory tract infection. Eur J Pediatr 146(3):293-95, 1987*).

Experimental Study: 6 young men consumed a semipurified diet providing 0.28 mg zinc and 0.8 kg protein daily. After 4-9 wks., there were significant decreases in plasma, whole blood, urinary, seminal and fecal zinc along with impairment of leukocyte chemotaxis and clinical signs indicative of decreased resistance to infection (*Baer MT et al. Nitrogen utilization, enzyme activity, glucose intolerance and leukocyte chemotaxis in human experimental zinc depletion. Am J Clin Nutr 41(6):1220-35, 1985*).

Plasma/serum zinc levels may decrease during acute infections (*Pras P et al. [The effect of various diseases on the zinc plasma level.]* <u>*Sem Hop Paris*</u> *59(20):1519-22, 1983*).

Observational Study: In a study of 53 pts. with acute bacterial and viral infections, plasma zinc levels were decreased in bacterial infections (septicemia, pneumonia, erysipelas and meningitis). Although plasma zinc was also decreased in viral infections, the change was not as pronounced. In viral infections, 60% of the zinc values were below the mean level of 12.8 µmol/L observed in healthy controls as compared with 90% of the values in pts. with sepsis or 92% of the values in pts. with pneumonia. The onset of change in zinc occurred within a few days and persisted for several weeks. The changes appeared to be non-specific and independent of the agent causing infection (*Srinivas U et al. Trace element alterations in infectious diseases.* <u>*Scand J Clin Lab Invest*</u> *48(6):495-500, 1988*).

Supplementation may improve resistance to infection even when not deficient.

Animal Experimental Study: When mice inbred to exhibit decreased cell-mediated immunity were fed diets that were high in zinc, their resistance to infection with candida albicans as well as their release of migration inhibitory factor (MIF) increased dramatically (*Salvin SB, Rabin BS. Resistance and susceptibility to infection in inbred murine strains. IV. Effects of dietary zinc.* <u>*Cellular Immunol*</u> *87(2):546-52, 1984*).

Supplementation may be effective for <u>trichomonal</u> infections even when metronidazole is ineffective (*Willmott F et al.* <u>*Lancet*</u> *1:1053, 1983*).

Supplementation may be effective for the <u>common cold</u>.

Experimental Double-blind Studies: 1.) 57 volunteers received lozenges of either zinc gluconate (23 mg elemental Zn) or placebo every 2 hr. while awake during 4 1/2 days. They were challenged with human rhinovirus 2 on the second day. Zinc reduced the total mean clinical score from 8.2 in the placebo gp. to 5.7; the reduction of the mean clinical score was significant on the second day after virus challenge. 2.) 69 volunteers were inoculated with human rhinovirus 2 and those who developed cold symptoms were randomly allocated to receive either zinc gluconate lozenges or placebo every 2 hrs. while awake for 6 days. Zinc reduced the mean daily clinical score; this was significant on the fourth and fifth days. Similarly, zinc reduced the mean daily nasal secretion weight and total tissue count; these reductions were significant on days 2 and 6 for nasal secretion weights, and days 4-6 for tissue counts when compared with placebo (*Al-Nakib W et al. Prophylaxis and treatment of rhinovirus colds with zinc gluconate lozenges.* <u>*J Antimicrob Chemother*</u> *20(6):893-901, 1987*).

Negative Experimental Double-blind Study: 55 pts. with upper respiratory tract illnesses received either zinc acetate lozenges (10 mg elemental zinc) or placebo. Mean symptom duration was 12.1 days for zinc users compared to 7.7 days for those on placebo (*Douglas RM et al. Failure of effervescent zinc acetate lozenges to alter the course of upper respiratory tract infections in Australian adults.* <u>*Antimicrob Agents Chemother*</u> *31:1263, 1987*).

Negative Experimental Blinded Studies: Lozenges containing either zinc gluconate (23 mg elemental zinc) or placebo were randomly given 36 hr. after nasal inoculation of rhinovirus type 39 and administered 8 times daily. After 5 days, all the volunteers had early cold symptoms. In trial 2, the same lozenge regimen was used, starting 2 hr. after nasal inoculation with rhinovirus type 13. After 7 days, zinc therapy failed to reduce the severity or duration of cold symptoms. In addition, zinc therapy failed to reduce the frequency or duration of viral shedding in either trial (*Farr BM et al. Two randomized controlled trials of zinc gluconate lozenge therapy of experimentally induced rhinovirus colds.* <u>*Antimicrob Agents Chemother*</u> *31(8):1183-87, 1987*).

Experimental Double-blind Study: 146 volunteers were given a 7 day supply of zinc gluconate tablets 180 mg (each containing 23 mg elemental zinc) or placebo tablets. Adults and youngsters at least 60 lbs. were told to to suck on 2 tabs for at least 10 min. at the outset of a cold, followed by 1 tab every 2 waking hrs. up to a maximum of 12 daily for adults and 9 daily for youngsters. Smaller children were limited to a maximum of 6 daily. Treatment was to stop 6 hrs. after symptoms ceased, and no other treatments were permitted. While cold sufferers receiving zinc completely recovered in an ave. of 3.9 days, those receiving placebo took 10.8 days to become symptom-free. The treatment was equally effective for both mild and severe infections, and was beneficial even if supplementation was delayed. Many subjects became asymptomatic within hrs. and 1/5 of the zinc-treated gp. fully recuperated within one day (*Eby GA, Davis DR, Halcomb WW. Reduction in duration of common colds by zinc gluconate lozenges in a double-blind study.* <u>*Antimicrob Agents Chemother*</u> *25(1):20-4, 1984*).

Note: This study has been criticized because of the higher rate of side effects in the zinc gp. and the lack of any confirmatory evidence of blinding efficacy. It is noted that unflavored zinc gluconate tablets can be easily distinguished from the relatively tasteless, unflavored calcium lactate tablets (Farr BM, Gwaltney JM Jr. The problems of taste in placebo matching: an evaluation of zinc gluconate for the common colds. J Chronic Dis 40(9):875-9, 1987).

Zinc-impregnated dressings are widely used to reduce bacterial counts and promote healing (*Soderberg T et al. The effects of an occlusive zinc medicated dressing on the bacterial flora in excised wounds in the rat. Infection 17:81-5, 1989*).

Zinc to Copper ratio:

May be inversely correlated with the risk of bronchitis.

Observational Study: In a study of 9,074 white and black adult Americans aged 30 yrs. and older, after controlling for age, race, sex, calories, and pack-years of cigarette smoking, the zinc to copper ratio was negatively associated with bronchitis (*Schwartz J, Weiss ST. Dietary factors and their relation to respiratory symptoms. The Second National Health and Nutrition Examination Survey. Am J Epidemiol 132(1):67-76, 1990*).

- -

OTHER NUTRITIONAL FACTORS

Essential Fatty Acids:

General Review Article: The oils of evening primrose, fish and linseed are rich in linoleic, linolenic and eicosapentaenoic acid, essential fatty acids which appear to have anti-bacterial, anti-fungal and anti-viral actions (*Das UN. Antibiotic-like action of essential fatty acids. Letter. Can Med Assoc J 132(12):1350, 1985*).

- Omega-3 Fatty Acids:

Eicosapentaenoic acid (EPA) and docosahexaenoic acid (DHA).

Highest in cold water fish. Available in a refined form as 'MaxEPA' (18% EPA).

Suggested MaxEPA dosage: 3 - 9 grams daily in divided doses (or 10 ml. concentrate twice daily)

WARNING: Supplementation may require additional vitamin E intake to prevent increased membrane peroxidation and cellular damage (*Laganiere S, Fernandes G. High peroxidizability of subcellular membrane induced by high fish oil diet is reversed by vitamin E. Clin Res 35:A565, 1987*).

Administration of fish oils may protect against infection with endotoxin-producing gram-negative bacteria.

Experimental Controlled Study: 18 gm of fish oil (3.2 gm EPA) was added to the diet of healthy volunteers. After 6 wks., subjects were injected with an endotoxin. Consumption of the oil decreased fever and diminished other symptoms, such as feeling cold, nausea, and shivering (*Endres S et al. Effects of dietary omega-3 fatty acids on the acute phase response during endotoxin fever in humans. J Leuk Biol 42:591, 1987*).

Lactic Acid:

The predominant acid in normal vaginal fluid as lactate producers (lactobacillus and streptococcus species) are the predominant organisms (*Spiegel CA et al. Anaerobic bacteria in nonspecific vaginitis. N Engl J Med 303(11):601-7, 1980*).

Decreased levels are associated with Gardnerella vaginitis as organisms which produce other acids predominate (*Spiegel CA et al. Anaerobic bacteria in nonspecific vaginitis. N Engl J Med 303(11):601-7, 1980*).

Supplementation may be beneficial in <u>Gardnerella vaginitis</u>.

> **Experimental Controlled and Observational Study:** Anaerobes dominated the flora in 62 bacterial vaginosis pts., while lactobacilli were the predominant organisms in 42 controls. Lactate-gel (pH 3.5, 5 ml) inserted into the vagina daily for 7 days was as effective as oral metronidazole 500 mg twice daily for 7 days. The women in both gps. became symptom-free and objectively improved. Anaerobes were significantly reduced (p<0.0001) in both gps. after treatment but Gardnerella was not significantly reduced. Results suggest that lactate-gel is an ideal treatment (*Andersch B et al. Treatment of bacterial vaginosis with an acid cream: A comparison between the effect of lactate-gel and metronidazole. <u>Gynecol Obstet Invest</u> 21(1):19-25, 1986*).

<u>Quercetin</u>:

May inhibit the infectiousness and/or replication of both RNA and DNA viruses (*Kaul TN et al. Antiviral effect of flavonoids on human viruses. <u>J Med Virol</u> 15:71-79, 1985*).

- -

OTHER FACTORS

Rule out <u>cadmium</u> toxicity.

May have adverse effects on host resistance to bacterial and viral infections (*Gainer JH. Effects of heavy metals and of deficiency of zinc on mortality rates in mice infected with encephalomyocarditis virus. <u>Am J Vet Res</u> 38:869-72, 1977; Cook JA et al. Influence of lead and cadmium on the susceptibility of rats to bacterial challenge. <u>Proc Soc Exp Biol Med</u> 150:741-47, 1975*).

Rule out <u>lead</u> toxicity.

Subtoxic oral doses may reduce host resistence to bacterial and viral infections (*Gainer JH. Effects of heavy metals and of deficiency of zinc on mortality rates in mice infected with encephalomyocarditis virus. <u>Am J Vet Res</u> 38:869-72, 1977; Cook JA et al. Influence of lead and cadmium on the susceptibility of rats to bacterial challenge. <u>Proc Soc Exp Biol Med</u> 150:741-47, 1975*).

Rule out <u>hydrochloric acid deficiency</u>.

> **Review Article:** The available data support the concept that gastric hypochlorhydria or achlorhydria increases both susceptibility to and severity of bacterial (and perhaps also of certain parasitic) enteric infections (*Giannella RA et al. Influence of gastric acidity on bacterial and parasitic enteric infections. <u>Ann Intern Med</u> 78:271-76, 1973*).

<u>Lactobacillus Acidophilus</u>:

May have antibacterial action.

> **In vitro Experimental Study:** Acidophyllin, the antibacterial component of acidophilus, caused a 50% inhibition in growth of 27 different types of bacteria in lactic-acid-free preparations, 10 of which were common pathogens (*Shahani KM et al. <u>Cultured Dairy Prod J</u> 12:8-11, 1977*).

Administration of hydrogen-peroxide-producing strains may inactivate <u>Clostridium difficile</u> cytotoxin, the major cause of antibiotic-induced diarrhea (*Ooi W et al. <u>J Infect Diseases</u> 149:215-19, 1984*).

Administration has been ineffective for the treatment of <u>traveler's diarrhea</u> (*Pozo-Olando J de Dios et al. <u>Gastroenterology</u> 74:829-30, 1978*) and <u>infantile diarrhea</u> (*Pearce JL, Hamilton JR. <u>J Pediatrics</u> 24:261-62, 1974*). However, administration may prevent the onset of illness - which is usually associated with enterotoxigenic strains of <u>Escherichia coli</u> (*Alm L. <u>Prog Food Nutr Sci</u> 7:19-28, 1983; Merson MH et al. <u>N Engl J Med</u> 294:1299-1305, 1976; Shore EG et al. <u>J Infect Dis</u> 129:577-82, 1974*).

Decrease in quantity (along with a decrease in lactate acid) is associated with <u>Gardnerella-associated ("non-specific") vaginitis</u> (*Fredricsson B et al. Gardnerella-associated vaginitis and anerobic bacteria. <u>Gynecol Obstet Invest</u>*

17(5):236-41, 1984; Spiegel CA et al. Diagnosis of bacterial vaginosis by direct gram stain of vaginal fluid. J Clin Microbiol 18(1):170-77, 1983).

Oral administration may be beneficial in recurrent candida vaginitis.

> **Experimental Study:** 11 women with recurrent candida vaginitis (at least 5 episodes within a yr.) ingested 1 cup of yogurt containing L. acidophilus daily. The number of infections fell from a mean of 3 to <1 during 6 mo. of daily yogurt consumption (*Hilton, Eileen, Long Island Jewish Medical Center, N.Y. - reported in Med World News, October 23, 1989*).

Local administration may be beneficial in vaginitis of various causes.

> **Experimental Study:** 25 pts. with recurrent, non-specific vaginal discharge and/or vaginitis (after exclusion of trichomoniasis, candidiasis and bacterial vaginosis), received vaginal LA therapy $(1 \times 10^{10}/\text{gm}$ lyophilized Doderlein bacilli). After 12 wks., 60% had a marked decrease in vaginal discharge, usually within 1 week. The combined improvement and cure rate was 60-80% (*Gerstner GJ, Muller G. Intravaginale lyophilisierte Laktobazillen zur therapie des unspezifischen fluor vaginalis. Gynak Rdsch 27:71-78, 1987*).

> **Experimental Study:** 444 women with trichomoniasis vaginalis were treated with lactobacillus acidophilis (SolcoTrichovac/Gynatren). One year after the first vaccination, 427 (96.2%) were followed up, and 92.5% of them were found to be cured of clinical symptoms, while the remaining 7.5% had either a positive slide or culture (*Litschgi MS et al. [Effectiveness of a lactobacillus vaccine on trichomonas infections in women. Preliminary results.] Fortschr Med 98(41):1624-27, 1980*).

> **Clinical Report:** 20 pts. reported that they cured their candidia vulvovaginitis with preparations containing viable LA cultures (*Will TE. Lactobacillus overgrowth for treatment of moniliary vulvovaginitis. Letter. Lancet 2:482, 1979*).

> - with oral Vitamin B Complex:

> > **Experimental Study:** Pts. whose vaginal infections had failed to respond to treatment with various antimicrobial agents received daily vaginal douches with LA and oral vitamin B complex. Inflammation disappeared in most pts. and they reported feeling better (*Friedlander A et al. Lactobacillus acidophillus and vitamin B complex in the treatment of vaginal infection. Panminerva Med. 28(1):51-3, 1986*).

Pancreatic enzymes:

Deficiency is associated with an increased risk of intestinal infection (*Rubinstein E et al. Antibacterial activity of the pancreatic fluid. Gastroenterol 88:927-32, 1985*).

Propolis:

A resinous substance produced by bees from the buds and twigs of trees.

May have antibacterial properties.

> **In vitro Experimental Study:** Propolis was found to have antibacterial properties against a range of commonly encountered cocci and Gram-positive rods, including human tubercle bacillus, but only limited activity against Gram-negative bacilli. These findings are possibly attributable to its high flavonoid content (*Grange JM, Davey RW. Antibacterial properties of propolis (bee glue). J R Soc Med 83(3):159-60, 1990*).

INFERTILITY

DIETARY FACTORS

Avoid <u>caffeine</u>.

Intake may be correlated with decreased female fertility.

Negative Observational Study: Data from a previous study (*Wilcox AJ, Weinberg CR, Baird DD. <u>Lancet</u> 2:1453-6, 1988*) were re-analyzed. Non-coffee beverages were separated into tea and caffeinated soft drinks (there were no data on non-caffeinated beverages) prior to analysis. While tea had a negligible association with fertility, caffeinated soft drinks were strongly related to lower fertility. When modelled as a linear variable, one caffeinated soft drink per day was associated with a 50% reduction in the monthly chance of conception (p=0.01) after coffee consumption, frequency of intercourse, and age were controlled for. The strength of the association exceeds what would be predicted from the coffee data were caffeine the responsible agent (*Wilcox AJ, Weinberg CR. Tea and fertility. Letter. <u>Lancet</u> 337:1159-60, 1991*).

Observational Study: For 3010 women, times to conception were longest for the 129 women who drank 4 or more cups of coffee per day; these women were consistently less likely to become pregnant than women who did not drink coffee. The estimated adjusted relative risk of failure to conceive within 1 yr. among consumers of 4 or more cups of coffee was 1.8 (95% CI 1.1-3.0) compared to non-coffee drinkers. As coffee consumption during the first trimester was used as a proxy measurement for caffeine exposure during attempted conception, if many women reduced their coffee intake during pregnancy, this misclassification of coffee consumption would underestimate the true risk of exposure to coffee while attempting to conceive (*Williams MA et al. Coffee and delayed conception. Letter. <u>Lancet</u> 335:1603, 1990*).

Negative Observational Study: In a study which interviewed 2817 fertile women who had recently had a live-born child, there was no evidence that the intake of caffeinated beverages was associated with the time until conception. For levels of consumption ranging from <1 cup of coffee/wk. (501 mg/mo.) to >2 cups/d (7000 mg/mo.), the ave. time to conceive was similar. The fecundability ratio adjusted for known risk factors for time to conceive was 1.03 between those who consumed >7000 mg caffeine/mo. and those who consumed 500 mg or less per month. Furthermore, caffeine consumption was not associated with infertility in 1818 infertile women and their primiparous controls (*Joesoef MR et al. Are caffeinated beverages risk factors for delayed conception? <u>Lancet</u> 1:136-37, 1990*).

Note: Caffeine consumption, unlike most other risk factors, is easily changed; thus the correlation between caffeine intake reported after delivery and actual intake a year earlier during the attempt to conceive could be poor. In addition, women having difficulty conceiving may tend to adopt healthier habits which would make a caffeine effect harder to detect (Weinberg CR, Wilcox AJ. Caffeine and infertility. Letter. <u>Lancet</u> 1:792-3, 1990).

Theoretical Discussion: Caffeine is known to reduce the concentration of serum prolactin, and low serum prolactin is known to be associated with infertility. Caffeine-associated prolactin reduction may be mediated by dopamine in the central nervous system (*Casas M et al. Dopaminergic mechanism for caffeine induced decrease in fertility? Letter. <u>Lancet</u> 1:731, 1989*).

Avoid <u>alcohol abuse</u>.

Excessive alcohol ingestion in women may provoke hyperprolactinemia which may cause menstrual cycle dysfunction and infertility (*Mendleson JH. Alcohol effects on reproductive function in women. <u>Psychiatry Letter</u> 4(7):35-38, 1986*).

Alcohol is a is a male reproductive tract toxin; the degree of reproductive impairment varies with the amount of ethanol ingested, and the duration of ethanol exposure (*Anderson RA Jr et al. Ethanol-induced male infertility: impairment of spermatozoa. J Pharmacol Exp Ther 225(2):47 9-86, 1983; Anderson RA Jr et al. Male reproductive tract sensitivity to ethanol: a critical overview. Pharmacol Biochem Behav 18 Suppl 1:305-10, 1983*). The results of animal research suggest that male alcoholic patients with reproductive disorders could have at least partial recovery following moderate periods of abstinence (*Anderson RA Jr et al. Spontaneous recovery from ethanol-induced male infertility. Alcohol 2(3):479-84, 1985*).

- -

VITAMINS

Folic Acid:

If deficient, supplementation may be beneficial to women.

> **Case Reports:** 3 women (2 aged 29 yrs., 1 aged 32 yrs.) with infertility for several yrs. had RBC macrocytosis together with low serum and RBC folate levels. 2/3 were gluten-intolerant and, upon jejunal biopsy, showed subtotal villous atrophy. Folic acid 5 mg 3 times daily returned hematologic indices to normal and all became pregnant during the following 3-15 mo. (*Dawson DW, Sawers AH. Infertility and folate deficiency. Case reports. Br J Obstet Gynaecol 89:678-80, 1982*).

Vitamin B$_6$:

Supplementation may be beneficial to women.

> **Experimental Study:** 6 pts. with amenorrhea, 5 of whom had galactorrhea and elevated prolactin levels, received 600 mg pyridoxine daily for 3-4 months. 2/6 pts. began having regular menses (*Kidd GS et al. The effects of pyridoxine on pituitary hormone secretion in amenorrhea-galactorrhea syndromes. J Clin Endocrinol Metab 54(4):872-75, 1982*).

> **Experimental Study:** 12/14 women (ages 23-31) with premenstrual syndrome who had been infertile from 18 mo. - 7 yrs. were able to conceive following pyridoxine supplementation 100 - 800 mg daily depending upon the dosage needed to relieve PMS for at least 6 months. Of the 13 pregnancies (1 woman conceived twice), 11 occurred within the first 6 mo. of therapy, 1 occurred in the seventh mo. and the last occurred following 11 mo. of supplementation. In 5/7 women studied, there was a significant increase in progesterone levels with B$_6$ supplementation (*Abraham GE, Hargrove JT - reported in Med World News March 19, 1979*).

Vitamin B$_{12}$:

Supplementation may be beneficial to men.

> **Experimental Double-blind Study:** 375 infertile men received mecobalamin 6,000 μg/d, mecobalamin 1,500 μg/d, or placebo. After 12 wks., there were no significant differences among the 3 gps. in relation to sperm count or motility rate. However, in cases with a sperm count of 20×10^6/ml or less, a motility rate of 50% or less and a serum LH level of ≤13.5 mIU/ml but within the normal range, the number of pts. whose sperm count became normal as a result of treatment was significantly (p<0.05) larger in the gps. administered mecobalamin than in the placebo group. On further analysis, a therapeutic effect was noted in a somewhat broader gp., with the total responders amounting to 57.1% of pts. with a sperm count of 20×10^6/ml or less (*Kumamoto Y et al. Clinical efficacy of mecobalamin in treatment of oligozoospermia: Results of double-blind comparative clinical study. Acta Urol Jpn 34:1109-32, 1988*).

Pernicious anemia, which is rare during childbearing ages, usually leads to infertility in men and women which is reversible with vitamin B$_{12}$ supplementation (*Marty H. [Pernicious anemia as cause of secondary sterility.] Schweiz Med Wochenschr 114(5):178-79, 1984*).

Vitamin C: 200 - 1000 mg daily

May protect against endogenous oxidative DNA damage to sperm (*Fraga CG et al. Ascorbic acid protects against endogenous oxidative DNA damage in human sperm. Proc Natl Acad Sci U S A 88(24):11003-6, 1991*).

Supplementation may be beneficial to men.

Experimental Placebo-controlled Study: Male heavy smokers (1 pack/d) received either 0, 200 or 1000 mg vitamin C daily. After 1 mo., sperm quality improved proportional to the level of vitamin supplementation; the placebo gp. showed no changes (*Dawson E, Harris W, Powell L. Effect of vitamin C supplementation on sperm quality of heavy smokers. FASEB J 5(4):A915, 1991*).

Experimental Placebo-controlled Study: 30 infertile but otherwise healthy men received either 200 mg vitamin C, 1,000 mg vitamin C or placebo daily. There were weekly measures of sperm count, viability, motility, agglutination, abnormalities and immaturity. While the placebo gp. showed few changes, after one wk. the 1,000 mg gp. showed a 140% increase in sperm count as well as improvements in all other measures. The 200 mg gp. showed a 112% increase in sperm count as well as less improvement than the 1,000 mg gp. on all other measures. After 3 wks., both treatment gps. continued to improve, and the men in the 200 mg gp. caught up to those in the 1,000 mg gp., suggesting that the lower dosage may be as effective in enhancing fertility. After 60 days, all of the vitamin C gp. had impregnated their wives, compared to none of the unsupplemented group. Results suggest that vitamin C supplementation is effective for male infertility characterized by sperm agglutination in excess of 25% (*Dawson EB et al. Effect of ascorbic acid on male fertility. Ann N Y Acad Sci 498:312-23, 1987*).

Supplementation may enhance the effect of clomiphene in anovulatory women.

Experimental Study: When ascorbic acid 400 mg/d was combined with therapeutic doses of clomiphene, menses and ovulation were induced in 17/42 women who were not responsive to clomiphene alone (*Igarashi M. Augmentative effect of ascorbic acid upon induction of human ovulation in clomiphene-ineffective anovulatory women. Int J Fertility 22:168-73, 1977*).

- -

MINERALS

Iron:

Conception may be prevented in women with depleted iron stores. If so, supplementation may restore fertility.

- with Vitamin C:

Experimental Study: 113 women aged 18-54 with increased scalp hair shedding were evaluated. In response to reduced serum ferritin values (≤40 ng/ml) compared to women without hair loss, daily oral iron 35 mg and vitamin C 200 mg supplementation was provided. 7 pts. became pregnant within 28 weeks. 3/7 had been investigated for infertility for 5-9 yrs. without success and the remaining 4 did not become preganant during the previous 30 mo. despite regular menses and unprotected sexual intercourse (*Rushton DH et al. Ferritin and fertility. Letter. Lancet 337:1554, 1991*).

Selenium:

Deficiency may impair male reproductive function.

Review Article: In a study presented at the Fourth Int. Sympos. on Selenium in Biol. and Med., Tubingen U., Germany, July, 1988, 12 different selenium-containing proteins were identified in the testes; 2 of these proteins are structually important in sperm. Severe selenium deficiency in rats led to a 60% reduction in testes weight, and selenium deficiency is well known to produce infertility in farm animals (*Schrauzer GN. Benefits of natural selenium. Anabolism 7(4):5, 1988*).

Negative Animal Experimental Study: 24 crossbred boars were fed a low selenium diet. 12 of them were injected every 2 wks. with sodium selenite while 12 served as saline-treated controls. Although concentrations of selenium in serum, semen and reproductive tissues were much lower in control boars than in treated boars, no apparent impairment of sperm morphology or viability resulted from low selenium status (*Segerson EC et al. Selenium and reproductive function in boars fed a low selenium diet. J Anim Sci 53(5):1360-67, 1981*).

Serum selenium may be <u>inversely</u> correlated with male fertility.

Observational Study: In a study of 142 men with variable semen quality and fertility, the serum selenium level was significantly higher (p<0.001) in infertile men than in fertile men (*Saaranen M et al. Lead, magnesium, selenium and zinc in human seminal fluid: comparison with semen parameters and fertility. Hum Reprod 2(6):475-79, 1987*).

Semen selenium may be an indicator of male reproductive function.

Negative Observational Study: Semen samples from 211 normozoospermic, oligozoospermic, asthenozoospermic, and azoospermic men failed to reveal significant correlations between the selenium level in the seminal plasma and sperm count or motility. However, in view of the known poor correlation between these 2 sperm parameters and the incidence of pregnancy, the assessment of the fertilizing potential of normozoospermic ejaculates with low semen selenium levels is suggested (*Roy AC et al. Lack of correlation of selenium level in human semen with sperm count/motility. Arch Androl 25(1):59-62, 1990*).

Observational Study: Selenium in seminal plasma is mainly derived from the prostate and the seminal content of selenium is dependent on the proportion of prostatic secretion in seminal plasma and on the sperm count. Provisional measurements suggest lower sperm selenium levels at abnormally low or high sperm counts (*Behne D. Selenium, rubidium and zinc in human semen and semen fractions. Int J Androl 11(5):415-23, 1988*).

Negative Observational Study: In a study of 142 men with variable semen quality and fertility, no significant difference in seminal plasma selenium was found between fertile and infertile men, and there was no correlation between seminal plasma selenium and sperm density or motility (*Saaranen M et al. Lead, magnesium, selenium and zinc in human seminal fluid: comparison with semen parameters and fertility. Hum Reprod 2(6):475-79, 1987*).

Observational Study: Semen selenium was measured in 125 men from couples complaining of infertility. There was a significant positive correlation between sperm count and semen selenium, and sperm motility was maximal at semen selenium levels ranging from 50-69 mg/ml. A follow-up 4.5-5 yrs. later revealed that low semen selenium levels were associated with male infertility (*Bleau G et al. Semen selenium and human fertility. Fertil Steril 42(6):890-94, 1984*).

Zinc:

Deficiency may be associated with oligospermia, decreased sperm motility and decreased serum testosterone levels.

Observational Study: Zinc levels in the granulocytes and platelets were significantly decreased in 1/3 of of 23 randomly selected elderly subjects aged 65-85 compared to younger age controls. Lower zinc levels were associated with decreased serum testosterone and dihydrotestosterone levels in the males (*Prasad AS. Zinc in growth and development and spectrum of human zinc deficiency. J Am Coll Nutr 7(5):377-84, 1988*).

Observational Study: Compared to 40 controls, the zinc levels in the seminal plasma of 105 infertile azoospermic men were significantly lower. Seminal plasma zinc levels were also reduced in oligospermic pts., but the difference was not statistically significant (*Mbtizvo MT et al. Seminal plasma zinc levels in fertile and infertile men. S Afr Med J 71:266, 1987*).

Experimental Study: Dietary zinc restriction for normal subjects resulted in a slight decrease in sperm count during restriction; oligospermia became significant during the early phase of zinc repletion. There was also a significant decrease in serum testosterone and dihydrotestosterone levels (*Abbasi AA et al. Experimental zinc deficiency in man: Effect on testicular function. J Lab Clin Med 96(3):544-50, 1980*).

Observational Study: Zinc levels in seminal plasma of normals were compared to those of oligospermic, asthenospermic and azoospermic subjects. A linear direct relationship was found between zinc levels and motility of spermatozoans (*Skandhan KP et al. Semen electrolytes in normal and infertile subjects. II. Zinc. Experientia 34(11):1476-77, 1978*).

Supplementation may be beneficial to men.

Experimental Study: 14 infertile males age 24-45 with idiopathic oligospermia (<40 million/ml) received zinc sulfate 220 mg/d. After 4 mo., seminal zinc levels significantly increased and there was significant improvement in sperm count, number of progressively motile and normal spermatozoa, and acid phosphatase activity. Serum zinc levels were unchanged. Wives of 2 pts. conceived (*Tikkiwal M et al. Effect of zinc administration on seminal zinc and fertility of oligospermic males. Indian J Physiol Pharmacol 31(1):30-34, 1987*).

Experimental Study: 100 infertile men with low seminal plasma zinc concentrations received zinc sulfate 440 mg daily for 60 days to 2 years. 2 mo. after starting treatment, seminal zinc levels were significantly higher; there were significant changes in sperm count and motility only in a sub-gp. of 36 men who started treatment after varicocelectomy. Of that sub-gp., only those who impregnated their wives showed a significant increase in sperm motility at that time; those who remained infertile showed a significant increase in sperm motility after 12 months. 18/65 men (28%) without varicocelectomy successfully impregnated their wives, while 18/36 (50%) of the post-surgical pts. did so (*Takihara H et al. Zinc sulfate therapy for infertile males with or without varicocelectomy. Urology 29(6):638-41, 1987*).

Experimental Study: 37 males with infertility of >5 yrs. duration whose sperm counts were <25 million (and, if >15 million, whose sperm motility was under 30%) who had no other known cause of infertility received zinc sulfate 120 mg twice daily (60 mg elemental zinc daily) for 40-50 days. In pts. with initially low plasma testosterone (#22), mean sperm count increased significantly from 8-20 million. Testosterone also increased significantly and 9/22 wives became pregnant. In the 15/37 with initially normal plasma testosterone, sperm count increased, though not significantly, plasma testosterone did not change, and no pregnancies occurred (*Netter A et al. Effect of zinc administration on plasma testosterone, dehydrotestosterone and sperm count. Arch Androl 7(1):69-73, 1981*).

- -

OTHER NUTRITIONAL FACTORS

L-Arginine: 4 gm daily

Deficiency may be associated with a decreased sperm count and motility.

Experimental Study: The sperm count of normal men given an arginine-deficient diet for 9 days was decreased. It returned to normal within several wks. after the restoration of arginine to the diet (*Holt et al cited in Tanimura J. Studies on arginine supplementation in human semen. Part I: the arginine contents of normal and sterile human semen. Bull Osaka Med Sch 13:76-83, 1967*).

Observational Study: Measurement of free and bound arginine in the semen of normal and infertile men showed a positive correlation between sperm count and bound arginine as well as between sperm motility and free arginine content (*Tanimura J. Studies on arginine supplementation in human semen. Part I: the arginine contents of normal and sterile human semen. Bull Osaka Med Sch 13:76-83, 1967*).

Abnormal arginine metabolism is associated with pathospermia (*Papp Gy et al. The importance of arginine content and arginase activity in fertility. Andrologia 11:37, 1979; Papp Gy et al. The role of arginine and arginase activities in fertility. Urol Nephrol Szle 5:189, 1978; Tanimura J. Studies on arginine in human sermen. Bull Osaka Med Sch 12:90, 1967*).

Observational Study: 15.7% of 47 pts. with pathospermia had mean seminal arginine concentrations which were significantly lower (p<0.01) by 57.3% than normozoospermic pts. (#28), while arginine values in the remainder of the pathospermia gp. were similar to those of the normozoospermic group. The mean seminal arginine concentrations of the azoospermic gp. (#29) were 27.5% lower (p<0.02) than those of the normozoospermic gp., while the arginine concentrations of the oligozoospermic gp. (#57) corresponded to those of the normozoospermic group. There were similar findings in regard to ornithine. Results indicate that the reduced basic amino acid concentrations found in a number of these pts. are primarily due to a reduction in the arginine and ornithine levels of the seminal plasma, and suggest that pts. should be selected for arginine supplementation based on seminal plasma arginine concentrations (*Papp G et al. The role of basic amino acids of the seminal plasma in fertility. Int Urol Nephrol 15(2):195-203, 1983*).

Supplementation may be beneficial to men.

Negative Experimental Double-blind Study: Supplementation with arginine 4 gm daily for 3 mo. failed to improve sperm count density or motility in infertile men with severe oligospermia (<10 million sperm per ejaculate) and there was no difference in conception rates between the 2 groups (*Pryor JP et al. Controlled clinical trial of arginine for infertile men with oligospermia. Br J Urol 50:47-50, 1978*).

In vitro Experimental Study: The addition of L-arginine increased human sperm motility (*Keller DW, Polakoski KL. L-arginine stimulation of human sperm motility in vitro. Biol Reprod 13:154-7, 1975*).

Experimental Study: 178 men with mild to severe problems with sperm count and motility received L-arginine 4 gm daily. After 3 mo., 111 (62%) had a marked improvement, 21 (12%) had a moderate improvement, and 46 (26%) had no improvement. 11/93 (12%) of men with sperm counts below 20 million per ejaculate increased their sperm count at least 100%, compared to 31/85 (36%) of men with sperm counts of 20-50 million per ejaculate, suggesting that men with mild oligospermia may have a better response. There were no side effects (*Schachter A et al. Treatment of oligospermia with the amino acid arginine. J Urol 110(3):311-13, 1973*).

- with aspartic acid:

Supplementation may be beneficial to men.

Experimental Controlled Study: 130 hypofertile men aged 22-43 (61 with asthenospermia, 69 with oligoasthenospermia) were treated with gonadotropins, antibiotics and/or arginine aspartate; 89 of the 130 men received arginine aspartate 9-18 g/d. Arginine aspartate was very effective when there was asthenospermia due to reduction of the nemaspermic cellular energy without cytostructural damage; it increased the effect of antibiotic and/or anti-inflammatory therapy in asthenospermia due to or associated with phlogosis of the seminal tract, and also increased the effect of gonadotropin therapy in cases of oligoasthenospermia which were not associated with seminal phlogosis. Higher dosages than 9 gm/d did not further improve the outcome. Results suggest that arginine aspartate may be considered the best therapy in cases of male hypofertility caused by a reduction in sperm motility; it has also been proven extremely effective when associated with gonadotropin therapy in many cases of alterations of spermatogenetic function (*De Aloysio D et al. The clinical use of arginine aspartate in male infertility. Acta Eur Fertil 13(3):133-67, 1982*).

- -

OTHER FACTORS

Avoid being excessively underweight or overweight.

Review Article: Low body weight is a risk factor for amenorrhea and infertility. In some studies, over half of all women seeking treatment for infertility were amenorrheic following a period of weight loss. While body weight and BMI are valuable risk indicators, the effects of composition of the diet override the effects of body weight, the hypothalamus being more sensitive to blood composition resulting from nutrients in the diet. It is wise to defer all attempts at conception for at least 3-4 mo. on a good diet following recovery from amenorrhea (*Wynn A, Wynn M. The need for nutritional assessment in the treatment of the infertile patient. J Nutr Med 1:315-24, 1990*).

Observational Study: 276 infertile women in whom there was evidence of ovulatory dysfunction were compared to fertile controls. In 204 nulligravid women, body weight for height 85% or less than "ideal" was associated with a 4.7-fold increase in risk of infertility associated with ovulatory dysfunction, while nulligravid women who were 120% or more over their ideal wt. had a relative risk of 2.1 for ovulatory infertility. Neither association was seen among women who had been previously pregnant. Results suggest that about 6% of primary infertility in which ovulatory dysfunction is present results from being excessively underweight, and another 6% from being excessively overweight (*Green BB et al. Risk of ovulatory infertility in relation to body weight. Fertil Steril 50(9);621-26, 1988*).

INFLAMMATION

See Also: ALLERGY

VITAMINS

Vitamin B12:

Supplementation may be beneficial.

    Animal Experimental Study: A minimum of 5 μgm/kg oral vitamin B12 administered to rats was shown to have a significant anti-inflammatory effect which was less pronounced than 20 mg oral phenylbutazone (*Hanck A, Weiser H. Analgesic and anti-inflammatory properties of vitamins. Int J Vitam Nutr Res (suppl)27:189-206, 1985*).

    Experimental Study: 40 pts. with acute bursitis (mostly sub-deltoid) received vitamin B12 1000 micrograms IM daily for 7-10 days; then 3 times weekly for 2-3 wks.; then 1-2 times weekly for 2-3 wks. (depending upon their rate of progress). All but 2 or 3 improved with rapid relief of pain and subjective symptoms, sometimes within a few hours. Complete relief was often noted in several days. Follow-up x-rays of cases of calcific bursitis showed considerable resorption of calcium deposits (*Klemes IS. Vitamin B12 in acute subdeltoid bursitis. Indust Med Surg 26:20-2, 1957*).

Vitamin C:

Inflammation may enhance degradation and excretion.

    In vitro Experimental Study: While resting human neutrophils did not oxidize ascorbic acid, the vitamin was effectively oxidized when added to suspensions of activated human neutrophils. Since oxidation favors degradation and excretion, inflammatory reactions could cause significantly accelerated losses of the vitamin (*Roberts P et al. Vitamin C and inflammation. Med Biol 62:88, 1984*).

Supplementation may be beneficial.

    Animal Experimental Study: When foot pad inflammation was induced in rats, vitamin C given 10 min. prior to the induction of inflammation was ineffective, while vitamin C given 2 1/2 hrs. afterwards significantly decreased swelling (*Spillert C et al. Inhibitory effect of high dose ascorbic acid on inflammatory edema. Agents Actions 27:401-02, 1989*).

    Animal Experimental Study: Oral vitamin C administered to rats was shown to have a significant dose-dependent anti-inflammatory effect comparable to phenylbutazone 20 mg at a minimum of 125 mg/kg; by comparison a minimum of 500 mg/kg was required for a significant dose-dependent analgesic effect comparable to phenylbutazone 20 mg (*Hanck A, Weiser H. Analgesic and anti-inflammatory properties of vitamins. Int J Vitam Nutr Res (suppl)27:189-206, 1985*).

    Animal Experimental Study: Vitamin C (20 mg/kg) was as effective as phenylbutazone (50 mg/kg) and twice as effective as ASA (100 mg/kg) in inhibiting induced peritonitis-polyarthritis swelling in rats. It was also 60% as effective as phenylbutazone and 300% as effective as ASA in inhibiting adjuvant arthritis at the same dose (*Dolbreare FA, Martlage KA. Some anti-inflammatory properties of ascorbic acid. Proc Soc Exp Biol Med 139:540-43, 1972*).

- and <u>Bioflavonoids</u>:

Supplementation may be beneficial.

Case Report: 38 year-old male presented with severe <u>subpatellar bursitis</u> with extensive local swelling and heat, extreme tenderness, severe pain and limitation of motion. He was treated with vitamin C along with citrus bioflavonoids 200 mg 3 times daily. Within 24 hrs. there was noticable diminuation in swelling and pain, and in 72 hrs. the lesion had subsided almost completely, leaving only slight local tenderness (*Biskind MS, Martin WC. The use of citrus flavonoids in infection. II. Am J Digest Dis 22:41-45, 1955*).

<u>Vitamin E</u>:

May reduce inflammation.

In vitro Experimental Study: D-alpha-tocopherol was found to inhibit both chemotaxis and chemiluminescence of activated neutrophilic granulocytes (*Blankenhorn G. Vitamin E: Clinical research from Europe. Nutr Dietary Consult, June, 1988*).

Supplementation may be beneficial.

Review Article: Animal studies suggest that vitamin E has an anti-inflammatory action. This may be due to its strong action to protect lysosome and other membranes which may inhibit histamine liberation from granules of mast cells and serotonin liberation from inside the tissue cells. Supporting this theory is that fact that vitamin E acts slowly, protects enlargement of inflammation, shortens its prognosis, and has lesser effects in suppressing inflammation already existing (*Kamimura M. Antiinflammatory effect of vitamin E. J Vitaminol 18:204-09, 1972*).

Experimental Studies: Vitamin E was effective in treating various inflammatory skin diseases (*Kamimura M. Shinyaku to Rinsho 5:363, 1956; Yasuda T et al. Theor Dermatol Urol (Japan) 19:69, 1957*).

<u>Vitamin K</u>$_1$:

Supplementation may be beneficial.

Animal Experimental Study: Oral, IM and IV vitamin K$_1$ administered to rats was shown to have a significant anti-inflammatory effect. Oily solutions, as the vehicle, were more effective than water-dispersible ones (*Hanck A, Weiser H. Analgesic and anti-inflammatory properties of vitamins. Int J Vitam Nutr Res (suppl) 27:189-206, 1985*).

MINERALS

<u>Copper</u>:

Accumulation of the superoxide radical as a result of reduced Cu,Zn superoxide dismutase activity (which requires adequate copper) may contribute to the development of inflammatory diseases (*Sorenson JRJ. Copper complexes offer a physiological approach to treatment of chronic diseases. Progress in Medical Chemistry Vol. 26, 1989*).

<u>Zinc</u>:

Accumulation of the superoxide radical as a result of reduced Cu,Zn superoxide dismutase activity (which requires adequate zinc) may contribute to the development of inflammatory diseases (*Sorenson JRJ. Copper complexes offer a physiological approach to treatment of chronic diseases. Progress in Medical Chemistry Vol. 26, 1989*).

Important in the inflammatory response.

Review Article: Zinc in physiological concentrations can cause approx. a 40% inhibition of immunologically induced histamine and leukotriene release from both basophils and mast cells. In addition, zinc modulates serotonin release from platelets, macrophage and neutrophil phagocytosis, lymphocyte proliferation, and immune hemolysis (*Marone G et al. Physiological concentrations of zinc inhibit the release of histamine from human basophils and lung mast cells. Agents Actions 18:103-106, 1986*).

- -

OTHER NUTRITIONAL FACTORS

Amino Acids:

- Creatine:

Supplementation may be beneficial.

Animal Experimental Study: Oral supplementation was as effective as phenylbutazone in suppressing acute and chronic inflammatory responses in rats and did not produce GI ulceration at effective doses. It exhibited analgesic activity (*Khanna NK, Madan BR. Studies on the anti-inflammatory activity of creatine. Arch Int Pharmacodyn Ther 231(2):340-50, 1978*).

- D-Phenylalanine:

Supplementation may be beneficial.

Theoretical Discussion: D-phenylalanine and possibly other enkephalinase inhibitors may protect peripheral enkephalin or other endorphins generated from the adrenal medulla where high concentrations of precursors are present and may also inhibit enkephalinases in joints. Both of these actions would result in accumulaton of endorphins in synovial fluid, counteracting the effects of prostaglandin-mediated inflammation (*Millinger GS. Neutral amino acid therapy for the management of chronic pain. Cranio 4(2):156-63, 1986*).

- L-Tryptophan or
  D,L-Tryptophan:

Supplementation may be beneficial.

Animal Experimental Study: Oral supplementation was as effective as phenylbutazone in suppressing acute and chronic inflammatory responses in rats, but not by exerting a counter-irritant effect as do almost all anti-inflammatory drugs (*Madan BR, Khanna NK. Anti-inflammatory activity of L-tryptophan and DL-tryptophan. Indian J Med Res 68:708-13, 1978*).

- D,L-Valine:

Supplementation may be beneficial.

Animal Experimental Study: Oral supplementation of rats was effective in suppressing acute and chronic inflammatory responses, although it had no analgesic activity. Its effect was not via counter-irritation (*Khanna NK, Madan BR. Anti-inflammatory activity of DL-valine. Indian J Exp Biol 16:834-36, 1978*).

Bioflavonoids:

May inhibit arachidonic acid metabolism.

Animal Experimental Study: Flavonoids that are selective inhibitors of lipoxygenase activity *in vitro* administered orally to mice inhibited dose-dependently the development of paw edema after carrageenin injection and induced a dose-dependent inhibition of inflammatory exudates following intraperitoneal injection of carrageenin. The selectivity of flavonoids towards lipoxygenase is not retained *in vivo* since they behave as dual inhibitors and PGE_2 and leukotriene B_4 formation in peritoneal exudates (*Ferràndiz ML, Alcaraz MJ. Anti-inflammatory activity and inhibition of arachidonic metabolism by flavonoids. Agents Actions 32(3-4):283-8, 1991*).

- Quercetin:

Inhibits the lipoxygenase pathway of arachidonic acid metabolism (which produces some of the most potent inflammatory mediators) while exerting a lesser inhibitory effect on the cyclooxygenase pathway which, in addition to producing less potent activators of inflammation, also produces anti-inflammatory prostaglandins (*Bauman J et al. Prostaglandins 20(4):627-37, 1980*).

Inhibits histamine release from basophils and mast cells (*Middleton E, Drzewieki G. Naturally occurring flavonoids and human basophil histamine release. Arch Allergy Appl Immunol 77:155-57, 1985; Amella M et al. Inhibition of mast cell histamine release by flavonoids and bioflavonoids. Planta Medica 51:16-20, 1985*).

Decreases neutrophil lysosomal enzyme secretion to stabilize cell membranes and decrease lipid peroxidation, leukotriene release, and collagen breakdown by hyaluronidase (*Busse WW et al. Flavonoid modulation of human neutrophil function. J Allergy Clin Immunol 73:801-9, 1984*).

Omega-3 Fatty Acids: minimum 8 week trial

Eicosapentaenoic acid (EPA) and docosahexaenoic acid (DHA).

Highest in cold-water fish such as herring, mackerel, salmon, bluefish and tuna (or EPA and DHA can be derived in the body from α-linolenic acid).

Suggested dosage: 4 g/d in divided doses

WARNING: Supplementation may require additional vitamin E intake to prevent increased membrane peroxidation and cellular damage (*Laganiere S, Fernandes G. High peroxidizability of subcellular membrane induced by high fish oil diet is reversed by vitamin E. Clin Res 35:A565, 1987*).

Supplementation may reduce inflammation by changing the balance of prostaglandins and leukotrienes (which are powerful mediators of inflammation) (*Moncada S et al. Leucocytes and tissue injury: The use of eicosapentaenoic acid in the control of white cell activation. Wien Klin Wochenschr 98(4):104-6, 1986*).

Animal Experimental Study: Rats received either their normal diet or a diet enriched with fish-oil-derived fatty acids. Acute and chronic phases of inflammation were induced by antigenic challenge and examined in the rat air-pouch model. In rats receiving the enriched diet, there was reduced production of arachidonic acid metabolites, prostaglandin E_2 and leukotriene B_4 in the exudate in the chronic phase of inflammation, but not in the acute phase, associated with increased leukocyte infiltration. Carrageenin-induced paw edema was not influenced by the diet; however, the diet appeared to suppress a delayed-type skin reaction (*Yoshino S, Ellis EF. Effect of a fish-oil-supplemented diet on inflammation and immunological processes in rats. Int Arch Allergy Appl Immunol 84(3):233-40, 1987*).

Animal Experimental Study: Supplementation of a standard rat diet with 240 mg/kg/day EPA for 4 wks. significantly decreased the concentration of PGE_2 and TXE_2 in inflammatory exudate derived from implantation of carrageenin impregnated sponges. In addition, edema induced by injection of carrageenin into rat paws was significantly reduced in animals fed an EPA-rich diet. Results suggest that supplementation with EPA could, mainly by reducing prostaglandin synthesis, offer a novel and non-toxic approach to the modulation of an inflammatory response (*Terano T et al. Eicosapentaenoic acid as a modulator of inflammation. Biochem Pharmacol 35(5):779-85, 1986*).

Experimental Study: The diets of 7 normal subjects were supplemented with 3.2 gm EPA or 1.8 gm MaxEPA daily for 6 weeks. EPA in neutrophils was increased 7 fold without any increase in arachidonic acid. When the neutrophils were activated, there was a 37% reduction in the release of arachidonic acid and a 48% reduction in the inflammatory products of this pathway. In addition, the adherence of neutrophils to bovine epithelial cells as monolayers treated with leukotriene B_4 was completely inhibited. The results suggest that diets enriched with fish oil-derived fatty acids have anti-inflammatory effects by inhibiting the 5-lipoxygenase pathway, thus causing a reduction in the release of leukotrienes along with a reduction in the release of superoxide from neutrophils (*Lee TH et al. Effect of dietary enrichment with eicosapentaenoic acid and docosahexaenoic acids on in vitro neutrophil and monocyte leukotriene generation and neutrophil function. N Engl J Med 312:1217-23, 1985*).

<u>Omega-6 Fatty Acids</u>:

linoleic acid → GLA → DGLA → prostaglandin E_1

Evening primrose oil is a rich source of GLA and has been used in many studies. Although borage and blackcurrent oils are richer in GLA, it is not known how their effectiveness compares.

Supplementation may be beneficial in reducing acute inflammatory reactions.

Experimental Placebo-controlled Study: 12 healthy volunteers received olive oil supplements for a 2-wk. baseline period and were then randomly divided into 3 gps. One gp. received borage oil 0.48 g/d with vitamin E, one gp. received black current oil 0.48 g/d with vitamin E, and the third gp. continued on olive oil. After 6 wks., there was a significant elevation of DGLA in the experimental gps. compared to controls (p<0.05) and a decreased capacity of polymorphonuclear cells to general pro-inflammatory leukotriene B_4 which paralleled the increase in DGLA. An increase in doage of borage oil to 1.5 g/d failed to significantly increase the inhibition of leukotriene B_4 (*Ziboh VA, Fletcher MP. Dose-response effects of dietary γ-linolenic acid-enriched oils on human polymorphonuclear-neutrophil biosynthesis of leukotriene B4. <u>Am J Clin Nutr</u> 55:39-45, 1992*).

In vitro Experimental Study: Rats were given EPO 0.75 ml daily in addition to their regular diets. After 2 wks., their neutrophils demonstrated a >60% reduction in chemotaxis compared to controls, suggesting that EPO influences the responsiveness of inflammatory cells involved in acute immune reactions (*Kunkel SL et al. Suppression of chronic inflammation by evening primrose oil. <u>Prog Lipid Res</u> 20(1-4):885-88, 1981*).

Supplementation may be beneficial in reducing chronic inflammatory reactions.

Animal Experimental Study: Rats whose diets were supplemented with EPO 0.75 ml daily 2 wks. before adjuvant challenge demonstrated both a delay in the onset and suppression of the polyarthritis response (*Kunkel SL et al. Suppression of chronic inflammation by evening primrose oil. <u>Prog Lipid Res</u> 20(1-4):885-88, 1981*).

<u>Proteolytic Enzymes</u>:

Administration may speed healing of injuries.

Experimental Double-blind Study: 64 college football players randomly received 10 pills daily containing either a concentrated proteolytic enzyme mixture or placebo. The experimental gp. sustained fewer time-loss injuries and were able to return to performance sooner than the control group. The number of minor time-loss injuries sustained in the control gp. greatly exceeded the number sustained by the experimental gp., while the number of major injuries sustained in each gp. was of equal number (*Cichoke AJ, Marty L. The use of proteolytic enzymes with soft tissue athletic injuires. <u>Am Chiropractor</u>, October 1981, p. 32*).

- <u>Chymotrypsin</u>:

Animal Experimental Study: Following experimentally-induced pleural effusions in rats, injections of chymotrypsin increased the rate of lymphatic flow from the pleural space without increasing capillary permeability (*Gabler WL, Fosdick LS. <u>Proc Soc Exp Biol Med</u> 120:160-63, 1965*).

Note: Oral doses have been shown to raise plasma levels:

Experimental Study: Plasma chymotrypsin levels significantly increased in 27 pts. receiving oral supplementation (*Avakian S. <u>J Clin Pharm Therapeut</u> 5:712-15, 1964*).

- <u>Trypsin</u>:

May reduce edema.

Animal Experimental Study: Suppressed experimentally induced egg white edema in rats (*Martin GJ et al. <u>Proc Soc Exp Biol Med</u> 86:636-38, 1954*).

Supplementation may be beneficial.

> **Experimental Study:** In a study of 538 pts., 428 of whom had acute thrombophlebitis, there was "a dramatic subsidence of all signs and symptoms of acute inflammation in 99.3% when trypsin was administered IV" (*Innerfield I et al. Proc Soc Exp Biol Med 112:189-90, 1963*).

- -

COMBINED SUPPLEMENTATION

Proteolytic Enzymes and
Bioflavonoids and
Vitamin C:

Combined supplementation may be at least as effective as non-steroidal anti-inflammatory drugs.

> **Animal Experimental Study:** In a rat study, when compared against the action of 7 non-steroidal anti-inflammatory drugs by 4 tests (histamine-induced wheal, dextran and carrageenin induced edemas, and permeability to Evans blue in the peritoneal cavity), a combination of oral proteolytic enzymes (chymotrypsin & trypsin), flavonoids (hesperidin-methyl-chalcone & methyl-4-esculetol sodium monoethanoate) and ascorbic acid showed a "more complete spectrum of action than the non-steroid anti-inflammatory substances against the initial symptoms of inflammation" as only the combination was effective in decreasing the effects of histamine and dextran (*Taraye JP, Lauressergues H. Advantages of a combination of proteolytic enzymes, flavonoids and ascorbic acid in comparison with non-steroid inflammatory drugs. Arzneim Forsch 27(1):1144-49, 1977*).

- -

OTHER FACTORS

Rule out gluten sensitivity.

May cause pericarditis.

> **Case Reports:** 2 pts. with celiac disease presented with recurrent pericarditis. Treatment with a gluten-free diet led to clinical and EKG improvement of the pericarditis (*Dawes PT, Atherton ST. Coeliac disease presenting as recurrent pericarditis. Lancet 1:1021-2, 1981*).

INNER EAR DYSFUNCTION

(including HEARING LOSS, MENIERE'S SYNDROME, TINNITUS and VERTIGO)

See Also: ATHEROSCLEROSIS
"HYPOGLYCEMIA" (FUNCTIONAL)

DIETARY FACTORS

Reduce <u>fat</u> and <u>cholesterol</u> to combat hyperlipidemia.

Animal Experimental Study: Some of a gp. of chinchillas rendered hyperlipidemic by a 1% cholesterol diet or maintained on a normal diet were exposed to bandpass noise. Compared to normal diet animals, the hyperlipidemic animals exhibited elevated hearing thresholds whether not not they were exposed to noise. Also, the hyperlipidemic animals exposed to noise exhibited a greater hair cell loss in the first turn of the cochlea than did similarly exposed normal animals. Results suggest that maintenance on a high-cholesterol diet can cause a high-frequency hearing loss and can increase susceptibility to noise-induced hearing loss (*Sikora MA et al. Diet-induced hyperlipidemia and auditory dysfunction. <u>Acta Otolaryngol (Stockh)</u> 102(5-6):372-81, 1986*).

Animal Experimental Study: Rats bred to become spontaneously hypertensive and normal controls were subjected to intermittent noise with and without an atherogenic diet. The noise-exposed hypertensive rats fed the atherogenic diet had greater hearing losses than those on the normal diet, with significantly decreased cochlear blood flow. Results suggest that, although hypertension plus an atherogenic diet alone do not produce significant hearing loss, hypertension, a chronic atherogenic diet, and chronic noise are devastating, even when the noise is of a moderate intensity (*Pillsbury HC. Hypertension, hyperlipoproteinemia, chronic noise exposure: Is there synergism in cochlear pathology? <u>Laryngoscope</u> 96(10): 1112-38, 1986*).

Observational Study: 33% of 90 pts. with fluctuant sensorineural hearing loss had hyperlipoproteinemia and 13% were borderline (*Gosselin EJ, Yanick P Jr. Audiologic and metabolic findings in 90 patients with fluctuant hearing loss. <u>J Am Audiol Soc</u> 2(1):15-18, 1976*).

Hyperlipidemia may cause hearing impairment by increasing erythrocyte aggregation (*Spencer J. Hyperlipoproteinemia and inner ear disease. <u>J Int Acad Metabology</u> 4:38-42, 1975*) and rigidity (*Browning GG et al. Blood viscosity as a factor in sensorineural hearing impairment. <u>Lancet</u> 1:121-23, 1986*); thus reducing the flow of oxygen and nutrients to the inner ear.

For hyperlipidemic patients, reduction in saturated fats may be beneficial.

Experimental Study: Several children with bilateral fluctuating sensorineural hearing losses and hyperlipidemia demonstrated a positive correlation between hearing and lipid levels. With dietary controls, the cholesterol levels returned to near normal and hearing returned to near baseline (*Strome M et al. Hyperlipidemia in association with childhood sensorineural hearing loss. <u>Laryngoscope</u> 98(2):165-9, 1988*).

Experimental Study: Over 1400 pts. with inner ear symptoms and hyperlipoproteinemia were put on individualized diets and given nutritional counseling. In most pts., dizziness cleared promptly, the sensation of pressure in the ears and associated headache was quickly relieved, hearing improved and stabilized (as demonstrated in the pure tone audiogram and in speech discrimination scores) and tinnitus often lessened in severity and sometimes disappeared (*Spencer JT Jr. Hyperlipoproteinemia, hyperinsulinism and Meniere's disease. <u>South Med J</u> 74:1194-97, 1981*).

Experimental Controlled Crossover Study: Gp. on low saturated fat diet had superior hearing after 5 yrs. compared to gp. on their usual high saturated fat diet. 4 yrs. after gps. crossed over, hearing had improved in the gp. now on the restricted diet and had deteriorated in the gp. on the high saturated fat diet. The incidence of coronary heart disease followed the same pattern. Hearing losses which occurred were usually of the sensorineural type. Audiological findings indicated that the diet may well arrest, if not reverse, hearing loss (*Rosen S et al. Dietary prevention of hearing loss. Acta Otolaryngol (Stockh) 70(4):242-47, 1970*).

Avoid sugar.

Said to cause inner ear dysfunction by promoting reactive hypoglycemia and consequent adrenalin release which, in turn, causes vasoconstriction.

Patients may have hyperinsulinemia and hypoglycemia; if so a low carbohydrate (or a low simple carbohydrate) diet may be beneficial.

Observational Study: 59 pts. with audio-vestibular disturbances and 22 controls received a prolonged oral glucose tolerance test. 67.7% of pts. had a pathologic GTT; of these, 16.9% had glucose intolerance and 50.8% had reactive hypoglycemia. In the latter case, a statistically significant difference with the control gp. was found (*Carrillo V et al. [Disorders of glucose tolerance and pathology of the labyrinth.] Acta Otorhinolaryngol Belg 38(5):474-84, 1984*) (*in French*).

Experimental Study: Nearly 75% of 50 Meniere's pts. had either an abnormal glucose tolerance test or high insulin levels. They were placed on a low carbohydrate, high protein diet. Nearly all controlled their vertigo, and a few with concurrent tinnitus or hearing loss also overcame those symptoms. Findings suggest that impaired ear circulation, possibly caused by abnormal glucose and insulin levels, may be the primary cause of Meniere's disease. The standard glucose tolerance test is of little value unless it is done concurrently with insulin levels (*Proctor B, Proctor C. Metabolic management in Meniere's disease. Ann Otol Rhinol Laryngol 90(6 Pt 1):615-18, 1981*).

Clinical Observations: 1,400 pts. were evaluated with both inner ear symptoms and lipid abnormalities. It has become increasingly apparent that most pts. seen by otolaryngologists because of Meniere's disease come from the same population gp. who are prone to obesity, maturity-onset diabetes, coronary heart disease, and atherosclerosis, and share the common problem of being unable to handle refined carbohydrates well. They were helped by replacing refined carbohydrates with complex carbohydrate having increased fiber. When Meniere's pts. have this condition, dietary management has been found to be the most effective therapy (*Spencer JT Jr. Hyperlipoproteinemia, hyperinsulinism and Meniere's disease. South Med J 74:1194-97, 1981*).

Observational Study: 58% of of 90 pts. with sensorineural hearing loss had abnormal 5 hour glucose tolerance curves (*Gosselin EJ, Yanick P Jr. Audiologic and metabolic findings in 90 patients with fluctuant hearing loss. J Am Audiol Soc 2:15-18, 1976*).

Observational Study: 42% of 19 pts. with Meniere's syndrome showed hypoglycemia at some point in a 5 hr. glucose tolerance test compared to 15% of pts. with other diseases (*Weille FR. Hypoglycemia in Meniere's disease. Arch Otol 87:129, 1968*).

- -

VITAMINS

Vitamin A:

The cochlea has a high concentration of vitamin A and all special sensory receptor cells contain, or are functionally dependent upon, vitamin A (*Chole Q. Vitamin A in the cochlea. Arch Otorhinolaryngol 124:379-82, 1978*).

Deficiency may be associated with inner ear dysfunction.

Animal Experimental Study: After feeding young rats a vitamin-A deficient diet, changes in the cuticle of the outer and inner hair cells of the cochlea were seen on electron microscopy (*Lohle E. The influence of chronic vitamin A deficiency on human and animal ears. Arch Otorhinolaryngol 234:167-73, 1982*).

Observational Study: Low serum vitamin A levels were associated with decreased auditory function (*Lohle E. The influence of chronic vitamin A deficiency on human and animal ears. Arch Otorhinolaryngol 234:167-73, 1982*).

Supplementation may be beneficial in the treatment of hearing loss and tinnitus.

Experimental Study: 249/300 pts. (83%) with hearing loss had an ave. gain of hearing in the left ear of 18.9% and in the right ear of 17.3% with very definite gains in hearing of conversational tones following a series of twice weekly IV injections of 2 cc of vitamin A. Amelioration and cessation of tinnitus occurred in the same proportions (*Lobel MJ. Is hearing loss due to nutritional deficiency? Arch Otolaryngol May, 1951, pp. 515-26*).

- with Vitamin E:

Review Article: A number of studies have demonstrated the clinical and therapeutic efficacy of supplementation with the combination of vitamin A and vitamin E for pts. with sensorineural hearing loss, particularly when the symptom is due to presbyaccusis, with a 5-15 decibel improvement of the pure-tone auditory threshold following supplementation (*Romeo G. The therapeutic effect of vitamins A and E in neurosensory hearing loss. Acta Vitaminol Enzymol 7 Suppl:85-92, 1985*).

Vitamin D:

Deficiency may cause hearing loss by depressing the concentration of ionized calcium in the perilymph (*Ikeda K et al. The effect of vitamin D deficiency on the cochlear potentials and the perilymphatic ionized calcium concentration of rats. Acta Otolaryngol Suppl (Stockh) 435:64-72, 1987*).

Serum levels may be deficient in cases of hearing loss.

Observational Study: Abnormally low 25-hydroxyvitamin D levels were found in 10/47 pts. with otosclerosis (mean age = 46 yrs.) and borderline low levels in 2. Raised serum alkaline phosphatase levels were present in 32.6%, calcium in 6.5% and inorganic phosphate in 4.3% (*Brookes GB. Vitamin D deficiency and otosclerosis. Otolaryngol Head Neck Surg. 93(3):313-21, 1985*).

Supplementation with calcium and vitamin D may correct a vitamin D deficiency and reverse hearing loss.

Experimental Study: Calcium and vitamin D replacement therapy for 16 pts. (mean age: 46 yrs.) with otosclerosis along with an abnormally low 25-hydroxyvitamin D level and/or a raised alkaline phosphatase level resulted in significant hearing improvement in 3/16 pts. (*Brookes GB. Vitamin D deficiency and otosclerosis. Otolaryngol Head Neck Surg 93(3):313-21, 1985*).

Experimental Study: 4 pts with bilateral cochlear deafness and vitamin D deficiency (abnormally low 25-hydroxyvitamin D levels) were supplemented with calcium and vitamin D 500-1000 IU daily resulting in unilateral hearing improvement in 2/4 (*Brookes GB. Vitamin D deficiency - A new cause of cochlear deafness. J Laryngol Otol 97(5):405-20, 1983*).

- -

MINERALS

Calcium:

Both Meniere's Syndrome (*Meyer zum Gottesberge AM. Imbalanced calcium homeostasis and endolymphatic hydrops. Acta Otolaryngol Suppl (Stockh) 460:18-27, 1988*) and sensorineural hearing loss (*Ikeda K et al. The effect of vitamin D deficiency on the cochlear potentials and the perilymphatic ionized calcium concentration of rats. Acta Otolaryngol Suppl (Stockh) 435:64-72, 1987*) may be due to a shift in Ca^{++} homeostasis towards a higher concentration of free Ca^{++} in the fluid compartments and adjacent intracellular spaces.

Fluoride: 16 - 60 mg daily (sodium fluoride)

> WARNINGS: Damages the surface of the gastric mucosa at therapeutic dosages (*Spak C-J et al. Tissue response of gastric mucosa after ingestion of fluoride. Br Med J 298:1686-87, 1989*) and, in animal studies, inhibits the enzyme phosphatase which is critically important for the assimilation of calcium and other minerals (*Yanick P. Solving problematic tinnitus. A clinical scientific approach. Townsend Letter for Doctors. February - March, 1985, p. 31*).

Administration may slow the progression of otosclerosis.

> **Experimental Double-blind Study:** 95 pts. with otospongiosis received either sodium fluoride 40 mg daily or placebo. There was a statistically significant greater deterioration of hearing loss in the placebo gp. compared to the treated group (*Bretlau P et al. Otospongiosis and sodium fluoride. A clinical double-blind, placebo-controlled study on sodium fluoride treatment in otospongiosis. Am J Otol 10(1):20-22, 1989*).

> **Experimental Study:** 93 relatives of pts. with surgically confirmed otosclerosis either received sodium fluoride 6-16 mg (in relation to age) or served as controls. After 2 yrs., the incidence of stable stapedius reflex findings was 91.5% in the treated ears and 77% in the controls (p<0.05). Results suggest a stabilizing effect of sodium fluoride on the disease process (*Colletti V, Fiorino FG. Stapedius reflex in the monitoring of NaF treatment of subclinical otosclerosis. Acta Otolaryngol (Stockh) 104(5-6):447-53, 1987*).

> **Experimental Study:** 94 pts. with cochlear otosclerosis and 98 pts. with stapedial otosclerosis and sensorineural hearing loss received treatment with sodium fluoride. The drug halted or slowed the progression of sensorineural hearing impairment in 63% of the pts. with cochlear otosclerosis and 46% of the pts. with stapedial otosclerosis. Pts. with more rapid rates of progression responded most favorably (*Forquer BD et al. Sodium fluoride: Effectiveness of treatment for cochlear otosclerosis. Am J Otol 7(2):121-25, 1986*).

Iron:

Deficiency may be associated with the development of hearing loss.

> **Animal Experimental Study:** 32% of 141 growing rats raised on an iron-deficient diet showed a raised auditory threshold. There was no auditory threshold elevation in controls or in non-iron-deficient rats made chronically anemic by injection of phenylhydrazine hydrochloride. Histologic changes were seen in the cochleas of iron-deficient animals. Results suggest that iron deficiency may lead to auditory impairment which is unrelated to the hypoxia of anemia (*Sun AH et al. Iron deficiency and hearing loss. ORL 49:118-22, 1987*).

> **Observational Study:** In a Chinese study, serum iron levels of pts. with sensorineural deafness were significantly lower than those of pts. with normal hearing (*Sun AH. A preliminary report on combined traditional Chinese and Western medicine in sensorineural hearing loss. An analysis of 108 cases. J Tradit Chin Med 2:215-222, 1982; Sun AH et al. [Probing the TCM theory of oto-kidney relationship by the changes of serum iron in sensorineural deafness.] Zhongyi Zazhi, Beijing 23:546-48, 1982*) (*in Chinese*).

If serum iron levels are reduced, patients with sensorineural deafness may benefit from supplementation.

> **Experimental Study:** Following iron supplementation of a gp. of pts. with sensorineural deafness and reduced serum iron levels, most pts. whose hearing improved had raised serum iron levels, while pts. whose hearing failed to improve showed no change in serum iron (*Sun AH. A preliminary report on combined traditional Chinese and Western medicine in sensorineural hearing loss. An analysis of 108 cases. J Tradit Chin Med 2:215-222, 1982; Sun AH et al. [Probing the TCM theory of oto-kidney relationship by the changes of serum iron in sensorineural deafness.] Zhongyi Zazhi, Beijing 23:546-48, 1982*) (*in Chinese*).

Magnesium:

Deficiency may cause ototoxicity.

> **Clinical Observation:** "Magnesium imbalance may cause tinnitus" (*DeBartolo HM Jr. Zinc and diet for tinnitus. Am J Otol 10(3):256, 1989*).

Animal Experimental Study: Guinea pigs on a magnesium-deficient diet were more susceptible to noise-induced hearing loss than were animals on a diet rich in magnesium (*Ising H et al. Increased noise trauma in guinea pigs through magnesium deficiency. Arch Otorhinolaryngol 236:139-46, 1986*).

Animal Experimental Study: Rats on a magnesium-deficient diet were more susceptible to noise-induced hearing loss than were animals on a diet rich in magnesium (*Joachims Z et al. Dependence of noise-induced hearing loss upon perilymph magnesium concentration. J Acoust Soc Am 74:104-08, 1983*).

Theoretical Discussion: It is postulated that aminoglycoside drugs cause ototoxicity by depleting magnesium in the hair cells of the cochlea (*Dolev E et al. Is magnesium depletion the reason for ototoxicity caused by aminoglycosides? Med Hypotheses 10(4):353-58, 1983*).

Potassium and
Sodium:

Electrolyte imbalances may affect the inner ear, since endolymph is higher in potassium and perilymph is higher in sodium (*Yanick P. Holistic applications to ear disorders. J Int Acad Prev Med 1983, pp. 24-27*).

Clinical Observation: "We have produced and taken away tinnitus with potassium iodide" (*DeBartolo HM Jr. Zinc and diet for tinnitus. Abstract. Am J Otol 10(3):256, 1989*).

Experimental and Observational Study: On the basis of a 24 hr. urinary electrolyte clearance test, pts. with sensorineural hearing loss and hypoglycemia were found to have higher levels of potassium than of sodium and a negative nitrogen balance. Increased salt improved their sodium-potassium balance as well as their nitrogen balance (*Goldman HB. Metabolic causes of fluctuant hearing loss. Otolaryngol Clin No Am 8:369, 1975; Tintera JW, Goldman HB. Stress and hypoadrenocorticism: The implications in otolaryngology. Ann Otol Rhinol Laryngol 67:185, 1958*).

Zinc: Zinc Sulfate 600 mg. daily

Serum zinc levels may decrease with age.

Clinical Observation: Assays on 1500 office pts. revealed a tendency towards decreasing serum zinc levels, especially after age 60 (*Shambaugh GE Jr. Zinc for tinnitus, imbalance, and hearing loss in the elderly. Am J Otol 7(6):476-7, 1986*).

Tissue zinc concentrations are highest in the sensory tissues of the labyrinth (*Shambaugh GE Jr. Zinc for tinnitus, imbalance, and hearing loss in the elderly. Am J Otol 7(6):476-7, 1986*).

Continuous, rather than intermittent, tinnitus, may be associated with hypozincemia (*Gersdorff M et al. A clinical correlation between hypozincemia and tinnitus. Arch Otorhinolaryngol 244(3):190-3, 1987*).

Supplementation may be beneficial, especially if deficient.

Negative Experimental Double-blind Study: 48 tinnitus pts., only one of whom was hypozincemic, randomly received either zinc 22 mg (as zinc sulfate 100 mg) 3 times daily or placebo. After 8 wks., no favorable effect of zinc treatment could be demonstrated even though serum zinc rose significantly, probably because serum zinc levels were normal (*Paaske PB et al. [Zinc therapy of tinnitus. A placebo-controlled study.] Ugeskr Laeger 152(35):2473-75, 1990*) (*in Danish*).

Clinical Observation: Tinnitus pts. were found to require 6 times more zinc than the US RDA (*DeBartolo HM Jr. Zinc and diet for tinnitus. Am J Otol 10(3):256, 1989*).

Experimental Study: Pts. with tinnitus with hypozincemia were overloaded with zinc sulfate. 52% of cases reported positive results, 15% reported good amelioration, and 37% reported a slight but significant amelioration of their symptoms. Males responded better than females and pts. with continuous tinnitus responded better than those with intermittent tinnitus (*Gersdorff M et al. [The zinc sulfate overload test in patients suffering from tinnitus associated with low serum zinc. Preliminary report.] Acta Otorhinolaryngol Belg 41(3):498-505, 1987*).

Clinical Observations: Pts. with hypozincemia (serum zinc <0.69 µg/g) received 4-10 times the US RDA for zinc as the sulfate, gluconate, aspartate, picolinate or other absorbable form for 3-6 mo. or longer. In addition to improvement in tinnitus, 35% had a 10% or more improvement in discrimination and a 5 dB or more improvement in pure-tone hearing. Imbalance improved occasionally (*Shambaugh GE Jr. Zinc for tinnitus, imbalance, and hearing loss in the elderly. Am J Otol 7(6):476-7, 1986*).

Clinical Observatons: 20% of a gp. of elderly pts. with progressive hearing deterioration, most of whom had symptoms of zinc deficiency or a low serum zinc, experienced a slight noticeable improvement, especially in discrimination, with zinc supplementation, while 25% of those with tinnitus noted reduction or sometimes elimination following supplementation. Often it took 3 mo. to 1 yr. to bring low serum zinc levels up to normal. After 3 mo., zinc was omitted for 1 wk. and a serum zinc was drawn. If the level was well above 1.0 (normal range 0.69-1.10 µg/ml), the supplement was reduced to a maintenance dosage. The most frequent side-effect was nausea and gastric distress, but this is rare if a combination of zinc gluconate and zinc sulfate with vitamin synergists ('Z-Plex' or 'Bronson 72'/ Bronson Pharm.) was used (*Shambaugh GE Jr. Zinc: An essential trace element. Clin Ecology 2(4):203-06, 1984*).

Clinical Observation: 20 pts. with sensorineural hearing loss, tinnitus, or both are described who benefited from supplementation with zinc sulfate 600 mg daily (*Shambaugh GE Jr - interviewed in Geriatrics 38(4):21, 1983*).

- -

OTHER NUTRITIONAL FACTORS

Coenzyme Q$_{10}$:

Supplementation may combat acute hearing loss due to hypoxia.

Animal Experimental Study: Acute sensorineural hearing loss was induced in guinea pigs artificially by creating hypoxia which, when repeated, caused a gradual disappearance of the ABR. Examination of the inner ear after the animals were sacrificed showed that CoQ$_{10}$ was effective in promoting recovery from damage to auditory hairs as well as in preventing respiratory metabolic impairment of hair cells due to hypoxia (*Sato K. Pharmacoklinetics of coenzyme Q$_{10}$ in recovery of acute sensorineural hearing loss due to hypoxia. Acta Otolaryngol Suppl (Stockh) 458:95-102, 1988*).

Hydroxyethylrutoside:

A bioflavonoid related to rutin.

Administration may be beneficial in sudden deafness of vascular origin.

Case Reports: 4 pts. with sudden deafness of vascular origin had improved hearing and disappearance of tinnitus following administration of O-(beta-hydroxyethyl)-rutoside (Venoruton) (*Madej S. [Treatment of sudden deafness of vascular etiology with venoruton.] Otolaryngol Pol 43(3):214-7, 1989*) (*in Polish*).

Administration may be beneficial in Meniere's syndrome.

Experimental Double-blind Crossover Study: 39 pts. with well-defined Meniere's disease first received placebo for 1 month. They then received in random order O-(beta-hydroxyethyl)-rutoside (HR) 2 gm/d and placebo for 3 months each. Despite a marked tendency to a "carryover" effect from the first sequence with HR into the second placebo sequence, there was a clear trend to greater symptomatic improvement with HR compared to placebo. Audiometric findings showed a very clear, uniform superiority under HR treatment for both air and bone conduction at all 5 frequencies studied (p=0.002-0.05). There were no significant changes in vestibulometry (calorie test). The incidence of side effects were similar with HR and placebo (*Moser M et al. A double-blind clinical trial of hydroxyethylrutosides in Meniere's disease. J Laryngol Otol 98(3):265-72, 1984*).

Omega-3 Fatty Acids (Fish Oils):

Eicosapentaenoic acid (EPA) and docosahexaenoic acid (DHA).

Highest in cold water fish. Available in a refined form as 'MaxEPA' (18% EPA).

Suggested MaxEPA dosage: 3 - 9 grams daily in divided doses (or 10 ml. concentrate twice daily)

> WARNING: Supplementation may require additional vitamin E intake to prevent increased membrane peroxidation and cellular damage (*Laganiere S, Fernandes G. High peroxidizability of subcellular membrane induced by high fish oil diet is reversed by vitamin E. Clin Res 35:A565, 1987*).

Increasing red-cell deformability may reduce <u>sensorineural hearing impairment</u> (*Browning GG et al. Blood viscosity as a factor in sensorineural hearing impairment. Lancet 1:121-23, 1986*). (*See "Reduce fat and cholesterol" above*).

Administration of fish oils may increase red-cell deformability.

> **Experimental Study:** Normal subjects received 'MaxEPA,' a fish oil concentrate, 3 gm daily. By 6 wks. there was a significant increase in red-cell deformability and a concomitant reduction in whole blood viscosity but no change in plasma viscosity or hematocrit, suggesting that the effects on blood rheology were mediated by changes in RBC lipid fluidity (*Cartwright IJ et al. The effects of dietary omega-3 polyunsaturated fatty acids on erythrocyte membrane phospholipids, erythrocyte deformability and blood viscosity in healthy volunteers. Atherosclerosis 55(3):267-81, 1985*).

- -

COMBINED TREATMENT

Experimental Controlled Study: 14 adults (8 women, 6 men) aged 29-67 (mean age 40) with confirmed sensorineural hearing loss (cochlear origin) and tinnitus of at least 1 year's duration unresponsive to medical treatment who were not on any drugs for the condition were studied. 6 had recurrent vertigo (Meniere's disease). Hearing loss was bilateral in 10 and unilateral in 2. All subjects had seen at least 3 otologists over 1-32 yrs. and were told that nothing more could be done for their conditions. 4/14 pts. chose to become controls. The 10 experimental subjects were given the following dietary goals:
1. Use distilled drinking water.
2. Reduce sodium intake to 250-400 mg/d.
3. Reduce intake of acid ash foods (meats, grains, etc.) and increase intake of alkaline ash foods (fruits, vegetables).
4. Reduce intake of saturated fats, substituting mostly polyunsaturated fats from cold-pressed oils and non-animal, high-fat proteins (avocado, nuts, coconuts).
5. Eat less animal protein, replacing it with vegetable protein.
6. Eliminate or reduce intake of processed and refined sugars.
7. Increase consumption of complex carbohydrates and naturally occurring sugars.
8. Reduce intake of high phosphorus foods by 20-50% (meats, grains).
9. Increase intake of whole foods in their raw, natural state (fresh fruits, vegetables, nuts, seeds).

They were also given digestive enzymes providing pepsin 30 mg, betaine HCl 125 mg, protease 20,000 NF units, amylase 20,000 NF units, and lipase 1,600 NF units daily. In some cases, this dosage was doubled to eliminate digestive symptoms such as bloating, gas or constipation. In addition, general recommendations were made for exercise and stress reduction. After 1 yr., the feeling of ear fullness improved in all experimental subjects, but in none of the controls. 8/10 reported decreased loudness of their tinnitus, 7/10 a decrease in the interference of tinnitus with their daily routine, and 8/10 a decrease in the severity of the tinnitus. None of the controls reported improvements in tinnitus. On objective testing, 10/17 ears in the treated gp. improved, with a decrease in tinnitus intensity. 5/8 ears in the control gp. were unchanged, while tinnitus worsened in 2. In regard to pure tone thresholds, improvement in treated subjects was statistically highly significant. While the thresholds of subjects and controls were similar prior to treatment, after treatment the mean change in hearing thresholds was significantly higher for the treated subjects than for the controls. Speech discrimination scores at +15dB and +40dB sensation levels revealed statistically significant improvements in treated subjects compared to small decreases for the controls. Total cessation of vertigo was reported by all 3 subjects with Meniere's disease, while 3 controls with Meniere's disease noted no change. Intracellular magnesium and both salivary and urinary pH increased more in the experimental gp. than in controls ($p<0.05-<0.005$) (*Yanick P, Jr. Dietary and lifestyle influences on cochlear disorders and biochemical status: A 12-month study. J Appl Nutr 40(2):75-84, 1988*).

Clinical Observation: The authors treat pts. with progressive sensorineural hearing loss due to cochlear otosclerosis without stapedial fixation by prescribing sodium fluoride, calcium and vitamin D (*Balle V, Linthicum FH Jr. Histologically proven cochlear otosclerosis with pure sensorineural hearing loss. Ann Otol Rhinol Laryngol 93(2 Pt 1):105-11, 1984*).

Clinical Observation: Results after individualized diet, nutrition, exercise and stress-reduction program for 130 pts. with hearing loss due to cochlear pathology of unknown etiology:
    85% (111/130) had dramatic improvements in hearing levels and in speech understanding ability.
    91% (74/82) of those with tinnitus reported dramatic relief.
(*Yanick P Jr. Holistic applications to ear disorders. J Int Acad Prev Med 1983, pp. 24-7*)

– –

OTHER FACTORS

Rule out aluminum toxicity.

Said to be common in otosclerosis causing reduced serum phosphate levels and abnormal calcium metabolism (*Yanick P. Solving problematic tinnitus: A clinical scientific approach. Townsend Letter for Doctors February - March, 1985, p. 31*).

Rule out lead toxicity.

May indirectly affect the ear by causing malfunction in the brain and/or symphathetic nervous system, by inhibiting the enzymatic oxidative processes dependent upon zinc and copper in the mitochondria of the cells of the inner ear, or by depleting the cochlea of phosphorus by forming insoluble salts (*Yanick, P. Nutritional aspects of tinnitus and hearing disorders, in P Yanick Jr, JG Clark, Eds. Tinnitus and its Management. Springfield, Illinois, Charles C. Thomas, 1984*).

Rule out food sensitivities:

Clinical Observation: "For the last 12 years we have identified certain individuals who are hypersensitive to salicylates and have improved or relieved tinnitus with a salicylate-free diet" (*DeBartolo HM Jr. Zinc and diet for tinnitus. Am J Otol 10(3):256, 1989*).

Experimental Study: 23 pts. that presented with incapacitating vertigo plus one or more of the other Meniere's disease symptoms (e.g. tinnitus, low frequency hearing loss, fullness of the ears) without evidence of metabolic, infective, or tumor-related etiologies, and who had failed to respond to anti-vertiginous drugs, received RAST food and inhalent testing. Positive foods according to RAST results were then tested with intradermal provocation. Foods that produced any ear symptoms were completely eliminated and immunotherapy started. All pts. were better within 2 weeks. Audiograms at 3 mo. showed improvement in sensorineural hearing losses, especially in the low frequencies (*Hoover SN. Food allergy and Meniere's disease. Annual Meeting Abstracts, AAOA News, 5(4):10, 1987*).

Clinical Observation: Dietary management in allergic pts. was often found to result in relief from tinnitus and other ear symptoms (*Shambaugh G. Allergy and the inner ear. Ear Clin Int 1:166-67, 1981*).

Case Reports: 2 pts. with Meniere's syndrome whose symptoms were so severe that they would fall helpless to the ground obtained relief of symptoms by avoiding specific foods. Ingestion of the offending food, or injection of the food extract, reproduced their symptoms (*Duke WW. Meniere's syndrome caused by allergy. JAMA 81:2179, 1923*).

IRRITABLE BOWEL SYNDROME

See Also: CONSTIPATION
DIARRHEA

DIETARY FACTORS

Reduce fat.

The major dietary stimulant of the gastrocolonic response (*Wright SH et al. Effect of dietary components on the gastrocolonic response.* Am J Physiol *238(3):G228-32, 1980*).

Experimental Study: 8 pts. with predominantly constipation, 8 age- and sex-matched pts. with predominantly diarrhea and 8 age-and sex-matched normals received a small intestinal infusion of a fatty meal. Compared to controls, the pts. responded excessively to the fatty meal. Pts. with diarrhea tended to be more sensitive than pts. with constipation and the ileum responded more to stimulation than the jejunum. The stimulus appeared to unmask intestinal dysmotility which was often accompanied by abdominal symptoms, suggesting that small bowel dysfunction contributes to symptoms of irritable bowel syndrome (*Kellow JF et al. Dysmotility of the small intestine in irritable bowel syndrome.* Gut *29(9):1236-43, 1988*).

Increase dietary fiber   example: unprocessed wheat bran: 8 -10 tsp. daily

The pentose-containing polysaccharides have a great capacity to hold water. Wheat bran has more pentose-containing polysaccharides than carrots, cabbage or apples, and thus is a preferable source of fiber (*Cummings JH et al. Colonic response to dietary fibre from carrot, cabbage, apple, bran.* Lancet *1:5-9, 1978*).

Supplementation may increase stool weight and decrease intestinal transit time.

Review Article: In all studies reviewed, bran increased stool weight and decreased transit time in pts. with IBS (*Müller-Lissner SA. Effect of wheat bran on weight of stool and gastrointestinal transit time: A meta analysis.* Br Med J *296:615-17, 1988*).

Supplementation may reduce symptoms.

Negative Experimental Double-blind Crossover Study: 9 pts. received 4 cookies daily containing 20 mg corn fiber or placebo for 7 months. Symptoms significantly improved during both fiber and placebo treatments including pain severity, stool frequency, stool consistency, and total symptom score (*Cook IJ et al. Effect of dietary fiber on symptoms and rectosigmoid motility in patients with irritable bowel syndrome. A controlled, crossover study.* Gastroenterology *98(1):66-72, 1990*).

Negative Experimental Double-blind Crossover Study: 28 pts. received either 12 bran biscuits or placebo biscuits daily, each for 3 months. Symptoms improved in both gps., with no significant difference between bran and placebo (*Lucei MR et al. Is bran efficacious in irritable bowel syndrome? A double-blind placebo controlled cross-over study.* Gut *28:221, 1987*).

Negative Experimental Double-blind Crossover Study: 38 pts. received either wheat bran 10-30 gm daily or placebo. Both bran and placebo significantly reduced the severity of most of the symptoms. Constipation only improved significantly with bran, while pain and urgency were significantly more frequent with bran (*Cann P et al. What is the benefit of coarse wheat bran in patients with irritable bowel syndrome?* Gut *25:168-73, 1984*).

Experimental Controlled Study: 14 pts. on wheat bran 20 gm daily showed a significant reduction in abdominal pain and "improvement in bowel habit" on bran compared to controls who excluded wholegrain cereal products (*Manning AP et al. Wheat fibre and irritable bowel syndrome: A controlled trial. Lancet 2:417, 1977*).

Negative Experimental Double-blind Study: The effect of biscuits containing wheat bran (30 gm daily) was compared to biscuits without bran in a mixed gp. of pts. including pts. with diverticular disease and pts. taking laxatives. Results failed to support the use of bran (*Soltoft J et al. A double-blind trial of the effect of wheat bran on symptoms of irritable bowel syndrome. Lancet 1:270-2, 1976*).

Avoid refined carbohydrates.

Experimental Study: 24 pts. were given fructose, sorbitol, fructose-sorbitol mixtures, and sucrose, and evaluated for malabsorption by the hydrogen breath test and GI symptoms. Malabsorption and pronounced GI distress was provoked by fructose, sorbitol and the fructose-sorbitol mixture. Sucrose did not cause malabsorption, and provoked less GI distress (*Rumessen JJ, Gudmand-Hÿer E. Functional bowel disease: Malabsorption and abdominal distress after ingestion of fructose, sorbitol, and fructose-sorbitol mixtures. Gastroenterology 95(3):694-700, 1988*).

Experimental Study: Subjects were placed on a 2-wk. baseline diet followed by a test diet of the same composition, but with an added 120 gm sugar. With the addition of sugar, fecal bile acid concentrations increased and the oro-anal transit time decreased. Bacterial fermentation activity also increased, which was thought to partially explain the increase in total and secondary bile acids in the feces. Since these alterations in colonic activity are associated with elevated risk for irritable bowel syndrome, sugar may increase the disease risk (*Kruis W et al. Influence of diets high and low in refined sugar on stool qualities, gastrointestinal transit time and fecal bile acid excretion. Gastroenterology 92:1483, 1987*).

Review Article: A diet high in refined carbohydrate is implicated in the etiology of irritable bowel syndrome and certain other diseases of the colon. It is suggested that spasm of the smooth muscle is the common pathogenetic mechanism, and the strength of the spasm producing increased pressure in the colonic lumen or wall and the length of time for which the colon has been affected are believed to determine the type of disease resulting. A diet high in refined carbohydrate allows the intense muscle spasm to occur because the physical buffering effect of fecal bulk is considerably reduced (*Grimes DS. Refined carbohydrate, smooth-muscle spasm and disease of the colon. Lancet 1:395-97, 1976*)

OTHER FACTORS

Rule out food sensitivities.

Review Article: "There appears to be a subset of IBS patients who have a strong history of atopy and immunologically linked food allergy. Many of these patients experience improvement of their IBS on an elimination diet; however, the underlying mechanism has not been explained on an immunologic basis and remains unknown" (*Mullen GE. Questions and Answers: Food allergy and irritable bowel syndrome. JAMA 265(13):1736, 1991*).

Experimental Study: 17 children with clinical symptoms of IBS were challenged with foods selected on the basis of history or on a positive RAST or prick test. Intestinal permeability was evaluated by analyzing the differential urinary elimination of lactulose and mannitol. As compared to controls, 9/17 pts. demonstrated modified intestinal permeability following specific food ingestion. All 9 children had a personal and/or family history of allergy and/or raised total IgE. Symptoms disappeared after food exclusion either alone (7 pts.) or together with cromolyn (*Barau E, Dupont C. Modifications of intestinal permeability during food provocation procedures in pediatric irritable bowel syndrome. J Pediatr Gastroenterol 11(1):72-77, 1990*).

Experimental Study: 91/189 pts. (48.2%) improved following 3 wks. on a food elimination diet. Subsequent challenge with individual foods showed that 73/91 were able to identify one or more food intolerances, and 50% of them identified 2-5 foods (range 1-14). The foods most commonly implicated were dairy products (40.7%) and grains (39.4%). 72/91 remained well on a modified diet during the follow-up period (mean: 14.7 mo; SD: 7.98 mo.) Of the 98/189 pts. who failed to improve, only 3 were symptomatically well at follow-up (mean: 12.48 mo.; SD 9.09 mo.) (*Nanda R et al. Food intolerance and the irritable bowel syndrome. Gut 30(8):1099-104, 1989*).

Negative Experimental Study: 10 pts. underwent an open elimination diet for 2 wks. followed by a 48-hr. challenge of each food considered suspicious on the basis of the patient's diary, a positive skin prick test, and/or positive IgG antibodies. 6/10 pts. had positive skin scratch test results and only 1 pt. had RAST IgG food antibodies markedly increased above normal. None had symptoms exacerbated by food challenges. Results suggest that positive skin tests and IgG serum antibodies are not reliable indicators of food hypersensitivity in IBS, and that food hypersensitivity does not seem to play a role in IBS symptoms (*Zwetchkenbaum J, Burakoff R. The irritable bowel syndrome and food hypersensitivity. Ann Allergy 61(1):47-49, 1988*).

Observational Study: Compared to controls, 58 pts. demonstrated an increased incidence of skin reactivity (48.3%; p<0.05) as well as increased serum IgG antibodies reactive to chicken, albumin, bovine milk or wheat gliadin (52.6%; p<0.01) (*Finn R et al. Immunological hypersensitivity to environmental antigens in the irritable bowel syndrome. Br J Clin Pract 41(12), 1987*).

Experimental Single-blind Study: 17 pts. who had failed to respond to standard therapy were placed on a strict diet eliminating foods commonly associated with hypersensitivity. After 1 mo., 9/17 (53%) were free of symptoms. Foods were individually re-introduced and 7/17 (41%) identified reactions to specific foods which they continued to avoid. These pts. remained well for the following year when naso-gastric tubes were inserted, and they were fed either known safe or test (excluded) foods. They correctly identified test foods on 10/12 occasions and safe foods on 10/12 occasions, a significant result (p<0.01). The test foods also caused an elevation of rectal prostaglandin E2 levels. In a separate study, 17/28 pts. (60%) were found to be atopic compared to 6/26 (23%) matched controls (*Finn R et al. Expanding horizons of allergy and the total allergy syndrome. Clin Ecology 3(3):129-131, 1985*).

Experimental Blinded Study: 12/24 pts. were found to be atopic (positive skin tests, positive IgE RAST, positive histories) and 9/12 had elevated total serum IgE levels. All 24 pts. were placed on an exclusion diet and blind challenged 1-2 wks. later with 18 different foods and 6 food additives. 17 improved on the diet and 14/17 exacerbated during challenges. Of the 6 additives tested, sodium benzoate, sodium nitrite, erythrosine and carminic acid were symptom-producing. All pts. with elevated IgE were food-sensitive. In only 10 cases did the IgE RAST correlate with the results of provocation. Six mo. after starting an exclusion diet based on test results, 10/14 pts. with positive provocative test results were asymptomatic, while the other 4 had only mild symptoms. The presence of yeast in the stools (Candida albicans and Geotrichum candidum) appeared to be related to their food sensitivities as treatment with nystatin was followed by improvement in most of the affected patients (*Petitpierre M et al. Irritable bowel syndrome and hypersensitivity to food. Ann Allergy 54:538-40, 1985*).

Negative Experimental Double-blind Study: Foods believed to provoke symptoms were first eliminated as were skin-test positive foods (i.e. foods such as wheat were not usually eliminated). About half the subjects reacted to an open trial of the remaining foods who were then subjected to double blind challenges. Reactions to the "placebo" capsules (which contained lactose, food coloring and beef- or pork-derived gelatin) were as frequent as reactions to the actual foods, suggesting that skin testing is unreliable as a method of identifying provoking foods (*Alun-Jones VA et al. Food intolerance and the irritable bowel. Lancet 2:633, 1983*).

Note: Subjects sensitive to milk, food coloring, beef or pork could have reacted to the "placebo" capsules, thus throwing the results into question.

Experimental Double-blind Study: 14/21 were found to be provoked by specific food challenges following 1 week on a single meat, a single fruit, and distilled or spring water. These reactions were confirmed in the 6 who were challenged double-blind. 9 reacted to wheat, 5 to corn, 4 to dairy products, 4 to coffee, 3 to tea and 2 to citrus. Rectal prostaglandin E2 was significantly increased after positive challenges and sometimes remained elevated for more than 24 hours (*Alun-Jones VA et al. Food intolerance: A major factor in the pathogenesis of irritable bowel syndrome. Lancet 2:1115-7, 1982*).

Lactobacillus Acidophilus: (may require weeks to months for beneficial effects)

Administration may be beneficial.

Experimental Study: Successful implantation of LA was followed by symptom relief in mucous colitis, irritable colon, idiopathic ulcerative colitis, and various other disorders causing constipation (*Rettger LF et al. Lactobacillus Acidophilus. Its Therapeutic Application. New Haven, Yale U. Press, 1935*).

KIDNEY STONES
(CALCIUM OXALATE)

See Also: OSTEOPOROSIS

DIETARY FACTORS

Adequate <u>fluid</u> intake (2-2.5 liters daily).

Fluid deprivation or loss of fluid from the body may predispose to stone formation by reducing the urinary output and increasing the concentration of stone-forming minerals in the urine (*Rao PN. Dietary habit and urolithiasis, in DLJ Freed, Ed. <u>Health Hazards of Milk</u>. London, Baillière Tindall, 1984*).

Drink <u>hard</u> water.

Note: Dietary calcium, which is related to water hardness, precipitates oxalate to form calcium oxalate which is not absorbed from the intestines.

Observational Study: In an American study, there was a negative correlation between the hospital incidence of kidney stones and local water hardness (*Sierakowski R et al. Stone incidence as related to water hardness in different geographical regions in the United States. <u>Urol Res</u> 7:157-60, 1979*).

The advantage of hard water may not be entirely due to its higher calcium content.

Observational Study: Home tap water samples were analyzed from the Carolinas (which has soft water and a high stone incidence) and the Rockies (which has hard water and a low stone incidence). The calcium content of water between these 2 areas was not significantly different (*Shuster J et al. Water hardness and urinary stone disease. <u>J Urol</u> 128:422-25, 1982*).

<u>Vegetarian</u> diet.

The intake of animal protein is correlated with calcium oxalate stone formation as well as with the urinary output of calcium.

Review Article: By increasing intestinal calcium absorption, meat intake induces hypercalciuria. The metabolic products include oxalate and uric acid, both of which are excreted in the urine. In addition, the urinary pH is reduced after a meat-containing meal. Animal protein can thus induce calcium oxalate supersaturation. Uric acid can also encourage calcium oxalate stones by interfering with the action of naturally occurring inhibitors in the urine (*Rao PN. Dietary habit and urolithiasis, in DLJ Freed, Ed. <u>Health Hazards of Milk</u>. London, Baillière Tindall, 1984*).

The hypercalciuria induced by a high meat diet appears to be mainly due to its high content of sulfur-containing amino acids (*Kaneko K et al. Urinary calcium and calcium balance in young women affected by high protein diet of soy protein isolate and adding sulfur-containing amino acids and/or potassium. <u>J Nutr Sci Vitaminol (Tokyo)</u> 36(2):105-16, 1990*).

Increase <u>dietary fiber</u>.

Patients with renal stones have a lower fiber intake than normals (*Fellström B et al. Dietary history and dietary records in renal stone patients and control. <u>Urol Res</u> 12:58, 1984; Griffith HM et al. A control study of dietary factors in renal stone formation. <u>Br J Urol</u> 53:416-20, 1981*).

Renal stones are rare in Third World countries where the fiber intake is still high (*Modlin M et al. Dietary structure and urinary composition in a stone free population, in LH Smith et al., Eds. Urolithiasis: Clinical and Basic Research. New York, Plenum Press, 1981:337-42; Modlin M. Urinary phosphorylated inositols and renal stone. Lancet 2:1113-14, 1980*).

Phytic acid (found in whole grain wheat, corn, rye, millet and barley and in beans) chelates calcium and magnesium to prevent their mucosal passage and thus may impede the formation of calcium stones (*Modlin M. Urinary phosphorylated inositols and renal stone. Lancet 2:1113-14, 1980*).

Increased dietary fiber intake may lower calcium excretion.

Experimental Study: 10 pts. with recurrent nephrolithiasis and hypercalciuria were given rice bran for 60 days. Hypercalciuria was reduced in all pts. by an ave. of 40%; the decrease averaged 65% in absorptive hypercalciuria and 33% in renal hypercalciuria. Urinary oxalate was increased in 28% of pts., and urinary magnesium was decreased in 28% (*Noronha IL et al. [Rice bran in the treatment of idiopathic hypercalciuria in patients with urinary calculosis.] Rev Paul Med 107(1):19-24, 1989*).

Experimental Study: 24 g of wheat bran daily lowered calcium excretion by 20-25% in 73% of stone formers (*Shah PJR. Unprocessed bran and its effect on urinary calcium excretion in idiopathic hypercalciuria. Br Med J 281:426, 1980*).

Restrict dietary fat.

Observational Study: Compared to healthy controls, urinary stone formers had a higher fat consumption (*Griffith HM et al. A control study of dietary factors in renal stone formation. Br J Urol 53:416-20, 1981*).

Review Article: Improper digestion of fats resulting in steatorrhea causes intraluminal calcium binding to these fatty acids, reducing the availability of calcium to bind oxalate and therefore increasing urinary oxalate excretion (*Smith IH et al. Nutrition and urolithiasis. N Engl J Med 298:87-89, 1978*).

Limit sodium intake in hypercalciuria.

High sodium intake may cause a rise in calcium excretion.

Experimental Study: Daily urinary calcium excretion in stone-forming subjects was shown to vary directly with moderate changes in dietary sodium intake. Reducing dietary sodium from 200 to 80 mMol/d was sufficient to normalize hypercalciuria. Results suggest that habitual high sodium intake may be an etiological factor in the generation of excessive excretion of calcium, sodium and phosphate (the hypercalciuria syndrome) (*Muldowney FP et al. Importance of dietary sodium in the hypercalciuria syndrome. Kidney Int 22:292-95, 1982*).

Avoid high oxalate foods:

Foods with 25 mg/100 gm oxalate (highest concentration):

Beans, Cocoa, Instant Coffee, Parsley, Rhubarb, Spinach, Tea

Other frequently eaten foods relatively high in oxalates:

Beet tops, Carrot, Celery, Chocolate, Cucumber, Grapefruit, Kale, Peanut, Pepper, Sweet Potato

Dietary oxalate may contribute to urinary oxalate excretion, although the increase in excretion between a low and high oxalate diet is relatively small.

Experimental Study: Oral loads of 400 mg sodium oxalate daily significantly increased urinary oxalate excretion in both 14 normals and 22 stone formers; however, 130 mg daily failed to produce significant increases and the degree of oxaluria did not differ at either dosage between normals and stone formers (*Butz M et al. Dietary influence on serum and urinary oxalate in healthy subjects and oxalate stone formers. Urol Int 35:309-15, 1980*).

Stone formers may have an increased tendency to absorb oxalate and excrete it in the urine.

Experimental Study: The effects of 6 days of low oxalate intake followed by 6 days of high oxalate intake on urinary oxalate excretion in 4 normals and 6 stone formers was compared. In the normals, the average 24-hour oxalate excretion increased from 19.3 mg to 30.3 mg, only 3.4% of the increase in dietary intake. In the stone formers, excretion increased from 14.5 mg to 24.4 mg (10.3% of the increase in dietary intake), suggesting that stone formers have a greater tendency to absorb oxalate and to excrete it in the urine (*Zarembski PM, Hodgkinson. Some factors increasing the urinary excretion of oxalate in man. Clin Chim Acta 25:1-10, 1969*).

In normals, about 40% of urinary oxalate is believed to be derived from glycine (*Crawhall JC et al. Conversion of glycine to oxalate in a normal subject. Lancet 2:810, 1959*) and 40% from ingested ascorbic acid (*Atkins GL et al. Quantitative aspects of ascorbic acid metabolism in man. J Biol Chem 239:2975-80, 1964*), with only 20% coming from dietary oxalate.

Hyperoxaluria does not necessarily cause kidney stones.

Case Report: A healthy man ingested 490 mg oxalate as beetroot extract for 5 yrs and was found to have both hyperoxaluria and oxalate crystalluria but no evidence of kidney stones (*Butz M et al. Dietary influence on serum and urinary oxalate in healthy subjects and oxalate stone formers. Urol Int 35:309-15, 1980*).

Most stone formers do not have hyperoxaluria.

Observational Study: 16.3% of 392 stone formers were found to have hyperoxaluria (*Rao RN et al. Dietary management of urinary risk factors in renal stone formers. Br J Urol 54:578-83, 1982*).

Observational Study: The daily excretion of oxalic acid by 39 normal adults and by 80 pts. was compared. The majority of pts. showed normal oxalic acid excretion. A few pts. with calcium oxalate stones excreted increased quantities of oxalic acid, but marked hyperoxaluria appeared to be rare, and only one case was found in this series (*Hodgkinson A. The urinary excretion of oxalic acid in nephrolithiasis. Proc R Soc Med 51:970-1, 1958*).

Avoid sugar.

Sugar ingestion may foster stone formation and, especially in stone-formers, is associated with increased urinary calcium concentration.

Experimental Study: Following an intake of 100 g glucose, renal excretion of calcium, magnesium and oxalate significantly increased and urinary pH decreased in 44 pts. and in 28 healthy controls. Before glucose administration, urine was supersaturated with calcium oxalate in stone formers (median 0.55) and healthy subjects (0.24; p<0.05). Carbohydrate intake caused a significant increase in the degree of urine saturation with calcium oxalate and uric acid, while the degree of urine saturation with brushite and sodium urate did not change. These data suggest that an excess of simple carbohydrate consumption may increase the degree of urine saturation with some of the compounds important in stone formation (*Güszek J. The effect of glucose intake on urine saturation with calcium oxalate, calcium phosphate, uric acid and sodium urate. Int Urol Nephrol 20(6):657-64, 1988*).

Review Article: There is evidence that, when sucrose is consumed, one-third of a normal population and over 70% of idiopathic stone formers respond in a exaggerated manner in respect to increased excretion of urinary risk factors: urine volume, pH and the excretion rates of calcium, oxalate, uric acid and glycosaminoglycans. In addition, sucrose induces nephrocalcinosis in rat kidney and similar calcific lesions have been found in human kidney. There is clear evidence that sucrose adversely influences urinary electrolyte composition, producing oversaturation with calcium oxalate, and there is evidence for a sucrose-induced mechanism whereby calcific lesions occur within the kidney on which crystal aggregation may first take place as a preliminary to stone formation (*Blacklock NJ. Sucrose and idiopathic renal stone. Nutr Health 5(1/2):9-17, 1987*).

Sugar (sucrose or glucose) may provoke an excessive insulin response in stone-formers (*Rao PHN et al. Metabolic response to refined carbohydrates in idiopathic urolithiasis. Urol Int 39(3):165-69, 1984; Rao PN et al. Are stone formers maladapted to refined carbohydrates? Br J Urol 54(6):575-77, 1982*). Insulin increases renal calcium output; thus sugar may increase calcium output in stone formers because of its effect upon insulin (*DeFronzo RA et al. The effect of insulin on renal handling of sodium, potassium, calcium and phosphate in man. J Clin Invest 55:845-55, 1975*).

Sugar increases the urinary output of n-acetyl-glucosaminidase (NAG) which is only present in patients with renal disease (*Dance N et al. The excretion of N-acetyl-beta-glucosaminidase and B-galactosidase by patients with renal disease. Clin Chem Acta 27:87-92, 1970*), suggesting that high sugar intake may cause renal damage which would contribute to the nephrocalcific foci believed necessary for the initiation of crystallization of supersaturated solutes from the urine (*Anderson CK. Renal histological changes in stone formers and non-stone formers, in A Hodgkinson, BEC Nordin, Eds. Proc Renal Stone Res Sympos. London, Churchill, 1969:133-36*).

Restrict <u>alcohol</u> consumption.

Intake may be correlated with stone formation.

Observational Study: In West Germany, the rise in the incidence in urinary calcium oxalate stones is more closely correlated with the rise in alcohol consumption than with other trends. 53% of pts. stated that they drank alcohol daily, and 43% drank beer daily. Of these, 55% drank up to 700 ml daily, 29% drank 1 liter exactly and 16% drank 1-2 liters (*Vahlensieck W et al. Nutrition history of recurrent calcium oxalate stone formers pre- and post-dietary, in R Ryall et al, Eds. Urinary Stone. London, Churchill Livingstone, 1984:41-46*).

Observational Study: Pts. with urinary stones consumed almost twice as much alcohol as healthy controls (*Fellström B et al. Dietary history and dietary records in renal stone patients and control. Urol Res 12?58, 1984*).

Avoid <u>caffeine</u>.

May increase urinary calcium excretion.

Experimental Study: 31 women ingested decaffeinated coffee at different times to which caffeine had been added. 3 hrs. afterwards, urinary calcium excretion increased significantly, but only in women taking estrogen, suggesting that caffeine ingestion may offset the beneficial effect of estrogen on calcium metabolism (*Hollingbery PW et al. Effect of dietary caffeine and aspirin on urinary calcium and hydroxyproline excretion in pre- and postmenopausal women. Fed Proc 44:1149, 1985*).

Experimental Study: 15 males drank decaffeinated coffee to which 0, 150 or 300 mg caffeine had been added. Total urinary 3 hr. excretion of calcium, magnesium, sodium and chloride increased significantly after caffeine intake, while zinc, phosphorus, potassium, creatinine and volume were unchanged (*Massey LK, Berg TA. The effect of dietary caffeine on urinary excretion of calcium, magnesium, phosphorus, sodium, potassium, chloride and zinc in healthy males. Nutr Res 5:1281-84, 1985*).

Observational Study: The caffeine intake of 168 women (ages 36-45) was studied over the long term. Subjects averaged about 2 cups of regular coffee daily and suffered from a net calcium loss of 22 mg daily. The addition of only 1 cup of regular coffee resulted in an additional 6 mg of daily calcium loss. In addition, women who consumed a high amount of caffeine also consumed fewer calcium-rich foods. The authors note that a negative calcium balance of only 40 mg daily is quite sufficient to explain the 1-1.5% loss in skeletal mass annually in postmenopausal women (*Heaney RP, Recker RR. Effects of nitrogen, phosphorus, and caffeine on calcium balance in women. J Lab Clin Med 99:46-55, 1982*).

– –

COMBINED DIETARY CHANGES

Review Article: Results of epidemiological and biochemical studies suggest that a <u>vegetarian-oriented, less energy-rich</u> diet would probably reduce the risk of kidney stone formation (*Robertson WG. Diet and calcium stones. Miner Electrolyte Metab 13:228-34, 1987*).

Experimental Study: Over an ave. period of 5 yrs., 60% of idiopathic calcium stone formers achieved freedom from recurrences by high fluid intake and stopping excessive consumption of foodstuffs which encourage urinary stone formation (*Hosking DH et al. The stone clinic effect in patients with idiopathic calcium urolithiasis. J Urol 130:1115-18, 1983*).

Experimental Study: While the dietary habits of 392 stone formers did not differ significantly from controls, dietary advice to <u>increase fiber</u> and <u>reduce sugar</u>, <u>refined carbohydrates</u> and <u>animal protein</u> produced a significant reduction in the urinary excretion of calcium, oxalate and uric acid, suggesting that this is the first line of management of idiopathic stone formers (*Rao PN et al. Dietary management of urinary risk factors in renal stone formers. Br J Urol 54(6):578-83, 1982*).

- -

VITAMINS

<u>Vitamin A:</u>

Deficiency may promote the formation of kidney stones (*Bichler KH et al. Influence of vitamin A deficiency on the excretion of uromucoid and other substances in the urine of rats. Clin Nephrol 20:32-39, 1983; Gershoff SN, McGandy RB. The effects of vitamin A-deficient diets containing lactose in producing bladder cacluli and tumors in rats. Am J Clin Nutr 34:483, 1981*).

Negative Observational Study: The rate of dark adaptation, the thresholds of the completely dark adapted eye and blood vitamin A levels were determined for 20 pts. and compared to normal controls. In addition, in 78 autopsy cases with urolithiasis, the respiratory and urinary tracts were examined for the epithelial metaplasia characteristic of vitamin A deficiency. None of these cases showed evidence of vitamin A deficiency, suggesting that urolithiasis in humans is not usually associated with vitamin A deficiency (*Jewett HJ et al. Does vitamin A deficiency exist in clinical urolithiasis? JAMA 121:566-69, 1943*).

<u>Vitamin B6:</u>

May be deficient.

Experimental Study: 90 pts. with calcium oxalate urolithiasis were loaded with L-tryptophan 5 g and the 24 hr. urinary excretion of xanthurenic acid and kynurenine was measured. In 10/90 cases (11%), there were abnormal findings with an excretion pattern similar to hereditary vitamin B6-dependent xanthurenic aciduria in homozygous or heterozygous form (*Grimm U et al. [Studies on tryptophan metabolism in calcium oxalate urolithiasis.] Z Urol Nephrol 81(5):299-303, 1988*).

Experimental Controlled Study: Following loading with D,L-tryptophan 10 mg for 2 days, 18 stone formers excreted more xanthurenic acid than 12 normals, suggesting a marginal B6 deficiency (*Gershoff SN, Prien EL. Excretion of urinary metabolites in calcium oxalate urolithiasis: Effect of tryptophan and vitamin B6 administration. Am J Clin Nutr 8:812, 1960*).

Deficiency is associated with a metabolic block in the degradation of oxalic acid resulting in increased urinary oxalic acid and stone precipitation; thus supplementation may benefit at certain hyperoxaluric patients.

Experimental Study: 12 pts. with recurrent calcium oxalate renal calculi and idiopathic hyperoxaluria received pyridoxine 250-500 mg daily. Urinary oxalate excretion was significantly decreased (p<0.025) during the 18 mo. of treatment. In that period, 8 pts. showed no evidence of active stone disease, 3 showed a slight increase in the size of old stones, and 1 formed one new stone. None developed any significant complications from the therapy (*Mitwalli A et al. Control of hyperoxaluria with large doses of pyridoxine in patients with kidney stones. Int Urol Nephrol 20(4):353-59, 1988*).

Experimental Study: Out of a gp. of 90 pts. with calcium oxalate urolithiasis, those with an excretion of >300 μmol xanthurenic acid after a 5 gm tryptophan load responded favorably to pyridoxine 60 mg/d over 2 yrs. of follow-up (*Grimm U et al. [Studies on tryptophan metabolism in calcium oxalate urolithiasis.] Z Urol Nephrol 81(5):299-303, 1988*).

Supplementation may be beneficial even in the absence of an abnormal tryptophan load study for vitamin B6 deficiency.

Experimental Study: 4 stone formers with primary hyperoxaluria in whom tryptophan load studies failed to suggest vitamin B6 deficiency were supplemented with pyridoxine 75-600 mg daily. Doses of 150 mg were found to cause a sustained maximal reduction in urinary oxalate excretion in 2/4 pts. at levels intermediate between normal and their pre-treatment baseline (*Gibbs DA, Watts RWE. The action of pyridoxine in primary hyperoxaluria. Clin.Sci 38:277-86, 1970*).

<u>Vitamin C</u>:

WARNING: As ascorbate can be metabolized to oxalate, megadoses may increase urinary oxalate levels and thus contribute to the formation of calcium oxalate stones in predisposed individuals.

Note: Most lab methods for measuring urinary oxalate involve overnight precipitation of calcium oxalate at a pH of around 7. Since ascorbate is unstable in urine at room temperature at pH 7 and above, it may be converted overnight to oxalate in amounts directly proportional to its concentration, and thus persons taking large amounts might erroneously be found to have large amounts of urinary oxalate. Conversion of urinary ascorbate to oxalate can be prevented by collecting the urine in disodium EDTA (Chalmers AH et al. Stability of ascorbate in urine: relevance to analyses for ascorbate and oxalate. Clin Chem 31:1703, 1985).

Note: When megadose vitamin C is otherwise indicated, concurrent supplementation with pyridoxine may prevent increased oxaluria (see "Vitamin B6" above).

Review Article: Urinary oxalate excretion generally does not increase significantly for both normal subjects and stone-formers with ascorbic acid supplementation unless doses exceed 6 gm daily; however, oxalate excretion even at those high doses is still usually in the range achievable by dietary influences alone. The exceptions derive from anecdotal reports of a small number of cases and from one poorly-controlled trial with unstated methodology and questionable assay techniques (*Piesse JW. Nutritional factors in calcium containing kidney stones with particular emphasis on vitamin C. Int Clin Nutr Rev 5(3):110-129, 1985*).

Observational Study: 51 healthy males not receiving supplemental vitamin C were found to have a range of urinary oxalic acid of 16-64 mg (ave. 38 mg). The ave. increased by 3 mg when they were supplemented with 2 gm daily of vitamin C, and by 12 mg following supplementation with 4 gm vitamin C. An additional intake of 8 gm/d increased ave. oxalic acid excretion by 45 mg, while an additional intake of 9 gm/d resulted in a 68 mg ave. increase, with one subject demonstrating a 150 mg increase (*Lamden MP, Chrystowski GA. Urinary oxalate excretion by man following ascorbic acid ingestion. Proc Soc Exp Biol Med 85:190-92, 1954*).

- -

MINERALS

<u>Calcium</u>:

While about 30-50% of patients have idiopathic hypercalciuria, calcium restriction is usually not indicated as:

1. some patients will continue to have high urinary calcium excretion rates and lose bone due to overproduction of 1,25-dihydroxyvitamin D which stimulates bone resorption along with intestinal calcium absorption (*Coe FL et al. Effects of low-calcium diet on urine calcium excretion, parathyroid function and serum 1,25 (OH)2D3 levels in patients with idiopathic hypercalciuria and normal patients. Am J Med 72:25-32, 1982; Maierhofer WJ et al. Bone resorption stimulated by elevated serum 1,25-(OH)2-vitamin D concentrations in healthy men. Kidney Int 24:555-60, 1983; Maierhofer WJ et al. Dietary calcium and serum 1,25-(OH)2-vitamin D concentrations as determinants of calcium balance in healthy men. Kidney Int 26:752-59, 1984*);

2. the lower the calcium intake, the higher the urinary oxalate excretion (*Brockis JG et al. The effects of vegetable and animal protein diets on calcium, urate and oxalate excretion. Br J Urol 54(6):590-93, 1982*) - perhaps because dietary calcium precipitates oxalate in the intestines to form calcium oxalate which is not absorbed;

3. hypercalciuria in perimenopausal women with renal calculi and osteoporosis may be due to excessive bone resorption consequent to estrogen deficiency; in that case estrogen replacement is the indicated treatment (*Wasserstein A. The calcium stone former with osteoporosis. JAMA 257(16):2215, 1987*).

However, it is possible that a sub-group of idiopathic hypercalciuric patients may reduce stone formation without increasing bone resorption following calcium restriction. Such restriction would have to be shown to significantly reduce the calciuria while both oxaluria and serum 1,25-dihydroxyvitamin D levels remain low.

Case Report: A pt. with frequently recurrent kidney stones was found to have 7 mg/kg/day urinary calcium excretion when drinking tap water. When, however, he began to boil his water for 10 min. (to lower calcium content by precipitating calcium carbonate), urinary calcium excretion decreased to 3 mg/kg/day and he remained free of symptoms for 3 yrs. of follow-up (*Popovtzer MM et al. Letter. N Engl J Med 310(11):721, 1984*).

Chronic high calcium intake in subjects with normal vitamin D levels does not significantly increase urinary calcium, presumably because of a parathormone-mediated decrease in 1,25 dihydroxyvitamin D levels. This in turn decreases the fraction of calcium absorbed. However, either the combination of high calcium intake and supplementation with vitamin D causing elevated vitamin D levels (25-hydroxyvitamin D >30 ng/ml), or extreme calcium intake alone (>2000 mg/day), significantly increases urinary calcium and thus the risk of kidney stones (*Pacifici R et al. Effect of Ca and vitamin D supplementation on urinary calcium excretion in an adult female population. Abstract. J Am Coll Nutr 6(5):430, 1987*).

Negative Experimental Study: Calcium supplementation (600 mg/d) induced hypercalciuria in 11 pts. which caused a significant fall in the urinary inhibitory activity against calcium oxalate precipitation, as shown by a decline in the formation product ratio from 12.6 to 9.6 (p<0.005) (*Zerwekh JE et al. Modulation by calcium of the inhibitor activity of naturally occurring urinary inhibitors. Kidney Int 33(5):1005-08, 1988*).

Observational Study: Calciuria in osteoporosis pts. who were on supplementatary calcium (250-1,500 mg/d) was similar to that of other osteoporosis pts. who took no supplementary calcium (*Licatta AA et al. Effect of supplemental calcium on serum and urinary calcium in osteoporotic patients. Abstract. J Am Coll Nutr 7(5):419, 1988*).

When calcium supplementation is indicated to prevent bone resorption, it may be given in the form of carbonate, citrate, gluconate or lactate, all of which tend to alkalinize the urine and thereby decrease urine calcium excretion (*Wasserstein A. The calcium stone former with osteoporosis. JAMA 257(16):2215, 1987*). The risk of stone formation may be further reduced by increasing fluid intake (10-20 oz/dose) during the first 3 mo., after which, if urinary calcium levels are high (250 mg/day), the possibility of hypercalciuria should be investigated (*Pak CY et al. Nephrolithiasis from calcium supplementation. J Urol 137:1212-13, 1987*).

Magnesium: 200 mg. twice daily

Kidney stones have repeatedly been produced in magnesium-deficient animals (*Hodgkinson A. Proc Roy Soc Med 51:970, 1958*).

The urine of stone formers has a lowered magnesium/calcium ratio (*Takahasi E. The magnesium:calcium ratio in the concentrated urines of patients with calcium oxalate calculi. Invest Urol 10:147, 1972*).

Patients may be hypomagnesiuric.

Observational Study: 5.1% of 1116 pts. had hypomagnesiuria (urinary magnesium <50 mg/d) (*Preminger G et al. Hypomagnesiuric hypocitraturia. An apparent new entity for calcium nephrolithiasis. J Lithotripsy Stone Dis, 1990*).

Hypomagnesiuria appears to be dietary in origin (*Preminger G et al. Hypomagnesiuric hypocitraturia. An apparent new entity for calcium nephrolithiasis. J Lithotripsy Stone Dis, 1990*), since intestinal magnesium has been shown to be normal in nephrolithiasis (*Johansson G et al. Biochemical and clinical effects of the prophylactic treatment of renal calcium stones with magesium hydroxide. J Urol 124:770-74, 1980*).

Supplementation may inhibit calcium oxalate stone formation.

Note: Magnesium salts (magnesium oxide; magnesium citrate) decrease the urinary saturation of calcium oxalate and increase its formation product (metastability) only if they are administered with meals; thus they should not be given on an empty stomach (Lindberg J et al. Effect of magnesium citrate and magnesium oxide on the crystallization of calcium salts in urine: changes produced by food-magnesium interaction. J Urol 143(2):248-51, 1990).

Review Article: "Urinary magnesium concentrations are abnormally low in relation to urinary calcium concentrations in more than 25% of patients with kidney stones. A supplementary magnesium intake corrects this abnormality and prevents the recurrence of stones. Magnesium seems to be as effective against stone formation as diuretics" (*Labeeuw M et al. [Magnesium in the physiopathology and treatment of renal calcium stones.] Presse Med 16(1):25-27, 1987).*

Review Article: Once excreted, urinary oxalic acid rapidly forms a complex with the multiple cationic salts and ions available and becomes oxalate salt. Oxalate is soluble when combined with most components of urine such as magnesium. Only when it forms a complex with calcium in high concentrations does it become insoluble; then crystalline precipitation of calcium oxalate occurs. Magnesium has been positively identified as an inhibitor of calcium oxalate/calcium phosphate crystallization (*Goldwasser B et al. Calcium stone disease: An overview. J Urol 135:1, 1986).*

In vitro Experimental Study: Magnesium decreased both the growth rate and nucleation rate of calcium oxalate crystals in a simulated renal environment (*Li MK et al. Effects of magnesium on calcium oxalate crystallization. J Urol 133:123, 1985).*

Experimental Controlled Study: 55 pts. who had an ave. of 0.8 stones annually (460 stones in 10 previous yrs.) without evidence of magnesium deficiency (normal serum and urinary magnesium; normal intracellular magnesium in muscle biopsies, normal GI absorption of ^{28}Mg; normal magnesium loading test) were treated with 500 mg elemental magnesium in the form of magnesium hydroxide. The magnesium/calcium ratio in the urine increased due to increased magnesium excretion and approached a value earlier found in healthy subjects, and urinary citrate increased. After 2-4 yrs., only 8/55 developed stones and the ave. rate of stone development decreased 90% to 0.08 stones per person per year and 85% of pts. remained free of recurrence during follow-up. Side effects were few. Over 4 yrs., a control group of 43 pts. averaged a much higher formation rate and, after 4 yrs., 59% of them had developed new stones (*Johansson G et al. Effects of magnesium hydroxide in renal stone disease. J Am Coll Nutr 1(2):179-85, 1982).*

Experimental Controlled Study: 56 consecutive pts. with renal calcium stones received prophylatic treatment with magnesium hydroxide 200 mg twice daily. After most pts. had received supplementation for at least 2 yrs., 45 were free of recurrences or formations of new stones. The mean stone episode rate during treatment was 0.03 stones/yr. compared to 0.8 stones/yr. before treatment. Of 34 pts. who served as controls, 15 experienced recurrences after 2 years. The only side-effect was minor GI discomfort (*Johansson G et al. Biochemical and clinical effects of prophylactic treatment of renal calcium stones with magnesium hydroxide. J Urol 124(6):770-4, 1980).*

- with <u>Vitamin B$_6$</u>:   10 mg. daily

Combined supplementation may inhibit calcium oxalate stone formation.

Experimental Study: 149 pts. who had had at least 1 stone annually for 5 years (total of 871 stones) were placed on magnesium oxide 300 mg and pyridoxine 10 mg daily. In the next 4 1/2-6 yrs., only 17/149 (11%) developed stones (a total of 71 stones). The rate of stone production decreased from an ave. of 1.3 stones/pt./yr. to 0.10 stones/pt./yr. during therapy (*Prien EL, Gershoff S. Magnesium oxide-pyridoxine therapy for recurring calcium oxalate urinary calculi. J Urol 112:509-12, 1974).*

Experimental Study: After 1 yr., stone formers (ave. 1.1 stones/yr.) receiving magnesium oxide 300 mg and pyridoxine 10 mg daily had a >90% reduction in stone formation (<0.1 stones/yr.), an increased capacity to maintain calcium oxalate in solution, a raised citric acid level and a decreased xanthurenic acid level (*Gershoff S, Prien EL. Effect of daily MgO and vitamin B$_6$ administration to patients with recurring calcium oxalate kidney stones. Am J Clin Nutr 20:393-99, 1967).*

<u>Phosphorus</u>:

In patients, urinary phosphorus excretion may be elevated and may correlate with calcium excretion (*Kitamura T et al. [Urinary calcium and phosphorus excretion and their relationship in calcium-containing urinary stone formers.] Nippon Hinyokika Gakkai Zasshi 80(2):197-203, 1989).*

In patients, the kidney may fail to transform orthophosphate to pyrophosphate (*Conte A et al. The relation between orthophosphate and pyrophosphate in normal subjects and in patients with urolithiasis. Urol Res 17(3):173-75, 1989*).

Supplementation with orthophosphate may be beneficial.

Negative Experimental Study: In a study of 802 pts. with calcium stone disease, orthophosphate administration failed to significantly affect urine supersaturation of calcium oxalate and, compared to treatment with thiazide, magnesium or alkaline citrate, resulted in a higher recurrence rate (*Tiselius HG, Sandvall K. How are urine composition and stone disease affected by therapeutic measures at an outpatient stone clinic? Eur Urol 17(3):206-12, 1990*).

Experimental Study: 32 pts. received orthophosphate 1.0-1.5 g/d for a median treatment period of 3.1 years. Urine composition with respect to calcium oxalate supersaturation was favorably affected. There were reductions of urinary calcium (p<0.01) and calcium/citrate quotients (p<0.001). Although there was no difference in the rate of stone formation during treatment compared to a similar period of time following diagnosis, during the follow-up period, 31 stones were formed by 12 pts. compared to 73 stones in a similar period of time prior to treatment. 4/11 pts. treated for a period longer than that expected for new stone formation continued to form stones, as did 8/15 pts. with a shorter follow-up. In summary, despite favorable biochemical effects, the clinical result with orthophosphate at these dosages was disappointing (*Palmqvist E, Tiselius HG. Phosphate treatment of patients with renal calcium stone disease. Urol Int 43(1):24-28, 1988*).

Experimental Study: 38 male recurrent idiopathic stone formers received orthophosphate (1 g phosphorus) daily. Urinary calcium excretion decreased (p<0.001) and inorganic phosphate increased (p<0.001). These changes resulted in a small decrease in urine supersaturation of calcium oxalate, and a small increase in the supersaturation of calcium phosphate. The stone episode rate fell in 35/38 pts. from a mean of 0.66 episodes/yr. to 0.22 episodes/yr.; however, the 3 initially most prolific stone formers increased their rate of stone formation during treatment (*Heyburn PJ et al. Phosphate treatment of recurrent calcium stone disease. Nephron 32(4):314-19, 1982*).

- with <u>dietary restrictions</u>:

Experimental Crossover Study: 36 pts. with absorptive hypercalciuria were initially treated with diet alone follwed by either oral neutral phosphate (1,500 mg elemental phosphorus daily) or trichlormethiazide 4 mg daily. After 6 wks., pts. were crossed over to the other treatment for another 6 weeks. In response to dietary treatment, urinary calcium decreased from 346 ± 63 mg/24 hrs. to 308 ± 90 mg/24 hours. Oral phosphate therapy caused a further decrease to 218 ± 85 mg/24 hrs., and an over-all decrease of 37%. Pretreatment renal phosphate threshold did not correlate with the response to oral phosphate administration (*Insogna KL et al. Trichlormethiazide and oral phosphate therapy in patients with absorptive hypercalciuria. J Urol 141(2):269-74, 1989*).

<u>Potassium</u>:

Hypokalemia causes hypocitraturia and makes the urine more alkaline.

The ingestion of potassium-rich foods reverses the hypercalciuria caused by a high meat diet (*Kaneko K et al. Urinary calcium and calcium balance in young women affected by high protein diet of soy protein isolate and adding sulfur-containing amino acids and/or potassium. J Nutr Sci Vitaminol (Tokyo) 36(2):105-16, 1990*).

<u>Sodium</u>:   *See "DIETARY FACTORS" above.*

– –

OTHER NUTRITIONAL FACTORS

<u>Citrate</u>:   potassium citrate 60 mEq daily
                     (available by prescription)

Stone formers may have <u>hypocitraturia</u> - which correlates with hypercalciuria (*Conte A et al. On the relation between citrate and calcium and normal and stone-former subjects. Int J Nephrol 21(4):369-73, 1989*) and, in most cases, with a urinary pH above 6 (*François B et al. Inhibitors of urinary stone formation in 40 recurrent stone formers. Br J Urol 58(5):479-83, 1986*).

> **Observational Study:** 11/40 pts. (27.5%) had hypocitraturia (*François B et al. Inhibitors of urinary stone formation in 40 recurrent stone formers. Br J Urol 58(5):479-83, 1986*).

> **Observational Study:** 7/46 pts. (15.2%) had hypocitraturia (*Menon M, Mahle CJ. Urinary citrate excretion in patients with renal calculi. J Urol 129(6):1158-60, 1983*).

> **Observational Study:** Stone formers were found to excrete less citric acid than normals (*Gershoff SN. Excretion of urinary metabolites in calcium oxalate urolithiasis: Effect of tryptophan and vitamin B6 administration. Am J Clin Nutr 8:812, 1960*).

Supplementation may benefit stone formers with hypocitraturia, as citrate augments inhibitor activity against calcium oxalate crystallization (*Harvey JA et al. Calcium citrate: Reduced propensity for the crystallization of calcium oxalate in urine resulting from induced hypercalciuria of calcium supplementation. J Clin Endocrinol Metabol 61(6):1223-25, 1985*).

> **Experimental Study:** With a dose of sodium-potassium (alkali) citrate of 11 mmol 3 times daily, the crystal growth rate of calcium oxalate in the urine of 6 healthy volunteers decreased by 70%. This could have been due to the decrease of calcium excretion, which caused 50% of the total change, and to the increase of citrate and pH, each contributing about 20-25% to the decline (*Achilles W et al. The in-vivo effect of sodium-potassium citrate on the crystal growth rate of calcium oxalate and other parameters in human urine. Urol Res 18(1):1-6, 1990*).

> **Experimental Study:** Potassium citrate prophylaxis (30-80 mEq/d) in 37 idiopathic hypocitraturic pts. over a 2-yr. period normalized citrate excretion, increased urinary pH to pH 6.5-7, and reduced urinary saturation of calcium oxalate. Further stone formation ceased in 89.2% of pts. and the stone formation rate declined from 2.11 ± 5.68 to 0.28 ± 1.30 stones/pt-yr. (p<0.01). In these pts., renal tubular acidosis, chronic diarrhea, urinary tract infection and hypokalemia, the main causes of hypocitraturia, had been excluded (*Pak CY, Fuller C. Idiopathic hypocitraturic calcium-oxalate nephrolithiasis successfully treated with potassium citrate. Ann Intern Med 104(1):33-37, 1986*).

> **Experimental Study:** Treatment of 89 recurrent calcium stone-forming pts. with potassium citrate 20 mEq 3 times daily over 1-4 yrs. resulted in a decrease in individual stone formation in 97.8% of pts. and remission in 79.8% (*Pak CYC et al. Long term treatment of calcium nephrolithiasis with potassium citrate. J Urol 134(1):11-19, 1985*).

Supplementation may benefit patients with hyperuricosuria in addition to hypocitraturia.

> **Experimental Study:** 19 hyperuricosuric pts. with recurrent calcium oxalate kidney stones were treated with potassium citrate 60-80 mEq daily. Urinary citrate levels, which were initially below normal, increased into the normal range, while the urinary uric acid and the saturation of monosodium urate remained elevated. Stones ceased to form in 16/19 pts., and stone formation declined from a mean of 1.55/pt.-yr. to 0.38/pt.-yr. (mean reduction of about 75%) during a mean observation period of 2.35 years (*Pak CY, Peterson R. Successful treatment of hyperuricosuric calcium oxalate nephrolithiasis with potassium citrate. Arch Intern Med 146(5):863-67, 1986*).

Administration of potassium citrate may prevent recurrent calcium stone formation in patients with distal renal tubular acidosis.

> **Experimental Study:** 6 pts. with incomplete distal renal tubular acidosis and recurrent calcium nephrolithiasis randomly received potassium citrate 80 mEq/d and sodium citrate 80 mEq/d in either order. Potassium citrate decreased urinary calcium and significantly increased urinary citrate resulting in a significant decrease in the urinary saturation of calcium oxalate. The saturation of brushite and sodium urate was unchanged. While sodium citrate also increased the urinary citrate level, owing to the increased sodium load, it failed to decrease urinary calcium; thus urinary saturation of calcium oxalate did not decrease as much as with potassium citrate, and brushite saturation increased significantly. Moreover, due to enhanced sodium excretion, the urinary saturation of sodium urate increased significantly. Results suggest that potassium citrate may retard the crystallization of calcium oxalate and may not cause calcium phosphate crystallization, while sodium citrate may have no effect or

may accentuate the crystallization of calcium salts (*Preminger GM et al. Alkali action on the urinary crystallization of calcium salts: contrasting responses to sodium citrate and potassium citrate. J Urol 139(2):240-42, 1988*).

Experimental Study: During the 3 yrs. prior to treatment, 9 calcium stone-forming pts. with distal renal tubular acidosis formed an ave. of 39.3 stones each. Treatment with oral potassium citrate 60-80 mEq daily over a 34 mo. period resulted in complete inhibition of new stone formation in all pts. (*Preminger GM et al. Prevention of recurrent calcium stone formation with potassium citrate therapy in patients with renal tubular acidosis. J Urol 134(1):20-23, 1985*).

L-Glutamic acid:

Note: As oral supplemental glutamic acid is metabolized, it is not yet known how to effectively increase urinary glutamic acid levels.

Low or absent in the urine of many stone formers (*McGeown MG. The urinary excretion of amino acids in calculus patients. Clin Sci 18:185, 1959*).

Effective *in vitro* in retarding calcium oxalate precipitation in the urine of stone formers, although this effect may be superfluous when vitamin B6 levels are adequate (*Azoury R et al. May enzyme activity in urine play a role in kidney stone formation? Urol Res 10:185, 1982; Azoury R et al. Retardation of calcium oxalate precipitation by glutamic-oxaloacetic-transaminase activity. Urol Res 10:169, 1982*).

Glycosaminoglycans:

There is evidence suggesting that glycosaminoglycans are potent inhibitors of growth and aggregation of calcium oxalate crystals *in vitro* (*Michelacci YM et al. Urinary excretion of glycosaminoglycans in normal and stone forming subjects. Kidney Int 36(6):1022-8, 1989*).

Stone formers may excrete less glycosaminoglycans than normals (*Michelacci YM et al. Urinary excretion of glycosaminoglycans in normal and stone forming subjects. Kidney Int 36(6):1022-28, 1989; Nikkilä MT. Urinary glycosaminoglycan excretion in normal and stone-forming subjects: significant disturbance in recurrent stone formers. Urol Int 44(3):157-9, 1989*).

The lower concentrations of glycosaminoglycans in stone formers may impede their inhibitory activity on the heterogeneous nucleation of uric acid in calcium stone formation (*Conte A et al. Uric acid and its relationship with glycosaminoglycans in normal and stone-forming subjects. Nephron 52(2):162-5, 1989*).

Supplementation may reduce renal clearance of oxalates.

Experimental Study: 40 pts. with idiopathic calcium-oxalate nephrolithiasis received 30 mg twice daily of a mixture of glycosaminoglycans. By day 15 there were significant reductions from baseline in urinary oxalate excretion (p<0.005) as well as in RBC oxalate self-exchange and RBC membrane protein phosphorylation. These changes had reversed by 15 days after withdrawal of treatment. Acute IV administration of glycosaminoglycans 60 mg induced a fall in carbon-14-labelled oxalate renal clearance (p<0.005), which strongly suggests the participation of the kidney. However, reduced oxalate absorption from the intestine, and even decreased synthesis of oxalate, cannot be ruled out (*Baggio B et al. Correction of erythrocyte abnormalities in idiopathic calcium-oxalate nephrolithiasis and the reduction of urinary oxalate by oral glycosaminoglycans. Lancet 338:403-5, 1991*).

Lysine:

Dietary deficiency may increase urinary calcium (*Wolinsky I, Fosmire GJ. Calcium metabolism in aged mice ingesting a lysine-deficient diet. Gerontol 28(3):156-62, 1982*

- -

OTHER FACTORS

Rule out cadmium toxicity.

Cadmium exposure has been associated with increased prevalence of urolithiasis (*Scott R et al. The importance of cadmium as a factor in calcified upper urinary tract stone disease - A prospective 7-year study. Br J Urol 54:584, 1982*).

Cadmium causes renal tubular damage which can lead to calcific foci in the kidneys (*Axellson B, Piscator M. Renal change after prolonged exposure to cadmium. Arch Environ Health 12:360-72, 1969*) and may encourage oxalate crystallization (*Eusebio E, Elliot JS. Effect of trace metals on the crystallisation of calcium oxalate. Invest Urol 4:431, 1967*).

Stone formers excrete significantly more cadmium than normals (*Elliot JS, Ribeiro ME. The urinary excretion of trace metals in patients with calcium oxalate urinary stone. Invest Urol 10:253-55, 1973*).

LUPUS

See Also: AUTO-IMMUNE DISORDERS (GENERAL)

DIETARY FACTORS

Low calorie, low fat diet.

Review Article: Studies of diet in the mouse model of SLE have established the beneficial effects of a low calorie, low fat diet in these animals and suggest that a similar diet would be of benefit to humans (*Corman LC. The role of diet in animal models of systemic lupus erythematosus: Possible implications for human lupus. Semin Arthritis Rheum 15(1):61-69, 1985*).

Animal Experimental Study: The results of this study performed on lupus-prone mice suggest that diets high in fat may influence immune responses and thus may affect the onset and severity of auto-immune disease, and that a low-fat diet can reduce the development of the disease by maintaining normal immune responses (*Morrow J et al. Dietary fat and immune function. J Immunol 135(6):3857, 1985*).

Limit beef and dairy products.

Review Article: Studies of diet in the mouse model of SLE have established the beneficial effects of limiting proteins with a high content of phenylalanine and tyrosine, such as beef and dairy products, and suggest that a similar diet would be of benefit to humans (*Corman LC. The role of diet in animal models of systemic lupus erythematosus: Possible implications for human lupus. Semin Arthritis Rheumatol 15(1):61-69, 1985*).

- -

VITAMINS

Niacin:

Intravenous supplementation may improve the skin lesions.

Clinical Observation: Daily IV injections of nicotinamide 20 cg rapidly improves skin lesions in lupus erythematosis. The day after the first injection the lesions are already less intense. After some days this improvement is very marked. They subsequently remain stationary and never completely disappear despite the continuation of treatment (*Daïnow I. Recherches cliniques sur certaines propriétés anti-allergiques de la nicotinamide. Z Vitaminforsch 15:245-50, 1944*).

Pantothenic Acid: example: calcium pantothenate 6-10 gm daily initially
followed by 2-4 gm daily for "some months"

Supplementation may be beneficial.

Negative Experimental Study: 35 pts. with subacute or chronic lupus were unchanged or worse following supplementation with 2-600 mg daily of calcium pantothenate for 2-14 wks., as were 9 pts. supplemented with panthenol 1-4 mg daily for 4-16 wks. No other treatment was given concomitantly (*Cochrane T, Leslie G. The treatment of lupus erythematosus with calcium pantothenate and panthenol. J Invest Dermatol 18:365-67, 1952*).

Experimental Study: 30/37 pts. with subacute or chronic discoid lupus improved with massive panthenol therapy (*Goldman L. Preliminary and short report: Intensive panthenol therapy for lupus erythematosus. J Invest Dermatol 15:291, 1950*).

Experimental Study: Pts. with subacute and chronic discoid lupus showed satisfactory improvement with massive calcium pantothenate therapy (*Goldman L. Treatment of subacute and chronic discoid lupus erythematosus with intensive calcium pantothenate therapy. J Invest Dermatol 11:95, 1948*).

Vitamin A:

WARNING: Excessive tissue levels may be harmful.

Theoretical Discussion: Several lines of indirect evidence suggest that SLE could reflect a toxicity reaction to excessive tissue levels of vitamin A and that the remission often associated with long-term hemodialysis in pts. with end-stage renal disease may be due to a gradual reduction in vitamin A levels at the sites of SLE activity (*Mawson AR. Systemic lupus erythematosus, renal disease, hemodialysis and vitamin A. Med Hypotheses 18(4):387-98, 1985*).

Deficiency may accelerate the disease process.

Animal Experimental Study: Mice susceptible to a lupus-like disease were fed a vitamin-A deficient diet or a normal control diet. The vitamin-A deficient animals were found to manifest more severe hyper-gammaglobulinemia and an earlier onset of both NTA and IgM anti-erythrocyte antibodies (*Gershwin ME et al. Nutritional factors and autoimmunity. IV. Dietary vitamin A deprivation induces a selective increase in IgM autoantibodies and hypergammaglobulinemia in New Zealand Black mice. J Immunology 133(1):222-26, 1984*).

Vitamin B$_{12}$:   1000 µg IM twice weekly

Intramuscular supplementation may be beneficial.

Experimental Study: After 6 wks. of IM supplementation with B$_{12}$, 3/3 pts. with SLE who had failed to respond to oral and IM vitamin E had complete clearing of the lesions (*Block MT. Vitamin E in the treatment of diseases of the skin. Clin Med January 1953, pp. 31-34*).

Vitamin E: 1200 - 1600 IU daily
(may also be applied locally to skin lesions)

Supplementation may be beneficial.

Experimental Study: 4 pts. with discoid lupus receiving vitamin E 900-1600 IU daily of vitamin E showed complete or almost complete clearing, while 2 pts. receiving 300 IU daily had no benefit (*Ayres S, Mihan R. Is vitamin E involved in the autoimmune mechanism? Cutis 21:321-25, 1978*).

Experimental Study: 12 pts. with SLE were treated with 100-150 mg orally 3 times daily after meals plus 150 mg IM in an aqueous solution 2-3 times weekly. 8 had excellent results, 1 had good results and 3 had poor results (*Block MT. Vitamin E in the treatment of diseases of the skin. Clin Med January 1953, pp. 31-34*).

- and Pantothenic Acid:

Supplementation may be beneficial.

Experimental Study: 67 pts. with biopsy-confirmed LE were treated with pantothenic acid (ex. calcium pantothenate) 10-15 gm daily and vitamin E 1-2000 mg daily. All pts. showed marked improvement. Pts. with chronic discoid lupus began to show objective improvement in 4-6 months. Pts. with disseminated discoid lupus improved in 2 mo., while pts. in the subacute disseminated gp. improved in 1 month. The 3 pts. in the acute disseminated gp. also received steroid hormones initially and subsequently were maintained on the supplements without relapse for 7-19 months. The only side effects were transient nausea and gastric distress from the pantothenate (*Welsh AL. Lupus erythematosus: Treatment by combined use of massive amounts of pantothenic acid and vitamin E. Arch Dermatol Syphilol 70:181-98, 1954*).

- -

MINERALS

Selenium:

- and Vitamin E:

Combined supplementation may be beneficial.

Experimental Study: 1 pt. with SLE was found to have a low level of of glutathione peroxidase compared to normal controls, while 5 pts. with discoid lupus had levels similar to the controls. The SLE pt. was treated with tab containing 0.2 mg selenium as Na_2SeO_3 and 10 mg tocopheryl succinate. Glutathione peroxidase levels increased slowly within 6-8 wks. and the clinical effect was encouraging (*Juhlin L et al. Blood glutathione-peroxidase levels in skin diseases: Effect of selenium and vitamin E treatment. Acta Derm Venereal (Stockh) 62(3):211-14, 1982*).

Sulfur:

Sulfur oxidation may be impaired in lupus erythematosus.

Observational Study: 25/35 pts. (71%) with SLE showed impaired sulfur oxidation and 21 (60%) produced virtually no sulfoxides, compared with 17/47 (36%) and 2 (4%), respectively, of healthy controls. This impairment was unrelated to disease activity or drug therapy and is likely to be clinically important, since supply of inorganic sulfate limits the rate of formation of readily excreted non-toxic sulfate conjugates of compounds such as xenobiotics and steroids, and the synthesis of sulfated biocomponents. The alternative pathway of sulfur metabolism, S-methylation, was not impaired. These findings contrast with those of rheumatoid arthritis, since both pathways are impaired in the latter disorder (*Gordon C et al. Abnormal sulphur oxidation in systemic lupus erythematosus. Lancet 339:25-6, 1992*).

- -

OTHER NUTRITIONAL FACTORS

Beta Carotene:

Supplementation may be beneficial in discoid lupus.

Case Reports: 3 pts. with treatment-resistent chronic discoid lupus are described whose lesions flared with sun exposure. Beta-carotene 50 mg 3 times daily resulted in clearing of all lesions starting in one week (*Newbold PCH. Beta-carotene in the treatment of discoid lupus erythematosus. Br J Dermatol 95:100-101, 1976*).

Essential Fatty Acids:

WARNING: An essential fatty acid-deficient diet has been found beneficial for the autoimmune disease which develops spontaneously in NZB/NZW F1 mice (an experimental animal model for human lupus) (*Hurd ER, Gilliam JN. Beneficial effect of an essential fatty deficient diet in NZB/NZW F1 mice. J Invest Dermatol 77(5):381-84, 1981*). The implications of this finding for human lupus patients are unknown.

- Omega-3 Fatty Acids (Fish Oils):

Most important member: eicosapentaenoic acid (EPA) which is particularly high in cold-water   fish.

Available in a refined form as "MaxEPA" (18% EPA).

Suggested MaxEPA dosage: 3 - 9 grams daily in divided doses (or 10 ml. concentrate twice daily)

WARNING: Supplementation may require additional vitamin E intake to prevent increased membrane peroxidation and cellular damage (*Laganiere S, Fernandes G. High peroxidizability of subcellular membrane induced by high fish oil diet is reversed by vitamin E. Clin Res 35:A565, 1987*).

Supplementation may be beneficial.

Animal Experimental Study: Disease development was strikingly slowed in lupus-prone mice fed a fish oil-containing diet. By 10 mo. of age, 94% of the mice fed fish oil were still living, while all the mice fed a saturated fat diet had died, and 35% of those fed a corn oil diet were alive. Long after the other 2 gps. had succumbed to glomerulonephritis, the fish oil gp. had negligible proteinuria. While the fish oil-supplemented mice had no or minimal arteritis in the spleen, arteritis was found in the spleens of nearly all the mice in the other 2 gps. (*Alexander NJ et al. The type of dietary fat affects the severity of autoimmune disease in NZB/NZW mice. Am J Pathol 127(1):106-21, 1987*).

Animal Experimental Study: The effect of fish oil on autoimmune lupus in mice showed that the substance "had the most striking protective effect seen thus far in any animal model of inflammatory disease" (*Robinson DR - reported in Med World News July 14, 1986; Robinson DR et al. The protective effect of dietary fish oil on murine lupus. Prostaglandins 30(1):51-75, 1985*).

Animal Experimental Study: Dietary supplementation of fish oil suppressed autoimmune lupus in mice, both delaying the onset of renal disease and prolonging survival (*Kelley VE et al. A fish oil diet rich in eicosapentaenoic acid reduces cyclooxygenase metabolites, and suppresses lupus in MRL-lpr mice. J Immunol 134(3):1914-19, 1985*).

- Omega-6 Fatty Acids:

Example: evening primrose oil 3 gm daily

Precursors of prostaglandin E$_1$, which has been shown to reduce kidney damage in an animal model of systemic lupus erythematosus (*Krakauer K et al. Prostaglandin E$_1$ treatment of NZB/W mice, III. Immunol Immunopathol 11:256, 1978; Zurier RB et al. Prostaglandin E$_1$ treatment of NZB/W mice, I. Arth Rheum 20:723-8, 1977*).

Administration of evening primrose oil may be beneficial.

Negative Animal Experimental Study: Although PGE$_1$ successfully controlled the auto-immune inflammatory disease, including kidney damage, which spontaneously develops in New Zealand black/white mice (believed to be an excellent model of human systemic lupus erythematosus), evening primrose oil failed to do so (*Zurier RB. Use of prostaglandins and evening primrose oil (Efamol) in experimental models of inflammation, in DF Horrobin, Ed. Clinical Uses of Essential Fatty Acids. Montreal, Eden Press, 1982:113-24*).

L-Tryptophan:

WARNING: Supplementation may be harmful.

Patients are said to have decreased serotonin levels, perhaps due to deficient conversion of tryptophan to serotonin. The tryptophan breakdown products may lead to auto-antibody production (*McCormick JP et al. Characterization of a cell-lethal product from the photooxidation of tryptophan: Hydrogen peroxide. Science 191:468-9, 1976*).

Review Article: In SLE, abnormal tryptophan metabolism is present with high excretion particularly of kynurenines and xanthurenic acid (*Cardin de' Stefani E, Costa C. [Changes in the metabolism of tryptophan in erythematosus.] Boll Soc Ital Bio Sper 60(8):1535-40, 1984*).

- -

OTHER FACTORS

Rule out <u>food and chemical sensitivities</u>.

Food allergies and other allergies may be more common in lupus patients than in normals (*Carr RI et al. Antibodies to bovine gamma globulin (BCG) and the occurrence of a BCG-like substance in systemic lupus erythematosus sera. <u>J Allergy Clin Immunol</u> 50(1):18-30, 1972*).

Observational Study: The frequency of a history of clinical manifestations of urticaria, pharyngitis, conjunctivitis and food allergy was significantly increased in 63 SLE pts. compared to pts. with other autoimmune diseases and normals, and SLE pts. had the highest incidence of different types of clinical manifestations per individual (*Diumenjo MS et al. [Allergic manifestations of systemic lupus erythematosus.] <u>Allergol Immunopathol (Madr)</u> 13(4):323-26, 1985*).

Food and chemical exposures may influence disease activity in sensitive patients.

Experimental Study: 4 pts. with SLE developed remissions following food eliminations and nutritional supplementation, while another 70 pts. with lupus and lupus-like syndromes showed a similar trend (*Cooke HM, Reading CM. Dietary intervention in systemic lupus erythematosus: 4 cases of clinical remission and reversal of abnormal pathology. <u>Int Clin Nutr Rev</u> 5(4):166-76, 1985*).

Case Report: 36 year-old female developed episodic vomiting at age 5 and migraine at age 11. At age 16 she developed a polyarthritis and a diagnosis of SLE was made. Her disease progressed over the years with further involvement of the GI, GU, respiratory and vascular symptoms. Spontaneous bruising and petechiae occurred, together with peripheral edema. Antinuclear antibodies and LE preparations were positive repeatedly and she was placed on cortisone and cytotoxic drugs. Following admission to an environmental control unit, all meds were stopped. Joint stiffness and swelling gradually disappeared and her sed rate fell from 63 to 15 mm in 1 week, the lowest value in years. Food and chemical challenges precipitated a return of her symptoms (*Rea WJ, Brown OD. Mechanisms of environmental vascular triggering. <u>Clin Ecology</u> 3(3):122-8, 1985*).

Rule out <u>hydrochloric acid deficiency</u>.

If deficient, supplementation may be beneficial.

Note: While gastric anacidity had been reported in the past to be a relatively common condition which was associated with a number of illnesses, the presence of achlorhydria is no longer accepted unless a potent parietal-cell stimulant (such as histamine) is employed in gastric analysis. More recent studies suggest that histamine-fast anacidity is uncommon before the fifth decade of life and, although it probably does not occur in a normal stomach, its presence is not necessarily associated with symptoms (Rappaport EM. Achlorhydria: Associated symptoms and response to hydrochloric acid. <u>N Engl J Med</u> 252(19):802-5, 1955).

Experimental Study: Of 9 pts. with lupus erythematosus, none had normal hydrochloric acid levels and 2 had no detectable hydrochloric acid. Signs of vitamin B complex deficiency seemed to correlate to the extent of the hydrochloric acid deficiency and improvement followed supplementation with hydrochloric acid and vitamin B complex (*Allison JR. The relation of hydrochloric acid and vitamin B complex deficiency in certain skin diseases. <u>South Med J</u> 38:235-241, 1945*).

MACULAR DEGENERATION

PATHOPHYSIOLOGY

Age-related macular degeneration (AMD) is an advanced stage of a deteriorative process that takes place in all eyes and involves a progressive impairment of the outer layers in the center of the retina. Its primary lesion appears to reside in the retinal pigment epithelium (RPE), possibly resulting from its high rate of molecular degradation. Throughout the life span, cells of the RPE gradually accumulate sacs of molecular debris. These residual bodies (lipofuscin) are remnants of the incomplete degradation of abnormal molecules which have been damaged within the RPE cells or derived from phagocytized rod and cone membranes. Progressive engorgement of RPE cells with these residues is associated with the extrusion of aberrant materials which accumulate in Bruch's membrane and aggregate in the form of drusen and basal laminar deposits. These extrusions contribute to the further deterioration of the RPE. Loss of vision results from death of visual cells due to degeneration of RPE cells, or the effects of leakage from neovascular membranes that invade the region of abnormal extracellular deposits (*Young RW. Pathophysiology of age-related macular degeneration. Surv Ophthalmol 31(5):291-306, 1987*).

- -

VITAMINS

Vitamin A:

Intake is negatively correlated with the risk of age-related macular degeneration.

Observational Study: Using data from the first National Health and Nutrition Examination Survey (US), the frequency of consumption of fruits and vegetables rich in vitamins A and C suggested a negative association with the prevalence of macular degeneration after stratified adjustment for age. In a logistic regression analysis, adjusting for demographic and medical factors, only the frequency of consumption of fruits and vegetables rich in vitamin A remained negatively correlated with age-related macular degeneration even after adjustment for demographic and medical factors (*Goldberg J et al. Factors associated with age-related macular degeneration. An analysis of data from the first National Health and Nutrition Examination Survey. Am J Epidemiol 128(4):700-10, 1988*).

Deficiency may be associated with retinal degeneration.

Animal Experimental Study: Retinas of monkeys made deficient in vitamin A showed disruption of photoreceptors (*Hayes KC. Retinal degeneration in monkeys induced by deficiencies of vitamin E or A. Invest Ophthalmol 13(7):499-510, 1974*).

Vitamin C:

WARNING: Excessive exposure to high-energy light, especially as focused in the vitreum, as in undercompensated myopia, combined with excessive supplemental ascorbic acid, may be associated with vitreopathy-induced age-related macular degeneration (odds ratio 95% confidence interval = 2.5-35.4) (*Lane BC. Evidence for a dietary/environmental etiological classification of several macular degenerations. Abstract. J Am Coll Nutr 10(5):550, 1991*).

As an antioxidant, supplementation may protect the retina against cellular damage.

Animal Experimental Study: Ascorbate supplementation prior to exposure protected rat retinas from damage due to oxidative insult by light (*Li ZY et al. Amelioration of photic injury in rat retina by ascorbic acid: a histopathologic study. Invest Ophthalmol Vis Sci 26(11):1589-98, 1985; Organisciak DT et al. The protective effect of ascorbate in retinal light damage of rats. Invest Ophthalmol Vis Sci 26(11):1580-8, 1985*).

Note: Experimental studies have demonstrated that bright light preferentially damages precisely the region that degenerates in age-related macular degeneration (Young RW. Solar radiation and age-related macular degeneration. Surv Ophthalmol 32(4):252-69, 1988).

Vitamin E:

Deficiency may be associated with retinal degeneration.

Animal Experimental Study: Compared to controls, rats on vitamin-E free diets with higher vitamin A levels exhibited marked disruption of photoreceptor outer segment membranes and a fivefold increase in the number of lipofuscin granules in the pigment epithelial cells which ingest these membranes. Rats on vitamin-E free diets with lower vitamin E levels also exhibited significant loss of photoreceptor cells with a pattern of loss different from that of vitamin A deficiency. Normal vitamin A levels probably protect photoreceptor membranes from oxidative damage and retard the accumulation of their remnants and other products of lipid breakdown in the pigment epithelium *(Robison WG Jr et al. Vitamin E deficiency and the retina: photoreceptor and pigment epithelial changes. Invest Ophthalmol Vis Sci 18(7):683-90, 1979).*

Animal Experimental Study: Retinas of monkeys made deficient in vitamin E showed disruption of photoreceptors *(Hayes KC. Retinal degeneration in monkeys induced by deficiencies of vitamin E or A. Invest Ophthalmol 13(7):499-510, 1974).*

Supplementation may be beneficial.

Clinical Observations: Over 90% of a gp. of more than 20 pts. improved following treatment with vitamin E and the replacement of table salt with mineral-rich sea salt. 4 pts. whose vision had deteriorated to mere hand movements improved sufficiently to read a newspaper (20/50). Only 1 pt. had deterioration of vision while under treatment, but a few deteriorated after stopping, only to improve again when supplementation was reinstituted. Improvement may be very slow, taking up to 12 months *(Todd GP. Nutrition, Health & Disease. Norfolk, Virginia, The Donning Company, 1988).*

- and Vitamin A:

In other tissues, vitamin E deficiency has been shown to lower vitamin A levels, and it is widely accepted that this effect is due to autoxidative destruction of vitamin A. In the retina, however, results of studies done on rats suggest that vitamin E may not regulate vitamin A levels by acting as an antioxidant, but rather may act as an inhibitor of vitamin A uptake and/or storage *(Katz ML et al. Dietary vitamins A and E influence retinyl ester composition and content of the retinal pigment epithelium. Biochim Biophys Acta 924(3):432-41, 1987; Katz ML et al. Relationship between dietary retinol and lipofuscin in the retinal pigment epithelium. Mech Ageing Dev 35(3):291-305, 1986).*

Vitamin A deficiency may increase the extent of retinal damage induced by vitamin E deficiency.

Note: However, vitamin A deficiency also caused greater retinal damage in rats supplemented with vitamin E (Katz ML et al. Dietary vitamins A and E influence retinyl ester composition and content of the retinal pigment epithelium. Biochim Biophys Acta 924(3):432-41, 1987).

Animal Experimental Study: Studies were performed on rats fed vitamin E-deficient diets. It was found that their vitamin A nutritional status significantly influenced the extent of retinal damage induced by vitamin E deficiency, with a poor vitamin A status being associated with greater damage *(Robison WG Jr et al. Vitamin E deficiency and the retina: photoreceptor and pigment epithelial changes. Invest Ophthalmol Vis Sci 18(7):683-90, 1979).*

– –

MINERALS

<u>Copper</u>:

The pigmented epithelium is a copper-rich tissue.

Serum levels may be elevated (*Silverstone BZ et al. Zinc and copper metabolism in patients with senile macular degeneration. <u>Ann Ophthalmol</u> 17(7):419-22, 1985*).

Ceruloplasmin, a copper-binding alpha-globulin, may be elevated in the serum (*Newsome DA et al. Macular degeneration and elevated serum ceruloplasmin. <u>Invest Ophthalmol Vis Sci</u> 27(12):1675-80, 1986*).

Excessive copper may be toxic to the retina (*Gahlot DK, Ratnakar KS. Effect of experimentally induced chronic copper toxicity on retina. <u>Indian J Ophthalmol</u> 29(4):351-3, 1981*).

<u>Zinc</u>:

Human retinal zinc concentration is higher than any other normal organ (*Underwood EJ. <u>Trace Elements in Human and Animal Nutrition</u>, 4th Edition. London, Academic press, 1977:198*).

Retinal zinc deficiency may reduce the activity of catalase, an antioxidant metalloenzyme found in the macular human retinal pigment epithelium (*Newsome D et al. The trace element and antioxidant economy of the human macula: can dietary supplementation influence the course of macular degeneration? Abstract. <u>J Am Coll Nutr</u> 10(5):536, 1991*).

Macular degeneration is associated with reduced catalase activity (*Newsome D et al. The trace element and antioxidant economy of the human macula: can dietary supplementation influence the course of macular degeneration? Abstract. <u>J Am Coll Nutr</u> 10(5):536, 1991*).

Retinal zinc deficiency may impair the utilization of vitamin A.

> **Animal Experimental Study:** When the retinal zinc concentration in rats was reduced due to dietary inadequacy, the zinc metalloenzyme alcohol dehydrogenase was significantly lowered, and the retinol-retinal conversion was significantly reduced (*Huber AM, Gershoff SN. Effects of zinc deficiency on the oxidation of retinol and ethanol in rats. <u>J Nutr</u> 105(11):1486-90, 1975*).

> *Note: Retinol is a substrate for alcohol dehydrogenase.*

Serum levels may be elevated (*Silverstone BZ et al. A metabolic analysis of high myopia and senile macular degeneration. <u>Metab Pediatr Syst Ophthalmol</u> 11(3):122-5, 1988; Silverstone BZ et al. Zinc and copper metabolism in patients with senile macular degeneration. <u>Ann Ophthalmol</u> 17(7):419-22, 1985*).

Supplementation may be beneficial.

> **In vitro Experimental Study:** Alpha mannosidase activity in cultured human retinal pigment epithelial cells significantly decreased with age, and cells from older donors could be activated almost 2-fold by the addition of zinc. Since alpha-manniosidase is probably required for the degradation of rhodopsin in the phagolysosomal system of the retinal pigment epithelium, a decrease in enzyme activity may lead to accumulation of undigested rod outer segments and drusen, both of which are associated with age-related macular degeneration (*Wyszynski RE et al. A donor-age-dependent change in the activity of alpha-mannosidase in human cultured RPE cells. <u>Invest Ophthalmol Vis Sci</u> 30(11):2341-7, 1989*).

> **Experimental Double-blind Study:** 151 subjects with drusen or macular degeneration randomly received either zinc supplementation (100 mg/d) or placebo with meals. Although some eyes in the zinc-treated gp. lost vision, this gp. had significantly less loss of visual acuity than the placebo gp. after a follow-up of 12-24 mo. (p<0.05). In vision testing, 33% of the placebo pts. lost 10 or more letters of vision compared to 10% of the zinc-treated gp.;

66% of the placebo gp. and 86% of the zinc gp. lost 9 or fewer letters of vision (*Newsome DA et al. Oral zinc in macular degeneration. Arch Ophthalmol 106(2):192-8, 1988*).

Note: A very little, and an extremely variable, amount of zinc is absorbed when taken with food, as substances in many foods bind zinc and prevent its absorption; thus perhaps only 10% or even less of the zinc administered was actually absorbed. This suggests that even more dramatic results could be obtained if zinc were administered in an effective manner and in a higher delivered dose (Yazbasiyan-Gurkan V, Brewer GJ. The therapeutic use of zinc in macular degeneration. Letter. Arch Ophthalmol 107(12):1723-4, 1989).

- -

OTHER NUTRITIONAL FACTORS

Taurine:

Necessary for normal vision, taurine is released from the retina following light exposure and is actively transported from retina to choroid by the retinal pigment epithelium (*Scharschmidt BF et al. Effect of taurine on the isolated retinal pigment epithelium of the frog: electrophysiologic evidence for stimulation of an apical, electrogenic Na^+-K^+ pump. J Membr Biol 106(1):71-81, 1988*).

Deficiency may be associated with retinal degeneration (*Hayes KC et al. Retinal degeneration associated with taurine deficiency in the cat. Science 188:949-51, 1975; Imaki H et al. Retinal degeneration in 3-month-old rhesus monkey infants fed a taurine-free human infant formula. J Neurosci Res 18(4):602-14, 1987; Lake N, Malik N. Retinal morphology in rats treated with a taurine transport antagonist. Exp Eye Res 44(3):331-46, 1987*).

- -

COMBINED NUTRITIONAL INTERVENTIONS

Riboflavin, Vitamin C, Vitamin E, Copper, Manganese, Selenium and Beta-carotene:

Experimental Controlled Studies: Pts. who ordered ICAPS plus, a multivitamin/mulimineral formula, regularly were compared with those who generally ordered only their first bottle. After 6 mo., 15/38 (40%) regular users compared to 6/37 (16%) drop-outs improved in vision by a line or more (p=0.025), and 3/38 regular users vs. 13/37 drop-outs lost a line or more or more of vision (p=0.004). In the second study, regularly treated pts. were compared to untreated controls. After 6 mo., visual acuity was the same or better in 168/192 (88%) treated pts. compared to 36/61 (59%) controls (p=0.028) (*Olson RJ. Supplemental dietary antioxidant vitamins and minerals in patients with macular degeneration. Abstract. J Am Coll Nutr 10(5):550, 1991*).

Vitamin A, Vitamin C, Vitamin E and Selenium:

Clinical Observations: Close to 1,000 pts. with senile macular degeneration or diabetic retinopathy were treated with antioxidant therapy (vitamin A, vitamin C, vitamin E and selenium). In about 70%, the diseases were retarded. The earlier the treatment was started, the better the response (*Ely J. Crary, Smyrna, Georgia, USA - quoted in Zarrow S. Keep your eyes young and sharp. Prevention March, 1985, pp. 74-80*).

Vitamin E, Selenium, Zinc, and Taurine:

Clinical Observations and Case Reports: Pts. were treated with a series of IV injections of selenium 400 μg and zinc 10 mg in 150 cm³ of 0.5 N saline or Ringer's lactate (infused over 30 min. twice weekly) along with oral selenium (selenomethionine or selenous acid liquid 2-300 μg daily), zinc (zinc picolinate or citrate 60 mg daily), vitamin E 800 IU daily and taurine 1 gm twice daily (with avoidance of protein for 1 hr. before or after). All pts. except one (first seen 8 yrs. after diagnosis) improved. After 8 wks., most pts. were able to stop the injections and rely on oral supplementation (selenium 800 μg and zinc 20 mg once weekly) which, if possible, was slowly tapered off (*Wright JV et al. Improvement of vision in macular degeneration associated with intravenous zinc and selenium therapy: two cases. J Nutr Med 1:133-8, 1990*).

MENOPAUSAL SYMPTOMS

VITAMINS

<u>Vitamin E</u>:   results in 2 wks. - 3 mo.

Supplementation may be beneficial.

Negative Experimental Placebo-controlled Study: 82 menopausal pts. received vitamin E 50-100 mg daily, 280 received estrogens, 88 received phenobarbital 15 mg 3 times daily and 298 received placebo during a 3-year period. Based on the Menopausal Index, a numerical conversion of the severity of the 11 most common menopausal symptoms, estrogens were most effective, while vitamin E was no more effective than placebo, with 25% of pts. reporting a moderate to excellent response (*Blatt MHG et al. Vitamin E and climacteric syndrome: Failure of effective control as measured by menopausal index. <u>Arch Intern Med</u> 91:792-9, 1953*).

Experimental Placebo-controlled Study: 66 pts. with vasomotor symptoms were given 20-100 mg (ave. 30 mg) alpha tocopherol in divided doses daily for 10 days-7 mo (ave. 31 days). 31 had good to excellent results and 16/66 had fair results, with prompt recurrence of symptoms after discontinuation of the vitamin. Placebo was substituted in 17 pts. followed by recurrence of symptoms which remitted again when vitamin E was resumed (*Finkler RS. The effect of vitamin E in the menopause. <u>J Clin Endocrinol Metab</u> 9:89-94, 1949*).

Experimental Placebo-controlled Study: 14/17 pts. who attained complete relief with estrogens but did not respond to barbiturates or placebos showed adequate improvement on vitamin E 75 mg/d, and 6 of these pts. attained complete relief (*Rubenstein BB. Vitamin E diminishes the vasomotor symptoms of menopause. Abstract. <u>Fed Proc</u> 7:106, 1948*).

- -

OTHER NUTRITIONAL FACTORS

<u>Bioflavonoids</u>:

The structural formulae of certain bioflavonoids resemble that of estradiol (*Clemetson CAB et al. Capillary strength and the menstrual cycle. <u>Ann N Y Acad Sci</u> 93:277-300, 1962*).

Bioflavonoids in the capillary wall may maintain the integrity of the capillary endothelium with an additional contribution from estrogen (*Clemetson CAB et al. Capillary strength and the menstrual cycle. <u>Ann N Y Acad Sci</u> 93:277-300, 1962*).

- with <u>vitamin C</u>:

Combined supplementation may be beneficial.

Experimental Study: 94 pts. with hot flashes (36 had had surgical castration; 58 had undergone physiological menopause) received Peridin-C (hesperidin complex 150 mg, hesperidin methyl chalcone 50 mg, ascorbic acid 200 mg) 6 tabs daily for 1 mo. as well as calcium carbonate, salicylamide and an estrogenic substance (at a minimal dosage as almost half the pts. had treated malignancies), each for 1 month. The drugs were indistinguishable from one another in appearance. Compared to the control drugs, Peridin-C was markedly superior. Symptoms were relieved in 50 pts. (53%) and moderated in 32 (34%). The only adverse effect was a slightly offensive perspiration odor with a tendency for perspiration to discolor the clothing (*Smith CJ. Non-hormonal control of vaso-motor flushing in menopausal patients. <u>Chic Med</u> 67(5):193-5, 1964*).

Experimental Study: 40 menopausal women, mean age 51, were treated. 14 had nocturnal leg cramps, 15 easy bruising, and 11 spontaneous nosebleeds. In all cases, symptoms worsened during the time of the month in which their menses had formerly occurred. They received hesperidin 200 mg and vitamin C 200 mg after each meal and at bedtime for 2 wks. followed by 100 mg of each 4 times daily for 4 weeks. Once symptoms had disappeared, the dosage was reduced to 200 mg of each daily and then supplementation was discontinued. 4/14 with nocturnal leg cramps noted that symptoms were under control within 2 wks., and the rest within an ave. of 7 weeks. 11/15 pts. with easy bruising improved after 8 wks., while the other 4 responded by 16 weeks. Nosebleeds stopped in 6-11 wks. in the 8/11 cases which were moderate, and the dosage was successfully reduced to 400 mg/d of hesperidin and vitamin C for a year. Of the remaining 3/11 cases, 1 was under control in 3 mo., and remained so on 400 mg of each daily. The other 2 pts. improved but their nosebleeds were never completely controlled until they stopped spontaneously in the 4th year (*Horoschak A. Nocturnal leg cramps, easy bruisability and epistaxis in menopausal patients: Treated with hesperidin and ascorbic acid. Del State Med J, January, 1959, pp. 19-22*).

Gamma-Oryzanol:

An extract of rice bran oil.

Supplementation may be beneficial.

Experimental Study: 40 pts. over 40 yrs. old with vasomotor problems, weakness, arthralgia, myalgia, headaches, insomnia, nervousness and/or melancholia received gamma-oryzanol 100 mg 3 times daily. After 4-8 wks., 16 pts. (40%) reported excellent results; 14 pts. (35%) reported good results; 6 pts. (15%) said treatment was "effective"; and 4 pts. (10%) were unchanged. According to Kupperman's index of menopausal symptoms, the symptoms of climacteric disturbance were successfully treated in 85% of the cases (*Ishihara M. Effect of gamma oryzanol on serum lipid peroxide level and climacteric disturbances. Asia-Oceania J Obstet Gynaecol 10(3):317, 1984; Ishihara M et al. Effect of gamma-oryzanol on serum lipid peroxide level of patients with climacteric disturbance. J Aichi Med Univ Assoc 11(3):278-85, 1983*).

Experimental Study: 8 menopausal women aged 39-52 and 13 women aged 30-61 who had undergone bilateral oophorectomies received gamma-oryzanol daily. After 38 days, there was a 50% or greater reduction in the Kupperman's index of menopausal symptoms in 67% of all pts. and in 75% of the menopausal women, indicating reduction of their subjective complaints. While improvements in vaginal secretions were reported, vaginal smears showed no changes. There were no untoward side effects (*Murase Y et al. Clinically cured cases by per os gamma oryzanol of menopausal disturbances or menopausal-like disturbances. Sanfujinka no Jissai 12(2):147, 1963*).

Experimental Study: 18 menopausal women with climacteric autonomic imbalance, 17 women with postmenopausal syndrome and 5 women with postcastration autonomic imbalance received gamma-oryzanol 30 mg daily. After 2 wks., 70% had moderate to marked clinical improvement and 20% had slight improvement. Both the disappearance of symptoms (headaches, low back pain, anorexia, fatigability, lassitude, dizziness, etc.) and normalization of the galvanic skin response were used as outcome measures. There was a "transient perturbation" of autonomic nervous system function following the start of treatment which coincided with symptom relief (*Okuda N et al. Mechanism of action of gamma oryzanol and clinical experience. Sanka to Fujinka 29:1488, 1962*).

- with vitamin E:

Combined administration may be beneficial (*Sotonishi T et al. Treatment of climacteric complaints with gamma oryzanol plus tocopherol. Folha Med (Brazil) 77(2):235, 1978*).

Phyto-estrogens:

Estrogenic compounds found in plants.

Dietary intake may affect the severity of the menopause.

Experimental Study: After a 14 day baseline, 25 post-menopausal women aged 51-70 who were not on drugs known to affect estrogen state supplemented their diets with soya flour (45 g/d), red clover sprouts (10 g dry seed/d), and linseed (25 g/d), each for 2 weeks. After 6 wks., there were significant increases in vaginal cell maturation (p<0.01) which persisted for 2 wks. after supplementation was stopped, but had disappeared after 8 weeks. There was a cumulative effect on serum concentrations of follicle stimulating hormone (p<0.05) but not on luteinizing hormone over the 6-wk. supplementation period. Up to half of the diet of some populations may comprise foods containing phyto-estrogens, while in this study such foods comprised only about 10% of energy intake for a fairly short time (*Wilcox G et al. Oestrogenic effects of plant foods in postmenopausal women. Br Med J 301:905-6, 1990*).

L-Tryptophan:

Reduced plasma estrogen may make less tryptophan available for conversion to brain serotonin.

Observational Study: In 3 perimenopausal women with climacteric symptoms including hot flushes, insomnia and depression, there was a significant positive correlation between total plasma estrogen concentration and the concentration of free plasma tryptophan (but not with total plasma tryptophan) during the night. The majority of tryptophan is bound to albumin, and plasma estrogens can bind to albumin. It thus seems likely that this relationship is due to a direct action of estrogen on the tryptophan binding site of albumin. Since the metabolism of brain serotonin depends partly on the concentration of free plasma tryptophan, these results suggest a possible means by which estrogens might influence cerebral serotonin metabolism and perhaps mood in perimenopausal women (*Thomson J et al. Relationship between nocturnal plasma oestrogen concentration and free plasma tryptophan in perimenopausal women. J Endocrinol 72(3):395-6, 1977*).

Observational Study: A positive correlation was found between low blood levels of tryptophan and estrogen in depressed women who had recently gone through menopause (*Editorial: Tryptophan and depression. Br Med J 1:242-3, 1976*).

- -

COMBINED NUTRITIONAL SUPPLEMENTATION

Vitamin C,
Vitamin E and
Calcium:

Clinical Observations: In a survey of hundreds of menopausal women, many reported relief from hot flashes in 2 days after starting vitamin E complex 800 IU daily. Hot flashes may disappear completely when the vitamin E is accompanied by vitamin C 2-3 g/d and calcium 1 g/d, both in divided doses. When the hot flashes have subsided, usually after 1 wk., vitamin E can be reduced to 400 IU/d (*Reitz R. Menopause: A Positive Approach. New York, Penguin Books, 1979*).

MENORRHAGIA

VITAMINS

Vitamin A: 25,000 I.U. twice daily for 15 days

If deficient, supplementation may be beneficial.

> **Experimental and Observational Study:** 71 women with menorrhagia were found to have significantly lower serum vitamin A levels than healthy controls. 40 of these women were treated with vitamin A 25,000 IU twice daily for 15 days. Menstruation returned to normal in 57.5% and diminished in an additional 35%. 17-β-estradiol production was increased more than 100% (*Lithgow DM, Politzer WM. Vitamin A in the treatment of menorrhagia. S Afr Med J 51:191-3, 1977*).

- -

MINERALS

Iron: 100 mg daily

Patients may be iron-deficient despite the absence of iron-deficiency anemia.

> **Observational Study:** Serum ferritin of menorrhagic pts. was significantly lower than that of controls despite the lack of significant differences in hemoglobin concentration, mean corpuscular volume and mean corpuscular hemoglobin (*Lewis GJ. Do women with menorrhagia need iron? Br Med J 284:1158, 1982*).

Chronic iron deficiency can cause menorrhagia.

> **Experimental Double-blind Study:** 75% of a gp. of pts. on iron improved compared to 32.5% on placebo, a significant difference (*Taymor ML et al. The etiological role of chronic iron deficiency in production of menorrhagia. JAMA 187:323-27, 1964*)

> **Experimental Study:**
> 1. 74/83 pts. (in whom organic pathology had been excluded) responded to iron supplementation.
> 2. Pts. who failed to respond to iron had a high rate of organic pathology (fibroids, polyps, adenomyosis, etc.).
> 3. 44/57 responding pts. had an associated rise in serum iron.
> 4. When initial iron levels were high, there was a decreased response to supplementation.
> 5. Menorrhagia correlated with depleted bone marrow iron stores irrespective of serum iron level.
> (*Taymor ML et al. The etiological role of chronic iron deficiency in production of menorrhagia. JAMA 187:323-27, 1964*)

Supplementation may prevent iron deficiency.

> **Experimental Study:** 15 pts. received iron 100 mg daily in connection with the menstrual period. Mean menstrual blood loss was 117 ml (range 21-117 ml), corresponding to 53 mg of iron (range 21-117 mg). The mean absorption was 81 mg (range 49-145 mg), with 14/15 absorbing more iron than was lost by menstrual bleeding (*Arvidsson B et al. Iron prophylaxis in menorrhagia. Acta Obstet Gynecol Scand 60:157-60, 1981*).

Manganese:

Deficiency may be associated with menorrhagia.

Experimental Study: 15 young women were placed on a low-manganese diet (1 mg/d - 1/2 of the US ave.). After 5.5 mo., menstrual fluid increased about 50% in volume. Also, between 50% and 100% more iron, copper, zinc and manganese were lost in the menstrual fluid (*Phyllis Johnson, Human Nutrition Center, US Dept. of Agriculture, Grand Forks, N. Dakota - reported in Townsend Letter for Doctors, May, 1991*).

- -

OTHER NUTRITIONAL FACTORS

Bioflavonoids plus
Vitamin C: 200 mg of each 3 times daily

Combined supplementation may be beneficial.

Experimental Study: Supplementation reduced symptoms in 14/16 pts. Of the 2 failing to respond, 1 had endometriosis and the other had metrorrhagia (*Cohen JD, Rubin, HW. Functional menorrhagia: Treatment with bioflavonoids and vitamin C. Curr Ther Res 2:539, 1960*).

MITRAL VALVE PROLAPSE

VITAMINS

Vitamin C:

Deficiency may contribute to the development of the valvular changes.

>**Review Article:** An ascorbic acid deficit may contribute to the development of the valvular lesions of MVP by altering collagen metabolism (*Zeana CD. Recent data on mitral valve prolapse and magnesium deficit. Magnes Res 1(3-4):203-11, 1988*).

- -

MINERALS

Magnesium:

May be deficient.

>**Review Article:** Idiopathic mitral valve prolapse is widespread and superimposed with the clinical picture of latent tetany. It appears as a late complication of latent tetany due to magnesium deficit. The high prevalence in women is mainly due to ovarian hormones. Palpitations and precordial pain are the most frequent cardiac symptoms (*Zeana CD. Recent data on mitral valve prolapse and magnesium deficit. Magnes Res 1(3-4):203-11, 1988*).

>**Observational Study:** 17 magnesium-depleted pts. with echocatrdiographically proven MVP showed a strong positive correlation between urinary magnesium and lactate. The strong correlation over all the range of urinary magnesium values and the significantly increased excretion of lactate suggest urinary magnesium loss in this syndrome (*Cohen L et al. Renal excretion of lactate and magnesium in mitral valve prolapse. Magnes Res 1(1-2):75-8, 1988*).

>**Observational Study:** 17 pts. with echocardiographically proven MVP were found to have below normal mean lymphocyte magnesium concentration and above normal magnesium retention following an IV magnesium loading test (*Cohen L et al. Idiopathic magnesium deficiency in mitral valve prolapse. Am J Cardiol 57(6):486-7, 1986*).

>**Observational Study:** 40 pts. were investigated and hypomagnesemia was a statistically significant finding, suggesting that it has an important role in causing the rhythm and neuropsychic disturbances (*Zeana C et al. Considerations on the pathogenesis of mitral valve prolapse. Med Interne 23(3):165-70, 1985*).

>**Observational Study:** Compared to 36 matched controls, 42 MVP pts. had significantly lower mean RBC magnesium (p<0.01), but there were no significant differences in serum magnesium or serum ionized calcium (*Galland L. Magnesium deficiency in mitral valve prolapse, in Halpern and Durlach, Eds. Magnesium Deficiency. First European Congress on Magnesium. Karger, Basel, 1985*).

>**Observational Study:** Out of a gp. of 170 pts. with neuromuscular hyperexcitability, 26% of the 143 pts. with latent tetany on the basis of Chvostek's sign, EEG or EMG findings were found to have MVP, compared to none of the 27 pts. without latent tetany. Although there were no significant differences in plasma and RBC magnesium levels between the non-tetanic nervous pts., the tetanic pts. and the MVP pts., these values were all significantly lower than normal reference values (p<0.001) (*Durlach J et al. Latent tetany and mitral valve prolapse due to chronic primary magnesium deficit, in Halpern and Durlach, Eds. Magnesium Deficiency. First European Congress on Magnesium. Karger, Basel, 1985*).

Observational Study: EMG in 64/75 (85.3%) MVP pts. showed changes suggestive of spasmophilia with symptoms typical of this condition. The specific clinical signs of spasmophilia were elicited with a positive Chvostek sign in 73.3%. Radiological, echo-cardiographical and hemodynamic studies underlined the hyperkinetic state of the left ventricle. There was a high incidence of low RBC magnesium levels. It is noted that chest pain suggestive of angina pectoris, mitral valve prolapse and spasmophilia are frequently associated (*Gërard R et al. [Mitral valve prolapse and spasmophila in the adult.]* Arch Mal Coeur *72(7):715-20, 1979*).

Supplementation may be beneficial.

Review Article: The histopathology, somatic morphology and genetics of MVP support the leading theory that it results from a hereditary disorder of connective tissue. Latent tetany due to chronic magnesium deficit occurs in over 85% of cases, and MVP complicates 26% of cases of latent tetany. Magnesium deficiency hinders the mechanism by which fibroblasts degrade defective collagen, increases circulating catecholamines, predisposes to arrhythmias, thromboembolic phenomena and dysregulation of the immune and autonomic nervous systems; magnesium therapy relieves MVP symptoms (*Galland LD et al. Magnesium deficiency in the pathogenesis of mitral valve prolapse.* Magnesium *5(3-4):165-74, 1986*).

Experimental Study: 12 pts. with MVP, ventricular hyperkinesia (LVH) and latent tetany received magnesium salts (pyrrolidone carboxylate 4.5 gm/day, lactate 3 gm/day) either alone or with a beta-blocker for a mean of 36.5 mo. (range 12-72 mo.). Following treatment, MVP and LVH were still present in 50%. Mean RBC magnesium was below normal prior to therapy and normal after therapy but no relationship was found between the increase in RBC magnesium and the disappearance or persistence of MVP and LVH (*Frances Y et al. Long-term follow-up of mitral valve prolapse and latent tetany. Preliminary data.* Magnesium *5(3-4):175-81, 1986*).

Review Article: To the list of signs of latent tetany due to magnesium deficit, MVP should be added as an irreversible neuromuscular sign. When MVP is found, it should be described as a common local sign of tetany which will help determine treatment in pts. with dyskinetic but normal, unthickened valves and not those associated with heart disease. Magnesium therapy is the essential specific element of treatment. Beta-blockers or phenytoin are suggested as first time treatment. The effects of magnesium therapy on the symptoms of MVP are even more dramatic when the signs of latent tetany have been controlled. Early control of tetany-producing magnesium deficit ensures the prevention of MVP. After at least 1 yr. of magnesium treatment, the symptoms may be partially or even totally reversed in about 1/3 of cases (*Durlach J et al. Latent tetany and mitral valve prolapse due to chronic primary magnesium deficit, in Halpern and Durlach, Eds.* Magnesium Deficiency. First European Congress on Magnesium. *Karger, Basel, 1985*).

Experimental Placebo-controlled Study: 35 pts. with symptomatic MVP and latent tetany attributed to a primary magnesium deficit received magnesium lactate 3 gms daily. 24 received magnesium for 16 wks., while 11 received placebo for 8 wks. followed by magnesium for 8 wks. Symptoms which improved during magnesium supplementation included palpitations, atypical chest pain, peripheral vascular spasms, psychological symptoms and muscle cramps. Trousseau's sign disappeared in the 10 cases in whom it was positive. No improvement occurred during placebo administration, but improvement did occur when pts. on placebo were switched to magnesium. Of those treated for 16 wks. with magnesium, 29.2% became asymptomatic after 4-12 wks., 45.8% had persistence of only 1-2 psychic symptoms (e.g. anxiety, depressive tendency), and the remaining 25% showed improvement, but it was less marked. Auscultatory signs of MVP were unchanged. Serum magnesium levels tended to rise during supplementation (*Fernandes JS et al. Therapeutic effect of a magnesium salt in patients suffering from mitral valvular prolapse and latent tetany.* Magnesium *4:283, 1985*).

- -

OTHER NUTRITIONAL FACTORS

Carnitine:

May be deficient and, if deficient, supplementation may be beneficial.

Case Reports: A pt. with MVP and numerous associated symptoms that were resistant to drug therapy was found to have below normal values for free plasma and urinary carnitine. After treatment with L-carnitine, 1 gm 3 times daily for 4 mo., symptoms resolved. In addition, in a random sampling of 4 pts., all 4 were found to have low levels of plasma and urinary carnitine (*Trivellato M et al. Carnitine deficiency as the possible etiology of idiopathic mitral valve prolapse: Case study with speculative annotation. Texas Heart Inst J 11(4):370, 1984*).

Coenzyme Q₁₀:

Supplementation may be beneficial.

Experimental Study: 400 children with MVP aged 8-16 received CoQ10 0.6-3.4 mg/kg/day. CoQ10 was found to be definitely effective for symptomatic MVP and improved stress-induced cardiac dysfunction if the appropriate dose was given. No side effects were noted. When the supplement was withdrawn, symptoms returned. Rapid normalization could be usually be achieved in 1 wk. on doses of 3.0-3.4 mg/kg/day, with gradual decreases to a patient-dependent stabilization dose (*Oda T. Effect of coenzyme Q10 on stress-induced cardiac dysfunction in paediatric patients with mitral valve prolapse: A study by stress echocardiography. Drugs Exp Clin Res 11(8):557-76, 1985*).

Experimental Placebo-controlled Study: All of 194 children with symptomatic MVP showed an abnormal response to a standard isometric hand grip test as a measure of cardiac performance. 8 were given coeynzme Q10 2 mg/kg/d, while 8 controls were given placebo. After 8 wks., hand grip testing had normalized in 7/8 treated children compared to none of the controls. Relapse to their former condition was frequently noted if pts. discontinued CoQ10 within 1 yr. to 17 mo., but rarely occurred in those who continued to take the supplement for 18 mo. or longer (*Oda T, Hamamoto K. Effect of coenzyme Q-10 on the stress-induced decrease of cardiac performance in pediatric patients with mitral valve prolapse. Jpn Circ J 48:1387, 1984*).

MULTIPLE SCLEROSIS

See Also: AUTO-IMMUNE DISORDERS (GENERAL)

DIETARY FACTORS

Low fat diet with a high polyunsaturate to saturate ratio.

> (*See Also: "Fatty Acids" below*)

A high fat diet impairs the conversion of linoleic acid to prostaglandin E_1 (PGE$_1$) (*Brenner RR. The oxidative desaturation of unsaturated fatty acids in animals. Mol Cell Biochem 3:41-52, 1974*). PGE$_1$ levels may have a relationship to disease activity (*see "Omega-6 Fatty Acids" below*).

Experimental Study: 144 pts. followed a low-fat diet for 34 years. At each level of severity of disability, pts. who adhered to the diet showed significantly less deterioration and much lower death rates than did those who consumed more fat than prescribed (>20g/d). The greatest benefit was seen in those with minimum disability at the start of the trial; in this gp., when those who died from non-MS diseases were excluded, 95% survived and remained physically active. Defaulting from the diet even after 5-10 yrs. was, in almost all cases, followed by reactivation of the disease. Pts. consuming 10-15g/d or less had even better improvement in energy and fatigue levels (*Swank RL, Dugan BB. Effect of low saturated fat diet in early and late cases of multiple sclerosis. Lancet 336:37-39, 1990*).

> *Note: Since pts. who are well are more likely to continue on treatment than those who deteriorate, "good compliers" are likely to be self-selected from those who do well, giving the predictable "positive" result (Editorial: Lipids and multiple sclerosis. Lancet 336:25-26, 1990).*

Experimental Study: The pts. in this 36-yr.-old study all reduced their saturated fat intake markedly from an ave. of 125 g/d prior to the start of the study. Only oils which were fluid at room temperature were allowed as a source of fats. All experienced a marked decrease in exacerbations. The best clinical results were in pts. who reduced daily fat intake to <20 g. For this gp., deterioration was slight, and only 31% died. Above 20 g fat per day, the level of disability was serious, and the death rate increased to 80%. Females tended to do better than males. The response to the diet was more marked if made early in the course of the disease. While oil consumption was found to be indirectly beneficial, the authors believe that this was the result of the replacement of saturated fats by unsaturated oils, rather than by a direct benefit from the essential fatty acids in the oils (*Swank RL, Grimsgaard A. Multiple sclerosis: The lipid relationship. Am J Clin Nutr 48:1387-93, 1988*).

Experimental Controlled Study: 83 pts. increased the P:S ratio of the diet from 0.8 to 1.5 after 6 mo. and 1.34 at 36 months. There were significant correlations between linoleic, eicosapentaenoic and docosahexaenoic acid levels and the diet. Not only was there a reduction in the exacerbation rate, but there was also an improvement in the neurological status of compliant pts., while matched controls continued to deteriorate in terms of rate and severity of exacerbations and neurological status (*Fitzgerald G et al. The effect of nutritional counselling on diet and plasma EFA status in multiple sclerosis patients over 3 years. Hum Nutr Appl Nutr 41(5):297-310, 1987*).

Observational Study: On the basis of an examination of the statistical correlations between the main foodstuff and nutrient intakes and the chief causes of mortality in 20 different countries, findings suggested a causal interpretation between total fat intake and multiple sclerosis (*Knox EG. Foods and diseases. Br J Prev Soc Med 31(2):71-80, 1977*).

Observational Study: Cow's milk contains only 1/5 the linoleic acid (an essential polyunsaturate) of human milk and there is none in skim milk. People who were fed cow's milk as children were found to be more susceptible to MS as adults than people who were breast fed (*Agranoff BW, Goldberg D. Diet and the geographical distribution of multiple sclerosis. Lancet 2:1061-66, 1974*).

Experimental Study: 146 pts. were placed on a low fat diet and followed up to an ave. of 17 years. The course of the disease was less rapidly progressive than in untreated cases. If treated before significant disability developed, a high percentage of cases remained unchanged for up to 20 years. When treated later, the disease was slowly progressive. Pts. consuming the least fat and the largest amount of fluid (mono- and polyunsaturated) oils deteriorated the least (*Swank RL. Multiple Sclerosis: Twenty years on low fat diet. Arch Neurol 23:460-74, 1970*).

Observational Study: The brain tissue of pts. was found to have a higher saturated fat content than controls (*Baker R. Lancet 1:26, 1963*).

- -

VITAMINS

Thiamine:

Supplementation by injection may be beneficial.

> **Case Reports:** Intraspinal injections led to dramatic, though transient, improvements (*Stern EI. The intraspinal injection of vitamin B₁ for the relief of intractable pain, and for inflammatory and degenerative diseases of the central nervous system. Am J Surg 34:495, 1938*).

- with Niacin:

> **Case Reports:** Pts. benefited from IV injections containing nicotinic acid 100 mg and thiamine 60 mg in each 10 cc solution (*Moore MT. Treatment of multiple sclerosis with nicotinic acid and vitamin B₁. Arch Intern Med 65:18, 1940*).

Vitamin B_6:

Deficiency may predispose to multiple sclerosis.

> **Theoretical Discussion:** Carbon monoxide pollution of the air is the one environmental factor present only in the localities where MS is common. Of 21,000 non-fatal cases of CM poisoning, a number developed a demyelinating condition. Similarly, animals exposed to CM develop CNS degeneration. It has been shown that CM exposure increases the need for pyridoxine, suggesting that a relative B_6 deficiency may cause MS in susceptible persons (*Mitchell DA, Schandl EK. Am J Clin Nutr August, 1973*).

Vitamin B_{12}:

Deficiency may be associated with multiple sclerosis.

> **Case Report:** A 46-year-old woman had painful paresthesias associated with progressive rt. leg wekaness. Myelography was normal. MS was diagnosed. During the following 15 yrs. she was admitted about every 18 mo. for symptom exacerbation and responded each time to ACTH infusions. In June, 1987, a brain MRI showed bilateral high-signal-intensity white matter abnormalities. About 2 mo. later, a MCV of 100.8 fl was recorded. When evaluated in 1988, she had severe spastic monoparesis of the rt. leg associated with distal wasting. Vibration appreciation was bilaterally absent in the feet, with decreased pinprick appreciation the the mid-thigh on the right. Reflexes were symmetrically depressed with bilateral plantor extensor responses. HGb was 14.4 g/dL, MCV was 98.3 fl. The blood smear contained rare hypersegmented polymorphonuclear leucocytes. Serum B_{12} was <100 pg/ml and folic acid was 8.2 ng/ml. Plasma concentrations of vitamin B_{12}-dependent metabolites were normal (total serum homocystine and serum methymalonic acid). Rheumatoid factor was raised with an antinuclear factor titer of 20. Serum intrinsic factor antibodies were present. She was treated with vitamin B_{12} injections 1000 μg daily for 1 wk. followed by weekly injections. Initial improvement was such that she could climb stairs without circumduction of the rt. leg. After 6 mo., she showed evidence of increased rt. leg strength. Blood count was normal with a decreased in MCV to 92.7 fl and no hypersegmented polymorphonuclear cells. Serum B_{12} was 210 pg/ml. Since pernicious anemia has an autoimmune basis, both ACTH and steroids produce amelioration of the disease with hematological remission. It is suggested that ACTH produced temporary remissions, giving rise to the mistaken impression that she had a classic clinical course for MS (*Ransohoff RM et al. Vitamin B₁₂ deficiency and multiple sclerosis. Letter. Lancet 335:1285-86, 1990*).

Case Reports: 3 pts. with convincing evidence of MS also had vitamin B12 deficiency of an unusual or obscure kind. One had juvenile pernicious anemia which preceded the onset of MS; the other 2 had unexplained deficiency. 2 of the pts., including the man with juvenile PA, had persistent macrocytosis despite vitamin B12 therapy. None had any of the usually recognized neurological or psychiatric complications of B12 deficiency. While the relationship between vitamin B12 deficiency and MS in these pts. is unclear, depletion of RBC cobalamin levels in one pt. suggests that there is a defect in transport of B12 into the cells, perhaps due to a disturbance in protein binding (*Reynolds EH, Linnell JC. Vitamin B12 deficiency, demyelination, and multiple sclerosis. Letter. Lancet 2:920, 1987*).

Review Article: During the 1950's and 1960's there were several studies of serum and CSF vitamin B12 levels in MS because of the suspected role of B12 in myelin formation. Because of equivocal results, the interest waned (*Chanarin I. The Megaloblastic Anemias. Oxford, Blackwell, 1982*).

- -

MINERALS

Calcium:

- and VitaminD:

Deficiency during puberty has been theorized to predispose to multiple sclerosis. If so, supplementation during puberty may be preventative.

Theoretical Discussion: Based on epidemiologic, biochemical and genetic evidence, it is hypothesized that demyelination in MS results from a breakdown due to abnormal lipid composition and structure produced during the period of brain development. Altered lipid concentrations and fatty acid profiles result from genetic deficiencies in enzymes that govern myelin synthesis and membrane asssembly which may occur because of inadequate supplies of vitamin D and calcium at times of rapid myelination and growth, especially adolescence. If this theory is correct, it may be possible to suppress the disease by dietary supplementation with vitamin D and calcium during puberty (*Goldberg P. Multiple sclerosis: Vitamin D and calcium as environmental determinants of prevalence. Int J Environ Stud 6:19-27 & 121-29, 1974*).

- and Magnesium , Vitamin D and Cod Liver Oil:

Supplementation may be beneficial.

Experimental Study: 16 pts. aged 22-37 who exhibited unambiguous exacerbations within 12-24 mo. prior to the trial received dolomite sufficient to furnish 16 mg/kg calcium and 10 mg/kg magnesium daily. Also, in order to promote mineral absorption, they received 20 g/d cod liver oil to furnish 5,000 IU daily of vitamin D. After 1-2 yrs., the number of exacerbations was <1/2 the number expected from case histories. Results tend to support the theory that calcium and magnesium are important in the development, structure and stability of myelin (*Goldberg P et al. Multiple sclerosis: decrease relapse rate through dietary supplementation with calcium, magnesium and vitamin D. Med Hypotheses 21(2):193-200, 1986*).

Note: Swank and Dugan state that increasing oil intake is normally accompanied by a decrease in saturated fat intake which may be as much as 2 g for every 1 g increase, which suggests that decreased saturated fat intake was another factor contributing to improvement (Swank RL, Dugan BB. Effect of low saturated fat diet in early and late cases of multiple sclerosis. Lancet 336:37-39, 1990).

Copper:

Deficiency is associated with defects in myelination in animal studies (*Underwood EJ. Trace Elements in Human and Animal Nutrition, 4th Ed. New York, Academic Press, 1971*).

Serum levels may be normal (*Wikström J et al. Selenium, vitamin E and copper in multiple sclerosis. Acta Neurol Scand 54(3):287-90, 1976*).

Tissue levels may be depressed.

Observational Study: Compared to 42 controls, hair copper levels were significantly lower in 40 pts. (*Ryan DE et al. Trace elements in scalp-hair of persons with multiple sclerosis and of normal individuals. Clin Chem 24, 1978*).

Ceruloplasmin levels may be elevated.

Observational Study: Compared to controls, ceruloplasmin levels of 27 pts. were higher, but not significantly (*Smith DK et al. Trace element status in multiple sclerosis. Am J Clin Nutr 50:136-40, 1989*).

Observational Study: Ceruloplasmin was found to be increased during acute exacerbations of MS (*Becus T et al. Study of serum and cerebrospinal fluid ceruloplasmin in multiple sclerosis and nother neurologic diseases. Rev Roum Neurol 8:3-12, 1971*).

Selenium:

The prevalence of multiple sclerosis may be inversely related to selenium levels in the soil.

Observational Study: The prevalence of MS is high in Ostrobothnia, a low selenium district in Finland, while in Lapland, a high selenium district, the prevalence is low (*Wikstrom J et al. Selenium, vitamin E and copper in multiple sclerosis. Acta Neurol Scand 54(3):287-90, 1976*).

Glutathione peroxidase activity may be reduced.

Observational Study: Compared to controls, pts. had lower glutathione peroxidase (GSH-px) activity (*Mai J et al. High dose antioxidant supplementation to MS patients. Biol Trace Element Res 24:109, 1990*).

Negative Observational Study: Compared to controls, concentrations of glutathione peroxidase in 27 pts. were similar (*Smith DK et al. Trace element status in multiple sclerosis. Am J Clin Nutr 50:136-40, 1989*).

Negative Observational Study: Normal activity of glutathione peroxidase (both selenium-depdendent and selenium-independent) was found in lymphocytes, granulocytes and platelets of MS patients (*Szeinberg A et al. Glutathione peroxidase activity in various types of blood cells in multiple sclerosis. Acta Neurol Scand 63(1):67-75, 1981*).

Observational Study: Lymphocyte and granulocyte glutathione peroxidase activity in Danish pts. was significantly reduced by 35-50% compared to controls (*Jensen GE et al. Leucocyte glutathione peroxidase activity and selenium level in multiple sclerosis. J Neurol Sci 48(1):61-67, 1980*).

If selenium-dependent glutathione-peroxidase activity is low, selenium supplementation may increase it.

Case Report: A 34 year-old primipara (weight 50 kg) had suffered from MS for 9 yrs. and her condition had deteriorated considerably during the first 5 mo. of lactation. Prior to selenium supplementation she was, due to fatigue and vertigo, unable to lift and carry her baby, or to walk with snow boots due to ataxia. Because of a low glutathione peroxidase level and short Se[75] half-life (58 days), it was decided to administer supplemental selenium. The pt. received oral sodium selenite 0.02 mg/kg body weight for 1 mo. and then 0.04 mg/kg. Plasma and breast milk selenium rose, and RBC glutathione peroxidase levels increased. After 3 mo., her condition clearly improved, and she was able to handle her baby and to walk normally. After about 1 1/2 yrs. of treatment, however, she had a relapse. Because of the natural history of exacerbations and remissions of MS, it is not possible to know whether selenium supplementation was related to her temporary improvement (*Westermarck T et al. Selenium level in milk during long-term supplementation with sodium selenite to a patient with multiple sclerosis. Nutr Res Suppl 1:S232-34, 1985*).

- with vitamin C and vitamin E:

Experimental Study: Following 5 wks. of supplementation with sodium selenite 6 mg/d, vitamin C 2 g/d and vitamin E 480 g/d, GSH-px levels increased 5-fold in a gp. of pts. with reduced glutathione peroxidase (GSH-px) activity, while side effects were minimal. Also, 2 mg of sodium selenite was shown to increase selenium concentrations by 24% (*Mai J et al. High dose antioxidant supplementation to MS patients. Biol Trace Element Res 24(2):109-17, 1990*).

Zinc:

May be abnormalities in its compartmentalization.

Observational Study: Compared to controls, plasma and RBC zinc levels were higher in MS patients and, during periods of relapse, RBC zinc levels decreased dramatically. RBC zinc levels were increased specifically in the extracts of the lipid fraction of the erythrocyte membrane (*Ho S-Y et al. Zinc in multiple sclerosis. II. Correlation with disease activity and elevated plasma membrane-bound zinc in erythrocytes from patients with multiple sclerosis. Ann Neurol 20:712-15, 1986*).

Note: Altered levels of cholesterol in plasma and erythrocytes may contribute to the increased RBC membrane zinc (Cunnane SC et al. Essential fatty acid and lipid profiles in plasma and erythrocytes in patients with multiple sclerosis. Am J Clin Nutr 50:801-06, 1989).

Observational Study: Compared to normal controls, plasma zinc levels were slightly increased in pts. with MS (and significantly increased in pts. with other neurological impairments), while albumin-bound and protein-bound zinc were normal. The alpha 2 macroglobulin-bound zinc was significantly lower in pts. than in controls, while RBC-bound zinc was significantly increased (p<0.05) in MS pts. but not in pts. with other neurological impairments. As RBC-bound zinc levels are relatively independent of daily dietary flucuations, this increase may suggest alterations in the control mechanisms governing zinc compartmentalization (*Dore-Duffy P et al. Zinc in multiple sclerosis. Ann Neurol 14(4):450-54, 1983*).

- -

OTHER NUTRITIONAL FACTORS

Fatty Acids:

70% of myelin is lipid and the unsaturated lipids, predominately oleic acid, may be subject to peroxidation insult (*Norton WT. Formation, structure, and biochemistry of myelin, in GJ Seigel et al, Eds. Basic Neurochemistry. 2nd Edition. Boston, Little, Brown, and Company, 1976:74-79*).

Note: Nutritional factors capable of influencing lipid peroxidation include vitamins with known antioxidant activity, such as vitamins C and E, and the trace element-dependent enzymes glutathione peroxidase (selenium), ceruloplasmin (copper), and superoxide dismutases (zinc, copper, and manganese) (Halliwell B, Gutteridge JM. Lipid peroxidation: A radical chain reaction, in B Halliwell, JM Gutteridge JM, Eds. Free Radicals in Biology and Medicine. Oxford, Clarendon Press, 1985:139-89).

Epidemiologic studies have shown a negative correlation between the prevalence of the disease and the intake of polyunsaturated fatty acids (*Alter M et al. Arch Neurol (Chicago) 31:267-72, 1974*).

Polyunsaturates may be deficient in the brain, serum and erythrocytes of patients (*Gul S et al. J Neurol Neurosurg Psychiatry 33:506-10, 1970; Baker RWR et al. J Neurol Neurosurg Psychiatry 33:506, 1970; Gerstl B et al. Brain 84:310-19, 1961*).

- Omega-3 Fatty Acids (Fish Oils):

Example: 'MaxEPA' 3 capsules three times daily (9 gms)

WARNING: Supplementation may require additional vitamin E intake to prevent increased membrane peroxidation and cellular damage (*Laganiere S, Fernandes G. High peroxidizability of subcellular membrane induced by high fish oil diet is reversed by vitamin E. Clin Res 35:A565, 1987*).

May be reduced.

Observational Study: Although levels of omega-3 fatty acids in the total phospholipids in plasma were not different from those of 14 healthy controls, the sum of the omega-3 fatty acids derived from α-linolenic acid was 19% lower in 12 MS pts. (p<0.01) (*Cunnane SC et al. Essential fatty acid and lipid profiles in plasma and erythrocytes in patients with multiple sclerosis. Am J Clin Nutr 50:801-06, 1989*).

Review Article: Of the 2 essential fatty acids, linoleic (omega-6) and α-linolenic (omega-3), the evidence points more to a dietary deficiency of α-linolenic acid as an etiologic factor. Epidemiologic information seems to indicate that the geographical distribution of MS is inversely related to the intake of foods such as fish which are rich in α-linolenic acid and its derivatives. For example, there is a relatively low incidence of MS in the Faroe Islands, compared to the Shetlands. The Islanders come from the same Danish genetic backgrounds but the Faroe Islanders remained as fishermen while the Shetlanders adopted a British agricultural practice. Similar contrasts are apparent in Scandinavia (*Bernsohn J, Stephanides LM. Aetiology of multiple sclerosis. Nature 215:821-23, 1967*).

Supplementation may be beneficial.

Experimental Study: 12 pts. with clinically definite MS according to the criteria of McAlpine received MaxEPA (R.P. Scherer) 25 ml/d (4.2 g EPA, 2.8 g DHA) (range 20-30 ml) with 1/3 of the daily dose taken with each meal. Pts. continued on vitamins and rehabilitation services; 2 pts. also supplemented their diets with sunflower seed oil. After 1-4 mo., 5 pts. with acute remitting MS, showed evidence of a slight, but significant reduction of total neurologic score from Kurtzke's Expanded Disability Status Scale (EDSS) of 16.5 to 13.5, mean EDSS degree from 3.3 to 2.7, and of Cendrowski's progression index from 0.59 to 0.44. In 7 pts. with slowly progressive MS, clinical parameters continued to deteriorate. Results suggest that, with a longer period of treatment, it may be possible to demonstrate clearly that the differences observed did not arise by chance (*Cendrowski W. Multiple sclerosis and MaxEPA. Br J Clin Prac 40:365-67, 1986*).

- Omega-6 Fatty Acids:

$$\text{linoleic acid} \rightarrow \text{GLA} \rightarrow \text{DGLA} \rightarrow \text{PGE}_1$$

Linoleic acid, a polyunsaturate which is the main essential fatty acid in the diet, tends to be low in the blood of patients and to fall further during relapses (*Mertin H, Meade CJ. Relevance of fatty acids in MS. Br Med Bull 33:67-71, 1977; Sanders H et al. Further studies on platelet adhesiveness and serum cholesteryl linoleate levels in MS. J Neurol Neurosurg Psychiatry 31:321-5, 1968; Thompson RHS. Proc Roy Soc Med 59:269, 1966*).

Negative Observational Study: Compared to 33 controls, 30 pts. showed no significant decrease in serum linoleic acid, suggesting that a disturbance in linoleic acid metabolism is not inevitably associated with this disease (*Wolfgram F et al. Serum linoleic acid in multiple sclerosis. Neurology 25(8):786-88, 1975*).

Epidemiologic studies of the relationship between the prevalence of MS and diet are consistent with the hypothesis that linoleic acid intake is negatively associated with MS (*Alter M et al. Multiple sclerosis and nutrition. Arch Neurol 31:267-72, 1974; Agranoff BW, Goldberg D. Diet and geographical distribution of multiple sclerosis. Lancet 2:1061-66, 1974*).

Supplementation with linoleic acid may be beneficial.

Review Article: Data from 3 double-blind trials of linoleic acid in pts. with a remitting-relapsing course were reanalyzed to determine whether inconsistency in the results was due to a relationship between pt. characteristics and treatment response. The combined data consisted of neurologic assessments over 2 1/2-year trials for 87 treated pts. and 85 control patients. Treated pts. with minimal or no disability at entry had a smaller increase in disability than did controls (p<0.05). In addition, treatment reduced the severity and duration of relapses at all levels of disability and duration of illness at entry to the trials. The authors suggest that treatment benefits compared to controls may have failed to demonstrate the full extent of potential benefits as oleic acid, the placebo used, may itself ameliorate MS-like illnesses (*Dworkin RH et al. Linoleic acid and multiple sclerosis: A reanalysis of three double-blind trials. Neurology 34:1441-45, 1984; Dworkin RH. Linoleic acid and multiple sclerosis. Lancet 1:1153-4, 1981*).

Note: David Horrobin has suggested that the results of these studies were not optimal due to inadequate dosages and the use of dyes which his group has shown to block the conversion of EFA's to prostaglandins (Horrobin D. Multiple sclerosis: The rational basis for treatment with colchicine and evening primrose oil. Med Hypotheses 5:365-78, 1979).

Supplementation with safflower oil (high in linoleic acid) may be beneficial.

> **Experimental Double-blind Crossover Study:** 20 pts. received daily doses of safflower oil (high in polyunsaturates) for 5 wks. and daily doses of olive oil (low in polyunsaturates) for 5 weeks. Only the safflower oil diet appeared to help some of the pts. *(Utermohlen, Virginia, nutrition scientist at Cornell University - reported in Science 9/4/82).*

In the event that there is a block in the conversion of linoleic acid to GLA, supplementation with evening primrose oil, which has a high concentration of GLA, may be beneficial.

> **Experimental and Observational Study:** 16 pts. were found to have abnormal blood rheology (whole blood filterability) and were supplemented with primrose oil 4 gm daily. After 3 wks., both blood rheology and hand grip strength were improved, suggesting that there was improved capillary perfusion in muscles *(Simpson LO et al. Dietary supplementation with Efamol and multiple sclerosis. N Z Med J 98(792):1053-54, 1985).*

> **Experimental Study:** Electrophoretic mobility studies of red cells from MS pts. indicate that treatment with unsaturated fatty acids must continue for at least 2 yrs. before normal reactivity is restored. Assuming this also applies to myelin, clinical trials need to last longer than 2 yrs. if treatment is to be effective *(Field EJ, Joyce G. Multiple sclerosis: Effect of gamma-linolenate administration upon membranes and the need for extended clinical trials of unsaturated fatty acids. Eur Neurol 22:78, 1983).*

> **Experimental Study:** 8 seriously disabled pts. were assessed using the Kurtzke disability score, the B-M manual dexterity test and a dynamometer and were treated with undyed EPO in capsules. After 6 mo., 3 showed some improvement on the Kurtzke score. While there was no improvement in grip strength, there was a significant improvement in manual dexterity *(Horrobin DF. Multiple sclerosis: The rational basis for treatment with colchicine and evening primrose oil. Med Hypotheses 5:365-78, 1979).*

D-Phenylalanine:

Supplementation may be beneficial.

> **Experimental Double-blind Study:** 12 men and 38 women were treated with DPA and TENS (transcutaneous electrical nerve stimulation). 49/50 improved. Improvements included better bladder control, greater mobility and less depression *(Winter A. New treatment for multiple sclerosis. Neurol Orthoped J Med Surg 5:1, April, 1984).*

Tryptophan:

Supplementation may be beneficial.

> **Experimental Study:** 12 pts. received tryptophan. After 30 days, there was a modest improvement in mood and neurological symptoms *(Hyyppä MT et al. Effect of L-tryptophan treatment on central indoleamine metabolism and short-lasting neurologic disturbances in multiple sclerosis. J Neural Trans 37:297-304, 1975).*

- -

COMBINED SUPPLEMENTATION

Case Reports: Pts. improved following daily supplementation (much of it by injection) of massive doses of various B complex vitamins, vitamin C, vitamin E, choline, lecithin, magnesium, calcium gluconate and pantothenate, aminoacetic acid-glycine, adenosine-5-monophosphoric acid and crude liver *(Klenner FR. Response of peripheral and central nerve pathology to mega-doses of the vitamin B-complex and other metabolites. J Appl Nutr 25:16-40, 1973).*

Experimental Study: 15 pts. received intraspinal B_1 & B_6 injections combined with mixed tocopherols and vitamin B complex orally. 4 of the 6 pts. with advanced disease improved, and 1 of them relapsed after stopping all vitamin therapy for 1 year. Arrest of the progress of the disease was noted in the other 9 cases with improvement in symptoms, recession of neurologic signs and diminution of reflex overactivity (*Stone S. Pyridoxine and thiamine therapy in disorders of the nervous system. Dis Nerv Sys 11:131-138, 1950*).

OTHER FACTORS

Rule out food sensitivities.

Review Article: Literature suggesting that MS may be caused by an allergic or other adverse reaction to certain foods, mostly cocoa products, cola and coffee is reviewed. Epidemiology studies have documented a correlation between high cocoa consumption and high MS incidence. When cocoa is introduced to an area, MS incidence rises sharply. Some dogs develop muscle weakness, twiching, loss of sphincter function and myocardial damage when fed chocolate. Cases are reported in which chocolate ingestion by MS pts. was followed by exacerbations (*Maas AG, Hogenhuis LAH. Multiple sclerosis and possible relationship to cocoa: A hypothesis. Ann Allergy 59:76-79, 1987*).

Observational Study: In a survey of about 26,000 pts. in the US, the incidence of MS correlated most strikingly with milk consumption. A similar correlation was found in 21 other countries (*Agranoff B, Goldberg D. Diet and the geographical distribution of multiple sclerosis. Lancet 2:1061-66, 1974*).

Observational Study: In a survey of 2000 pts. with MS and related diseases, those with the most severe cases were food sensitive, those with moderate symptoms were sensitive to molds or fungi, and the least affected were strongly sensitive to pollens (*Jonez HD. Calif Med 79:376-80, November, 1953*).

Rule out mercury amalgam toxicity.

There is an epidemiological correlation between multiple sclerosis and dental caries.

Observational Study: Death rates from MS were "linearly related to the numbers of decayed, missing and filled teeth in six Australian and 48 American states and in 45 Asian and European countries," suggesting that dental caries "may be a precursor of one form of MS" (*Craelius W. Comparative epidemiology of multiple sclerosis and dental caries. J Epidemiol Comm Health 32:155-65, 1972*).

The correlation between multiple sclerosis and rates of dental caries may be due to the placement of mercury amalgams.

Theoretical Discussion: When silver amalgam fillings are exposed to gingival action and oxidation, inorganic mercury in the fillings (especially class V fillings and root canals) may be converted to an organic form which may act as a neurotoxin (*Ingalls TH. Epidemiology, etiology and prevention of multiple sclerosis. Am J Forensic Med Pathol 4:55-61, 1983*).

Case Report: The author, an MS pt., was found to have lead toxicity (lead line in his gums, positive blood and urine studies) 4 yrs. after symptom-onset. Extraction of a suspicious tooth showed it to be grossly blackened from its amalgam interior, and a biopsy section of the adjacent gingiva stained for heavy metal depositions. Recently he abruptly developed diplopia following the pulverising of 50-year-old amalgam fillings which, he is convinced, was due to released mercury vapor which reached the oculomotor nerves (probably via the mandibular branch of the trigeminal) (*Ingalls TH. Triggers for multiple sclerosis. Letter. Lancet 2:160, 1986*).

MUSCLE CRAMPS

See Also: "HYPOGLYCEMIA" (FUNCTIONAL)
PAIN
PREGNANCY AND ILLNESS

DIETARY FACTORS

Sugar-free, high protein diet.

Symptoms may be a manifestation of reactive hypoglycemia.

Clinical Observations: In a gp. of over 350 pts. who presented with either spontaneous leg cramps (SLC) or restless legs (RL), approx. 2/3 pts. had SLC alone, while 1/3 experienced both SLC and RL. Although the calf and foot musculature usually was involved, occasionally pts. suffered cyclic cramps primarily in the upper thighs, low back or hands. There were also several cases of severe nocturnal carpal spasm and the "stiff man syndrome." With few exceptions, these pts. also experienced typical features of recurrent hypoglycemia which was confirmed by afternoon glucose tolerance testing and an attack of muscle cramps occasionally was precipitated concomitantly with a hypoglycemic episode during testing. Institution of a sugar-free, high protein diet with frequent nibling and at least one night feeding was followed by prompt and persistent remission or striking alleviation of longstanding symptoms in the vast majority of pts., while symptom recurrence could usually be attributed to some dietary indiscretion within the preceeding 12 hours (*Roberts HJ. Spontaneous leg cramps and "restless legs" due to diabetogenic (functional) hyperinsulinism: A basis for rational therapy. J Fla Med Assoc 60(5):29-31, 1973*).

- -

VITAMINS

Riboflavin:

Supplementation may reduce neuromuscular irritability in normals.

Experimental Study: Oral supplementation with riboflavin 10 mg resulted in moderate lowering of neuromuscular irritability in athletes, particularly for 0.1 msec rectangular stimuli (*Haralambie G. Vitamin B2 status in athletes and the influence of riboflavin administration on neuromuscular irritability. Nutr Metab 20(1):1-8, 1976*).

Supplementation may be effective for cramps of pregnancy as well as muscle cramps secondary to other disorders.

NOTE: The pts. should be warned that the urine may be colored red or orange (Morgan AA. Treatment of cramp. Letter. J R Soc Med 76(8):712, 1983).

Clinical Observation: Many women suffering from cramps of pregnancy were relieved by supplementation with riboflavin 18 mg daily (*Morgan AA. Treatment of cramp. Letter. J R Soc Med 76(8):712, 1983*).

Clinical Observation: In a series of cases of cramps of pregnancy, only 3 pts. failed to respond to oral riboflavin (*Thoyer-Rozat J et al. La semaine des hôpitaux 36:1991-3, 1960*).

Clinical Observation: 80 women with cramps of pregnancy were all successfully treated with either oral or IV riboflavin (*Kleine HO. Zentralblatt für Gynäkologie 76:344-56, 1954*).

Clinical Observation: Riboflavin supplementation was effective for treating muscle cramps due to diabetes, circulatory disturbances, infections and intoxications (*Perrault M et al. Paris médicale 36:549-54, 1946*).

<u>Vitamin B6</u>:

Carpal tunnel syndrome, which can often be relieved by supplementation with pyridoxine, may be associated with <u>nocturnal muscle spasms in the extremities</u> (*Ellis JM, Presley J. Vitamin B6: The Doctor's Report. New York, Harper & Row, 1973*).

<u>Vitamin B12</u>:

Supplementation by injection may be effective for <u>night cramps</u>.

Clinical Observation: 16 consecutive middle-aged and elderly pts. with night cramps all had dramatic relief for 4-6 wks. or even longer following an injection of 500 μg of vitamin B12. By far the great majority spontaneously requested another injection within the 6-wk. period (*Aitchison WR. Nocturnal cramps. Letter. N Z Med J 80:137, 1974*).

<u>Vitamin E</u>:   200 IU four times daily after meals
(50 IU four times daily for children with "growing pains" or if there is a history of cardiovascular or renal disorder.)
Minimum trial: 4 weeks
Dosage can usually be reduced after maximal results are achieved.

Supplementation may be beneficial.

Clinical Observation: Supplementation with vitamin E 450 IU daily controlled most cramping for approx. 50 pts. with muscle cramps. As soon as pts. stopped the supplement, the cramps recurred, and if they used less than 450 IU daily, they got cramps of varying degree (*Lotzof L. Vitamin E controls muscle cramps. Letter. Med J Aust June 11, 1977, p. 904*).

Experimental Study: 103/125 pts. with nocturnal leg and foot cramps, over half of whom had suffered for over 5 yrs., reported complete or nearly complete relief following vitamin E supplementation, 20/125 had a moderate to good response and only 2 failed to respond. Half responded to 300 IU or less, while half required 400 IU or more. Many had to continue vitamin E to prevent cramps from recurring. Response was usually within 1 week. Similar success was obtained with nocturnal rectal cramps, abdominal muscle cramps and cramps following heavy exercise (*Ayres S, Mihan R. Nocturnal leg cramps (systremma): A progress report on response to vitamin E. South Med J 67(11):1308-12, 1974*).

Clinical Observation: Almost 100 pts. complaining of leg cramps, other types of idiopathic cramps, or pains in the neck or low back received vitamin E 300 IU daily. Supplementation was almost universally effective for idiopathic nocturnal leg cramps. Pts. who reduced the dosage to 100 IU daily often found it to be inadequate; others who settled at 200 IU daily found, after several months, that they had to increase the dosage to maintain benefits (*Cathcart RF 3rd. Leg cramps and vitamin E. Letter. JAMA 219(2):216-17, 1972*).

Experimental Study: 24 pts. with nocturnal leg cramps ranging from mild to severe received d-alpha tocopheryl acetate 100 IU 3 times daily before meals. Nearly all received relief in the first week or two. One pt. with leg and foot cramps also had severe nocturnal rectal cramps which were also relieved. 2 pts. who had obtained almost complete relief discontinued the vitamin after about 2 months. There was a gradual return of symptoms within 4-5 wks. in both pts., but the cramps disappeared again on resumption of vitamin E (*Ayres S Jr., Mihan R. Leg cramps (systremma) and "restless legs" syndrome. Response to vitamin E (tocopherol). Calif Med 111(2):87-91, 1969*).

- -

MINERALS

<u>Calcium</u>:

Alterations in calcium metabolism may affect leg cramps during pregnancy (*Pitkin RM. Endocrine regulation of calcium homeostasis during pregnancy. Clin Perinatol 10(3):575-92, 1983*).

Negative Observational Study: 42 pregnant women with leg cramps failed to demonstrate any differences in total serum or ionized calcium concentrations compared to pregnant women without leg cramps (*Hammar M et al. Calcium treatment of leg cramps in pregnancy. Effect on clinical symptoms and total serum and ionized serum calcium concentrations.* <u>Acta Obstet Gynecol Scand</u> *60(4):345-47, 1981*).

Supplementation may relieve leg cramps.

Clinical Observations: While prophylactic quinine has been recommended for the treatment of nocturnal leg cramps, it often fails at a dose of 600 mg at bedtime. Calcium gluconate 4800 mg fails less often, but some pts. seem to need the combination, and even then their cramps may be incompletely suppressed (*Knowles FW. Fluoride and leg cramps. Letter.* <u>N Z Med J</u> *93:60, 1981*).

Supplementation (or reduction in <u>phosphorus</u>) may prevent or relieve leg cramps during pregnancy.

Negative Experimental Double-blind Study: 60 pregnant women with leg cramps received either calcium or ascorbic acid 1 g twice daily. There was no significant difference between the 2 treatment gps. with respect to clinical improvement. No biochemical differences were found between the different treatment regimens or between those pts. relieved or not relieved of their symptoms (*Hammar M et al. Calcium and magnesium status in pregnant women. A comparison between treatment with calcium and vitamin C in pregnant women with leg cramps.* <u>Int J Vitam Nutr Res</u> *57(2):179-83, 1987*).

Experimental Study: 21 pregnant women with leg cramps were treated with calcium 1 gm orally twice daily for 2 weeks. Leg cramps ceased in 9/21 and improved in 11/21 while only 3/21 matched controls improved. Treatment increased total serum calcium concentration but did not alter ionized serum calcium (*Hammar M et al. Calcium treatment of leg cramps in pregnancy. Effect on clinical symptoms and total serum and ionized serum calcium concentrations.* <u>Acta Obstet Gynecol Scand</u> *60(4):345-47, 1981*).

Negative Experimental Placebo-controlled Study: 48/64 pts. with leg cramps responded to calcium compared to 50/65 pts. given placebo (*Odendahl HJ.* <u>S Afr Med</u> *48:780, 1974*).

Experimental Study: Calcium supplementation, reduction of milk intake or aluminum hydroxide (to decrease phosphorus absorption) was effective in relieving leg cramps in a gp. of pregnant women. Effective treatment was accompanied by a rise in ionizable calcium and a reduction in blood phosphorus (*Page EW, Page EP. Leg cramps in pregnancy: Etiology and treatment.* <u>Obstet Gynecol</u> *1(94):1953*).

<u>Fluorine:</u>

Supplementation may be beneficial.

Clinical Observations: When the author was in practice in South India, where fluorine levels are very high, pts. did not present with nocturnal leg cramps as they did in New Zealand, where fluorine levels are sometimes deficient. Therefore, a number pts. underwent a trial of sodium fluoride 6.6 mg at bedtime which was so successful that several of them could cease taking the previously indispensable quinine and calcium (*Knowles FW. Fluoride and leg cramps. Letter.* <u>N Z Med J</u> *93:60, 1981*).

<u>Magnesium:</u>

Reduced serum levels may be associated with muscle cramps.

Observational Study: 5 pts. with Crohn's disease and recurrent low serum magnesium levels had symptoms of muscle cramps, tetany and bone pain (*Russell RI. Magnesium requirements in patients with chronic inflammatory disease receiving intravenous nutrition.* <u>J Am Coll Nutr</u> *4(5):553-58, 1985*).

Supplementation may be beneficial.

Review Article: The favorable effects of magnesium on nocturnal leg cramps during pregnancy are due to the compensation of a combined magnesium and calicum deficiency and/or magnesium-induced membrane stabilization (*Classen HG, Helbig J. [Magnesium therapy in pregnancy. Pharmacologic and toxicologic aspects of mag-*

nesium supplementation and use in pre-eclampsia and threatened premature labor.] Fortschr Med 102(34):841-4, 1984).

Case Report: Leg cramps in a pt. with severe cardiac decompensation and hypomagnesemia improved after the infusion of magnesium sulfate 25 mmol IV (*Johansson BW. Magnesium infusion in decompensated hypomagnesemic patients. Acta Pharmacol Toxicol (Copenh) 54 (Suppl 1):125-28, 1984*).

Experimental Controlled Study: 21 pregnant women with muscle cramps received 1.8 g/d of monomagnesium aspartate twice daily, while another 21 received no therapy. After 4 wks., 19/21 treated women were free of symptoms, compared to only 7/21 controls (*Riss P et al. [Clinical aspects and treatment of calf muscle cramps during pregnancy.] Geburtshilfe Frauenheilkd 43(5):329-31, 1983*).

Potassium:

When muscle cramps are associated with hypokalemia, supplementation with potassium chloride may be beneficial (*Portier C. [Muscle cramps and hypokalemia.] Letter. Nouv Presse Med 2(25):1717, 1973*).

Sodium:

Supplementation with sodium chloride may be beneficial in treating nocturnal calf cramps (*Glatzel H. [Nocturnal calf cramps.] Letter. Dtsch Med Wochenschr 105(20):736, 1980*).

— —

OTHER NUTRITIONAL FACTORS

Bone meal:

Administration may be beneficial.

WARNING: Bone meal may contain a significant amount of lead.

- with vitamin A and vitamin D:

Experimental Study: 112 children with "growing pains" or who kicked and screamed at night were given either dicalcium phosphate or bone meal (which contains calcium and phosphorus in addition to other minerals) 20 gr daily along with vitamins A and D. Over a 2-year period, all 57 children on bone meal were completely relieved, while 22/56 of the children on dicalcium phosphate were relieved. When the remaining children were switched to bone meal, all of them were completely relieved (*Martin EM. Report on the clinical use of bone meal. Can Med Assoc J 50:562, 1944*).

MYOPATHY

See Also: ALCOHOLISM
         AUTO-IMMUNE DISORDERS (GENERAL)
         CARDIOMYOPATHY
         NEUROMUSCULAR DEGENERATION

VITAMINS

Riboflavin:

Supplementation may be beneficial in mitochondrial myopathies.

Case Report: At the age of 14 mo., a girl presented with general muscle weakness, muscle hypotonia and motor retardation. The level of blood lactate and pyruvate was consistently increased and enzymatic studies showed impairment of NADH-dehydrogenase activity (complex I of the respiratory chain) in skeletal muscle. Electron microscopic findings were consistent with a mitochondrial myopathy. She was treated with riboflavin and, at age 30 mo., she showed mild muscle hypotonia and weakness, but good motor progress and normal cognitive development. Lactate and pyruvate levels were normal (*Griebel V et al. A mitochondrial myopathy in an infant with lactic acidosis. Dev Med Child Neurol 32(6):528-31, 1990*).

Case Report: A man with a painful proximal myopathy had excess lipid deposition in skeletal muscle, excretion of dicarboxylic acids in urine, and low acyl-coA dehydrogenase activities in skeletal muscle mitochondria. In addition he had little immunoreactive short-chain and medium-chain acyl-coA dehydrogenase enzyme protein compared to normal controls. Following riboflavin treatment, there was considerable improvement in his clinical condition which was confirmed by further biochemical and morphological investigations (*Turnbull DM et al. Lipid storage myopathy associated with low acyl-coA dehydrogenase activities. Brain 111(Pt 4):815-28, 1988*).

Vitamin A:

May be depressed in alcoholic myopathy (*Ward RJ et al. Reduced antioxidant status in patients with chronic alcoholic myopathy. Biochem Soc Trans 16:581, 1988*).

Vitamin B6:

In myasthenia gravis, supplementation may be beneficial.

Clinical Observation: 3 pts. with myasthenia gravis showed pronounced improvement within 24-48 hrs. after IV vitamin B6 (*Spies TD et al. Some recent advances in vitamin therapy. JAMA 115(4):292-97, 1940*).

Vitamin C and
Vitamin K:

In mitochondrial myopathy, combined supplementation may be beneficial.

Case Report: A 15-year-old girl presented with progressive muscular weakness, mitochondrial myopathy and lactic acidosis. She was found to have low levels of reducible cytochrome b and deficient activity of ubiquinol-cytochrome c reductase complex (complex III) in isolated muscle mitochondria. The adminstration of ascorbic acid 4 g and menodione (vitamin K3) 40 mg daily provided a shunt around the metabolic block in electron transport, resulting in clinical improvement. Dramatic further improvement occurred after 1 yr. when the menodione was doubled to 80 mg daily (*Lactic acidosis and mitochondrial myopathy in a young woman. Nutr Rev 46(4):157-63, 1988*).

Vitamin E:

Deficiency may be associated with myopathy.

Observational Study: 2/3 of chronic alcoholics develop atrophy of type II skeletal muscle. In this study, 10/21 chronic alcoholic pts. showed atrophy of the type II fibers in their quadriceps muscle on biopsy. The mean plasma alpha tocopherol concentration was significantly lower in alcoholics with myopathy than in those with normal muscle structure or in non-alcoholic controls. Plasma vitamin E and vitamin A levels were significantly correlated, and the mean plasma selenium level was significantly reduced in alcoholics with myopathy compared to those with normal muscle structure and to normal controls, suggesting impaired antioxidant status (*Ward RJ et al. Reduced antioxidant status in patients with chronic alcoholic myopathy. Biochem Soc Trans 16:581, 1988*).

Review Article: Vitamin E deficiency causes a myopathy in a number of animal species but the mechanism of the damage is obscure. Muscles from vitamin E-deficient mice and rats are more prone than normal to damage during contractile activity. In this situation, the tissue rather than the plasma level of the vitamin is probably the more important factor (*Jackson MJ et al. Vitamin E and skeletal muscle. CIBA Found Symp 101:224-39, 1983*).

Case Report: A 7-year-old boy with severe malabsorption since birth showed pathological signs similar to those seen in vitamin E-deficient animals. Treatment with vitamin E 400-800 IU daily for 16 mo. resulted in the gradual decrease of serum muscle enzyme levels as blood vitamin E levels rose (*Tomasi LG. Reversibility of human myopathy caused by vitamin E deficiency. Neurology 29:1182, 1979*).

Muscular dystrophy may be caused by tocopherol deficiency.

Theoretical Discussion: Progressive muscular dystrophy in humans closely resembles the muscular dystrophy induced in animals by deprivation of tocopherol which is reversed by oral but not parenteral tocopherol (*Milhorat AT, Bartels WE. The defect in utilization of tocopherol in progressive muscular dystrophy. Science 101:93-4, 1945*).

In muscular dystrophy, plasma levels may be depressed (*Hunter MI, Mohamed JB. Plasma antioxidants and lipid peroxidation products in Duchenne muscular dystrophy. Clin Chim Acta 155(2):123-31, 1986*).

In muscular dystrophy, supplementation may be beneficial.

Experimental Study: Pts. were supplemented with up to 300 mg of tocopherols daily, mainly in the form of wheat germ oil. Symptoms were arrested in 5/25 with progressive muscular dystrophy and moderate to marked improvement occurred. 3/5 with menopausal muscular dystrophy showed "remarkable" improvement (*Rabinovitch R et al. Neuromuscular disorders amenable to wheat germ oil therapy. J Neurol Neurosurg Psychiatry 14:95-100, 1951*).

- with inositol:

Experimental Study: 7 pts. with progressive muscular dystrophy given tocopherol or inositol alone showed no reduction in creatinuria, but 5 of them responded with reduced creatinuria when both substances were given in equimolar amts. for 1 or 2 days. This suggests that there is an inherited deficiency in muscular dystrophy preventing the formation of a condensation product of the 2 substances in the GI tract (*Milhorat AT, Bartels WE. The defect in utilization of tocopherol in progressive muscular dystrophy. Science 101:93-4, 1945*).

- -

MINERALS

Magnesium:

Intracellular magnesium depletion can cause a myopathy which responds rapidly to supplementation (*Pall HS et al. Hypomagnesaemia causing myopathy and hypocalcaemia in an alcoholic. Postgrad Med J 63:665-67, 1987*).

Selenium:

Deficiency may be associated with <u>alcoholic myopathy</u>.

Observational Study: 2/3 of chronic alcoholics develop atrophy of type II skeletal muscle. In this study, 10/21 chronic alcoholic pts. showed atrophy of the type II fibers in their quadriceps muscle on biopsy. The mean plasma selenium concentration was significantly lower in alcoholics with myopathy than in those with normal muscle structure or in non-alcoholic controls. Plasma vitamin E and vitamin A levels were significantly correlated, and the mean plasma tocopherol level was significantly reduced in alcoholics with myopathy compared to those with normal muscle structure and to normal controls, suggesting impaired antioxidant status (*Ward RJ et al. Reduced antioxidant status in patients with chronic alcoholic myopathy. Biochem Soc Trans 16:581, 1988*).

May be reduced in <u>myotonic dystrophy</u> (*Örndahl G et al. Selenium therapy of myotonic dystrophy. Acta Med Scand 213(3):237-39, 1983*).

Observational Study: In a study of 22 pts. with myotonic dystrophy, serum selenium concentration was inversely correlated with the severity of the illness, and decreased in parallel with progression of the illness (*Örndahl G et al. Myotonic dystrophy and selenium. Acta Medica Scand 211:493-99, 1982*).

May be reduced in <u>Duchenne muscular dystrophy</u> and <u>Becker X-linked muscular dystrophy</u>.

Experimental and Observational Study: 15 boys with <u>Duchenne MD</u> and 5 with <u>Becker X-linked MD</u> were evaluated. 12/20 pts. had pretreatment serum selenium levels that were within the 95% confidence limit of unsupplemented control children. 2/20 pts. with Duchenne MD fell below this level. Supplementation with selenium 6 μg/kg/d along with vitamin E for 6 mo. caused a substantial rise in both serum and RBC selenium, suggesting suboptimal pretreatment body contents, with the greatest increases observed in pts. with initially low selenium levels. In only 4/20 pts., supplementation resulted in a significant rise in RBC glutathione peroxidase activity. An increase in dosage to 20 μg/kg/d resulted in a further rise in both serum and RBC selenium, but not in RBC glutathione peroxidase activity (*Gebre-Medhin M et al. Selenium supplementation in X-linked muscular dystrophy. Effects on erythrocyte and serum selenium and on erythrocyte glutathione peroxidase activity. Acta Paediatr Scand 74(6):886-90, 1985*).

Supplementation may be beneficial for <u>muscular dystrophy</u>.

Review Article: In experimental animals, all the major symptoms of myotonic dystrophy (muscle dystrophy, infertility, alopecia, cataract and myocardial degeneration) can be cured or prevented by selenium supplementation (*Örndahl G et al. Selenium therapy of myotonic dystrophy. Acta Med Scand 213(3):237-39, 1983*).

- with <u>Vitamin E</u>:

Experimental Study: 16 boys, 9 with Duchenne MD and the rest with more benign variants, received selenium 6 μg/kg for 6 mo. and 20 μg/kg for 6 mo. along with vitamin E followed by 1 yr. of no treatment. The decrease in muscle strength was slightly more rapid during the yr. of no treatment than during the treatment year. The difference was, however, slight and could conceivably be explained by the increase in age. No boy showed any practically usable increase of muscle strength during treatment (*Gamstorp I et al. A trial of selenium and vitamin E in boys with muscular dystrophy. J Child Neurol 1(3):211-14, 1986*).

Case Report: A pt. was treated with 228 μg selenium (as 0.5 mg sodium selenite) and 10 mg vitamin E daily which was increased over 2 yrs. to 3 mg sodium selenite and 125 mg vitamin E daily. After 6 mo., gradual improvements were observed with regression of all symptoms (muscular weakness, myopathic facies, bilateral ptosis and mental tiredness) except active myotonia. After 2 yrs., there was marked subjective and objective improvement with increased muscular strength and regression of pathological electromyographic findings (*Örndahl G et al. Selenium therapy of myotonic dystrophy. Acta Med Scand 213(3):237-39, 1983*).

- -

OTHER NUTRITIONAL FACTORS

Carnitine:

Deficiency may be associated with a lipid storage myopathy presenting with muscle weakness and elevated triglycerides (*Angelini C et al. Carnitine deficiency of skeletal muscle: Report of a treated case. Neurology 26:633-7, 1976*).

- with <u>Riboflavin</u>:

Combined supplementation may be beneficial in <u>mitochondrial myopathies</u>.

> **Case Report:** A 6-year-old boy with progressive muscle weakness was diagnosed with myopathy and pure motor neuropathy. Biochemical investigation of muscle tissue revealed a defect in NADH dehydrogenase activity (complex I). Treatment with L-carnitine and riboflavin dramatically improved symptoms. 7 mo. after the start of supplementation, lab tests showed normalization of NADH dehydrogenase activity (*Bernsen P et al. Successful treatment of pure myopathy, associated with complex I deficiency, with riboflavin and carnitine.* <u>Arch Neurol</u> *48:334-8, 1991*).

<u>Coenzyme Q10</u>:

In <u>muscular dystrophy</u>, supplementation may be beneficial.

> **Experimental Double-blind Crossover Study:** 12 pts. with progressive muscular dystrophies and neurogenic atrophies were treated with CoQ10 or placebo. Solely by the presence or absence of significant change in stroke volume and cardiac output, all 8 pts. on blind CoQ10 and all 4 on blind placebo were correctly assigned ($p < 0.003$). After 3 mo., improved physical well-being was observed in 4/8 treated pts. and for 0/4 placebo patients. One with Becker dystrophy was able to increase physical exercise from 30 min. to 45 minutes. A second with Duchenne dystrophy fell less frequently. A third with Charcot-Marie-Tooth disorder could walk further, while the last, who had the same diagnosis, became more energetic and less tired. Of the pts. first given placebo and then crossed over, 3/4 improved on CoQ10. 5/6 on CoQ10 in crossover to placebo (2 resigned before crossover) maintained improved cardiac function, while 1/6 relapsed (*Folkers K et al. Biochemical rationale and the cardiac response of patients with muscle disease to therapy with coenzyme Q10.* <u>Proc Natl Acad Sci U S A</u> *82(13):4513-16, 1985*).

<u>Phosphatidyl Choline</u>:

Synthesis may be impaired in <u>muscular dystrophy</u>.

> **Theoretical Discussion:** An analysis of published data suggests an impaired synthesis of 4,7,10,13,16,19-docosahexaenoic phosphatidylcholine as the primary defect in <u>Duchenne muscular dystrophy</u>. This phosphatidylcholine species is postulated to be required for optimum sarcoplasmic Ca^{++} transport activity. It is proposed that this impairment initiates the secondary series of events which lead to the observed pathology (*Infante JP. Impaired biosynthesis of highly unsaturated phosphatidylcholines: a hypothesis on the molecular etiology of some muscular dystrophies.* <u>J Theor Biol</u> *116(1):65-88, 1985*).

Supplementation may be beneficial in <u>muscular dystrophy</u>.

> **Case Report:** A pt. with progressive muscular dystrophy ingested 20 gm soy lecithin daily. After day 15 the creatinuria dropped slowly. When lecithin was discontinued, the creatine output remained at a low level for 6 days and then slowly rose to its previous level (*Milhorat AT et al. Effect of wheat germ on creatinuria in dermatomyositis and progressive muscular dystrophy.* <u>Proc Soc Exp Biol Med</u> *58:40-1, 1945*).

- -

OTHER FACTORS

Rule out <u>gluten</u> sensitivity.

May cause a secondary myopathy.

> **Case Report:** An 8-year-old girl with signs and symptoms of myopathy was found to have celiac disease. The myopathy disappeared on a gluten-free diet. It is suggested that the acquired myopathy may have been caused by a deficiency in the fat-soluble vitamins D or E as a result of protracted steatorrhea (*Hardoff D et al. Myopathy as a presentation of coeliac disease.* <u>Dev Med Child Neurol</u> *22(6):781-3, 1980*).

NEURALGIA AND NEUROPATHY

See Also: **CARPAL TUNNEL SYNDROME**
DIABETES MELLITUS
HERPES ZOSTER
PAIN

VITAMINS

Folic Acid:

Deficiency may be associated with peripheral neuropathy.

Observational Study: 7/34 pts.(21%) with severe folate deficiency and megaloblastosis due to GI or dietary causes had clinical or electrophysiological evidence of peripheral neuropathy that was usually mild and predominantly sensory. The presence of neuropathy was unrelated to age, sex, hemoglobin, mean cell volume, serum or red cell folate, or serum vitamin B_{12}. It is concluded that the neuropathy is at least in part the result of folate deficiency, although a contributing role of other deficiencies cannot be excluded (*Shorvon SD, Reynolds EH. Folate deficiency and peripheral neuropathy, in MI Botez, EH Reynolds, Eds. Folic Acid in Neurology, Psychiatry, and Internal Medicine. New York, Raven Press, 1979*).

If deficient, supplementation may be beneficial.

Case Report: A pt. developed dementia and peripheral neuropathy 16 yrs. after partial gastrectomy. Symptoms failed to respond to vitamin B_{12} alone, but improved following the addition of folic acid (*Enk C et al. Reversible dementia and neuropathy associated with folate deficiency 16 years after partial gastrectomy. Scand J Haematol 25:63, 1980*).

Review Article: Several clinical clues may lead to the suspicion of a folate-responsive polyneuropathy in a pt. with a long-standing low serum folate level: (a) hematological abnormalities; however, their absence does not rule out folate deficiency as an etiological factor; (b) chronic GI dysfunction with evidence of an irritable colon for years, sometimes with atrophy of the jejunal mucosa; (c) chronic low-residue diet; (d) a neurological picture indicative of a mild and predominantly sensory demyelinating type of polyneuropathy, at times associated with signs of posteroloateral cord involvement (*Botez MI et al. Polyneuropathies responsive to folic acid therapy, in MI Botez, EH Reynolds. Folic Acid in Neurology, Psychiatry, and Internal Medicine. New York, Raven Press, 1979*).

Niacin:

Supplementation may be beneficial.

Note: Neuropathy in pellagra may worsen if patients are given niacin alone without the rest of the vitamin B complex (Wadia NH, Swami RK. Pattern of nutritional deficiency disorders of nervous system in Bombay. Neurology India 18:207, 1970).

Experimental Study: 74 consecutive Bell's palsy pts. were treated with nicotinic acid 100-250 mg with "excellent results" noted in all pts. within 2-4 weeks (*Kime CE. Bell's palsy: A new syndrome associated with treatment by nicotinic acid. Arch Otolaryngol 68:28-32, 1958*).

Experimental Study: 8 pts. with trigeminal neuralgia received nicotinic acid 1-200 mg IV daily. 4 were completely cured, 3 were partial cures and 1 was a treatment failure. In successful cases, a few injections were followed by complete pain relief lasting for months, and when an injection was given during an actual paroxysm, the relief was immediate (*Furtado D, Chicorro V. Rev Clin Espan Madrid 5:416, 1942*).

Thiamine:

Deficiency is known to cause a polyneuropathy (the essential feature of dry beriberi) in addition to other neurologic disorders.

> **Observational Study:** 31% of 176 pts. with various neurologic disorders were deficient in thiamine as estimated by RBC transketolase activation. More than 1/2 of these pts. had been addicted to alcohol; the remainder had the following diagnoses: polyneuropathy of malabsorption, polyneuropathy of diabetes mellitus, optic atrophy of unknown etiology, cerebellar ataxia, neoplasm-related neurologic disorders, B_{12} neuromyelopathy, myelopathy of unknown origin, and Thévenard's syndrome (*Langohr HD et al. Vitamin B-1, B-2 and B-6 deficiency in neurological disorders. J Neurol 225:95-108, 1981*).

Alcoholic polyneuropathy may be due either to deficiency or to a defect in thiamine utilization.

> **Observational Study:** Plasma thiamine levels in 30 alcoholic pts. with peripheral neuropathy were comparable to those of normal subjects, although RBC transketolase activity was lower. In pts. with Wernike's-Korsakoff's Syndrome, both measures were lower than those of normals. Results suggest that, in peripheral neuropathy, pts. have a defect in thiamine utilization rather than a lack of thiamine itself (*Paladin F, Russo Perez G. The haematic thiamine level in the course of alcoholic neuropathy. Eur Neurol 26(3):129-33, 1987*).

> **Experimental Study:** 12 pts. with alcoholic polyneuropathy were deprived of alcohol and given only a vitamin B-free diet. After a maximum of 5 days, neuritic symptoms worsened in most of the patients. With the addition of thiamine, there was improvement in all cases. After a maximum of 2 wks., the improvement was purely symptomatic with no measurable effect on the neuritic signs in 10/12 patients. In 2 pts. who were maintained on a vitamin B-deficient diet plus thiamine alone for 8 full wks., a definite improvement occurred in motor and sensory signs and there was a return of ankle jerks. 4 of the 10 pts. who improved suffered a worsening of symptoms and signs initially for the first 2-3 days after the addition of thiamine (*Victor M, Adams RD. On the etiology of the alcoholic neurologic diseases. Am J Clin Nutr 9(4):379-97, 1961*).

> **Experimental Study:** 10 alcoholic pts. who continued their daily whiskey consumption while eating a well balanced diet supplemented with yeast and vitamin B concentrates made an adequate recovery from alcoholic polyneuritis, suggesting that the polyneuritis was nutritional in origin (*Strauss MB. Etiology of "alcoholic" polyneuritis. Am J Med Sci 189:378, 1935*).

If deficient, supplementation may be beneficial for acute neuropathy.

> **Review Article:** Treatment of acute thiamine deficiency neuropathy consists of thiamine 50 mg IM daily for several days followed by 2.5-5 mg orally (*Skelton WP III, Skelton NK. Thiamine deficiency neuropathy: It's still common today. Postgrad Med 85(8):301-06, 1989*).

Supplementation may be beneficial for trigeminal neuralgia.

> - with liver extract:

> > **Experimental Study:** 37/58 pts. with trigeminal neuralgia were markedly improved following treatment with thiamine chloride 10 mg daily IM or IV, liver extract by injection 3 times weekly (total of 22.5 USP units), and a high vitamin, low carbohydrate diet with 30 cc orally of an aqueous concentrate of rice polishings daily, providing 1500 IU B_1 as well as other components of the vitamin B complex. Treatment had to be continued for as long as 6 mo. before maximal benefits were obtained (*Borsook H et al. The relief of symptoms of major trigeminal neuralgia (tic douloureux) following the use of vitamin B₁ and concentrated liver extract. JAMA April 13, 1940, p. 1421*).

Vitamin B$_6$:

WARNING: Pyridoxine supplementation may cause a sensory neuropathy in doses as low as 200 mg daily over 3 years (usually 2-5 gm daily). The neurotoxicity is believed to be due to exceeding the liver's ability to phosphorylate pyridoxine to the active coenzyme, pyridoxal phosphate. The resulting high pyridoxine blood level could be directly neurotoxic or may compete for binding sites with pyridoxal phosphate resulting in a relative deficiency of the active metabolite (*Parry GJ. Sensory neuropathy with low-dose pyridoxine. Neurology 35:1466-68, 1985*). Supplementation in the form of pyridoxal phosphate should thus avoid this danger.

Experimental Study: 172 women had raised serum B_6 levels; 60% of them presented with neurological symptoms which disappeared when B_6 was withdrawn. In 4 cases, the symptoms reappeared when B_6 was restarted. The mean B_6 dose in the 103 pts. was 117 ± 92 mg compared with 116.2 ± 66 mg in the control group. The ave. duration of B_6 ingestion in the neurotoxic gp. was 2.9 ± 1.9 yrs. compared to 1.6 ± 2.1 yrs. in controls ($p<0.01$). Symptoms consisted of paresthesia, hyperesthesia, bone pain, muscle weakness, numbness and fasciculation, most marked in the extremities and predominantly bilateral unless there was a history of limb trauma (*Dalton K, Dalton MJT. Characteristics of pyridoxine overdose neuropathy syndrome. Acta Neurol Scand 76:8-11, 1987*).

Deficiency may cause a vitamin B_6-responsive neuropathy.

Experimental Study: Using electrodiagnostic criteria, pts. with carpal tunnel syndrome (CTS) were categorized into 4 groups of at least 7 subjects each: CTS, peripheral neuropathy (PN), CTS and PN, and normal. Based on RBC glutamine oxaloacetic acid transaminase (EGOT) activity with vs. without pyridoxal phosphate, a significant difference in pyridoxine metabolic activity (PMA) was found between gps. by both chi square ($p<0.05$) and analysis of variance ($p<0.05$) which was associated with the presence or absence of PN. There was no difference in PMA when gps. were separated on the basis of CTS, suggesting that a PMA abnormality is highly correlated, not with CTS, but with PN, and that pts. with CTS responding to pyridoxine may have an unrecognized PN (*Byers CM et al. Pyridoxine metabolism in carpal tunnel syndrome with and without peripheral neuropathy. Arch Phys Med Rehabil 65(11):712-16, 1984*).

Case Report: 51 year-old non-alcoholic, non-diabetic female developed a sensorimotor peripheral neuropathy and pyridoxine deficiency associated with long-term phenelzine therapy (*Heller CA, Friedman PA. Pyridoxine deficiency and peripheral neuropathy associated with long-term phenelzine therapy. Am J Med 75(5):887-88, 1983*).

Review Article: Isoniazid, which competitively inhibits the actions of the coenzymes derived from pyridoxine, can produce a peripheral neuropathy. The routine use of pyridoxine supplementation to prevent peripheral neuropathy in high risk populations receiving isoniazid is recommended (*Snider DE Jr. Pyridoxine supplementation during isoniazid therapy. Tubercle 61(4):191-96, 1980*).

Intraspinal injections may be effective in sciatic neuritis and Korsakoff's polyneuritis.

Experimental Study: 8/8 cases of sciatic neuritis without evidence of nerve root compression (most of whom had failed to improve after prolonged bed rest and local sciatic nerve infiltration) improved with intraspinal B_6 injections. 2/2 cases of Korsakoff's polyneuritis unresponsive to large doses of B complex orally and IV also responded rapidly to 2 intraspinal B_6 injections along with the addition of oral natural mixed tocopherols (*Stone S. Pyridoxine and thiamine therapy in disorders of the nervous system. Dis Nerv Sys 11:131-8, 1950*).

Vitamin B_{12}: 1000 µg IM as needed

Deficiency may cause a peripheral neuropathy, even in the absence of the classic findings of pernicious anemia, which responds to supplementation.

Placebo-controlled Case Reports: Vitamin B_{12} 15 gamma IM was rapidly effective in relieving pain in 3 pts. believed to have neuritis due to malnutrition but not in pts. with other painful illnesses, including 2 with brachial neuritis. It was also ineffective in reducing pain threshold in 2 normal controls, suggesting that it did not have an analgesic effect:
1. A 43-year-old male alcoholic with an 8 wk. history paresthesias of legs and feet with pain preventing ambulation. BP was 165/105 and his heart was slightly enlarged. Both feet were sweating excessively and were acutely painful spontaneously and to touch. Calves were tender and atrophic. Tendon reflexes were hypoactive, and there was decreased touch and vibratory sensation in the legs and feet. Gait was unsteady but the Romberg was negative. HGb was 10 gms and RBC count was 3.9 million. He failed to improve in 1 wk. on a control vitamin B-poor diet and was then given 1 cc normal saline IM without effect. When given a similar injection containing 15 gamma vitamin B_{12}, all spontaneous pain vanished with 1/2 hour, he could walk normally and pain to touch was gone. With a good diet and vitamin B supplementation, the neuritis entirely disappeared.
2. A 17-year-old female was completely disabled by pain, weakness and numbness of the extremities following an 11 wk. siege of vomiting. She had the pigmentation of pellagra, absent tendon reflexes, absent pallesthesia and position sense in legs and arms, tender skin and muscles and generalized weakness. Anemia and leukopenia were found. She failed to respond to the control diet and placebo injection, but had relief of pain within 45 min. after the vitamin B_{12} injection and gradually improved with proper diet and supplementation.

3. A 58-year-old male alcoholic diabetic had a 5 yr. history of gradually increasing neuritis of legs and feet. He had mild cirrhosis or fatty liver. IM vitamin B$_{12}$ stopped the pain within 1 hour (*Bean BB et al. An effect of vitamin B$_{12}$ on pain in nutritional neuropathy. Am J Med Sci 220:431-4, 1950*).

Supplementation may be beneficial even without evidence of deficiency.

Experimental Study: Pts. with pain due to degenerative neuropathy received 10,000 µg vitamin B$_{12}$ (cobamide) daily. After 2 wks., 80% reported marked and prompt pain relief (*Dettori AG, Ponari O. Effetto antalgico della cobamamide in corso di neuropatie periferiche di diversa etiopatogenesi. Minerva Med 64:1077-82, 1973*).

Case Reports: 2 cases of Bell's palsy, one of about 1.5 yrs. duration and the other of about 4 yrs. duration were treated with "massive" doses of cyanocobalamin (500-1000 µg daily to every other day for a total of 2000-20,000 µg) with complete recovery (*Mitra M, Nandi AK. Cyanocobalamin in chronic Bell's palsy. J Indian Med Assoc 33:129-31, 1959*).

Experimental Study: 18 pts. with trigeminal neuralgia and 1 pt. with glossopharyngeal neuralgia were treated with IM cyanocobalamin with the later cases receiving 1000 µg daily for 10 days. 15/18 showed considerable improvement or complete relief of pain (including the pt. with glossopharyngeal neuralgia), 1 showed moderate improvement and 3 showed little or no immediate improvement (*Surtees SJ, Hughes RR. Treatment of trigeminal neuralgia with vitamin B$_{12}$. Lancet 1:439-41, 1954*).

Experimental Study: 17 pts. with trigeminal neuralgia received vitamin B$_{12}$ IM daily for 10 days. 6 obtained complete relief lasting 2-8 mo., and 2 obtained satisfactory relief (*Alexander E, Davis CH Jr. Trigeminal neuralgia: Conservative management with massive vitamin B$_{12}$ therapy. N Carolina Med J 14:206-07, 1953*).

Experimental Study: 13 pts. with trigeminal neuralgia received cyancobalamin with the later cases receiving 100 µg IM daily for 10 days. All achieved "remarkable relief." While 9/13 experienced a prompt and complete remission, 4 pts. who had previously been treated with surgery or alcohol nerve blocks took longer to achieve pain relief (*Fields WS, Hoff HE. Relief of pain in trigeminal neuralgia by crystalline vitamin B$_{12}$. Neurology 2:131-39, 1952*).

Vitamin E:

Deficiency (as observed, for example, in patients with lipid malabsorption syndromes) is a known cause of peripheral neuropathy (*Traber MG et al. Lack of tocopherol in peripheral nerves of vitamin E-deficient patients with peripheral neuropathy. N Engl J Med 317:262-65, 1987*).

If deficient, may also be deficient in peripheral nerves, and the deficiency in the nerves may precede histologic degeneration.

Observational Study: The alpha-tocopherol content in biopsy specimens of sural nerve and adipose tissue from 5 pts. with symptomatic vitamin E deficiency (due either to homozygous hypobetalipoproteinemia or to familial isolated vitamin E deficiency) was compared to that of 34 pts. with neurologic diseases without vitamin E deficiency. A significant reduction in tissue vitamin E content was present in the vitamin E-deficient pts. in both sural nerve and adipose tissue compared to the controls. In addition, the low tocopherol content of the nerves preceded histologic degeneration in 3 vitamin E-deficient pts., suggesting that the nerve injury resulted from the low tocopherol content (*Traber MG et al. Lack of tocopherol in peripheral nerves of vitamin E-deficient patients with peripheral neuropathy. N Engl J Med 317:262-65, 1987*).

If deficient, supplementation may improve neurologic functioning, or at least prevent further neurologic deterioration (*Traber MG et al. Lack of tocopherol in peripheral nerves of vitamin E-deficient patients with peripheral neuropathy. N Engl J Med 317:262-65, 1987*).

Supplementation may be beneficial for muscular lesions due to leprous nerve involvement.

Experimental Study: Five pts. with neuritic pain due to lepromatous, tuberculoid, and indeterminate leprosy who symptoms had failed to respond to sulfone therapy experienced striking pain relief following supplementation with vitamin E (*Floch H, Horth R. La vitaminothérapie E dans la lèpre: Névrites et troubles trophiques. Bull Soc Pathol Exot 45:157-60, 1952*).

Experimental Study: Eight pts. with muscular lesions caused by nerve involvement due to leprosy received vitamin E. All had good to moderate results (*De Mello HA. Contribuição à terapeutica das lesões tróficas na lepra. Arq Min Leprol 11:148-51, 1951*).

- -

MINERALS

Zinc:

Deficiency may cause a neuropathy which may be reversible in its early stages.

Animal Experimental Study: Guinea pigs fed a zinc-deficient diet showed decreased motor nerve conduction velocity (NCV) which correlated to the degree of deficiency and was associated with abnormal posture and loco-motion, and hypersensitivity to touch. Altered NCV appeared to be caused by zinc-induced defects of Na,K-AT-Pase activity of the peripheral nerves. Increased zinc intake reversed the neuropathy (*O'Dell B et al. Zinc status and peripheral nerve function in guinea pigs. FASEBJ 4:2919-22, 1990*).

- -

OTHER NUTRITIONAL FACTORS

Coenzyme Q$_{10}$:

Supplementation may be beneficial.

Case Report: A 16 year-old male student complained of difficulty in walking and of muscle atrophy of the lower legs. He noticed his gait disturbance at about 12 yrs. of age and his symptoms gradually increased. On examination, he was unable to walk on his heels and on his toes. He had mild pes cavus and marked muscle wasting of the lower legs. The weakness was limited to the feet, lower legs, and hands. Mild sensory losses were demonstrated inside of the feet. Autonomic dysfunction was not present. The deep tendon reflexes were diminished. On lab testing, pyruvate and lactate were elevated in both serum and cerebrospinal fluid, and the serum level of CoQ$_{10}$ was low. Nerve conduction velocities were normal or just below normal except for the sural nerves, and the amplitudes of M waves were decreased. Sural nerve biopsy revealed marked reduction in the number of large myelinated fibers and no onion bulb formation, while the teased myelinated fiber analysis suggested ongoing axonal degeneration. Electron microscopy showed no mitochondrial abnormalities in muscle and nerve. He was treated with CoQ$_{10}$ 120 mg/d which was dramatically effective at about the third wk. after starting treatment. After about 16 mo., his gait disturbance disappeared. These findings suggest that an alteration of mitrochondrial function was involved (*Yamanaka N et al. [A case of motor and sensory neuropathy with elevated serum lactate and pyruvate which responded to a large dose of coenzyme Q$_{10}$ therapy.] Rinsho Shinkeigaku 29(7):885-9, 1989*) (*in Japanese*).

Essential Fatty Acids:

Supplementation may be beneficial in Guillain-Barre Syndrome.

Case Reports: Two children who had been severely disabled for 6 and 12 mo. respectively with idiopathic polyneuritis (Guillain-Barre Syndrome) began to recover within a week of starting on a polyunsatuated fatty-acid diet consisting of avoidance of fatty foods and supplementation with sunflower-seed oil 10 ml 3 times daily. They subsequently recovered virtually completely (*Bower BD, Newsholme EA. Treatment of idiopathic polyneuritis by polyunsaturated fatty acid diet. Lancet 1:583-5, 1978*).

- -

OTHER FACTORS

Cadmium:

Exposure may cause a peripheral neuropathy (*Blum LW et al. Peripheral neuropathy and cadmium toxicity. Pa Med 92(4):54-56, 1989*).

NEUROMUSCULAR DEGENERATION

See Also: AUTO-IMMUNE DISORDERS (GENERAL)
MULTIPLE SCLEROSIS
MYOPATHY

DIETARY FACTORS

Patients with amyotrophic lateral sclerosis are frequently malnourished (*Kasarskis E et al. Malnutrition in amyotropic lateral sclerosis patients. Abstract. J Am Coll Nutr 10(5):548, 1991*).

- -

VITAMINS

Folic Acid:

Deficiency may cause subacute combined systems degeneration which responds to supplementation in its earlier stages.

Review Article: The clinical signs of subacute system degeneration of the spinal cord can exist in the absence of vitamin B_{12} deficiency in pts. that are severely deficient in folate, and these neurological signs remit during therapy with folate. Although neuropathological and experimental verifications of the relationship between folate deficiency and myelopathy are lacking, a causal relationship appears to be highly probable (*Pincus JH. Folic acid deficiency: A cause of subacute combined system degeneration, in MI Botez, EH Reynolds, Eds. Folic Acid in Neurology, Psychiatry, and Internal Medicine. New York, Raven Press, 1979*).

Case Reports: Two pts. with subacute combined degeneration of the spinal cord and polyneuropathy had low serum folate levels compared to controls, long-standing GI disease, and deficient folate intake. The D-xylose absorption test gave low values in all pts., while none displayed the classical malabsorption syndrome. They had substantial improvement or recovered after periods ranging from 9-39 mo. of supplementation with oral folic acid 5-15 mg daily (*Botez MI et al. Polyneuropathy and folate deficiency. Arch Neurol 35:581-84, 1978*).

Vitamin B_6:

Supplementation may be beneficial in senile corea.

Case Report: A 71 year-old housewife had a 12-yr. history of gross, bizarre, purposeless, involuntary movements which began first in the arms and later spread to the rest of her musculature. She had been totally incapacitated for 3 years. Her mother had been similarly afflicted, but to a lesser degree, and her brother, aged 67, had noted similar mild twitching during the past few years. The other 5 siblings were unaffected. She was treated with pyridoxine hydrochloride 50 mg daily IV which was increased to 100 mg after the second week. After 3 wks. the regimen was discontinued and she was switched to oral pyridoxine hydrochloride 40 mg weekly. She began to improve following the first few injections. After 3 wks., she was walking unassisted and with ease, and her gait showed no observable abnormality. The choreiform movements were greatly reduced, and she could now sit quietly in a chair, whereas previously she had presented a rather bizarre picure. She felt stronger and her appetite and sleeping improved (*Baker AB. Treatment of paralysis agitans with vitamin B_6 (pyridoxine hydrochloride). JAMA 116:2484-7, 1941*).

Supplementation may be beneficial in amyotrophic lateral sclerosis.

Clinical Observation: Improvement was seen in pts. with ALS following IV administration of vitamin B_6 (*Spies TD et al. Some recent advances in vitamin therapy. JAMA 115(4):292-97, 1940*).

Vitamin B₁₂:

Deficiency is well-known to result in <u>subacute combined degeneration of the spinal cord</u> along with dementia, peripheral neuropathy, and optic neuritis which responds to supplementation in its earlier stages.

If deficient, supplementation may be beneficial.

Experimental Study: 141 consecutive pts. with neuropsychiatric abnormalities and low or low-normal serum cobalamin levels responded to IM cyanocobalamin. Characteristic features in these pts. included paresthesias, sensory loss, ataxia, dementia, and psychiatric disorders; longstanding neurologic symptoms without anemia; and markedly elevated serum concentrations of methylmalonic acid and total homocysteine. 40 (28%) had no anemia or macrocytosis. The hematocrit was normal in 34, the mean cell volume was normal in 25, and both tests were normal in 19. "Results suggest that neuropsychiatric disorders due to cobalamin deficiency occur commonly in the absence of anemia or an elevated mean cell volume and that measurements of serum methylmalonic acid and total homocytsteine both before and after treatment are useful in the diagnosis of these patients" (*Lindenbaum J et al. Neuropsychiatric disorders caused by cobalamin deficiency in the absence of anemia or macrocytosis. N Engl J Med 318:1720-28, 1988*).

Vitamin E:

May protect lipid components of neuronal tissue from free radical reactions and peroxidation.

Animal Experimental Study: Vitamin-E deficient one-month-old rats had a significant reduction in vitamin E concentrations in all 4 brain regions (cerebrum, cerebellum, mid-brain and brain stem). Lipid peroxidation in brain homogenates incubated under air for 2 hrs. was inhibited by vitamin E supplementation and increased by vitamin E deficiency. The magnitude of lipid peroxidation was inversely correlated with vitamin E content. Selenium supplementation or deficiency failed to significantly affect either vitamin E concentrations or lipid peroxidation (*Meydani M et al. Effect of dietary vitamin E and selenium on susceptibility of brain regions to lipid peroxidation. Lipids 23:405-09, 1988*).

Deficiency (which may be caused by defective absorption of fat-soluble vitamins) is associated with <u>progressive neurologic deterioration</u>, probably due to disordered intracellular peroxidation. Diseases associated with vitamin E deficiency include <u>abetalipoproteinemia</u> and <u>chronic cholestatic liver disease</u>.

Observational Study: 43.% of 42 female pts. with biopsy-confirmed primary biliary cirrhosis were deficient in vitamin E, and vitamin E status was directly related to the severity of hepatic dysfunction. Compared to normal controls and vitamin E-sufficient pts., the vitamin E-deficient pts. performed more poorly on a battery of neuropsychologic tests of psychomotor capacity (p<0.01) (*Arria AM et al. Vitamin E and neurologic function in adults with chronic cholestatic liver disease. Abstract. J Am Coll Nutr 6(5):442, 1987*).

Observational Study: Of 93 children (ages 1 mo.-17 yrs.) with prolonged neonatal cholestatic disorders due to either intrahepatic neonatal cholestasis or to extrahepatic biliary atresia, 64% of the intrahepatic and 77% of the extrahepatic cholestasis gps. were vitamin E-deficient based on serum concentrations and the ratios of serum vitamin E concentration to total serum lipid concentration. While neurologic function was normal in vitamin E-sufficient children, between the ages of 1-3 yrs., neurologic abnormalities were present in approx. 50% of the vitamin E-deficient children. By the ages of 8-10 yrs., neurologic dysfunction in the majority of vitamin E-deficient children had progressed to a disabling combination of findings (*Sokol RJ et al. Frequency and clinical progression of the vitamin E deficiency neurologic disorder in children with prolonged neonatal cholestasis. Am J Dis Child 139(12):1211-15, 1985*).

If deficient, supplementation may result in clinical improvement.

Case Report: A 72 year-old male had severe malabsorption, progressive retinopathy, and spinocerebeller degeneration 32 yrs. after gastric surgery, blind loop formation, and intestinal bacterial overgrowth. Clinical and pathologic features were typical of vitamin E deficiency; vitamin E was nearly undetectable in serum and profoundly low in adipose tissue. Vitamin E blood levels initially improved on treatment with antibiotics; after additional vitamin E supplementation, there was clinical improvement (*Brin MF et al. Blind loop syndrome, vitamin E malabsorption, and spinocerebeller degeneration. Neurology 35(3):338-42, 1985*).

Experimental Study: Vitamin E deficiency in 14 children with chronic cholestasis was corrected with either oral supplementation of up to 120 IU/kg daily or IM supplementation of 0.8-2.0 IU/kg daily. Neurologic function remained normal in 2 asymptomatic children below age 3 after 15 and 18 mo. of supplementation, while neurologic function became normal in 3 symptomatic chldren below age 3 after 18-32 mo. of supplementation. Restitution of neurologic function was more limited in 9 symptomatic children 5-17 yrs. old (*Sokol RJ et al. Improved neurologic function after long-term correction of vitamin E deficiency in children with chronic cholestasis. N Engl J Med 313(25):1580-86, 1985*).

Case Report: 23 year-old female with specific vitamin E malabsorption who, starting at age 13, suffered from increasing ataxia and a disturbance of proprioception. There was neither fat malabsorption nor deficiencies of fat-soluble vitamins A,D or K. Serum vitamin E was undetectable, and fasting lipid and lipoprotein concentrations were abnormal. After an initial treatment of alpha-tocopheryl acetate 2 g/d for 2 wks., serum vitamin E rose to the normal range. A maintenance dose of 800 mg/d was continued. After 10 wks., there was marked clinical improvement. After 15 mo., proprioception (with appreciation of vibration) had marginally improved (*Harding AE et al. Spinocerebellar degeneration associated with a selective defect of vitamin E absorption. N Engl J Med 313(1):32-35, 1985*).

Experimental Study: 4 children (ages 6-17) with chronic cholestasis who developed a slowly progressive neuromuscular disease characterized by ataxia, dysmetria, areflexia, loss of vibratory sensation, and a variable ophthalmoplegia were found to have low serum vitamin E concentrations. Muscle histochemical findings were similar to those described in vitamin E-deficient animals. Alpha tocopherol 0.55-1.42 mg/kg daily IM was required to achieve normal serum vitamin E levels in 3 pts., while 1 pt. achieved normal levels with an oral dosage of 32 mg/kg daily. After normalization of serum concentrations for 12-20 mo., the neurologic disease improved in all 4 pts. (*Guggenheim MA et al. Progressive neuromuscular disease in children with chronic cholestasis and vitamin E deficiency: Diagnosis and treatment with alpha tocopherol. J Pediatr 100(1):51-58, 1982*).

Supplementation may be beneficial in amyotrophic lateral sclerosis.

Case Reports: 11/20 cases of ALS improved on 60-75 IU daily of alpha tocopheryl acetate. The author suggests 300 IU for maximal effectiveness (*Wechsler IS. The treatment of amyotrophic lateral sclerosis with vitamin E (tocopherols). Am J Med.Sci 200:765-778, 1940*).

Clinical Observation: In occasional ALS pts. with malnutrition, especially those with vitamin E deficiency, the injection of synthetic alpha tocopherol 500 mg in oil is effective, at least temporarily, in relieving neuromuscular symptoms, roaring sensations in the ears, anorexia, and insomnia. Occasionally the improvement is striking, but it is difficult to measure objectively (*Spies TD, Vilter RW. A note on the effect of alpha-tocopherol (Vitamin E) in human nutrition. South Med J 33:663, 1940*).

- with thiamine:

Case Reports: 8/9 cases of ALS improved on up to 375 IU of alpha tocopheryl acetate "enhanced" with thiamine (*Rosenberger AI. Observations on the treatment of amyotrophic lateral sclerosis with vitamin E. Med Rec 154:97-100, 1941*).

Not deficient in spinal muscular atrophy (Werdnig-Hoffmann disease) (*Sokol RJ, Iannaccone ST. Normal vitamin E status in spinal muscular atrophy. Ann Neurol 13(3):328-30, 1983*).

Supplementation may be beneficial in Charcot-Marie-Tooth disease.

Experimental Single-blind Study: 20 pts. with type I Charcot-Marie-Tooth disease received supplementation with vitamin E 81.6 IU daily and placebo (paraffin oil). After 3 mo., improvement was demonstrated by neuropsychological testing and neurologic examination. Linoleic and gamma-linolenic acids 3 gms daily were then substituted for placebo. After 1 yr., the previous level of improvement was maintained, suggesting that vitamin E may have a membrane stabilization effect (*Williams LL et al. Dietary essential fatty acids, vitamin E, and Charcot-Marie-Tooth disease. Neurology 36(9):1200-05, 1986*).

- -

MINERALS

Calcium:

Deficiency may cause amyotrophic lateral sclerosis.

> **Animal Experimental Study:** In an attempt to duplicate the low calcium, high aluminum and high manganese in the soil and drinking water in the western Pacific where there is an increased risk for ALS and parkinsonism-dementia, monkeys were maintained for 41-46 mo. on a low-calcium diet with or without supplemental aluminum and manganese. Mild calcium and aluminum deposition and degenerative changes, compatible with those of early ALS and parkinsonism-dementia, were found in motor neurons of the substantia nigra, cerebrum, brain stem and spinal cord. The magnitude and extent of these lesions far exceeded those found in normal aged monkeys (*Garruto RM et al. Low-calcium, high-aluminum diet-induced motor neuron pathology in cynomolgus monkeys. Acta Neuropathol (Berl) 78(2):210-9, 1989*).

> **Observational Study and Theoretical Discussion:** There has been a decline in the high incidence rate of ALS and parkinsonism-dementia among the Chamorros of Guam which has occurred principally among males, especially those born after 1920 and living in areas where calcium and magnesium levels are low in soil in water. The decline is consistent with the hypothesis that the previously high incidence resulted from defects in mineral metabolism and secondary hyperparathyroidism, provoked by nutritional deficiencies of calcium and magnesium, with resultant deposition of calcium and aluminum in neurons (*Garruto RM et al. Disappearance of high-incidence amyotrophic lateral sclerosis and parkinsonism-dementia on Guam. Neurology 35(2):193-98, 1985*).

> **Theoretical Discussion:** In old age, low calcium and vitamin D intake, short solar exposure, decreased intestinal absorption, and falling renal function with insufficient 1,25-dihydroxyvitamin D synthesis all contribute to calcium deficiency, secondary hyperparathyroidism, bone loss and possibly calcium shift from the bone to soft tissue, and from the extracellular to the intracellular compartment, blunting the sharp concentration gap between these compartments. Consequences may include amyotrophic lateral sclerosis and senile dementia due to calcium deposition in the central nervous system (*Fujita T. Aging and calcium as an environmental factor. J Nutr Sci Vitaminol (Tokyo) 31 Suppl S15-9, 1985*).

> **Observational Study:** 16 Guamanian Chamorros with ALS were evaluated. The serum immunoreactive parathyroid hormone was mildly elevated in 6/16 patients. Intestinal calcium absorption was decreased in 2/16 pts., all of whom had low levels of serum 1,25-dihydroxyvitamin D. Reductions in cortical bone mass were striking. A significant negative correlation was found between the percentage of cortical area of the second metacarpal bone and muscle atrophy and weakness, and significant positive correlations were found between degree of immobility and ratio of urinary hydroxyproline to creatinine. In general, abnormalities in calcium metabolism were subtle, suggesting that, if the deposition of calcium and aluminum in CNS tissues is a cause of the disease and of the early appearance of neurofibrillary tangles in neurons, the accumulation had occurred long before onset of symptoms, and detectable abnormalities of calcium and vitamin D metabolism may already have been corrected (*Yanagihara R et al. Calcium and vitamin D metabolism in Guamanian Chamorros with amyotrophic lateral sclerosis and parkinsonism-dementia. Ann Neurol 1591):42-8, 1984*).

- -

OTHER NUTRITIONAL FACTORS

Amino Acids:

- Branched-chain (Leucine, Isoleucine, Valine):

> Glutamate metabolism is abnormal in amyotrophic lateral sclerosis (*Plaitakis A, Caroscio JT. Abnormal glutamate metabolism in amyotrophic lateral sclerosis. Ann Neurol 22:575-79, 1987*), and increased concentrations of branched-chain amino acids in plasma may activate and thus modify glutamine metabolism (*Dennis S, Clark JB. The synthesis of glutamate by rat brain mitochondria. J Neurochem 46:1811-19, 1986*).

Supplementation may be beneficial in amyotrophic lateral sclerosis.

> **Experimental Double-blind Study:**   18 ALS pts. randomly received either 3 gm L-leucine, 2 gm L-iso-leucine, and 1.6 gm L-valine 4 times daily between meals or placebo. During the 1-year trial, pts. in the placebo gp. showed a linear decline in functional status; those treated with amino acids showed significant benefit in terms of maintenance of extremity muscle strength and continued ability to walk. Repeated-measures analysis of the spinal scores for all pts. who completed the trial revealed significant differences in the rate of progression of the disease between the 2 groups, although the changes in bulbar scores did not differ significantly. 5/9 placebo gp. pts. lost their ability to walk, 2 subsequently dying and another becoming respirator-dependent, while only 1/9 AA-treated pts. became unable to walk (*Plaitakis A et al. Pilot trial of branched-chain aminoacids in amyotrophic lateral sclerosis. Lancet 1:1015-18, 1988*).

- Glycine:

Increased plasma concentration may be associated with neurodegenerative disease (*Bank WJ, Morrow G III. A familial spinal cord disorder with hyperglycaemia. Arch Neurol 27:136-44, 1972; De Belleroche J, Recordati A, Clifford Rose F. Elevated levels of amino acids in the CSF of motor neurone disease patients. Neurochem Pathol 2:1-6, 1984; Lane RJM, Dick JPR, de Belleroche J. Glycine and neurodegenerative disease. Letter. Lancet 337:732-3, 1991; Lane RJM et al An abnormality of glycine metabolism in ALS patients. J Neurol Neurosurg Psychiatry 52:180, 1990*).

- L-Threonine:

May increase the cerebrospinal content of glycine.

Supplementation may be beneficial in amyotrophic lateral sclerosis.

> **Experimental Placebo-controlled Study:**   15 ALS pts. received L-threonine 2-4 gm daily. 7/15 had definite symptom improvement in regard to speech, swallowing, energy, and spasticity, and 3/15 showed minor improvement. There were no adverse effects. Improvement occurred within 48 hrs. and was most dramatic in the seriously afflicted patients. By contrast, 2 unrelated amino acid placebos had no effect (*BM Patten, Baylor College of Medicine - reported in Am Fam Physician 37(6):312, 1988*).

Carnitine:

In patients with neuromuscular diseases, there is a positive correlation between creatinine excretion and carnitine excretion (*Carroll JE et al. Carnitine intake and excretion in neuromuscular diseases. Am J Clin Nutr 34:2693-8, 1981*).

Coenzyme Q10:   100 mg daily in divided doses

Supplementation may be beneficial for neurogenic atrophies.

> **Case Report:**   65 year-old male with 2 yr. history of a walking disability due to upper motor neuron disease was initially placed on a complex nutrient treatment program which emphasized the B-complex vitamins. 1 yr. later he reported that he had been able to greatly decrease the dose of their nutrients while maintaining a stable state. His weight was unchanged, and he could walk 1 mile slowly with difficulty, and was able to climb a small hill in 1 hr., but could not hold his head erect due to weak back muscles. He was placed on Coenzyme Q10 30 mg 3 times daily. 2 1/2 mo. later, he reported that, after 3 wks. on CoQ10, there was a dramatic improvement, He was able to walk 8 miles, and faster, although he still had a slight limp. He climbed the same hill in 30 minutes. He was able to hold his head erect and had less neck pain. He also stated that this was the first time in 8 yrs. that he had felt so well (*Hoffer A. Vitamin Q10. Int Clin Nutr Rev 9(2):62-63, 1989*).

> **Experimental Double-blind Crossover Study:**   12 pts. with progressive muscular dystrophies and neurogenic atrophies were treated with CoQ10 or placebo. Solely by the presence or absence of significant change in stroke volume and cardiac output, all 8 pts. on blind CoQ10 and all 4 on blind placebo were correctly assigned (p<0.003). After 3 mo., improved physical well-being was observed in 4/8 treated pts. and for 0/4 placebo patients. One with Becker dystrophy was able to increase physical exercise from 30 min. to 45 minutes. A second with Duchenne dystrophy fell less frequently. A third with Charcot-Marie-Tooth disorder could walk further, while the last, who had the same diagnosis, became more energetic and less tired. Of the pts. first given placebo and then crossed

over, 3/4 improved on CoQ$_{10}$. 5/6 on CoQ$_{10}$ in crossover to placebo (2 resigned before crossover) maintained improved cardiac function, while 1/6 relapsed (*Folkers K et al. Biochemical rationale and the cardiac response of patients with muscle disease to therapy with coenzyme Q$_{10}$. Proc Natl Acad Sci U S A. 82(13):4513-16, 1985*).

- -

OTHER FACTORS

Rule out heavy metal toxicity.

May predispose to amyotrophic lateral sclerosis.

Observational Study: The standard mortality ratios (1968-78) for motor neuron disease were calculated for those counties in England and Wales which had the highest and lowest aluminum concentrations in the water. Results suggest that mortality from motoneuron disease, like the incidence of Alzheimer's disease, varies with the local water aluminum concentration, especially among women (*Lindegard B. Aluminium and Alzheimer's disease. Letter. Lancet 1:267-68, 1989*).

Observational Study: In Guan and on Kii (Japan) where a 100-fold increased prevalence of amyotrophic lateral sclerosis was observed 2 decades earlier, high levels of heavy and/or trace metals, such as manganese and aluminum, and low levels of minerals such as calcium and magnesium, were detected in soil and water samples (*Yase Y. Environmental contribution of the amyotrophic lateral sclerosis process, in G Serratrice et al, Eds. Neuromuscular Diseases. New York, Raven Press, 1984:335-39; Yase Y. The pathogenesis of amyotrophic lateral sclerosis. Lancet 2:292-96, 1972*).

Rule out gluten sensitivity.

May cause a progressive pancerebellar syndrome.

Case Report: A 57-year-old man developed a progressive pancerebellar syndrome with ataxia, palatal myoclous and marked speech impairment. Malabsorption studies and jejunal biopsy established the diagnosis of celiac disease. Postmortum examination demonstrated characteristic GI and cerebral abnormalities (*Finelli PF et al. Adult celiac disease presenting as cerebellar syndrome. Neurology 30(3):245-49, 1980*).

OBESITY

DIETARY FACTORS

Homeostatic caloric requirement at an average activity level can be estimated by multiplying a person's ideal weight in pounds by 12-14 for a woman or by 14-16 for a man. To lose 1 pound, intake must be 3,500 kcal less than energy expenditure (500 kcal less per day to lose 1 lb/wk). Increasing energy expenditure through exercise should be combined with dietary measures. Most people will begin to lose weight if they decrease their calorie intake to below 1,500 kcal/d, although some reach a point at which they may require less than 1,000 kcal/d to continue to lose weight. Most obese people are unable to achieve their ideal weight; of those who do, the overwhelming majority regain the weight in 1-2 years (*Friedman RB. Fad diets: Evaluation of five common types. Postgrad Med 89(1):249-58, 1986*).

Low calorie balanced diet.

These diets are the safest, generally provide 800-1500 kcal/d using a wide variety of foods, and usually provide the Recommended Dietary Allowances for vitamins and minerals. Examples are variations of the American Dietetics Association/American Diabetes Association pattern diets, the Prudent Diet, the La Costa Spa Diet, and the TOPS (Take Off Pounds Sensibly) and Weight Watchers diets. The Setpoint Diet is similar; however, the author's theory that each person has a setpoint that the body will try to maintain despite changes in calorie consumption has not been well proven. For optimum results, the diet should be combined with exercise and psychological/behavioral interventions (*Friedman RB. Fad diets: Evaluation of five common types. Postgrad Med 89(1):249-58, 1986; Morgan SL. Rational weight loss programs: A clinician's guide. J Am Coll Nutr 8(3):186-94, 1989; Weinsier RL et al. Recommended therapeutic guidelines for professional weight control programs. Am J Clin Nutr 40:865-72, 1984*).

References for typical balanced diets:

Bennett L, Simon M. The Prudent Diet. New York, David White, 1972

Leveille GA. The Setpoint Diet. New York, Ballantine, 1985

Smith RP. The La Costa Spa Diet and Exercise Book. New York, Grosset & Dunlap, 1977

Low Fat Diet.

Reducing fat intake even without restricting calories may result in weight loss.

Experimental Controlled Study: 303 women were randomly assigned to an intervention gp. that received intensive instruction in maintaining a low-fat diet or to a control group. After 1 yr., intervention-gp. women had decreased fat intake by 45.3 g (from 39.2% to 21.6% energy from fat) and weight by 3.1 kg (all p<0.0001); control-gp. women decreased fat intake by 8.8 g (from 38.9% to 37.3% energy from fat) and weight by 0.4 kg. In both univariate analyses and multivariate models, weight loss was more strongly associated with change in percent energy from fat than with change in total energy intake. These data, which are consistent with both epidemiologic and clinical studies, suggest that body adiposity is a function both of energy balance and the proportion of energy derived from fat (*Sheppard L, Kristal AR, Kuski LH. Weight loss in women participating in a randomized trial of low-fat diets. Am J Clin Nutr 54:821-8, 1991*).

Experimental Controlled Study: 18 premenopausal women with body mass index (BMI) of 18-44 were fed a 37% fat control diet for 4 wks. followed by a 20% fat (low-fat) diet for 20 weeks. Despite adjustments in energy intake to maintain weight throughout the study, subjects exhibited a 2.8% decrease in total body weight (p<0.0006), an 11.3% decrease in fat weight (p<0.0001), and a 2.2% increase in lean body weight (p<0.0149) by the end of the low fat period. Similar changes were observed in obese (BMI>30) and non-obese (BMI<30) women. By the end of the low-fat period, energy intake had increased significantly in comparison with the high-fat diet (119% of the high-fat intake, p<0.0001). Results could not be explained by changes in daily activity levels and suggest that macronutrient composition plays a role in energy requirements for weight maintenance

(*Prewitt TE et al. Changes in body weight, body composition, and energy intake in women fed high- and low-fat diets. Am J Clin Nutr 54:304-10, 1991*).

Experimental Controlled Crossover Study: 13 females randomly received either a low-fat diet (20-25% of calories as fat) or a control diet (35-40% fat) for 11 weeks. After a 7-wk. washout period, the conditions were reversed for another 11 weeks. Energy intake on the low-fat diet gradually increased, resulting in a total caloric compensation of 35% by the end of the 11-wk. treatment period and a weight loss of 2.5 kg in 11 wks., twice the amt. of weight lost on the control diet (*Kendall A et al. Weight loss on a low-fat diet: consequence of the imprecision of the control of food intake in humans. Am J Clin Nutr 53:1124-9, 1991*).

High Carbohydrate Diet.

These diets generally induce weight loss through limited food choices (*Morgan SL. Rational weight loss programs: A clinician's guide. J Am Coll Nutr 8(3):186-94, 1989*). Most contain enough sweets to satisfy sugar cravings, and their high water content appeases hunger by increasing bulk. The Pritikin Maximum Weight Loss Diet (*Pritikin N, McGrady P, Jr. The Pritikin Program for Diet and Exercise. New York, Grosset & Dunlap, 1979*) provides up to 85% of its calories in the form of complex carbohydrates and is extremely low in fat (5-10% of calories) and low in protein (about 10% of calories). It has both a 600 kcal and 1,000 kcal version and is supposed to be combined with exercise. A more recent version, described in The Pritikin Permanent Weight Loss Manual (*Pritikin N. New York, Grosset & Dunlap, 1981*), presents a more palatable diet with an increased protein content.

Several versions of the high carbohydrate diet tend to be nutritionally unbalanced in terms of proteins, vitamins and minerals. Examples are the Beverly Hills diet (*Mazel J. The Beverly Hills Diet. New York, Macmillin, 1981*) which has been severely criticized (*Mirkin GB, Shore RN. The Beverly Hills diet: Dangers of the newest weight loss fad. JAMA 246(19):2235-37, 1981*) and the Rice diet (*Moscovitz J. The Rice Diet Report*), as well as some versions of the Zen macrobiotic diet (*Morgan SL. Rational weight loss programs: A clinician's guide. J Am Coll Nutr 8(3):186-94, 1989*). Possible adverse side effects include diarrhea, muscle wasting, and hair loss (*Council on Foods and Nutrition. Zen macrobiotic diets. JAMA 218:397, 1971*). The current macrobiotic diet, however, appears to be nutritionally adequate if the mix of foods proposed is carefully followed (*House of Representativies, Subcommittee on Health and Long-Term Care. Quackery: A $10 Billion Scandal. Washington DC, US Gov't. Print. Off. 1984:66-68, 187; Committee publication No. 98-435*).

Low Carbohydrate Diet.

These diets have high satiety value because of their high protein and fat contents. Examples are the Dr. Atkins, Dr. Stillman, and Scarsdale diets. Ketosis (incomplete oxidation of fats resulting in the accumulation of intermediary acetyl-CoA molecules) caused by the low carbohydrate composition of these diets is responsible for a diuresis causing a rapid initial weight loss. Potential risks are hyperuricemia, sodium and potassium loss, diarrhea, glucose intolerance, hyperlipidemia, constipation, postural hypotension, fatigue, euphoria and, unless they are added to the diet, nutritional inadequacy of vitamins and minerals (*Friedman RB. Fad diets: Evaluation of five common types. Postgrad Med 89(1):249-58, 1986; Morgan SL. Rational weight loss programs: A clinician's guide. J Am Coll Nutr 8(3):186-94, 1989*).

References for typical low carbohydrate diets:

Atkins RC, Linde SM. Dr. Atkins' Superenergy Diet. New York, Arlington House (Crown), 1976

Stillman IM, Baxter SS. The Doctor's Quick Weight-Loss Diet. New York, Dell, 1968

Tarnower H, Baker SS. The Complete Scarsdale Medical Diet. New York, Rawson-Wade, 1978

If total calorie intake is equal, greater weight loss may occur on a low carbohydrate diet than on a high carbohydrate diet.

Experimental Study: 45 pts. were placed on a 1000 kcal diet which contained either 170 gm carbohydrate and 11 gm fat or 25 gm carbohydrate and 75 gm fat. After 1 mo., the low-carbohydrate gp. had lost an mean of 14 ± 7.2 kg with a mean daily weight loss of 362 ± 91 g/d, while the high-carbohydrate gp. had lost only 9.8 ± 4.5 kg and 298 ± 80 g/d, respectively; thus the weight loss was 20% greater on the low carbohydrate diet (*Rabast U et al. Comparative studies in obese subjects fed carbohydrate-restricted and high carbohydrate 1,000-calorie formula diets. Nutr Metab 22(5):269-77, 1978*).

Experimental Study: Pts. were placed on a 1800 kcal diet containing 30-104 gm carbohydrate. While 25% of the weight lost on the high carbohydrate (104 gm) diet was nonfat tissue, only 5% of the weight lost was nonfat tissue on the low carbohydate (30 gm) diet. After 9 wks., pts. on the low carbohydrate diet lost an ave. of 32.7 lb, while the pts. on the high carbohydrate diet lost 17.5 lb (*Young CM et al. Effect of body composition and other parameters in obese young men of carbohydrate level of reduction diet. Am J Clin Nutr 24(3):290-96, 1971*).

Exclusion of dietary carbohydrate maintains a high degree of ketosis and low levels of plasma insulin. Ketones replace much of the glucose used by the brain; thus reducing gluconeogenesis. The low plasma insulin levels are associated with increased release of free fatty acids from adipose tissue and, thus, with enhanced fat mobilization (*Flatt JP, Blackburn GL. The metabolic fuel regulatory system: Implications for protein-sparing therapies during caloric deprivation and disease. Am J Clin Nutr 27:175-87, 1974*).

Experimental Study: 6 matched gps. of pts. underwent 3-week selective hypocaloric diets which consisted of 240-800 kcal and 19-112 g/d carbohydrate. The rate of ketogenesis which developed during each nutritional treatment was inversely related to the amt. of dietary carbohydrates (*Pasquali R et al. Interrelationships between dietary carbohydrates, B cell function and rate of ketogenesis during underfeeding in obese patients. Ann Nutr Metab 31(4):219-30, 1987*).

Isocaloric substitution of carbohydrate for protein in hypocaloric diets decreases protein sparing (*Blackburn GL et al. Mechanisms of nitrogen sparing with severe calorie restricted diets. Int J Obes 5:215-16,1981*).

Negative Experimental Study: In a study of severely obese pts. subjected to very-low-calorie diets (<500 kcal/d), nitrogen balance, labile protein concentrations and plasma amino acid profile were not significantly affected by adding carbohydrate to proteins (*Scalfi L et al. Protein balance during very-low-calorie diets for the treatment of severe obesity. Ann Nutr Metab 31(3):154-59, 1987*).

High Protein Diet.

High protein diets can be effective for weight loss, but tend to be montonous and are frequently high in cholesterol. Simlar to low carbohydrate diets, they require a great deal of water to wash away ketone bodies and can cause fatigue and bad breath. Deficiencies of vitamins and minerals are common. They should be avoided by persons with gout, diabetes, kidney or liver disease or who are pregnant (*Friedman RB. Fad diets: Evaluation of five common types. Postgrad Med 89(1):249-58, 1986*).

References for typical high protein diets:

Berger S, Cohen M. Southampton Diet. New York, Simon & Shuster, 1982

Berkowitz GM, Neimark P. The Berkowitz Diet Switch. Westport CT, Arlington House, 1981

Simmons R. Richard Simmons' Never-Say-Diet Book. New York, Warner, 1980

Very-low-calorie Diet:

WARNINGS: Dehydration and postural hypotension are common. Cold intolerance is invariable after 3 wks.; beyond 14 wks., a diminished metabolic rate can cause temporary hair loss (*Prasad N. Very-low-calorie diets. Postgrad Med 88(3):179-88, 1990*). Headaches, muscle cramps, diarrhea, halitosis and abdominal cramps may also occur. Uric acid levels peak in 1-2 wks., then usually return to normal (*Atkinson RL. Low and very low calories diets. Med Clin North Am 73(1):203-15, 1989*). After several wks., a normocytic normochromic anemia or leukopenia can occur (*Fisler JS, Drenick EJ. Starvation and semi-starvation diets in the the management of obesity. Annu Rev Nutr 7:465-84, 1987*). Gallstone formation has been reported (*Liddle RA et al. Gallstone formation during weight-reduction dieting. Arch Intern Med 149(8):1750-53, 1989*). Other possible adverse effects include ketosis, negative nitrogen balance, brittle nails, and dry skin (*Morgan SL. Rational weight loss programs: A clinician's guide. J Am Coll Nutr 8(3):186-94, 1989*). In diabetics, serum and fasting blood glucose levels may be reduced, and serum lipid levels may be lowered (*Bistrian BR et al. Nitrogen metabolism and insulin requirements in obese diabetic adults on a protein-sparing modified fast. Diabetes 25:494-504, 1976*).

These diets generally contain 3-400 kcal/d. Women lose an ave. of 1.5 kg/wk, while men lose an ave. of 2.0 kg/wk. The greater weight loss noted on liquid protein diets, when compared to balanced diets of equal calorie content, is attributed solely to the large amount of water loss (*Yang MU, Van Itallie TB. A composition of weight loss during short-term weight reduction. J Clin Invest 58:722-30, 1976*). They should be limited to persons who are a minimum of 30% and 18 kg overweight, have received a recent medical examination and electrocardiogram with satisfactory results, and are free of contraindications (recent MI; cardiac conduction disorder; history of cerebrovascular, renal or hepatic disease; cancer; type I diabetes; significant psychiatric disturbance) (*Wadden TA et al. Responsible and irresponsible use of very-low-calorie diets in the treatment of obesity. JAMA 263(1):83-85, 1990*).

- with fiber:

May reduce hunger and improve bowel function.

> **Experimental Controlled Crossover Study:** 22 obese pts. were placed on a 366-466 kcal diet with or without the addition of dietary fiber 30 g/d for 2 wks. and then crossed over to the other diet for another 2 weeks. Both gps. showed similar weight loss; however, pts. consumimg supplemental fiber reported less hunger and constipation (*Astrup A et al. Dietary fibre added to very low calorie diet reduces hunger and alleviates constipaton. Int J Obes 14:105-112, 1990*).

Early "liquid protein" diets, popularized by Dr. Robert Linn (*Linn R, Stuart SL. The Last Chance Diet. Secaucus, NJ, Lyle Stuart, 1976*) often contained protein of poor biological quality and were responsible for a number of deaths (*Van Itallie TB. Liquid protein mayhem. Editorial. JAMA 240:140-45, 1978*). Cardiac dysfunction appeared to be the immediate cause of death, but the cause of death has not been clearly determined (*Lantigua RA et al. Cardiac arrhythmias associated with a liquid protein diet for the treatment of obesity. N Engl J Med 303:735-38, 1980*).

Contemporary versions are based on the Protein-sparing Modified Fast developed by Drs. Alan Howard and McLean Baird (*Howard A, Baird IM. The treatment of obesity by low calorie semisynthetic diets, in G Bray, Ed. Recent Advances in Obesity Research. London, Newman, 1975*). These researchers reported that, if carbohydrate is added to a low-calorie, high-quality protein mixture, less protein is needed to maintain nitrogen balance. Diets based on their work usually provide 1.0-1.5 g of high biological value protein daily per kilogram of ideal body weight. 20-40 g of carbohydrate is provided daily, and the diet is generally supplemented with vitamins and minerals. A one-day portion of the Cambridge Diet, for example, contains 330 kcal, 31 g of high biological value protein, 44 g of carbohydrate, 2 g of fat, and 100% of the RDA for vitamins and minerals. (*The Cambridge diet. Med Lett 24:91, 1982*).

> *Note: At least 6 deaths have been reported on the Cambridge Diet (Wadden TA et al. The Cambridge Diet: more mayhem? JAMA 2540:2833-34, 1983). It has therefore been suggested that this diet be restricted to patients who are at least 30-40% above ideal weight and who are under medical supervision (Felig P. Very low calorie protein diets: An editorial retrospective. N Engl J Med 310:589-91, 1984; Lee RB, Lindner PG. The ulta-low calorie diet revisited. Obes Bariatr Med 1(11):4, 1982).*

High Fat Diet:

High fat diets taste good. In addition, since fats take longer to digest, people usually feel full longer than on other diets containing a similar amount of calories. These advantages, however, are strongly counterbalanced by the unhealthy effects of a high fat intake as well as by the dangers of inadequate nutrition. Dr. Robert Atkins' high-fat, low-carbohydrate diet (*Atkins RC. Dr. Atkins' Diet Revolution: The High Calorie Way to Stay Slim Forever. New York, David McKay, 1972*) has been repeatedly criticized in the professional literature (*A critique of low-carbohydrate ketogenic weight reduction regimens: A review of Dr. Atkins' Diet Revolution. JAMA 224:1415-19, 1973; Dr. Atkins' Diet Revolution. Med Lett 15(May 1):41-42, 1973*). Calories Don't Count by Dr. Herman Taller (*New York, Simon & Shuster, 1961*) is an earlier example of a high fat diet.

"Fit for Life" diet.

This best-selling popular diet, designed by Harvey and Marilyn Diamond, is based on a number of generally unaccepted and unproven claims - such as "eating two concentrated foods simultaneously will cause the food to rot" (*Trubo R. Fad diets: Unqualified hunger for miracles. Med World News August 11, 1986*).

Fasting:

These programs produce variable results (*Fisler JS, Drenick EJ. Starvation and semistarvation diets in the management of obesity. Annu Rev Nutr 7:465-84, 1987*) and are not useful for long-term weight maintenance (*Newmark SR, Williamson B. Survey of very-low-calorie weight reduction diets. II. Total fasting, protein-sparing modified fasts, chemically defined diets. Arch Intern Med 143:1423-27, 1983*). About 1/3 of the weight lost during a 24-day fast is fluid and lean body mass (*Apfelbaum M et al. [The composition of weight lost during the water diet. Effects of protein supplementation.] Gastroenterologia 108(3):121-34, 1967*).

Possible adverse effects include ketosis, electrolyte imbalance, hyperuricemia, gouty arthritis, abdominal cramps, orthostatic hypotension, muscle wasting, hepatic and renal impairment, and negative nitrogen balance (*Blackburn GL. Fad reducing diets: Separating fads from facts. Contempr Nutr 8(7), 1983; Duncan GG et al. Contraindications and therapeutic results of fasting in obese patients. Ann N Y Acad Sci 131:632-36, 1965; Runcie J, Thomson TJ. Prolonged starvation - dangerous procedure? Br Med J 3:432-35, 1970*). Several deaths have been reported (*Wadden TA et al. Very low calorie diets: Their efficacy, safety, and future. Ann Intern Med 99:675-84, 1983*).

Increase dietary fiber.

Increases non-caloric bulk to cause satiety with less intake.

Experimental Double-blind Study: 52 overweight men and women (body mass index of 25 or greater) consumed a low-calorie diet providing 25-30% fewer calories than were consumed prior to the study. In addition, they randomly received either a fiber supplement or placebo taken as 7 tabs 3 times daily with 120 ml water 20-30 min before meals. The fiber supplements provided 7 g dietary fiber/d from beet, barley and citrus, and about 90% of it was insoluble. After 6 mo., the experimental gp. lost an ave. of 5.5 kg whereas the placebo gp. lost an ave. of 3.0 kg. While the fiber gp. had reduced feelings of hunger, the placebo gp. had increased feelings of hunger (*Rigaud D et al. Overweight treated with energy restriction and a dietary fibre supplement: A 6-month randomized, double-blind, placebo-controlled trial. Int J Obes 14:763-9, 1990*).

Review Article: Supplementing a normal diet with gel-forming fibers, such as guar gum, leads to an increased satiation probably due to a slower gastric emptying. Recent long-term studies have confirmed the usefulness of viscous fibers. Apart from a beneficial effect during calorie restriction, dietary fiber may improve some of the metabolic aberrations seen in obesity (*Smith U. Dietary fibre, diabetes and obesity. Int J Obes 11 Suppl 1:27-31, 1987*).

Experimental Double-blind Studies: 1.) 60 females were treated with general dietary advice, providing a mean daily energy intake of 1,400 kcal. In addition, some randomly received a daily 5 gm fiber supplement while the others took placebos. After 2 mo., mean weight loss in the fiber gp. (7.0 kg) was significantly higher than that of the control gp. (6.0 kg) (p<0.05). 2.) 45 females were treated similarly, with a recommended mean daily energy intake of 1,600 kcal and a daily 7 gm fiber supplement. After 3 mo., mean weight loss in the fiber gp. (6.2 kg) was significantly higher than that of the control gp. (4.1 kg) (p<0.05). No significant difference in hunger feelings was found between the fiber and non-fiber groups (*Rössner S et al. Weight reduction with dietary fibre supplements. Results of two double-blind randomized studies. Acta Med Scand 222(1):83-88, 1987*).

Ingestion of high-fiber breakfast cereals may reduce food intake at lunchtime.

Experimental Study: At 0730, 14 subjects ingested 1 of 5 cereals, plus milk and orange juice. At 1100 they were presented with a buffet lunch. There was a significant inverse correlation between fiber content of the cereals and energy intake at lunch (*Levine AS et al. Effect of breakfast cereals on short-term food intake. Am J Clin Nutr 50:1303-07, 1989*).

- Bean Husk Powder: 400 mg with breakfast, 600 mg with lunch, and 600 mg with supper.
Take with a glass of water at the start of the meal.

Experimental Double-blind Study: 60 women, all overweight by at least 20% of their ideal weight, were divided into 2 matched groups. They were placed on an 1800 calories diet and received either bean husk power in capsules (Arkocaps) as noted above or placebo. After 15 days, weight loss in the treatment gp. was double that of controls (1.73 kg vs. 0.86 kg). After 30 days, weight loss in the treatment gp. was triple that of controls (3.11 kg vs. 0.935 kg). Similarly, reduction in waist measurement was twice as great in the treatment gp. by day 15 and 3.5 times as great by day 30. 3 pts. in the treatment gp. reported flatulence and the number of stools increased from 1 to 1.7 daily (*Lecomte A. A double-blind study confirms the effects on weight of bean husk Arkocaps. Revue de L'association Mondiale de Phytotherapie 1:41-44, 1985*).

- Glucomannan: 3 grams daily

Unabsorbable carbohydrate derived from Konjak root. Absorbs 50 - 200 times its weight of water.

Supplementation may be beneficial.

Experimental Placebo-controlled Study: 31 hypertensive pts. on hypotensive agents received either glucomannan 3 gm daily, glucomannan plus a restricted calorie diet, or placebo. Body weight decreased by about 1.4 kg in the glucomannan gp. and 2.4 kg in the glucomannan plus diet group (*Reffo GC et al. Glucomannan in hypertensive outpatients. Curr Ther Res 44(1):22-27, 1988*).

Experimental Double-blind Study: 20 obese subjects received either glucomannan 1 gm or placebo with 8 oz water 1 hr. prior to each meal. Eating and exercise patterns were unchanged. After 8 wks., there was a significant mean weight loss in subjects using glucomannan and no side-effects were reported (*Walsh DE et al. Effect of glucomannan on obese patients: A clinical study. Int J Obes 8(4):289-93, 1984*).

- Guar Gum:

Supplementation may be beneficial.

Experimental Study: 12 overweight women (115%-140% ideal body weight) aged 20-60 randomly received either 14, 21, or 28 g of guar product per day; each 7 g packet contained 4.2 g of soluble fiber. The guar product was mixed with 6-8 oz water and ingested 30-60 min. before meals. Subjects were placed on a low-fat, high-fiber diet (60% CHO, 24% PRO, 16% fat, 25-30 g fiber), with guar supplementation prior to 2 or 3 meals. While there was significant weight loss (p<0.0001), no correlation was seen between guar dosage gps. and weight loss. At wks. 2 and 10, >72% reported enhanced adherence to the diet program, and >63% reported that adherence was a little to a lot better with the addition of the guar as compared to previous weight loss attempts (*Spielman A et al. The effect of guar granules as an adjuvant to a self-help weight loss program. Abstract. Am J Clin Nutr 51:524, 1990*).

Experimental Study: Guar gum reduced hunger in obese subjects and seemed to influence carbohydrate and lipid metabolism in a beneficial way (*Krotkiewski M. Effect of guar gum on body-weight, hunger ratings and metabolism in obese subjects. Br J Nutr 52(1):97-105, 1984*).

- Xanthum Gum:

Supplementation may be beneficial.

Experimental Placebo-controlled Study: 20 females (ages 20-50) received either xanthum gum 1100 mg 3 times daily at the start of each meal or starch placebo. Experimental subjects lost a mean of 2.9 kg at 30 days and 7.7 kg at 60 days, with results significantly different from those of controls. 9/10 noted a short-term (after 90 min.) sensation of satiety, and 3/10 also noted a long-term (after 5 hrs.) sensation of satiety (*Cairella M, Godi R. Clinical observations on the use of xanthum gum in obesity. Clin Dietol 13(1):37-40, 1986*).

Increase intake of raw foods.

Benefits may be due to increased dietary fiber or to the reduction in energy intake resulting from substituting raw foods for other foods of higher caloric value.

Experimental Study: 32 hypertensive pts., 28 of whom were obese, received an ave. of 62% of ingested calories as raw foods for a mean duration of 6.7 months. There was a significant mean weight loss of 3.8 kg (*Douglass J et al. Effects of a raw food diet on hypertension and obesity. South Med J 78(7):841, 1985*).

Avoid sugar.

May stimulate increased calorie consumption, especially in patients with a genetic predisposition to obesity.

Animal Experimental Study: Weanling genetically obese mice and lean mice were given either a standard laboratory diet or the standard diet plus a 32% sucrose solution. Both obese and lean mice given access to sucrose consumed approximately 30% more calories per day than animals given access to the standard diet alone, and obese animals consumed significantly more calories from the sucrose solution than the lean animals (*Marks-Kaufman R et al. The effects of dietary sucrose on opiate receptor binding in genetically obese (ob/ob) and lean mice. J Am Coll Nutr 8(1):9-14, 1989*).

Review Article: "Results of a number of studies have suggested that hyperinsulinemia and resultant hypoglycemia are part of a sequence of responses that can lead to hunger and to sugar-induced hyperphagia. However, it is argued . . . that neither hyperinsulinemia, hypoglycemia, nor any other factor *per se* is solely responsible for the hyperphagic effect of sugar . . . " (*Geiselman PJ. Sugar-induced hyperphagia: is hyperinsuliemia, hypoglycemia, or any other factor a 'necessary' condition? Appetite 11 Suppl 1:26-34, 1988*).

Review Article: Animal research suggests that nutrients, particularly sugar, affect opiate-mediated feeding behavior. Clinical experience with humans suggests that carbohydrates, particularly sugar, play a role in binge eating and obesity. Many binge eaters preferentially eat sweats during a binge, and sweet snacking is a frequent behavior at times of stress. Recent evidence suggests that sugar can lead to increased beta-endorphin production in obese subjects (*Fullerton DT et al. Sugar, opioids and binge eating. Brain Res Bull 14(6):673-80, 1985*).

Review Article: The results of several studies suggest that sucrose ingestion can lead to calorie overconsumption and obesity. There is insufficient evidence, however, to conclude that obese people consume a higher proportion of carbohydrates compared to lean people (*Vasselli JR. Carbohydrate ingestion, hypoglycemia and obesity. Appetite 6:53-59, 1985*).

Substitute fructose for glucose or sucrose.

May result in greater thermogenesis.

Experimental Study: The thermogenesis induced by pure fructose was found to be significantly greater than that of an equivalent amt. of glucose when it was combined with lipids and protein in a mixed meal (*Schwarz J-M et al. Thermogenesis in men and women induced by fructose vs glucose added to a meal. Am J Clin Nutr 49:667-74, 1989*).

Experimental Studies: The thermogenesis induced by pure fructose has been found to be significantly greater than that of an equivalent amt. of glucose (*Macdonald I. Differences in dietary-induced thermogenesis following the ingestion of various carbohydrates. Ann Nutr Metab 28:226-30, 1984; Tappy L et al. Comparison of thermogenic effect of fructose and glucose in normal humans. Am J Physiol 250:E718-24, 1986*).

May reduce subsequent calorie and fat consumption compared to glucose, aspartame or water.

Experimental Single-blind Study: 24 obese and normal weight males and females were randomly assigned to a given counterbalanced order of presentation of each of 4 preloads: 50 g of either fructose or glucose or 0.25 g of aspartame in 500 mL of lemon-flavored water, or 500 mL of unflavored, unsweetened water. When subjects drank the fructose preload, they subsequently ate fewer overall calories and fewer grams of fat than when they drank any of the other preloads (*Rodin J. comparative effects of fructose, aspartame, glucose, and water preloads on calorie and macronutrient intake. Am J Clin Nutr 51:428-35, 1990*).

Drink occasional beverages containing caffeine:

A thermogenic defect may contribute to the development of obesity (*Dullo AG, Miller DS. Obesity: A disorder of the sympathetic nervous system. World Rev Nutr Diet 50:1-56, 1987*).

Caffeine consumption at commonly consumed doses may have a significant effect on energy balance and may promote thermogenesis in the treatment of obesity.

Experimental Study: Repeated caffeine administration (100 mg) at 2 hr. intervals over a 12-h day period increased the energy expenditure (EE) of postobese volunteers by 8-11% (p<0.01) during that period, but had no influence on the subsequent 12-h night EE. The net effect was a significant increase (p<0.02) in daily EE of 79 kcal in the postobese subjects (*Dulloo AG et al. Normal caffeine consumption: Influence on thermogenesis and daily energy expenditure in lean and postobese human volunteers. Am J Clin Nutr 49:44-50, 1989*).

– –

VITAMINS

Vitamin C:

May theoretically reduce obesity by increasing cellular energy consumption through increasing sodium pump activity (*Naylor GJ et al. A double blind placebo controlled trial of ascorbic acid in obesity. Nutr Health 4:25-8, 1985*).

Supplementation may be beneficial.

Experimental Double-blind Study: 38 females who were about 50% above ideal body weight and who had failed to lose weight on various reducing programs received either ascorbic acid 1 gm 3 times daily or placebo. There was no calorie restriction. After 6 wks., mean weight loss in the experimental gp. was 2.53 kg compared to only 0.95 kg in the control gp. (p<0.012). This difference became significant by the second week (*Naylor GJ et al. A double blind placebo controlled trial of ascorbic acid in obesity. Nutr Health 4:25-8, 1985*).

Experimental Double-blind Study: Large doses of acorbic acid led to wt. loss in obese pts., particularly those who were >33.3% above ideal body wt. (*Naylor GJ et al. A double blind placebo controlled trial of ascorbic acid in obesity. IRCS Med Sci 10:848, 1982*).

Vitamin D:

Serum levels may be reduced.

Observational Study: Serum vitamin D levels were found to be significantly lower in obese than in non-obese subjects. Lower vitamin D levels may contribute to the lower serum 25-hydroxyvitamin levels which earlier studies have found in obese individuals (*Liel Y et al. Low circulating vitamin D in obesity. Calcif Tissue Int 43(4):199-201, 1988*).

- -

MINERALS

Copper:

May be elevated (*Atkinson RL et al. Plasma zinc and copper in obesity and after intestinal bypass. Ann Intern Med 89(4):491-93, 1978; Bhattacharya SK et al. Significantly altered copper and zinc levels in serum, urine, liver and skeletal muscle of morbidly obese patients. Abstract. J Am Coll Nutr 7(5):401, 1988*).

Zinc:

May be reduced (*Bhattacharya SK et al. Significantly altered copper and zinc levels in serum, urine, liver and skeletal muscle of morbidly obese patients. Abstract. J Am Coll Nutr 7(5):401, 1988; Ming-Der Chen, MA et al. Zinc in hair and serum of obese individuals in Taiwan. Am J Clin Nutr 48:1307-9, 1988*).

- -

OTHER NUTRITIONAL FACTORS

Coenzyme Q_{10}:

May be reduced (*van Gaal L et al. Exploratory study of coenzyme Q_{10} in obesity, in K Folkers, Y Yamamura, Eds. Biomed & Clin Aspects of Coenzyme Q. Vol. 4. Amsterdam, Elsevier Science Publishers, 1984:369-73*).

If reduced, supplementation may increase weight loss during dieting.

Experimental Study: 9 subjects, 5 of whom were deficient in coenzyme Q_{10}, received 100 mg daily of CoQ_{10} along with a 650 kcal diet. After 8-9 wks., mean weight loss in the deficient gp. was 13.5 kg compared to 5.8 kg in the other group (*van Gaal L et al. Exploratory study of coenzyme Q_{10} in obesity, in K Folkers, Y Yamamura, Eds. Biomed & Clin Aspects of Coenzyme Q. Vol. 4. Amsterdam, Elsevier Science Publishers, 1984:369-73*).

Omega-6 Fatty Acids:

Example: evening primrose oil: 2 - 4 grams daily

By normalizing decreased brown fat activity, may promote weight loss in obese patients who have been unable to lose weight despite appropriate dieting.

Experimental Double-blind Study: 47 pts., each with one or more obese parents, received either evening primrose oil or placebo. In the EPO gp., there was significant weight loss, reduction in skin thickness, and lowered BP

(*Garcia CM et al. Gamma linolenic acid causes weight loss and lower blood pressure in overweight patients with family history of obesity. Swed J Biol Med 4:8-11, 1986*).

Negative Experimental Double-blind Study: 74 women with substantial obesity received either EPO or placebo. After 12 wks., there was no significant difference in weight loss achieved by those taking EPO compared to placebo (*Haslett C et al. A double-blind evaluation of evening primrose oil as an antiobesity agent. Int J Obes 7(6):549-53, 1983*).

Experimental Study: Extremely obese pts. investigated on a metabolic unit lost large amts. of weight with evening primrose oil supplementation. Brown fat activation was measured using thermography, since activated brown fat has a higher temperature than ordinary fat or inactive brown fat. In addition, the amt. of brown fat in reserve was evaluated by injecting ephedrine. Very obese people had minimal resting brown fat activity and a poor response to ephedrine. In those who lost weight on primrose oil, both resting brown fat activity and the response to ephedrine were dramatically increased after 3-4 weeks. Primrose oil also activated Na^+-K^+-ATPase activity in those for whom enzyme activity was low (*Lowndes RH, Mansel RE. The effects of evening primrose oil (Efamol) on serum lipid levels of normal and obese subjects, in DF Horrobin, Ed. Clinical Uses of Essential Fatty Acids. Montreal, Eden Press, 1982:37-52*).

Experimental Study: 32 normals supplemented their regular diets with 2 gm primrose oil daily and 6 took 4 gms daily. In addition, 6 schizophrenics took 4 gms daily. After 6-8 weeks, about half of those who were more than 10% above ideal weight noted a reduction in appetite and had lost weight without dieting. The higher the starting weight, the greater the weight loss. There was a dose/response effect in that those taking 8 gms daily lost more weight than those taking 4 gms daily. People within 10% of ideal body weight showed no weight change (*Vaddadi KS, Horrobin DF. Weight loss produced by evening primrose oil administration in normal and schizophrenic individuals. IRCS J Med Sci 7:52, 1979*).

L-Glutamine:

Said to blunt carbohydrate craving (*Frederick Goodwin, director of intramural research, Natl. Instit. of Mental Health (USA) - quoted in APA Psychiatric News December 5, 1986*).

Note: Glutamic acid, like glucose, is a source of energy for the brain, but poorly penetrates the blood-brain barrier. Glutamine, on the other hand, readily penetrates the blood-brain barrier where it is transformed to glutamic acid (Williams, Roger J. Nutrition Against Disease. New York, Pitman Publishing Co., 1971).

L-Tryptophan:

Plasma concentration may be reduced by weight-reducing diets.

Experimental Study: 8 men and 8 women who were on a weight-reducing diet showed decreased plasma tryptophan concentrations compared to baseline and a reduction in the ratio of the mean plasma concentrations of tryptophan to branched chain amino acids. Irritability and early morning awakening were common in the third wk. of the diet, perhaps due to decreased brain serotonin because of reduced tryptophan availability (*Goodwin GM et al. Plasma concentrations of tryptophan and dieting. Br Med J 300:1499-500, 1990*).

Supplementation said to reduce the urge for late-night binges (*Goodwin, Frederick, director of intramural research, Nat. Instit. of Mental Health (USA) - quoted in APA Psychiatric News December 5, 1986*).

Supplementation may reduce carbohydrate cravings.

Negative Animal Experimental Study: Rats were allowed access to 2 levers, one of which, when pressed, supplied a carbohydrate-rich pellet, while the other, when pressed, supplied a protein-rich pellet. When injected with tryptophan, brain serotonin levels increased, but carbohydrate consumption was unchanged (*Holder M, Huether G. Role of prefeedings, plasma amino acid ratios and brain serotonin levels in carbohydrate and protein selection. Physl Behav 47:113-19, 1990*).

Animal Experimental Study: Animals fed a diet supplemented with tryptophan consumed less food, especially carbohydrate-rich foods, than did controls fed a standard diet (*Morris P et al. Food intake and selection after peripheral tryptophan. Physl Behav 40:155-63, 1987*).

Supplementation, in combination with psychopharmacologic drugs, may lead to weight loss in obese depressed patients.

Case Reports: 3 obese depressed pts. successfully lost weight and noted an improved mental state following treatment with psychopharmacologic drugs and tryptophan 500-2000 mg 4 times daily 1 hr. before meals and at bedtime. The most common side-effects were nausea, sedation, diarrhea, or painful muscle spasms in the lower extremities; these usually occurred when the fasting a.m. tryptophan level was >3.0 mg/dL. In 2 cases, maximum weight loss was correlated with fasting serum tryptophan levels of 2.0 mg/dL or greater (*Caston JC. Clinical applications of L-tryptophan in the treatment of obesity and depression. Adv Ther 4(2):78-83, 1987*).

Xylitol:

The pentose-sugar alcohol.

May reduce food intake, possibly by delaying gastric emptying.

Experimental Study: After ingesting 25 gm xylitol, gastric emptying was markedly prolonged in normal volunteers. After preloading with water, food intake was 920 ± 60 kcal; preloading with glucose, fructose, or sucrose failed to suppress food intake. After xylitol preloading, however, food intake was reduced to 690 ± 45 kcal, suggesting that xylitol may potentially be an important agent in dietary control (*Shafer RB et al. Effects of xylitol on gastric emptying and food intake. Am J Clin Nutr 45:744-47, 1987*).

- -

OTHER FACTORS:

Rule out food sensitivities.

Case Report: A 33-year-old chronically obese woman also had a history of depression, migraine headaches, irritability, perceptual and learning problems, periodic motor problems, and childhood hyperactivity. Upon repeated testing, several foods were found to produce consistent irregular behavioral and physiological states. By avoiding these substances, she was more effective in controlling her weight and greatly improved in other problem areas. Although calorie intake remained constant during her evaluative period, she gained weight during 6-day phases when sensitive foods were eaten and lost weight during phases when nonsensitive foods were eaten (*O'Banion D, Greenberg M. Behavioral effects of food sensitivity, in DR O'Banion, Ed. An Ecological and Nutritional Approach to Behavioral Medicine. Springfield, IL, Charles C. Thomas, 1981*).

Clinical Observations: If an allergenic food is eaten several times daily, a masked or chronic allergic reaction may develop characterized by improvement in chronic symptoms immediately after eating a specific allergen - lasting 2 hrs. and followed by a progressive increase in symptoms. These pts. learn to avoid sharp reactions by eating such foods frequently, including between meals and occasionally even during the night. Without such interval feedings, they may develop symptoms of gnawing hunger, nasal stuffiness, inability to concentrate, somnolence, extreme fatigue, tenseness, or nervousness. Corn, wheat and milk are most frequently implicated. For these pts., it is exceedingly difficult to adhere to a weight reduction diet; however, avoidance of masked food allergens is often followed by a diuresis, the disappearance of edema, and a sudden decrease in weight, all of which are associated with the cessation of the abnormal appetite and an improved ability to follow through on a weight reduction diet (*Randolph TG. Masked food allergy as a factor in the development and persistence of obesity. Abstract. J Lab Clin Med 32:1547, 1947*).

OSTEOARTHRITIS

See Also: PAIN
"RHEUMATISM"

VITAMINS

<u>Niacinamide</u>:   1 gram three times daily (Taper once effective.)
(Start with 500 mg. twice daily.)
(Take with 100 mg. vitamin B complex.)

WARNING: May cause nausea or affect liver function studies.

May enhance glucocorticoid secretion (*Shneïder AB. [Stereometric evaluation of the myocardial cardiomyocyte-capillary ratio of thiamine and nicotinamide.] Kardiologiia 29(4):97-9, 1989*).

Effects of decreased pain and increased mobility may start to be noted in 2 - 6 weeks. Said to be particularly effective for degenerative arthritis of the knee.

Experimental Controlled Study: 663 pts. receiving niacinamide were shown to have superior scores on an index of joint range of movement than 842 untreated age-matched pts. (*Kaufman W. The use of vitamin therapy to reverse certain concomitants of aging. J Am Geriatr Soc 3:927, 1955*).

<u>Pantothenic Acid</u>:

Deficiency may be associated with OA.

Animal Experimental Study: Acute deficiency of PA in the rat resulted in pathologic joint changes which closely resembled those of osteoarthrosis (osteoporosis, calcification of cartilage, and the formation of osteophytes and of lipping) (*Nelson MN et al. Proc Soc Exp Biol 73:31, 1950*).

Supplementation may be beneficial.

Negative Double-blind Experimental Study: 47/94 pts. with arthritic conditions (63% with osteoarthrosis) who were previously untreated or who had not responded to previous drug treatment were randomly chosen to receive 2 gm daily of oral calcium pantothenate (starting with 500 mg daily and gradually increasing to 500 mg 4 times daily by day 10), while the rest received placebo. Pts. were permitted to take paracetamol to relieve pain but no other medications were permitted. After 2 mo., daily records kept by pts. failed to show significant reductions in the duration of morning stiffness or degree of disability in either the experimental or control groups. Both gps. reported significant pain relief but neither resulted in any significant reduction in requirements for pain medication. There were no significant between-group differences, and overall assessments by the doctors at the end of the trial gave similar results for active and placebo medication. There was, however, evidence that the sub-gp. of pts. with rheumatoid arthritis may have benefited (*Calcium pantothenate in arthritic conditions. A report from the General Practitioner Research Group. Practitioner 224:208-11, 1980*).

- with <u>Vitamin B Complex</u>:

Experimental Study: 20/26 (77%) pts. treated with pantothenic acid 12.5 mg twice daily along with vitamin B complex demonstrated a significant symptomatic improvement starting in 1-2 weeks. 10/20 (50%) responding pts. relapsed on stopping treatment and improved upon resumption. There was no measurable improvement in joint crepitus. It appeared that a reasonable response could be expected if treatment is begun before signs of advanced disease have developed (*Annand JC. Pantothenic acid and osteoarthritis. Letter. Lancet 2:1168, 1963; Annand JC. Osteoarthrosis and pantothenic acid. Letter. J Coll Gen Pract 5:136-37, 1962*).

Vitamin C:

Supplementation may be beneficial.

Review Article: In the treatment of OA, "certainly vitamin C is always indicated and is harmless in adequate doses" (*Bland JH, Cooper SM. Osteoarthritis: A review of the cell biology involved and evidence for reversibility. Management rationally related to known genesis and pathophysiology. Semin Arthritis Rheum 14(2):106-33, 1984*).

Animal Experimental Study: Cartilage taken from guinea pigs with experimental OA fed 2-4 mg vitamin C daily showed classic signs of advanced osteoarthritis while cartilage taken from control guinea pigs who consumed a diet containing 150 mg daily showed only minor arthritic changes with much less cartilage erosion and milder histologic and biochemical changes in and around the OA joint (*Schwartz ER. The modulation of osteoarthritic development by vitamins C and E. Int J Vitam Nutr Res Suppl 26, 141-6, 1984*).

Vitamin E:

May be a prostaglandin inhibitor (as are non-steroidal anti-inflammatory drugs) (*White G. Vitamin E inhibition of platelet prostaglandin biosynthesis. Fed Proc 36:350, 1977*).

Supplementation may be beneficial.

Experimental and Observational Study: 62 pts. with primary degenerative osteoarthrosis had high concentrations of malonic dialdehyde and acylhydroperoxide when at the initial stage of the disease, when reactive synovitis was present, or when there was multiple joint involvement. Antioxidants were given to correct enhanced lipid peroxidation. Vitamin E 100 mg/d as part of a multimodality therapy caused a decrease in the the blood level of both primary and secondary products of lipid peroxidation (*Rubyk BI et al. [Change in lipid peroxidation in patients with primary osteoarthrosis deformans.] Ter Arkh 60(9):110-13, 1988*) (*in Russian*).

Experimental Double-blind Study: 50 pts. randomly received either 400 IU d-alpha-tocopheryl acetate or placebo. After 6 wks., vitamin E was superior to placebo with respect to pain relief (pain at rest, pain during movement, pressure-induced pain) and the necessity of additional analgesic treatment (p<0.05 to p<0.01). Improvement of mobility was better in the experimental gp., but not significantly. Adverse side-effects were practically identical in both groups (*Blankenhorn G. [Clinical effectiveness of Spondyvit (vitamin E) in activated arthroses. A multicenter placebo-controlled double-blind study.] Z Orthop 124(3):340-43, 1986*) (*in German*).

Experimental Double-blind Crossover Study: 29 pts. received 600 mg. of tocopherol and placebo for 10 days each in randomized order. 15 (52%) had a "good analgesic effect" while on tocopherol as compared to 1 (4%) during placebo administration (*Machtey I, Ouaknine, L. Tocopherol in osteoarthritis: A controlled pilot study. J Am Geriatr Soc 26:328, 1978*).

- -

MINERALS

Boron:

Intake may be inversely related to the risk of osteoarthritis.

Review Article: Epidemiologic studies from a number of countries have shown an inverse relationship between soil boron levels and the prevalence of osteoarthritis (*de Fabio A. Treatment & prevention of osteoarthritis. Townsend Letter for Doctors, February-March, 1990:143-48*).

Supplementation may be beneficial.

Experimental Double-blind Study: 15 pts. with radiographically confirmed OA randomly received either boron 6 mg daily (as borax 50 mg) or placebo. After 8 wks., 5/7 pts. in the experimental gp. rated themselves as subjectively improved compared to 1/8 pts. on placebo. There was a significantly greater improvement in the condition of all joints on boron than on placebo (p<0.01) as well as significantly less pain on passive movement on boron (p<0.001). However, since 3 boron and 2 placebo pts. had dropped out, when data from all 20 pts. starting the trial was included, 5/10 pts. on boron vs. 1/10 pts. on placebo improved (results n.s.). There were no side effects; however it is now believed that the pts. on boron who dropped out were probably showing a typical Herxheimer reaction. Although OA pts. do not show this reaction, rheumatoid arthritis pts. may, and the 2 women who dropped out may have had RA which degenerated to OA. If so, they were likely to have improved if they had remained in the study (*Travers RL et al. Boron and arthritis: the results of a double-blind pilot study. J Nutr Med 1:127-32, 1990; Travers RL, Rennie GC. Clinical trial - boron and arthritis. The results of a double blind pilot study. Townsend Letter for Doctors. June 1990, pp. 360-62*).

Clinical Observations: Boron supplementation was effective for about 90% of arthritis pts., including those with osteoarthritis, most with complete remission of symptoms. Pts. normally took 6-9 mg elemental boron daily to achieve symptom relief followed by a maintenance dose of 3 mg daily (*Newnham RE. Arthritis or skeletal fluorosis and boron. Letter. Int Clin Nutr Rev 11(2):68-70, 1991; Newnham RE. Boron beats arthritis. Proceedings of the ANZAAS, Australian Academy of Science, Canberra, Australia, 1979*).

Selenium:

Levels of glutathione peroxidase, a selenium-containing enzyme, may be low.

Observational Study: Compared to 54 healthy controls from the same region, Swedish pts. with osteoarthrosis had significantly lower mean blood glutathione peroxidase levels (*Jameson S et al. Pain relief and selenium balance in patients with connective tissue disease and osteoarthrosis: A double-blind selenium tocopherol supplementation study. Nutr Res Suppl 1:391-97, 1985*).

- with Vitamin E:

Supplementation may be beneficial.

Experimental Double-blind Study: 81 pts. with disabling muscular pain, stiffness and aching of long duration, many of whom had osteoarthrosis, received sodium selenite (140 µg Se) and α-tocopherol 100 mg daily or placebo. Following supplementation, glutathione peroxidase levels increased in 75% of the patients. Mean pain score reduction was significantly more frequent and more marked among pts. whose glutathione peroxidase levels increased than among those whose levels decreased. While pain score reduction was more pronounced among treated pts., the reduction as compared to pts. on placebo were not significant (*Jameson S et al. Pain relief and selenium balance in patients with connective tissue disease and osteoarthrosis: A double-blind selenium tocopherol supplementation study. Nutr Res Suppl 1:391-97, 1985*).

Experimental Study: Following treatment with selenium and vitamin E, a correlation was found between pain relief and increased blood levels of glutathione peroxidase (*Bruce A et al. The effect of selenium and vitamin E on glutathione peroxidase levels and subjective symptoms in patients with arthrosis and rheumatoid arthritis, in Proceedings New Zealand Workshop on Trace Elements in New Zealand. Dunedin, U. of Otago, 1981:92*).

Sulfur:

May be reduced.

Observational Study: While the cystine content of fingernails in normals is 12%, in arthritics it is only 8.9% (*Sullivan MX, Hess WC. Cystine content of finger nails in arthritis. J Bone Joint Surg 16:185, 1935*).

Supplementation may be beneficial.

> **Experimental Study:** 100 "arthritics" received I.V. colloidal sulfur. Pain and effusions disappeared in many cases with a return of the cystine fingernail test to normal (*Woldenberg SC. The treatment of arthritis with colloidal sulphur. J South Med Assoc 28:875-81, 1935*).

Sulfur baths may increase blood sulfur levels.

> **Observational Study:** Following sulfur baths, there was an increase in patients' blood sulfur levels (*Osterberg AE et al. Absorption of sulphur compounds during treatment by sulphur baths. Arch Dermatol Syphilol 20:156-66, 1929*).

<u>Zinc</u>:

> Serum levels may be depressed (*Grennan DM et al. Serum copper and zinc in rheumatoid arthritis and osteoarthritis. N Z Med J 91(652):47-50, 1980*).

- -

OTHER NUTRITIONAL FACTORS

<u>Glucosamine Sulfate</u>:

Glucosamine is the building block of the proteoglycans, the ground substance of articular cartilage, while sulfate, another important component, appears to potentiate its therapeutic effect (*D'Ambrosio E et al. Glucosamine sulphate: A controlled clinical investigation in arthrosis. Pharmatherapeutica 2(8):504-08, 1981*).

Inhibits the degradation of proteoglycans while non-steroidal anti-inflammatory drugs inhibit proteoglycan synthesis (*Vidal y Plana RR et al. Articular cartilage pharmacology: I. In vitro studies on glucosamine and non-steroidal anti-inflammatory drugs. Pharmacol Res Commun 10(6):557-69, 1978*).

Rebuilds experimentally damaged cartilage (*Eichler J, Nöh E. Behandlung der Arthrosis Deformans durch Beeinflussung des Knorpelstoffwechsel. Orthop Praxis 9:225, 1970*).

Administration may be beneficial.

> **Experimental Double-blind Study:** 30 in-patients with chronic degenerative osteoarthrosic disorders (mean age 70.5 ± 3.2 yrs.) randomly received either glucosamine sulfate 400 mg IM or IV daily for 7 days followed by 0.5 gm orally 3 times daily or placebo delivered in a similar fashion for 14 days. During both initial parenteral treatments, each symptom (pain at rest, pain during active movement, pain during passive movement, restricted function and time to walk 20 metres) significantly improved, but to a faster and greater extent in the treated gp., mainly in restricted function. During the period of oral maintenance, a further improvement was recorded in pts. treated with glucosamine, while those on placebo indicated increased symptom scores which almost reached the pre-treatment level. A similar pattern was shown in the measurement of walking speed. Despite the short treatment period, 3/15 treated pts. became symptom-free after parenteral treatment and 1/15 (total of 27% of pts.) became symptom-free after the maintenance period, while none of the controls became symptom-free. No drug-related complaints were recorded (*D'Ambrosio E et al. Glucosamine sulphate: A controlled clinical investigation in arthrosis. Pharmatherapeutica 2(8):504-08, 1981; Crolle G, D'Este E. Glucosamine sulphate for the management of arthrosis: A controlled clinical investigation. Curr Med Res Opin 7(2):104-09, 1980*).

> **Experimental Double-blind Study:** 24 out-patients with established osteoarthrosis of the knee randomly received either glucosamine sulfate 500 mg 3 times daily or placebo. After 6-8 wks., significant alleviation of symptoms was associated with the active treatment (pain, joint tenderness, swelling, restricted movement). Compared to controls, treated pts. experienced earlier symptom alleviation and a significantly larger proportion of them experienced lessening or disappearance of symptoms within the trial period. No adverse reactions were reported (*Pujalte JM et al. Double-blind clinical evaluation of oral glucosamine sulphate in the basic treatment of osteoarthrosis. Curr Med Res Opin 7(2):110-14, 1980*).

Experimental Double-blind Study: 80 in-patients with established osteoarthrosis randomly received either glucosamine sulfate (Viartril-S®, Rotta, Italy) 500 mg 3 times daily before meals or placebo. After 30 days, all symptoms (articular pain, joint tenderness, swelling, restriction of active movements, restriction of passive movements) decreased in both groups. Treated pts. experienced a significantly larger reduction in overall symptoms (73% vs. 41%) which was also significantly faster (20 vs. 36 days) as those on placebo. For placebo pts., improvement in autonomous mobility was relatively less compared to improvement in other symptoms; for treated pts., by contrast, such improvement was as great and as fast as that of the other symptoms. On electron microscopy, sample of articular cartilage from pts. on placebo showed established osteoarthritis, while cartilage from treated pts. showed a picture more similar to healthy cartilage (*Drovanti A et al. Therapeutic activity of oral glucosamine sulfate in osteoarthrosis: A placebo-controlled double-blind investigation. Clin Ther 3(4):260-72, 1980*).

Administration may be more effective in relieving pain than non-steroidal anti-inflammatory drugs, although pain relief may be slower.

Experimental Double-blind Study: 40 out-patients with unilateral osteoarthrosis of the knee randomly received orally either 1.5 gm glucosamine sulfate or 1.2 gm ibuprofen daily for 8 weeks. Pain scores decreased faster during the first 2 wks. with ibuprofen. Despite the slower rate of pain reduction, the decrease in pain scores with glucosamine sulfate continued throughout the trial period. At week 8, the difference in pain between the 2 gps. turned significantly in favor of glucosamine. No significant differences were noted in swelling or in any of the other parameters monitored. Minor complaints were noted by 2 pts. on glucosamine and 5 pts. on ibuprofen (*Lopes Vaz A. Double-blind clinical evaluation of the relative efficacy of ibuprofen and glucosamine sulphate in the management of osteoarthrosis of the knee in out-patients. Curr Med Res Opin 8:145-49, 1982*).

Glycosaminoglycans: one month trial

(*See also: "Calf Tracheal Cartilage" and "Shark Cartilage" below*)

- Glycosaminoglycan-peptide Complex (Rumalon®): 2 ml IM for 15 injections or 1 ml IM for 25 injections (2-3/wk.)

A high molecular weight GAG-peptide association complex isolated from bovine cartilage and bone marrow.

Administration may be beneficial.

> WARNING: Intramuscular injections of Rumalon or Arumalon have caused nephrotic syndrome and severe hepatotoxicity as well as other untoward reactions (*Berg PA et al. Bovine cartilage and marrow extract. Letter. Lancet 1:1275, 1989*).

Review Article: The therapeutic value of Rumalon has been clearly shown in controlled studies, summaries of clinical experience in large European hospitals, and in a large number of other reports covering about 10,000 patients. There is evidence that the progression of radiologically visible joint change is inhibited by Rumalon in OA pts. receiving 2 series of injections annually for some years compared to pts. treated only symptomatically with NSAIDs (*Rejholec V. Long-term studies of antiosteoarthritic drugs: An assessment. Semin Arth Rheum 17:2:Suppl 1:35-53, 1987*).

Experimental Controlled Study: 60 pts. with OA of the knee received either GP-C (2 series of 24 injections of 2 ml each twice annually) and ibuprofen or ibuprofen alone. After 3 yrs., in the GP-C gp., various pain parameters showed significantly greater improvement, with approx. half the initial ibuprofen dosage required at the end of the study. In addition, joint space width narrowed significantly less in the GP-C gp. than in the controls (*Lopes Vaz A. Estudo aberto, controlado, com um complexo glicosaminoglicano peptido na artrose da articulação do joelho. Reumatol Med Int 20:24-28, 1986*).

Experimental Double-blind Study: 55 pts. with OA of the knee or hip received NSAIDs and physiotherapy. In addition, some of them randomly received CP-C (24 injections of 2 ml twice annually). After 2 yrs., pts. who received Rumalon had significant reductions in pain with decreasing use of NSAIDs and improved mobility compared to the other pts. (*Dorn R, Kluge F. Effects of Arumalon® in the treatment of cox- and gonarthrosis - An ambulatory 2-year trial. EULAR Symposium, Vienna, 1985, abstr.163*).

In vitro Experimental Study: Rumalon was found to stimulate sulfate metabolism in human osteoarthritic cartilage (*Bollet AJ. Stimulation of protein-chondroitin sulfate synthesis by normal and osteoarthritic articular cartilage. Arthrit Rheum 11:663-73, 1968*).

- <u>Glycosaminoglycan polysulphate (Arteparon®)</u>: 50 mg IA or IM, usually twice weekly, for 10-15 injections

Prepared by extraction from bovine lung and tracheal tissues followed by sulfate esterification of certain sugar hydroxy groups resulting in glycosaminoglycan polysulphuric esters.

Administration may be beneficial.

Experimental Double-blind Study: 140 pts. with medium-grade OA of the knee or hip received either 15 IM injections of 50 mg Arteparon or placebo. After 8 wks., pain and joint mobility were significantly improved in the treated pts. (*Siegmeth W, Radi I. Vergleich von Glykosaminoglykanpolysulfat (Arteparon®) und physiologischer Kochsalzlösung bei Arthrosen grosser Gelenke. Ergebnisse einer multizentrichen Doppelblindstudie. Zschr Rheumatol 42:223-28, 1983*).

Experimental Double-blind Study: 40 pts. with stages I and II OA of the knee received either 15 IM injections of 50 mg Arteparon or placebo. After 8 wks., joint mobility and walking ability were significantly improved in the treated pts. (*Ishikawa K et al. Clinical evaluation of the intraarticular injection of glycosaminoglycan polysulfate for osteoarthrosis of the knee joint. A multi-centric double-blind controlled study. Zschr Orthop 120:708-16, 1982*).

Experimental Double-blind Study: 120 pts. with OA of the knee randomly received either ten 50 mg Arteparon IA injections or placebo injections with isotonic NaCl. After 6 mo., there was significant improvement in pain and joint mobility in the treated pts. (*Anderson IF. Intramuskuläre Behandlung der Arthrose des Kniegelenks mit Arteparon® (Doppelblind-Versuch). Akt Rheumatol 7:164-66, 1982*).

Experimental Double-blind Study: 74 pts. with OA of the knee randomly received either ten 50 mg Arteparon IA injections or placebo injections with isotonic NaCl. After 6 mo., there was significant improvement in pain and joint mobility in the treated pts. (*Wagenhäuser FJ. Die medikamentöse Basisbehandlung der Arthrosen. Fortbildungkurse Rheumatol 5:75-80, 1978*).

<u>Omega-3 Fatty Acids</u>:

Most important member: eicosapentaenoic acid (EPA), which is particularly high in cold water fish.

Administration may be beneficial.

Experimental Blinded Study: 21 women and 5 men aged 52-85 were studied with a clinical diagnosis of OA which was confirmed by radiology in 22 (85%). These pts. had symptoms after taking ibuprofen 1200 mg daily for at least 2 wks. prior to entering the study. They were given 10 ml EPA or placebo daily in addition to ibuprofen. After 6 mo., the ave. visual analog scores for both pain and interference with everyday activities were strikingly lower in the EPA than the placebo group; however, the results were not significant (*Stammers T et al. Fish oil in osteoarthritis. Letter. Lancet 2:503, 1989*).

<u>S-Adenosyl-L-Methionine (SAMe)</u>:   1,200 mg daily

Produced from L-methionine and ATP through the action of methionine-adenosyl-transferase (MAT).

May be as effective as non-steroidal anti-inflammatory drugs, but with less side-effects.

Review Article: SAMe is a physiologic compound that ranks with ATP as a pivotal molecule in biology. Studies, including cinical trials on about 22,000 pts., suggest that it exerts analgesic and antiphlogistic activities and stimulates the synthesis of proteoglycans by articular chondrocytes with minimal or absent side-effects. The intensity of its therapeutic activity is similar to that of the nonsteroidal anti-inflammatory drugs, but its tolerability is higher (*di Padova C. S-adenosylmethionine in the treatment of osteoarthritis. Review of the clinical studies. Am J Med 83(5A):60-65, 1987*).

Experimental Double-blind Study: 36 pts. with OA of the knee, hip and/or spine randomly received either 1,200 mg SAMe of 1,200 mg ibuprofen. After 4 wks., The total score for clinical parameters (morning stiffness, pain at rest, pain on motion, crepitus, swelling, and limitation of motion of the affected joints) improved to the same extent in both pt. groups. Both treatments were well tolerated and no pt. from either gp. withdrew from the study (*Müller-Fassbender H. Double-blind clinical trial of S-adenosylmethionine versus ibuprofen in the treatment of osteoarthritis. Am J Med 83(5A):81-83, 1987*).

Experimental Double-blind Study: 36 pts. with OA of the knee, hip and/or spine randomly received either SAMe 1,200 mg or indomethacin 150 mg daily. After 4 wks., SAMe significantly improved the total score obtained by the sum of all clinical findings. Indomethacin-treated pts. similarly improved. 2 pts. in the SAMe gp. reported slight nausea after 2 wks., while 7 pts. in the indomethacin gp. developed adverse effects (*Vetter G. Double-blind comparative clinical trial with S-adenosylmethioninine and indomethacin in the treatment of osteoarthritis. Am J Med 83(5A):78-80, 1987*).

Experimental Double-blind Study: 45 pts. with OA of one knee randomly received either SAMe 1,200 mg daily or piroxicam 20 mg daily. Both SAMe and piroxicam were effective in inducing a significant improvement in the total pain score after 28 days. Improvement in other clinical parameters started from about day 56 in both groups. No significant difference was found between the 2 treatments in terms of efficacy and tolerability, although pts. treated with SAMe maintained clinical improvement achieved at the end of treatment longer (*Maccagno A et al. Double-blind controlled clinical trial of oral S-adenosylmethionine versus piroxicam in knee osteoarthritis. Am J Med 83(5A):72-77, 1987*).

Experimental Double-blind Study: 734 pts. received either SAMe 1,200 mg daily, naproxen 750 mg daily, or placebo. SAMe exerted the same analgesic activity as naproxen, and both drugs were more effective than placebo (p<0.01). Tolerability of SAMe was significantly better than that of naproxen (*Caruso Ik, Pietrogrande V. Italian double-blind multicenter study comparing S-adenosylmethionine, naproxen, and placebo in the treatment of degenerative joint disease. Am J Med 83(5A):66-71, 1987*).

Superoxide Dismutase:

The ability of oral SOD to be absorbed is controversial.

Experimental Study: 10 elderly adults received 6 tablets daily of SOD/CAT®, a wheat-sprout-derived, enteric-coated product containing superoxide dismutases and catalases. After 10 days, the erythrocyte superoxide dismutase levels were increased in all 10 subjects (*Effect of oral antioxidant enzyme supplementation upon erythrocyte superoxide dismutase (ESOD) level of 10 persons over 65 years of age. Unpublished study. Biotec Food Corporation, 1215 Center St., Honolulu, HI 96816-3226, 1989*).

Double-blind Experimental Study: 60 subjects received 6 tablets daily of SOD/CAT®, a wheat-sprout-derived enteric-coated product containing superoxide dismutases and catalases, or the same product which had been heat inactivated. After 14 days, the experimental gp. had an ave. increase in serum SOD levels of 40%, while the levels in the placebo gp. were unchanged (*Ordonez L, Rothschild PR. Absorption study with SOD/CAT® whole food antioxidant enzyme complex. Unpublished study. Biotec Food Corporation, 1215 Center St., Honolulu, HI 96816-3226, 1988*).

Negative Animal Experimental Study: Both radiolabeled ^{65}Zn-superoxide dismutase (purified) and crude SOD (pills dissolved in normal saline) were intubated into mice. Most of the radioactivity was found in the fecal material, and feeding SOD pills did not affect the plasma and liver levels, suggesting that oral SOD is of no therapeutic value (*Giri SN, Misra HP. Fate of superoxide dismutase in mice following oral route of administration. Med Biol 62(5):285-89, 1984*).

Negative Animal Experimental Study: Mice received a complete purified diet either with or without the addition of 0.004% superoxide dismutase. There were no differences in the activity of CuZn superoxide dismutase or Mn superoxide dismutase in intestine, liver, kidney or blood. While these data show that ordinary oral SOD has no effect on tissue levels, it is conceivable that an enteric-coated pill could escape digestion (*Zidenberg-Cherr S et al. Dietary superoxide dismutase does not affect tissue levels. Am J Clin Nutr 37:5, 1983*).

Oral supplementation may be beneficial.

Experimental Study: 228/253 pts. (90%) with non-infectious joint inflammation improved following oral treatment with a enteric-coated, whole food (wheat sprout-derived) antioxidant enzyme complex emphasizing superoxide dismutase and catalase (SOD/CAT®) or SOD and CAT along with glutathione peroxidase and methionine reductase (AOX/PLX®). Pts. who responded demonstrated increased mobility, with decreased pain and swelling in the affected areas. The ave. response time was 14 days, although 47 pts. did not improve until the fourth week. After the initial response, a maintenance dosage of 1/2 the initial dosage was adequate to sustain improvement (*Rothschild PR et al. Effect of oral antioxidant enzyme supplementation upon musculo-skeletal inflammation. Unpublished study. Biotec Food Corporation, 1215 Center St., Honolulu, HI 96816-3226, 1989*).

Animal Experimental Study: 340/387 dogs (88%) with osteoarthritis due to injury, stress, developmental conditions or aging improved following treatment with an enteric-coated, wheat-sprout-derived, whole food antioxidant enzyme complex emphasizing superoxide dismutase and catalase (Dismutase®). Improvement consisted of increased mobility, function and range of motion, with decreased pain and swelling. The ave. response time was 8 days, although 63 animals did not improve until the fourth week. In most cases, the minimum effective dosage was 1 tablet/20 lb/d. After the initial response, a maintenance dosage of 1/2 the initial dosage was adequate to sustain improvement (*Randall D et al. Effect of oral Dismutase® enzyme supplementation upon musculo-skeletal inflammation. Unpublished study. Biotec Food Corporation, 1215 Center St., Honolulu, HI 96816-3226, 1989*).

Parenteral administration may be beneficial.

Review Article: In 3 placebo-controlled and 1 steroid-controlled double-blind trials, bovine SOD applied intra-articularly at a dosage of 2-16 mg proved to be effective in OA of the knee joint (*Flohë L. Superoxide dismutase for therapeutic use: clinical experience, dead ends and hopes. Mol Cell Biochem 84(2):123-31, 1988*).

Experimental Study: Intra-articular injection of bovine-derived Zn,Cu superoxide dismutase (Orgotein) appeared to be effective in reducing swelling in pts. with different forms of hydrarthrosis of the knee, except in the presence of marked exudative synovitis processes (chronic primary polyarthritis) when it was of limited value (*Terlizzi N et al. [Evaluation of the efficacy of orgotein in a series of patients with hydrarthrosis of the knee.] Minerva Med 77(21):947-51, 1986*).

Experimental Double-blind Study: Orgotein (2 mg every 2 wks. for 6 wks. or 4 mg/wk. for 4 wks.) or placebo was injected into the knee joints. Pts. in the orgotein gp. noted greater pain relief and had greater functional improvement (*Manander-Huber KB. Double-blind controlled clinical trials in man with bovine copper-zinc superoxide dismutase. New York, Elsevier/North-Holland, 1980:299-317*).

Experimental Double-blind Study: Orgotein 4 mg/wk or placebo was injected into the knee joints. After 8 wks., Orgotein significantly improved the pain and disability scores, as well as reduced the joint circumference and synovial thickening (*Flohë L et al. Effectiveness of superoxide dismutase in osteoarthritis of the knee joint. Results of a double blind multicenter clinical trial, in WH Bannister, JV Bannester, Eds. Biological and Clinical Aspects of Superoxide and Superoxide Dismutase. New York, Elsevier/North Holland, 1980:424-30*).

- -

TISSUE EXTRACTS

Beche-de-Mer (Sea Cucumber):

Administration of an extract may be beneficial.

Experimental Double-blind Study: 30 pts. with various forms of arthritis received either C-Cure (Aldgate Grove Pty., Ltd., Australia) or placebo. After 3 mo., about half found the product to be of subjective benefit, while none found benefit from placebo. No side effects were reported (*MJE McPhillips, MacKay, Queensland, Australia. Unpublished manuscript, 1985*).

Experimental Study: 13 OA pts. were treated with Beche de Mer extract 2 tabs daily for 2 wks. followed by 1 tab daily. After 6 mo., 7/13 (54%) showed improvement. Improvement was moderate in two, and significant in five. The other 5/13 pts. showed worsening of their symptoms. One pt. had diarrhea on the first day of medication, another developed GI upset; both symptoms abated when it was stopped. There were no other side effects (*Mori Schwartzberg, Neptune, New Jersey. Unpublished manuscript.*)

<u>Cartilage Extracts</u>:

Animal cartilage contains a protein which may inhibit tumor growth by inhibiting angiogenesis (*Folkman J et al. Induction of angiogenesis during the transition from hyperplasia to neoplasia. <u>Nature</u> 339:58-61, 1989; Langer R et al. Isolations of a cartilage factor that inhibits tumor neovascularization. <u>Science</u> 193:70-2, 1976; Moses MA, Subhalter J, Langer R. Identification of an inhibitor of neovascularization from cartilage. <u>Science</u> 248:1408-10, 1990*).

In osteoarthritis, neovascularization is involved in the reinitiation of cartilage growth and mineralization (*Brown RA, Weiss JB. Neovascularisation and its role in the osteoarthritic process. <u>Ann Rheum Dis</u> 47(11):881-5, 1988*).

Administration may be beneficial.

Experimental Study: 6 elderly pts. aged 65-85 who failed to benefit from standard anti-inflammatory agents stopped taking all prescriptions for pain and inflammation and received a shark cartilage preparation (Cartilade™) 740 mg capsules. For 3 wks. they received twelve 740 mg caps which was reduced to six caps afterwards. Improvement began to be noted by the end of the third week. At the fourth wk., they demonstrated greater motility, less inflammation, and reduced pain. The 3 pts. who completed the study required lower doses of non-steroidal anti-inflammatory drugs and achieved greater pain relief from them. There were no adverse side effects (*Jose A. Orcasita, assistant clinical professor of internal medical, Center for Advanced Therapeutics and Clinical Research, Division of Clinical Pharmacology, U. of Miami School of Medicine - reported in Walker M. Therapeutic effects of shark cartilage. <u>Townsend Letter for Doctors</u>, June, 1989, pp. 288-91*).

Animal Experimental Study: 3 dogs with severe secondary OA due to hip dysplasia confirmed by x-ray received one 740 mg capsule of a shark cartilage preparation (Cartilade™) per 5 kg/d for 21 days. Lameness diasppeared, capacity for moving around obstacles improved and there was excellent restoration of function. In addition there was decreased evidence of pain on palpation, decreased immobilization, and decreased crepitation and swelling of joints. The study was then expanded to include 16 dogs of various ages, breeds and weights, all affected by lameness due to secondary OA confirmed by x-rays. After 21 days 70% showed improvement in local swelling and pain in response to manipulation, and half showed improvement in all functional signs. The cartilage was discontinued and, 15 days later, all dogs regressed by losing about half of the improvement they had achieved (*Jacques Rauis, Institut Jules Bordet Centre Des Tumeurs de L'Universite libre de Bruxelles & faculty of medicine, University of Liege - presented to the British Small Animal Veterinary Assoc Congress, Manchester, UK, 1991 and reported in Lane IW. Shark cartilage: Its potential medical applications. <u>J Advance Med</u> 4(4):263-71, 1991*).

Experimental Double-blind Study: 147 pts. received one of two cartilage extracts or placebo. The placebo gp. was encouraged to use various non-steroidal anti-inflammatory drugs during active episodes. After 5 yrs., ave. pain scores dropped 85% in the cartilage-treated gps. compared to only a 5% decrease in the controls. Moreover, joint deterioration was significantly less in the cartilage-treated gps. (37% that of the control gp.) and the treated gps. lost significantly less time from work (*Rejholec V. Long-term studies of antiosteoarthritic drugs: an assessment. <u>Semin Arthritis Rheum</u> 17(2) (Suppl 1):35-53, 1987*).

Experimental Study: 28 pts. with severe OA received sub-cut. injections of 300-800 cc of a solution of activated acid-pepsin-digested calf tracheal cartilage (Catrix-S). After 3-8 wks., 19 had excellent results, 6 good results, 2 fair results and 1 no benefit. Relief lasted from 6 wks. to over 1 year. There was no evidence of toxicity as assessed both clinically and from lab studies (*Prudden JF, Balassa LL. The biological activity of bovine cartilage preparations. <u>Semin Arthritis Rheum</u> 3(4):287-321, 1974*).

<u>Perna canaliculus</u> (New Zealand Green-lipped mussel):

A rich source of glycosaminoglycans, although it is not known if its glycosaminoglycan content is the explanation for its therapeutic benefits.

Administration of the extract may be beneficial.

Experimental Double-blind Study: 33 pts. (mean age 68.8 yrs.) with clinical and radiological evidence of severe osteoarthritis who had failed to respond to non-steroidal anti-inflammatory drugs for several months to several yrs. randomly received either an extract of Perna canaliculus (Seatone, McFarlane Labs, NZ) 1050 mg daily or placebo in addition to their NSAIDs. After 3 mo., 6/12 (50%) of the treated pts. improved compared to 3/21 (14%) of the controls. Comparison of their pain as scored by visual analog scales, functional index, and the time taken to walk 50 ft. showed improvements in the treated gp. which were significant at the 95%, 99%, and 95% confidence levels, respectively, compared to controls. All pts. then received treatment with active extract. After an additional 3 months, 29% of pts. switched from placebo to active treatment were improved. Side-effects were limited to nausea, flatulence, fluid retention and, in 2 pts., increased stiffness lasting 2-3 wks. (*Gibson RG et al. Green-lipped mussel extract in arthritis. Letter. Lancet 1:439, 1981; Gibson RG et al. Perna canaliculus in the treatment of arthritis. Practitioner 224:955-60, 1980*).

Experimental Study: 31 pts. received NZ Green Mussel Extract (Seatone, McFarlane, Aukland) for 6 mo. to 4 1/2 years. 35% benefited. Adverse side-effects were uncommon and generally mild (*Gibson RG et al. Perna canaliculus in the treatment of arthritis. Practitioner 224:955-60, 1980*).

OTHER FACTORS

Rule out food sensitivities.

Non-steroidal anti-inflammatory medications (NSAIDs) may increase intestinal permeability to food antigens.

Experimental Controlled Study: Pts. with rheumatoid arthritis receiving non-steroidal anti-inflammatory medication excreted significantly more radioactively labeled EDTA, while untreated pts. did not differ from controls. Studies in pts. with osteoarthritis showed that the permeabiity abnormalities were due to the effect of the drugs on both the proximal and the distal intestine and that the effect was systemically mediated. This suggests that NSAIDs are associated with increased intestinal permeability to food antigens (*Bjarnason I et al. Intestinal permeability and inflammation in rheumatoid arthritis: Effects of non-steroidal anti-inflammatory drugs. Lancet 2:1171-74, 1984*).

Rule out hydrochloric acid deficiency.

Observational Study: In a gp. of 35 female pts. (ave. age 52), 9 (25.7%) were achlorhydric, while 1 (3%) was hypochlorhydric. By comparison, 2 studies of normal females of similar ages reported an incidence of achlorhydria of 12% and 15.5% (*Hartung EF, Steinbrocker O. Gastric acidity in chronic arthritis. Ann Intern Med 9:252-7, 1935*).

Note: While gastric anacidity had been reported in the past to be a relatively common condition which was associated with acne rosacea and a number of other illnesses, the presence of achlorhydria is no longer accepted unless a potent parietal-cell stimulant (such as histamine) is employed in gastric analysis. More recent studies suggest that histamine-fast anacidity is uncommon before the fifth decade of life and, although it probably does not occur in a normal stomach, its presence is not necessarily associated with symptoms (Rappaport EM. Achlorhydria: Associated symptoms and response to hydrochloric acid. N Engl J Med 252(19):802-5, 1955).

OSTEOPOROSIS

(including OSTEOMALACIA)

See Also: KIDNEY STONES
PERIODONTAL DISEASE

DIETARY FACTORS

Low <u>fat</u> diet.

High dietary fat decreases calcium absorption as fatty acids form calcium soaps (*Weiser NM, in NW Solomons, IH Rosenberg, Eds. <u>Absorption and Malabsorption of Mineral Nutrients</u>. New York, Alan R. Liss, 1984:15*).

Low <u>carbohydrate</u> diet.

Intake of carbohydrates may be inversely correlated to trabeular bone density.

Observational Study: For 11 normal women aged 19-21, trabecular bone density was inversely related to dietary carbohydrate independently of sex steroid hormones (*Leuenberger PK et al. Determination of peak trabecular bone density: Interplay of dietary fiber, carbohydrate, and androgens. <u>Am J Clin Nutr</u> 50:955-61, 1989*).

Low <u>sucrose</u> diet.

Sucrose ingestion may increase urinary calcium losses.

Experimental Study: 13 fasting subjects consumed a beverage containing 2 g sucrose/kg. There were significant increases in serum insulin, and urine calcium was significantly increased between 1 and 2.5 hrs. afterwards. While sucrose-induced increases in serum insulin and urine calcium were highly variable among subjects, within the gp. these measures were significantly correlated ($p<0.01$). The effect of sucrose on urinary calcium is consistent with the hypothesis that insulin inhibits renal calcium absorption (*Holl MG, Allen LH. Sucrose ingestion, insulin response, and mineral metabolism in humans. <u>J Nutr</u> 117(7):1229-33, 1987*).

A high fat, high sugar diet may reduce bone strength.

Animal Experimental Study: Young rats were fed either a high fat, high sugar diet or a control diet. After 10 wks., the strength and stiffness of the bones of the rats in the experimental gp. were reduced compared to controls (*Ronald Zernicke, professor of kinesiology, UCLA - reported at the 12th Int. Congress on Biomechanics, UCLA, 1989*).

<u>Alkaline ash</u> diet.

A high acid ash diet (meat and other high protein foods, most cereal grains and other starches) increases calcium excretion and may foster bone loss (*Barzel US. Acid loading and osteoporosis. Letter. <u>J Am Geriatr Soc</u> 30(9):613, 1982*).

Restrict <u>meat</u>.

Lacto-ovo-vegetarian and vegetarian females have less bone mineral loss than omnivorous females, perhaps due to the lower calcium intake, the higher protein intake, or to the higher phosphorus intake among omnivores.

Negative Observational Study: In a study of 146 elderly Methodist omnivores and 144 Seventh-day Adventist vegetarians, bone mineral content/bone width (BMC/BW) was not different in omnivores vs. vegetarians, and there were no significant relationships or trends between current or early dietary intakes and BMC/BM in either group (*Hunt IF et al. Bone mineral content in postmenopausal women: comparison of omnivores and vegetarians. Am J Clin Nutr 50:517-23, 1989*).

Observational Study: For men on a high meat diet, long-term calcium and phosphorus balances were 4 and 184 mg, respectively, while for men on a control diet, balances were -15 and 12 mg. The difference was not significant for calcium, but was for phosphorus (*Spencer H et al. Further studies of the effect of a high protein diet as meat on calcium metabolism. Am J Clin Nutr 37:924-9, 1983*).

Observational Study: Bone mineral mass in lacto-ovo-vegetarian women was compared with that of omnivorous women. While no significant differences were found in the 20's, 30's or 40's, there was a significant difference in the 50's and older, accelerating with age. At each decade past 50, the omnivorous women had more osteoporosis (*Marsh AG. Cortical bone density of adult lacto-ovo-vegetarian and omnivorous women. J Am Diet Assoc Feb. 1980, pp. 148-51*)

Observational Study: Bone mineral mass in 48 lacto-ovo-vegetarian women was compared with that of 48 omnivorous women. Before age 60 there was no significant difference. Between the ages of 60 and 89, however, lacto-ovo-vegetarian women had lost 18% of their bone mass compared to 35% in the omnivorous women (*Sanchez IV et al. Bone mineral mass in elderly vegetarian females. Am J Roentgenol 131:542-, 1978*).

Avoid excessive, <u>protein</u>.

A high protein diet may be associated with increased calcium loss.

Experimental Study: Women aged 50-64 were placed on a diet containing either 58 or 92 grams of protein. Dietary intakes and fecal and urinary output were monitored and analyzed for nitrogen, calcium, and phosphorus. 5/8 were in negative calcium balance by >100 mg/d on the high-protein diet. Phosphorus intake was 46% greater on the high-protein diet than on the moderate-protein diet. This increment was reflected in a reduction in serum calcium and a rise in urinary cyclic AMP, both indicators of elevated parathyroid activity. Results suggest that even adequate calcium intake in the presence of high protein intake could result in negative calcium balance (*Draper H, Piche L, Gibson R. Effects of high protein intake from common foods on calcium metabolism in a cohort of postmenopausal women. Nutr Res 11:273-81, 1991*).

Review Article: A high protein diet has a calciuretic effect which may promote osteoporosis (*Blank RP et al. Calcium metabolism and osteoporotic ridge absorption: A protein connection. J Prosthet Dent 58(5):590-95, 1987*).

Low <u>fiber</u> diet.

Dietary fiber may depress serum androgens which, in turn, increase bone density.

Observational Study: For 11 normal women aged 19-21, trabecular bone density was inversely related to dietary fiber and directly related to serum free-and-albumin-bound testosterone and total testosterone. Dietary fiber was inversely related to free-and-albumin-bound testosterone, total testosterone, and androstenedione (*Leuenberger PK et al. Determination of peak trabecular bone density: Interplay of dietary fiber, carbohydrate, and androgens. Am J Clin Nutr 50:955-61, 1989*).

Low <u>salt</u> diet.

Review Article: A number of studies measuring either urinary or dietary sodium have indicated that there is a positive correlation between salt intake and osteoporosis. By reducing the ave. sodium consumption in New Zealand to 70 mmol, urinary calcium would be decreased by 33% which could have significant implications for the development of osteoporosis (*Goulding A. Osteoporosis: Why consuming less sodium chloride helps to conserve bone. N Z Med J 103:120-2, 1990*).

Review Article: Due to impaired synthesis of 1,25-$(OH)_2$ vitamin D following stimulation by parathyroid hormone, sodium-induced hypercalciuria fails to produce an adequate compensatory rise in intestinal calcium absorption in postmenopausal women, suggesting that excessive sodium intake should be avoided (*Pak CYC. Calcium metabolism. J Am Coll Nutr 8(S):46S-53S, 1989*).

Avoid caffeine.

Consumption may increase urinary and fecal calcium loss.

Observational Study: In a study of 84,484 American women aged 34-59, there was a positive relation between caffeine intake and risk of hip but not forearm fracture. After potential risk factors were controlled for, the relative risk of hip fracture for women in the top quintile of caffeine consumption (≥817 mg/d) was 2.95 (95% CI = 1.18-7.38). Of the dietary sources of caffeine, coffee was the only significant predictor of the risk of hip fracture. When compared with women who almost never consumed coffee, women with a high consumption (>4 cups/d) had a threefold increase in the risk of hip fractures (*Hernandez-Avila M et al. Caffeine, moderate alcohol intake, and risk of fractures of the hip and forearm in middle-aged women. Am J Clin Nutr 54:157-63, 1991*).

Negative Experimental Double-blind Crossover Study: 16 healthy premenopausal women randomly received either caffeine 200 mg twice daily or placebo, each with decaffeinated coffee, in either order for 19 days each. There were no significant effects of caffeine on fractional calcium absorption, endogenous fecal calcium, or urine calcium. Although the mean calcium balance shift was negative, the change was not significantly different from zero. There was evidence of altered bone remodeling, with slight decreases in bone accretion, bone resorption, and calcium pool turnover. The findings add weight to the opinion that moderate caffeine intake does not increase osteoporosis risk, at least for those women with higher calcium intakes (*Barger-Lux MJ et al. Effects of moderate caffeine intake on the calcium economy of premenopausal women. Am J Clin Nutr 52:722-25, 1990*).

Observational Study: In a study of women aged 31-78 who consumed 200 mg caffeine daily (1-2 cups coffee), only women who also consumed <600 mg calcium daily had low blood calcium levels and signs of bone loss, suggesting that moderate caffeine intake increases the rate of bone loss only when calcium intake is also low (*Bergman E et al. Effects of dietary caffeine on calcium metabolism and bone turnover in adult women. Fed Proc 46:632, 1987*).

Experimental Study: 31 women ingested decaffeinated coffee at different times to which caffeine had been added. 3 hours afterwards, urinary calcium excretion increased significantly, but only in women taking estrogen, suggesting that caffeine ingestion may offset the beneficial effect of estrogen on calcium metabolism (*Hollingbery PW et al. Effect of dietary caffeine and aspirin on urinary calcium and hydroxyproline excretion in pre- and postmenopausal women. Fed Proc 44:1149, 1985*).

Consumption may be directly correlated with decreased bone minerals in adult women (*Yano K et al. The relationship between diet and bone mineral content of multiple skeletal sites in elderly Japanese-American men and women living in Hawaii. Am J Clin Nutr 42:877-88, 1985*).

Consumption may be directly correlated with an increased risk of hip fractures.

Observational Study: In a study of 3,170 people, heavy caffeine drinkers (>2 cups of coffee or the equivalent caffeine in tea daily) were 53% more likely to suffer hip fractures, probably because caffeine promotes calcium loss (*Kiel D et al. Caffeine and the risk of hip fracture: The Framingham Study. Am J Epidemiol 132:675-84, 1990*).

Restrict alcohol.

Ethanol may cause osteoblastic dysfunction resulting in diminished bone formation and bone demineralization.

Observational Study: In a study of 84,484 American women aged 34-59, alcohol intake was independently associated with increased risk of both hip and forearm fractures and with a dose-response relation. Compared to nondrinkers, women consuming ≥25 g alcohol/d had a relative risk of 2.33 (95% CI = 1.18-4.57) for hip fractures and a relative risk of 1.38 (95% CI = 1.09-1.74) for forearm fractures (*Hernandez-Avila M et al. Caffeine, moderate alcohol intake, and risk of fractures of the hip and forearm in middle-aged women. Am J Clin Nutr 54:157-63, 1991*).

Observational Study: 28 pts. currently drinking ethanol and 12 claiming not to have consumed ethanol for at least 6 mo. along with 35 controls were studied. Forearm bone mineral densities, spinal bone mineral densities, and iliac crest cancellous bone areas were significantly lower in the alcoholic pts. compared to controls (p<0.01), but these values did not differ between the "drinkers" and "abstainers." The drinkers, however, had significantly less osteoblastic activity than the abstainers (p<0.001) (*Diamond T et al. Ethanol reduces bone formation and may cause osteoporosis. Am J Med 86(3):282-88, 1989*).

– –

VITAMINS

<u>Folic acid</u>:   5 mg daily

Coenzyme for the conversion of homocysteine (toxic) to methionine. Homocysteine, which is increased in post-menopausal women, interferes with collagen crosslinking leading to a defective bone matrix and osteoporosis. (The incidence of heterozygous homocystinuria due to cystathionine synthase deficiency is about 1 in 70.)

Note: See also "<u>Vitamin B6</u>" below.

Supplementation may reduce homocysteine concentrations.

Experimental Study: Supplementation with folic acid 5 mg daily for 4 wks. substantially reduced homocysteine concentrations (p<0.01) both before a methionine load and afterwards (despite the fact that subjects had normal levels of serum and RBC folate) in normal men and pre- and post-menopausal women, suggesting that folic acid may have a prophylactic action against postmenopausal osteoporosis if moderate homocysteinemia promotes its development (*Brattström LE et al. Folic acid responsive postmenopausal homocysteinemia. <u>Metabolism</u> 34(11):1073-7, 1985*).

<u>Vitamin B6</u>:

Promotes the conversion of homocysteine (toxic) to cystathionine (*Seashore, MR et al. Studies on the mechanism of pyridoxine-responsive homocystinuria. <u>Pediatr Res</u> 6:187-96, 1972*). Homocysteine, which is increased in post-menopausal women, interferes with collagen crosslinking leading to a defective bone matrix and osteoporosis. (The incidence of heterozygous homocystinuria due to cystathionine synthase deficiency is about 1 in 70.)

Note: See also "<u>Folic acid</u>" above.

Deficiency may be associated with osteoporosis.

Animal Experimental Study: Rats receiving a pyridoxine-deficient diet developed osteoporosis (*Benke PH et al. Osteoporotic bone disease in the pyridoxine-deficient rat. <u>Biochem Med</u> 6:526-35, 1972*).

<u>Vitamin B12</u>:

Deficiency may impair osteoblast activity.

Observational Study: Compared to 5 non-deficient and 5 iron-deficient control subjects, 12 cobalamin-deficient pts. had lower mean blood skeletal alkaline phosphatase levels, and significantly lower osteocalcin levels. The degreee of megaloblastic anemia correlated with the reduction in skeletal alkaline phosphatase (p<0.01). With cobalamin therapy, skeletal alkaline phosphatase and osteocalcin levels rose in pts. but not in controls. Findings suggest that osteoblast activity depends on cobalamin and that bone metabolism is affected by cobalamin deficiency, but do not indicate whether cobalamin deficiency produces clinically important bone disease (*Carmel R et al. Cobalamin and osteoblast-specific proteins. <u>N Engl J Med</u> 319:70-75, 1988*).

<u>Vitamin C</u>:

Deficiency may cause osteoporosis (*Hyams DE, Ross EJ. Scurvy, megaloblastic anaemia and osteoporosis. <u>Br J Clin Pract</u> 17:332-40, 1963*).

<u>Vitamin D</u>:   10-20 µg/d (400-800 IU/d)

Known to be necessary for calcium absorption.

Deficiency may be associated with osteomalacia, osteoporosis and increased risk of hip fractures.

Reviw Article: Several reports have indicated an increased prevalence of osteomalacia in elderly people, including some with hip fracture, sugesting that osteomalacia might increase the risk of hip fracture in such patients. Prolonged, severe vitamin D deficiency causes osteomalacia, and lesser degrees of deficiency may stimulate parathyroid hormone secretion, resulting in increased bone turnover and accelerated bone loss. While the evidence of vitamin D deficiency in elderly pts. with hip fracture is conflicting, a strong case can be made for supplementation in the elderly, at least for high-risk groups (*Editorial: Vitamin supplementation in the elderly. Lancet 1:306-7 1987*).

Osteoporotic patients may have a deficit in converting vitamin D to its active form (1,25-dihydroxy vitamin D).

Observational Study: 24/153 men aged 48-96 residing in a nursing home for an ave. of 6.3 yrs. had one or more fractures during the preceding 1-5 yrs. of residence. After the effect of age was partialed out, the fracture cases had significantly higher blood urea nitrogen and 25-OH-D, and significantly lower 1,25-(OH)-D, than their non-fracture counterparts, suggesting that impaired renal production of the latter vitamin D metabolite contributed to the excessive rate of fractures (*Rudman D et al. Fractures in the men of a Veterans Administration nursing home: Relation to 1,25-dihydroxyvitamin D. J Am Coll Nutr 8(4):324-34, 1989*).

Experimental and Observational Study: The level of 25-hydroxy vitamin D was not found to decrease with age but 1,25 dihydroxy vitamin D was lower in elderly women both with and without hip fractures than it was in normal premenopausal women and normal women within 20 yrs. after menopause. Infusion with a tropic agent for the converting enzyme (bovine parathyroid fragment 1-34) resulted in a higher increase in 1,25 dihydroxy vitamin D for the younger women than for the other gps. and the least increase for the elderly women with hip fractures, suggesting that an age-related decrease in the kidney's ability to synthesize 1,25 dihydroxy vitamin D is a contributing factor to the development of senile osteoporosis (*Tsai KS et al. Impaired vitamin D metabolism in women: Possible role in pathogenesis of senile osteoporosis. J Clin Invest 73:1668-1672, 1984*).

Deficiency and resultant disease can be caused by hepatic or renal disease as the vitamin is initially metabolized to 25-hydroxyvitamin D (vitamin D_2) in the liver and subsequently converted to 1,25-dihydroxyvitamin D (calcitriol), the active form, in the kidney. Hypoparathyroidism can also be a cause, as parathyroid hormone is necessary for renal activation. (Calcitriol is available by prescription.)

Postmenopausal women have an impaired synthesis of 1,25-$(OH)_2$ vitamin D following stimulation by parathyroid hormone (*Slovik DM et al. Deficient production of 1,25-dihydroxyvitamin D in elderly osteoporotic patients. N Engl J Med 305:372-74, 1981*). This impairment depresses fractional calcium absorption, especially at low calcium intakes, causing a negative calcium balance. In addition, sodium-induced hypercalciuria fails to produce an adequate compensatory rise in intestinal calcium absorption (*Pak CYC. Calcium metabolism. J Am Coll Nutr 8(S):46S-53S, 1989*).

Supplementation may be effective in raising serum vitamin D levels.

Experimental Study: 500 IU daily given to older people with low vitamin D levels resulted in a significant increase by 2 mo. and levels approaching those of healthy young adults by 6 mo. (*MacLennan WJ, Hamilton JC. Vitamin D supplements and 25-hydroxy vitamin D concentrations in the elderly. Br Med J 2:859-61, 1977*).

Supplementation may be effective in normalizing calcium absorption.

Experimental and Observational Study: 56 pts. had significantly lower mean fractional calcium absorption than 20 age-matched controls (p<0.001). Long-term treatment with calcitriol 0.5-0.75 µg daily (6-24 mo.) significantly increased calcium absorption (p<0.001). After treatment, only 1 pt. still had subnormal calcium absorption. Results suggest that insufficient endogenous production of calcitriol may be the major cause of decreased calcium absorption in postmenopausal OP (*Riggs BL, Nelson KI. Effect of long term treatment with calcitriol on calcium absorption and mineral metabolism in postmenopausal osteoporosis. J Clin Endocrinol Metab 61(3):457-61, 1985*).

Supplementation may be beneficial.

Review Article: The optimal dose of vitamin D or its derivative that will promote calcium absorption without causing bone reabsorption has yet to be established. Until more data are available, elderly pts. should ingest 6-800 IU of vitamin D daily and pharmacologic doses are not indicated. Vitamin D supplementation is unlikely to be beneficial in postmenopausal osteoporosis (type I), in which pts. have a calcium excess caused by estrogen-related bone calcium loss, but may be effective in senile osteoporosis (type II) in which pts. are usually calcium deficient due to decreased calcium absorption resulting from decreased synthesis of 1,25 dihydroxyvitamin D by the kidney (*Eufemio MA. Vitamin D: Advances in the therapy of osteoporosis - Part VIII. Geriatr Med Today 9(11):37-49, 1990*).

Review Article: The data supporting the use of cholecalciferol are conflicting and based largeley on calcium absorption and balance studies. While vitamin D treatment clearly increases intestinal absorption of calcium, it increases bone resorption as well (*Resnick NM, Greenspan SL. 'Senile' osteoporosis reconsidered. JAMA 261:1025-29, 1989*).

Negative Experimental Double-blind Study: 86 postmenopausal women with vertebral compression fractures randomly received either calcitriol (mean dose 0.43 μg/d) or placebo. Dietary calcium was 1000 mg/d (24.9 mmol/day). Both medication dose and dietary calcium were adjusted for hypercalcicuria or hypercalcemia. After 2 yrs., no significant differences between gps. were seen in percent change in total body calcium, single photon absorptiometry or dual photon absorptiometry. New fractures were seen in 16% of the placebo gp. and 26% of the calcitriol group. Bone biopsies did not show changes in either group. While the calcitriol gp. had significantly higher serum and urinary calcium, renal function was not worse than in the placebo group (*Ott SM, Chesnut CH 3rd. Calcitriol treatment is not effective in postmenopausal osteoporosis. Ann Intern Med 110(4):267-74, 1989*).

Experimental Double-blind Study: After 1 yr., vitamin D_3 was more effective than estradiol, estradiol with vitamin D_3, or placebo in treating 28 women with post-menopausal OP (*Caniggia A et al. Clinical, biochemical and histological results of a double-blind trial with 1,25-dihydroxyvitamin D_3, estradiol and placebo in post-menopausal osteoporosis. Acta Vitaminol Enzymol 6:117-30, 1984*).

Vitamin K:

The vitamin K cycle plays a significant role in calcification (*Hauschka PV et al. Vitamin K and mineralization. Trends in Biochemical Science 3:75, 1978*) and antagonists of the cycle retard the formation of new bone in experimental fractures (*Dodds RA et al. Effects on fracture healing of an antagonist of the vitamin K cycle. Calcif Tissue Int 36:233, 1984*).

Deficiency may be associated with increased urinary calcium excretion (*Robert D et al. Hypercalciuria during experimental vitamin K deficiency in the rat. Calcif Tissue Int 37:143-47, 1985*).

Reduced plasma vitamin K may be associated with fractures in osteoporotic patients.

Observational Study: 16 osteoporotic pts. with fractures of the femoral neck or spinal crush fractures had significantly less plasma vitamin K_1 than age-matched controls (*Hart JP et al. Electrochemical detection of depressed circulating levels of vitamin K_1 in osteoporosis. J Clin Endocrinol Metab 60(6):1268-69, 1985*).

Supplementation may be associated with reduced urinary calcium excretion.

Experimental Study: Healthy postmenopausal women were supplemented with vitamin K. There was a decrease in urinary calcium levels and and increase in the calcium-binding capacity of serum osteocalcin, suggesting that vitamin K may play a role in preventing postmenopausal bone loss (*Knapen MHJ et al. The effect of vitamin K supplementation on circulating osteocalcin (bone Gla protein) and urinary calcium excretion. Ann Intern Med 111:1001-05, 1989*).

Supplementation may be associated with accelerated healing of experimental fractures (*Bouckaert JH, Said AH. Fracture healing by vitamin K. Nature 185:849, 1960*).

- -

MINERALS

Boron:

Deficiency may foster calcium loss and bone demineralization.

Experimental Study: 12 postmenopausal women aged 48-82 received a boron supplement of 3 mg daily after 119 days on a conventional low-boron diet supplying about 0.25 mg boron which was either low or adequate in magnesium. Boron supplementation markedly reduced urinary calcium and magnesium excretion, especially when dietary magnesium was low, and depressed the urinary excretion of phosphorus in subjects on the low-magnesium diet. It also markedly elevated the serum levels of 17 β-estradiol and testosterone, especially when dietary magnesium was low. Results suggest that supplementation of a low-boron diet with an amt. of boron commonly found in diets high in fruits and vegetables induces changes consistent with the prevention of calcium loss and bone demineralization (*Nielsen FH et al. Effect of dietary boron on mineral, estrogen, and testosterone metabolism in postmenopausal women. Fed Am Soc Exp Biol 1(5):394-97, 1987*)

Calcium: 1.5 gm. daily for postmenopausal women
(1 gm. daily for premenopausal women over 35)

Women over age 35 who ingest less than the above amounts are in negative calcium balance (*Heaney RP et al. Menopausal changes in calcium balance performance. J Lab Clin Med 92(6):953-63, 1978*), most likely due to impaired calcium absorption (*Spencer H et al. Absorption of calcium in osteoporosis. Am J Med 37:223, 1964*).

> *Note: Calcium balance studies have been criticized as being subject to inaccuracies:*
> *1. It is unknown to what extent the minimal obligatory calcium loss in the different age and sex groups is related to an intrinsic skeletal calcium loss and/or a lack of external calcium preservation through kidney, skin, and intestine (Charles P et al. Dermal, intestinal, and renal obligatory losses of calcium: relation to skeletal calcium loss. Am J Clin Nutr 54:266S-73S, 1991).*
> *2. Incomplete recovery of calcium output can produce the artefact of a positive shift in calcium balance (Stevenson JC et al. Dietary intake of calcium and postmenopausal bone loss. Br Med J 297:15-17, 1988).*
> *3. Dermal calcium losses are commonly neglected (Charles P et al. Dermal, intestinal, and renal obligatory losses of calcium: relation to skeletal calcium loss. Am J Clin Nutr 54:266S-73S, 1991).*
> *4. Since these studies are unable to distinguish between unabsorbed calcium in the feces and that which has been absorbed, utilized, and reexcreted into the GI tract, it is questionable whether they provide a useful measure of absorption (Mertz W. Use and misuse of balance studies. J Nutr 117:1811-13, 1981).*
> *5. Since exercise may influence calcium balance, results of studies using subjects whose exercise has been restricted may not extend to the general population (Westrich BJ. Effect of physical activity on skeletal integrity and its implications for calcium requirement studies. Nutr Health 5(1/2):53-60, 1987).*

Experimental Study: 48 pts. (ave. age 67) were followed over an ave. of 3.5 years. Gp. 1 consisted of 24 postmenopausal women and 1 man over 60 with "typical" causes for their OP. Gp. 2 consisted of men and women (ave. age 47) with OP due to uncommon causes. Initially each pt. received calcium lactate or gluconate supplements according to his or her individual needs; then a particular sex hormonal regimen was added; then a second sex hormonal regimen was substituted for the first; then all hormone therapy was stopped. At each stage, calcium balance studies were conducted. Results indicated that both calcium and sex hormone supplementation improved calcium balance, suggesting that the first line of treatment for most osteoporotic pts. is a high calcium intake, while hormone therapy should be reserved for those pts. with continuing vertebral fractures after 1 yr. of calcium supplementation (*Thalassinos NC et al. Calcium balance in osteoporotic patients on long-term oral calcium therapy with and without sex hormones. Clin Science 62(2):221-26, 1982*).

Observational Study: 171 early postmenopausal women (ave. age 54 yrs.) who were estrogen-deprived and non-osteoporotic were evaluated. Calcium intake averaged 802 ± 0.419 mg/day, urine calcium output was 144 ± 62 mg/day and fractional absorption (estimated using a double tracer method) was 0.266 ± 0.096. Absorption of calcium in 55% was inadequate at an intake of 800 mg/day and, in 75%, an intake of even 1.5 gm of calcium daily could not maintain a positive calcium balance. Results suggest that poor absorptive performance was due to defective absorption rather than to bone breakdown since urine calcium was positively correlated with absorbed calcium (*Heaney RP, Recker RR. Distribution of calcium absorption in middle-aged women. Am J Clin Nutr 43:299-305, 1966*).

Hair calcium levels may be reduced.

Observational Study: In a study of 14 hair mineral levels of 20 osteoporotic women, 50% were normal. Only calcium levels correlated with the disease state, with calcium levels significantly lower (99% confidence level) in pts. than in normals (*Stephens-Newsham LG et al. Comparison of elemental composition of hair between osteoporotic and normal women by instrumental neutron activation analysis. J Radioanal Nucl Chem 113(2):495-500, 1987*).

Osteoporosis is more common in lactose intolerance due, possibly, to decreased calcium intake due to avoidance of milk products.

Experimental Study: 11/33 women with idiopathic OP had a history of milk intolerance compared to 4/33 matched controls. Although their calcium intakes were comparable, the daily intake of calcium from milk was significantly lower in the OP patients, while their fasting glucose concentrations were significantly higher. OP pts. who demonstrated lactose malabsorption also exhibited a significantly flatter glucose concentration curve during the lactose tolerance test than did the normal women with lactose malabsorption, and lactose tolerance curves were generally flatter in the "normal" OP pts. compared to normal controls. These findings suggest that a disturbance of glucose homeostasis may coincide with asymptomatic minor changes in lactose malabsorption that may predispose to OP (*Finkenstedt G et al. Lactose absorption, milk consumption, and fasting blood glucose concentrations in women with idiopathic osteoporosis. Br Med J 292:161-62, 1986*).

Both acute and chronic hypocalcemia stimulate the release of parathyroid hormone which, in turn, stimulates the osteoclasts to resorb calcified bone (*Hahn TJ. Parathyroid hormone, calcitonin, vitamin D, mineral and bone: Metabolism and disorders, in EL Mazzaferri, Ed. Textbook of Endocrinology. Third Edition. New York, Elsevier Science Publishing Co., 1986*).

High calcium intake, primarily during childhood and adolescence, may reduce the risk of osteoporosis (*Cauley JA et al. Endogenous estrogen levels and calcium intakes in postmenopausal women. JAMA 260(21):3150-55, 1988*).

Review Article: From what is currently known about the calcium requirement in childhood and adolescence, an intake of $\approx$1000 mg/d in males and $\approx$850 mg/d in females would not appear to satisfy these needs, particularly during adolescence. In children and adolescents consuming lower amts., it is unlikely that optimal bone mass is being achieved (*Peacock M. Calcium absorption efficiency and calcium requirements in children and adolescents. Am J Clin Nutr 54:261S-5S, 1991*).

Experimental Controlled Study: 20 premenopausal women aged 30-42 increased their dietary calcium intake an ave. of 610 mg/d (p<0.03) by increasing their intake of dairy products for 3 yrs., while 17 age- and weight-matched women served as controls. While vertebral bone density in the experimental gp. failed to change, vertebral bone density in the controls declined (p<0.001) and was significantly lower than that in the supplemented gp. at 30 and 30 mo., suggesting that increased calcium intake in estrogen-replete premenopausal women may prevent age-related bone loss (*Baran D et al. Dietary modification with dairy products for preventing vertebral bone loss in premenopausal women: a three-year prospective study. J Clin Endocrinol Metab 70(1):264-70, 1990*).

In postmenopausal women, impaired synthesis of 1,25-$(OH)_2$ vitamin D following stimulation by parathyroid hormone depresses fractional calcium absorption, especially at low calcium intakes, causing a negative calcium balance. In addition, sodium-induced hypercalciuria fails to produce an adequate compensatory rise in intestinal calcium absorption (*Pak CYC. Calcium metabolism. J Am Coll Nutr 8(S):46S-53S, 1989*).

It is uncertain whether calcium supplementation following menopause reduces bone loss at clinically important sites (*Consensus on preventing osteoporosis. International Symposium on Osteoporosis, Aalborg, Denmark. Br Med J 295:914, 1987; Editorial: Calcium supplements and osteoporosis. Lancet 1:370, 1987; NIH Consensus Conference: Osteoporosis. JAMA 252(6):799-802, 1984; Kanis JA, Passmore R. Regular Review: Calcium supplementation of the diet: Not justified by present evidence. Br Med J 298:137-40 & 205-08, 1989*).

Note: Part of the reason for the controversy is due to the fact that the loss of cortical *bone (as measured, for example, in a phalanx) may fail to correlate with the loss of* trabecular *bone (for example, in the vertebrae). Calcium supplementation appears to be more effective in preventing loss of cortical bone than of trabecular bone, where most osteoporotic fractures occur (Trachtenbarg DE. Treatment of osteoporosis: What is the role of calcium? Postgrad Med 87(4):263-70, 1990).*

Note: Absorption of different calcium preparations varies greatly, thus the efficacy of calcium supplementation may vary greatly according to the preparation used:

Experimental Controlled Study: 53 post-menopausal women with seriously impaired calcium absorption and accelerated bone loss due to primary biliary cirrhosis received either vitamin D_2 100,000 IU IM monthly alone, or vitamin D_2 along with 1000 mg of either calcium gluconate or hydroxyapatite. After 14 mo., the control gp. showed significant loss of cortical bone, the calcium gluconate gp. showed no change in bone status, and the hydroxyapatite gp. showed a significant increase in bone thickness (*Epstein O et al. Vitamin D, hydroxyapatite, and calcium gluconate in treatment of cortical bone thinning in postmenopausal women with primary biliary cirrhosis. Am J Clin Nutr 36:426-30, 1982*).

Review Article: "The responsiveness of postmenopausal women to supplementation with calcium appears to depend upon their menopausal age. In women who are within the first 5 y of menopause, bone loss from the radius is attenuated but not arrested by added calcium. The maximal effect appears to occur with daily supplemental dosages of ≈1000 mg elemental calcium. In contrast, the spine is unresponsive to supplementation with calcium even at higher doses in early postmenopausal women. In late postmenopausal women, bone loss from the radius is attenuated by increasing calcium intake. Loss from the spine can be retarded by increasing calcium intake to the current recommended dietary allowance in older women with low usual calcium diets. The effect of supplementation with higher doses of calcium in this segment of the population is unknown. Finally, the effect of added calcium on hip density of postmenopausal women is not yet established" (*Dawson-Hughes B. Calcium supplementation and bone loss: a review of controlled clinical trials. Am J Clin Nutr 54:274-80S, 1991*).

Supplementation may be most effective when given in the evening.

Experimental Study: In a previous study, calcium carbonate 2 g daily over 2 yrs. failed to affect urinary hydroxyproline excretion, a reliable indicator of calcium resorption from bone. In the present study, 15 post-menopausal women with osteoporosis but normal calcium absorption received 1 g calcium (5.23 g calcium lactate gluconate and 0.8 g calcium carbonate) at 2100 hr daily. Urinary hydroxyproline decreased, indicating a significant decrease in bone resorption (*Horowitz M et al. Biochemical effects of calcium supplementation in postmenopausal osteoporosis. Eur J Clin Nutr 42:775-78, 1988*).

Supplementation may prevent bone loss in <u>breastfeeding mothers</u>.

Experimental Study: In a study of young breastfeeding mothers, those who consumed a high-calcium diet (>1,600 mg daily) had stronger bones than those who consumed 900 mg calcium daily. Results suggest that bone loss is common during breastfeeding and can be prevented with adequate calcium intake (*Chan G et al. Effects of increased dietary calcium intake upon the calcium and bone mineral status of lactating adolescent and adult women. Am J Clin Nutr 46:319-23, 1987*).

Since post-menopausal women often suffer from achlorhydria which inhibits the absorption of calcium salts under fasting conditions, supplementation with an acidified form of calcium, or taking calcium supplements with meals, may enhance absorption.

Experimental Controlled Study: Compared to normal controls, absorption of calcium from a pH-adjusted solution of calcium citrate under fasting conditions resulted in enhanced calcium absorption for pts. with achlorhydria (*Recker RR. Calcium absorption and achlorhydria. N Engl J Med 313(2):70-73, 1985*).

- with <u>Vitamin D</u>:

Combined supplementation may be beneficial.

Experimental and Observational Study: Almost 2/3 of older French adults studied consumed <500 mg calcium daily compared to the US RDA of 800 mg daily as well as less than the RDA for vitamin D. Blood levels of calcium and vitamin D were low and blood indicators of tissue and bone loss were high. When their diets were supplemented with calcium and vitamin D, blood levels increased and bone loss was reversed (*Chapuy M et al. Calcium and vitamin D supplements: Effect on calcium metabolism in elderly people. Am J Clin Nutr 46:324-28, 1987*).

Experimental Placebo-controlled Study: 67 women (ages 37-73) were divided into two groups. One received 750 mg. calcium and 375 mg. vitamin D daily in addition to their regular diet while the other received placebo. After 3 yrs., bone density increased in gp. I 12.5% and decreased in gp. II 6% (*Albanese AA et al. Osteoporosis: Effects of calcium. Am Fam Physician 18(4):160-67, 1978*).

Combined supplementation may be more effective than calcium or vitamin D alone in osteoporosis when it is associated with calcium malabsorption.

Experimental Study: The effects of calcitriol and calcium, combined or separately, were studied in 45 pts. with OP and calcium malabsorption. Results suggest that calcitriol and calcium suppress bone resorption in OP associated with calcium malabsorption and may be more effective than either given alone (*Need AG et al. 1,25-Dihydroxycalciferol and calcium therapy in osteoporosis with calcium malabsorption. Dose response relationship of calcium absorption and indices of bone turnover. Miner Electrolyte Metab 11(1):35-40, 1985*).

<u>Copper</u>:

Deficiency may enhance bone resorption.

> **Review Article:** Many western diets are low in copper. Osteoporotic lesions attributable to copper deficiency have been described in both man and animals and the hypothesis that a mild dietary copper deficiency may be implicated in the onset and progression of osteoporosis is consistent with epidemiological evidence (*Strain JJ. A reassessment of diet and osteoporosis: Possible role for copper.* <u>Med Hypotheses</u> *27(4):333-38, 1988*).

Serum copper levels may be directly associated with bone mass density (*Strause L et al. Dietary calcium intake, serum copper concentration and bone density in postmenopausal women. Abstract.* <u>FASEBJ</u> *5:A576, 1991*).

<u>Fluoride</u>:   25-40 mg sodium fluoride twice daily

> **WARNINGS:** Damages the surface of the gastric mucosa at therapeutic dosages (*Spak C-J et al. Tissue response of gastric mucosa after ingestion of fluoride.* <u>Br Med J</u> *298:1686-87, 1989*) and, in animal studies, inhibits the enzyme phosphatase which is critically important for the assimilation of calcium and other minerals (*Yanick P. Solving problematic tinnitus. A clinical scientific approach.* <u>Townsend Letter for Doctors</u>. *February - March, 1985, p. 31*).

Clinical studies suggest that sodium fluoride is one of the most potent agents for increasing bone volume in OP patients. Skeletal responses to supplementation include increases in the rate of bone formation, increases in the number of osteoblasts, and heightening of the serum activity of skeletal alkaline phosphatase. Some controlled studies, however, suggest that its effectiveness may be more limited than previously thought (*Editorial: Fluoride and the treatment of osteoporosis.* <u>Lancet</u> *1:547, 1984; Fluoride/calcium in osteoporosis. Letter.* <u>N Engl J Med</u> *307(7):441-43, 1982*).

> *Note: The unanimous opinion of the US FDA endocrinologic and metabolic drugs advisory committee is that fluoride has yet to prove its worth (*<u>Med World News</u> *November 13, 1989).*

> **Negative Experimental Double-blind Study:** 135 postmenopausal women with osteoporosis and vertebral fractures randomly received either sodium fluoride 75 mg/d or placebo. As compared to the placebo gp., the treatment gp. had increases in median bone mineral density of 45% in the lumbar spine (predominantly cancellous bone), 12% in the femoral neck, and 10% in the femoral trochanter (sites of mixed cortical and cancellous bone), but the bone mineral density decreased by 4% in the shaft of the radius (predominantly cortical bone). The number of new vertebral fractures was similar in the treatment and placebo gps., but the number of nonvertebral fractures was higher in the treatment gp. (72 vs. 24; p<0.01). 54 women in the fluoride gp. and 24 in the placebo gp. had side effects sufficiently severe to warrant dosage reduction, especially GI symptoms and lower-extremity pain. Results suggest that fluoride therapy increases cancellous but decreases cortical bone mineral density and increases skeletal fragility. Under the conditions of this study, it is thus not effective (*Riggs BL et al. Effect of fluoride treatment on the fracture rate in postmenopausal women with osteoporosis.* <u>N Engl J Med</u> *322:802-09, 1990*).

> **Review Article:** "Sodium fluoride was been shown unequivocally to increase trabecular bone density and may well be the drug of choice in patients with adequate amounts of cortical bone, but the significance of its adverse effect on cortical bone and the risk of hip fractures remain, to date, not totally elucidated" (*Eufemio MA. Fluoride therapy: Advances in the therapy of osteoporosis, Part III.* <u>Geriatr Med Today</u> *8(9):79-88, 1989*).

- with <u>calcium</u> and <u>vitamin D₂</u>:

Combined supplementation may be beneficial.

> **Experimental Study:** 251 pts. received slow-release sodium fluoride (Mission Pharm.) and calcium citrate. In addition, some of the pts. received 1,25-dihydroxyvitamin D. In the 5-yr. study, treatment stabilized or increased bone mass in all but the pts. who also received vitamin D. In the majority of pts., most of them postmenopausal females, lumbar bone density increased 3-6% annually for up to 4 years. Only 2 pts. had stress fractures. GI and rheumatologic complications, which have occurred in up to 40% of pts. given conventional sodium fluoride formulations, were limited to 3.2% and 1.6%, respectively. The optimal regimen appeared to be 25 mg sodium fluoride and 400 mg calcium citrate twice daily for 1 yr., followed by 1 mo. of calcium citrate alone to avoid development of resistance or toxicity to sodium fluoride (*CYC Pak, chief of mineral metabolism, U. of Texas Southwestern Medical Center - reported in* <u>Med World News</u>, *February 13, 1989*).

Experimental Blinded Study: 257 pts. randomly received enteric-coated sodium fluoride 25 mg twice daily plus elemental calcium 1 gm daily and vitamin D_2 800 IU daily, while 209 received alternative treatments (calcium and vitamin D_2; calcitonin and phosphorus; calcitonin and calcium; calcium and phosphorus; or phosphorus and sodium etidronate). After 24 mo., the fluoride-calcium gp. showed a significantly lower rate of new vertebral fractures, the main adverse effect being a higher incidence of osteoarticular pains in the ankle and foot (*Mamelle N et al. Risk-benefit ratio of sodium fluoride treatment in primary vertebral osteoporosis. Lancet 2:361-65, 1988*).

Germanium:

Administration of carboxyethyl germanium sesquioxide (Ge-132) may be beneficial.

Experimental Study: After 12 mo., the bone mass of controls tended to decrease, while the bone mass of pts. receiving Ge-132 demonstrated a slight increase. Significant differences began to be noted 1-3 mo. after initiating treatment. Administration of Ge-132 was associated with a significant decrease in parathyroid hormone levels, and these levels are known to be negatively correlated with bone mass (*Mizushima M et al. Some pharmacological and clinical aspects of a novel organic germanium compound Ge-132, in Lekim & Samochowiec, Eds. 1st Int Conf on Germanium. Semmelweis-Verlag, 1985*).

Iron:

Intake may be correlated with bone mineral density.

Observational Study: In 159 Caucasian women aged 23-75, iron intake was a positive predictor of bone mineral density in the femoral neck and of forearm bone mineral content (*Angus RM et al. Dietary intake and bone mineral density. Bone Mineral 4(3):265-78, 1988*).

Magnesium:

Required for the activation of alkaline phosphatase, an enzyme involved in forming calcium crystals in bone (*Iseri LT, French JH. Magnesium: Nature's physiologic calcium blocker. Am Heart J 108:188-93, 1984*) and for the conversion of vitamin D into 1,25-dihydroxyvitamin D_3, its biologically active form (*Rude RK et al. Low serum concentrations of 1,25-dihydroxyvitamin D in human magnesium deficiency. J Clin Endocrinol Metab 61:933-40, 1985*).

Magnesium promotes and regulates parathormone (PTH) (*Mahaffee D et al. Magnesium promotes both parathyroid hormone secretion and adenosine $3^1,5^1$-monophosphate production in rat parathyroid tissues and reverses the inhibitory effects of calcium on adenylate cyclase. Endocrinol 110:487-95, 1982*) which, in turn, stimulates the osteoclasts to resorb calcified bone (*Hahn TJ. Parathyroid hormone, calcitonin, vitamin D, mineral and bone: Metabolism and disorders, in EL Mazzaferri, Ed. Textbook of Endocrinology. Third Edition. New York, Elsevier Science Publishing Co., 1986:467*). While <u>acute</u> hypomagnesemia stimulates PTH release, <u>chronic</u> hypomagnesemia is associated with an inappropriately <u>low</u> level of PTH secretion (*Anast CS et al. Impaired release of parathyroid hormone in magnesium deficiency. J Clin Endocrinol Metab 42:707, 1976*).

Clinical magnesium deficiency is common in OP patients.

Observational Study: 16/19 OP pts. had lower than normal trabecular bone magnesium content (by infrared spectrophotometry) and clinical magnesium deficiency (based on Thoren's magnesium loading test) (*Cohen L, Kitzes R. Infrared spectroscopy and magnesium content of bone mineral in osteoporotic women. Isr J Med Sci 17:1123-5, 1981*).

Magnesium intake may be correlated with bone mineral density.

Observational Study: In 159 Caucasian women aged 23-75, magnesium intake was a significant predictor of forearm bone mineral content by multiple regression analysis in all women, and was positively correlated with forearm bone mineral content in premenopausal women (*Angus RM et al. Dietary intake and bone mineral density. Bone Mineral 4(3):265-78, 1988*).

The plasma of osteoporotic patients is often supersaturated with octocalcium phosphate which appears to control the solubility of bone mineral. Magnesium decreases octocalcium phosphate saturation. In this way, as well as by suppressing hyperparathyroidism, it may stabilize bone in pts. (*Muenzenberg KJ, Koch W. Mineralogic aspects in the treatment of osteoporosis with magnesium. Abstract. J Am Coll Nutr 8(5):461, 1989*).

Supplementation may reduce the adverse side effects of sodium fluoride treatment.

Experimental Controlled Study: The addition of magnesium 400-600 mg/day to sodium fluoride 20 mg daily resulted in far fewer adverse effects, especially arthalgia which is due, probably, to deposition of calcium phosphate particles in periarticular tissues (p=0.01) (*Muenzenberg KJ, Koch W. Mineralogic aspects in the treatment of osteoporosis with magnesium. Abstract. J Am Coll Nutr 8(5):461, 1989*).

Manganese:

Necessary for bone mineralization (*Amdur MO et al. The need for manganese in bone development by the rat. Proc Soc Exp Biol Med 59:254-55, 1945*).

Deficiency may be associated with decreased bone density and resistance to fractures (*Amdur MO et al. The need for manganese in bone development by the rat. Proc Soc Exp Biol Med 59:54-55, 1945*).

Blood levels may be reduced.

Observational Study: Blood manganese levels in osteoporotic women were found to be only 25% that of controls (*study cited in Raloff J. Reasons for boning up on manganese. Sci News 1986(Sept 27):199*).

Phosphorus:

High phosphorus intakes may increase calcitriol levels.

Experimental Study: Increases and reductions in oral phosphorus intake in healthy men were found to induce rapidly occurring, large, inverse, and persisting changes in serum 1,25-dihydroxyvitamin D levels due to phosphorus-induced changes in the rate of vitamin D production (*Portale A. Oral intake of phosphorus can determine the serum concentration of 1,25-dihydroxyvitamin D by determining its production rate in humans. J Clin Invest 77:7-12, 1986*).

High phosphorus intakes may increase calcium retention by reducing urinary calcium while having little, if any, effect on calcium absorption (*Hegsted M et al. Urinary calcium and calcium balance in young men as affected by level of protein and phosphorus intake. J Nutr 111:553-62, 1981; Spencer H et al. Effect of phosphorus on the absorption of calcium and on the calcium balance in man. J Nutr 108:447-57, 1978*).

High phosphorus intakes may decrease fracture healing time in normals.

Experimental Study: Pts. with fractures of the femur and ankle were supplemented with phosphorus 1 gm daily. The time required for clinical union of the fracture was reduced, as was the amt. of deminieralization in the immobilized limb (*Goldsmith RS et al. Effect of phosphate supplements in patients with fractures. Lancet 1:687-90, 1967*).

High phosphorus intakes may enhance osteoporotic changes.

Experimental Study: 7 pts. were supplemented with 1 gm phosphorus daily. Histologic examination of bone biopsies showed a decrease in the bone-forming surface and an increase in bone surface involved in resorption. There was no evidence of soft tissue calcification. Calcium balance was enhanced and serum calcium, phosphorus, alkaline phosphatase and parathyroid levels, as well as urinary hydroxyproline, were unchanged (*Goldsmith RS et al. Effect of phosphorus supplementation on serum parathyroid hormone and bone morphology in osteoporosis. J Clin Endocrinol Metab 43:523-32, 1976*).

Calcium to
Phosphorus ratio:

Note: References to the Ca/P ratio are confusing as some authors refer to increases in the denominator as a raising, rather than a lowering, of the ratio. For uniformity, the abstracts have been modified so that "lowering" the ratio refers to increasing phosphorus in relation to calcium and vice versa.

Calcium balance is significantly affected by the dietary calcium/phosphorus ratio. The optimal Ca/P ratio is estimated to be 1:1, while the typical American diet yields a ratio of 1:2-1:4 (*Worthington-Roberts B. Contemporary Developments in Nutrition. St. Lewis, Mo., C.V. Mosby Co., 1981:240-53*).

Review Article: Calcium intake that may be adequate for adults consuming a low protein, low phosphorus, neutral or alkaline cereal-based diet is not necessarily adequate for subjects consuming a high protein, high phosphorus, acidic mixed Western diet. Although the Ca:P ratio for the ave. diet consumed in the U.S. and Canada (about 1:1.6) appears to be satisfactory, a low intake of dairy foods, coupled with a high intake of other foods rich in natural and added phosphorus, may lower the ratio below 1:2 (*Draper HH, Scythes CA. Calcium, phosphorus, and osteoporosis. Fed Proc 40(9):2434-38, 1981*).

Observational Study: In the U.S. Dept. of Agriculture longitudinal surveys (1971-1979), it was found that, beyond the age range of 19-22, the daily calcium intake of 3,438 females fell from 800 to 500 mg/day while phosphorus consumption remained at approx. 1000 mg/day. As a result, Ca:P ratios of 1:1.4 to 1:1.8 prevailed (*Chinn HI. Effects of dietary factors on skeletal integrity in adults: Calcium, phosphorus, vitamin D and protein. Life Sciences Research Office, Federation of American Societies for Experimental Biology, Bethesda, Md., 1981*).

A lowered Ca/P ratio may enhance bone resorption.

Observational Study: In a study of 158 females (ages 20-75), their ave. calcium intake was 600 mg/day with age-related decrements of dietary Ca:P ratios (all of which were <1:1.4) and marked loss of bone densities (*Albanese AA et al. Effects of dietary calcium:phosphorus ratios on utilization of dietary calcium for bone synthesis in women 20-75 years of age. Nutr Rep Int 33(6):879-91, 1986*).

Experimental Controlled Study: 38 females, ages 43-65, increased their habitual daily calcium intake from 448 mg/day to 1100 mg/day which increased Ca:P ratios from 1:1.65 to 1:1.20 and increased bone density increments from 80 mils of aluminum (the high fracture risk zone) to 110 mils after 25-38 months. By contrast, in an unsupplemented control gp. of 42 females, ages 43-67, whose calcium intake was 463 mg/day with a Ca:P ratio of 1:1.70 and whose ave. bone density was 80 mils of aluminum, there was a minimal change in Ca:P ratio after 26-42 mo. and the coefficient of bone density fell to 75 mils of aluminum. Results suggest that the treatment of osteoporosis may be fruitless so long as dietary Ca:P ratios are <1:1.25 (*Albanese AA et al. Effects of dietary calcium:phosphorus ratios on utilization of dietary calcium for bone synthesis in women 20-75 years of age. Nutr Rep Int 33(6):879-91, 1986*).

Review Article: Data from animal studies suggest that Ca/P ratios of <1:2 enhance bone resorption regardless of calcium intake (*Worthington-Roberts B. Contemporary Developments in Nutrition. St. Lewis, Mo., C.V. Mosby Co., 1981:240-53*).

The low Ca/P ratio of the Western diet (relatively low in calcium for the amount of phosphorus; <1:1.2) is associated with increased secretion and action of parathyroid hormone.

Experimental Study: 8 men and 8 women aged 18-25 ingested a control diet that had calcium (820 mg) and phosphorus (930 mg) contents near the recommended daily intakes for 8 days. They were then switched to a test diet with calcium (420 mg) and phosphorus (930 mg) contents typical of the moderately low calcium, high phosphorus intake of U.S. teenagers and young adults. The 24 hr. mean serum immunoreactive PTH levels increased significantly in both men and women during the test diet. In both sexes, the test diet significantly increased serum phosphorus and plasma 1,25-dihydroxyvitamin D; in women only it decreased serum ionized and total calcium levels (*Calvo MS et al. Elevated secretion and action of serum parathyroid hormone in young adults consuming high phosphorus, low calcium diets assembled from common foods. J Clin Endocrinol Metab 66(4):823-29, 1988*).

Review Article: Animal experiments, as well as acute studies in men involving an oral phosphorus load, suggest that parathyroid secretion might be increased by a low calcium/phosphorus ratio. Therefore it is possible that a diet too low in calcium could contribute to the pathogenesis of periodontal disease (*Rottka H et al. The influence of the calcium/phosphorus ratio in the diet on human bone disease: The role of nutritive secondary hyperparathyroidism. Int J Vitam Nutr Res 51:373, 1981*).

Strontium:

Supplementation may be beneficial.

WARNING: May block calcium absorption unless high doses of vitamin D are given (*Rousselet F et al. [Strontium and calcium metabolism. Interaction of strontium and vitamin D.]   C R Soc Biol (Paris) 169(2):322-29, 1975*).

Animal Experimental Study: The addition of 0.27% strontium to the drinking water of mice increased the osteoid surface and reduced the number of acid phosphatase-stained osteoclasts, but failed to augment trabecular calcified bone volume (*Marie PJ, Hott M. Short-term effects of fluoride and strontium on bone formation and resorption in the mouse. Metabolism 35(6):547-51, 1986*).

Experimental Study: 27/32 (84%) pts. who received strontium lactate 1.7 gm daily (10 also received estrogen and testoterone) experienced marked reduction in bone pain after 3 mo. - 3 years of supplementation, and radiologic examination showed possible improvement in 78% (*McCaslin FE Jr, Janes JM. The effect of strontium lactate in the treatment of osteoporosis. Proc Staff Mtgs Mayo Clin 34:329-34, 1959*).

Zinc:

Essential for normal bone formation (*Calhoun NR et al. The effects of zinc on ectopic bone formation. Oral Surg 39:698-706, 1975*).

Enhances vitamin D activity (*Yamaguchi M, Sakashita T. Enhancement of vitamin D3 effect on bone metabolism in weanling rats orally administered zinc sulphate. Acta Endocrinol 111:285-88, 1986*).

Serum and bone levels may be low in elderly OP patients (*Atik OS. Zinc and senile osteoporosis. J Am Geriatr Soc 31:790-91, 1983*).

Intake may be positively correlated with bone mineral density.

Observational Study: In 159 Caucasian women aged 23-75, zinc intake was positively correlated with forearm bone mineral content in premenopausal women (*Angus RM et al. Dietary intake and bone mineral density. Bone Mineral 4(3):265-78, 1988*).

- -

COMBINED NUTRITIONAL INTERVENTIONS

Experimental Controlled Study: 19/26 postmenopausal women receiving hormonal replacement therapy were given dietary counseling and supplemented with Gynovite® Plus (Optimox, USA), a multivitamin/multimineral supplement, 6 tabs daily, while the other 7 women were only given dietary counseling. After 6-12 mo., there was a mean increase of 11% in calcaneous bone density (p<0.01) in the women who received the supplement compared to a non-significant increase of 0.7% in the controls (*Abraham GE. The importance of magnesium in the management of postmenopausal osteoporosis. J Nutr Med 2:165-78, 1991; Abraham GE, Grewel H. A total dietary program emphasizing magnesium instead of calcium. J Reprod Med 35(5):503-7, 1990*).

- -

OTHER FACTORS

Avoid even minimal aluminum ingestion.

Aluminum absorption is enhanced in the presence of elevated circulating parathyroid hormone, and elevated parathyroid hormone leads to preferential deposition of aluminum in brain and bone. Dialysis pts. with aluminum-related vitamin D-resistant osteomalacia may be euparathyroid, however, because parathyroid hormone excess also seems to lead to aluminum deposition in the parathyroid gland, and aluminum has been shown *in vitro* to inhibit parathyroid hormone release. Since impaired renal function is not a prerequisite for increased tissue aluminum burdens, it is likely that aluminum-related osteomalacia will be observed in people with normal renal function (*Burnatowska-Hledin MA et al. Aluminum, parathyroid hormone, and osteomalacia. Spec Top Endocrinol Metab 5:201-26, 1983*).

Even small amounts, such as in aluminum-containing anacids, bind inorganic phosphorus in the intestines resulting in phosphorus depletion which, in turn, increases fecal calcium excretion causing a negative calcium balance. Fecal fluoride is also significantly increased, thus decreasing the intestinal absorption of fluoride (*Spencer H et al. Effect of small doses of aluminum-containing antacids on calcium and phosphorus metabolism. Am J Clin Nutr 36:32-40, 1982; Spencer H, Kramer L. Osteoporosis: Calcium, fluoride, and aluminum interactions. J Am Coll Nutr 4(1):121-28, 1985*).

Rule out <u>hydrochloric acid deficiency</u>.

40% of post-menopausal women have no basal gastric acid secretion (*Grossman M et al. Basal and histalog-stimulated gastric secretion in control subjects and in patients with peptic ulcer or gastric cancer. Gastroenterology 45:15-26, 1963*).

Deficiency impairs calcium absorption and increases urinary calcium excretion.

Experimental Study: Absorption of calcium carbonate was compared to the absorption of calcium in a pH-adjusted citrate form in 11 fasting achlorhydric pts. and 9 fasting controls. For the achlorhydric pts., mean calcium absorption was 0.452 for the citrate and 0.042 for the carbonate. For the controls, absorption was 0.243 for the citrate and 0.225 for the carbonate, suggesting that pH and/or the form of calcium salt affects calcium absorption in achlorhydric pts. (*Recker RR. Calcium absorption and achlorhydria. N Engl J Med 313(2):70-73, 1985*).

Negative Experimental Study: A large dose of cimetidine was given to increase intragastric pH but calcium absorption was unaffected, suggesting that gastric acid secretion and gastric acidity do not normally play a role in the absorption of dietary calcium (*Bo-Linn G et al. An evaluation of the importance of gastric acid secretion in the absorption of dietary calcium. J Clin Invest 73:640-7, 1983*).

Note: This study has been criticized on the following grounds:
1. Patients, with the exception of one, were not achlorhydric and thus may have had adequate acidity to dissolve the calcium load.
2. The test meal (pH 5.4) used lowered stomach pH, possibly increasing calcium solubilization.
3. The absorption method required lavage of the GI tract with 7.2 liters of a balanced solution that could have dissolved some of the calcium or increased absorption.
(Calcium absorption and the achlorhydric patient. Capsulations Number 2, August, 1985).

Experimental Study: 4 men with achlorhydria absorbed 0-2% of radiolabelled calcium carbonate. After histalog stimulation in 1 subject, gastric pH dropped from 6.5 to 1.0 and calcium absorption increased from 2% to 10% (*Ivanovich P et al. The absorption of calcium carbonate. Ann Intern Med 66:917-23, 1967*).

PAIN

See Also: **DYSMENORRHEA**
HEADACHE
MUSCLE CRAMPS
NEURALGIA AND NEUROPATHY
"RHEUMATISM"

DIETARY FACTORS

High fiber diet.

May be beneficial in cases of non-pathological, recurrent abdominal pain, perhaps because of its efficacy in irritable bowel syndrome.

Experimental Double-blind Study: Either high- or low-fiber cookies were randomly added to the diets of children with non-pathological, recurrent attacks of abdominal pain. 50% of the children who received the high-fiber cookies, but none of the children who received the low-fiber cookies, improved (*Christensen MF. Recurrent abdominal pain and dietary fiber. Letter. Am J Dis Child 140(8):738-39, 1986*).

Avoid coffee.

Has powerful opiate receptor binding activity.

In vitro Experimental Study: Instant coffee powders were found to compete with naloxone for binding to opiate receptors in rat brain membrane preparations irregardless of whether or not they contained caffeine. Instant tea, cocoa, soup powders, stock cubes and extracts of yogurt and cream cheese were without activity. The receptor binding activity resembled that seen with opiate antagonists and its concentration suggests that drinking coffee may be followed by effects mediated via opiate receptors (*Boublik JH et al. Coffee contains potent opiate receptor binding activity. Nature 301:246-48, 1983*).

Reduction in caffeine intake may reduce breast pain in fibrocystic breast disease.

Experimental Study: 138 pts. with symptoms of fibrocystic breast disease, including breast pain, were counseled to abstain from or reduce caffeine consumption. After 1 yr., 113 pts. (81.9%) had reduced their caffeine intake substantially and, of those, 69 (61%) reported a decrease or absence of breast pain (*Russell LC. Caffeine restriction as initial treatment for breast pain. Nurse Pract 14(2):36-37,40, 1989*).

- -

VITAMINS

Thiamine:

Massive IV doses (10-30 gm) produce ganglionic blockade and suppress the transmission of neural stimuli to skeletal muscles (*Lenot G. Note sur l'aneurine, anesthésique général. Ann Anesthésiol Franc 7(suppl 1):173-75, 1966; Mazzoni P, Valenti F. Un nuovo anestetico generale per via endovenosa - la tiamina. Acta Anesth (Padova) 15:815-28, 1964*).

Supplementation may be beneficial.

Experimental Study: 133 pts. who had failed to respond to physical therapy or analgesics received oral thiamine 1-2 gms daily to twice daily as needed. 54/69 (78%) of headache pts. improved; 8/69 complained of nausea. 40/56 (71/%) of pts. with joint or spine pain improved, and 5/8 pts. with neuralgia reported satisfactory or very good results. All 8 pts. who had used analgesics habitually (6 of whom had analgesic nephropathy) were satisfied with the pain-relief effect of thiamine and stopped abusing analgesics (*Quirin H. Pain and vitamin B₁ therapy. Bibl Nutr Dieta (38):110-1, 1986*).

Experimental Study: Thiamine was shown to have an analgesic effect. Analgesia from oral doses, however, failed to reach statistical significance (*Charonnat R, Lechat P. Sur le phénomène de réveil de l'anesthésie cornéenne. Thérapie 8:704, 1953*).

Note: The dosage used in this study was too low to show a significant effect (Quirin H. Pain and vitamin B₁ therapy. Bibl Nutr Dieta (38):110-1, 1986).

Vitamin B₆:

Supplementation may be beneficial.

Review Article: Chronic pain pts. have decreased pain thresholds and decreased serotonin levels. Also, after prolonged analgesic use, there appears to be a reduction in analgesic receptor sites which leads to a paradoxical increase in pain associated with increasing use of analgesics. Withdrawal of analgesics may produce rebound pain so that the use of serotonin-stimulating agents such as pyridoxine improves patient comfort. The use of pyridoxine is increasing as an adjunct in the treatment of chronic pain, especially for pts. being taken off all pain medication and for chronic pain associated with temporomandibular joint dysfunction. A dose of 100-150 mg/d appears to improve tolerance for drug withdrawal if started 4 wks. earlier (*Bernstein AL. Vitamin B₆ in neurology. Ann N Y Acad Sci 585:250-60, 1990*).

Vitamin B₁₂:

Supplementation may be beneficial.

Animal Experimental Study: Oral vitamin B₁₂ administered to rats was shown in 3 independent trials to have a dose-dependent analgesic effect. 5-10 μg/kg was comparable to 20 mg oral phenylbutazone (*Hanck A, Weiser H. Analgesic and anti-inflammatory properties of vitamins. Int J Vitam Nutr Res (suppl)27:189-206, 1985*).

Experimental Study: 400 pts. with vertebral pain and sensory disturbances received vitamin B₁₂ (hydroxycobalamin) 5000 μg IM or IV daily. After 6-16 days, the analgesic effect was "very good" or "good" in about 50% of the cases and, with the exception of 10 pts. who failed to respond, "satisfactory" in the rest (*Hieber H. Die behandlung vertebragener schmerzen und sensibilitätsstörungen mit hochdosiertem hydroxocobalamin. Med Monatsschr 28:545-48, 1974*).

Experimental Studies:
1. Pts. with pain due to degenerative neuropathy received 10,000 μg vitamin B₁₂ (cobamamide) daily. After 2 wks., 80% reported marked and prompt pain relief.
2. Pts. with pain due to cancer received 10,000 μg vitamin B₁₂ (cobamamide) daily. After 2 wks., 27% of pts. reported disappearance of pain, while 33% reported improvement (*Dettori AG, Ponari O. Effetto antalgico della cobamamide in corso di neuropatie periferiche di diversa etiopatogenesi. Minerva Med 64:1077-82, 1973*).

- and Thiamine and Vitamin B₆:

Combined supplementation may be beneficial.

Experimental Double-blind Study: 376 pts. with acute pain of the lumbar vertebrae randomly received either diclofenac 25 mg or a combination of diclofenac 25 mg plus thiamine nitrate 50 mg, pyridoxine hydrochloride 50 mg and cyanocabalamin 0.25 mg as 2 caps 3 times daily until pain was totally relieved or for a maximum of 2 weeks. 53/184 (29%) receiving the combination compared to 48/192 (25%) receiving diclofenac alone could stop treatment after 1 week. Results of the Hoppe Pain Questionnaire and the data concerning pain intensity also revealed better results with the combination. The differences in favor of the combination were significant in pts. with severe pain at the start of therapy. There were no significant differences in side effects (*Brüggemann G et al. [Results of a double-blind study of diclofenac + vitamin B₁, B₆, B₁₂ versus declofenac in patients with acute pain of the lumbar vertebrae. A multicenter study.] Klin Wochenschr 68(2):116-20, 1990*).

Animal Experimental Study: The effect of a compound of vitamins B_1, B_6 and B_{12} on the nociceptive responses of single neurons in the spinal cord dorsal horn in anesthetized cats was studied. Results indicate that the therapeutic effect of vitamin B compounds in the clinical management of pain may involve a suppression of nociceptive transmission at the spinal level (*Fu QG et al. B vitamins suppress spinal dorsal horn nociceptive neurons in the cat. Neurosci Lett 95(1-3):192-7, 1988*).

Vitamin C:

Supplementation may be beneficial.

Experimental Study: 21 adults aged 18-59 complaining of "sensitivity at the gum line" were tested for sensitivity to a jet of air directed at the facial surface of each exposed root. They then received 1 tsp (about 2.4 g) sodium ascorbate dissolved in juice or water every 15 min. until watery diarrhea occurred. The amt. was recorded, and 1 tsp less than that amt. was ingested on day 2 in divided doses. Treatment was continued for 4 days, and each day the dose was reduced by 1 teaspoon. Teeth which had previously beeen found to be sensitive were then retested. The median intake of sodium ascorbate the first day was 19 g (9-47 g; 4-20 tsp). After treatment, 10/21 reported that their sensitivity was completely gone, including 3/8 whose sensitivity had been continuous. 9/21 were improved and 2/21 were unchanged. Initially 306/525 teeth were air-sensitive and 125/525 were water-sensitive. Upon retesting, only 110/206 (36%) remained sensitive to air, and 53/125 (42%) remained sensitive to water ($p<10^{-5}$). Subsequent experience suggests that 1 tsp sodium ascorbate with meals and at bedtime (about 10g/d) may be adequate for pain relief while avoiding diarrhea (*Lytle RL. Chronic dental pain: Possible benefits of food restriction and sodium ascorbate. J Appl Nutr 40(2):95-98, 1988*).

Clinical Observation: Breast cancer pts. who no longer responded to the usual analgesics sometimes became pain-free when the analgesic was administered together with 10-25 gm vitamin C IV (*Hanck A, Weiser H. Analgesic and anti-inflammatory properties of vitamins. Int J Vitam Nutr Res (suppl) 27:189-206, 1985*).

Animal Experimental Study: Oral vitamin C administered to rats was shown to have a significant dose-dependent analgesic effect at a minimum of 500 mg/kg comparable to phenylbutazone 20 mg; by comparison a minimum of 125 mg/kg was required for a significant dose-dependent anti-inflammatory effect comparable to phenylbutazone 20 mg (*Hanck A, Weiser H. Analgesic and anti-inflammatory properties of vitamins. Int J Vitam Nutr Res (suppl)27:189-206, 1985*).

Experimental Double-blind Study: Severely ill cancer pts. receiving vitamin C 10 gm/day showed a significant reduction in pain (*Creagan ET et al. Failure of high-dose vitamin C (ascorbic acid) therapy to benefit patients with advanced cancer. N Engl J Med 301:687-90, 1979*).

Experimental Controlled Study: Vitamin C supplementation for pts. with post-suxamethonium pains following procedures such as esophagoscopy, bronchoscopy and direct laryngoscopy significantly reduced muscle pain (p=0.01). In addition, pain severity was greater in the control gp. compared to the supplemented patients (*Gupte SR, Savant NS. Post suxamethonium pains and vitamin C. Anaesthesia 26:436-40, 1971*).

Vitamin E:

Supplementation may reduce pain by activating the endorphin system.

Experimental Study: Pts. with algomenorrhea studied while in pain were supplemented with vitamin E until an analgesic effect was reached; 9 pts. had resumption of pain following naloxone administration. Compared to baseline, beta-endorphin-like immunoreactivity was increased in 7 pts. studied 15 min. after vitamin E administration. There was evidence that the efficacy of vitamin E depended upon the pathogenesis of the algomenorrhea. In some pts. for whom vitamin E had a strong analgesic effect, naloxone failed to cause the pain to return (*Kryzhanovskiĭ GN et al. [Endogenous opioid system in the realization of the analgesic effect of alpha-tocopherol.] Biull Eksp Biol Med 105(2):148-50, 1988*).

Vitamin K₁:

Supplementation may be beneficial.

> **Animal Experimental Study:** Oral, IM and IV vitamin K$_1$ administered to rats was shown to have a significant analgesic effect. Oily solutions, as the vehicle, were more effective than water-dispersible ones (*Hanck A, Weiser H. Analgesic and anti-inflammatory properties of vitamins. Int J Vitam Nutr Res (suppl)27:189-206, 1985*).

- -

MINERALS

Copper:

If deficient, may lower enkephalin levels to affect the endogenous control of pain perception.

> **Experimental Study:** 24 men were placed on a copper-deficient diet. As serum copper concentration decreased, enkephalin levels lowered. When copper levels were replenished, enkephalin levels in the pituitary and central nervous system rose (*Bhathena S et al. Decreased plasma enkephalins in copper deficiency in man. Am J Clin Nutr 43:42-46, 1986*).

Germanium sesquioxide:

May enhance morphine analgesia.

> **Animal Experimental Study:** As measured by the Tail-Flick test, Ge-132 enhanced morphine analgesia both following oral and intraperitoneal injection. The effect was completely abolished by Naloxone. Ge-132 alone intraperitoneally failed to show any antinociceptive action (*Hachisu M et al. Analgesic effect of novel organogermanium compound, Ge-132. J Pharmacobiodyn 6(11):814-20, 1983*).

Selenium:

A deficient intake may be associated with muscle pain (*van Rij AM et al. Selenium deficiency in total parenteral nutrition. Am J Clin Nutr 32:2076-85, 1979*).

Serum levels may be reduced.

> **Observational Study:** Compared to healthy controls, middle-aged women with sustained pains in the back and shoulder had lower serum selenium levels (*Jameson S et al. Effekter av selenvitamin E-behandling till kvinnor med lång variga arbetsrelaterade nack-och skuldersmärtor. En dubbelblindstudie. Läkaresällskapets Riksstämma, 1985*) (*in Swedish*).

- and Vitamin E:

Supplementation may be beneficial.

> **Experimental Double-blind Study:** 81 pts. with disabling muscular pain, stiffness and aching of long duration, received sodium selenite (140 μg Se) and α-tocopherol 100 mg daily or placebo. Following supplementation, glutathione peroxidase levels increased in 75% of the patients. Mean pain score reduction was significantly more frequent and more marked among pts. whose glutathione peroxidase levels increased than among those whose levels decreased. While pain score reduction was more pronounced among treated pts., the reduction as compared to pts. on placebo was not significant (*Jameson S et al. Pain relief and selenium balance in patients with connective tissue disease and osteoarthrosis: A double-blind selenium tocopherol supplementation study. Nutr Res Suppl 1:391-97, 1985*).

> **Experimental Double-blind Study:** Middle-aged women with sustained pains in the back and shoulder received selenium 200 μg and vitamin E or placebo in addition to physiotherapy. Women with initially high serum selenium or increasing levels were more often improved by the physiotherapy than the other women,

particularly if they were in the experimental group, suggesting that a relative selenium deficiency may have contributed to their pains (*Jameson S et al. Effekter av selenvitamin E-behandling till kvinnor med lång variga arbetsrelaterade nack-och skuldersmärtor. En dubbelblindstudie. Läkaresällskapets Riksstämma, 1985) (in Swedish)*.

- -

OTHER NUTRITIONAL FACTORS

D-Phenylalanine: 250 mg 15-30 minutes before meals 3 times daily (2 - 21 days for results)
                          Double the dose for up to another 3 wks. if ineffective.

Side effects: "jitters" or anxiety, headache, hypertension

Inhibits carboxypeptidase A which is involved in enkephalin degradation.

Potentiated in 50% of patients by ASA 325 mg. (or other prostaglandin inhibitor).

Supplementation may be effective for chronic pain, even when standard medications have provided limited or no relief.

Experimental Study: In a study of 8 healthy volunteers using the submaximal effort tourniquet test, DPA attenuated the increase of the intensity of the ischemic and pressure pain components with increasing ischemia duration, but only the effect on the pressure pain component was significant (*Nurmikko T et al. Attenuation of tourniquet-induced pain in man by D-phenylalanine, a putative inhibitor of enkephalin degradation. Acupunct Electrother Res 12(3-4):185-91, 1987)*.

Negative Experimental Double-blind Crossover Study: 30 pts. with chronic pain unrelieved by various treatments received either D-phenylalanine 250 mg 4 times daily or lactose placebo. After 4 wks., the gps. were crossed over for an additional 4 weeks. Pain was quantified using a visual analog pain scale and a cold pressor test. Results suggest that DPA is no better than placebo in chronic pain pts. (*Walsh NE et al. Analgesic effectiveness of D-phenylalanine in chronic pain patients. Arch Phys Med Rehabil 67(7):436-9, 1986)*.

Negative Animal Experimental Study: DPA was not found to exhibit opiate receptor-mediated analgesia in monkeys (*Halpern LM, Dong WK. D-phenylalanine: A putative enkephalinase inhibitor studied in a primate acute pain model. Pain 24:223-7, 1986)*.

Experimental Study: 43 pts. (most with osteoarthritis) were supplemented with DPA 250 mg 3-4 times daily for 4-5 weeks. Significant pain relief was achieved in the last 2 wks., especially in the osteoarthritis patients. The effectiveness of DPA increased with decreasing severity of pain (*Balagot RC et al. Analgesia in mice and humans by D-phenylalanine: Relation to inhibition of enkephalin degradation and enkephalin levels. Adv Pain Res Ther 5:289-92, 1983)*.

Note: A statistical analysis of the data using a binomial probability distribution revealed the effect of DPA to be insignificant (Walsh NE et al. Letter. Pain 409-10, 1986).

Experimental Double-blind Crossover Study: After 2 wks. of DPA 250 mg 3 times daily, 7/21 chronic pain pts. taken off all other medications noted over 50% pain relief which was not seen or maintained while on placebo. One pt. improved while on placebo as the second medication, while 13 pts. noted no significant pain relief from either DPA or placebo. Side effects on DPA and placebo were essentially the same (*Budd K. Use of D-phenylalanine, an enkephalinase inhibitor, in the treatment of intractable pain. Adv Pain Res Ther 5:305-308, 1983)*.

Note: The Balagot study (see above) suggests that a longer study period may have resulted in greater therapeutic effects.

Note: A statistical analysis of the data using McNamar's test for the significance of changes revealed the effect of DPA to be insignificant (Walsh NE et al. Letter. Pain 409-10, 1986).

Supplementation may potentiate acupuncture analgesia.

Experimental Placebo-controlled Studies:
1.) 30 pts. with chronic low back pain were treated with acupuncture 30 min. after the oral administration of DPA 4 g or of placebo. The anesthetic effect was increased 26% in the DPA gp., but failed to reach significance ($p < 0.1$).
2.) 18/56 pts. who had tooth extractions under acupuncture anesthesia had received DPA orally 30 min. earlier while the rest of the gp. received placebo. The cases with excellent and good results (14/18) were compared to controls and the pain-relieving effect was significantly increased by 35% ($p < 0.01$) (*Kitade T et al. Studies on the enhanced effect of acupuncture analgesia and acupuncture anesthesia by D-phenylalanine (2nd report) — schedule of administration and clinical effects in low back pain and tooth extraction.* Acupunct Electrother Res *15(2):121-35, 1990*).

Experimental Studies:
1.) In all 5 subjects whose pain threshold (PT) was raised after acupuncture anesthesia (respondents), the rise in PT was significantly prolonged by the pre-administration of DPA.
2.) In 5/10 subjects whose PT remained almost unchanged by acupuncture anesthesia (non-respondents), the PT was increased by DPA.
3.) The rise in PT was most prominent when DPA was administered 30 min. prior to acupuncture anesthesia.
4.) In all 4 respondents in whom the rise in PT persisted after DPA and acupuncture anesthesia, their raised PT dropped after an IV naloxone injection.
(*Kitade T et al. Studies on the enhanced effect of acupuncture analgesia and acupuncture anesthesia by D-phenylalanine (first report): effect on pain threshold and inhibition by naloxone.* Acupunct Electrother Res *13(2-3):87-97, 1988*).

Experimental Placebo-controlled Study: 15 pts. were divided into acupuncture responsive and non-responsive groups and pre-treatment with DPA or placebo was given. In the responsive group, all showed increases in pain threshold and greater analgesic persistence. In the non-responsive group, half showed increases. Placebo preadministration was ineffective (*Hyodo M et al.* Adv Pain Res Ther *5:577-82, 1983*).

Animal Experimental Study: After DPA, acupuncture non-responsive animals became responsive with enhanced analgesic persistence (*Takeshirge M et al. Parallel individual variations in effectiveness of acupuncture, morphine analgesia, and dorsal PAG-SPA and their abolition by D-phenylalanine.* Adv Pain Res Ther *5:563-8, 1983*).

Potentiates morphine analgesia and antagonizes morphine tolerance and dependence in rats (*Hachisu M et al. Relationship between enhancement of morphine analgesia and inhibition of enkephalinase by 2S, 3R 3-amino-2-hydroxy-4 - phenylbuanoic acid derivatives.* Life Sci. *30:1739-46, 1982*), perhaps because chronic morphine administration increases enkephalinase activity which results in reduced endorphin levels (*Malfroy B et al. High-affinity enkephalin-degrading pepidase in brain is increased after morphine.* Nature *276:523-26, 1978*).

L-Tryptophan: 2 - 4 grams daily (1 month trial)
                 Take with sugar.
                 Avoid protein for 90 min. before and afterwards.

Serotonin (5-hydroxytryptamine), which is derived from dietary tryptophan, is one of the many neurotransmitters involved in modulating pain perception and may be involved in opiate-produced analgesia.

WARNING: May reduce the efficacy of morphine analgesia (*Franklin KB et al. Tryptophan-morphine interactions and postoperative pain.* Pharmacol Biochem Behav *35(1):157-63, 1990*).

Supplementation may be beneficial.

Review Article: Clinical applications for tryptophan may be as (a) a mild analgesic similar to ASA or acetaminophen which can be used in combination with one of them; (b) in combination with diazepam or similar compound to avoid narcotic use; (c) treatment of a possible sub-class of chronic pain pts. with a disorder of serotonergic transmission (*Liberman HR et al. Mood, performance and pain sensitivity: Changes induced by food constituents.* J Psychiatr Res *17:135-45, 1983*).

Specific effects of supplementation:

1. May raise pain tolerance threshold.

Experimental Double-blind Study (chronic maxillofacial pain): 30 chronic pain pts. were placed on a high carbohydrate, low fat, low protein diet and were randomly assigned to a tryptophan (3 gm daily) or placebo group. After 4 wks., there was a a greater increase in pain tolerance threshold in the tryptophan group, while both gps. noted lower anxiety and depression (*Seltzer S et al. The effects of dietary tryptophan on chronic maxillofacial pain and experimental pain tolerance. J Psychiatr Res 17:181-6, 1982-3*).

Experimental Double-blind Study (dental pulp stimulation): 30 normal subjects received either L-tryptophan 2 gms daily in divided doses or placebo. On the eighth day, pain induction through dental pulp stimulation showed pain perception threshold levels to be similar in both groups, while pain tolerance thresholds were significantly higher in the experimental group. Side-effects such as nausea, skin itching, weight loss and mood elevation were more common in the experimental than in the control group (*Seltzer S et al. Alteration of human pain thresholds by nutritional manipulation and L-tryptophan supplementation. Pain 13(4):385-93, 1982*).

Experimental Placebo-controlled Study: 30 healthy subjects were placed on a high carbohydrate, low protein, low fat diet which was supplemented with tryptophan 2 gms daily or placebo. While pain perception thresholds (as measured by electrical stimulation of dental pulps) were the same in both gps., pain tolerance levels were significantly higher in the experimental group (*Seltzer S et al. Alteration of human pain thresholds by nutritional manipulation and L-tryptophan supplementation. Pain 13:385-93, 1982*).

2. May restore post-op analgesia in patients with dorsal rhizotomies and/or cordotomies for intractable pain.

Experimental Study: 5 pts. who had previously undergone dorsal rhizotomy and/or cordotomies for intractable pain, with resulting initial but temporary postoperative sensory deficits leading to the return of pain, were supplemented with L-tryptophan 2 gm daily. After 1 month the analgesic and anesthetic areas began to spread or reappear. In 3-4 months, the maximum sensory deficit imposed by surgery was re-established, and the pts. were essentially pain-free. In addition, 6 pts. with recurrent or persistent facial pain following denervation procedures had a similar result, while 8 pts. with pain due to a peripheral nerve injury showed no change in sensory deficit or pain relief (*King RB. Pain and tryptophan. J Neurosurg 53(1):44-52, 1980*).

3. May reverse tolerance to opiates.

Experimental Study: 5 pts. with low back and leg pain on chronic opiate medication were determined to have developed opiate tolerance. Following 2-9 wks. of supplementation with L-tryptophan 4 gm daily, they achieved significant pain relief during the opiate tolerance test and were able to lead more active lives by reducing opiate intake (*Hosobuchi Y et al. Tryptophan loading may reverse tolerance to opiate analgesics in humans: A preliminary report. Pain 9:161-169, 1980*).

4. May reduce reports of clinical pain.

Negative Experimental Controlled Study (chronic myofascial pain): No significant reduction in pain was noted in pt. gps. receiving tryptophan with dietary manipulation compared to control groups (*Stockstill JW et al. The effect of L-tryptophan supplementation and dietary instruction on chronic myofascial pain. J Am Dent Assoc 118(4):457-60, 1989*).

Experimental Placebo-controlled Study (acute pain following root-canal therapy): Subjects given tryptophan 3 gm in 6 divided doses over the first 24 hrs. following the procedure (the period of worst pain) recorded a significantly lower level of pain at 24 hrs. after surgery than those taking placebo (p<0.01) (*Shpeen SE et al. The effect of tryptophan on postoperative endodontic pain. Oral Surg Oral Med Oral Pathol 58(4):446-449, 1984*).

- with a <u>high carbohydrate, low fat, low protein</u> diet.

Experimental Double-blind Study (chronic maxillofacial pain): 30 chronic pain pts. were placed on a high carbohydrate, low fat, low protein diet and were randomly assigned to a tryptophan (3 gm daily) or placebo group. After 4 wks., there was a greater reduction in reported clinical pain in the tryptophan group, while both gps. noted lower anxiety and depression (*Seltzer S et al. The effects of dietary tryptophan on chronic maxillofacial pain and experimental pain tolerance. J Psychiatr Res 17:181-6, 1982-3*).

OTHER FACTORS:

Rule out food sensitivities.

Abdominal Pain:

May be due to lactose intolerance.

Negative Experimental Double-blind Study: 40 children with recurrent abdominal pain of at least 3 months' duration were studied. Although 12 children (30%) were lactose malabsorbers, only 3 malabsorbed part of a smaller, more physiologic, lactose load (12.5 g vs. 2 g/kg). Improvement rates of lactose malabsorbers and absorbers during lactose elimination were not significantly different (*Wald A et al. Lactose malabsorption in recurrent abdominal pain of childhood. J Pediatr 100(1):65-8, 1982*).

Negative Experimental Double-blind Study: 103 white children aged 6-14 with recurrent abdominal pain were evaluated. 21/69 (30.4%) had abnormal lactose tolerance tests and 8/26 (31%) were lactase deficient. However, 16/61 (26.4%) of controls matched for age and ethnic background were also lactase deficient. 38 pts. completed 3 successive 6-wk. double-blind diet trials. An increase above baseline value in pain frequency was seen in 10/21 (48%) lactose malabsorbers and 4/17 (24%) lactose absorbers. After a 12-mo. milk elimination diet, 6/15 (40%) malabsorbers and 5/13 (38%) absorbers had elimination of their pain. This result compares with improvement in 5/12 (42%) absorbers who received a regular diet for 1 yr. and suggests that lactose elimination will not affect the overall frequency of improvement in recurrent abdominal pain (*Lebenthal E et al. Recurrent abdominal pain and lactose absorption in children. Pediatrics 67(6):828-32, 1981*).

Experimental Study: 80 schoolchildren with recurrent abdominal pain were studied prospectively. Malabsorption was documented in 40% on the basis of elevated breath hydrogen. Those with lactose malabsorption were not clinically distinguishable on the basis of past milk ingestion (p>0.05), weekly pain frequency (median, 5 vs. 6 times), presence of diarrhea (40 vs. 27%) or symptom response to a lactose load. In children with malabsorption who completed a 6-wk. diet trial, 70% reported increased pain frequency (p<0.002) when placed on their usual lactose-containing diet (*Barr RG et al. Recurrent abdominal pain of childhood due to lactose intolerance. N Engl J Med 300(26):1449-52, 1979*).

Experimental Study: In a study of 166 hospitalized male pts., abnormal lactose tolerance tests were found in 81% of 98 blacks, 12% of 59 whites of Scandinavian or Northwestern European extraction, and 33% of 9 non-European whites. 72% of the lactose-intolerant pts. had previously realized that milk drinking could induce abdominal and bowel symptoms. 240 ml of low-fat milk produced gaseousness or cramps in 59% of 44 lactose-intolerant men, and 68% were symptomatic with the equivalent amt. of lactose. None of the 18 lactose-intolerant men noted symptoms with milk or lactose. Refusal to drink 240 ml of low-fat milk served with meals correlated significantly with lactose-intolerance: 31.4% vs. 12.9% among lactose-tolerant patients (*Bayless TM et al. Lactose and milk intolerance: Clinical implications. N Engl J Med 292(22):1156-9, 1975*

Dental Pain:

Clinical Observations: Pts. with dental pain were instructed to eat a single food for 4 days (usually watermelon, fresh vegetable juice or orange juice). In case of poor compliance, lightly steamed vegetables were added or substituted. All pts. used only distilled or spring water. After 4 days, pts. added 1 food at a time. If a reaction occurred, that food was avoided 60-90 days and an attempt was made to reintroduce it no more often than every 4 days. In addition to the chronic dental pain from exposed roots and temporomandibular joint discomfort, food intolerances were found to trigger or exacerbate sinus problems and toothache and to affect the depth or profoundness of local dental anesthesia (*Lytle RL. Chronic dental pain: Possible benefits of food restriction and sodium ascorbate. J Appl Nutr 40(2):95-98, 1988*).

Muscle and Joint Pain:

Case Reports: 2 women with severe intractable back pain of several yrs. duration together with other musculoskeletal and systemic symptoms were found to be sensitive to a number of foods, chemicals and inhalants. Both improved rapidly on fasting and were treated with oligoantigenic diets and neutralization therapy. On follow-up, they remained well, apart from infrequent reactions due to dietary lapses (*Maberly DJ, Honor MA. A reversible back pain syndrome: report of two cases. J Nutr Med 2:83-7, 1991*).

Clinical Observations and Case Reports: Pts. with allergic toxemia may present with aching and soreness in muscles and joints along with allergic fatigue, mental confusion, dopiness, inability to concentrate, irritability, depression, etc. A food elimination diet will reveal the diagnosis (*Rowe AH. Allergic fatigue and toxemia. Ann Allergy 17:9-18, 1959*).

PARKINSON'S DISEASE

DIETARY FACTORS

Low protein diet.

WARNING: May require reduction of L-dopa dosage.

May control the daily fluctuations in efficacy of L-dopa.

Experimental Study: 5 pts. with motor fluctuations on L-dopa were placed on a high protein diet (1.6 g/kg) (which represents the standard American protein intake), or a low protein diet (0.8 g/kg) (which is the US RDA of protein) with protein evenly distributed between meals, and a low protein diet with 90% of protein consumed at the evening meal. Symptoms such as tapping and tremor improved during the low protein diet and pts. were able to walk for greater amts. of time. Both reducing the dietary protein content and eating most protein in the evening significantly improved their symptoms; these effects were unrelated to L-dopa absorption, but appeared to be due to variation in the plasma large amino acids (*Carter J et al. Amount and distribution of dietary protein affects clinical response to levodopa in Parkinson's disease. Neurology 39:552-56, 1989*).

Experimental Double-blind Study: 10 pts. aged 48-81 on L-dopa and carbidopa randomly received a high protein diet (80g for men; 70g for women) and a low protein diet (50g for men; 40g for women) for one wk. each in either order. Patients' symptoms were found to be significantly better while on the low-protein diet. These results did not correlate with L-dopa levels, which had higher peaks in 3 pts. while they were on the high protein diets despite inferior performance and increased number of "off" hours; thus high dietary protein probably affects the efficacy of L-dopa at a central level (*Tsui J et al. The effect of dietary protein on the efficacy of L-dopa: A double-blind study. Neurology 39:549-52, 1989*).

- -

VITAMINS

Folic Acid:

Deficiency may be associated with Parkinsonism (*Clayton P et al. Subacute combined degeneration of the cord, dementia and parkinsonism due to an inborn error of folate metabolism. J Neurol Neurosurg Psychiatry 49:920-7, 1986*).

Niacin:

Treatment with L-dopa, especially when given concurrently with a decarboxylase inhibitor such as carbidopa or benserazide, places patients at risk for niacin deficiency.

Review Article: Decarboxylase inhibitors inhibit the enzyme kyurenine hydrolase in rat and mouse liver, resulting in reduced synthesis of nicotinamide coenzymes from tryptophan and an increased reliance on dietary niacin. Also, the urinary excretion of 1-N-methyl-nicotinamide, a product of nicotinamide nucleotide metabolism, is considerably reduced in pts. treated with L-dopa alone or L-dopa in combination with a decarboxylase inhibitor (*Bender DA et al. Niacin depletion in Parkinsonian patients treated with L-dopa, benserazide and carbidopa. Clin Sci 56(1):89-93, 1979*).

Supplementation with niacin or 1-N-methylnicotinamide, its metabolite, may extend the period of elevated brain dopamine levels with L-dopa treatment (*Black MJ, Brandt RB. Nicotinic acid or N-methyl nicotinamide prolongs elevated brain dopa and dopamine in L-dopa treatment. Biochem Med Metab Biol 36(2):244-51, 1986*).

Tetrahydrobiopterin is the cofactor for the enzyme tyrosine hydroxylase which catalyzes the conversion of tyrosine to L-dopa, and nicotinamide adenine dinucleotide (NADH), a coenzyme formed from niacin, is involved in its synthesis.

Supplementation with NADH may be beneficial.

> **Experimental Study:** 34 pts. received NADH parenterally. All improved, and 21/34 (62%) had a better than 30% improvement of disability. The best therapeutic dose was 25-50 mg/d. Clinical improvement was more pronounced after IV than after IM administration (*Birkmayer W et al. Nicotinamidadenindinucleotide (NADH): The new approach in the therapy of Parkinson's disease. Ann Clin Lab Sci 19:38-43, 1989*).

Thiamine:

May help to prevent Parkinson's and other diseases involving neurotransmitter loss.

> **In vitro Experimental Study:** Out of a wide range of compounds studied for their ability to inhibit dopamine oxidation at pH 7.5 in phosphate buffer, thiamine was one of the most effective inhibitors and completely inhibited oxidation both in the presence and absence of manganese (*Florence TM, Stauber JL. Neurotoxicity of manganese. Letter. Lancet 1:363, 1988*).

Vitamin B$_6$:

The enzyme dopa decarboxylase, which catalyzes the conversion of dopa to dopamine, is dependent upon pyridoxal phosphate.

> WARNING: Supplementation may counteract the effects of L-dopa unless L-dopa is given currently with carbidopa (*AMA Drug Evaluations, Fifth Edition. Chicago, American Medical Association, 1983*).

Treatment with L-dopa alone may enhance plasma and RBC pyridoxal-5-phosphate concentrations.

> **Experimental Study:** Compared to 8 controls, after both 10 mg and 100 mg pyridoxine, plasma and RBC pyridoxal-5-phosphate concentrations of 8 chronic levodopa-treated pts. were significantly higher (*Mars H. Effect of chronic levodopa treatment on pyridoxine metabolism. Neurology 25(3):263-6, 1975*).

Treatment with L-dopa plus a decarboxylase inhibitor may provoke a marginal vitamin B$_6$ deficiency.

> **Experimental Study:** Pts. treated with L-dopa plus a decarboxylase inhibitor, but not those treated with L-dopa alone, show a reduced excretion of xanthurenic acid, and an increased excretion of kynurenine, as would be expected after inhibition of the kynurenine pathway, and possibly indicative of a marginal vitamin B$_6$ deficiency (*Bender DA et al. Niacin depletion in Parkinsonian patients treated with L-dopa, benserazide and carbidopa. Clin Sci 56(1):89-93, 1979*).

Supplementation may be beneficial.

> **Experimental Study:** 60 pts. with parkinsonism of various etiologies with pronounced tremor were effectively treated with IM doses of vitamin B$_6$. Single doses were 1-400 mg; total doses were 3-6000 mg. EMG, tremorographic and myotonometric findings correlated with the clinical picture. Vitamin B$_6$ is recommended irrespective of the etiology of the disease and of the patient's age, and can be given either alone or in combination with anti-parkinsonian drugs except DOPA. High doses of B$_6$ are not recommended, however, for pts. with angina or exacerbations of coronary insufficiency (*Vaïnshtok AB. [Treatment of parkinsonism with large doses of vitamin B$_6$.] Sov Med (7):14-9, 1979*) (*in Russian*).

> **Experimental Study:** 15 pts. received pyridoxine 10-100 mg IV daily for 2-4 wks. supplemented in most cases by oral brewers' yeast. 4/9 with idopathic or arteriosclerotic parkinsonism improved, as well as 2 of the other 6 patients. Those who improved developed bladder control and a steadier gait, while cramps, trembling and rigidity decreased. The improved pts. noted decreased fatigability, better sleeping and increased appetite. In addition, 4 pts. with arteriosclerotic or idiopathic parkinsonism received oral pyridoxine hydrochloride 50 mg daily for 3 wks. supplemented by 54 gr of brewers' yeast. 2/4 believed themselves to have improved; however only in one was there an observable decrease in tremor and rigidity (*Baker AB. Treatment of paralysis agitans with vitamin B$_6$ (pyridoxine hydrochloride). JAMA 116:2484-7, 1941*).

Negative Experimental Study: 7 pts. (4 with arterioclerotic parkinsonism; 3 with post-encephalitic parkinsonism; 1 with idopathic parkinsonism) received pyridoxine hydrochloride 50-100 mg IV for 1-2 weeks. Care was taken to explain the experimental nature of the procedure to minimize placebo effects. None showed objective improvement; one noted subjective improvement. The later pt. responded equally well to saline injections (*Barker WH et al. Failure of pyridoxine (vitamin B6) to modify the Parkinsonian syndrome. Bull Johns Hopkins Hosp 69:266-75, 1941*).

Negative Experimental Study: 10 pts. with post-encephalitic parkinsonism and 5 pts. with arteriosclerotic parkinsonism received daily IV injections of 50-100 mg pyridoxine hydrochloride without benefit (*Zeligs MA. Use of pyridoxine hydrochloride (vitamin B6) in parkinsonism. JAMA 116:2148, 1941*).

Experimental Study: 15 pts. with severe involvement received 50-100 mg pyridoxine hydrochloride IV. 4/15 showed definite objective improvement. The best results were in the idopathic or arteriosclerotic type of the disease (*Jolliffe N. Clinical aspects of vitamin B deficiencies. Minn Med 23:542, 1940*).

Thiamine and
Vitamin B6:

Combined treatment by intraspinal injection may be beneficial.

Experimental Study: 5 pts. with postencephalitic Parkinsonism obtained temporary relaxation of rigidity following 2-3 intraspinal injections of pyridoxine 5-25 mg and thiamine 5-10 mg. The severity of their tremors, however, was unchanged (*Stone S. Pyridoxine and thiamine therapy in disorders of the nervous system. Dis Nerv Sys 11(5):131-8, 1950*).

Vitamin C: one month trial

May be decreased in the amygdaloid nucleus (*Riederer P et al. Transition metals, ferritin, glutathione, and ascorbic acid in parkinsonian brains. J Neurochem 52(2):515-20, 1989*).

May help to prevent Parkinson's and other diseases involving neurotransmitter loss.

In vitro Experimental Study: Out of a wide range of compounds studied for their ability to inhibit dopamine oxidation at pH 7.5 in phosphate buffer, ascorbic acid was one of the most effective inhibitors and completely inhibited oxidation both in the presence and absence of manganese (*Florence TM, Stauber JL. Neurotoxicity of manganese. Letter. Lancet 1:363, 1988*).

Supplementation may counteract the adverse side-effects of L-dopa.

Experimental Double-blind Crossover Study: Pts. who experience "on-off" effects on levodopa have higher RBC catechol-o-methyltransferase (COMT) activities and plasma 3-o-methyldopa concentrations than do pts. without these levodopa-related motor fluctuations. Since ascorbic acid is a weak competitive inhibitor of COMT, 6 pts. with on-off effects were given ascorbic acid. Although supplementation produced a modest improvement in functional performance, no fundamental change was observed in the pattern of on-off effects, severity of parkinsonism/dyskinesia, or self-assessment ratings. Ascorbic acid reduced plasma concentrations of levodopa and 3-o-methyldopa but did not alter RBC COMT activity (*Reilly DK et al. On-off effects in Parkinson's disease: a controlled investigation of ascorbic acid therapy. Adv Neurol 37:51-60, 1983*).

Experimental Double-blind Case Study: 62 year-old male had stopped levodopa because of intolerable nausea and salivation. Levodopa was re-instituted along with ascorbic acid. After 4 wks, his ability to move his head increased, salivation decreased, and speech and handwriting improved considerably. Hand coordination improved so markedly that he began to play the organ for the first time in several years. Several times placebo was substituted for vitamin C on a double-blind basis. Each time his condition deteriorated on placebo and improved with vitamin C (*Sacks W, Simpson GM. Ascorbic acid in levodopa therapy. Letter. Lancet 1:527, 1975*).

<u>Vitamin E</u>:

Dietary intake in early life is negatively associated with the risk of Parkinson's disease.

> **Observational Study:** The early-life intake of vitamin E-rich foods of 106 pts. were compared to their spouses who served as controls. Female pts. were less likely than spouses to have eaten peanuts and peanut butter (p<0.05) which are high in vitamin E. The male-predominant pt. gp. was more likely than spouses to have eaten salad with dressing (p<0.05), which is also high in vitamin E. Separate comparison of male controls with female controls ruled out sex-related preferences to explain the findings (*Golbe LI et al. Follow-up study of early-life protective and risk factors in Parkinson's disease. <u>Mov Disord</u> 5(1):66-70, 1990*).

> **Observational Study:** A retrospective case-control study on the early life dietary habits of Parkinson's pts. revealed an unexpected association between the absence of Parkinson's disease and the preference for nuts, salad oil or dressing, and plums, all of which have a higher vitamin E content than the other items on the dietary questionnaire (*Golbe LI et al. Case-control study of early life dietary factors in Parkinson's disease. <u>Arch Neurol</u> 45:1350-53, 1988*).

Supplementation may be beneficial.

> **Theoretical Discussion:** There is scientific evidence supporting the hypothesis that oxidative mechanisms in dopaminergic neurons may contribute to cell death and the progression of Parkinson's disease. Clinical trials are now underway to assess the protective effect of augmenting the free radical scavenging system with vitamin E (*Grimes JD et al. Prevention of progression of Parkinson's disease with antioxidative therapy. <u>Prog Neuropsychopharmacol Biol Psychiatry</u> 12(2-3):165-72, 1988*).

> **Observational Study:** In a retrospective study, pts. who were taking vitamin E 400-3200 IU daily for an ave. of 7 yrs. showed significantly less symptoms than age-matched unsupplemented pts. and were better able to carry out activities of daily living (*Factor SA. Retrospective evaluation of vitamin E therapy in Parkinson's disease. Presented at: Vitamin E: Biochemistry and Health Implications. N Y Academy of Sciences Meeting, New York, November, 1988*).

> **Negative Case Report:** A pt. developed Parkinson's disease at the age of 56 after taking at least 400 IU vitamin E daily. There was no evidence that the supplement materially altered the history of his illness or his response to levodopa and selegiline (*Stern GM. Vitamin E and Parkinson's disease. Letter. <u>Lancet</u> 1:508, 1987*).

> **Theoretical Discussion:** The devleopment of a Parkinson-like syndrome in addicts who were using the compound methyl-phenyl-pyridine has refocused attention on the possible participation of free radicals in the etiology of PD. It is postulated that the use of the free radical scavengers, vitamin E and selenium, might be effective in the early treatment of PD and might help to circumvent some of the complications associated with agonist therapy (*Cadet JL. The potential use of vitamin E and selenium in parkinsonism. <u>Med Hypotheses</u> 20(1):87-94, 1986*).

<u>Vitamin C</u> and
<u>Vitamin E</u>:

> In Parkinson's disease, dopamine-containing cells in the substantia nigra may be damaged by increased lipid peroxidation.

>> **Observational Study:** Compared to controls, lipid peroxidation was increased in parkinsonian nigral tissue, adversely affecting dopamine-containing cells, perhaps because of continued exposure to excess free radicals derived from some endogenous or exogenous neurotoxic species (*Dexter DT et al. Basal lipid peroxidation in substantia nigra is increased in Parkinson's disease. <u>J Neurochem</u> 52(2):381-9, 1989; Dexter DT et al. Lipid peroxidation as cause of nigral cell death in Parkinson's disease. Letter. <u>Lancet</u> 2:639-40, 1986*).

> Supplementation with antioxidants (such as vitamins C and E) may be beneficial.

>> **Experimental Study:** 15 pts. were given vitamin C 3000 mg and vitamin E 3,200 IU in gradually increasing doses. Compared to unsupplemented pts., they were able to delay starting standard drug treatment for 2 1/2 yrs. longer (*Fahn S. An open trial of high-dosage antioxidants in early Parkinson's disease. <u>Am J Clin Nutr</u> 53:380S-1S, 1991*).

- -

MINERALS

Copper:

Levels may be elevated in the cerebrospinal fluid and may exert a pro-oxidative effect.

Observational Study: CSF copper concentration was significantly higher in 24 pts. with untreated, idiopathic Parkinson's disease than in 34 controls ($p<0.001$). The diffference in the *in vitro* capacity of copper to damage DNA, measured by the phenanthroline assay, was even greater. The high phenanthroline-copper concentration correlated with disease severity ($p=0.02$) and with the rate of progression of the disease ($p<0.05$). Results suggest a possible role for copper-catalyzed oxidative mechanisms in the pathogenesis of Parkinson's disease and raise the possibility of treatment with copper-chelating agents, which have been successful in the treatment of Wilson's disease (*Pall HS et al. Raised cerebrospinal-fluid copper concentration in Parkinson's disease. Lancet 2:238-41, 1987*).

Levels in the substantia nigra may be depressed (*Dexter DT et al. Increased nigral iron content and alterations in other metal ions occurring in brain in Parkinson's disease. J Neurochem 52(6):1830-6, 1989; Uitti RJ et al. Regional metal concentrations in Parkinson's disease, other chronic neurological diseases, and control brains. Can J Neurol Sci 16(3):310-4, 1989*).

Iron:

WARNING: The administration of iron (ferrous sulfate) together with levodopa and carbidopa may reduce the drugs' efficacies, at least in some patients, due to the formation of chemical complexes with iron (*Cambpell NR et al. Sinemet-ferrous sulphate interaction in patients with Parkinson's disease. Br J Clin Pharmacol 30(4):599-605, 1990*).

Excessive exposure may promote the development of Parkinson's disease.

Observational Study: 42 pts. were compared to 84 matched controls. An increased risk for PD seems to be associated with occupational exposure to manganese, iron and aluminum (odds ratio: 2.28; $p=0.07$) especially when the exposure is longer than 30 yrs. (odds ratio: 13.64; $p≤0.05$) (*Zayed J et al. [Environmental factors in the etiology of Parkinson's disease.] Can J Neurol Sci 17(3):286-91, 1990*).

Levels in substantia nigra pars compacta may be elevated.

Observational Study: There was a significant selective increase of iron (III) and ferritin in substantia nigra zona compacta but not in zona reticulata of Parkinsonian, but not in Alzheimer's, brains (*Jellinger K et al. Brain iron and ferritin in Parkinson's and Alzheimer's diseases. J Neural Transm Park Dis Dement Sect 2(4):327-40, 1990*).

Increased iron in substantia nigra pars compacta is not solely the consequence of neuronal degeneration (*Hirsch EC et al. Iron and aluminum increase in the substantia nigra of patients with Parkinson's disease: an X-ray microanalysis. J Neurochem 56(2):446-51, 1991*).

Increased iron in substantia nigra pars compacta may promote the generation of hydrogen peroxide and oxygen free radicals by participating in the autooxidation of dopamine (*Sofic E et al. Selective increase of iron in substantia nigra zona compacta of parkinsonian brains. J Neurochem 56(3):978-82, 1991*).

Review Article: The evidence that iron accumulates in substantia nigra pars compacta of pts. is compatible with changes in the respiratory chain activity, increased malondialdehyde concentration (a measure of lipid peroxidation), decreased activity of the enzymes involved in the detoxification of hydrogen peroxide and oxygen radical species, increased MAO-B activity, etc. All of these data suggest that oxidative stress may play a role in the pathobiochemistry of PD (*Youdim MB et al. The role of monamine oxidase, iron-melanin interaction, and intracellular calcium in Parkinson's disease. J Neural Transm Suppl 32:239-48, 1990*).

Levels in the globus pallidus may be decreased (*Dexter DT et al. Increased nigral iron content and alterations in other metal ions occurring in brain in Parkinson's disease. J Neurochem 52(6):1830-6, 1989*).

The activity of tyrosine hydroxylase, an enzyme which is involved in the production of dopa from tyrosine which requires iron as coenzyme, is reduced in Parkinson's disease and can be stimulated by iron supplementation, which may reduce the "off-effects" of levodopa in Parkinsonism.

> **Experimental Study:** Oxyferriscarbone, an iron complex, was given IV to 8 male and 2 female pts. (ages 54-77) who were in akinetic crisis. Disability scores decreased from an ave. of 70% before iron treatment to 42%. Posture and ability to walk improved remarkably. All pts. experienced considerable benefit, and no side effects were reported. In 3 pts. L-dopa treatment could be discontinued, while in 4 pts. drug treatment was reduced. The effects of iron supplementation were dose-dependent and lasted 24-48 hrs. (*Birkmayer W, Birkmayer JGD. Iron, a new aid in the treatment of Parkinson patients. J Neural Trans 67:287-92, 1986*).

Magnesium:

May be reduced in the caudate nucleus (*Uitti RJ et al. Regional metal concentrations in Parkinson's disease, other chronic neurological diseases, and control brains. Can J Neurol Sci 16(3):310-4, 1989*).

Manganese:

Excessive exposure increases the risk of Parkinsonism (or a Parkinson-like syndrome). When accumulated by inhalation, it is concentrated in the basal ganglia (*Mena I. Manganese, in F Bronner, JW Coburn, Eds. Disorders of Mineral Metabolism. I. Trace Minerals. New York, Academic Press, 1981:233-70; Mena I et al. Chronic manganese poisoning. Clinical picture and manganese turnover. Neurology 17:128-36, 1967; Zayed J et al. [Environmental factors in the etiology of Parkinson's disease.] Can J Neurol Sci 17(3):286-91, 1990*).

Neurotoxicity results from the depletion of dopamine and the production of the neurotoxins dopamine quinone and hydrogen peroxide (*Florence TM, Stauber JL. Neurotoxicity of manganese. Letter. Lancet 1:363, 1988*).

Levels in the medial putamen may be slightly decreased (*Dexter DT et al. Increased nigral iron content and alterations in other metal ions occurring in brain in Parkinson's disease. J Neurochem 52(6):1830-6, 1989*).

Zinc:

Levels in the substantia nigra, the caudate nucleus and lateral putamen may be increased (*Dexter DT et al. Increased nigral iron content and alterations in other metal ions occurring in brain in Parkinson's disease. J Neurochem 52(6):1830-6, 1989*).

— —

OTHER NUTRITIONAL FACTORS

L-Dopa: (L-dihydroxyphenylalanine)

Precursor to dopamine.

Parkinsonian brains show a massive deficit of striatal dopamine (*Hornykiewicz O. Parkinson's disease: from brain homogenate to treatment. Fed Proc 32:183-90, 1973*).

Currently used routinely in treatment.

> WARNING: Should be combined with a low-protein diet as it is a large, neutral amino acid that must compete with leucine, isoleucine, valine, tryptophan, tyrosine, phenylalanine and methionine for passage across the blood-brain barrier (*Pardridge WM. Regulation of amino acid availability to the brain, in R Wurtman, J Wurtman, Eds. Nutrition and the Brain, Vol. 1. New York, Raven Press, 1977:141-204*); thus even a single high protein meal will decrease its efficacy (*Mena I, Cotzias GC. Protein intake and treatment of Parkinson's disease with levodopa. N Engl J Med 292:181-84, 1975*).

L-Methionine:

An essential sulfur amino acid.

Readily crosses the blood-brain barrier where it can be converted into S-adenosyl methionine.

L-dopa supplementation reduces brain SAMe levels (*Catto E et al Brain monomine changes following the administration of S-adenosyl methionine (SAMe). Neuropharmacol 2:1978; Surtees R, Hyland K. L-3,4-dihydroxyphenylalanine (levodopa) lowers central nervous system S-adenosylmethionine concentrations in humans. J Neurol Neurosurg Psychiatry 53(7):569-72, 1990*).

Supplementation may be beneficial.

Experimental Study: 15 pts. who had had maximal improvement from standard medications received L-methionine starting with 1 gm/day and increasing gradually to 5 gm/day while medications were continued. After 2 mo., 10/15 were improved. Symptoms responding included activity level, ease of movement, rigidity and dyskinesia, mood, sleep, attention span, muscular strength, concentration, and voice. Tremor and drooling failed to improve in all cases. 2 pts. developed nausea and 1 developed diarrhea (*Smythies JR. Halsey JH. Treatment of Parkinson's disease with L-methionine. South Med J 77:1577, 1984*).

Experimental Study: 11 pts. with previously untreated PD were treated with L-methionine 5 g daily for periods from 2 wks. to 6 months. Within about 3 wks., clinical signs improved, particularly akinesia and rigidity, with a less marked effect on tremor. Therapeutic effects were similar to those observed with L-dopa treatment (*Meininger V et al. [L-methionine treatment of Parkinson's disease: preliminary results.] Rev Neurol (Paris) 138(4):297-303, 1982*) (*in French*).

Octacosanol: 1 - 2 mg daily   (6 wk. trial)

A long-chain alcohol extracted from wheat germ oil.

Administration may be beneficial.

Experimental Double-blind Crossover Study: 10 pts. with mild to moderate symptoms randomly received either octacosanol in a wheat germ oil base (Viobin) 5 mg 3 times daily with meals or placebo for 6 weeks. Based on a standard self-appraisal rating form, 3/10 significantly improved (p≤0.05) and none worsened on octacosanol. These 3 and 1 other correctly identified the octacosanol period, while 2 rated the placebo as the active substance and 4 were uncertain. The experimental gp. showed a small but significant ave. improvement in activities of daily living and mood ratings compared to placebo baselines. Side effects were mild and infrequent. It is possible that the dosage exceeded optimal as other nonstudy pts. reported that they improved without adverse effects with a daily dosage of 1-2 mg. (*Snider SR. Octacosanol in parkinsonism. Letter. Ann Neurol 16(6):723, 1984*).

Omega-6 Fatty Acids:

Linoleic acid → GLA → DGLA → Prostaglandin E₁

Several oils are rich in linoleic acid, while evening primrose oil is one of the richest sources of gammalinolenic acid (GLA). When, due to such factors as aging, the intake of *trans* fatty acids, pyridoxine, magnesium or zinc deficiencies, excessive alcohol consumption, etc., the conversion of linoleic acid to GLA is inhibited, primrose oil is superior to most oils as a PGE₁ precursor (*Horrobin DF. The importance of gamma-linolenic acid and prostaglandin E₁ in human nutrition and medicine. J Holistic Med 3:118-139, 1981*).

Note: Borage and blackcurrent oils are higher in GLA than evening primrose oil, although it is not known how they compare therapeutically.

Administration of evening primrose oil may reduce tremor.

Experimental Controlled Study: 6/11 pts. with tremor improved following administration of evening primrose oil (*Critchley EMR. Evening primrose oil (Efamol) in parkinsonian and other tremors: A preliminary study, in DF Horrobin, Ed. Clinical Uses of Essential Fatty Acids. Montreal, Eden Press, 1982:205-8*).

D-Phenylalanine:

Urinary phenylethylamine may be diminished (*Heller B, Fischer E. Arzneim-Forsch 23:884-5, 1973*).

Supplementation may be beneficial.

> WARNING: Phenylalanine should not be taken at the same time in the day as L-dopa since it competes with L-dopa for transport from plasma to the brain and thus could cause a fluctuating ("on-off") response to the drug (*Nutt JG et al. The "on-off" phenomenon in Parkinson's disease. Relation to levodopa absorption and transport. N Engl J Med 310(8):483-8, 1984*).

> **Experimental Study:** 10 days after suspending their medications, 15 pts. were neurologically evaluated and then received DPA 100-250 mg twice daily. After 4 wks., repeat exams revealed highly significant improvements in rigidity, walking disabilities, speech difficulties and psychic depression, but no improvement in tremor (*Heller B et al. Therapeutic action of D-phenylalanine in Parkinson's disease. Arzneim-Forsch 26:577-9, 1976*).

> **Animal Experimental Study:** D-phenylalanine (but not L-phenylalanine) had a therapeutic effect on drug-induced Parkinsonian-like states in animals (*Fernández Pardal J et al. Ann Psiq Biol 3:234-6, 1974*).

L-Tryptophan:

Supplementation may be beneficial for patients receiving L-dopa, as competition between tryptophan and L-dopa may result in tryptophan malabsorption in the gut leading to depression and other side-effects of levodopa treatment (*Lehmann J. Levodopa and depression in Parkinsonism. Lancet 1:140, 1971*). Reduced functioning of serotonergic pathways in Parkinsonism may also be involved (*Sandyk R, Fisher H. L-tryptophan supplementation in Parkinson's disease. Int J Neurosci 45(3-4):215-9, 1989*). In addition, competition between L-dopa and L-tryptophan for transport across the blood-brain barrier could cause a fluctuating ("on-off") response to L-dopa (*Nutt JG et al. The "on-off" phenoomenon in Parkinson's disease. Relation to levodopa absorption and transport. N Engl J Med 310(8):483-8, 1984*) and a further reduction in the availability of tryptophan for conversion to serotonin in the brain.

> **Case Reports:** Mental disturbances were observed in 7 pts. treated with levodopa who had extremely low serum tryptophan values. In 2 of the cases, tryptophan supplementation was followed by considerable improvement of mental symptoms, suggesting that prophylactic tryptophan or protein treatment during levodopa treatment may be beneficial (*Lehmann J. Tryptophan malabsorption in levodopa-treated parkinsonian patients. Acta Med Scand 194:181-89, 1973*).

> **Experimental Placebo-controlled Study:** 40 pts. received either levodopa and tryptophan 2 gm 3 times daily or levodopa and placebo. Levodopa produced striking improvement in ratings of tremor, rigidity, akinesia, gait and posture equally in both groups, while tests of functional ability to do certain tasks showed a significant improvement only in the tryptophan group. Also, only pts. in the tryptophan gp. showed a small but significant improvement in mood and drive (*Coppen A et al. Levodopa and L-tryptophan therapy in parkinsonism. Lancet 1:654-7, 1972*).

> - with niacin and pyridoxine:

>> **Case Reports:** 2 female pts. with levodopa-induced "on-off" responded dramatically to supplementation with L-tryptophan (2 and 8 g/d) along with niacin 25 mg/d and pyridoxine 50 mg/d (1 was also placed on a low-protein diet), suggesting that L-tryptophan may be useful in ameliorating motor complications of chronic levodopa therapy (*Sandyk R, Fisher H. L-tryptophan supplementation in Parkinson's disease. Int J Neurosci 45(3-4):215-9, 1989*).

L-Tyrosine: 100 mg/ kg daily

Deficiency may be due to reduced intake (major sources meats, dairy and eggs) or to diminished conversion from phenylalanine.

Parkinson's disease may be associated with decreased synthesis of biopterin, the cofactor for tyrosine hydroxylase.

Experimental Study: Serum biopterin is lower in pts. than in normal controls. After tyrosine administration, the increase in serum biopterin concentration was smaller in pts. (<2-fold) than in controls (3 to 7-fold) (*Yamaguchi T et al. Effects of tyrosine administration on serum biopterin in normal controls and patients with Parkinson's disease. Science 219:75-7, 1983*).

Increases dopamine turnover to enhance dopaminergic transmission.

WARNING: L-tyrosine should not be taken at the same time in the day as L-dopa since it competes with L-dopa for transport from plasma to the brain and thus could cause a fluctuating ("on-off") response to the drug (*Nutt JG et al. The "on-off" phenoomenon in Parkinson's disease. Relation to levodopa absorption and transport. N Engl J Med 310(8):483-8, 1984*).

Experimental Study: 5 untreated pts. diagnosed by sleep polygraphy and 5 L-dopa- and/or dopamine agonist-treated pts. were treated with L-tyrosine. For some pts., 3 yrs. of L-tyrosine treatment was associated with better clinical results and many fewer side effects than L-dopa or dopamine agonists (*Lemoine P et al. [L-tyrosine: a long-term treatment of Parkinson's disease.] C R Acad Sci [III] 309(2):43-7, 1989*).

Experimental Study: Supplementation with L-tyrosine 100 mg/kg/d increased CSF levels of tyrosine and homovanillic acid (the major dopamine metabolite) in 23 pts. pretreated with probenecid (a renal tubular blocking agent), suggesting that supplementation with L-tyrosine can increase dopamine turnover in pts. who may benefit from enhanced dopaminergic neurotransmission (*Growdon JH et al. Effects of oral L-tyrosine and homovanillic acid levels in patients with Parkinson's disease. Life Sci 30(10):827-32, 1982*).

_ _

OTHER FACTORS

Rule out aluminum toxicity.

Observational Study: Analysis of Lewy bodies in the substantia nigra of Parkinsonian brains revealed the presence of aluminum which, despite nigral cell death, was not found in progressive supranuclear palsy, suggesting that the detection of aluminum is not solely the consequence of neuronal degeneration (*Hirsch EC et al. Iron and aluminum increase in the substantia nigra of patients with Parkinson's disease: an X-ray microanalysis. J Neurochem 56(2):446-51, 1991*).

Observational Study: 42 pts. were compared to 84 matched controls. An increased risk for PD seems to be associated with occupational exposure to manganese, iron and aluminum (odds ratio: 2.28; p=0.07) especially when the exposure is longer than 30 yrs. (odds ratio: 13.64; p≤0.05) (*Zayed J et al. [Environmental factors in the etiology of Parkinson's disease.] Can J Neurol Sci 17(3):286-91, 1990*).

Rule out mercury toxicity.

Observational Study: 54 pts. with idiopathic PD were compared to 95 hospital-based controls, matched for age, sex and ethnicity. After adjusting for potential confounding factors, there was a clear monotonic dose-response distribution between PD and blood mercury levels. The odds ratios for the approximate subject terciles relative to the lowest tercile were 8.5 and 9.4. Similar associations were found using scalp hair and urinary mercury levels; however only the comparisons between the highest and lowest terciles were significant (p<0.05). When the body burden mercury indicators were mutually adjusted in addition to the 4 confounding factors (dietary fish intake, medications, smoking and alcohol consumption), blood and urinary mercury levels showed odds ratios of 21.0 and 81.65, respectively. These odds ratios were significant (p<0.05). After adjustment, scalp hair mercury was shown to be a poor predictor of PD risk (*Ngim CH, Devathasan G. Epidemiologic study on the association between body burden mercury level and idiopathic Parkinson's disease. Neuroepidemiology 8(3):128-41, 1989*).

PERIODONTAL DISEASE

See Also: INFLAMMATION
OSTEOPOROSIS

GENERAL REVIEW ARTICLE

"Virtually all unbiased reviews of nutrition in periodontal disease conclude, that although periodontal disease is not a nutritional deficiency disease, inadequate nutrition may either predispose the host to the disease, or modify the progress of a pre-existing disease" (*Pack ARC. A review of nutritional implications in periodontics. J N Z Soc Periodontol (65):6-10, 1988*).

- -

DIETARY FACTORS

Avoid sugar.

Increases plaque accumulation while decreasing chemotaxis and phagocytosis of polymorphonuclear leukocytes (*Ringsdorf W et al. Sucrose, neutrophil phagocytosis and resistance to disease. Dent Surv 52:46-8, 1976*).

Refined sugar may hasten the development of gingivitis; however, sugar avoidance fails to protect against the development of periodontal disease.

Experimental Double-blind Study: 21 dental students were provided with a 75 g glucose drink 3 times daily, while 21 controls were given an artificially sweetened drink. On the fifth day, mean sulcus depth in the experimental gp. (as measured by an examiner who was unaware of the initial findings) was found to have increased significantly ($p<0.01$) while the mean sulcus depth in the controls was unchanged. Similarly, based on a 4-point scale of gingival inflammation, mean gingival inflammation in the experimental gp. increased significantly ($p<0.01$) while mean gingival inflammation in the controls was slightly reduced ($p<0.05$) (*Cheraskin E. How quickly does diet make for change: A study in sulcus depth. Clin Prev Dent 10(4):20-2, 1988; Cheraskin E. How quickly does diet make for change? A study in gingival inflammation. N Y J Dent 58(4):133-5, 1988*).

Experimental Single-blind Study: 22 dental students were provided with a 50 g sucrose drink twice daily, while 14 controls received nothing. On the fifth day, mean sulcus depth in the experimental gp. (as measured by an examiner who was unaware of the initial findings) was found to have increased significantly ($p<0.01$) while the mean sulcus depth in the controls was unchanged. Similarly, based on a 4-point scale of gingival inflammation, mean gingival inflammation in the experimental gp. increased significantly ($p<0.01$) while mean gingival inflammation in the controls was unchanged (*Cheraskin E. How quickly does diet make for change: A study in sulcus depth. Clin Prev Dent 10(4):20-2, 1988; Cheraskin E. How quickly does diet make for change? A study in gingival inflammation. N Y J Dent 58(4):133-5, 1988*).

Experimental Single-blind Study: 40 dental students were instructed to avoid all refined carbohydrate foodstuffs as much as possible. On the fifth day, mean sulcus depth in the gp. (as measured by an examiner who was unaware of the initial findings) was found to have decreased significantly ($p<0.01$) from baseline (*Cheraskin E. How quickly does diet make for change: A study in sulcus depth. Clin Prev Dent 10(4):20-2, 1988*).

Experimental Controlled Study: 4 subjects consumed a sugar-reduced diet while 4 consumed a sugar-supplemented diet. 10 index teeth in each subject were completely free of dental plaque and without clinical signs of gingivitis. Subjects were instructed to refrain from oral hygiene. After 21 days, no significant differences in the amt. of plaque could be detected between the test and control groups. After 3 wks., gingivitis could be detected in 100% of index teeth in the sugar-reduced gp. and in 80% of the index teeth in the sugar-supplemented group, although identifiable gingivitis developed at a later date in subjects in the sugar-reduced group. Reulsts suggest that a low sugar diet does not prevent periodontal disease (*Gaengler P et al. The effects of carbohydrate-reduced diet on development of gingivitis. Clin Prev Dent 8(6):17-23, 1986*).

Experimental Single-blind Crossover Study: 20 normal young male subjects received a high and a low sugar diet in random order for 3 wks. each and experimental gingivitis was induced in the lower anterior area. At 3 wks., significantly higher bleeding scores at the 2 designated levels were found with the high sugar diet, but no significant differences were observed in crevicular fluid flow and plaque amount (*Sidi AD, Ashley FP. Influence of frequent sugar intakes on experimental gingivitis. J Periodontol 55(7):419-23, 1984*).

Experimental Controlled Study: Experimental gingivitis was induced in 21 volunteers in 21 days. Half received a sugar-enriched diet, and half received a sugar-reduced diet. The development of gingivitis was more rapid in subjects on the sugar-enriched diet (*Pfister W et al. [Bacteriological characterization of gingivitis-inducing plaque depending on different sugar levels of the diet.] Zentralbl Bakteriol Mikrobiol Hyg [A] 257(3):364-71, 1984*).

– –

VITAMINS

<u>Folic acid</u>:   1 mg. daily orally or local application of 0.1% solution

Supplementation or local application may reduce gingival exudate from inflamed and infected gums - which suggests improved tissue health. (Folate mouthwash appears to be more effective than oral folate.)

Experimental Double-blind Study: 60 pts with visible gingivitis rinsed for 1 min. twice daily with either 5 ml of 0.1% folate solution (1 mg/ml) or a placebo. After 4 wks., the folate gp. was significantly improved compared to the placebo group. Dietary folate did not correlate with treatment results, suggesting a local effect (*Pack ARC. Folate mouthwash: Effects on established gingivitis in periodontal patients. J Clin Periodontol 11:619-28, 1984*).

Experimental Double-blind Study: 30 women in their 32nd wk. of pregnancy randomly received either placebo mouthwash and placebo tablets (Gp. A), placebo mouthwash 1 min. twice daily and folate 5 mg/d (Gp. B), or a 1% folate mouthwash and placebo tablets (Gp. C). After 28 days, folate levels increased significantly in Gps. B and C. Gp. C showed a highly significant improvement in a gingival index despite no significant changes in a plaque index ($p<0.01$) while there were no significant changes in Gps. A or B (*Thomson ME, Pack ARC. Effects of extended systemic and topical folate supplementation on gingivitis of pregnancy. J Clin Periodontal 9(3):275-80, 1982*).

Experimental Double-blind Study: 30 women in their 4th or 8th mo. of pregnancy randomly received either placebo mouthwash 1 min. twice daily and placebo tablets (Gp. A), placebo mouthwash and folate 5 mg/d (Gp. B), or 1% folate mouthwash and placebo tablets (Gp. C). The gingival index tended to increase throughout pregnancy in all gps. except Gp C, for whom there was a highly significant improvement in the 8th mo. ($p<0.01$) despite no change in plaque index. Compared to Gps. A and B, dietary intake of folate was significantly higher in Gp. C in the 8th mo. ($p<0.01$) (*Pack ARC, Thomson ME. Effects of topical and systemic folic acid supplementation on gingivitis in pregnancy. J Clin Periodontol 7(5):402-14, 1980*).

Experimental Double-blind Study: 30 pts. with normal fasting blood folate levels rinsed their mouths daily with 5 cc of a 1 mg/cc folate solution or placebo. After 60 days, experimental subjects showed significant improvement in gingival health compared to controls (*Vogel RI et al. The effect of topical application of folic acid on gingival health. J Oral Med 33(1):20-22, 1978*).

Experimental Study: Contraceptive users with normal plasma folate levels demonstrated improved gingival health after receiving supplementation with folic acid 4 mg/d for 60 days (*Vogel RI et al. J Prev Dent 6:221, 1980*).

Experimental Double-blind Study: 30 pts. ingested either folic acid 2 mg twice daily or placebo. After 30 days, based on plaque and gingival indices, folic acid supplementation appeared to increase the resistance of the gingiva to local irritants leading to a reduction in inflammation. Plasma folate levels, which were normal, were unaffected by supplementation (*Vogel RI et al. The effect of folic acid on gingival health. J Periodontol 47(11):667-8, 1976*).

Vitamin A:

Deficiency known to predispose to periodontal disease as it is associated with:
1. keratinizing metaplasia of the gingival epithelium
2. early karyolysis of gingival epithelial cells
3. inflammatory infiltration and degeneration
4. periodontal pocket formation
5. gingival calculus formation
6. increased susceptibility to infection
7. abnormal alveolar bone formation
(*Carranza F. Glickman's Clinical Periodontology. Philadelphia, Pa., WB Saunders, 1984*).

Reduction may be associated with inflammatory periodontal changes.

Observational Study: 39 pregnant women in good general health were studied. Maximum inflammatory changes of periodontium occurred in the 8th mo. with amelioration shortly before delivery. Also during the 8th mo., the mean physiologic level of vitamin A declined and became markedly elevated shortly before delivery, raising the question whether this elevation contributes to the simultaneous improvement of periodontal inflammation (*Cernä H et al. Periodontium and vitamin E and A in pregnancy. Acta Univ Palacki Olomuc Fac Med 125:173-9, 1990*).

Vitamin C: 1000 mg. daily

Protects the mucosal barrier against the infiltration of antigenic material such as bacterial endotoxins.

In vitro Experimental Study: Prior treatment with ascorbic acid completely protected fibroblasts in a culture medium against endotoxin challenge (*Aleo JJ. Inhibition of endotoxin-induced depression of cellular proliferation by ascorbic acid. Proc Soc Exp Biol Med 164(3):248-51, 1980*).

Subclinical deficiency may increase susceptibility to periodontal disease and worsen established disease.

Review Article: Clinical trials providing vitamin C supplementation at the levels of 60-70 mg/d have shown decreased gingival bleeding, increased collagen-producing fibroblasts, enhanced WBC formation and increased number of epithelial attachments. However, the results of trials of megadoses of vitamin C on individuals consuming adequate intakes have not demonstrated a predictable response on gingival clinical parameters (*Rubinoff AB et al. Vitamin C and oral health. J Can Dent Assoc 55(9):705-7, 1989*).

Experimental Study: As demonstrated by biochemical indices of ascorbic acid (AA) nutriture, young men were brought into various states of AA depletion and repletion by varying their dietary AA intakes. The propensity of the gingiva to become inflamed or bleed on probing was reduced after normal AA intakes (65 mg/d) compared to deficient intakes (5 mg/d), and upon supplementary intakes (605 mg/d) compared to normal intakes. Results suggest that AA status may influence early stages of gingival inflammation and crevicular bleeding (*Jacob RA et al. Experimental vitamin C depletion and supplementation in young men. Nutrient interactions and dental health effects. Ann N Y Acad Sci 498:333-46, 1987*).

Experimental Study: 11 healthy non-smoking males (aged 19-28) ate a rotating 7-day diet deficient only in ascorbic acid (5 mg) which was supplemented with 60 mg/day ascorbic acid for 2 wks., 0 mg/day for 4 wks., 600 mg/day for 3 wks., and 0 mg/day for 4 weeks. No mucosal pathoses or changes in plaque accumulation or probing depths were noted during any of the periods of depletion or supplementation; however, measures of gingival inflammation were directly related to the ascorbic acid status, suggesting that ascorbic acid may influence early stages of gingivitis, particularly crevicular bleeding (*Leggott PJ et al. The effect of controlled ascorbic acid depletion and supplementation on periodontal health. J. Periodontol. 57(8):480-85, 1986*).

Review Article and Theoretical Discussion: Ascorbic acid deficiency has been shown to be a conditioning factor in the development of gingivitis. When humans are placed on ascorbic acid-deficient diets there is increased edema, redness and swelling of gingiva. While these changes have been attributed to deficient collagen production by gingival blood vessels, they may be due to the antihistaminic role of the vitamin (*Nakamoto T et al. The role of ascorbic acid deficiency in human gingivitis: a new hypothesis. J Theor Biol 108(2):163-71, 1984*).

Review Article: Scurvy and periodontitis both manifest gingival bleeding but constitute separate entities. While symptoms of scurvy are due to defective collagen, the various periodontal diseases are caused by oral plaque micro-organisms. The body's reaction to these micro-organisms is strongly influenced by leucocyte and monocyte function, and their functioning is reduced when ascorbic acid is deficient. Although certain infections and systemic diseases cause gingival bleeding, avitaminosis C does not cause commonly encountered periodontal diseae, but will aggravate established periodontitis. Vitamin C should not be used for prophylaxis or cure of periodontitis in healthy, well-nourished individuals (*Touyz LZ. Vitamin C, oral scurvy and periodontal disease. S Afr Med J 65(21):838-42, 1984*).

Negative Experimental Placebo-controlled Study: 10 nondeficient individuals, carefully matched according to age, periodontal status, and oral hygience level received either ascorbic acid 250 mg 4 times daily or placebo. After 1 wk. all pts. were scaled and root planed and received oral hygiene instructions. Repeated blood samples were taken and a gingival biopsy was taken at wk. 6. After 7 wks., there were no significant differences between the 2 gps. (*Woolfe SN et al. Relationship of ascorbic levels of blood and gingival tissue with response to periodontal therapy. J Clin Periodontol 11(3):159-65, 1984*).

Animal Experimental Study: Localized periodontal disease was induced in 2 gps. of monkeys by tying a silk thread around a single molar tooth at the gum line. In 2 wks., marginally vitamin C-deficient animals showed 36% greater inflammation in the gingival tissues and a 41% greater periodontal pocket depth around the encircled teeth than a gp. of pair-fed control animals. Also, 23 wks. after the experimental diet began, polymorphonuclear leukocytes of the marginally deficient animals showed a significant reduction in chemotaxis and in phagocytosis compared to pair-fed controls (*Alvares O et al. The effect of subclinical ascorbate deficiency on periodontal disease in nonhuman primates. J Periodontal Res 16:628-36, 1984*).

Supplementation may increase gingival ascorbic acid levels.

Experimental Controlled Study: 11/18 pts. (ages 17-24) with "little" or "slight" periodontal disease received either vitamin C 1 gm daily or placebo. At the end of the trial, ascorbic acid levels were up to 15-20 times higher in the gums of the experimental gp. (*Mallek HM. J Dent Res March, 1979*).

Supplementation may decrease gingival flow (which is directly related to gingival inflammation) (*Mallek HM Doctoral Thesis, Inst Arch, MIT, Cambridge, 1978*).

Vitamin D:

Deficiency is known to impair calcium absorption (*Migicovsky BB, Jamieson JWS. J Biochem Physiol 33:202, 1955*).

Vitamin E: 800 mg. daily for 3 weeks (capsules bitten and vitamin applied locally before swallowing)

May be reduced.

Observational Study: 39 pregnant women in good general health were studied. Maximum inflammatory changes of periodontium occurred in the 8th mo. with amelioration shortly before delivery. Also during the 8th mo., the mean physiologic level of vitamin E declined and became markedly elevated shortly before delivery, raising the question whether this elevation contributes to the simultaneous improvement of periodontal inflammation (*Cernä H et al. Periodontium and vitamin E and A in pregnancy. Acta Univ Palacki Olomuc Fac Med 125:173-9, 1990*).

Negative Observational Study: Vitamin E levels in pts. with and without periodontal disease were measured. There was no significant difference between the 2 groups (*Slade EW Jr et al. Vitamin E and periodontal disease. J Periodontol 47(6):352-54, 1976*).

Supplementation and local application may reduce inflammation.

Experimental Double-blind Study: 244 pts. received an ointment either containing 2% vitamin E or placebo. The vitamin E ointment was found effective in curing and improving local inflammatory symptoms such as flare and swelling (*Kimura Y et al. J Japan Assoc Periodontol 19:413, 1977*).

Experimental Controlled Study: 14 pts. received 800 mg vitamin E daily which they were told to bite open and swish in their mouths before swallowing. After 21 days, treated pts. had significantly reduced fluidity of the sulcus fluid (indicating reduced inflammation) while the control gp. was unchanged (*Goodson JM, Bowles D. IRDR Abs 633, 1973*).

- -

COMBINED VITAMIN THERAPY

Vitamin A,
Vitamin E and
Vitamin K:

Supplementation and oral application may be beneficial.

Experimental Study: In pts., glutathione reductase is activated and the content of glutathione sulfhydryl gps. is increased in the gingival tissue. Administration of antioxidants (vitamins A, E and K) locally and by ingestion normalized these parameters and improved the status of the periodontium (*Khmelevski:i, IuV et al. [Effect of vitamins A, E and K on the indices of the glutathione antiperoxidase system in gingival tissues in periodontosis.] Vopr Pitan (4):54-56, July-Aug., 1985*).

- -

MINERALS

Calcium: 1000 - 1500 mg. daily

Dietary deficiency is associated with alveolar bone loss.

Observational Study: Among denture wearers, those with good underlying bone had a daily calcium intake of about 900 mg while those with bone deterioration had a daily intake of about 500 mg (*Wical KE, Swoope CC. Studies of residual ridge resorption. Part II. The relationship of dietary calcium and phosphorus to residual ridge resorption. J Prosthet Dent 32(1):13-22, 1974*).

Animal Experimental Study: Beagles were fed a low calcium/high phosphorus diet to elicit secondary hyperparathyroidism. Osteolytic demineralization of bone followed which seemed to involve alveolar bone more than other bones (*Henrikson PA. Periodontal disease and calcium deficiency. An experimental study in the dog. Acta Odontol Scand 26:Suppl 50:1-132, 1968*).

Alveolar bone loss induced by nutritional secondary hyperparathyroidism may not be associated with periodontitis if the teeth are cleaned frequently to prevent plaque accumulation.

Review Article: "Bone destruction in periodontal disease is caused principally by local factors. It may also be caused by systemic factors, but their role has not been clearly defined. Chronic inflammation is the most common cause of bone destruction in periodontal disease" (*Goodman SF. Periodontal disease is not a metabolic disease. N Y State Dent J 47(8):462-4, 1981*).

Animal Experimental Study: Rats were placed on a hypocalcemic diet. Results suggest that a hypocalcemic diet alone has no significant effect on the degree or spread of gingival inflammation, migration of the epithelial attachment or the height of the alveolar bone (*Bissada NF, DeMarco TJ. The effect of a hypocalcemic diet on the periodontal structures of the adult rat. J Periodontol 45:739-45, 1974*).

Animal Experimental Study: 4 dogs were fed a calcium-deficient, phosphorus-rich diet while 2 controls were fed an adequate but soft diet for 18 months. The teeth of the right jaws were subjected regularly to thorough cleaning. While nutritional secondary hyperparathyroidism and osteopenia of the alveolar process were induced in the test jaws, tooth mobility or gingivitis did not develop in the absence of plaque. In the areas where dental deposits were allowed to accumulate, pathologic pockets gradually developed in all 6 animals, but the degree of attachment was the same in both groups. X-rays failed to show evidence of reduction of the marginal alveolar bone height in any of the dogs, and the lamina dura could be distinguished around all teeth at all periods of observation (*Svanberg G et al. Effect of nutritional hyperparathyroidism on experimental periodontitis in the dog. Scand J Dent Res 81:155-62, 1973*).

Supplementation may reverse the course of periodontal disease.

Negative Experimental Placebo-controlled Study: 59 pts. randomly received calcium 1 g/d or placebo. After 6 mo., their periodontal status was re-evaluated using the following parameters: Plaque index, gingival index, probing depth, mobility and furcaton involvement. Both gps. showed a slight improvement in plaque index, gingival index and probing depth; however, there was no difference between the 2 groups. Dietary analysis established a low calcium consumption (<800 mg/d) in 1/3 of the pts.; however, this sub-gp. of pts. also failed to benefit from calcium supplementation (*Uhrbom E, Jacobson L. Calcium in periodontitis: clinical effect of calcium medication. J Clin Periodontol 11(4):230-41, 1984*).

Negative Experimental Study: Animal experiments, as well as acute studies in men involving an oral phosphorus load, suggest that parathyroid secretion might be increased by a lowered calcium/phosphorus ratio; thus it is possible that a diet too low in calcium could contribute to the pathogenesis of periodontal disease. 60/100 pts. suffering from severe periodontal disease received supplementation with calcium 1 or 2 g/d for 9 or 12 months. Different investigations such as parathormone levels and serum parameters were unaffected, suggesting that other factors are more important for the development of this disorder (*Rottka H et al. The influence of the calcium/phosphorus ratio in the diet on human bone disease: the role of nutritive secondary hyperparathyroidism. Int J Vitam Nutr Res 51(4):373-9, 1981*).

Review Article: It is unlikely that nutritional secondary hyperparathyroidism (caused by a reduced calcium to phosphorus ratio) is the primary etiological factor in periodontal disease, although this process may contribute significantly to the progression of the disease process (*Alfano MC. Controversies, perspectives and clinical implications of nutrition in periodontal disease. Dent Clin N Am 20:519, 1976*).

Experimental Study: 10 pts. were found to have an ave. daily calcium intake of 325 milligrams. 6 mo. after supplementation with calcium 500 mg. twice daily, 8/10 had reduction in the size of the pockets of inflammation around the roots of their teeth and all 8 with loose or woobly teeth had some improvement. X-rays revealed that the pattern of jawbone loss was reversed in 7/10, with the appearance of new bone (*Krook L et al. Human periodontal disease: Morphology and response to calcium therapy. Cornell Vet 62(1):32-53, 1972*).

- with <u>Vitamin D</u>:

Supplementation may decrease the rate of alveolar bone loss.

Experimental Double-blind Study: 46 denture pts. received calcium 750 mg and vitamin D2 (ergocalciferol) 375 USP units daily or a placebo. After 1 year, the experimental gp. had 34% less bone loss in their upper jaws and 39% less in their lower jaws (*Wical KE, Brussee P. Effects of a calcium and vitamin D supplement on alveolar ridge resorption in immediate denture patients. J Prosthet Dent 41(1):4-11, 1979*).

<u>Magnesium</u>:

Supplementation may increase bone density.

Experimental Study: A 1% increase in bone magnesium following supplementation was associated with a 100% increase in alveolar bone density (*Louis Barnett - reported in Huggins HA. The influence of calcium in the periodontal patient. J Holistic Med 2(1):32-9, 1980*).

<u>Phosphorus</u>:

Excess dietary phosphorus impairs calcium absorption (high in meat, grains, potatoes and soft drinks).

It has been theorized that periodontal disease results from a decreased calcium to phosphorus ratio by causing secondary hyperparathyroidism in order to maintain normal serum calcium levels (*Krook L et al Human periodontal disease and osteoporosis. Cornell Vet 62(3):371-91, 1972*).

Zinc:

Deficiency may increase the permeability of gingival tissues to foreign substances.

Animal Experimental Study: Compared to controls, a significant increase in local ^{14}C-bovine serum albumin intake was found in the gingiva, sulcular connective tissue and periosteum and a significant increase in ^{14}C-phenytoin uptake was found in the sulcular connective tissue and periosteum of zinc-deficient rabbits, suggesting that zinc deficiency increases molecular uptake by a number of periodontal tissues. Since these 2 tracer molecules are similar in size and molecular weight to substances known to be cytotoxic originating from oral bacteria, zinc deficiency may decrease host resistance to inflammatory periodontal disease by allowing greater penetration of bacterial products from the gingival sulcus into the adjacent periodontal tissues (*Joseph CE et al. Zinc deficiency changes in the permeability of rabbit periodontium to ^{14}C-phenytoin and ^{14}C-albumin. J Periodontol 53:251-56, 1982*).

Serum levels are negatively correlated with marginal alveolar bone loss.

Observational Study: Serum zinc levels were assayed for 51 pts. of varying age and varying degrees of alveolar bone loss as recorded on roentgenograms and found to negatively correlate with marginal alveolar bone loss (*Frithiof L et al. The relationship between marginal bone loss and serum zinc levels. Acta Med Scand 207(1):67-70, 1980*).

Topical application may be beneficial.

Experimental Study: A zinc mouthwash containing 18-30 mM soluble zinc markedly reduced plaque extension along the gingival margin over 16 hrs., while oral supplementation was ineffective (*Harrap GJ et al. Inhibition of plaque growth by zinc salts. J Periodont Res 18:634-42, 1983*).

COMBINED VITAMIN AND MINERAL SUPPLEMENTATION

Experimental Double-blind Study: 22 dental students were provided with an over-the-counter multivitamin/trace mineral tablet daily, while 21 controls were given an indistinguishable lactose placebo. On the fifth day, mean sulcus depth in the experimental gp. (as measured by an examiner who was unaware of the initial findings) was found to have decreased significantly ($p<0.01$) while the mean sulcus depth in the controls was unchanged. Similarly, based on a 4-point scale of gingival inflammation, mean gingival inflammation in the experimental gp. decreased significantly ($p<0.01$) while mean gingival inflammation in the controls was unchanged (*Cheraskin E. How quickly does diet make for change: A study in sulcus depth. Clin Prev Dent 10(4):20-2, 1988; Cheraskin E. How quickly does diet make for change? A study in gingival inflammation. N Y J Dent 58(4):133-5, 1988*).

OTHER NUTRITIONAL FACTORS

Coenzyme Q$_{10}$:   25 mg twice daily (2 month minimum trial)

May be deficient.

Observational Study: 29/29 periodontal pts. had a gingival deficiency of CoQ$_{10}$, and 86% also had a leucocytic deficiency (*Folkers K, Watanabe T. Bioenergetics in clinical medicine. X. Survey of the adjunctive use of coenzyme Q with oral therapy in treating periodontal disease. J Med 8(5):333-48, 1977*).

Supplementation may be beneficial.

Experimental Double-blind Study: 56 pts. received either CoQ$_{10}$ or placebo. There was a significant difference in the mean depth of significant pockets (>4 mm) between the CoQ$_{10}$ gp. and the control gp. and, at certain stages of the study, the score of tooth mobility was significantly lower in the CoQ$_{10}$ gp. (*Iwamoto Y et al. Clinical effect of Coenzyme Q$_{10}$ on periodontal disease, in K Folkers, Y Yamamura, Eds. Biomed & Clin Aspects of Coenzyme Q, Vol 3. Amsterdam, Elsevier/North-Holland Biomedical Press, 1981:109-19*).

Review Article: A review of 7 studies found 70% of 332 pts. to respond favorably to supplementation (*Folkers K, Yamamura Y. Biomed & Clin Aspects of Coenzyme Q Vol. 1. Amsterdam, Elsevier/North Holland Biomedical Press, 1977:294-311*).

Experimental Study: 8 pts. who had undergone the initial phase of periodontal treatment (debridement, plaque control, etc.) but whose conditions merited periodontal surgery were given CoQ10 25 mg twice daily. 126 teeth and 504 pocket depths were surveyed. After 21 days, a significant overall reduction of 0.61 mm of pocket depth was found (p<0.05), and a periodontal score based on gingival pocket depth, swelling, bleeding, redness, pain, exudate, and looseness of teeth was significantly decreased (p<0.01). 8 dentists viewed transparencies of pre- and post- gingival biopsies and were asked to estimate the period of time between the 2 biopsies for that amt. of healing to occur. They overestimated and therefore agreed that healing was "very impressive" (*Wilkinson EG et al. Treatment of periodontal and other soft tissue diseases of the oral cavity with coenzyme Q, in K Folkers, Y Yamamura, Eds. Biomed & Clin Aspects of Coenzyme Q. Vol. 1. Amsterdam, Elsevier/North Holland Biomedical Press, 1977*).

Experimental Double-blind Study: 18 pts. received either CoQ10 25 mg twice daily or placebo. After 21 days, all 8 supplemented pts. were rated as improved compared to only 3/10 pts. on placebo (p<0.01) (*Wilkinson EG et al. Bioenergetics and clinical medicine. VI. Adjunctive treatment of periodontal disease with Coenzyme Q10. Res Commun Chem Pathol Pharmacol 14:715, 1976*).

- -

OTHER FACTORS

Rule out mercury toxicity from silver amalgams.

Symptoms of chronic mercury exposure include bleeding gums, increased salivation and metallic taste (*Mateer RS, Reitz CD. Corrosion of amalgam restorations. J Dent Res 49:339, 1970*).

Silver amalgams may be associated with periodontal disease.

Observational Studies: 50 subjects with amalgams (ave. 10) and 51 subjects without amalgams were matched for sex and age. Urine mercury levels were 201% higher (p=0.0002) in the amalgam gp. and the number of fillings correlated directly with the amt. of urine mercury (p=0.001). Hair mercury levels were 26.56% higher in the amalgam gp. (p=0.008) with direct correlation to the number of fillings (p=0.08). The amalgam gp. had 32 oral cavity symptoms compared to 9 in the non-amalgam gp., with significant differences in symptoms of foul breath and metallic taste. In a separate survey of 86 subjects who had amalgams removed (ave. 11) and responded to a questionnaire, 32% of their oral cavity symptoms were eliminated within 10 mo. after removal and 54% of symptoms improved, while only 4% of symptoms worsened (*Siblerud RL. The relationship between mercury from dental amalgam and oral cavity health. Ann Dent 49(2):6-10, 1990*).

Observational Study: In a study of 100 subjects who had their amalgams removed, gingivitis, mouth dryness and metallic taste disappeared after amalgam removal (*Raue H. Resistance to therapy: Think of tooth fillings. Med Prac 32: 2203-9, 1980*).

Rule out cadmium and lead toxicity (*Baranska-Gachowska M et al. [The effect of toxic substances emitted by zinc and lead processing plants on the periodontal status of school children.] Czas Stomatol 39(4):235-41, 1986*).

Rule out hydrochloric acid deficiency.

Reduced gastric acidity impairs calcium absorption which may cause alveolar bone resorption.

Experimental Study: 4 men with achlorhydria absorbed 0-2% of radiolabelled calcium carbonate. After histalog stimulation in 1 subject, gastric pH dropped from 6.5 to 1.0 and calcium absorption increased from 2% to 10% (*Ivanovich P et al. The absorption of calcium carbonate. Ann Intern Med 66:917-23, 1967*).

Experimental Controlled Study: 42 pts with alveolar bone resorption had a mean free gastric acidity of 12.4 meq/l and total acidity of 23 meq/l compared to 27.4 meq/l and 44 meq/l respectively in 32 controls (*Brechner J, Armstrong WD. Relation of gastric acidity to alveolar bone resorption. Proc Soc Exp Biol Med 48:98-100, 1941*).

PERIPHERAL VASCULAR DISEASE
(including THROMBOPHLEBITIS)

See Also: ATHEROSCLEROSIS
ULCERS (SKIN)

DIETARY FACTORS

<u>Low fat</u> diet.

Saturated fat intake is at least as closely related to <u>arterial and venous thrombosis</u> as it is to atherosclerosis and is more closely related to the clotting activity of platelets and their response to thrombin than serum cholesterol (*Renaud S. Dietary fatty acids and platelet function.* <u>Proc Nutr Soc Aust</u> *10:1-13, 1985*).

Reduction in fat intake may be beneficial.

Experimental Double-blind Study: 45 pts. were randomly assigned to either the Am. Heart Assoc. Hyperlipidemia Diet C (n=20) or a low-fat, high-fiber, complex carbohydrate diet similar to the Pritikin Maintenance Diet (n=25). After 1 yr., walking distance increased significantly in both gps., with no difference between groups. No vascular parameters changed significantly, suggesting that increased walking distance was due to improved metabolic capacity of the muscle. A trend toward lower lipids values was observed, with no significant differences within or between groups. Results suggest no advantage to the more difficult complex carbohydrate diet (*Hunchinson K et al. Effects of dietary manipulation on vascular status of patients with peripheral vascular disease.* <u>JAMA</u> *259(24):3326-30, 1983*).

Avoid <u>sucrose</u>.

Sucrose consumption may correlate with both platelet adhesiveness and serum insulin levels in patients.

Observational Study: 27 men with PVD (mean age 59) were compared with 27 healthy men (mean age 51). In pts., but not in normals, there was a significant correlation between sucrose consumption and both serum insulin levels and platelet adhesiveness. Ave. sucrose consumption was 123 gm in pts. compared to 119 gm in normals (*Yudkin J et al. Sugar intake, serum insulin and platelet adhesiveness in men with and without peripheral vascular disease.* <u>Postgrad Med J</u> *45:608, 1969*).

- -

VITAMINS

<u>Niacin</u>: *See "<u>Inositol Nicotinate</u>" below.*

<u>Vitamin A</u>:

Supplementation may be beneficial.

Theoretical Discussion: The major pathogenetic factors of the atherosclerotic diseases are: a) vasal endothelium distress; b) rheological disturbances; c) alterations in the plasma lipid pattern; d) dietary intake of saturated and polyunsaturated fatty acids; e) alteration of mitochondrial and microsomal membranes; f) vascular injury induced by immune complexes; g) increased lipid peroxidation. Many well-documented reports state a positive effect of vitamins A and E on some of these factors. Vitamins A and E have an endothelium-protective activity and an antiperoxidative effect; they act as antiaggregant factors, affect O_2 transport and utilization processes, increase

HDL-cholesterol, and potentiate the hypolipidemic action of nicotinic acid (*Butturini U. Vitamins E and A in vascular diseases. Acta Vitaminol Enzymol 4(1-2):15-9, 1982*).

Vitamin B$_6$:

Promotes conversion of homocysteine (toxic) to cystathionine; thus B$_6$ deficiency is theorized (originally by Kilmer McCully, M.D., Professor of Pathology, Harvard Medical School) to cause arterial damage due to build-up of homocysteine. (The incidence of heterozygous homocystinuria due to cystathionine synthase deficiency is about 1 in 70.)

> *Note: See also "Folic acid" and "Betaine" in "ATHEROSCLEROSIS"- as the addition of folate and betaine to pyridoxine may be beneficial.*

Observational Study: Hyperhomocysteinemia was detected in 16/38 pts. with cerebrovascular disease (42%), 7/25 pts. with peripheral vascular disease (28%), and 18/60 pts. with coronary vascular disease (30%) compared to none of 27 normal controls. After adjustment for the effects of conventional risk factors, the lower 95% confidence limit for the odds ratio for vascular disease among pts. with hyperhomocysteinemia as compared to normals was 3.2. The geometric-mean peak serum homocysteine level was 1.33 times higher in pts. with all vascular disease than in normals (p=0.002). The presence of cystathionine beta-synthase deficiency was confirmed n 18/23 pts. with vascular disease who had hyperhomocysteinemia. Results suggest that hyperhomocysteinemia is an independent risk factor for vascular disease, including coronary disease, which is probably due in most instances to cystathionine beta-synthase deficiency (*Clarke R et al. Hyperhomocysteinemia: an independent risk factor for vascular disease. N Engl J Med 324(17):1149-55, 1991*).

> *Note: The authors also found an inverse relation between both RBC folate and serum vitamin B$_{12}$ levels and hyperhomocysteinemia. They believe that there are probably multiple mechanisms involved in the pathogenesis of hyperhomocysteinemia and suggest that the relative contributions of genetic and nutritional factors require further study (Clarke R et al. Homocysteinemia: a risk factor for vascular disease. Letter. N Engl J Med 325(13):966-7, 1991).*

Observational Study: 72 pts. below age 55 with occlusive arterial disease of cerebral, carotid, or aorto-iliac vessels were studied. 20 pts. (36%) had basal homocysteinemia. Also, 20 pts. (36%) had abnormal increases of plasma homocysteine after peroral methionine loading, reaching levels which exceeded the highest value for 46 comparable controls and were within the range for 20 obligate heterozygotes for homocystinuria due to pyridoxal-5-phosphate-dependent cystathionine betasynthase deficiency. Basal plasma homocysteine content was strongly and negatively correlated to vitamin B$_{12}$ and folate concentrations. Plasma pyridoxal-5-phosphate (PLP) was depressed in most pts. but there was no correlation between PLP and homocysteine levels (*Brattström L et al. Impaired homocysteine metabolism in early-onset cerebral and peripheral occlusive arterial disease. Effects of pyridoxine and folic acid treatment. Atherosclerosis 81(1):51-60, 1990*).

Experimental Study: 20 pts. below age 55 with occlusive arterial disease of cerebral, carotid, or aorto-iliac vessels found to have impaired homocysteine metabolism were treated with pyridoxine hydrochloride 240 mg/d and folic acid 10 mg/d. After 4 wks., fasting homocysteine was reduced by a mean of 53%, and the increase in plasma homocysteine after methionine loading was reduced by a mean of 39%, suggesting that the impaired metabolism can be improved easily and without side effects (*Brattström L et al. Impaired homocysteine metabolism in early-onset cerebral and peripheral occlusive arterial disease. Effects of pyridoxine and folic acid treatment. Atherosclerosis 81(1):51-60, 1990*).

Experimental Study: 25 pts. developing occlusive peripheral arterial disease before the age of 50 were studied. Heterozygous homocystinuria was diagnosed on the basis of excessive homocysteine accumulation after methionine loading and by the presence of cystathionine synthetase deficiency in skin fibroblasts. The disorder was found in 7 of the pts. (28%). Abnormal homocysteine metabolism improved in 10/11 pts. with ischemic vascular disease supplemented with B$_6$ (*Boers GHJ et al. Heterozygosity for homocystinuria in premature peripheral and cerebral occlusive arterial disease. N Engl J Med 313:709-15, 1985*).

Animal Experimental Study: Arteriosclerotic plaques were found in the aorta and arteries of rabbits given homocysteine thiolactone, methionine or homocysteic acid. Pyridoxine prevented thrombosis and pulmonary embolism but did not prevent arteriosclerotic plaques (*McCully KS, Wilson RB. Homocysteine theory of arteriosclerosis. Atherosclerosis 22(2):215-27, 1975*

Vitamin C:

Supplementation may improve peripheral arterial circulation.

Experimental Study: 10 pts. with intermittent claudication received baseline arteriograms prior to supplementation with ascorbic acid 500 mg 3 times daily. After several months, repeat arteriograms revealed definite improvement in some of the involved arteries for 6/10 pts. (*Willis GC. The reversibility of atherosclerosis. Can Med Assoc J July 15, 1957, pp. 106-09; Willis GC et al. Serial arteriography in atherosclerosis. Can Med Assoc J December, 1954, pp. 562-68*).

Vitamin E: 300 - 1600 IU daily (6 month trial)

Theoretical Discussion: The major pathogenetic factors of the atherosclerotic diseases are: a) vasal endothelium distress; b) rheological disturbances; c) alterations in the plasma lipid pattern; d) dietary intake of saturated and polyunsaturated fatty acids; e) alteration of mitochondrial and microsomal membranes; f) vascular injury induced by immune complexes; g) increased lipid peroxidation. Many well-documented reports state a positive effect of vitamins A and E on some of these factors. Vitamins A and E have an endothelium-protective activity and an antiperoxidative effect; they act as antiaggregant factors, affect O_2 transport and utilization processes, increase HDL-cholesterol, and potentiate the hypolipidemic action of nicotinic acid (*Butturini U. Vitamins E and A in vascular diseases. Acta Vitaminol Enzymol 4(1-2):15-9, 1982*).

Supplementation may reduce intermittent claudication.

Review Article: In 7 controlled studies, 3 of which were double-blind, pts. receiving vitamin E exhibited significantly better outcome in walking distance, exertional leg pain, lower rates of surgical intervention and longer survival prognosis, when compared to controls. Maximal effectiveness is for femoro-popliteal arterial obstruction with poor distal circulation, and least effectiveness is for aorto-iliac arterial disease. Significant improvement in intermittent claudication may take 4-6 mo. and may not be seen sooner than 8 weeks (*Piesse JW. Vitamin E and peripheral vascular disease. Int Clin Nutr Rev 4(4):178-82, 1984*).

Experimental Single-blind Study: Of 158 pts. observed for 1-16 yrs. (mean of 4 yrs.), all instructed in active muscular exercise, standardized walking distances improved by 30% or more in 50% of those receiving D-α-tocopherol 300 mg daily and in 11% of controls. Arterial flow improved in 73.4% of treated pts. and 19.2% of controls. Maximum improvement in arterial flow occurred after 12-18 months. Walking distance worsened in 5% of treated pts. and in 10% of controls. (Evaluation of walking distance and of arterial flow was done 'blind' by an independent evaluator.) 17% of controls required surgery for intractable rest pain or manifest gangrene compared to 2.4% of the treated patients (*Haeger K. Long term study of α-tocopherol in intermittent claudication. Ann N Y Acad Sci 393:369-75, 1982*).

Experimental Controlled Study: 32/47 men with severe symptoms received 100 IU D-alpha-tocopherol 3 times daily while the control gp. received drugs. After about 3 mo., 54% of the men on vitamin E vs. 23% of the controls could walk 1 kilometer. After about 18 mo., 29/32 men on vitamin E demonstrated increased calf blood flow while 10/14 of the men in the control gp. demonstrated a decrease (*Haeger K. Long-time treatment of intermittent claudication with vitamin E. Am J Clin Nutr 27(10):1179-81, 1974*).

Review Article: Numerous studies and 4 controlled trials give a positive result for tocopherol at doses of at least 400 mg for periods of >12 weeks. By contrast, only 1 study had negative results (*Hamilton M et al. Lancet 1:367-70, 1953*), and this study is open to question because (1) wheat germ oil was given so that the actual daily dose of tocopherol appears to have been only 40 mg, and (2) supplementation was only provided for 12 wks. while the positive studies lasted longer (*Marks J. Critical appraisal of the therapeutic value of alpha-tocopherol. Vitam Hormones 20:573-98, 1962*).

Supplementation may help prevent the development of thromboembolic disease following surgical or other trauma.

Review Article: 6 controlled clinical trials were reviewed, none of which was double-blind. In the control gps., the risk of peripheral venous thrombosis was double that of the experimental gps., the risk of pulmonary embolism was six-fold greater, and the chances of fatal pulmonary embolism was nine-fold greater (*Kanofsky JD, Kanofsky PB. Prevention of thromboembolic disease by vitamin E. Letter. N Engl J Med 305(3):173-74, 1981*).

Negative Clinical Observation: In over 10 yrs. of clinical experience, 50 pts. taking >400 IU daily of vitamin E had clinical thrombophlebitis involving the lower extremeties, with or without associated edema and pulmonary embolism. In the majority of pts., symptoms disappeared when vitamin E was stopped; they reappeared in 2 cases when vitamin E was resumed (*Roberts HJ. Thrombophlebitis associated with vitamin E therapy. Angiology 30(3):169-77, 1979*).

- with Calcium:

    Clinical Observation: Pts. were given 200-600 IU alpha tocopherol daily either IM or orally along with 10 ml of a 10% solution of calcium gluconate every 24-48 hrs. beginning no later than the day of surgery and continuing through the post-operative period. In 15 yrs., no pt. developed a pulmonary embolism (*Ochsner A. Preventing and treating venous thrombosis. Postgrad Med 44(1):91-95, 1968*).

- -

MINERALS

Magnesium:

May be deficient.

    Observational Study: Compared to 20 normal controls, mean RBC magnesium and vascular function parameters were low in 138 patients. 102/138 had low RBC magnesium (1.54 ± 0.11 mmol/L vs. 1.88 ± 0.12 for controls). 12/20 pts. with PVD without occlusion had low RBC magnesium levels, as did 16/20 diabetic pts. with PVD and 9/10 pts. with severe PVD. Findings suggest that magnesium deficiency is a highly significant factor in peripheral vascular disease (*Howard JMH. Magnesium deficiency in peripheral vascular disease. J Nutr Med 1:39-49, 1990*).

May be deficient in deep thrombophlebitis (*Durlach J. Clinical aspects of chronic magesnium deficiency, in MS Seelig, Ed. Magnesium in Health and Disease. New York, Spectrum Publications, 1980*).

If deficient, supplementation may be beneficial.

    Clinical Observation: There are encouraging results regarding improvement in vascular functioning as magnesium deficiency is corrected (*Howard JMH. Magnesium deficiency in peripheral vascular disease. J Nutr Med 1:39-49, 1990*).

Zinc:

Supplementation may reduce intermittent claudication.

    Experimental Study: 24 pts. with severe intermittent claudication received 220 mg. zinc sulfate 3 times daily for 1 yr. or longer. 8 became able to live independently but continued to have limited exercise tolerance (*JH Henzel, U. of Missouri School of Med. - reported in Med Trib 10/26/70; Henzel JH et al. Trace elements in atherosclerosis: Efficacy of zinc medication as a therapeutic modality. Proc 2nd Ann Conf Trace Substances in Environ Health 1968:83-9*).

- -

OTHER NUTRITIONAL FACTORS

L-Carnitine:

Supplementation may increase walking distance in intermittent claudication.

    Experimental Double-blind Crossover Study: 20 pts. were randomly assigned to receive either L-carnitine 2 gm twice daily or placebo for 3 wks. before being crossed over to the other treatment for an additional 3 weeks. Absolute walking distance rose from 174 ± 63 m with placebo to 306 ± 122 m ($p<0.01$) with carnitine (*Brevetti G et al. Increases in walking distance in patients with peripheral vascular disease treated with L-carnitine: A double-blind, cross-over study. Circulation 77(4):767-73, 1988*).

<u>Hydroxyethylrutosides</u>:

May reduce red cell aggregation and whole blood viscosity at low shear rates, and may increase red cell deformability (*Schimdt-Schönbein H et al. Vasa 4:263, 1975; van Haeringen NJ et al. Bibl Anat 12:459, 1973*).

Administration may improve arterial blood flow in the extremities.

Experimental Study: 4 pts. with bilateral arterial insufficiency were treated with 1.5 grs twice daily of IV hydroxyethylrutosides. After 3 days, all pts. experienced relief of symptoms. In addition, a significant increase of nutritional blood flow in the foot averaging 33% could be demonstrated during the second and third hour (*Jelnes R et al. Improvement of subcutaneous nutritional blood flow in the forefoot by hydroxyethylrutosides in patients with arterial insufficiency: Case studies. Angiology 37(3 Pt 1):198-202, 1986*).

Administration may reduce clinical symptoms and swelling in the <u>post-thrombotic syndrome</u>.

Experimental Double-blind Study: 87 pts. randomly received either o-(beta-hydroxyethyl)-rutosides (HR) capsules 1,200 mg daily or placebo. Mean follow-up scores at the 4th and 8th wk. show that the HR pts. were feeling less tired than controls. Mean calf circumference for the HR gp. decreased from 390 (± 33) mm at visit one to 382 (± 33) mm at visit three, with a mean circumference reduction of 8.7 (± 8) mm, compared to a steady placebo circumference of 387 (± 31) mm at all 3 visits with a mean circumference reduction of only 2 mm (± 9). The estimated treatment effect at wk. 8 was -6.7 mm. Similar findings were noted in regard to mean ankle circumference (*de Jongste AB et al. A double blind three center clinical trial on the short-term efficacy of o-(beta-hydroxyethyl)-rutosides in patients with post-thrombotic syndrome. Thromb Haemost 62(3):826-29, 1989*).

Administration may be beneficial in <u>venous insufficiency</u> (*Pulvertaft TB. General practice treatment of symptoms of venous insufficiency with oxerutins. Results of a 660 patient multicentre study in the UK. Vasa 12(4):373-76, 1983*).

<u>Inositol</u>:

Administration of inositol nicotinate may be beneficial in treating <u>intermittent claudication</u>.

Experimental Double-blind Study: 120 pts. with disease severe enough to limit walking to 500 yards received either inositol nicotinate (Hexopal) 2 gms or placebo twice daily. After 3 mo., the experimental gp. had significantly larger changes in claudication times (p<0.05) and number of free-walking paces (p<0.05) than the placebo group. The subjective improvement in smokers was particularly marked. Side-effects were equally distributed between the 2 gps., and were minor and self-limiting (*O'Hara J et al. The therapeutic efficacy of inositol nicotinate (Hexopal) in intermittent claudication: a controlled trial. Br J Clin Pract 42:377-83, 1988*).

Experimental Double-blind Study: 80 pts. with stable IC received either inositol nicotinate (Hexopal) 2 gm twice daily or placebo. In pts. with unchanged smoking habits, improvement in maximum treadmill distance was greater in the treated gp. than in controls (p<0.05) (*Kiff RS. Does inositol nicotinate (Hexopal) influence intermittent claudication? - a controlled trial. Br J Clin Pract 42(4):141-45, 1988*).

Experimental Double-blind Study: In a 3-mo. study, 113 pts. with IC due to vascular insufficiency received either inositol nicotinate (Hexopal) 1 gm daily or placebo. Significantly more pts. receiving treatment (67%) than those receiving placebo (37%) reported an improvement in their walking ability (p<0.05), and treated pts. with moderately severe symptoms obtained a significantly greater improvement in the exercise test than controls (*Head A. Treatment of intermittent claudication with inositol nicotinate. Practitioner 230:49-54, 1986*).

Experimental Double-blind Study: 100 pts. with mild-moderate IC aged 50-75 who were not excluded for medical reasons received either inositol nicotinate (Hexopal) 2 gm twice daily or placebo for 3 months. There was a gradual increase in time to claudication pain in both gps.; however these changes were only significant in the treatment gp. compared to baseline after 3 mo. (p<0.05). After 3 mo., treated pts. reported significantly greater subjective improvement than did those on placebo, and symptomatic improvement was found to correspond significantly with functional improvement (p<0.005) (*O'Hara J. A double-blind placebo-controlled study of Hexopal in the treatment of intermittent claudication. J Int Med Res 13:322-27, 1985*).

Experimental Double-blind Study: Pts. selected for the study were able to walk a minimum of 50 yards before experiencing claudication, had no rest pain or claudication from other causes, were 30-75 yrs. old, were of ave.

weight and did not have diabetes mellitus. They received either inositol nicotinate (Hexopal) 2 tabs 4 times daily or placebo for 12 weeks. Of 104 pts. selected, 86 returned proper pedometer readings for analysis. By the ninth wk. of treatment, pts. in the severely affected gp. receiving inositol nicotinate were able to walk significantly further than controls (p<0.05). Also, visual analog scales rating leg discomfort causing problems in walking, after adjusting for the difference in initial values, showed a significantly greater improvement in treated pts. in the severely affected gp. at 8 wks. (p<0.05) and at 12 wks. (p<0.01). In regard to lower limb pulses, there was an improvement in both treated gps., with a greater improvement in the more severely affected group. While, among the more severely affected pts., the mean walking distance more than doubled in treated pts., it increased by only 50% in those on placebo (*Tyson VCH. Treatment of intermittent claudication. Practitioner 223:121-26, 1979*).

Omega-3 Fatty Acids:

Sardine oil is rich in eicosapentaenoic acid (an omega-3 essential fatty acid) and vitamin E.

Administration may increase RBC membrane fluidity, thus potentially reducing symptoms due to impaired red cell deformability (such as <u>intermittent claudication</u>).

Experimental Controlled Study: Dietary sardine oil 2.7 gm daily was given to diabetic and control subjects. Compared to controls, RBC membrane fluidity was lower in the diabetics prior to supplementation. After 4 wks., membrane fluidity was increased in both diabetics and controls, and remained elevated for the entire 8 wk. study, with disappearance of the difference in RBC membrane fluidity between diabetics and controls (*Kamada T et al. Dietary sardine oil increases erythrocyte membrane fluidity in diabetic patients. Diabetes 35:604, 1986*).

Omega-6 Fatty Acids:

$$\text{linoleic acid} \rightarrow \text{GLA} \rightarrow \text{DGLA} \rightarrow \text{prostaglandin E}_1$$

Supplementation with gamma-linolenic acid (GLA) may improve exercise tolerance in <u>intermittent caudication</u>.

Experimental Double-blind Study: GLA supplementation significantly improved exercise tolerance in pts. suffering from intermittent claudication (*Christie SBM et al. Observations on the performance of a standard exercise test by claudicants taking gamma-linolenic acid. J Atheroscler Res 8:83-90, 1986*).

PREGNANCY-RELATED ILLNESS

See Also: **DIABETES MELLITUS**
HYPERTENSION
MUSCLE CRAMPS

DIETARY FACTORS

Nutritious, well-balanced diet including 70-90 gm. protein and 2300-2800 kcal/day.

Low maternal albumin is associated with increased fetomaternal complications.

Observational Study: In a study of 450 women, a significant association was found between the total occurrence of fetomaternal complications and albumin levels in the lowest quartile (p<0.02), and low albumin was also associated with the specific complication of fetal distress (p<0.002) (*Mukherjee MD et al. Maternal zinc, iron, folic acid, and protein nutriture and outcome of human pregnancy. Am J Clin Nutr 40(3):496-507, 1984*).

Protein and energy intake during the first trimester may affect infant size.

Observational Study: In a study of 513 women living in London, there were positive correlations (p<0.001) between the maternal intake of protein and energy during 1 wk. towards the end of the first trimester of pregnancy and birthweight, newborn head circumference and newborn length for babies below the median weight (*Doyle W et al. The association between maternal diet and birth dimensions. J Nutr Med 1:9-17, 1990*).

Multi-vitamin, multi-mineral supplement.

Nutritional deficiencies during pregnancy are common.

Observational Study: Of 76 healthy pregnant women, 78% had one or more glaring nutritional deficiencies (*Dostálová L. Correlation of the vitamin status between mother and newborn during delivery. Dev Pharmacol Ther 4 Suppl:45-57, 1982*).

Supplementation with a multivitamin around the time of conception may reduce the risk of neural tube defects.

(See Also: "Folic Acid" below)

Experimental Controlled Study: English mothers known to have had one or more NTD pregnancies who were not pregnant but were considering a future pregnancy were asked to take Pregnavite Forte F (containing folic acid 0.36 mg daily along with vitamins A, B_1, B_2, B_3, B_6, C, D and E and calcium phosphate) for not less than 4 wks. before conception and to continue until they had missed 2 menstrual periods. Among 320 infants/fetuses born to 315 unsupplemented mothers, 18 (5.6%) had NTD, including an affected twin pair. Among 150 infants/fetuses born to 148 fully supplemented mothers, there was 1 NTD recurrence (0.7%) (p=0.006), and there were no NTD recurrences among 37 partly supplemented mothers (i.e. those who took vitamins for a shorter period) (*Smithells RW et al. Prevention of neural tube defect recurrences in Yorkshire: Final report. Letter. Lancet 2:498-99, 1989*).

Negative Observational Study: The periconceptual use of vitamin supplements was examined for 571 American women who had a conceptus with a neural-tube defect, 546 women who had had a stillbirth or a conceptus with another malformation, and 573 women who had had a normal conceptus. The rate of periconceptional multivitamin use among the mothers of infants with neural-tube defects (15.8%) was not significantly different from the rate among mothers in either the abnormal or the normal control group. After adjustment for potential confounding factors, the odds ratio for having an infant with an neural-tube defect among women classified as having had full supplementation with multivitamins was 0.95 as compared with the mothers of the abnormal infants and 1.00 as compared with the mothers of normal infants (*Mills JL et al. The absence of a relation between the periconceptional use of vitamins and neural-tube defects. N Engl J Med 321(7):430-35, 1989*).

> *Note: This study has been criticized as the interviews were performed several months after the deliveries; thus information on vitamin use in early pregnancy may not be completely accurate. Also women in their first 6 weeks of pregnancy who have not yet seen an obstetrician may have taken vitamins on their own and been misclassified as nonusers of supplements (Milunsky A. Periconceptual use of multivitamins and the prevalence of neural tube defects. Letter. N Engl J Med 322(15):1082-83, 1990). Comparisons among users and nonusers of multivitamins are meaningless, since multivitamins consist of varied mixtures and amounts of vitamins, each of which has a specific biologic function. Also, the data appear to be skewed toward a marginally malnourished population; thus the question of whether a normal folate intake and folate status might have prevented neural-tube defects remains unanswered (Halsted CH. Periconceptual use of multivitamins and the prevalence of neural tube defects. Letter. N Engl J Med 322(15):1082, 1990). Finally, selection biases may have distorted the results (Mulinare J et al. Periconceptual use of multivitamins and the prevalence of neural tube defects. Letter. N Engl J Med 322(15):1083, 1990).*

Observational Study: American mothers of 347 babies with born with neural tube defects were compared with mothers of 2829 randomly-selected control babies. There was a overall apparent protective effect of periconcpetional multivitamin use on the occurence of neural tube defects, with a crude estimated relative risk of 0.40; however, it is not possible to determine whether this apparently lower risk is the direct result of multivitamin use (*Mulinare J et al. Periconceptional use of multivitamins and the occurrence of neural tube defects. JAMA 260(21):3141-45, 1988*).

Experimental Study: Half of several hundred women who had delivered children with spina bifida or anencephaly were found to have had a poor diet during the pregnancy which ended with a child with a NTD. 103 of these women received dietary counseling prior to their next pregnancy while 71 controls received no counseling. Of those who improved their diet, all delivered normal children, while all 8/186 newborns with NTD were born to women who ate a poor diet during their first 6 mo. of pregnancy (*Laurence KM. Nutr Health 2(3/4), 1983*).

Combined supplementation during pregnancy may reduce the risk of pre-eclampsia.

Review Article: One controlled clinical trial found that women receiving several different vitamins and minerals had less pre-eclampsia and fewer deliveries before the 40th week of gestation, while another showed that women receiving a polyvitamin concentrate had less pre-eclampsia (*Hemminki E, Starfield B. Routine administration of iron and vitamins during pregnancy: review of controlled clinical trials. Br J Obstet Gynaecol 85(6):404-10, 1978*).

Avoid alcohol.

Even mild alcohol ingestion during pregnancy is said to result in hyperactivity, short attention span and emotional lability in children (*Gold S, Sherry L. Hyperactivity, learning disabilities, and alcohol. J Learn Disabil 17(1):3-6, 1984*).

Alcohol consumption during pregnancy contributes to birth abnormalities.

Observational Study: Over 1000 pregnant women were questioned about alcohol consumption at 3 mo. gestation, outcomes of pregnancies were assessed at birth, and offspring were assessed at 3 mo. of age. 10/96 reported abnormalities were alcohol-related. One alcohol-related abnormality was found in 23.9% of offspring and 2 or more in 15.3% of offspring. No significant difference in abnormality rate was found between abstainers, light and heavy drinkers. When the abnormalities were analyzed with respect to 30 possible causative agents, it was found that 94% of abnormalities were non-alcohol related (*Plant ML. Drinking in pregnancy and foetal harm: Results from a Scottish prospective study. Midwifery 2(2):81-85, 1986*).

Avoid caffeine.

Observational Study: Data on caffeine consumption was obtained from 1,230 women with live births. Results showed increased uterine growth retardation in infants of women who consumed >300 mg of caffeine daily. The odds ratio for low birth weight and high maternal caffeine consumption also was elevated to 2.05 compared to 1.0 for women who did not consume caffeine. Women who restricted their otherwise high caffeine consumption during the early stages of pregnancy had lower risks of delivering growth-retarded or low birth weight infants. Caffeine consumption was unrelated to preterm deliveries (*Fenster L et al. Caffeine consumption during pregnancy and fetal growth. Am J Public Health 81:458-61, 1991*).

Observational Study: The association between the annual ave. national coffee consumption per person and the age - standardized incidence of insulin-dependent diabetes (age gp. 0-14 yrs.) was investigated. The simple correlation between coffee consumption and insulin-dependent diabetes was 0.74. A linear regression analysis showed that 53% of the geographic variation in incidence could be attributed to differences in coffee consumption. The countries with the highest coffee consumption per head also had the the highest incidence of insulin-dependent diabetes (*Tuomilehto J et al. Coffee consumption as trigger for insulin dependent diabetes mellitus in childhood. Br Med J 300:642-43, 1990*).

Review Article: A review of studies suggests that, until more information is available, it might be prudent to limit caffeine intake to approx. 300 mg/d during pregnancy in view of decreases in birth weight that might occur above that level of consumption. Since caffeine is known to enter breast milk, that level might also be appropriate for nursing mothers (*Berger A. Effects of caffeine consumption on pregnancy outcome. A review. J Reprod Med 33(12):945-56, 1988*).

- -

VITAMINS

Folic Acid:

> WARNING: High plasma folate has been significantly associated with total occurrence of complications (p<0.008) and with fetal distress (p<0.002), perhaps because of its competition with zinc for intestinal absorption sites (*Mukherjee MD et al. Maternal zinc, iron, folic acid, and protein nutriture and outcome of human pregnancy. Am J Clin Nutr 40(3):496-507, 1984*).

Folate is the only vitamin whose requirement doubles in pregnancy. Serum and RBC folate levels decline during pregnancy and some degree of megaloblastic change can be found in substantial minorities of women in late pregnancy (*Truswell AS. ABC of nutrition. Nutrition for pregnancy. Br Med J 291:263-6, 1985*).

Dietary intake may be inadequate.

> **Observational Study:** Dietary folate intakes were well below the Recommended Dietary Allowance for 332 pregnant women of different ethnic gps. attending a Parisian antenatal clinic. Only 23% had a daily folacin intake of 400 μg or more (*Herberg S et al. Iron and folacin status of pregnant women: Relationships with dietary intakes. Nutr Rep Int 35(5):915-30, 1987*).

Low serum levels may be associated with low birth weight.

> **Observational Study:** The ave. birthweight at all gestational ages of 100 infants with erythroblastosis was lower than that of 200 controls, and there was a strong correlation between low maternal serum folate and the incidence of small-for-dates babies as well as a strong correlation between maternal and cord blood serum folate values, suggesting that a shortage of folic acid available for fetal growth may be the cause (*Gandy G, Jacobson W. Influence of folic acid on birthweight and growth of the erythroblastotic infant. I. Birthweight. Arch Dis Child 52(1):1-6, 1977*).

Supplementation may reduce the risk of a low-birth-weight infant (*Goyal U et al. Effects of folic acid supplementation on birth weight of infants. J Obstet Gyn India 30:104, 1980*

Supplementation around the time of conception may prevent neural tube defects.

> **Experimental Double-blind Study:** 1817 women at high risk of having a pregnancy with a neural tube defect, because of a previous affected pregnancy, randomly received either folic acid 4 mg daily, other vitamins (A, B₁, B₂, B₃, B₆, C, D), both or neither. 1195 had a completed pregnancy in which it was known whether the fetus or infant had a neural tube defect; 27 of these had a known neural tube defect - 6 in the folic acid gps. and 21 in the two other gps., a 72% protective effect (relative risk 0.28; 95% confidence interval 0.12-0.71). The other vitamins

showed no significant protective effect. There was no demonstrable harm from the folic acid supplementation (*MRC Vitamin Study Research Group. Prevention of neural tube defects: Results of the Medical Research Council Vitamin Study. Lancet 338:131-7, 1991*).

Note: While the high dosage of folic acid used in this study was effective, the possibility of it having an adverse effect on the fetus cannot be ruled out. On the other hand, a dose of 2-400 μg folate daily would be safe but has yet to be proven to be effective (Scott JM et al. Folic acid to prevent neural tube defects. Letter. Lancet 338:505, 1991).

Experimental Controlled Study: While fasting whole-blood pyridoxal 5^1-phosphate, serum vitamin B_{12} and serum and RBC folate levels were similar to those of controls, 5/16 women (31.3%) who had previously given birth to a baby with a neural tube defect showed evidence of methionine intolerance, suggesting heterozygous homocystinuria which can be corrected with high doses of pyridoxine or folic acid (*Steegers-Theunissen RPM et al. Neural-tube defects and derangement of homocysteine metabolism. Letter. N Engl J Med 324(3):199-200, 1991*).

Observational Study: Using a food frequency questionnaire, the dietary intakes of mothers of 77 cases of neural tube defect children in Australia were assessed for their free and total folate content. 77 subjects with other types of birth defects and 184 subjects with no birth defects were investigated as controls. Several confounding factors were controlled for. An increased maternal intake of free folate during the first 6 wks. of pregnancy was found to be associated with a decreased risk of bearing offspring with neural tube defects (*Bower D, Stanley FJ. Dietary folate as a risk factor for neural-tube defects: Evidence from a case-control study in Western Australia. Med J Aust 150:613-19, 1989*).

Note: This study has been criticized as the food frequency questionnaire used has not not been validated for its ability to accurately indicate dietary folate intake. Also the food tables used to determine folate content are unreliable for this nutrient (Mann J. Dietary folate and neural-tube defects. Editorial. Med J Aust 150:609, 1989).

Observational Study: In a cohort of 22,776 pregnancies, the prevalence of neural tube defect was 3.5/100 among American women who never used multivitamins before or after conception or who used multivitamins before conception only. For women who either used multivitamins without folic acid during the first 6 wks. of pregnancy or who used multivitamins containing folic acid beginning after 7 or more wks. of pregnancy, the prevalences were similar to that of the nonusers and the prevalence ratios were close to 1.0; however, the prevalence of neural tube defects for women who used folic acid-containing multivitamins during the first 6 wks. of pregnancy was substantially lower compared to never-users (0.9/1000; prevalence ratio 0.27; 95% confidence interval, 0.12-0.59) (*Mulinsky A et al. Multivitamin/folic acid supplementation in early pregnancy reduces the prevalence of neural tube defects. JAMA 262(20:2847-52, 1989*).

Negative Observational Study: The periconceptual use of vitamin supplements was examined for 571 American women who had a conceptus with a neural-tube defect, 546 women who had had a stillbirth or a conceptus with another malformation, and 573 women who had had a normal conceptus. There were no differences among the gps. in the use of folate supplements. The adjusted odds ratio for having an infant with an neural-tube defect among those receiving the recommended daily allowance of folate was 0.97 as compared with the mothers of abnormal infants and 0.98 as compared with the mothers of normal infants (*Mills JL et al. The absence of a relation between the periconceptional use of vitamins and neural-tube defects. N Engl J Med 321(7):430-35, 1989*).

Experimental Double-blind Study: 60 of 109 women who previously had delivered a NTD infant were randomly given folic acid 4 mg daily prior to conception and during early pregnancy and 44 complied, while 51 received placebo. None of the supplemented mothers delivered an NTD infant compared to 2/16 non-compliers and 6/51 placebo controls. The difference between the supplemented and unsupplemented gps. was significant (p=0.04) (*Laurence KM et al. Double-blind randomized controlled trial of folate treatment before conception to prevent recurrence of neural-tube defects. Br Med J 282:1509, 1981*).

Niacin:

Maternal intake early in pregnancy may be directly associated with infant birthweight and size.

Observational Study: In a study of 513 women living in London, there was a positive correlation between the maternal intake of niacin during 1 wk. towards the end of the first trimester of pregnancy and birthweight, newborn head circumference and newborn length for babies below the median weight (*Doyle W et al. The association between maternal diet and birth dimensions. J Nutr Med 1:9-17, 1990*).

Niacin supplementation in the second and third trimesters may fail to affect birth dimensions of the infant.

Experimental Controlled Study: Vitamin/mineral supplementation of mothers during the last 2 trimesters had no significant effect on birth dimensions compared to unsupplemented mothers (*Doyle W et al. The association between maternal diet and birth dimensions. J Nutr Med 1:9-17, 1990*).

Riboflavin:

Riboflavin depletion is common during pregnancy, although the riboflavin nutritional status of mothers may be unrelated to the course or outcome of pregnancy.

Observational Study: Based on the RBC glutathione reductase activation test, 25% of 651 pregnant women were riboflavin-depleted in the first trimester - increasing to 40% at term as compared to >300 male and female blood donors. Although no correlation between riboflavin status and the course or outcome of pregnancy could be demonstrated, riboflavin supplementation is recommended to prevent subclinical metabolic disturbances of thiamine-dependent enzyme systems (*Heller S et al. Riboflavin status in pregnancy. Am J Clin Nutr 27:1225-30, 1974*).

Thiamine:

Maternal intake early in pregnancy may be directly associated with infant birthweight and size.

Observational Study: In a study of 513 women living in London, there was a positive correlation between the maternal intake of thiamine during 1 wk. towards the end of the first trimester of pregnancy and birthweight, newborn head circumference and newborn length for babies below the median weight (*Doyle W et al. The association between maternal diet and birth dimensions. J Nutr Med 1:9-17, 1990*).

Thiamine supplementation in the second and third trimesters may fail to affect birth dimensions of the infant.

Experimental Controlled Study: Vitamin/mineral supplementation of mothers during the last 2 trimesters had no significant effect on birth dimensions compared to unsupplemented mothers (*Doyle W et al. The association between maternal diet and birth dimensions. J Nutr Med 1:9-17, 1990*).

Thiamine depletion is common during pregnancy, although the thiamine nutritional status of mothers may be unrelated to the course or outcome of pregnancy.

Observational Study: Based on the RBC transketolase activation test, 25-30% of 599 pregnant women were thiamine-depleted throughout gestation as compared to >300 male and female blood donors. Although no correlation between thiamine status and the course or outcome of pregnancy could be demonstrated, thiamine supplementation is recommended to prevent subclinical metabolic disturbances of thiamine-dependent enzyme systems (*Heller S et al. Vitamin B₁ status in pregnancy. Am J Clin Nutr 27:1221-24, 1974*).

Vitamin A: 5000 IU daily

WARNING: Daily doses of 40,000 IU or more during pregnancy may be teratogenic (*Martinez-Frias ML, Salvador J. Megadose vitamin A and teratogenicity. Letter. Lancet 1:236, 1988*), while doses lower than 10,000 IU appear to be safe (*Smithell RW. Spina bifida and vitamins. Br Med J 286:388-89, 1983*).

Vitamin A deficiency during pregnancy may be teratogenic (*Schardein JL. Chemically Induced Birth Defects. New York, Marcel Dekker, Inc., 1985:704-09*).

Often deficient in preterm infants, for whom deficiency may predispose to the development of chronic lung disease.

Observational Study: 64% of 91 preterm infants had retinol values <20 μg/l, which is suggestive of vitamin A deficiency. Retinol binding proteins were lower on the third day of life in babies with respiratory distress syndrome, and babies who developed bronchopulmonary dysplasia had lower concentrations of retinol at birth (p<0.05) on day 21 (p<0.05) despite receiving recommended intakes of vitamin A (*Hustead VA et al. Relationship of vitamin A (retinol) status to lung disease in the preterm infant. J Pediatrics 105(4):610-15, 1984*).

Lower levels may be associated with increased risk of pre-eclampsia.

Observational Study: Plasma vitamin E and retinol levels, but not beta-carotene levels, were significantly lower at 28 weeks gestation for healthy pregnant women who subsequently developed pre-eclampsia compared to others with normal preganancies, and remained significantly lower until delivery (*Jendryczko A, Drozdz M. Plasma retinol, beta-carotene and vitamin E levels in relation to the future risk of pre-eclampsia. Zent bl Gynakol 111:1121-23, 1989*).

Vitamin B₆: 20 mg. daily

WARNING: Higher doses may shut off breast milk and thus must be reduced before delivery in nursing mothers (*Marcus RG. Suppression of lactation with high doses of pyridoxine. S Afr Med J December 6, 1975, pp. 2155-56; Foukas MD. An antilactogenic effect of pyridoxine. J Obstet Gynaecol Br Commonw August, 1973, pp. 718-20*). Also, the baby could have withdrawal seizures if there is inadequate pyridoxine in commercial formula. Therefore, it is suggested that the mother nurse while continuing to take 20-30 mg. pyridoxine daily.

Note: A case has been reported in which an infant with a partially formed leg (phocomelia) was born to a mother who ingested 50 mg "doses" of B₆ daily for 7 months of pregnancy before stopping as they "made her sick." She was also ingesting various other supplements including a multivitamin, vitamin B₁₂ tablets and lecithin and there was no evidence that her supplementation had any connection with the fetal malformation (Gardner LI et al. Phocomelia in an infant whose mother took large doses of pyridoxine during pregnancy. Lancet 1:636, 1985).

Supplementation has been shown in a number of studies to be necessary to keep the laboratory measurements of vitamin B₆ (RBC glutamate-oxaloacetate transaminase) for pregnant women in the normal range, since it is marginally deficient in about 50% of pregnant women (*Heller S et al. Vitamin B₆ status in pregnancy. Am J Clin Nutr 26(12):1339-48, 1973*).

Note: Plasma pyridoxal-5-phosphate (PLP) levels may be reduced during pregnancy. The sum of PLP and pyridoxal, its hydrolysis product and the ultimate transport form of B₆, may still be normal, however, and thus PLP alone is not an adequate measure of B₆ status (Barnard HC et al. A new perspective in the assessment of vitamin B₆ nutritional status during pregnancy in humans. J Nutr 117(7):1303-06, 1987).

Given during labor, it may prevent many postnatal adaptation problems by increasing the oxygen-carrying capacity of the blood.

Experimental Study: Vitamin B₆ 100 mg given orally or IM at term resulted in greater oxygen affinity *in vitro* (p50) in the newborn's cord blood (*Temesvari P et al. Effects of an antenatal load of pyridoxine (vitamin B₆) on the blood oxygen affinity and prolactin levels in newborn infants and their mothers. Acta Paediatrica Scand. 72(4):525-9, 1983*).

Local application as a lozenge may reduce maternal caries which are more common during pregnancy.

Experimental Study: 540 pregnant women received a multiple vitamin with or without 20 mg. pyridoxine as a capsule once daily or as a lozenge (available from Alacer, US) divided into 3 doses. Although women who received pyridoxine developed less cavities, the difference was significant only for those who received the lozenges (*Hillman RW et al. Am J Clin Nutr 10:512, 1962*).

May be deficient in women with hyperemesis gravidarum (nausea and vomiting).

Negative Observational Study: When 180 pregnant women were evaluated to ascertain the relationship between B₆ status (pyridoxal 5-phosphate, RBC aspartate aminotransferase activity and stimulation of the latter by PLP) and the incidence of morning sickness, no correlation was found (*Schuster K et al. Morning sickness and vitamin B₆ status of pregnant women. Hum Nutr Clin Nutr 39C:75-79, 1985*).

Observational Study: Serum pyridoxal 5-phosphate level was low in 20 women with hyperemesis gravidarum as compared to 22 healthy pregnant women during the first trimester, 18 healthy pregnant women during the last trimester, and 29 healthy non-pregnant women of comparable age (*Gant H et al. [Vitamin B6 depletion in women with hyperemesis gravidarum.] Wein Klin Wochenschr 87(16):510-13, 1975*) (*in German*).

Supplementation is said to sometimes be effective in hyperemesis gravidarum (nausea and vomiting).

Protocol: Start with 25 mg three times daily. If no relief within 48 hours, increase as needed to 200 mg three times daily or give IM.

Experimental Double-blind Study: 31 pregnant women suffering from nausea and vomiting of pregnancy received vitamin B6 25 mg every 8 hrs., while another 28 women received a placebo. After 3 days, there was a significant difference in nausea after supplementation in women with initially severe nausea as compared to the control group. While almost half of the women in this gp. had vomited prior to supplementation, only 8/31 supplemented women had any vomiting after supplementation. In contrast, the number of women who vomited increased in the control gp. from 10/28 to 15/28 (*Sahakian V et al. Vitamin B6 is effective therapy for nausea and vomiting of pregnancy: A randomized double-blind placebo-controlled study. Obstet Gynecol 78:33-36, 1991*).

Experimental Placebo-controlled Study: 31 out-pts. randomly received pyridoxine 25 mg every 8 hrs. for 3 days while 28 others received placebo. Among women with initially severe nausea, pyridoxine significantly reduced the number of vomiting episodes and the mean nausea score, while placebo was without benefit. Among women with mild or moderate nausea, there was no significant difference between groups (*Anonymous. Vitamin B6 curbs severe nausea, emesis in gravida. Fam Pract News 21(11):10, 1991*).

Experimental Study: Vitamin B6 alone was compared to B6 plus meclozine (an antihistamine). In both gps., approx. 75% experienced complete relief (*Baum G et al. Meclozine and pyridoxine in pregnancy. Practitioner 190:251, 1963*).

Supplementation may prevent toxemia of pregnancy.

Observational Study: In pts. with toxemia, both pyridoxine levels and pyridoxal kinase activity are reduced in the placenta. Inasmuch as most observers consider the administration of pyridoxine to the pt. with toxemia to be of little or no demonstrable therapeutic value, the "deficiency" may be related to a failure to phosphorylate pyridoxine via pyridoxal kinase to its utilizable tissue form (*Klieger JA et al. Abnormal pyridoxine metabolism in toxemia of pregnancy. Ann N Y Acad Sci 166:288-96, 1969*).

Experimental Study: 4.4% of women on multivitamins without pyridoxine developed toxemia versus 1.1% of women on multivitamins with 10 mg pyridoxine (*Wachstein M, Graffeo LW. Influence of vitamin B6 on the incidence of preeclampsia. Obstet Gynecol 8:177, 1956*).

Vitamin C: 500-1000 mg daily

WARNING: Unless supplemented with vitamin C, infants born of mothers on megadoses of vitamin C may develop rebound scurvy.

Case Reports: Women taking more than 5000 mg of vitamin C throughout pregnancy delivered healthy infants which soon thereafter developed scurvy (*Rhead WJ, Schrauzer GN. Risks of long-term ascorbic acid overdosage. Nutr Rev 29:(11)262-63, 1971*).

Supplementation may be as effective as calcium for the treatment of leg cramps.

Experimental Double-blind Study: 60 pregnant women with leg cramps received either calcium or ascorbic acid 1 gm twice daily. There was no significant difference between the 2 gps. with respect to clinical improvement. In 14/60 pts., the symptoms were totally abolished; in 27/60 symptoms were significantly decreased; in 17/60 symptoms were unaffected; while in 2/60 symptoms increased in frequency (*Hammar M et al. Calcium and magnesium status in pregnant women: A comparison between treatment with calcium and vitamin C in pregnant women with leg cramps. Int J Vitam Nutr Res 57(2):179-83, 1987*).

Vitamin E: 200 IU daily

Vitamin E status may be low.

Observational Study: Plasma tocopherol levels increased gradually and significantly during pregnancy to twice the level of early pregnancy. These levels correlated with increasing plasma lipid levels, so that the plasma tocopherol/lipid ratio remained almost constant. RBC tocopherol levels did not change during the first trimester but decreased gradually through the remainder of the pregnancy and continued at the minimal level five days prior to delivery. Since previously studies have shown that changes in RBC tocopherol closely reflect changes in liver tocopherol concentrations, bioavailable tocopherol may be passively carried off into the increasing plasma lipids. Results suggest that vitamin E status declines during pregnancy in spite of increased plasma tocopherol levels due to elevated blood lipid levels. This explains the common finding that fetal vitamin E levels are usually low even though plasma vitamin E levels of mothers are higher during pregnancy (*Mino M, Nagamatu M. An evaluation of nutritional status of vitamin E in pregnant women with respect to red blood cell tocopherol level. Int J Vitam Nutr Res 56:149-53, 1986*).

Lower plasma levels may be associated with increased risk of pre-eclampsia.

Observational Study: Plasma vitamin E and retinol levels, but not beta-carotene levels, were significantly lower at 28 weeks gestation for healthy pregnant women who subsequently developed pre-eclampsia compared to others with normal preganancies, and remained significantly lower until delivery (*Jendryczko A, Drozdz M. Plasma retinol, beta-carotene and vitamin E levels in relation to the future risk of pre-eclampsia. Zent bl Gynakol 111:1121-3, 1989*).

Deficiency is associated with an increased risk of <u>premature</u> and <u>low birth weight infants</u>.

Observational Study: Pregnant Indian women who were poorly nourished with respect to vitamin E had more premature infants, more low birth weight infants , and greater hemolysis of maternal red blood cells (*Shah RS et al. Vitamin E status of the newborn in relation to gestational age, birth weight, and maternal vitamin E status. Br J Nutr 58:191-8, 1987*).

Supplementation may be effective in preventing <u>habitual abortion</u>.

Review Article: There is reasonable evidence of the prophylactic value of vitamin E in habitual abortion. Conclusive proof is lacking because it would require a controlled study comparing vitamin E against a placebo with no other therapy to rule out interactional effects; however it is difficult to ethically justify withholding all other treatments in habitual aborters (*Marks J. Critical appraisal of the therapeutic value of alpha-tocopherol. Vitam Hormones 20:573-98, 1962*).

Vitamin K:

Subclinical deficiency is common.

Observational Study: 33/99 pregnant women were found to have evidence of deficiency (*Family Pract News 14(5):27, 1984*).

Supplementation (along with vitamin C) may be effective for <u>nausea and vomiting of pregnancy</u>. Theorized to work by decreasing placental capillary permeability to prevent transport of a toxin into the maternal circulation.

Experimental Study: Vitamin K_1 (menadione) 5 mg daily along with vitamin C 25 mg daily was effective for 64/70 women within 72 hrs. (*Merkel RL. The use of menadione bisulfite, and ascorbic acid in the treatment of nausea and vomiting of pregnancy: A preliminary report. Am J Obstet Gynecol 64(2):416-18, 1952*).

Supplementation may reduce the risk of <u>intraventricular hemorrhage</u> in premature infants.

Experimental Controlled Study: 92 women destined to deliver infants less than 32 weeks gestation were randomized into 2 gps., one of which received vitamin K 10 mg IM every 5 days until delivery. Vitamin K therapy resulted in a significant reduction in prothrombin time (12.7 vs. 15.2 seconds) and partial thromboplastin time (42.6 vs. 58.9 seconds) in cord blood. In addition, the gp. receiving vitamin K had a lower incidence of total (16% vs. 36%) and severe (0% vs. 11%) grades of intraventricular hemorrhage (*Morales WJ et al. The use of antenatal vitamin K in the prevention of early neonatal intraventricular hemorrhage. Am J Obstet Gynecol 159:774-79, 1988*).

- -

MINERALS

Calcium: 1 - 1.5 gm. daily during pregnancy
2 gm. daily during lactation
(give 1/2 the amount of magnesium)

Hypercalcemia may be associated with puerperal psychosis.

> **Observational Study:** The serum calcium levels of 53 recently delivered mothers with severe puerperal psychosis were compared to those of 35 female psychiatric pts. and 49 normal postnatal women. The mean corrected and ionized serum calcium values of the PP pts. with no personal or family history of psychiatric illness were markedly elevated and were significantly higher than those of the PP pts. with personal or family histories and those of the 2 control groups. Follow-up of 16 PP pts. indicated that the fall in ionized serum calcium levels correlated positively and significantly with improvement in rated symptomatology (*Riley DM, Walt DC. Hypercalcemia in the etiology of puerperal psychosis. Biol Psychiatry 20:479, 1985*).

Calcium is the only mineral whose requirement doubles during pregnancy (*Truswell AS. Nutrition for pregnancy. Br Med J July, 1985*).

Low dietary intake may be associated with eclampsia.

> **Observational Study:** The eclampsia incidence and calcium intake for 3 countries, Guatemala (low eclampsia, high calcium), Colombia (high eclampsia, low calcium) and the U.S. (low eclampsia, high calcium) were compared. Crude rates for eclampsia incidence were adjusted to control for age, parity, and prenatal care. Results support an association between calcium intake and the development of eclampsia (*Villar J et al. Epidemiologic observations on the relationship between calcium intake and eclampsia. Int J Gynaecol Obstet 21(4):271-78, 1983*).

Hypocalciuria may be associated with pre-eclampsia.

> **Observational Study:** In a study of 40 women in the third trimester, the mean 24 hr. urinary calcium excretion in those with pre-eclampsia or hypertension with superimposed pre-eclampsia was significantly lower (42 ± 29 and 78 ± 49 mg/24 hrs.) than that in normal pregnant women (313 ± 140 mg/24 hrs.), women with transient hypertension (248 ± 139 mg/24 hrs.), or women with chronic hypertension (223 ± 41 mg/24 hrs.) ($p<0.0001$). The hypocalciuria in pts. with pre-eclampsia was associated with a decreased fractional excretion of calcium. Although their mean creatinine clearance was reduced, the range of values overlapped with those in other groups, while there was little or no overlap with respect to calcium excretion. These results suggest that determination of urinary calcium excretion may be useful in differentiaing pre-eclampsia from the more benign forms of gestational hypertension (*Taufield PA et al. Hypocalciuria in preeclampsia. N Engl J Med 316(12):715-18, 1987*).

Placental calcium level may be positively correlated with birth weight.

> **Observational Study:** In a study of the levels in the placenta of 26 elements as related to birthweight for 79 randomly selected live births, there was a significant positive correlation between calcium levels and birthweight. Results suggest that the dietary intake of calcium is too low for optimal fetal development in this population gp. (*Ward NI et al. Elemental factors in human fetal development. J Nutr Med 1:19-26, 1990*).

Supplementation may reduce the risk of preterm delivery.

> **Experimental Double-blind Study:** 189 healthy, pregnant, female adolescents age 17 or less were enrolled by the 23rd wk. of gestation and randomly received 2 g/d of elemental calcium as calcium carbonate or placebo. The mean duration of supplementation was about 14 weeks. The calcium gp. had a lower incidence of preterm deliv-

ery (<37 wks.: 7.4% vs. 21.1%; p=0.007); spontaneous labor and preterm delivery (6.4% vs. 17.9%; p=0.01); and low birth weight (9.6% vs. 21.1%; p=0.03). Life-table analysis demonstrated an overall shift to a higher gestational age in the calcium gp. compared to controls (p=0.02) (*Villar J, Repke JT. Calcium supplemention during pregnancy may reduce preterm delivery in high-risk populations. Am J Obstet Gynecol 163:1124-31, 1990*).

Supplementation may prevent <u>hypertensive disorders of pregnancy</u>.

> *Note: Pregnancy is associated with absorptive hypercalciuria. The addition of 2 g/d of calcium will increase the degree of calciuria and may theoretically increase the danger of renal calculi which occur in about 1 in 500 pregnancies (Ferris TF. Pregnancy, preeclampsia, and the endothelial cell. Editorial. N Engl J Med 325(20):1439-40, 1991).*

Experimental Double-blind Study: 1194 nulliparous women in the 20th wk. of gestation randomly received either calcium carbonate (2 g/d elemental calcium) or placebo. The rates of hypertensive disorders during pregnany were lower in the calcium gp. than in the placebo gp. (9.8% vs. 14.8%; odds ratio, 0.63; 95% confidence interval, 0.44-0.90). The risk of these disorders was lower at all times during gestation, particularly after the 7trh week, in the calcium gp., and the risk of both gestational hypertension and preeclampsia was also lower in the calcium group. Among the women who had low ratios of urinary calcium to urinary creatinine (≤0.62 mmol/mmol) during the 20th wk. of gestation, those in the calcium gp. had a lower risk of hypertensive disorders of pregnancy (odds ratio, 0.56; 95% confidence interval, 0.29-1.09) and less of an increase in diastolic and systolic BP than the placebo group. The pattern of response was similar among the women with a high ratio of urinary calcium to urinary creatinine during the 20th wk. of gestation, but the differences were smaller (*Belizán JM et al. Calcium supplementation to prevent hypertensive disorders of pregnancy. N Engl J Med 325:1399-405, 1991*).

Experimental Double-blind Study: 56 healthy nulliparous women (ave. age 19.4 yrs.) had a positive roll-over test (rise in diastolic BP of 20 mm Hg or more) at 28-32 weeks gestation and were therefore at risk for pregnancy-induced hypertension (PIH). They were randomly assigned to receive either elemental calcium 2 g daily or placebo. None of the 3 women on calcium in whom PIH developed had proteinuria of >20 mg/dL, whereas 8/24 women on placebo had such proteinuria. Results show a much lower frequency of PIH, a longer duration of pregnancy and higher birthweights in the experimental gp. (*Lopez-Jaramillo P et al. Dietary calcium supplementation and prevention of pregnancy hypertension. Letter. Lancet 335:293, 1990*).

Experimental Double-blind Study: 52 healthy pregnant women received either 1.5 gm elemental calcium or placebo daily after the 26th wk. of gestation. The incidence of pregnancy-induced hypertension was 11.1% in the placebo gp. and 4.0% in the calcium gp., a non-significant difference; however, subjects in the calcium gp., after adjustment for race and initial BP, had a term mean systolic and diastolic BP which was 4.5 mm Hg lower than those in the placebo gp. (p<0.05). Combining these values with previous data, there was a dose-effect relationship between calcium intake and BP reduction in the third trimester of pregnancy (*Villar J et al. Calcium supplementation reduces blood pressure during pregnancy: Results of a randomized controlled clinical trial. Obstet Gynecol 70(3 Pt. 1):317-22, 1987*).

Supplementation may prevent <u>premature delivery</u>.

- with <u>Magnesium</u>:

Experimental Double-blind Study: 190 pregnant teenagers received either calcium carbonate 1.5 g or placebo daily along with prenatal vitamins containing 200 mg calcium and 100 mg magnesium per day. Supplementation was begun before the 23rd wk. of gestation and continued for a mean duration of 14 weeks. The calcium gp. had a 65% lower incidence of preterm deliveries (7.4% vs. 21.1%; p=0.007) and a 55% lower incidence of low-birth-weight-infants (9.6% vs. 21.1%; p=0.03) than the placebo group. The effect of calcium may be mediated by a reduction in uterine smooth muscle contractability (*Villar J, Repke JT. Calcium supplementation during pregnancy may reduce preterm delivery in high-risk populations. Am J Obstet Gynecol 163:1124-31, 1990*).

<u>Chromium</u>:

Placental chromium level may be positively correlated with birth weight.

Observational Study: In a study of the levels in the placenta of 26 elements as related to birthweight for 79 randomly selected live births, there was a significant positive correlation between chromium levels and birthweight. Results suggest that the dietary intake of chromium is too low for optimal fetal development in this population gp. (*Ward NI et al. Elemental factors in human fetal development. J Nutr Med 1:19-26, 1990*).

Cobalt:

Placental cobalt level may be positively correlated with birth weight.

Observational Study: In a study of the levels in the placenta of 26 elements as related to birthweight for 79 randomly selected live births, there was a significant positive correlation between cobalt levels and birthweight. Results suggest that the dietary intake of cobalt is too low for optimal fetal development in this population gp. (*Ward NI et al. Elemental factors in human fetal development. J Nutr Med 1:19-26, 1990*).

Copper:

Pregnant women may be in negative copper balance unless supplemented.

Experimental Study: 24 women in their second trimester were found to ingest less than the RDA of copper. Copper retention was -0.02 mg/day until they were supplemented with copper which raised copper retention to 0.89 mg/day (*Taper L et al. Am J Clin Nutr 41:1184-1192, 1985*).

Placental copper level may be positively correlated with birth weight.

Observational Study: In a study of the levels in the placenta of 26 elements as related to birthweight for 79 randomly selected live births, there was a significant positive correlation between copper levels and birthweight. Results suggest that the dietary intake of copper is too low for optimal fetal development in this population gp. (*Ward NI et al. Elemental factors in human fetal development. J Nutr Med 1:19-26, 1990*).

Iron: 60 mg daily

Supplement if deficient.

> *Note: In pregnancy, physiological alterations in plasma volume and red-cell mass diminish the reliability of hemoglobin or hematocrit as a measure of iron status. Some of the established measurements of iron status such as serum iron and transferrin concentrations are altered in pregnancy independently of iron status, while othere are not sensitive to iron deficiency of recent onset. Serum ferritin <12 mg/L indicates absent iron stores but not necessarily iron-deficient erythropoiesis. Since it is low in the majority of pregnant women, it should be combined with measurements of circulating serum transferrin receptor to evaluate the entire spectrum of iron status in pregnancy (Carriaga MT et al. Serum transferrin receptor for the detection of iron deficiency in pregnancy. Am J Clin Nutr 54:1077-81, 1991).*

WARNING: Iron supplementation may exacerbate subclinical zinc depletion (*Meadows NJ et al. Lancet 2:1135, 1981*).

Dietary need is known to be increased during pregnancy and amenorrhea and increased iron absorption may not be adequate to make up for the extra demands if storage iron is low.

Experimental Controlled Study: 24 healthy young women <16 wks. pregnant and with normal hemoglobin status randomly received either a multivitamin/multimineral with 65 mg iron or one without iron. Those who did not receive iron had significantly lower mean serum ferritin levels (p<0.05) during pregnancy and the puerperium. 9/21 (43%) of these women, but none of the women on iron, failed to maintain an acceptable hemoglobin level (>11 gm/dl) and were medicated with 110 mg ferrous iron daily. Results suggest that iron supplementation is essential during pregnancy and for 3 mo. post-partum in order to maintain adequate maternal iron stores (*Dawson EB, McGanity WJ. Protection of maternal iron stores in pregnancy. J Reprod Med 32(6 Suppl):478-87, 1987*).

Experimental Controlled Study: 21 pregnant women received supplementation while 21 controls did not. Ferritin fell to 70% of its value at week 16 of amenorrhea in those supplemented versus only 30% in controls. Six and twelve week post-partum levels were still low in the controls (*Wallenburg HCS et al. Effect of oral iron supplementation during pregnancy on maternal and fetal iron status. J Perinat Med 12(1):7-12, 1984*).

Maternal intake early in pregnancy may be directly associated with infant birthweight and size.

Observational Study: In a study of 513 women living in London, there was a positive correlation between the maternal intake of iron during 1 wk. towards the end of the first trimester of pregnancy and birthweight, newborn head circumference and newborn length for babies below the median weight (*Doyle W et al. The association between maternal diet and birth dimensions. J Nutr Med 1:9-17, 1990*).

Iron supplementation in the second and third trimesters may fail to increase birth dimensions of the infant.

Experimental Controlled Study: Vitamin/mineral supplementation of mothers during the last 2 trimesters had no significant effect on birth dimensions as compared to those of unsupplemented mothers (*Doyle W et al. The association between maternal diet and birth dimensions. J Nutr Med 1:9-17, 1990*).

Placental iron level may be positively correlated with birth weight.

Observational Study: In a study of the levels in the placenta of 26 elements as related to birthweight for 79 randomly selected live births, there was a significant positive correlation between iron levels and birthweight. Results suggest that the dietary intake of iron is too low for optimal fetal development in this population gp. (*Ward NI et al. Elemental factors in human fetal development. J Nutr Med 1:19-26, 1990*).

Routine iron supplementation during pregnancy is not clearly indicated.

Experimental Controlled Study: 2912 pregnant women were randomized into 2 groups. The routine iron gp. was advised to take iron alone (not in combination preparations) throughout pregnancy, starting no later than in the 17th week as a single daily dose of elemental iron in the dosage and form determined by midwives; a mean dose of 124 mg was provided. In the selective gp., if the hematocrit of the mothers was <0.30 (hemoglobin <100g/L) after the 14th wk. of gestation on 2 consecutive visits and the lab confirmed anemia, 50 mg of ferrous sulfate was prescribed in slow release form twice daily for 2 mo. or until the hematocrit increased to 0.32 (hemoglobin = 110g/L). In the middle of the study, the limit for starting iron supplementation was raised to a hematocrit of <0.31. There were no significant differences in health outcomes between the 2 groups. Were routine iron supplementation a new practice, rather than customary, it would be easy to advise against it, because of the lack of firm evidence of its usefulness and because women in the selective gp. had less subjective adverse effects and fewer births after the 40th gestation week (*Hemminki E, Rimpelä U. A randomized comparison of routine versus selective iron supplementation during pregnancy. J Am Coll Nutr 10(1):3-10, 1991*).

<u>Magnesium:</u>   250-500 mg daily

The mean dietary intake of pregnant women is 35-58% of the recommended dietary allowance of 450 mg (*Franz KB. Magnesium intake during pregnancy. Magnesium 6:18-27, 1987*).

Serum levels may be lower than those of non-pregnant women, whether or not they are on birth control pills (*Stanton M et al. Serum magnesium in women during pregnancy, while taking contraceptives and after menopause. J Am Coll Nutr 6(4):313-20, 1987*). There is a steady fall in plasma concentrations during pregnancy and a rapid return to prepregnancy concentrations after delivery (*Sheldon WL et al. The effects of oral iron supplementation on zinc and magnesium levels during pregnancy. Br J Obstet Gynaecol 92:892-98, 1985*).

Induced deficiency may be associated with elevated blood pressure, reduced fetal weight, and pathologic placental and renal lesions (*Weaver K. Pregnancy-induced hypertension and low birth weight in magnesium-deficient ewes. Magnesium 5(3-4):191-200, 1986*).

Maternal intake early in pregnancy may be directly associated with infant birthweight and size.

Observational Study: In a study of 513 women living in London, there was a positive correlation between the maternal intake of magnesium during 1 wk. towards the end of the first trimester of pregnancy and birthweight, newborn head circumference and newborn length for babies below the median weight (*Doyle W et al. The association between maternal diet and birth dimensions. J Nutr Med 1:9-17, 1990*).

Serum and urinary magnesium may be low in <u>pre-eclampsia</u>.

Observational Study: Women without proteinuria who developed pre-eclampsia had low urinary magnesium even before pre-eclampsia developed (*Franz KB. Correlation of urinary magnesium excretion with blood pressure of pregnancy. Magesium Bull. 4:73-78, 1982*).

Observational Study: Women with pre-eclampsia were low in serum magnesium prior to therapy (*Weaver K. Magnesium in Health and Disease. Jamaica, N.Y., Spectrum Publications, 1980:833*).

Hypomagnesemia (1.4 mg/dl or less) may be a marker for true preterm labor.

Observational Study: Pts. in preterm labor have a significantly depressed serum magnesium level (mean 1.60 ± 0.46 mg/dl at 21-33 wks.; p<0.0005). This level was not dependent upon the etiology for the preterm labor (*Kurzel RB. Serum magnesium levels in pregnancy and preterm labor. Am J Perinatol 8:119-27, 1991*).

Magnesium supplementation in the second and third trimesters may fail to affect birth dimensions of the infant.

Experimental Controlled Study: Vitamin/mineral supplementation of mothers during the last 2 trimesters had no significant effect on birth dimensions as compared to unsupplemented mothers (*Doyle W et al. The association between maternal diet and birth dimensions. J Nutr Med 1:9-17, 1990*).

Supplementation may be beneficial in the treatment of pre-eclampsia.

Theoretical Discussion: Recent evidence suggests that cerebral vasospasm in involved in the pathogenesis of eclampsia. Magnesium may act by opposing calcium-dependent arterial vasoconstriction; it may also antagonize the increase in intracellular calcium caused by ischemia and thus prevent cell damage and death (*Sadeh M. Action of magnesium sulfate in the treatment of preeclampsia-eclampsia. Stroke 20(9):1273-75, 1989*).

Review Article: The drug of choice in the treatment of pre-eclampsia is magnesium sulfate 24-72 gm daily, with the dosage dependent upon urinary output (*Conradt A. [Pathophysiology and clinical aspects of pre-eclampsia.] Z Geburtshilfe Perinatol 189(4):149-61, 1985*).

Experimental Study: 6000 pregnant women at risk for pre-eclampsia and fetal growth retardation were given a magnesium supplement. Neither problem developed (*Conradt A et al. On the role of magnesium in fetal hypotrophy, pregnancy induced hypertension, and pre-eclampsia. Magnesium Bull 2:68-76, 1984*).

Parenteral magnesium sulfate is considered to be the treatment of choice for seizures associated with eclampsia (*Pritchard JAA, Pritchard SA. Standardized treatment of 154 consecutive cases of eclampsia. Am J Obstet Gynecol 123:543-52, 1975; Sabai GM, Anderson GD. Eclampsia, in P Goldstein, Ed. Neurological Disorders of Pregnancy. Mount Kisco, NY, Futura, 1986:1-18*).

Supplementation may reduce the complications of pregnancy and improve the health of the infant.

Negative Experimental Double-blind Study: 400 young pregnant women randomly received either 365 mg/d of elemental magnesium as magnesium aspartate HCl or aspartic acid. In addition, all pts. received a prenatal supplement containing 200 mg of calcium and 100 mg magnesium per day. There were no significant differences in pregnancy outcome or in perinatal outcome between gps. (*Sibai BM et al. Magnesium supplementation during pregnancy: a double-blind randomized controlled clinical trial. Am J Obstet Gynecol 161:115-119, 1989*).

Note: This study has been criticized as the incidence of severe pre-eclampsia was 41% lower and the incidence of small-for-gestational-age babies was 22% lower in the magnesium group. With such substantial differences, the lack of statistical difference may be a function of small sample size. Also, administration of 100 mg magnesium to the placebo group may have corrected a borderline deficiency in some women, thereby masking a beneficial effect of magnesium supplementation. In addition, since the aspartic acid "placebo" is a known mineral transporter, it may have further masked a beneficial effect of magnesium supplementation (Gaby AR. Magnesium and pregnancy: A poorly conceived study causes confusion. Townsend Letter for Doctors April, 1990, p. 166).

Experimental Double-blind Study: Pregnant women randomly received, as early in pregnancy as possible, either 15 mmol (365 mg) magnesium-aspartate-hydrochloride (n=278) or placebo (n=290) in 6 divided doses daily. In the magnesium gp., 15.8% had complications requiring hospitalization, compared to 22.4% in the placebo group. Magnesium-treated women had a 29.5% reduction in the risk of hospitalization and a 37% reduction in per capita hospital days. Hemorrhage, incompetent cervix and preterm labor were significantly less frequent and median length of gestation was significantly greater by one day in the magnesium group. Significantly fewer infants of mothers in the magnesium gp. required neonatal intensive care and, after exclusion of women who did not take magnesium as directed, the magnesium gp. had significantly fewer low-birth-weight infants as well as fewer infants with low Apgar scores (≤ 7) (*Spatling L, Spatling G. Magnesium supplementation in pregnancy. A double-blind study. Br J Obstet Gynaecol 95:120-25, 1988*).

Potassium:

May be reduced during pregnancy, especially in eclampsia.

Observational Study: Skeletal muscle concentrations of potassium were significantly lower in 17 women with normal pregnancies than in 11 female controls. Concentrations were lowest in 5 eclamptic women (*Sjögren A et al. Reduced concentrations of magnesium, potassium and zinc in skeletal muscle from women during normal pregnancy or eclampsia. Abstract. J Am Coll Nutr 7(5):408, 1988*).

Zinc: 10-30 mg daily

Pregnant women ingest only about 2/3 of the recommended dietary allowance of zinc (*Hambridge KM et al. Zinc nutritional status during pregnancy: A longitudinal study. Am J Clin Nutr 37:429-42, 1983*).

Plasma zinc declines about 30% during pregnancy; WBC and hair zinc also decline (*Truswell AS. Nutrition for pregnancy. Br Med J July, 1985*).

Note: Serum zinc is not a reliable indicator of zinc status in pregnancy due to an increase in protein-zinc binding capacity which causes an apparent, but falacious, decrease in available zinc (Argemi J et al. Serum zinc binding capacity in pregnant women. Ann Nutr Metab 32:121-26, 1988).

Low zinc intake is associated with spontaneous abortion and premature delivery.

Animal Experimental Study: Zinc intake of pregnant guinea pigs was reduced started on the 30th day of gestation. Poor zinc intake resulted in spontaneous abortion and premature delivery in 2 out of 3 experiments. In contrast, zinc-supplemented animals delivered living young at term (*Apgar J, Everett G. Low zinc intake affects maintenance of pregnancy in guinea pigs. J Nutr 121:192-200, 1991*).

Low maternal zinc levels may be associated with complications and labor abnormalities.

Observational Study: In a study of zinc status of 279 pregnant women at delivery, low levels of maternal plasma zinc were associated with more complications in the antenatal or intrapartum periods than maternal levels of either alkaline phosphatase or RBC zinc. Plasma zinc levels less than the median value were more commonly associated with mild toxemia (p=0.02), vaginitis (p=0.01) and postdates (p=0.01) in the antenatal period. During the intrapartum period, low plasma zinc levels were associated with a prolonged latent phase (p=0.05), a protracted active phase (p=0.04),. labor >20 hrs. (p=0.03), second stage >2.5 hrs. (p=0.01), and cervical and vaginal lacerations (p=0.0005). While a low maternal RBC zinc level was not associated with complications in either period, low levels of maternal alkaline phosphatase activity were strongly associated with a history of previous stillbirth (p=0.0005) (*Lazebnik N et al. Zinc status, pregnancy complications, and labor abnormalities. Am J Obstet Gynecol 158(1):161-66, 1988*).

Observational Study: In a study of 450 women, a significant association was found between the total occurrence of fetomaternal complications and zinc levels in the lowest quartile (p<0.02), and low zinc was also associated with the specific complication of fetal distress (*Mukherjee MD et al. Maternal zinc, iron, folic acid, and protein nutriture and outcome of human pregnancy. Am J Clin Nutr 40(3):496-507, 1984*).

Low maternal zinc levels may be associated with CNS abnormalities in infants including neural tube defects.

Observational Study: 259 pregnant women who were either over 40 years of age or had family histories of chromosomal abnormalities had their serum zinc measured during their second trimester. 15 pregnancies were abnormal and in 7/15, mean maternal serum zinc concentration was significantly lower than for the rest of the group (*Buamah PK et al. Maternal zinc status: A determinant of central nervous system malformation. Br J Obstet Gynaecol 91:788-90, 1984*).

Observational Study: Hair zinc of 17 mothers of infants with spina bifida was significantly higher than that of 30 unselected controls and rose during pregnancy while it decreased in the controls. There was a positive correlation between hair zinc in spina bifida mothers and that of their infants but no such correlation in controls. In addition, mean birth weight and length of spina bifida infants was significantly less than that of the control gp. (*Bergmann, KE et al. Abnormalities of hair zinc concentration in mothers of newborn infants with spina bifida. Am J Clin Nutr 33:2145, 1980*).

Note: Elevated hair zinc usually indicates decreased tissue zinc.

Low maternal zinc levels may be associated with low birth weight infants.

Observational Study: Zinc concentrations of placental tissue and cord blood were measured in mothers who gave birth to normal or low-birth-weight infants. Placental zinc concentrations were similar in both gps. and there were no correlations between birth weight and placental zinc, nor between head circumference and placental zinc. However, cord blood zinc levels of mothers producing normal-weight babies were significantly higher than those found in mothers of low-birth-weight infants (*Malhotra A et al. Placental zinc in normal and intra-uterine growth-retarded pregnancies. Br J Nutr 63:613-21, 1990*).

Observational Study: In a study of the levels in the placenta of 26 elements as related to birthweight for 79 randomly selected live births, there was a significant positive correlation between zinc levels and birthweight. Of all 26 elements, this was the strongest correlation. Results suggest that the dietary intake of zinc is too low for optimal fetal development in this population gp. (*Ward NI et al. Elemental factors in human fetal development. J Nutr Med 1:19-26, 1990*).

Observational Study: In a study of 250 healthy pregnant women who did not smoke or consume alcohol, mothers with serum zinc levels of <65 µg/dl in the last trimester showed a higher incidence of newborn birth weights below the 50th percentile, as well as below the 25th percentile, at term delivery (*Higashi A et al. A prospective survey of serial serum zinc levels and pregnancy outcome. J Ped Gastroenterol 7:430-33, 1988*).

Observational Study: Based on zinc status, healthy pregnant women were divided into normozincemia (ave. serum zinc: 933 µg/L) and hypozincemia gps. (ave. serum zinc 388 µg/L). 64.5% of the infants of the hypozincemia mothers were low in birth weight, compared to 42.6% of the normozincemic mothers, suggesting that serum zinc below 500 µg/L at the time of delivery is associated with an increased liklihood of delivering a low birth weight infant (*Singh P et al. Maternal hypozincemia and low-birth-weight infants. Clin Chem 33:1950, 1987*).

Low maternal zinc levels may be associated with toxemia of pregnancy.

Observational Study: Low plasma zinc levels were found in women with toxemia (*Cherry FF et al. Am J Clin Nutr 34:2367-75, 1981*).

Supplementation, especially if zinc levels are low, may reduce the risk of fetal and maternal complications.

Experimental Double-blind Study: Pregnant adolescents thought to be at risk for poor zinc nutriture were randomly assigned to receive 30 mg zinc gluconate daily or placebo. Zinc supplementation improved pregnancy outcome in normal-weight women and in underweight multiparas, but not in underweight primiparas, possibly due to multiple limiting factors (*Cherry FF et al. Adolescent pregnancy: Associations among body weight, zinc nutriture, and pregnancy outcome. Am J Clin Nutr 50:945-54, 1989*).

Negative Experimental Double-blind Study: 494 pts. randomly received either elemental zinc 20 mg daily or placebo starting when they booked for delivery prior to 20 wks. of gestation and lasting until delivery. Baseline leukocyte zinc levels were not significantly different between the 2 gps.; leuckocyte zinc levels were also not significantly different after 28-32 wks. gestation. There were no differences in outcome for either the mothers or the babies (*Mahomed K et al. Zinc supplementation during pregnancy: A double blind randomised controlled trial. Br Med J 299:826-29, 1989*).

Review Article: In studies done to date, supplementation with 15-45 mg/d of zinc failed to improve pregnancy outcome except for a possible reduction in the incidence of a dysfunctional labor pattern; thus the relationship between zinc status and pregnancy outcome remains an open question (*Swanson CA, King JC. Zinc and pregnancy outcome. Am J Clin Nutr 46(5):763-71, 1987*).

Experimental Controlled Study: 179 pts. received zinc aspartate 20 mg between the 12th and 34th wk. of pregnancy while 345 randomly selected controls did not. The control gp. was found to have a higher proportion of both large and small-for-date infants. Complications during labor (vaginal bleeding, fetal acidosis, uterine inertia) were also for frequent in the control gp. (*Kynast G, Saling E. Effect of oral zinc application during pregnancy. Gynecol Obstet Invest 21(3):117-22, 1986*).

Experimental Double-blind Study: 213 low-income Hispanic women were randomized to receive vitamin and mineral supplementation either with or without 20 mg zinc. The incidence of pregnancy-induced hypertension was lower (p<0.003) in the experimental gp. than in the controls; however, pregnancy-induced hypertension was not associated with low serum zinc levels at either the initial or final visit. Except for pregnancy-induced hypertension, there was a higher incidence of abnormal pregnancy outcomes in the noncompliers (those who failed to take their supplements) than in the compliers (*Hunt IF et al. Zinc supplementation during pregnancy: effects on selected blood constituents and on progress and outcome of pregnancy in low-income women of Mexican descent. Am J Clin Nutr 40(3):508-21, 1984*).

- -

OTHER NUTRITIONAL FACTORS

<u>Bioflavonoids</u>:   200 mg. three times daily

Supplementation may be effective in preventing <u>spontaneous abortion</u> and <u>premature labor</u>.

Experimental Study: Many chronic aborters stopped aborting after they were placed on citrus bioflavonoids 200 mg 3 times daily as soon as a period was missed. One pt. who developed uterine bleeding when 3 mo. pregnant began supplementation and delivered a normal baby (*Redman, JC. Letter. Med Trib April 16, 1980*).

Supplementation may prevent or reduce the severity of <u>erythroblastosis fetalis</u>.

Case Reports: 6 previously Rh immunized mothers treated with bioflavonoids (CVP six 600 mg caps daily) during their pregnancy delivered babies who were less erythroblastotic than expected (*Jacobs WM. The use of the bioflavonoid compounds in the prevention or reduction in severity of erythroblastosis fetalis. Surg Gynecol Obstet 103:233-36, 1956*).

<u>Omega-6 Fatty Acids</u>:

(Evening primrose oil is a source of GLA, precursor to prostaglandin E₁.)

Supplementation may be beneficial in pregnancy-induced <u>hypertension</u>.

Experimental Controlled Study: Pregnancy-induced hypertension is associated with diminished tissue production of E series prostaglandins and an enhanced pressor response to angiotension II (AII). 10 pregnant and 10 non-pregnant subjects were supplemented daily with 3 gm linoleic acid, 32 mg GLA and cofactors. After 1 wk., their pressor response to AII was compared to that of 40 pregnant and 24 non-pregnant unsupplemented controls. While supplementation was not associated with BP changes, the diastolic pressor response to AII in the pregnant subjects was significantly less after treatment and the systolic pressor response was significantly blunted at higher infusion doses, suggesting that supplementation may help to prevent or slow the development of pregnancy-induced hypertension (*O'Brien PMS et al. The effect of dietary supplementation with linoleic acid and linolenic acid on the pressor response to angiotension II: A possible role in pregnancy-induced hypertension? Br J Clin Pharmacol 19(3):335-42, 1985*).

- -

TOXIC MINERALS

Cadmium:

Body cadmium burden may be negatively correlated with birth weight.

Observational Study: In a study of the levels in the placenta of 26 elements as related to birthweight for 79 randomly selected live births, there was a significant negative correlation between cadmium levels and birthweight. Results suggest that the intake/body burden of cadmium is too high for optimal fetal development in this population gp. (*Ward NI et al. Elemental factors in human fetal development. J Nutr Med 1:19-26, 1990*).

Lead:

Elevated body lead burden may be associated with an increased risk of miscarriage.

Observational Study: In an informal survey, at least 13/36 women employees of USA Today who had been pregnant after December, 1987 suffered miscarriages. A subsequent study found excessively high amounts of lead and barium in the staff's drinking-fountain water (*Miscarriages prompt study of lead levels at USA Today. Am Med News April 14, 1989, p. 61*).

Elevated body lead burden may promote pre-eclampsia, perhaps by inhibiting calcium and magnesium metabolism.

Observational Study: Blood samples from 24 normal and 19 preeclampsia pregnancies which were 35-42 wks. of gestation were obtained. RBC magnesium levels were lower ($p \leq 0.05$) and lead levels were higher ($p \leq 0.001$) in the preeclamptic patients. Both the Pb/Mg and Pb/Ca ratios were higher ($p \leq 0.01$, 0.02) in the preeclamptic patients. Results suggest that pre-natal supplementation of calcium and/or magnesium, or reduction of exposure to lead, may prevent preeclampsia (*Dawson EB, Kelly R. Calcium, magnesium, and lead relationships in preeclampsia. Abstract. Am J Clin Nutr 51:512, 1990*).

Body lead burden may be negatively correlated with birth weight.

Observational Study: In a study of the levels in the placenta of 26 elements as related to birthweight for 79 randomly selected live births, there was a significant negative correlation between lead levels and birthweight. Results suggest that the intake/body burden of lead is too high for optimal fetal development in this population gp. (*Ward NI et al. Elemental factors in human fetal development. J Nutr Med 1:19-26, 1990*).

PREMENSTRUAL SYNDROME

See Also: "HYPERESTROGENISM"
"HYPOGLYCEMIA" (FUNCTIONAL)

OVERVIEW

Premenstrual syndrome has been divided into four subgroups:

PMT-A: ('Anxiety') anxiety irritability insomnia depression (late)	PMT-D: ('Depression') depression forgetfulness confusion lethargy

PMT-C: ('Craving')
craving for sweets
increased appetite;
sugar ingestion →
    headache
    palpitations
    fatigue or fainting
	PMT-H: ('Hyperhydration')
	weight gain above 1.4 Kg
	breast congestion & tenderness
	abdominal bloating & tenderness
	edema of face & extremities

PMT-A:

Characterized by elevated blood estrogens (CNS stimulants) and low progesterone (CNS depressant) during the luteal phase. A low progesterone/estradiol-17β ratio is the most consistent finding.

Patients consume excessive dairy products and refined sugars, the intake of which should be reduced. Caffeine-containing foods and drinks should be curtailed, and total fats limited to 30% of calories. Twice as much vegetable protein as animal protein should be consumed. Fiber intake should be increased to 20-40 g daily. Pyridoxine 2-800 mg daily reduces blood estrogen, increases progesterone and reduces symptoms under double-blind conditions.

PMT-C:

Caused primarily by the ingestion of large amounts of refined simple carbohydrates. During the luteal phase, there is increased carbohydrate tolerance, with a flat curve on glucose tolerance testing. RBC magnesium is low, and prostaglandin E_1 may be deficient.

Note: Although many patients experience hypoglycemic symptoms during glucose tolerance testing, the symptoms may not resemble PMT symptoms and may not be specific to the luteal phase of their menstrual cycles (Denicoff KD et al. Glucose tolerance testing in women with premenstrual syndrome. Am J Psychiatry 147(4):477-80, 1990).

Adequate magnesium replacement may result in improvement in glucose tolerance and symptoms, and chromium supplementation may be of value. Cis-linoleic acid (safflower oil is a good source) should be increased to 5-6% of total calories, while animal fat consumption should be limited. Unrefined complex carbohydrates should be increased to at least 40% of total calories, while simple carbohydrates should be limited to 15% of calories with elimination of refined sugar. Salt intake should be limted to 1 g/day.

PMT-D:

Mean blood progesterone may be higher than normal during the midluteal phase, and elevated adrenal androgens are observed in some hirsute patients. Other patients with normal progesterone and estrogens have chronic lead intoxication with elevated hair lead levels.

Treatment depends upon the individual findings. Tyrosine 3-6 gm daily in the morning may be helpful if hypotyrosinemia is found. Insomnia may be relieved with L-tryptophan 0.5-1 gm. Pyridoxine and magnesium, as with other PMT types, may be beneficial.

PMT-H:

Associated with symptoms of water and salt retention, and possibly by elevated serum aldosterone.

Methylxanthines should be avoided and sodium limited to 3 gm/day. Pyridoxine suppresses aldosterone resulting in diuresis, while magnesium increases the threshold response to stress, thus preventing ACTH-mediated aldosterone secretion. Vitamin E reduces breast symptoms.

(Abraham GE. Mangaement of the premenstrual tension syndromes: Rationale for a nutritional approach, in J Bland, Ed. 1986: A Year in Nutritional Medicine. New Canaan, Conn., Keats Publishing, 1986; Abraham GE. Nutritional factors in the etiology of the premenstrual tension syndromes. J Reprod Med 28(7):446-64, 1983; Abraham GE. Premenstrual tension. Prob Obstet Gynecol 3(12):1-39, 1980).

- -

DIETARY FACTORS

Low fat diet (PMT-H).

May reduce symptoms associated with fluid retention.

Experimental Controlled Study: 30 healthy premenopausal women were fed a high fat diet (40% of energy from fat) for 4 menstrual cycles, followed by a similar period on a low fat diet (20% of energy from fat). During both menses and the premenstrual wk. of the low fat dietary period there were significant decreases in self-reported symptoms associated with water retention (weight gain, bloating, breast tenderness). A decrease in "arousal" during the rest of the menstrual cycle was also reported (*Jones DV. Influence of dietary fat on self-reported menstrual symptoms. Physiol Behav 40(4):483-87, 1987*).

Animal fats stimulate the growth of intestinal bacteria which are capable of hydrolyzing conjugated estrogens into biologically active free estrogens which can be reabsorbed (*Adlercreutz H et al. Excretion of the lignans enterolactone and enterodiol and of equol in omnivorous and vegetarian postmenopausal women and in women with breast cancer. Lancet 2:1295-99, 1982; Goldin BR, Borback SL. The relationship between diet and rat fecal bacterial enzymes implicated in colon cancer. J Natl Cancer Inst 57:371-75, 1976*).

- with a high complex carbohydrate diet.

Experimental Controlled Study: 21 pts. with severe persistent cyclical mastopathy of at least 5 years' duration randomly received either training to reduce dietary fat to 15% of calories while increasing complex carbohydrate consumption to maintain calorie intake, or general dietary advice. After 6 mo., there was a significant reduction in the intervention gp. in the severity of premenstrual breast tenderness and swelling. Physical exam showed reduced breast swelling, tenderness, and nodularity in 6/10 pts. in the intervention gp. and 2/9 pts. in the control gp. (*Boyd NF et al. Effect of a low-fat high-carbohydrate diet on symptoms of cyclical mastopathy. Lancet 2:128-32, 1988*).

High complex carbohydrate, low refined sugar diet.

During the luteal phase, cells have an increased capacity to bind insulin which may be further modified by sugar (*De Pirro R et al. Insulin receptors during the menstrual cycle in normal women. J Clin Endocrinol Metabol 47(6):1387-89, 1978; Muggeo M et al. Change in affinity of insulin receptors following oral glucose in normal adults. J Clin Endocrinol Metabol 44:1206-9, 1977*). However, patients with PMS have normal 3-hr. glucose tolerance tests including normal insulin levels (*Spellacy WN et al. Plasma glucose and insulin levels during the menstrual cycles of normal women and premenstrual syndrome patients. J Reprod Med 3595):508-11, 1990*). Moreover, although patients often have hypoglycemic symptoms during testing, these symptoms do not resemble their PMS symptoms and are not specific to the luteal phase (*Denicoff KD et al. Glucose tolerance testing in women with premenstrual syndrome. Am J Psychiatry 147(4):477-80, 1990*).

Carbohydrate intake may be greater in patients than in normals.

Observational Study: In a study of 853 female university students, the consumption of foods and beverages that are high in sugar content or taste sweet was associated with prevalence of the premenstrual syndrome (*Rossignol AM, Bonnlander H. Prevalence and severity of the premenstrual syndrome. Effects of foods and beverages that are sweet or high in sugar content. J Reprod Med 36(2):131-6, 1991*).

Observational Study: Women with PMT have a significantly greater intake of refined carbohydrates than normals (*Goei GS et al. Dietary patterns of patients with premenstrual tension. J Appl Nutr 34(1):4-11, 1982*).

Observational Study (PMT-A): PMT-A pts. were found to consume 2 1/2 times the amt. of refined sugar than women with or without mild PMT (*Abraham GE. Magnesium deficiency in premenstrual tension. Magnesium Bull 1:68-73, 1982*).

Increased carbohydrate intake may reduce dysphoric symptoms (PMT-D).

Observational Study (PMT-D): In a study of the occurrence and coincidence of depressed mood and excessive carbohydrate intake in 19 pts. with severe premenstrual depression and 9 controls, pts. significantly increased carbohydrate intake during the late luteal phase by 24% from meals and by 43% from snacks. Calorie intake significantly rose without a change in protein intake, while fat intake rose in proportion to calorie intake. Consumption of a carbohydrate-rich, protein-poor evening test meal during the late luteal phase improved depression, tension, anger, confusion, sadness, fatigue, alertness, and calmness scores (p<0.01) among pts.; no effect was seen during the follicular phase among pts. or during either phase among controls. Because synthesis of brain serotonin, which is known to be involved in mood and appetite, increases after carbohydrate intake, PMS pts. may overconsume carbohydrates in an attempt to improve their dysphoric mood state (*Wurtman JJ et al. Effect of nutrient intake on premenstrual depression. Am J Obstet Gynecol 161(5):1228-34, 1989*).

Ingestion of large amounts of sugar abruptly increases insulin secretion, suppressing ketoacid formation. As ketoacids help the kidney clear excess sodium and water, sodium and water retention occurs causing expansion of extracellular fluid volume and PMT-H symptoms (*Abraham GE. Management of the premenstrual tension syndromes: rationale for a nutritional approach, in J Bland, Ed. 1986: A Year in Nutritional Medicine. New Canaan, CT, Keats Publishing, Inc., 1986*).

Refined sugar increases the urinary excretion of magnesium, a deficiency of which may contribute to PMT-C (*Seelig M. Human requirements of magnesium: Factors that increase needs, in J Durlach, Ed. First Int Sympos on Magnesium Deficiency in Human Pathol Paris, Springer, Verlag, 1973:11*).

High fiber diet (PMT-A).

Increases estrogen binding and excretion.

Observational Study: Peripheral and fecal estrogens were compared in 10 vegetarian and 10 omnivorous women who were menstruating regularly. The omnivorous women consumed 11-13 g/d of fiber compared to 25-33 g/d for vegetarian women. A significant negative correlation between fiber intake and fecal estrogens suggests that food fiber increases the clearance and fecal excretion of estrogens. Blood estrogen levels were significantly lower in the vegetarian women than in the omnivorous women (*Goldin BR et al. Estrogen excretion patterns and plasma levels in vegetarian and omnivorous women. N Engl J Med 307:1542-47, 1982*).

Reduce salt to 3 gm/day at least 3 days prior to symptom-onset (PMT-C, PMT-H).

Salt may aggravate PMT-C as it enhances glucose-induced insulin production by facilitating glucose absorption (*Ferrannini E et al. Sodium elevates the plasma glucose response to glucose ingestion in man. J Clin Endocrinol Metab 54:455, 1982*).

PMT-H is associated with a relative deficiency of dopamine at the renal level (*Kuchel D et al. Catecholamine excretion in 'idiopathic' edema: Decreased dopamine excretion, a pathologic factor. J Clin Endocrinol Metab 44:639, 1977*). Since dopamine is natiuretic and diuretic (*McDonald RH et al. Effects of dopamine in man: Augmentation of sodium excretion, glomerular filtration rate and renal plasma flow. J Clin Invest 43:1116, 1964*), a deficiency leads to sodium and water retention.

Reduce caffeine at least 3 days prior to symptom-onset.

Women who consume large amounts of caffeine are more likely to suffer from PMS.

Observational Study: In a survey of 841 unselected female university students, consumption of caffeine-containing beverages was strongly related to the prevalence of premenstrual syndrome. Among women with more severe symptoms, the relation between consumption of caffeine-containing beverages and premenstrual syndrome was dose-dependent, with prevalence odds ratios equal to 1.3 for consumers of 1 cup of a caffeine-containing beverage per day and increasing steadily to 7.0 for consumers of 8-10 cups per day. The observed effects were only slightly reduced when daily total fluid consumption was controlled (*Rossignol AM, Bonnlander H. Caffeine-containing beverages, total fluid consumption, and premenstrual syndrome. Am J Public Health 80(9):1106-10, 1990*).

Observational Study: 188 nursing students and tea factory workers in the People's Republic of China were evaluated. Tea consumption was found to be strongly related to the prevalence of premenstrual syndrome and the effects were dose-dependent (*Rossignol AM et al. Tea and premenstrual syndrome in the People's Republic of China. Am J Public Health 79(1):67-69, 1989*).

Observational Study: In a survey of 295 students, the prevalence of PMS, especially with moderate to severe symptoms, increased with greater consumption of caffeine-containing beverages. 61% of women who drank 4.5-15 caffeine-containing drinks daily experienced moderate to severe symptoms, while only 16% of women consuming no caffeine experienced moderate to severe symptoms (*Rossignol AM. Caffeine-containing beverages and premenstrual syndrome in young women. Am J Public Health 75(11):1335-37, 1985*).

Avoid alcohol.

Consumption may facilitate the development of PMT-C by inhibiting gluconeogenesis and promoting a fall in plasma glucose (*Rabin D. Hypoglycemia: Physiologic and diagnostic considerations, in GE Abraham, Ed. Radioassay Systems in Clinical Endocrinology. New York, Marcel Dekker, 1981:609-24*).

The increase in gastric acidity which follows alcohol ingestion might cause excessive release of gut secretagogues which augment beta-cell responsiveness to glucose fluctuations, leading to excessive insulin release (*Freinkel N, Getzger BE. Oral glucose tolerance curve and hypoglycemias in the fed state. N Engl J Med 280:820-8, 1969*).

- -

VITAMINS

Vitamin A: 100,000 - 300,000 IU daily (2nd half of cycle)

Although blood retinol levels appear to be normal (*Chuong CJ, Dawson EB, Smith ER. Vitamin A levels in premenstrual syndrome. Fertil Steril 54(4):643-7, 1990; Mira M et al. Vitamin and trace element status in premenstrual syndrome. Am J Clin Nutr 47:636-41, 1988*), supplementation may be beneficial.

WARNING: Close medical supervision is necessary due to possible adverse side effects.

Experimental Placebo-controlled Study: Pts. received vitamin A 2-300,000 IU daily premenstrually or placebo. All experimental subjects benefited, compared to 25% of those on placebo (*Block E. The use of vitamin A in premenstrual tension. Acta Obstet Gynecol Scand 39:586-92, 1960*).

Experimental Study: 218 pts. received vitamin A 2-300,000 IU daily. 48% had complete symptom relief, 41.2% had a partial effect and 10.8% failed to improve. Results were best for premenstrual headache and worst for PMT-A (*Block E. The use of vitamin A in premenstrual tension. Acta Obstet Gynecol Scand 39:586-92, 1960*).

Experimental Study: 100 pts. received vitamin A 50,000 IU twice daily during the second half of their cycles with good results (*Kleine HO. Vitamin A therapie bei pra menstruellen nervosen Beschwerden. Dtsch med Wschr 79:879-80, 1954*).

Experimental Study: 30 pts. received vitamin A 200,000 IU daily from day 15 of their cycles until symptom-onset. After 2-6 mo. the majority of pts. were considerably improved. PMT-H responded better than PMT-A. Symptoms did not recur in the year following cessation of vitamin A therapy (*Argonz J, Albinzano C. Premenstrual tension treated with vitamin A. J Clin Endocrinol 10:1579-89, 1950*).

<u>Vitamin B$_6$</u>:   500 mg. daily   (3 month trial)

Vitamin B$_6$ is <u>not</u> deficient.

Observational Study: In a study of the levels of RBC pyridoxine-dependent enzymes in 38 pts. and 23 controls both in the premenstrium and in the mid-follicular phase, there was no evidence of either an absolute or relative deficiency (*Mira M et al. Vitamin and trace element status in premenstrual syndrome. Am J Clin Nutr 47(4):636-41, 1988*).

Observational Study: There was no correlation between the severity of PMS symptoms in 210 healthy premenopausal women and plasma pyridoxal-5-phosphate levels (*Richie CD, Singkamani R. Plasma pyridoxal-5^1-phosphate in women with the premenstrual syndrome. Hum Nutr Clin Nutr 40C:75-80, 1986*).

Supplementation may be beneficial.

> *Note: Based on unpublished data, Abraham suggests that B$_6$ 500 mg daily in sustained release form will decrease symptoms of PMT-A, PMT-C and PMT-H. It will also benefit PMT-D, but only when combined with PMT-A (Guy Abraham - personal communication reported in Piesse JW. Nutrition factors in the premenstrual syndrome: A review. Int Clin Nutr Rev 4(2):54-81, 1984.*

Review Article: 12 controlled trials of vitamin B$_6$ were found. A major drawback of these trials was the limited number of patients included. The existing evidence of positive effects of vitamin B$_6$ is weak (*Kleijnen J, Ter Riet G, Knipschild P. Vitamin B$_6$ in the treatment of premenstrual syndrome - - a review. Br J Obstet Gynaecol 97(9):847-52, 1990*).

Negative Experimental Controlled Study: 28 women aged 21-28 received pyridoxine 250 mg to take each morning in addition to dietary instruction, while controls received only dietary instruction. No significant improvement in symptom cluster score was reported for either group (*Berman MK et al. Vitamin B-6 in premenstrual syndrome. J Am Diet Assoc 90(6):859-61, 1990*).

Experimental Double-blind Crossover Study: 32 women aged 18-49 with moderate to severe premenstrual symptoms randomly received either pyridoxine 50 mg daily or placebo. After 3 mo. the gps. were crossed over for another 3 months. A significant beneficial effect was only found in women with emotional-type symptoms (depression, irritability and tiredness) (p<0.05) (*Doll H et al. Pyridoxine (vitamin B$_6$) and the premenstrual syndrome: A randomized crossover trial. J R Coll Gen Pract 39:364-68, 1989*).

Experimental Double-blind Study: 55 women who reported mild to severe premenstrual mood changes randomly received daily supplements of 150 mg vitamin B$_6$ or placebo for 2 months. Analysis of covariance suggested that even though vitamin B$_6$ may have improved premenstrual symptoms related to autonomic reactions (e.g. dizziness, vomiting) and behavioral changes (e.g. poor performance, decreased social activities), a significant amount of physical and emotional symptomatology (e.g. anxiety, depression, pain, water retention) remained (*Ken-*

dall KE, Schnurr PP. The effects of vitamin B6 supplementation on premenstrual symptoms. Obstet Gynecol 70(2):145-49, 1987).

Review Article: Pyridoxine is the first-line drug for PMS, but should be discontinued if there is absolutely no response after 1 month. 5/7 studies show it to be superior to placebo; by contrast, no other drug has shown much efficacy (*David R. Rubinow, biological psychiatry branch, National Institute of Mental Health (USA) - quoted by Clin Psychiatry News, December, 1987).*

Supplementation with vitamin B6 may normalize deficient intracellular magnesium levels.

Experimental Controlled Study: Vitamin B6 intake of 10 premenopausal and 7 postmenopausal females with normal RBC and plasma magnesium levels was either 2.3 mg/d or supplemented to 10.4 mg/d, while dietary magnesium was kept at 240-70 mg/d. After 48 days, RBC and plasma magnesium levels were unchanged, suggesting that, at usual intakes, vitamin B6 does not influence normal RBC and plasma magnesium levels (*Lee CM, Leklem JE. Blood magnesium constancy with vitamin B-6 supplementation in pre- and post-menopausal women. Ann Clin Lab Sci 14(2):151-4, 1984).*

Experimental Study: 9 females with low RBC magnesium levels received vitamin B6 100 mg twice daily. After 4 wks., RBC magnesium levels had normalized (*Abraham GE et al. Effect of vitamin B6 on plasma and red blood cell magnesium levels in premenopausal women. Ann Clin Lab Sci 11(4):333-36, 1981).*

Deficiency may reduce the efficacy of estrogen by interfering with its binding to the estrogen receptors.

Animal Experimental Study (PMT-D): Even though vitamin B6-deficient rats showed a greater uptake of estrogens in their tissues, including the CNS, the biological activity of estrogen was decreased (*Holley J et al. Effect of vitamin B6 nutritional status on the uptake of [3H]-oestradiol into the uterus, liver and hypothalamus of the rat. J Steroid Biochem 18:161-66, 1983).*

A co-factor in the conversion of gamma-linoleic acid (GLA) to dihomogamma-linolenic acid (DGLA) and of DGLA to prostaglandin E1 (*See "Omega-6 Fatty Acids" below*).

<u>Vitamin E:</u>   300 IU daily (2 month trial)
    Increase to 600 IU daily if ineffective.

Although blood levels appear to be normal (*Chuong CJ et al. Vitamin E levels in premenstrual syndrome. Am J Obstet Gynecol 163 (5 Pt 1):1591-5, 1990),* supplementation may be beneficial.

Experimental Double-blind Study: Pts. randomly received D-alpha-tocopherol 400 IU or placebo daily for 3 cycles. Pts. receiving vitamin E reported a 33% reduction in physical symptoms (such as weight gain and breast tenderness), a 38% reduction in anxiety and a 27% reduction in depression. They were also less tired and had fewer headaches and cravings for sweets. By contrast, pts. on placebo only noted a 14% reduction in physical symptoms (*London RS et al. Efficacy of alpha-tocopherol in the treatment of the premenstrual syndrome. J Reprod Med 32(6):400-04, 1987).*

Experimental Double-blind Study (PMT-A,C,D,H): 75 pts. with benign breast disease and PMT randomly received either D,L-alpha-tocopherol 75 IU (#18), 150 IU (#19), or 300 IU (#19) twice daily or placebo (#19). After 2 mo., supplementation significantly improved PMT-A at the 150 IU twice daily dosage, and PMT-C and PMT-D at the 300 IU twice daily dosage, but not PMT-H. Post-menstrually there was a small but significant increase in PMT-H symptoms (*London RS et al. The effect of alpha-tocopherol on premenstrual symptomatology: A double-blind study. J Am Coll Nutr 2(2):115-122, 1983).*

_ _

MINERALS

<u>Calcium</u>:

In PMT-A:

1. Consumed in significantly higher quantities than by normals (*Goei GS et al. Dietary patterns of patients with premenstrual tension.* <u>*J Appl Nutr*</u> *34(1):4-11, 1982; Abraham GE. Magnesium deficiency in premenstrual tension.* <u>*Magnesium Bull*</u> *1:68-73, 1982*).

2. The dietary calcium to magnesium ratio is higher than it is for either normals or other PMT patients (*Abraham GE. Magnesium deficiency in premenstrual tension.* <u>*Magnesium Bull*</u> *1:68-73, 1982*).

3. Hair calcium levels are significantly more likely to be elevated than in normals (*Abraham GE. Nutritional factors in the etiology of the premenstrual syndrome.* <u>*J Reprod Med*</u> *28(7):446-464, 1983*).

> *Note: Elevated hair calcium merely suggests the possibility of a metabolic disturbance in calcium regulation; it is thus difficult to interpret its significance without more data.*

> *Note: Elevated hair calcium has been found to directly correlate with sugar intake (Maher CC. Dissertation. U. of Michigan, 1976:209).*

Supplementation may be beneficial.

> *Note: Since calcium impairs the absorption of magnesium, a deficiency of which may contribute to PMT (Seelig M. Human requirements of magnesium: Factors that increase needs, in J Durlach, Ed.* <u>*First Int Sympos on Magnesium Deficiency in Human Pathol*</u>. *Paris, Springer, Verlag, 1971:11), calcium should not be supplemented unless magnesium is also supplemented.*

Experimental Double-blind Crossover Study: 33 pts. randomly received calcium carbonate 1,000 mg daily and placebo for 3 mo. each in either order. On prospective daily ratings, there was a reduction in symptoms while on calcium supplementation during both their luteal (p=0.011) and menstrual phases (p=0.032), but not during their intermenstrual phase. On retrospective assessment, 73% reported fewer symptoms during calcium treatment, 15% preferred placebo, and 12% had no clear preference. 3 premenstrual factors: negative affect (p=0.045), water retention (p=0.003) and pain (p=0.036); and 1 menstrual factor: pain (p=0.02) were significantly alleviated by calcium (*Thys-Jacobs S et al. Calcium supplementation in premenstrual syndrome: a randomized crossover trial.* <u>*J Gen Intern Med*</u> *4(3):183-9, 1989*).

<u>Magnesium</u>:   400 mg. daily

Erythrocyte magnesium may be reduced despite normal plasma/serum levels.

Observational Study: Plasma and RBC magnesium levels were measured in 105 pts. and 50 normal premenopausal controls in the mid-luteal phase of the menstrual cycle. Plasma magnesium was not significantly different between the 2 gps., but RBC magnesium was significantly lower (mean 2.06 mmol/L) in the pt. gp. compared to controls (mean 2.47 mmol/L). 45% of the pt. gp. had RBC magnesium levels below the normal range. The authors note that they have tested many conditions, and PMS is the only one of them that is correlated with lower than normal population levels of magnesium (*Sherwood RA et al. Magnesium and the premenstrual syndrome.* <u>*Ann Clin Biochem*</u> *23(6):667-70, 1986*).

Deficiency causes depletion of brain dopamine (*Barbeau A et al. Deficience en magnesium et dopamine cerebrale, in J Durlach, Ed.* <u>*First Int. Symposium on Magnesium Deficit in Human Pathology*</u>. *Paris, F. Vittel, 1973:149-52*). Since PMT-A is believed to be associated with relative dopamine depletion by excess estrogen in the luteal phase (*Redmond DE et al. Menstrual cycle and ovarian hormone effects on plasma and platelet monamine oxidase (MAO) and plasma dopamine-hydroxylase activities in the Rhesus monkey.* <u>*Psychosom Med*</u> *37:417, 1975*), magnesium deficiency may contribute to the syndrome.

May reduce glucose-induced insulin secretion (*Curry DL et al. Magnesium modulation of glucose-induced insulin secretion by the perfused rat pancreas. Endocrinology 101:203, 1977*); thus a deficiency could favor the development of PMT-C.

Most B vitamins require phosphorylation to become activated, a process which is magnesium-dependent (*Abraham GE. Management of the premenstrual tension syndromes: Rationale for a nutritional approach, in J Bland, Ed. 1986: A Year in Nutritional Medicine. New Canaan, Conn., Keats Publishing, 1986*).

Required for the the conversion of cis-linoleic acid to gamma-linolenic acid by delta-6-desaturase (*Cunnane SC, Horrobin DF. Parenteral linoleic and gamma-linolenic acids ameliorate the gross effects of zinc deficiency. Proc Soc Exp Biol Med 164:583, 1980*). (*See "Omega-6 Fatty Acids" below*).

Deficiency causes hyperplasia of the adrenal cortex, elevated aldosterone levels and increased extracellular fluid volume (*Cantin M. Hyperaldosteronisme secondaire au cours de la carence en magnesium, in J Durlach, Ed. First Int Sympos on Magnesium Deficit in Human Pathol. Paris, F. Vittel, 1973:451-60*). Aldosterone also increases urinary magnesium excretion (*Horton R, Biglieri EG. Effect of aldosterone on the metabolism of magnesium. J Clin Endocrinol 22:1187, 1962*).

Increases the activity of glucuronyl transferase, an enzyme involved in the hepatic glucuronidation of estrogens (*Brown RC, Bidlack WR. Regulation of glucuronyl transferase by intracellular magnesium, in Proceed Int Sympos Magnesium and its Relationship to Cardioivascular, Renal and Metabolic Disorders. Los Angeles, 1985:24*).

Supplementation may be beneficial.

> **Experimental Double-blind Study:** 20 pts. with perimenstrual migraine received 360 mg/d of elemental magnesium as magnesium pyrrolidone carboxylic acid or a placebo. Treatments were started on the 15th day of the menstrual cycle and continued until menstruation. After 2 mo., the Pain Total Index, a measure of the intensity and duration of migraines, was significantly lower in the treatment gp. than in the controls and the number of days with migraines was significantly reduced only in the treatment group. Treatment was also associated with a significant reduction in Menstrual Distress Questionnaire scores. Pretreatment magnesium levels were reduced in lymphocytes and polymorphonuclear leukocytes compared to healthy controls. After treatment, these levels increased significantly (*Faccinetti F et al. Magnesium prophylaxis of menstrual migraine: effects on intracellular magnesium. Headache 31:298-304, 1991*).

> **Experimental Double-blind Study:** 32 pts. aged 24-39 randomly received either magnesium carboxylic acid (360 mg Mg) 3 times daily or placebo from the 15th day of their cycle to the onset of menstrual flow. After 2 cycles, both gps. received magnesium. The Menstrual Distress Questionnaire score of the cluster "pain" was significantly reduced during the second month in both gps., whereas magnesium treatment significantly affected both the total Menstrual Distress Questionnaire score and the cluster "negative affect." In the second month, the women assigned to treatment showed a significant increase in magnesium in lymphocytes and polymorphonuclear cells, but no changes in plasma and erythrocytes. Results suggest that magnesium supplementation could be effective for premenstrual symptoms related to mood changes (*Faccinetti F et al. Oral magnesium successfully relieves premenstrual mood changes. Obstet Gynecol 78(2):177-81, 1991*).

Zinc:

During the luteal phase, serum zinc levels in patients may be reduced (*Chuong CJ et al, Baylor College of Medicine, Houston - presented at the 46th Annual Mtg. of the Am. Fertility Society, Washington, DC, 1991*).

A zinc deficiency during the luteal phase may theoretically lead to decreased secretions of progesterone and endorphins (*Chuong CJ et al, Baylor College of Medicine, Houston - presented at the 46th Annual Mtg. of the Am. Fertility Society, Washington, DC, 1991*).

- -

OTHER NUTRITIONAL FACTORS

Omega-6 Fatty Acids:

$$\text{linoleic acid} \rightarrow \text{GLA} \rightarrow \text{DGLA} \rightarrow \text{prostaglandin E}_1$$

Example: Evening primrose oil (a source of GLA) 500 mg. three times daily

A functional deficiency of essential fatty acids, either due to inadequate linoleic acid intake or absorption or to failure of normal conversion of linoleic acid to GLA, has been postulated to cause abnormal sensitivity to prolactin and the features of PMS (*Horrobin DF. The role of essential fatty acids and prostaglandins in the premenstrual syndrome. J Reprod Med 28(7):465-68, 1983*).

Observational Study: Plasma concentrations of linoleic acid were consistently higher, and levels of linoleic acid metabolites were consistently lower, in 2 gps. of women with premenstrual syndrome, 2 gps. with cyclical breast disease and 2 gps. with non-cyclical breast disease compared to 2 gps. of normal controls. These findings suggest an abnormality in EFA metabolism, probably involving reduced conversion of linoleic acid to its EFA metabolites (*Horrobin DF et al. Abnormalities in plasma essential fatty acid levels in women with premenstrual syndrome and with non-malignant breast disease. J Nutr Med 2:259-64, 1991*).

Observational Study: In a study of 42 pts., the levels of linoleic acid were significantly elevated, while the levels of all its metabolites were significantly reduced, suggesting a defect in the conversion of linoleic acid to gamma-linolenic acid. Possibly in compensation, levels of omega-3 essential fatty acids were significantly elevated. As the same abnormalities were present in both follicular and luteal phases, the defect cannot be the direct cause of luteal phase symptoms, but it may sensitize tissues so that they respond abnormally to normal levels of reproductive hormones (*Brush MG et al. Abnormal essential fatty acid levels in plasma of women with premenstrual syndrome. Am J Obstet Gynecol 150(4):363-66, 1984*).

Supplementation may be beneficial.

Negative Experimental Double-blind Crossover Study: 38 pts. randomly received evening primrose oil (Efamol) and placebo in either order; the crossover was after 3 menstrual cycles. Although symptoms improved, no significant differences between the active and placebo gps. were found, and no "carry-over" effect of primrose oil was observed. The beneficial effect on all symptoms (psychological, fluid retention, breast) was rapid, the scores decreasing in the first cycle but increasing slightly at the changeover period after the third cycle, irrespective of whether the active or placebo medication was next given (*Khoo SK et al. Evening primrose oil and treatment of premenstrual syndrome. Med J Aust 153(4):189-92, 1990*).

Experimental Double-blind Study: 10/20 women with severe, treatment-resistant symptoms reported moderate to complete relief following 3 mo. of supplementation with EPO compared to 1/16 given placebo (p<0.01) (*Ockerman PA et al. Evening primrose oil as a treatment of the premenstrual syndrome. Recent Adv Clin Nutr 2:404-05, 1986*).

Experimental Double-blind Study: 30 pts. with severe PMS randomly received either EPO (Efamol) 1.5 gm twice daily or placebo. After 4 cycles, EPO slightly alleviated PMS, as assayed by PMS score or by the patients' own judgement. Depression was the only symptom which was significantly reduced (p<0.05) when compared to placebo (*Ylikorkala O et al. Prostaglandins and premenstrual syndrome. Prog Lipid Res 25:433-35, 1986; Puolakka J et al. Biochemical and clinical effects of treating the premenstrual syndrome with prostaglandin synthesis precursors. J Reprod Med 39(3):149-53, 1985*).

Experimental Placebo-controlled Study: 92 pts. with cyclical severe breast pain in whom breast cancer had been excluded were treated with evening primrose oil 3 g/d for 3-6 months. Following treatment, 45% had either no residual pain or residual pain which was easily bearable compared to 19% of a gp. of pts. on placebo. Side effects were minimal (*Pye JK et al. Clinical experience of drug treatments for mastalgia. Lancet 2:373-77, 1985*).

Experimental Double-blind Study: 73 pts. with mastalgia randomly received evening primrose oil or placebo. 19 pts. dropped out within the first 3 mo., 16 of whom were on placebo. After 3 mo., pain and tenderness were significantly reduced in both cyclical and non-cyclical groups as compared to baselines, while controls failed to significantly improve (*Pashby NL et al. A clinical trial of evening primrose oil in mastalgia. Abstract.* Br J Surg *68:801-24, 1981*).

Tyrosine: 3-6 grams daily in the morning

If the patient has hypotyrosinemia, supplementation may be beneficial (PMT-D) (*Abraham GE. Nutrition and the premenstrual tension syndromes.* J Appl Nutr *36:103-24, 1984*).

- -

COMBINED NUTRITIONAL SUPPLEMENTATION

Experimental Double-blind Study: 44 pts. randomly received either Optivite®, a multivitamin/multimineral supplement, 6 or 12 tabs daily, or placebo. After 3 menstrual cycles, significant treatment effects were noted in 3 sub-gps. for the 6 tab gp. and in all 4 sub-gps. for the 12 tab group (*London RS, Bradley L, Chiamori NY. Effect of a nutritional supplement on premenstrual symptomatology in women with premenstrual syndrome: a double-blind longitudinal study.* J Am Coll Nutr *10(5):494-9, 1991*).

Experimental Double-blind Study: 57 pts. randomly received either Optivite®, a multivitamin/multimineral supplement, 12 tabs daily, Optivite® 6 tabs daily, or placebo. Based on PMS questionnaires, the 12 tab daily gp. significantly reduced scores for Irritability, Tension, Dysphoria, Mental-Cognitive, Motor-Coordination, and Other Physical (p<0.05); the 6 tab daily gp. significantly reduced scores for Tension, Dysphoria, and Mental/Cognitive (p<0.05). The only significant reduction in the placebo gp. was for Irritability (p<0.05) (*Reynolds MA, London RS. Efficacy of a multivitamin/mineral supplement in the treatment of the premenstrual syndrome. Abstract.* J Am Coll Nutr *7(5):416, 1988*).

Experimental Double-blind Study: 119 pts. randomly received either Optivite®, a multivitamin/multimineral supplement, 12 tabs daily or placebo, while another 104 pts. randomly received either Optivite® 2 tabs daily during the first 2 wks. of their menstrual cycle and 4 tabs daily during the rest of the cycle or placebo. After 3 menstrual cycles, premenstrual symptoms were significantly improved in the women on the high-dose regimen compared to placebo (p<0.05) but not in women on the low-dose regimen (*Stewart A. Clinical and biochemical effects of nutritional supplementation on the premenstrual syndrome.* J Reprod Med *32(6):435-41, 1987*).

Experimental Double-blind Crossover Study: 31 pts. received Optivite® 6 tabs daily and placebo for 3 consecutive menstrual cycles each, in random order. Compared to placebo, treatment was associated with lower premenstrual symptoms for pts. with PMT-A and PMT-C but not for pts. belonging to the other 2 sub-gps. (*Chakmakjian ZH, Higgins CE, Abraham GE. The effect of a nutritional supplement, Optivite® For Women, on premenstrual tension syndromes: II. Effect on symptomatology, using a double blind, cross-over design.* J Appl Nutr *37(1):12-17, 1985*).

- and diet:

Experimental Study: 200 pts. were given dietary instruction and supplemented with Optivite® plus, in some cases, additional vitamin C, vitamin E, magnesium, zinc or evening primrose oil. On retrospective analysis, 96.5% reported a significant degree of improvement by 3 mo., with >30% rating themselves as asymptomatic (*Stewart A et al. Effect of a nutritional programme on premenstrual syndrome: a retrospective analysis.* Complement Med Res *5(1):8-11, 1991*).

Experimental Double-blind Study: Dietary guidelines and supplementation with Optivite® (Optimox, Torrance, CA, USA), a multivitamin/multimineral formula, 6 tablets daily decreased premenstrual tension syndrome symptom scores to significantly lower levels than did placebo. A significantly higher percentage of pts. reported feeling better on the dietary program than did those on the placebo. The program, implemented for 3-6 mo., decreased serum estradiol 17-β and increased serum progesterone levels during the midlutel phase (*Abraham GE, Rumley RE. Role of nutrition in managing the premenstrual tension syndromes.* J Reprod Med *32(6):405-22, 1987*).

OTHER FACTORS

Rule out vaginal candidiasis.

Experimental Controlled Study: 32 women with severe PMS and a history of vaginal candidiasis had previously failed to respond to various treatments including pyridoxine supplementation, drugs and psychotherapy. 10/15 who received a sugar-free, yeast-free diet and oral nystatin had significant relief from PMS symptoms, while symptoms were unchanged in the controls (*Schinfeld JS. PMS and candidiasis: Study explores possible link. Female Patient July 1987, p. 66*).

Rule out lead toxicity (PMT-D).

Chronic lead intoxication interferes with the binding of estrogen to its receptors, thus reducing its effect (*Young PCM et al. Effect of metal ions on the binding of 17β-estradiol to human endometrial cystol. Fertil Steril 28:312-18, 1972*).

Patients may have evidence of lead toxicity.

Observational Study: Hair samples from the nape of the neck were analysed in 56 pts. and 14 normal controls. Hair lead levels were 34% higher for the pt. gp. taken as a whole (p<0.05). For 2 pts. with severe PMT-D, hair lead levels were 11.3 times and 14 times, respectively, the levels for the normal women (*Hanson MA et al. Hair tissue concentration of minerals, trace elements, and toxic metals in normal women and patients with premenstrual tension syndromes, in M Abdulla et al, Eds. Health Effects and Interactions of Essential and Toxic Elements. New York, Pergamon Press, 1983:608-11*).

Since magnesium blocks the intestinal absorption of lead (*Fine BP, Barth A et al. Influence of magnesium on the intestinal absorption of lead. Environ Res 12:224, 1976*) and increases its urinary excretion (*Krall AR et al. Effects of magnesium infusions on the metabolism of calcium and lead, in M Cantin, MS Seelig, Eds. Magnesium in Health and Disease. Spectrum Publications, 1980:941-48*), a magnesium deficiency may predispose to lead intoxication.

PSORIASIS

See Also: RHEUMATOID ARTHRITIS

DIETARY FACTORS

High fiber diet.

Psoriasis is associated with high levels of circulating endotoxins, and a diet low in fiber is associated with increased levels of endotoxin-producing bacteria (*Rosenberg E, Belew P. Microbial factors in psoriasis. Arch Dermatol 118:1434-44, 1982*).

Low protein, low fat diet.

Clinical Observation: Pts. with psoriasis, being treated with the Kempner rice diet for kidney, hypertensive vascular and heart disease or diabetes, have shown a dramatic reduction in or disappearance of their skin lesions within 2-3 months and local steroid treatment was able to be discontinued. Many of these pts. had previously been treated unsuccessfully for years with systemic and/or local medications, and not a single pt. noted worsening of the lesions on the diet. The diet contains no more than 20 g protein and very little fat with a relatively large percentage of linoleic acid. The author suspects that improvement is due to a decrease in a harmful substance (*Newborg B. Disappearance of psoriatic lesions on the rice diet. N Carolina Med J 47:253-55, 1986*).

Experimental Study: Pts. were placed on a modified fast for 2 wks. followed by a vegan diet for 3 weeks. While their condition was unchanged during the fast, some of the pts. experienced an improvement on the vegan diet (*Lithell H et al. A fasting and vegetarian diet treatment trial on chronic inflammatory disorders. Acta Derm Venereol (Stockh) 63(5):397-403, 1983*).

Experimental Study: Pts. gave definite signs of abnormal nitrogen retention. When placed on diets containing no more than 4-5 g nitrogen daily (about 30 gm protein), with an adequate caloric intake, pts. experienced a gradual disappearance of the lesions while maintaining their weight. However, the lesions recurred when the diet was stopped. In 18 yrs., only 1 pt. failed to respond to this regimen (*Schamberg JF. The dietary treatment of psoriasis. JAMA 98:1633, 1932; Schamberg JF et al. Protein metabolism in psoriasis. J Cutan Dis 31:892-915, 1913; Schamberg JF et al. Research studies in psoriasis: A preliminary report. J Cutan Dis 31:698, 1913*).

Negative Experimental Study: 13 pts. were hospitalized for 4-17 wks. and maintained on varying levels of protein intake ranging from 4.0-162 gm daily. Local therapy was restricted to a bland cream. All pts. improved during the first 7 wks., and only 2 relapsed thereafter. No significant difference in the degree of rapidity of improvement on the various dietary protein levels was evident, and 3 pts. who improved while on a low-protein intake failed to flare when changed to a high-protein diet (*Zackheim HS, Farber EM. Low-protein diet and psoriasis. A hospital study. Arch Dermatol 99(5):580-6, 1969*).

Clinical Observations: 140 pts. were placed on a vegetarian diet. Results were often brilliant; often the eruption steadily faded and actually disappeared with absolutely no internal or local treatment. However, in general, the best results were obtained by combining the diet with other forms of treatment. Sometimes the rash will recur but, as a rule, the outbreak will not be nearly so severe or persistent as previous ones (*Bulkley LD. Diet and hygiene in diseases of the skin. JAMA 59:535, 1912; Bulkley LD. Report of 140 recent cases of psoriasis in private practice under a strictly vegetarian diet. JAMA 58:714, 1911*).

Avoid alcohol:

Observational Study: 144 men aged 19-50 with psoriasis and 295 unmatched male controls with other skin diseases reported their alcohol intake 12 mo. before the onset of skin disease and 12 mo. prior to examination. Recalled mean alcohol intake before the onset of skin disease was 42.9 g/d among psoriasis pts. and 21.0 g/d among controls. In logistic regression analysis psoriasis was associated with alcohol intake but not with coffee consumption, smoking, age, marital state, or social group. The odds ratio for psoriasis at an alcohol intake of 100 g/d compared to no intake was 2.2 (95% confidence interval 1.3 to 3.9). The controls decreased their alcohol intake after disease onset but the psoriasis gp. did not, suggesting that psoriasis sustains drinking (*Poikolainen K et al. Alcohol intake: a risk factor for psoriasis in young and midde aged men? Br Med J 300:780-83, 1990*).

Observational Study: Compared to 310 controls, the percentage of alchol abusers for a gp. of 326 pts. was higher (*Zanetti G et al. Enhanced prevalence of red blood cell macrocytosis in psoriatic patients. A sign of ethanol abuse? Acta Derm Venereol Suppl (Stockh) 146:196-8, 1989*).

Observational Study: In a study of 100 pts. with chronic plaque psoriasis, in male pts., heavy drinking was found significantly more commonly in those with severe psoriasis, and alcohol-related medical or social problems were frequent. By contrast, alcohol excess and alcohol-related problems were significantly less common in women irrespective of the severity of their psoriasis (*Monk BE, Neill SM. Alcohol consumption and psoriasis. Dermatologica 173(2):57-60, 1986*).

- -

VITAMINS

Folic Acid:

May be deficient (*Fry L et al. The mechanism of folate deficiency in psoriasis. Br J Dermatol 84:539-44, 1971*).

Vitamin A:

The polyamines (putrescine, spermidine and spermine) are increased in psoriasis and lowering of cutaneous and urinary levels is associated with clinical improvement (*Proctor M et al. Lowered cutaneous and urinary levels of polyamines with clinical improvement in treated psoriasis. Arch Dermatol 115:945-49, 1979*).

Vitamin A inhibits ornithine decarboxylase, the rate-limiting step in endogenous polyamine synthesis (*Haddox M et al. Retinol inhibition of ornithine decarboxylase induction and G1 progression in CHD cells. Cancer Res 39:4930-38, 1979*).

Serum levels may be reduced (*Günther S et al. [Serum carotene and serum retinol in psoriasis.] Z Hautkr 60(11):897-901, 1985; Majewski S et al. Decreased levels of vitamin A in serum of patients with psoriasis. Arch Dermatol Res 280:499-501, 1989*).

Supplementation may be beneficial (*Novotny F, Cerny J. [Vitamins and antivitamins in the treatment of psoriasis.] Cesk Dermatol 50(5):334-40, 1975 (in Czechoslovakian)*.

Administration of etretinate, a synthetic vitamin A analog, may be beneficial.

> WARNING: May have serious side effects.

Experimental Study: 20 pts. with psoriasis vulgaris were treated with etretinate. After 12 mo., etretinate was found to be an effective therapy for the skin disorder, and arthritis in 4/7 pts. was greatly improved. Side effects were dose-related and included mucocutaneous abnormalities as well as abnormalities of blood lipids and liver function tests. Maintainence therapy appeared to be required in nearly all pts. (*Kaplan RP et al. Etretinate therapy for psoriasis: clinical responses, remission times, epidermal DNA and polyamine responses. J Am Acad Dermatol 8(1):95-102, 1983*).

Vitamin B_{12}:

Supplementation by injection may be beneficial.

Experimental Placebo-controlled Study: Vitamin B_{12}, triamcinolone or normal saline was injected into lesions with a spring-loaded gun giving a concentration in the epidermis and penetration into the superficial and middle dermis. Triamcinolone caused rapid regression, while normal saline had no effect. Of the 8 pts. who received vitamin B_{12}, 6 showed regression of the lesion (*Carslaw RW, Neill J. Vitamin B_{12} in psoriasis. Letter. Br Med J 1:611, 1963*).

Negative Double-blind Experimental Study: 33 pts. with psoriasis for over 2 yrs. who had failed to respond to conventional treatments randomly received 21 IM injections of either vitamin B_{12} or placebo within 4 wks. Results were assessed at completion and 6 wks. later. There was no difference in results between B_{12} and placebo (*Sneddon JB. Vitamin B_{12} in psoriasis. Letter. Br Med J 1:328, 1963*).

Experimental Study: Good results were obtained with a series of 30 injections of vitamin B_{12} 1000 µg IM but a shorter series was ineffective. Improvement was often delayed up to 6 wks. after treatment was completed (*Cohen EL. Vitamin B_{12} in psoriasis. Letter. Br Med J 1:125, 1963*).

Negative Experimental Study: Treatment with a series of 15 IM injections of vitamin B_{12} 1000 µg was ineffective (*Baker H, Comaish JS. Br Med J December 29, 1962, p. 1729*).

Vitamin D:

Calcitriol (1,25-dihydroxyvitamin D_3) regulates terminal differentiation of basal cells of epidermal keratinocytes (*Morimoto S, Yoshikawa K. Psoriasis and vitamin D_3. A review of our experience. Arch Dermatol 125(2):231-4, 1989*).

Serum concentrations of 1,25-dihydroxyvitamin D may be low (*Staberg B et al. Abnormal vitamin D metabolism in patients with psoriasis. Acta Dermatol Venereol (Stockh) 67:65-68, 1987*).

Negative Observational Study: Levels of 1,25 $(OH)_2$ vitamin D was similar in 20 pts. and 15 controls (*Guilhou JJ et al. Vitamin D metabolism in psoriasis before and after phototherapy. Acta Dermatol Venereol (Stockh) 70(4):351-4, 1990*).

The efficacy of UV-B phototherapy may be due to increased 1,25 dihydroxyvitamin D.

Experimental Study: Although, at baseline, 1,25 dihydroxyvitamin D levels in 20 pts. were similar to those of 15 controls, after UV-B phototherapy, 15 (OH) D and 24,25 (OH) D_2 were dramatically increased in both pts. and controls; 1,25 $(OH)_2$ D was significantly increased in pts. but unmodified in controls (*Guilhou JJ et al. Vitamin D metabolism in psoriasis before and after phototherapy. Acta Dermatol Venereol (Stockh) 70(4):351-4, 1990*).

The topical or oral administration of 1,25-$(OH)_2$-D_3 may improve skin lesions.

Experimental Study: Of 40 pts. with psoriasis vulgaris, 17 received 1 alpha-hydroxyvitamin D_3 orally 1 µg/day for 6 mo., 4 pts. received 1 alpha-25-dihydroxyvitamin D_3 orally 0.5 µg/day for 6 mo., and 19 pts. recieved 1 alpha, 25-dihydroxyvitamin D_3 applied topically at a concentration of 0.5 µg/g of base for 8 weeks. At the end of the study periods, improvement was observed in 13/17 (76%) pts. in Gp. 1 with a mean treatment period of 2.7 mo., in 1/4 (25%) pts. in Gp. 2 at 3 mo., and in 16/19 (84%) pts. in Gp. 3 after a mean of 3.3 weeks. No side effects were observed (*Morimoto S, Yoshikawa K. Psoriasis and vitamin D_3. A review of our experience. Arch Dermatol 125(2):231-4, 1989; Morimoto S et al. An open study of vitamin D_3 in psoriasis patients. Br J Dermatol 115(4):421-29, 1986*).

Experimental Study: 5 pts. received topical administration of 1,25-dihydroxyvitamin D_3 and a control base. After 2-5 wks. of vitamin D application, all 5 pts. showed definite and in some cases remarkable improvement of the lesions. No systemic toxicity was detected (*Morimoto S et al. Therapeutic effect of 1,25-dihydroxyvitamin D_3 for psoriasis: Report of five cases. Calcif Tissue Inter 38:119-22, 1986*).

Topical application of the active vitamin D_3 analogue, 1 alpha, 24-dihydoxycholecalciferol, may improve skin lesions.

Experimental Study: 11 pts. were treated with 1 alpha, 24-dihydroxycholecalciferol, a synthetic analogue of active vitamin D_3. In 10/15 tests, the lesions cleared completely within 1-4 wks., although some relapses occurred shortly after cessation of treatment. There were no side-effects (*Kato T et al. Successful treatment of psoriasis with topical application of active vitamin D_3 analogue, 1 alpha, 24-dihydroxycholecalciferol. Br J Dermatol 115(4):431-33, 1986*).

Supplementation with oral 1,25 dihydroxyvitamin D₃ may improve psoriatic arthritis.

Experimental Study: 10 pts. with psoriatic arthritis received 1,25-dihydroxyvitamin D₃ 2 μg/d.   After 6 mo., there was a significant improvement in "tender joint count" (a composite indice reflecting joint tenderness in 66 sites).   4 showed over 50% improvement in the count and 3 had over 25% improvement, while 2 were unable to receive such therapeutic doses due to hypercalciuria.   There was also a significant improvement in "physician global assessment" (an index reflecting the overal extent of arthritis) and in physical activity (*Huckins D, Felson D, Holick M.   Treatment of psoriatic arthritis with oral 1,25-dihydroxyvitamin D₃: a pilot study.   Arth Rheum 33:1723-27, 1990*).

- and <u>Vitamin A</u>:

Combined administration may improve skin lesions.

Experimental Study: In a retrospective analysis, the records of 607 pts. who received treatment were reviewed.   Adult pts. initially received vitamin A 100,000 units and vitamin D 150,000 units daily, usually for 2-4 mo., followed by half the dosage for another 2 months.   11% had "++++" results, 23% had "+++" results, 27% had "++" results, 19% had "+" results and 20% had poor results.   Generally, the younger the pt. and the newer the lesions, the better the results.   8% had side effects.   Headache and GI side effects were the most common (*Dochao A et al.   [Therapeutic effects of vitamin D and vitamin A in psoriasis: A 20-year experiment].   Actas Dermosifiliogr 66(3-4):121-30, 1975*) (*in Spanish*).

Experimental Study: In a retrospective analysis, the records of 142 pts. were reviewed.   142 cases received 400,000 units of vitamin A and 600,000 units of vitamin D 3 wks. per month followed by weekly doses.   Treatment was for a total of 2 mo. for pts. experiencing their first outbreak and 3 mo. for pts. who had experienced more than one outbreak.   Of the 27 pts. with their first outbreak, 60% had very good results, 26% good results, 8% fair results and 8% poor results.   Of the pts. experiencing further outbreaks, 9% had very good results, 32% had good results, 40% had fair results, and 19% had poor results.   3 pts. had to stop treatment due to headaches or anorexia (*Marron Gasca J et al.   [General treatment of psoriasis.   Review of our cases.   Actas Dermosifiliogr 65(7-8):295-304, 1974*) (*in Spanish*).

- -

MINERALS

<u>Copper</u>:

Plasma levels may be elevated (*Dogan P et al.   Superoxide dismutase and myeloperoxidase activity in polymorphonuclear leukocytes, and serum ceruloplasmin and copper level, in psoriasis.   Br J Dermatol 120(2):239-44, 1989; Donadini A et al.   Plasma levels of Zn, Cu and Ni in healthy controls and in psoriatic patients.   Acta Vitaminol Enzymol 2:9-16, 1980*).

Serum copper and ceruloplasmin may be elevated in psoriatic arthritis (*Oriente P et al.   Supportive laboratory findings in psoriatic arthritis.   Clin Rheumatol 3(2):189-93, 1984*).

<u>Iron</u>:

Serum iron may be elevated in psoriatic arthritis (*Oriente P et al.   Supportive laboratory findings in psoriatic arthritis.   Clin Rheumatol 3(2):189-93, 1984*).

<u>Nickel</u>:

Plasma levels may be reduced (*Donadini A et al.   Plasma levels of Zn, Cu and Ni in healthy controls and in psoriatic patients.   Acta Vitaminol Enzymol 2:9-16, 1980*).

<u>Selenium</u>:

Required for activation of glutathione peroxidase, an inhibitor of the 5-lipoxygenase pathway which promotes formation of inflammatory leukotrienes (*White A et al. Role of lipoxygenase products in the pathogenesis and therapy of psoriasis and other dermatoses. <u>Arch Dermatol</u> 119:541-7, 1983*).

Blood selenium may be reduced (*Michaëlsson G et al. Selenium in whole blood and plasma is decreased in patients with moderate and severe psoriasis. <u>Acta Derm Venereol (Stockh)</u> 69(1):29-34, 1989*).

Oral administration appears to be ineffective.

Experimental Placebo-controlled Study: The mean whole blood and plasma selenium of a gp. of 69 pts. were reduced compared to healthy controls but their RBC glutathione peroxidase activity was normal. They received either 600 µg/d of selenium-enriched yeast, 600 µg/d of selenium-enriched yeast plus 600 IU of vitamin E or a placebo. After 12 wks., although their mean whole blood, plasma and platelet selenium concentrations, platelet glutathione peroxidase activity and plasma vitamin E concentration had risen significantly, their mean skin selenium concentration and RBC glutathione peroxidase activity remained unchanged. Neither supplement regimen reduced the severity of the psoriasis. The failure of the skin selenium content to increase may explain the failure of oral therapy (*Fairris GM et al. The effect of supplementation with selenium and vitamin E in psoriasis. <u>Ann Clin Biochem</u> 26(Pt 1):83-8, 1989*).

Topical application may be beneficial.

Experimental Study: Over 100 pts. were treated with Selson® shampoo (Abbott) which contains 25 mg/ml selenium sulfide. The shampoo was mainly used for scalp lesions, but lesions on the trunk, and in the axillae and groins were also treated. The shampoo was left on the skin surface for 15 min. and then washed off. Applications were made once daily for about 1-3 wks. and thereafter the frequency of application was reduced gradually. The overall results have been good and the shampoo is now frequently used in treatment. The best results are seen in scalp psoriasis; psoriasis of the slowly evolving, profuse dispersed guttate type; psoriasis of the inverse type and stable plaque psoriasis where itch is predominant; and in pts. with expanding nummular psoriatic lesions, especially if pruritic (*Broglund E, Enhamre A. Treatment of psoriasis with topical selenium sulphide. Letter. <u>Br J Dermatol</u> 117(5):665-6, 1987*).

<u>Zinc</u>:

Plasma level is inconsistent.

Observational Study: Plasma and cutaneous zinc were studied in 22 pts. (10 extensive psoriasis vulgaris, 5 palmoplantar psoriasis, 7 extensive pustular psoriasis) and 14 controls. Low plasma zinc and decreased *in vitro* chemotaxis of polymorphonuclear leukocytes was found only in pustular psoriasis, whereas zinc was elevated in the skin. This explains why conflicting results on plasma zinc have been previously reported in psoriasis (*Dreno B et al. Plasma zinc is decreased only in generalized pustular psoriasis. <u>Dermatologica</u> 173(5):209-12, 1986*).

Serum level may be normal (*Wasik F et al. [Zinc content of leukocytes and serum in psoriasis patients.] <u>Hautarzt</u> 36(10):573-6, 1985*).

Erythrocyte level may be reduced (*Leung RS et al. Neurophil zinc levels in psoriasis and seborrhoeic dermatitis. <u>Br J Dermatol</u> 123(3):319-23, 1990; Tsambaos D, Orfanos CE. [Zinc distribution disorder in psoriasis.] <u>Arch Dermatol Res</u> 259(1):97-100, 1977*).

Leukocyte level may be reduced (*Wasik F et al. [Zinc content of leukocytes and serum in psoriasis patients.] <u>Hautarzt</u> 36(10):573-6, 1985*).

Neutrophil level may be reduced (*Leung RS et al. Neurophil zinc levels in psoriasis and seborrhoeic dermatitis. <u>Br J Dermatol</u> 123(3):319-23, 1990*).

Epidermal level may be reduced (*Michäelsson G, Ljunghall K. Patients with dermatitis herpetiformis, acne, psoriasis and Darier's disease have low epidermal zinc concentrations. <u>Acta Derm Venereol (Stockh)</u> 70(4):304-8, 1990*).

Cutaneous level may be elevated (*Dreno B et al. Plasma zinc is decreased only in generalized pustular psoriasis. Dermatologica 173(5):209-12, 1986; Kurz K et al. PIXE analysis in different stages of psoriatic skin. J Invest Dermatol 88(2):223-6, 1987*).

Oral supplementation appears to be ineffective.

Experimental Study: Zinc 50 mg 3 times daily in the form of zinc sulfate was given to pts. with psoriasis vulgaris and psoriatic arthritis. After 6 wks., treatment had little or no effect on the course of the disease. However, it reduced both neutrophil random migration and directed chemotaxis to normal values, suggesting that neutrophils play only a secondary role in the pathogenesis of psoriasis (*Leibovici V et al. Effect of zinc therapy on neutrophil chemotaxis in psoriasis. Isr J Med Sci 26(6):306-9, 1990*).

- -

OTHER NUTRITIONAL FACTORS

Essential Fatty Acids:

Linoleic acid plays an important part in maintenance of epidermal integrity by intervening in the cohesion of the stratum corneum and in prevention of transepidermal water loss. Metabolites of arachidonic acid (mostly those obtained by the lipoxygenase pathway) are important agents in causing many inflammatory skin reactions concurrent with the development of skin diseases such as psoriasis (*Berbis P et al. [Essential fatty acids and the skin.] Allergy Immunol (Paris) 22(6):225-31, 1990*).

In psoriatic patients, the skin contains increased total lipid and phospholipid and extremely large amounts of free arachidonic acid (*Ellis CN, Gorsulowsky DC, Voorhess JJ. Experimental therapies for psoriasis. Semin Dermatol 4:414-19, 1985; Kragballe K, Voorhees JJ. Arachidonic acid and leukotrienes in clinical dermatology. Curr Probl Dermatol 13:1-10, 1985; Yardley HJ, Summerly R. Lipid composition and metabolism in normal and diseased epidermis. Clin Exp Dermatol 7:357-83, 1981*).

Fatty acid levels in plasma and adipose tissue may be abnormal.

Observational Study: Plasma phospholipid concentrations of arachidonic acid (20:4 omega 6) and docosapentaenoic acid (22:5 omega 6) were significantly lower, and concentrations of dihomogammalinolenic acid (DGLA) (20:3 omega 6) were significantly higher, in pts. compared to normal controls (*Grattan C et al. Essential-fatty acid metabolites in plasma phospholipids in patients with ichthyosis vulgaris, acne vulgaris and psoriasis. Clin Exp Dermatol 15(3):174-6, 1990*).

Observational Study: The fatty acid composition of plasma lipid esters (cholesterol esters, triglycerides and phospholipids) and adipose tissue of 20 male pts. and 36 matched controls were examined. In comparison to controls, patients' plasma lipid esters contained significantly lower levels of linoleic acid (18:2 omega 6) and alpha-linolenic acid (18:3 omega 3), and higher levels of dihomogammalinolenic acid (20:3 omega 6). In the patients' adipose tissue, the amt. of alpha-linolenic acid was significantly decreased, while that of arachidonic acid (20:4 omega 6) was increased (*Vahlquist C et al. The fatty-acid spectrum in plasma and adipose tissue in patients with psoriasis. Arch Dermatol Res 278(2):114-19, 1985*).

Supplementation may be beneficial.

Theoretical Discussion: Leukotriene B_4, a major proinflammatory metabolite of arachidonic acid, is known to accumulate in the lesions of psoriasis. Epidermal 15-lipoxygenase, on the other hand, metabolizes arachidonic acid into 15-hydroxyeicosatetraenoic acid (15-20:4 n-6), presumably serving as a negative feedback to inhibit the local generation of leukotriene B_4. Both eicosapentaenoic acid (in fish oil) and gamma-linolenic acid (in vegetable oils) are metabolized by epidermal 15-lipoxygenase into monohydroxy acids which are potent *in vitro* inhibitors of leukotriene B_4 generation. It seems reasonable, therefore, that adequate supplementation with eicosapentaenoic acid or gamma-linolenic acid may suppress cutaneous inflammation in psoriasis (*Ziboh VA. Implications of dietary oils and polyunsaturated fatty acids in the management of cutaneous disorders. Arch Dermatol 125(2):241-5, 1989*).

- <u>Omega-3 Fatty Acids</u>:   minimum 8 wk. trial

Eicosapentaenoic acid (EPA) and docosahexaenoic acid (DHA).

Highest in cold water fish. Available in a refined form as "MaxEPA" (18% eicosapentaenoic acid).

Suggested MaxEPA dosage: 3 - 9 grams daily in divided doses

WARNING: Supplementation may require additional vitamin E intake to prevent increased membrane per-oxidation and cellular damage (*Laganiere S, Fernandes G. High peroxidizability of subcellular membrane induced by high fish oil diet is reversed by vitamin E. <u>Clin Res</u> 35:A565, 1987*).

Eiscosapentaenoic acid (EPA) can substitute for arachidonic acid in cell membranes; its products may less biologi-cally active than those derived from arachidonic acid and at least one of them (leukotriene B5) inhibits leukotriene B4, an arachidonic acid metabolite which causes polymorphonuclear leukocyte infiltration. Theoretically, there-fore, EPA supplementation should be beneficial (*Ellis CN et al. Experimental therapies for psoriasis. <u>Sem Der-matol</u> 4(4):313-19, 1985*).

Greenland Eskimos, with a fishy diet high in omega-3 fatty acids, have a lower incidence of psoriasis than Euro-pean controls (*Kromann N, Green A. Epidemiological studies in the Upernavik District, Greenland. <u>Acta Med Scand</u> 208:401-6, 1989*).

Supplementation with fish oils may be beneficial.

Experimental Study: Pts. with psoriasis, 42% of whom also had psoriasis-related arthritis, received fish oil supplements containing 1,122 mg/d of EPA and 756 mg/d of DHA. Symptoms decreased progressively. Itching decreased rapidly, followed by scaling, hardening of the plaques, and reddening of the skin. After 2 mo., 7 pts. were completely healed, 13 pts. had 75% healing, and the majority of pts. reported improvements. Only 17.5% of pts. showed no response. The best results were seen in pts. with milder cases (*Lassus A et al. Effects of dietary supplementation with polyunsaturated ethyl-ester lipids (angiosan) in patients with psoriasis and psoriatic arthritis. <u>J Int Med Res</u> 18:68-73, 1990*).

Experimental Study: 26 pts. received fish oil supplementation. While none of the pts. with plaque-type psoriasis improved, a pt. with generalized pustular psoriasis showed a marked improvement (*Kettler AH et al. The effect of dietary fish oil supplementation on psoriasis. Improvement in a patient with pustular psoriasis. <u>J Am Acad Dermatol</u> 18(6):1267-73, 1988*).

Negative Experimental Double-blind Study: Pts. randomly received either 10 g/d fish oil containing 1.8 g EPA or olive oil. After 8 wks., there was no significant change (*Bjrneboe A et al. Effect of dietary supple-mentation with n-3 fatty acids on clinical manifestations of psoriasis. <u>Br J Dermatol</u> 118(1):77-83, 1988*).

Experimental Double-blind Study: 28 pts. with chronic stable plaque psoriasis randomly received either "MaxEPA" 10 caps daily (containing 1.8 gm eicosapentaenoic acid) or vegetable oil placebo. After 8 wks., there was a significant lessening of itching, erythema, and scaling as well as a trend towards a reduction in mean surface area affected in the experimental gp., but no change in the controls (*Bittiner SB et al. A double-blind, randomised, placebo-controlled trial of fish oil in psoriasis. <u>Lancet</u> 1:378-80, 1988; Bittiner SB et al. Fish oil in psoriasis - a double-blind randomized placebo-controlled study. <u>Br J Dermatol</u> 32(Suppl):25, 1987*).

- with a <u>low fat</u> diet:

Experimental Study: 26 pts. with psoriasis vulgaris received a low fat diet supplemented with Max EPA 30 ml daily. After 4 mo., 58% demonstrated moderate or excellent improvement, 19% demon-strated mild improvement and 23% were unchanged (*Kragballe K, Fogh K. A low-fat diet supplemented with dietary fish oil (Max-EPA) results in improvement of psoriasis and in formation of leukotriene B5. <u>Acta Derm Venereol (Stockh)</u> 69(1):23-8, 1989*).

- with a <u>low saturated fat</u>, <u>low arachidonic acid</u>, <u>low linoleic acid</u> diet:

> **Experimental Study:**   13 pts. with stable psoriasis vulgaris were placed on a diet that was low in arachidonic acid, linoleic acid, and saturated fats which was supplemented with MaxEPA 60-75 gm mixed in orange juice. In addition, all pts. applied an emolient (Unibase) twice daily to their entire body. After 8 wks., all pts. showed statistically significant improvements in scaling, inflammation and lesion thickness. 8/13 showed mild to moderate medical improvement in skin lesions. 2 pts. who also had moderately severe psoriatic arthritis reported symptom alleviation, and 5 pts. reported a marked decrease in itching (*Ziboh VA et al. Effects of dietary supplementation of fish oil on neutrophil and epidermal fatty acids.   Modulation of clinical course of psoriatic subjects.   <u>Arch Dermatol</u> 122(11):1277-82, 1986*).

Topical application may be beneficial.

> **Experimental Single-blind Study:**   11 pts. applied a topical preparation of 10% MaxEPA in a commercial vehicle to some of their lesions, and applied the vehicle alone to others. 8/11 had greater improvement in the EPA-treated lesions (p<0.05) (*Dewsbury CE et al. Topical eicosapentaenoic acid in the treatment of psoriasis. <u>Br J Dermatol</u> 120:581, 1989*).

- <u>Omega-6 Fatty Acids</u>:

$$\text{linoleic acid} \;\rightarrow\; \text{GLA} \;\rightarrow\; \text{DGLA} \;\rightarrow\; \text{prostaglandin } E_1$$

Example: <u>evening primrose oil</u> (a source of GLA) 500 mg. three times daily

Arachidonic acid and its metabolites are increased in lesional psoriasis compared to the skin of normals. The arachidonic level in uninvolved skin of psoriasis patients is in-between (*Ellis CN et al. Experimental therapies for psoriasis. <u>Sem Dermatol</u> 4(4):313-19, 1985*).

Glucocorticoids inhibit skin arachidonic acid release when applied topically or given systemically (*Black AK et al. The effect of systemic prednisolone on arachidonic acid, and prostaglandin E_2 and $F_2\alpha$ levels in human cutaneous inflammation. <u>Br J Clin Pharmacol</u> 14:391-94, 1982; Hammarstrom S et al. Glucocorticoid in inflammatory proliferative skin disease reduces arachidonic and hydroxyeicosatetrenoic acids. <u>Science</u> 197:994-96, 1977*).

Supplementation with linoleic acid or its metabolites may theoretically be beneficial as, although DGLA can be converted to arachidonic acid, there is some evidence that metabolites of DGLA may inhibit the formation of leukotrienes from arachidonic acid (*Ellis CN et al. Experimental therapies for psoriasis. <u>Semin Dermatol</u> 4(4):313-19, 1985*).

Topical application of arachidonic acid may be beneficial.

> **Experimental Double-blind Study:**   45 pts. with psoriasis vulgaris received topical applications of arachidonic solutions in concentrations of 0.1%-2% or of the vehicle alone. Topical arachidonic acid in concentrations of 0.5%-2% applied under occlusion every 24-48 hrs. 5-7 times produced marked improvement or complete resolution of lesions in about half of the pts. studied. The optimal concentration was 1%. Some pts. experienced skin irritation. Histologic exam showed polymorphonuclear leukocytes in the stratum corneum, with its eventual destruction. The parakeratotic horny layer became detached; this was followed by restoration of the granular layer and an apparently normal stratum corneum. Following discontinuation, the lesions recurred in most patients. While arachidonic metabolites can be proinflammatory and proproliferative, they may also be important in the healing process for psoriasis (*Hebborn P et al. Action of topically applied arachidonic acid on the skin of patients with psoriasis. <u>Arch Dermatol</u> 124:387-91, 1988*).

<u>Fumaric Acid</u>:

The *trans* isomer of malic acid (the *cis* isomer) and an intermediate in the Krebs citric acid cycle.

Formed in the skin upon exposure to sunlight.

Administration may be beneficial.

WARNINGS:

1. Transient hypoglycemia may occur.
2. Avoid penicillin.
3. Around days 10-14, there may be transient slight worsening.
4. Contraindicated during pregnancy.
5. Serious side effects, including kidney failure, have occasionally been reported; liver and kidney function testing and complete blood counts are advised.

Fumaric acid monoester regimen (minimum effective dosages):

First 4 wks.: 120 mg daily
Next 2 wks.: 120 mg twice daily
Next 2 wks.: 240 mg in AM; 120 mg in PM
Maintenance: 120-240 mg daily

Note: Doses up to 1500 mg daily are sometimes required. Because of potential toxicity, the lowest effective dose is recommended.

Take prior to breakfast with plenty of fluids.
After about 15 min., there will be a warm feeling in the shoulders and neck up to the ear lobes lasting 10-15 minutes.
Visible benefits in 3 weeks to 3 months.

- with dietary restrictions:

Foods Forbidden: Certain spices (pepper, cloves, nutmeg, mustard caraway seeds, anisette (licorice), cinnamon paprika, mixed seasoning, prespiced dishes, mayonnaise); certain nuts (filberts, peanuts, walnuts); certain citrus products (skins, artificial or canned citrus juice); and certain alcoholic beverages (wines, brandy, cognac, vermouth, sherry, orange liquor).

Experimental Double-blind Study: The effects of dimethylfumaric acid esters (DMFAE) and DMFAE combined with salts of monoethylfumaric acid esters (FAC), both in enteric-coated tablets, were compared in 22 pts and 23 pts., respectively. After 4 mo., about 50% in both gps. showed a considerable improvement; i.e. the initial score was more than halved. There were no significant differences in therapeutic effects with respect to the total psoriasis score or the different parameters. In the FAC gp. therapeutic effects were more rapid. The most frequent side effects were flushing, stomach ache and diarrhea which caused 3 pts. in the DMFAE gp. and 8 pts. in the FAC gp. to discontinue treatment. Eosinophilia, leukopenia and lymphopenia were the most frequently observed differences in lab tests. FAC was not significantly better than monotherapy with DMFAE, and enteric coating failed to prevent GI complaints. Until more information has been obtained about the pharmacokinetics, toxicity and optimal composition of the drug, fumaric acid therapy should be seen as experimental (*Nieboer C et al. Fumaric acid therapy in psoriasis: a double-blind comparison between fumaric acid compound therapy and monotherapy with dimethylfumaric acid ester. Dermatologica 181(1):33-7, 1990*).

Experimental Double-blind Study: 39 pts. randomly received tablets containing a combination of dimethylfumarate and different salts of monoethylfumarate, with octylhydrogen fumarate or with placebo tablets in addition to topical fumaric acid therapy and dietary restrictions. 34 completed the study; 5 pts. dropped out because of side effects or aggravation of skin lesions. Pts. treated with the combination of monoethyl- and dimethylfumarate showed a significantly better therapeutic response compared with those treated with placebo or octylhydrogen fumarate. Side effects of the fumarate-containing tablets were flushing, diarrhea, a reversible transaminase elevation, lymphocytopenia and eosinophilia. One pt. developed a disturbance of kidney function which normalized after discontinuation of the therapy (*Nugteren-Huying WM et al. [Fumaric acid therapy in psoriasis; a double-blind, placebo-controlled study.] Ned Tijdschr Geneeskd 134(49):2387-91, 1990*) (*in Dutch*).

Experimental Double-blind Studies: 36 pts. appeared to respond well to Schäfer's fumaric acid compound therapy (FACT) which consists of oral dimethylfumaric acid ester (DMFAE) and several salts of monoethylfumaric acid ester (MEFAE) in combination with topical fumaric acid (1-3% MEFAE) and dietary restrictions. Thereafter, several randomized double-blind studies with MEFAE sodium vs. placebo, and DMFAE vs. placebo, were done. MEFAE sodium was ineffective in dosages up to 240 mg daily, whereas dosages of 720 mg daily resulted in a significant decrease in scaling and itching but did not affect extension of the eruption. DMFAE 240 mg daily produced a significant amelioration and prevented extension. Side effects of treatment were nausea, diarrhea, general malaise, severe stomach ache, mild disturbances of liver and kidney function and, in 50% of pts. treated with DMFAE, a relative lymphopenia with a selective decrease of suppressor T lymphocytes (*Nieboer C et al. Systemic therapy with fumaric acid derivatives: new possibilities in the treatment of psoriasis. J Am Acad Dermatol 20(4):601-8, 1989*).

Glycosaminoglycans (mucopolysaccharides):

Urinary level may be elevated.

Observational Study: Urine from pts. with generalized plaque psoriasis contained substantially more precipitable glycosaminoglycans (GAG) and uronic acid than the urine of healthy controls. The difference was unrelated to sex, age, renal function, the hospital environment or the presence of arthritis. Cellulose acetate electrophoresis of the GAG from pts. and controls showed similar patterns dominated by chondroitin sulfate. Successful topical treatment did not affect the rate of GAG excretion. As there was no evidence to favor the skin lesions as the source of the additional GAG, the findings suggest that psoriasis is a generalized disease (*Priestley GC. Urinary excretion of glycaminoglycans in psoriaisis. Arch Dermatol Res 280(2):77-82, 1988*).

Supplementation may be beneficial.

Experimental Study: 38 pts. with severe total-body psoriasis received sub-cut. injections of an extract of activated acid-pepsin-digested calf tracheal cartilege ("Catrix-S"). 19/39 had total remissions within 2 mo. with complete disappearance of the lesions for 6 wks. to more than 1 yr., with the ave. being 5 months. 3/38 had an excellent response with little residual disease. 15/38 had a good result, and 1/38 a poor result. 11/16 who did not have a complete remission within 2 mo. went into a complete remission after receiving booster injections every 3 wks. and topical therapy with a 5% activated acid-pepsin-digested calf tracheal cartilege cream ("Psoriacin"). Responding pts. developed prompt descaling, although the dilated capillary bed beneath the lesions remained dilated and tender to touch. The authors believe that eventually the capillaries will return to normal and the skin will return to normal thickness (*Prudden JF, Balassa LL. The biological activity of bovine cartilege preparations. Semin Arthritis Rheum 3(4):287-321, 1974*).

Lecithin:

Supplementation may be beneficial.

Experimental Study: 118/155 pts. responded during a 10-year study with purified granulated soya phosphatides 15-45 gm daily orally which supplied 0.6 gm each of choline and inositol. Crude lecithin 3-6 gm daily was also given along with small amts. of vitamins A, D, B_1, B_2 and B_6 and calcium pantothenate. When appropriate, crude liver extract, thyroid and reducing diets were utilized, and local applications with various preparations were also provided (*Gross P et al. The treatment of psoriasis as a disturbance of lipid metabolism. N Y State J Med 50:2683-86, 1950*).

Undecylenic Acid:

An 11-carbon monounsaturated organic fatty acid (Mycocidin, Thorne, US).

Supplementation may be beneficial.

Negative Experimental Study: 1,100 cases were treated for at least 3 mo. by 75 dermatologists. Side effects, especially gastrointestinal, were frequent, and not a few cases experienced a flare-up and spread of the psoriasis. Only a few of the physicians regarded their results as at all favorable; on the whole, the overwhelming opinon was decidedly unfavorable (*Rattner H, Rodin H. Treatment of psoriasis with undecylenic acid by mouth. JAMA 146(2):1113-15, 1951*).

Experimental Study: 41 pts., mostly with recalcitrant disease, generally received 15 perles (0.44 cc each) of undecylenic acid 3 times daily. There were no serious or lasting toxic effects, although mild GI disturbances occurred. 12/40 pts. with cutaneous lesions showed unequivocal improvement, 15/40 were somewhat improved, 10 were unchanged and 3 had distinct aggravation of the disease. 7/8 pts. with psoriatic arthropathy noted relief from pain (*Perlman HH, Milberg IL. Peroral administration of undecylenic acid in psoriasis. JAMA 140(10):865-68, 1949*).

Experimental Study: 17 pts. with both localized and generalized psoriasis were given gradually increasing doses of undecylenic acid for varying periods of time, with definite improvement characterized by a disappearance of the lesions, permanent relief of itching and of, in several pts. with arthropathy, a definite disappearance or improvement in joint pains. The effective dose seems to be 15-20 0.5 gm perles (7.5-10 gm) given 3 times daily for many weeks. There were no harmful effects and no GI disturbances (*Perlman HH. Undecylenic acid given orally in psoriasis and neurodermatitis: A preliminary report. JAMA 139(7):444-47, 1949*).

- -

OTHER FACTORS

Rule out <u>food sensitivities</u>.

Experimental Study: Pts. improved on a fasting and vegetarian regime (*Lithell H et al. A fasting and vegetarian diet treatment trial in chronic inflammatory disorders. Acta Derm Venererol (Stockh) 63:397-403, 1983*).

Experimental Study: 6/6 pts. improved on elimination diets. One improved on a diet which avoided fruits (especially citrus), nuts, corn and milk; the others improved on a diet which avoided acidic foods such as coffee, tomato, soda and pineapple (*Douglass, JM. Psoriasis and diet. Letter. Calif Med 133(5):450, 1980*).

Rule out <u>hydrochloric acid deficienciy</u>.

Supplementation may be beneficial.

> *Note: While gastric anacidity had been reported in the past to be a relatively common condition which was associated with a number of illnesses, the presence of achlorhydria is no longer accepted unless a potent parietal-cell stimulant (such as histamine) is employed in gastric analysis. More recent studies suggest that histamine-fast anacidity is uncommon before the fifth decade of life and, although it probably does not occur in a normal stomach, its presence is not necessarily associated with symptoms (Rappaport EM. Achlorhydria: Associated symptoms and response to hydrochloric acid. N Engl J Med 252(19):802-5, 1955).*

Experimental and Observational Study: Of 9 pts., 5 had no hydrochloric acid and only 1 had a normal hydrochloric acid level. The severity of the condition seemed to correlate with the extent of the hydrochloric acid deficiency and also seemed to be associated with signs of B complex deficiency. Improvement seemed to be associated with supplemental hydrochloric acid and vitamin B complex (*Allison JR. The relation of hydrochloric acid and vitamin B complex deficiency in certain skin diseases. South Med J 38:235-241, 1945*).

Observational Study: 19 pts. underwent a fractional gastric analysis following a routine Ewald test meal. Hypoacidity was defined as values for total and free acids of 1/2 normal or less, while hyperacidity was defined as values 10-15 points above normal or values which were relatively high at the start of the test. 10/19 (52%) of the pts. were found to have hypoacidity, while 5/19 (26%) had normal acid and 4/19 (21%) had hyperacidity. For 5/19 (26%) of the pts., the severity of the eruption correlated with both the presence of GI symptoms and abnormal gastric acid levels (*Ayers S. Gastric secretion in psoriasis, eczema and dermatitis herpetiformis. Arch Dermatol Syphilol 20:854-57, 1929*).

RAYNAUD'S SYNDROME

See Also: AUTO-IMMUNE DISORDERS (GENERAL)

VITAMINS

Niacin:

Inositol Nicotinate 4 gm daily (Believed to act by the slow release of nicotinic acid.)

Administration of inositol nicotinate may be beneficial.

> **Experimental Double-blind Study:** 23 pts. with primary Raynaud's disease received either inositol nicotinate (Hexopal) 4 g/day or placebo in cold weather. After 84 days, the treatment gp. felt subjectively better and had demonstrably shorter and fewer attacks of vasospasm during the trial period. Serum biochemistry and rheology was not significantly different between the 2 groups (*Sunderland GT et al. A double blind randomised placebo controlled trial of hexopal in primary Raynaud's disease. Clin Rheumatol 7(1):46-49, 1988*).

> **Experimental Study:** 20 pts. with primary Raynaud's syndrome received inositol nicotinate (Hexopal) 1 gm 4 times daily. After 36 wks., there was objective improvement in the thermal gradient of the hand after cold challenge (p<0.05), and statistically significant improvements were noted on 4/5 subjective assessments. No drug-related adverse reactions were noted (*Ring EFJ et al. Quantitative thermal imaging to assess inositol nicotinate treatment for Raynaud's syndrome. J Int Med Res 9:393-99, 1981*).

> **Experimental Single-blind Study:** 30 pts. with primary and secondary Raynaud's phenomenon received either inositol nicotinate (Hexopal) 4 g/day in divided doses or placebo. After 12 wks., recording the time required to induce Raynaud's phenomenon as well as assessments of total and nutrient digital blood flow showed significant beneficial therapeutic effects upon the skin's microcirculation for treated patients (*Holti G. An experimentally controlled evaluation of the effect of inositol nicotinate upon the digital blood flow in patients with Raynaud's phenomenon. J Int Med Res 7:473-83, 1979*).

Vitamin E:

Supplementation may be beneficial.

> **Case Reports:**
> 1. A 45 year-old male with a 6 mo. history of rapidly deteriorating illness causing ulceration and gangrene was placed on 400 IU of D-alpha tocopherol acetate twice daily before meals and local application of emulsified vitamin E drops. The fingers were healed in 8 weeks and remained healed one year later.
> 2. A 37 year-old female with a 1 yr. history of numbness, tingling and discoloration of the left fifth finger was placed on 100 IU of D-alpha tocopherol acetate three times daily 15 min. before meals. Three wks. later, both the symptoms and the discoloration had improved. Three mo. later, only a trace of discoloration remained and she was symptom-free. Vitamin E was reduced to 100 IU daily and stopped after 6 months. Three years later she remained well.
> (*Ayres Jr. S et al. Raynaud's phenomenon, scleroderma and calcinosis cutis: Response to vitamin E. Cutis 11:54-62, 1973*).

- Alpha-tocopheryl Nicotinate: 400 mg daily

Supplementation may be beneficial, and may be superior to tocopheryl acetate.

Experimental Studies: In a series of studies on pts. who were suffering from "feeling cold" due to various diseases, one of which included 4 pts. with Raynaud's syndrome, the effectiveness of tocopheryl nicotinate was superior to tocopheryl acetate in both alleviation of clinical symptoms and in the cooling-rewarming test. In addition, when both agents were cross-administrated, tocopheryl nicotinate had a more rapid and higher effectiveness than tocopheryl acetate in repairing micorcirculatory deficiencies. It appears that the effectiveness of tocopheryl nicotinate is not due to the synergistic effect of tocopherol and nicotinic acid but to the independent effect of tocopheryl nicotinate on the micorcirulatory system (*Kamimura M. Comparison of alpha-tocopheryl nicotinate and acetate on skin microcirculation. Am J Clin Nutr 27:1110-16, 1974*).

- -

MINERALS

Magnesium:

Serum levels may be reduced by exposure to cold, causing vasospasm.

Experimental Study: After exposure to cold, mean serum magnesium levels in a gp. of 80 women with primary Raynaud's phenomenon was significantly lower than in 24 age- and sex-matched controls (p<0.05). One yr. later, without cold exposure, serum magnesium levels were identical in the 2 groups. The serum magnesium level was lower in 82% of the pt. gp. after cold exposure compared to 45% of the controls (p<0.001). No differences were found in the other electrolytes (*Leppert J et al. Lower serum magnesium level after exposure to cold in women with primary Raynaud's phenomenon. J Intern Med 228:235-9, 1990*).

- -

OTHER NUTRITIONAL FACTORS

Hydroxyethylrutosides:

May reduce red cell aggregation and whole blood viscosity at low shear rates, and may increase red cell deformability (*Schimdt-Schönbein H et al. Vasa 4:263, 1975; van Haeringen NJ et al. Bibl Anat 12:459, 1973*).

Administration may be beneficial.

Experimental Study: 7 pts. with severe Raynaud's syndrome (3 with primary Raynaud's; 1 with scleroderma; 1 with Buerger's disease, 1 with vibration-induced disease; 1 with a vasculitis and additional "vibration disease") were studied. All had severe pain in the digits and some degree of ulceration. 5/7 had organic arterial changes, while 2 had pronounced vasospastic tendencies. They received hydroxyethylrutosides (troxerutin) 2-3 g/d IV in 2 injections for 2-4 wks. followed by oral treatment with 3-6 g/d in 3-4 doses for maintenance. During parenteral treatment, all pts. showed clear improvement, with fewer episodes, healing of ulcers, and pronounced pain relief. Five pts. showed improvement in peripheral blood flow as shown by fluorescein angiography. During oral treatment, the increased blood flow was maintained or improved further. Tolerance to these high doses was excellent (*Lund F et al. Troxerutin in Raynaud's syndrome. Letter. Br Med J 280:334-35, 1980*).

Omega-3 Fatty Acids:

Most important member: Eicosapentaenoic acid - which is particularly high in cold-water fish.

Supplementation may be beneficial.

Experimental Double-blind Study: 32 pts. with primary or secondary Raynaud's phenomenon randomly received either 12 fish oil capsules daily containing a total of 3.96 g EPA and 2.64 g DHA or olive oil placebo. After 6 wks., the median time interval before the onset of Raynaud's phenomenon after their hands were submerged in a cold water bath increased significantly (p=0.04). 5/11 pts. with primary Raynaud's phenomenon could not be induced to develop Raynaud's at the 6- or 12-wk. visit compared with 1/9 primary Raynaud's pts. on placebo. The mean digital systolic pressures were also higher in treated pts. with primary Raynaud's than in similar pts. on placebo (p=0.02). Pts. with secondary Raynaud's failed to improve (*DiGiacomo RA et al. Fish-oil dietary supplementation in patients with Raynaud's phenomenon: a double-blind, controlled, prospective study. Am J Med 86:158-64, 1989*).

Experimental Double-blind Crossover Study: 13 normal males randomly received 5000 mg of omega-3 fatty acids (Promega™, Parke-Davis) or wheat germ oil placebo for 30 days per crossover arm with a 1-mo. washout between interventions. The time to peak pain during the cold pressor test (hand in ice water at $4°$ C for 5 min.) was prolonged when subjects were receiving omega-3 fatty acids, although the peak pain scores were not different (*Ringer TV et al. Fish oil blunts the pain response to cold pressor testing in normal males. Abstract. J Am Coll Nutr 8(5):435, 1989*).

<u>Omega-6 Fatty Acids</u>:

$$\text{linoleic acid} \rightarrow \text{GLA} \rightarrow \text{DGLA} \rightarrow \text{prostaglandin E}_1$$

Example: evening primrose oil (a source of GLA) 2 gm three times daily

Supplementation may be beneficial.

Experimental Double-blind Study: 21 pts. with either Raynaud's Phenomenon (RP) or RP and systemic sclerosis were given placebo for 2 wks. when they were split into 2 gps., with 10 pts. continuing on placebo and 11 on EPO (Efamol) 12 capsule daily. In the EPO gp., 6/11 pts. felt a definite benefit and 2 felt moderate benefit, with the results, based on visual analog scales, reaching significance after 6-8 weeks. With colder weather, the placebo gp. experienced more frequent and longer attacks, while the EPO gp. experienced decreased severity of attacks and decreased hand coldness. The majority of pts. on EPO also reported decreased depression and increased energy. Objective measurement of blood flow revealed no change on EPO (*Belch JJF et al. Evening primrose oil (Efamol) as a treatment for cold-induced vasospasm (Raynaud's phenomenon). Prog Lipid Res 25:335-40, 1986; Belch JJF et al. Evening primrose oil (Efamol) in the treatment of Raynaud's phenomenon: A double-blind study. Thromb Haemost 54(2):490-94, 1985*).

OTHER FACTORS

Rule out <u>food sensitivities</u>.

Case Report: 30 year-old female with 25 yr. history of severe recurrent headaches, sore throats and kidney infections developed right index finger pain diagnosed as Raynaud's disease which worsened despite vasodilators and analgesics. She was admitted to an environmental medical unit where, following a 6 day fast, her symptoms completely cleared and normal color returned to her finger. Digital spasm was provoked by challenge with foods and chemicals. Following discharge she remained almost symptom-free unless she was inadvertently exposed to chemicals. The authors report that they have also been able to identify triggering agents in 9 other patients (*Rea WJ, Suits CW. Cardiovascular disease triggered by foods and chemicals, in JW Gerrard, Ed. Food Allergy: New Perspectives. Springfield, Illinois, Charles C. Thomas, 1980*).

RESTLESS LEGS SYNDROME

DIETARY FACTORS

Avoid <u>caffeine</u> and other xanthine derivatives (coffee, tea, cola, cocoa).

Experimental Study: 62 pts. with restless legs syndrome and associated symptoms improved on a xanthine-free diet with the temporary addition of diazepam (*Lutz EG. Restless legs, anxiety and caffeinism. J Clin Psychiatry Sept. 1978, pp.693-8*).

<u>Sugar-free</u>, <u>high protein</u> diet.

Symptoms may be manifestations of reactive hypoglycemia.

Clinical Observations: In a gp. of over 350 pts. who presented with either spontaneous leg cramps (SLC) or restless legs (RL), approx. 2/3 pts. had SLC alone, while 1/3 experienced both SLC and RL. Although the calf and foot musculature usually was involved, occasionally pts. suffered cyclic cramps primarily in the upper thighs, low back or hands. There were also several cases of severe nocturnal carpal spasm and the "stiff man syndrome." With few exceptions, these pts. also experienced typical features of recurrent hypoglycemia which was confirmed by afternoon glucose tolerance testing and an attack of muscle cramps occasionally was precipitated concomitantly with a hypoglycemic episode during testing. Institution of a sugar-free, high protein diet with frequent nibling and at least one night feeding was followed by prompt and persistent remission or striking alleviation of longstanding symptoms in the vast majority of pts., while symptom recurrence could usually be attributed to some dietary indiscretion within the preceeding 12 hours (*Roberts HJ. Spontaneous leg cramps and "restless legs" due to diabetogenic (functional) hyperinsulinism: A basis for rational therapy. J Fla Med Assoc 60(5):29-31, 1973*).

- -

VITAMINS

<u>Folic Acid</u>: 5 mg. three times daily
        (WARNING: Should be under medical supervision.)

Dietary deficiency can result in a defect in the ability of intestinal cells to absorb folate when the diet is corrected (*Elsborg L. Reversible malabsorption of folic acid in the elderly with nutritional folate deficiency. Acta Haematology 55:140-7, 1976*).

Supplementation may be beneficial.

Review Article: There are at least 2 clinical forms of RLS: (1) the classic mixed sensorimotor form in which pain, numbness, and lightning stabs of pain in the lower or even the upper limbs are relieved by movement or local massage, and (2) the pure motor or myoclonic form which does not involve any sensory component. The folate-responsive form is exclusively of the mixed type (*Boutez MI et al. Neuropsychological correlates of folic acid deficiency: Facts and hypotheses, in MI Botez, EH Reynolds, Eds. Folic Acid in Neurology, Psychiatry, and Internal Medicine. New York, Raven Press, 1979*).

Case Reports:
1. Three women diagnosed has having acquired folate deficiency based on depressed serum folate concentrations had mild symptoms of restless legs, depression, muscular and mental fatigue, depressed ankle jerks, diminution of vibratory sensation in the legs, a stocking type hypoesthesia, and chronic constipation. All 3 recovered with adequate folate treatment..
2. Three women who were members of a family with restless legs syndrome, fatigability and diffuse muscular pain had folate deficiency based on depressed serum folate concentrations. One also had subacute combined degeneration of the spinal cord and kidney disease but no megaloblastosis; the other 2 had minor neurologic signs. All 3 responded to large doses of folic acid.

(Boutez MI et al. Neurologic disorders responsive to folic acid therapy. Can Med Assoc J 15:217-22, 1976).

Vitamin E:

Supplementation may be beneficial.

Experimental Study: Nine pts. recieved vitamin E supplementation. The response was completely controlled in 7, almost 75% controlled in one, and 50% controlled in one *(Ayres S, Mihan R. "Restless legs" syndrome: response to vitamin E. J Appl Nutr 25:8-15, 1973).*

Case Reports:
1. A 78 year-old female with a 20-year history of "jumpy" legs up to several times nightly was unresponsive to phenytoin and diphenhydramine. Following 2 months of 300 IU daily, she was completely cured.
2. A 37 year-old female with a 10-year history of severe nightly "restless legs" was placed on 300 IU daily for 6 wks. and 200 IU daily for the following 4 wks. with complete relief.
(Ayres S, Mihan R. Leg cramps and "restless leg" syndrome responsive to vitamin E. Calif Med 111:87-91, 1969).

- -

MINERALS

Iron:

Deficiency may be associated with RLS.

Observational Study: 25% of affected pts. were found to have a low serum iron; conversely, 24% of pts. with iron deficiency anemia were found to have RLS *(Ekbom KA. Restless legs syndrome. Neurology 10:868-73, 1960).*

Symptoms may sometimes improve dramatically following iron therapy.

Theoretical Discussion: Abnormalities of iron metabolism may be the common link between the widely varying clinical associations with RLS as well as with the equally variable therapeutic approaches *(Pall HS et al. Restless legs syndrome. Letter. Neurology 37(8):1436, 1987).*

Case Reports: Three pts. are described who obtained rapid relief of symptoms of RLS with oral iron supplementation: a women who, among other disabilities, had been unable to visit the theatre for 15 yrs. because she could not sit still; a 28 year-old man in whom restless legs was the only symptom of iron deficiency due to blood loss; and a women being treated for malignant disease whose symptoms had been misinterpreted as those of carcinomatous neuropathy *(Matthews WB. Iron deficiency and restless legs. Letter. Br Med J April 10, 1976, p. 898).*

Experimental Study: In cases of iron deficiency and RLS, iron supplementation cured the symptoms *(Nordlander NB. Acta Med Scand 145:453, 1953).*

- -

OTHER NUTRITIONAL FACTORS

L-Tryptophan:

Case Reports:
1. A 68 year-old male with chronic renal failure due to malignant hypertension had been on maintenance hemodialysis for 4 years. Three yrs. ago he developed symptoms of crawling, tingling, and burning sensations in his legs which were most prominent during the evening and on attempts to relax during the daytime. These symptoms led to chronic severe insomnia and depression. Neuro exam revealed no motor weakness or peripheral neuropathy. Clonazepam and hypnotics were ineffective; diazepam 20 mg and propoxyphene 2 tabs were mildly effective. L-tryptophan 1 gm twice daily produced amelioration of both the RLS and the insomnia within 3 days of administration without side effects.
2. A 64 year-old man with steroid-dependent chronic obstructive lung disease and steroid myopathy had a 2 yr. history of RLS causing severe insomnia and depression. Numerous medication trials were unsuccessful. L-tryptophan 2 gm at night produced dramatic amelioration of the insomnia and RLS after 4 nights without side effects.
(Sandyk R. L-tryptophan in the treatment of restless legs syndrome. Letter. Am J Psychiatry 143(4):554-5,1986).

"RHEUMATISM"
including ARTHRALGIA, "ARTHRITIS," FIBROSITIS and SYNOVITIS

See Also: CARPAL TUNNEL SYNDROME
MUSCLE CRAMPS
OSTEOARTHRITIS
PAIN

VITAMINS

Thiamine:

In fibrositis, may be deficient.

Observational Study: Thiamine pyrophosphate effect was significantly higher in 13 women with fibrositis than in 12 normal volunteers (p<0.01), suggesting a thiamine deficiency (*Eisinger J, Ayavou T. Transketolase stimulation in fibromyalgia. J Am Coll Nutr 9(1):56-57, 1990*).

Supplementation may be beneficial for fibrositis.

Experimental Study: 20/21 fibrositis pts. had good results from supplementation with thiamine pyrophosphate 50 mg IM 3 times weekly for 6 wks., while 5/13 pts. treated with thiamine hydrochloride 100 mg IM 3 times weekly for 6 wks. had good results. The better clinical response to thiamine pyrophosphate suggests that pts. have an abnormality in thiamime metabolism rather than a dietary thaimine deficiency (*Eisinger J et al. Données actuelles sur les fibromyalgies: traitement des fibromyalgies primitives par la cocarboxylase. Lyon Méditeranée Méd 24:11585-86, 1988; Eisinger J. Cocarboxylase et fibromyalgies, un rendezvous manqué. Lyon Méditerranée Méd 23:11526, 1987*

Vitamin B6:

Supplementation may be beneficial for tenosynovitis.

Experimental Study: Pts. with tenosynovitis producing numbness, tingling, pain, stiffness and weakness in the shoulders, arms and hands commonly improved in 8-12 wks. while on 100-150 mg pyridoxine hydrochloride daily, while RBC glutamic oxaloacetic transaminase (EGOT) levels (a functional measure of B6 nutriture) and the severity of rheumatic symptoms showed a close negative correlation, both prior to and following administration of pyridoxine (*Ellis JM. Vitamin B6 deficiency and rheumatism. Anabolism Winter 1985*).

Note: Carpal tunnel syndrome, in the majority of cases, is caused by tenosynovitis (Ellis JM, Folkers K. Clinical aspects of treatment of carpal tunnel syndrome with vitamin B6. Ann N Y Acad Sci 585:302-20, 1990).

Vitamin E:

Fibrositis is said to be common among menopausal women when, especially if estrogen is given, the need for vitamin E is tremendously increased (*Editorial. JAMA 167:1896, 1958*).

In fibrositis, the blood vitamin E level is usually normal, but the utlization curve is a plateau pattern, indicating difficulty in utilization (*Steinberg CL. Vitamin E and collagen in the rheumatic diseases. Ann N Y Acad Sci 52:380-9, 1949*).

Supplementation may be beneficial in <u>fibrositis</u>.

> **Clinical Observations:** 300 middle-aged pts. with generalized primary fibrositis received supplementation with mixed natural tocopherols 100 mg 3 times daily after meals. While sedation with a barbiturate was ineffective, supplementation was effective for the vast majority of cases. After clinical cure was obtained, a maintenance dose of 50-150 mg was required in most cases; in rare instances, 300 mg/d had to be continued indefinitely. There were no untoward symptoms except for mild gastric irritation on rare occasions (*Steinberg CL. Vitamin E and collagen in the rheumatic diseases. Ann N Y Acad Sci 52:380-9, 1949*).

- -

MINERALS

<u>Copper</u>:

Local application of elemental copper may be beneficial in <u>arthritis</u> and "<u>rheumatism</u>."

> **Experimental Single-blind Crossover Study:** 240 "arthritis/rheumatism" pts. were randomized into 3 groups. Gp. I wore a copper bracelet for 1 mo. followed by a "placebo" bracelet for 1 month. Gp. II wore the 2 bracelets in reverse order, while Gp. III wore no bracelets. Of those who noted a difference between the 2 bracelets, more perceived the copper to be more effective (p<0.01). Previous users of copper bracelets deterioriated while wearing the placebo. The ave. loss of copper from the bracelet was 13 mg (*Walker WR, Keats DM. An investigation of the therapeutic value of the "copper bracelet": Dermal assimilation of copper in arthritic/rheumatoid conditions. Agents Actions 6:454,1976*).

<u>Magnesium</u>:

May be decreased in <u>fibrositis</u>.

> **Negative Observational Study:** Compared to 12 normal controls, RBC magnesium was not significantly lower in 13 women with fibrositis (*Eisinger J, Ayavou T. Transketolase stimulation in fibromyalgia. J Am Coll Nutr 9(1):56-57, 1990*).

> **Observational Study:** Depressed RBC magnesium was found in fibrositis pts. compared to controls (*Eisinger J et al. Données actuelles sur les fibromyalgies: magnésium et transaminases. Lyon Méditerranée Méd 24:11585-86, 1988*).

<u>Selenium</u>:

A deficient intake may be associated with <u>muscle pain</u> (*van Rij AM et al. Selenium deficiency in total parenteral nutrition. Am J Clin Nutr 32:2076-85, 1979*).

Serum levels may be low.

> **Observational Study:** Compared to healthy controls, middle-aged women with sustained pains in the back and shoulder had lower serum selenium levels (*James S et al. Effekter av selenvitamin E-behandling till kvinnor med lång variga arbetsrelaterade nack-och skuldersmärtor. En dubbelblindstudie. Läkaresällskapets Riksstämma, 1985*) (*in Swedish*).

- with <u>Vitamin E</u>:

Supplementation may be beneficial.

> **Experimental Double-blind Study:** 81 pts. with disabling muscular pain, stiffness and aching of long duration, received sodium selenite (140 µg Se) and α-tocopherol 100 mg daily or placebo. Following supplementation, glutathione peroxidase levels increased in 75% of the patients. Mean pain score reduction was significantly more frequent and more marked among pts. whose glutathione peroxidase levels increased than among those whose levels decreased. While pain score reduction was more pronounced among treated pts., the reduction as compared to pts. on placebo were not significant (*Jameson S et al. Pain relief and selenium*

balance in patients with connective tissue disease and osteoarthrosis: A double-blind selenium tocopherol supplementation study. Nutr Res Suppl 1:391-97, 1985).

Experimental Double-blind Study: Middle-aged women with sustained pains in the back and shoulder received selenium 200 µg and vitamin E or placebo in addition to physiotherapy. Women with initially high serum selenium or increasing levels were more often improved by the physiotherapy than the other women, particularly if they were in the experimental gp., suggesting that a relative selenium deficiency may have contributed to their pains (*James S et al. Effekter av selenvitamin E-behandling till kvinnor med lång variga arbetsrelaterade nack-och skuldersmärtor. En dubbelblindstudie. Läkaresällskapets Riksstämma, 1985) (in Swedish*).

- -

OTHER NUTRITIONAL FACTORS

5-Hydroxytryptophan:

Supplementation may be beneficial for fibrositis.

Experimental Double-blind Study: Pts. with primary fibromyalgia syndrome received either 5-hydroxytryptophan or placebo. All the clinical parameters studied were significantly improved by treatment and only mild and transient side-effects were reported (*Caruso I et al. Double-blind study of 5-hydroxytryptophan versus placebo in the treatment of primary fibromyalgia syndrome. J Int Med Res 18(3):201-09, 1990*).

L-Tryptophan:

Serum levels may be reduced in fibrositis.

Observational Study: In 8 pts. with severe fibrositis syndrome, plasma free tryptophan levels were inversely related to the severity of subjective pain (*Moldofsky H, Warsh JJ. Plasma tryptophan and musculoskeletal pain in non-articular rheumatism ("fibrositis syndrome"). Pain 5(1):65-71, 1978*).

- -

OTHER FACTORS

Rule out food sensitivities.

Experimental Study: 9 pts. with episodic joint pain and sometimes swelling precipitated by certain foods or associated with allergic manifestations were studied. All were atopic; 3 had strong evidence of Type I (immediate) allergy and 3 "urticarial arthralgia," in which attacks of severe urticaria and joint pain occurred conincidentally. Food allergy appeared to be responsible for the joint symptoms in 3 pts.; in 1 it was possible to precipitate swelling in a knee due to synovitis with effusion by drinking milk a few hours beforehand (the synovial fluid having mildly inflammatory features and a relatively high eosinophil count). Allergy appears to be an occasional cause of episodic rheumatic pain or synovitis in certain atopic pts., whether or not they have an underlying arthritis. These are usually Type I hypersensitivity reactions, though some food-allergic reactions may be immune complex-mediated (*Golding DN. Is there an allergic synovitis? J R Soc Med 83(5):312-4, 1990*).

Experimental Study: 14 pts. with chronic arthralgias were re-challenged with foods already found to be offensive through dietary exclusion and challenges. 8/14 reacted to the re-challenges and 2/14 had doubtful reactions. 6/8 of the reactors developed IgE immune complexes after challenges (PEG precipitation method) while the remainder developed high levels of IgG immune complexes. None of the 4 non-reactors developed IgE or IgG immune complexes (*Brostoff J, Scadding GK. Complexes in food induced arthralgia. Paper presented at the XII International Congress of Allergy and Clinical Immunology, Washington, DC, October, 1985*).

Experimental Study: While inflammatory arthritis (e.g. rheumatoid arthritis) failed to be influenced by food exclusions and challenges, food challenges did provoke transient synovitis in some pts. with atopic allergy as part of their allergic symptomatology (*Denman AM et al. Joint complaints and food allergic disorders. Ann Allergy 51:260-3, 1983*).

Experimental Double-blind Study: 30 pts. with "<u>arthritis and rheumatism</u>" were each challenged sub-lingually with 25 foods and chemicals in a double-blind manner. Soy was the most commonly provoking substance (22/30 = 73.3% of pts.), while only 2/30 pts. (6.6%) reacted to placebo. Only 1 pt. had no subjective reactions. In 26 pts. (86%), musculoskeletal symptoms were evoked (*Mandell M, Conte AA. The role of allergy in arthritis, rheumatism and polysymptomatic cerebral, visceral and somatic disorders: A double blind study.* <u>J Int Acad Prev Med</u> *July, 1982, pp. 5-16*).

Experimental Study: In a study performed totally through the mail, over 5000 "<u>arthritis</u>" pts. agreed to avoid members of the nightshade family of plants which includes the white potato, the tomato, eggplant, all peppers (except black) and tobacco. Over 70% reported gradually increasing relief from aches and pains and from some disfigurement over a study period of 7 years (*Childers NF. A relationship of arthritis to the solanaceae (nightshades).* <u>J Int Acad Prev Med</u> *November 1982, pp. 31-7*).

Clinical Observations and Case Reports: Pts. with allergic toxemia may present with <u>aching and soreness in muscles and joints</u> along with allergic fatigue, mental confusion, dopiness, inability to concentrate, irritability, depression, etc. A food elimination diet will reveal the diagnosis (*Rowe AH. Allergic fatigue and toxemia.* <u>Ann Allergy</u> *17:9-18, 1959*).

RHEUMATOID ARTHRITIS

See Also: AUTO-IMMUNE DISORDERS (GENERAL)
PAIN
"RHEUMATISM"

OVERVIEW

1. Since malnutrition is common among patients, it should be ruled out.

2. A low fat diet may be beneficial, particularly if it is relatively high in polyunsaturates.

3. Copper salicylate has been found to be an effective anti-inflammatory agent which may be more potent than aspirin.

4. In regard to supplementation with micronutrients, pantothenic acid may be reduced, and there is preliminary evidence that supplementation may be beneficial. A controlled study suggests that vitamin E may be beneficial in ankylosing spondylitis. Iron supplementation, despite the common finding of a microcytic anemia, is controversial, as is zinc supplementation. While sulfur is an old-fashioned remedy, its use is still not validated by double-blind studies. On the other hand, the evidence is mounting that the omega-3 essential fatty acids may be beneficial.

5. There have been an increasing number of studies in the past few years, some double-blind, demonstrating improvement following food eliminations and worsening following provocation with particular foods.

- -

DIETARY FACTORS

Rule out malnutrition.

Observational Study: Nearly 3/4 of Alabama pts. showed evidence of malnutrition. It is suggested that these results are primarily due to changes in the way vitamins are handled and nutrients absorbed in RA (*FC McDuffie, Arthritis Foundation - reported in* Med World News *July 22, 1985*).

Observational Study: Compared to controls with other types of musculoskeletal disorders, 25% of a gp. of 50 RA pts. were malnourished. The adequacy of dietary intake did not correlate with their nutritional status, but the degree of malnourishment did correlate with the severity of the RA (*Helliwell M et al.* Ann Rheum Dis *43:386-90, 1984*).

Low fat diet.

Observational Study: Compared to healthy controls, pts. had high concentrations of total saturated fatty acids in both serum and adipose tissue, and the severity of this abnormality was associated with disease duration (*Jacobsson I et al. Correlation of fatty acid composition of adipose tissue lipids and serum phosphatidylcholine and serum concentrations of micronutrients with disease duration in rheumatoid arthritis.* Ann Rheum Dis *49:901-05, 1990*).

Case Reports: 2 pts. with obesity and active RA experienced remission of joint symptoms within days of going on a low-calorie, fat-free weight control formula and remained symptom-free for 9 and 14 mo. respectively. 24-48 hrs. after eating foods which contained a high proportion or all of its calories from fat they experienced short-term exacerbations. Subsequently 4 additional active rheumatoid factor-positive pts. who had fats and oils removed from their diets also experienced remissions. When, after 7 wks., either vegetable oil or animal fat was returned to their diets, they experienced exacerbations within 72 hours. When chicken, cheese, safflower oil, beef or coconut oil were added to the diet, they experienced inflammatory changes affecting joint count, joint swelling and morning stiffness (*Lucas C, Power L. Dietary fat aggravates active rheumatoid arthritis.* Clin Res *29(4):754A, 1981*).

- with <u>omega-3 fatty acids</u>:

Experimental Study: In 31 pts., a typical high-saturated fat diet was compared to a diet high in polyunsaturated fats, low in saturated fats, and supplemented with 1.8 g/d of eicosapentaenoic acid. By 12 wks., morning stiffness was significantly more severe in the control gp. as their symptoms had lengthened while symptoms in the study group were unchanged. In addition, the study gp. indicated a significantly greater decrease in the number of tender joints. Reintroduction of the typical diet was followed by substantial deterioration (*Kremer JM et al. Effects of manipulation of dietary fatty acids on clinical manifestations of rheumatoid arthritis. Lancet 1:184-7, 1985*).

<u>Vegan</u> diet.

May be beneficial due to its low cholesterol and saturated fat content or due to the removal of food antigens.

- with additional food eliminations:

Experimental Study: 20 pts. were placed on a vegan diet following a 7-10 day fast. Also excluded or used sparingly were refined sugar, corn flour, salt, strong spices, alcohol, tea and coffee. After 4 mo., 12 pts. reported some improvement, 5 reported no change, and 3 felt worse. Most felt less pain and were better able to function, although there were no changes in objective measures such as grip strength and joint tenderness (*Sköldstam L. Fasting and vegan diet in rheumatoid arthritis. Scand J Rheumatol 15(2):219-21, 1987*).

- -

VITAMINS

<u>Pantothenic Acid</u>:

Found to be reduced compared to normals, with an inverse correlation between its level and the severity of symptoms (*Barton-Wright EC, Elliott WA. The pantothenic acid metabolism of rheumatoid arthritis. Lancet 2:862-63, 1963*).

Supplementation may be beneficial.

Experimental Double-blind Study: 18 pts. with RA who were previously untreated or who had not responded to previous drug treatment were randomly chosen to receive 2 gm daily of oral calcium pantothenate (starting with 500 mg daily and gradually increasing to 500 mg 4 times daily by day 10), while the rest received placebo. Pts. were permitted to take paracetamol to relieve pain but no other medications were permitted. After 2 mo., daily records kept by pts. in the experimental gp. showed a significant subjective reduction in the duration of morning stiffness (p<0.01), degree of disability (p<0.04) and severity of pain (p<0.01) compared to baseline, while controls failed to report significant improvements. Analysis of co-variance between gps. revealed a significant difference in the reduction of disability (p<0.04), although the duration of morning stiffness and severity of pain differences were not significant (*Calcium pantothenate in arthritic conditions. A report from the General Practitioner Research Group. Practitioner 224:208-11, 1980*).

Experimental Study: 20 pts. received calcium-D-pantothenate 50 mg IM daily leading to temporary alleviation of symptoms after 7 days along with an increase in whole blood pantothenate. Another 21 days of injections failed to result in further improvement. After discontinuation, blood levels fell to their initial values by the end of 1 mo. with concomitant reappearance of symptoms, suggesting that abnormal pantothenate metabolism is due to some other factor. Since royal jelly is rich in pantothenic acid in its free state as well as in other 10-carbon straight chain fatty acids, 20 pts. received a mixture of royal jelly and pantothenic acid 50 mg of each IM daily. By 28 days, 14 pts. (70%) noted an improvement in general condition and joint mobility along with a fall in ESR coincident with rising blood levels which lasted until blood levels returned to previous values 2 mo. following discontinuation of the injections. 10 vegetarians with RA all improved on the same regime by 14 days with a greater rise in whole blood pantothenate levels than in the non-vegetarian arthritics. Preliminary results with oral supplementation has been encouraging (*Barton-Wright EC, Elliott WA. The pantothenic acid metabolism of rheumatoid arthritis. Lancet 2:862-63, 1963*).

<u>Vitamin A</u>:

Plasma/serum levels may be reduced (*Honkanen V et al. Vitamins A and E, retinol binding protein and zinc in rheumatoid arthritis. Clin Exp Rheumatol 7:465-69, 1989*).

Vitamin C:

Plasma/serum levels may be reduced.

Observational Study: Compared to healthy controls, pts. had reduced serum levels of vitamin C (*Jacobsson I et al. Correlation of fatty acid composition of adipose tissue lipids and serum phosphatidylcholine and serum concentrations of micronutrients with disease duration in rheumatoid arthritis. Ann Rheum Dis 49:901-05, 1990*).

Review Article: Leucocyte and plasma concentrations of ascorbate are significantly decreased in RA (*Mullen A, Wilson CWM. The metabolism of ascorbic acid in rheumatoid arthritis. Proc Nutr Sci 35:8A-9A, 1976; Sahud MA, Cohen RJ. Effect of aspirin ingestion on ascorbic-acid levels in rheumatoid arthritis. Lancet 1:937-38, 1971*) possibly because of increased degradation and excretion due to the greatly enhanced rates of oxidation of ascorbate in inflammation in activated neutrophils (*Roberts P et al. Vitamin C and inflammation. Med Biol 62:88, 1984*).

Deficiency may be associated with spontaneous bruising on the forearms and lower limbs as well as with cutaneous hemorrhages; these signs may resolve with supplementation.

Experimental Study: 3 elderly pts. with significant cutaneous hemorrhages were determined to be deficient in vitamin C. One of the 3 was on steroids; all had spontaneous bruising. Supplementation with vitamin C 500 mg daily produced complete resolution of the hemorrhages (*Oldroyd KG, Dawes PT. Clinically significant vitamin C deficiency in rheumatoid arthritis. Br J Rheumatol 24:362-63, 1985*).

Vitamin E:

Plasma/serum levels may be reduced (*Honkanen VEA et al. Serum cholesterol and vitamins A and E in juvenile chronic arthritis. Clin Exp Rheumatol 8:187-91, 1990; Honkanen V et al. Vitamins A and E, retinol binding protein and zinc in rheumatoid arthritis. Clin Exp Rheumatol 7:465-69, 1989*).

Supplementation may be as effective in ankylosing spondylitis as non-steroidal anti-inflammatory drugs.

Experimental Controlled Study: After 6 wks., pts. treated with vitamin E showed a similar significant (p<0.05) increase in motility of the spine as pts. treated with diclofenac. Differences in circumvention of the thorax in the inhaled vs. the exhaled state increased with either treatment which continued over the 12 wks. of the study, and there was no significant difference between them. In addition, subjective pain ratings were improved with either treatment, with maximal improvement after 6 wks. and slight reduction after 12 wks., suggesting that placebo effects contributed to the initial improvement. Ratings for general well-being showed a similar pattern. One pt. on diclofenac had to stop treatment due to GI bleeding; there were no significant side-effects in pts. receiving vitamin E (*Blankenhorn G. Vitamin E: Clinical research from Europe. Nutr Dietary Consult June, 1988*).

Vitamin K (menadione):   5 - 10 mg. three times daily

May stabilize the synovial linings of affected tissue.

In vitro Experimental Study: Hydrogen-accepting molecules, especially menadione, stabilized the lysosomal membranes of synovial lining cells of human rheumatoid tissue and decreased the excessively reductive cytoplasmic pH, while ascorbate, a hydrogen donor, did the opposite (*Chayen J et al. The effect of experimentally induced redox changes on human rheumatoid and non-rheumatoid synovial tissue in vitro. Beitr Path Bd 149:127, 1973*).

- -

MINERALS

Boron:

Supplementation may be beneficial.

Clinical Observations: Boron supplementation was effective for about 90% of arthritis pts., including rheumatoid arthritis, most with complete remission of symptoms. It was especially effective with juvenile arthritis. Pts. normally took 6-9 mg elemental boron daily to achieve symptom relief followed by a maintenance dose of 3 mg daily (*Newnham RE. Arthritis or skeletal fluorosis and boron. Letter. Int Clin Nutr Rev 11(2):68-70, 1991; Newnham RE. Boron beats arthritis. Proc ANZAAS, Australian Academy of Science, Canberra, Australia, 1979*).

<u>Copper</u>:   copper salicylate: 1-2 64 mg. tabs daily with meals
                        (maximum of 10 days per treatment)

Serum copper and ceruloplasmin concentrations are elevated (*Conforti A et al. Serum copper and ceruloplasmin levels in rheumatoid arthritis and degenerative joint disease and their pharmacological implications. <u>Pharmacol Res Commun</u> 15(9):859-676, 1983; Grennan DM et al. Serum copper and zinc in rheumatoid arthritis and osteoarthritis. <u>N Z Med J</u> 91(652):47-50, 1980; Youssef AA et al. Serum copper: A marker of disease activity in rheumatoid arthritis. <u>J Clin Pathol</u> 36(1):14-17, 1983*).

Serum copper levels are directly related to length and severity of the disease and return to normal with remission but do not reflect copper balance in the body. The rise in serum copper seen in RA is associated with a fall in liver copper stores as well as an increased rate of synthesis of ceruloplasmin and an increase of ceruloplasmin within synovial fluid (*Sorenson J, in <u>The Anti-inflammatory Activities of Copper Complexes. Metal Ions and Biological Systems</u>. Marcel Dekker, 1982:77-125*).

Plasma copper levels are directly correlated with disease activity (*Honkanen VEA et al. Plasma zinc and copper concentrations in rheumatoid arthritis: influence of dietary factors and disease activity. <u>Am J Clin Nutr</u> 54:1082-6, 1991*).

The changes in blood copper levels and in the activities of copper-dependent processes reflect a change in oxidative status of the blood which may have implications in the pathogenesis of the disease (*Banford JC et al. Serum copper and erythrocyte superoxide dismutase in rheumatoid arthritis. <u>Ann Rheum Dis</u> 41(5):458-62, 1982*).

Synovial fluid copper concentrations are 3 times that of normals due to elevated ceruloplasmin which may reflect both the elevated serum copper and increased permeability of the synovial membrane to ceruloplasmin (*Niedermeier W. Concentration and chemical state of copper in synovial fluid and blood serum of patients with rheumatoid arthritis. <u>Ann Rheum Dis</u> 24:544, 1965*).

Copper deficiency, due to its effects on ceruloplasmin, may contribute to the disease by increasing iron accumulation in storage tissues (*Watts DL. The nutritional relationships of copper. <u>J Orthomol Med</u> 4(2):99-108, 1989*).

> **Theoretical Discussion:** The low incidence of RA in Europe during pre-industrial times may have been due to the protection of copper which was commonly used in cooking and eating utensils. Industrialization brought increased production and use of copper antagonists such as cadmium, zinc, lead, etc. (*Rainsford KD. Environmental metal ion pertubations, especially as they affect copper status are a factor in the etiology of arthritic conditions: An hypothesis, in JRJ Sorenson, Ed. <u>Inflammatory Diseases and Copper</u>. New Jersey, Humana Press, 1982*).

Supplementation with <u>copper salicylate complex</u> may be beneficial and is more effective in animal models of inflammaton than aspirin alone.

> **Review Article:** Copper's anti-inflammatory effect appears to be related to its ability to form complexes which serve as selective antioxidants, thus reducing the localized tissue inflammation which has resulted from enhanced oxidant damage (*Sorenson J. Copper aspirinate: A more potent anti-inflammatory and anti-ulcer agent. <u>J Int Acad Prev Med</u> 1980, pp. 7-21*).

> **Review Article:** Copper salicylates are believed to be the best copper complex for the treatment of arthritic pain based on rat studies and uncontrolled human trials (*Sorenson JR, Hangarter W. Treatment of rheumatoid and degenerative diseases with copper complexes: A review with emphasis on copper-salicylate. <u>Inflammation</u> 2(3):217-38, 1977*).

> **Experimental Study:** 89% of 1140 pts. treated with short-term IV copper salicylate showed remission of fever, increased joint mobility, decreased swelling, and normalization of ESR for an ave. of 3 yrs. (*Sorenson JR, Hangarter W. Treatment of rheumatoid and degenerative diseases with copper complexes: A review with emphasis on copper-salicylate. <u>Inflammation</u> 2(3):217-38, 1977*).

Local application of elemental copper may have some therapeutic value.

> **Experimental Single-blind Crossover Study:** 240 "arthritis/rheumatism sufferers" were randomized into 3 groups. Gp. I wore a copper bracelet for 1 mo. followed by a "placebo" bracelet for 1 month. Gp. II wore the 2

bracelets in reverse order, while Gp. III wore no bracelets. Of those who noted a difference between the 2 bracelets, more perceived the copper to be more effective (p<0.01). Previous users of copper bracelets deteriorated while wearing the placebo. The ave. loss of copper from the bracelet was 13 mg. (*Walker WR, Keats DM. An investigation of the therapeutic value of the "copper bracelet": Dermal assimilation of copper in arthritic/rheumatoid conditions. Agents Actions 6:454,1976*).

Gold:

A non-essential mineral.

First introduced in the early part of this century, intramuscular injection of gold has become one of the standard treatment options (*Fifty years of gold in rheumatoid arthritis. Br Med J 1:289-90, 1979*).

However, toxicity is not uncommon, and controversy over the efficacy of gold therapy continues (*Editorial: Gold therapy in rheumatoid arthritis. Lancet 338:19-20, 1991*).

Iron:

While, compared to normals, serum iron is significantly reduced (*Niedermeier W, Griggs JH. Trace metal composition of synovial fluid and blood serum of patients with rheumatoid arthritis. J Chron Dis 23:527-36, 1971*), it is significantly elevated in both the synovial fluid and the synovial membrane and iron deposits in the membrane can regularly be seen histologically (*Muirden KD, Senator GB. Iron in the synovial membrane in rheumatoid arthritis and other joint diseases. Ann Rheum Dis 27:38-48, 1968; Niedermeier W, Griggs JH. Trace metal composition of synovial fluid and blood serum of patients with rheumatoid arthritis. J Chron Dis 23:527-36, 1971; Senator GB, Muirden KD. Concentration of iron in synovial membrane, synovial fluid and serum in rheumatoid arthritis and other joint diseases. Ann Rheum Dis 27:49-54, 1968*).

Microcytic anemia is common; however iron supplementation must be used with caution as the anemia may not be due to iron deficiency and supplementary iron can increase joint inflammation due to the formation of highly reactive hydroxyl radicals from hydrogen peroxide and iron salts by superoxide and ascorbate-dependent mechanisms (*Rawley DA, Halliwell B. Formation of hydroxyl radicals from hydrogen peroxide and iron salts by superoxide and ascorbate-dependent mechanisms: Relevance to the pathology of rheumatoid disease. Clin Sci 64:649-53, 1983*).

Experimental Study: 6 pts. with definite or classical RA and the anemia of chronic disease (ACD) (diagnosed by exclusion of other causes of anemia and by the presence of increased stainable bone marrow iron) received an oral iron chelator. After treatment, hemoglobin increased in 5/6 patients. Serum iron and iron excretion increased significantly whereas ferritin tended to decrease. Clinical and serological indices of RA were unchanged. Results suggest that the observed rise in Hb may be due to iron release from the mononuclear phagocyte system (which retains iron in ACD), resulting in increased bone-marrow iron availability or increased transferrin receptor expression in erythroblasts (*Vreugdenhil G et al. Efficacy and safety of oral iron chelator L1 in anaemic rheumatoid arthritis patients. Letter. Lancet 2:1398-99, 1989*).

Single-blind Case Report: A 39 year-old female pt. developed both subjective and objective worsening of her peripheral synovitis within 48 hrs. of ingesting ferrous sulfate 200 mg 3 times daily, while placebo caused no change. Serum ferritin rose from 30-50 µg/L while her symptoms exacerbated on iron, but returned to 15 µg/L one mo. after iron was stopped (*Blake D, Bacon P. Lancet 1:623, 1982*).

Serum or plasma ferritin level may be the most appropriate measure for determining whether to provide supplemental iron to patients with microcytic anemias although, since it is also an acute phase reactant, its level may also show some correlation with disease activity (*Rothwell RS, Davis P. Relationship between serum ferritin, anemia, and disease activity in acute and chronic rheumatoid arthritis. Rheumatol Int 1(2):65-67, 1981*).

Suggested criteria for iron supplementation:
   Serum ferritin: <60 µg/l
   Plasma ferritin: <110 µg/l

Experimental Study: 67 pts. with active RA received oral iron. A rise in hemoglobin was taken as evidence than iron deficiency anemia had been present. A pre-treatment serum ferritin level <60 µg/l was a good indicator of iron-responsive anemia, with a sensitivity of 83%, and was a superior indicator to plasma transferrin or MCV (*Hansen TM, Hansen NE. Serum ferritin as indicator of iron responsive anemia in patients with rheumatoid arthritis. Ann Rheum Dis 45:569, 1986*).

Experimental Study: The combination of microcytic anemia and a plasma ferritin concentration of <110 μg/l predicted that oral iron supplementation would result in increases in HGb concentration, red cell MCV and red cell ferritin contents (*Davidson A et al. Red cell ferritin content: A re-evaluation of indices for iron deficiency in the anaemia of rheumatoid arthritis. Br Med J 289:648-50, 1984*).

Experimental Study: 21/38 randomly selected anemic pts. with classical or definite RA had iron deficiency as estimated from the iron content in stained bone marrow aspiration. Serum ferritin concentrations <60 μg/l had a sensitivity for iron deficiency of 86% and a specificity of 88%. These results were superior to those obtained by measurements of serum iron, plasma transferrin, MCV or MCHC. Serum ferritin was not correlated to disease activity. During iron therapy, serum ferritin rose in 7/8 pts. (*Hansen TM et al. Serum ferritin and the assessment of iron deficiency in rheumatoid arthritis. Scand J Rheumatol 12(4):353-59, 1983*).

Manganese:

Total body turnover is low in pts. but is restored to normal with corticosteroid therapy. RBC manganese levels, however, are higher than in normals (*Cotzias GC et al. Slow turnover of manganese in active rheumatoid arthritis and acceleration by prednisone. J Clin Invest 47:992, 1968*).

Selenium:

Serum/plasma levels may be reduced (*Jacobsson I et al. Correlation of fatty acid composition of adipose tissue lipids and serum phosphatidylcholine and serum concentrations of micronutrients with disease duration in rheumatoid arthritis. Ann Rheum Dis 49:901-05, 1990; Johansson V et al. Nutritional status in girls with juvenile chronic arthritis. Hum Nutr Clin Nutr 40C:57-67, 1986*).

Supplementation may be beneficial.

Theoretical Discussion: Rheumatoid arthritis is characterized by increased macrophage activity causing production of toxic forms of oxygen which may mediate rheumatoid inflammation. Therapeutic induction of increased intracellular levels of glutathione or administration of selenium in such a form that it incorporates into glutathione peroxidase and increases the efficacy of the enzyme may lead to accelerated metabolism of toxic oxygen (*Munthe E et al. Trace elements and rheumatoid arthritis: Pathogenetic and therapeutic aspects. Acta Pharmacol Toxicol (Copenh) 59(Suppl 7):365-73, 1986*).

Negative Experimental Double-blind Study: 40 pts. with active RA received either selenium 256 μg in selenium-enriched yeast or placebo. Although concentrations of selenium in serum and erythrocytes increased considerably, no significant antirheumatic effect of selenium could be demonstrated (*Tarp U et al. Selenium treatment in rheumatoid arthritis. Scand J Rheumatol 14(4):364-68, 1985*).

- with **Vitamin E**:

Experimental Study: Following treatment with selenium and vitamin E, a correlation was found between pain relief and increased blood levels of glutathione peroxidase (*Bruce A et al. The effect of selenium and vitamin E on glutathione peroxidase levels and subjective symptoms in patients with arthrosis and rheumatoid arthritis, in Proc N Z Workshop on Trace Elements in N Z. Dunedin, U. of Otago, 1981:92*).

Sulfur:

Sulfur is metabolized by two pathways: oxidation and S-methylation. In rheumatoid arthritis, both pathways are impaired (*Gordon C et al. Abnormal sulphur oxidation in systemic lupus erythematosus. Lancet 339:25-6, 1992*).

Tissue and blood levels may be reduced.

Observational Study: Significantly lower sulfur values were found in type IIA and IIB muscle fibers of RA patients as compared to controls, perhaps because of a decreased amount of sulfur-rich proteins (*Wróblewski R et al. Electron probe X-ray microanalysis of human skeletal muscle involved in rheumatoid arthritis. Histochemistry 57(1):1-8, 1978*).

Observational Study: While the cystine content of fingernails in normals is 12%, in "arthritics" it is only 8.9% (*Sullivan MX, Hess WC. Cystine content of finger nails in arthritis. J Bone Joint Surg 16:185, 1935*).

Supplementation may be beneficial.

> **Experimental Study:** 100 "arthritics" received IV colloidal sulfur. Pain and effusions disappeared in many cases with a return of the cystine fingernail test to normal (*Woldenberg SC. The treatment of arthritis with colloidal sulphur. J South Med Assoc 28:875-81, 1935; See Also: Neligan AR, Salt HB. Sulphur in rheumatoid arthritis. Lancet 2:209, 1934*).

May be absorbed through the skin.

> **Experimental Study:** Blood sulfur levels rose following sulfur baths (*Osterberg AE et al. Absorption of sulphur compounds during treatment by sulphur baths. Arch Dermatol Syphilol 20:156-66, 1929*).

Zinc: 20 - 50 mg three times daily

Serum levels are significantly reduced (*Dijkmans BA et al. Serum aluminium concentrations in patients with rheumatoid arthritis. Scand J Rheumatol 16(5):361-64, 1987; Pandey SP et al. Zinc in rheumatoid arthritis. Indian J Med Res 81:618-20, 1985*).

The reduction in serum zinc level appears related to disease activity.

> **Observational Study:** In a study of 40 pts., 7-day food diaries were analyzed along with clinical and lab data by means of stepwise multiple linear regression analyses. The indices assessing the disease activity were the best predictors of serum zinc levels (*Honkanen VEA et al. Plasma zinc and copper concentrations in rheumatoid arthritis: influence of dietary factors and disease activity. Am J Clin Nutr 54:1082-6, 1991*).

> **Observational Study:** In a study of 60 pts., joint score index, rheumatoid factor titer, seropositivity, hemoglobin, and C reactive protein were among the 9 independent variables which together predicted 73% of the serum zinc variation, suggesting an association between the immune-inflammatory process and the serum zinc concentration (*Mussalo-Rauhamaa H et al. Predictive clinical and laboratory parameters for serum zinc and copper in rheumatoid arthritis. Ann Rheum Dis 47(10):816-19, 1988*).

Plasma zinc levels may be reduced, with the reduction inversely correlated with measures of inflammation.

> **Observational Study:** In a study of 40 pts., 7-day food diaries were analyzed along with clinical and lab data by means of stepwise multiple linear regression analyses. Plasma zinc levels appeared to be determined mostly by the activity and extent of the inflammatory process and not by dietary factors (*Honkanen VEA et al. Plasma zinc and copper concentrations in rheumatoid arthritis: influence of dietary factors and disease activity. Am J Clin Nutr 54:1082-6, 1991*).

> **Observational Study:** Plasma zinc was reduced in the majority of pts. compared to healthy controls, and was negatively correlated to the inflammatory activity as estimated by ESR and serum orosomucoid (*Svenson KL et al. Reduced zinc in peripheral blood cells from patients with inflammatory connective tissue diseases. Inflammation 9(2):189-99, 1985*).

> **Experimental Study:** Plasma zinc levels were significantly lower in pts. on NSAIDs than in those on levamisole and penicillamine. In addition, plasma zinc levels correlated positively with serum albumin, and negatively with both ESR and serum globulin, suggesting that it is one of the nonspecific features of inflammation (*Balogh Z et al. Plasma zinc and its relationship to clinical symptoms and drug treatment in rheumatoid arthritis. Ann Rheum Dis 39(4):329-32, 1980*).

Cellular zinc levels may be reduced (*Svenson KL et al. Reduced zinc in peripheral blood cells from patients with inflammatory connective tissue diseases. Inflammation 9(2):189-99, 1985*).

Synovial fluid zinc levels may be elevated (*Niedermeier W, Griggs JH. Trace metal composition of synovial fluid and blood serum of patients with rheumatoid arthritis. J Chron Dis 23:527-36, 1971*)

Urinary zinc levels may be elevated (*Pandey SP et al. Zinc in rheumatoid arthritis. Indian J Med Res 81:618-20, 1985*).

Zinc supplementation may lessen disease activity.

> **Theoretical Discussion:** Rheumatoid arthritis is characterized by increased macrophage activity causing production of toxic forms of oxygen which may mediate rheumatoid inflammation. Zinc is a component of superoxide dismutase which detoxifies oxygen. In high parenteral doses, it can immobilize macrophages and induce metallothionein-like proteins (*Munthe E et al. Trace elements and rheumatoid arthritis: Pathogenetic and therapeutic aspects. Acta Pharmacol Toxicol (Copenh) 59(Suppl 7):365-73, 1986*).

> **Negative Experimental Double-blind Study:** 22 pts. with severe long-standing RA received oral zinc sulfate 220 mg 3 times daily 1 hr. before meals or placebo. 6/22 had subjective but not objective improvement for 6 mo. but then deteriorated. In the whole gp., neither the number of affected joints, the ARA grading, the functional classification, ESR, hemoglobin, hematocrit, or platelet count changed significantly. The main side-effect was nausea (*Rasker JJ, Kardaun SH. Lack of beneficial effect of zinc sulphate in rheumatoid arthritis. Scand J Rheumatol 11:168-70, 1982*).

> **Review Article and Theoretical Discussion:** The conflicting results of studies researching the effect of zinc supplementation may be explained by its benefits being limited to pts. with zinc deficiency which is a sometime complication, not a cause of RA. Better ways to identify the zinc-deficient individual are needed (*Simkin PA. Treatment of rheumatoid arthritis with oral zinc sulfate. Agents Actions 8:587-96, 1981 (Suppl)*).

> **Experimental Double-blind Crossover Study (psoriatic arthritis):** 24 pts. with negative tests for rheumatoid factors, LE cells and antinuclear antibodies experienced reduction in signs and symptoms of RA following supplementation with zinc sulphate 220 mg 3 times daily for 6 wks. accompanied by reduction of serum immunoglobulins and an increase in serum albumin. Only joint pains were significantly reduced following the initial study; however, during a subsequent 24 wk. open trial, morning stiffness and improvement in their overall condition reached significance. There was no improvement in psoriatic lesions and severe side-effects were not seen (*Clemmensen OJ et al. Psoriatic arthritis treated with oral zinc sulphate. Br J Dermatol 103:411-15, 1980*).

> **Negative Experimental Blinded Study:** 18 pts. were treated for 4 mo. with zinc sulfate 600 mg/d while 17 well-matched control pts. received placebo. Careful evaluations of a number of clinical variables revealed no therapeutic response in the zinc-treated group. Lab studies also showed no improvement despite evidence of zinc absorption (*Job C et al. Zinc sulphate in the treatment of rheumatoid arthritis. Arthritis Rheum 23:1408, 1980*).

> **Experimental Double-blind Study:** 12/24 pts. with chronic, active disease received 50 mg. elemental zinc (zinc sulfate heptahydrate 250 mg) 3 times daily with meals for 12 wks. while the rest received placebo, then all 24 pts. received zinc for 12 more weeks. There were significant improvements in joint swelling, morning stiffness, walking time and subjective symptoms during the first part of the study with continuing, impressive improvement in the second part (*Simkin PA. Oral zinc sulphate in rheumatoid arthritis. Lancet 2:539-42, 1976*).

One effect of zinc that may explain its benefits is the lowering of serum copper levels (*Honkanen VEA et al. Plasma zinc and copper concentrations in rheumatoid arthritis: influence of dietary factors and disease activity. Am J Clin Nutr 54:1082-6, 1991*).

– –

OTHER NUTRITIONAL FACTORS

Catechin:

> A naturally occurring flavonoid.

> Able to inhibit the breakdown of collagen caused by either free radicals or enzymes (hyaluronidase, collagenase, and pepsin) as well as to crosslink directly with collagen fibers and inhibit procollagen biosynthesis (*Blumenkrantz N, Asboe-Hansen G. Effect of (+)-catechin on connective tissue. Scand J Rheumatol 7:55-60, 1978*).

Glycosaminoglycans (mucopolysaccharides):

> Concentrations are increased in blood cells and biological fluids of patients (*Volkova ZI et al. [Glucosaminoglycans and beta-glucuronidase in peripheral blood cells and biological fluids of patients with rheumatoid arthritis.] Vopr Med Khim 34(3):53-59, 1988*).

Supplementation may be beneficial.

> **Experimental Study:** 9 pts. received sub-cut. injections of an activated acid-pepsin-digested calf tracheal cartilege extract ("Catrix-S") over a period of 10-35 days followed by booster doses every 3-4 wks. depending upon pt. response. 3/9 had an excellent response, while the other 6 had a good response (*Prudden JF, Balassa LL. The biological activity of bovine cartilage preparations. Semin Arthritis Rheum 3(4):287-321, 1974*).

L-Histidine: 1000 mg. 2-3 times daily between meals (several month trial)

Markedly depressed (while other amino acids are normal) (*Gerber DA et al. Free serum histidine levels in patients with rheumatoid arthritis and control subjects following an oral load of free L-histidine. J Clin Inves 55:1164,1975; Gerber DA et al. Specificity of a low free serum histidine concentration for rheumatoid arthritis. J Chron Dis 30:115, 1977*).

Supplementation may be beneficial.

> **Experimental Double-blind Study:** Pts. were treated with oral L-histidine 4.5 gm daily or placebo. After 30 wks. no clinical measurement showed an advantage of histidine over placebo, although a small decrease in rheumatoid factor titer and a small increase in hematocrit were found only in the histidine group and there was suggestive evidence of a beneficial effect of histidine in pts. with more active and prolonged disease (*Pinals RS et al. Treatment of rheumatoid arthritis with L-histidine: A randomized, placebo controlled, double-blind trial. J Rheumatol 4(4):414-19, 1977*).

Supplementation may lower elevated levels of heavy metals such as copper and iron in affected joints (*Niedermeier W, Griggs JH. J Chronic Dis 23:527-536, 1971*

Essential Fatty Acids:

- General:

May be reduced in serum and adipose tissue (*Jacobsson I et al. Correlation of fatty acid composition of adipose tissue lipids and serum phosphatidylcholine and serum concentrations of micronutrients with disease duration in rheumatoid arthritis. Ann Rheum Dis 49:901-05, 1990*).

Supplementation may be beneficial.

> **Experimental Double-blind Study:** 49 pts., all on NSAIDs, received either evening primrose oil (Efamol) 12 caps daily (540 mg), 80% evening primrose oil and 20% fish oil rich in eicosapentaenoic acid (Efamol Marine) 12 caps daily (240 mg EPO, 450 mg GLA), or placebo. After 3 mo., efforts were made to reduce NSAID use in all patients. After an additional 9 mo., pts. on evening primrose oil rated themselves 94% better, those on evening primrose and fish oil rated themselves 100% better, while those on placebo rated themselves only 33% better. 83% of pts. on evening primrose oil and 94% on evening primrose and fish oils either completely eliminated NSAIDs or cut them in half, while on 34% of pts. on placebo were able to reduce their drug intake. All pts. were then placed on placebo for 6 months. During this time, the majority of pts. who had been on fatty acid supplements noted worsening of their condition (*Belch JJ et al. Effects of altering dietary essential fatty acids on requirements for non-steroidal andti-inflammatory drugs in patients with rheumatoid arthritis: A double blind placebo controlled study. Ann Rheum Dis 47(2):96-104, 1986*).

- Omega-3 Fatty Acids:

Eicosapentaenoic acid (EPA) and docosahexaenoic acid (DHA).

Highest in cold-water fish (mackerel, herring, salmon, bluefish, tuna, etc). Available in a refined form as "MaxEPA" (18% EPA).

Suggested dosage: 10 one gm MaxEPA (R.P. Scherer) capsules daily (1.8 g EPA & 1.2 g DHA) (2 mo. minimum trial)

> WARNING: Supplementation may require additional vitamin E intake to prevent increased membrane peroxidation and cellular damage (*Laganiere S, Fernandes G. High peroxidizability of subcellular membrane induced by high fish oil diet is reversed by vitamin E. Clin Res 35:A565, 1987*).

Supplementation may be beneficial.

Experimental Double-blind Study: 49 pts. with active RA randomly received either olive oil capsules containing 6.8 g oleic acid, or fish oil capsules containing either 54 mg/kg EPA and 36 mg/kg DHA (high dose) or 27 mg/kg EPA and 18 mg/kg DHA (low dose). Significant improvements from baseline in the number of tender joints were noted in the low-dose gp. at wk. 24 (p=0.05) and in the high-dose gp. at wk. 18 (p=0.04) and 24 (p=0.02). Significant decreases in the number of swollen joints were noted in the low-dose gp. at wks. 12 (p=0.003), 18 (p=0.002), and 24 (p=0.001) and in the high-dose gp. at wks. 12 (p=0.0001), 18 (p=0.008), and 24 (p=0.02). 5/45 clinical measures were significantly changed from baseline in the olive oil gp., 8/45 in the low-dose fish oil gp., and 21/45 in the high-dose fish oil gp. (p=0.0002) (*Kremer JM et al. Dietary fish oil and olive oil supplementation in patients with rheumatoid arthritis. Clinical and immunologic effects.* Arthritis Rheum *33(6):810-20, 1990*).

Experimental Double-blind Crossover Study: 16 pts. with active, stable RA received 12 caps fish oil (2g EPA & 1.3g DHA) or placebo daily for 12 wks. each in random order. The fish oil produced a statistically significant improvement in clinical disease, but the biochemical measures of disease activity, such as the levels of C-reactive protein and the RBC sedimentation rate, were unchanged (*Tulleken JE et al. N-3 polyunsaturated acids, interleukin-1 and tumor necrosis factor. Letter.* N Engl J Med *321(1):55, 1989*).

Experimental Double-blind Study: Fish oil supplementation (18 g/d) was compared with olive oil supplementation in pts. receiving conventional therapies. After 12 wks., an improvement in tender joint score and grip strength was seen only in the fish oil-treated gp., while the more subjective measures of mean duration of morning stiffness and analog pain score improved similarly in both groups - although statistical significance was only achieved in paired analyses in the olive oil-treated group. Production of leukotriene B4 by isolated neutrophils stimulated *in vitro* was reduced 30% in the fish oil, but not in the olive oil, group (*Cleland LG et al. Clinical and biochemical effects of dietary fish oil supplements in rheumatoid arthritis.* J Rheumatol *15(10):1471-75, 1988*).

Review Article: While fish oil supplementation appears to have a favorable effect on morning stiffness, number of tender joints, and grip strength, the magnitude of these effects is modest and there is as yet no evidence that it will slow the progression of the disease (*Editorial. Fish oils in rheumatoid arthritis.* Lancet *2:720-21, 1987*).

Experimental Double-blind Crossover Study: 33 pts. with active, definite, or classical RA received either EPA 2.7 gm and DHA 1.8 gm daily in 15 MaxEPA capsules or placebo. After 14 wks., mean time to onset of fatigue improved by 156 min., and number of tender joints decreased by 3.5 in treated patients. Other clinical measures also favored fish oil over placebo but did not reach statistical significance. There were no adverse effects, and the effect from fish oil persisted beyond the 4-week washout period (*Kremer JM et al. Fish-oil fatty acid supplementation in active rheumatoid arthritis. A double-blinded, controlled, crossover study.* Ann Intern Med *106(4):497-503, 1987*).

Experimental Controlled Study: 12/17 pts. randomly received 10 fish oil capsules daily for 14 wks., while 7 received placebo. During the first 6 wks., all 19 also received a NSAID. After 6 wks., the fish-oil cohort showed a significant reduction in the number of painful joints compared to controls. This relief disappeared after withdrawal of NSAID therapy, although pts. did not regress from their baseline status as usually happens when NSAIDs are withdrawn, suggesting that fish oil has an anti-inflammatory effect (*RI Sperling - reported in* Med. World News *July 14, 1986*).

Experimental Double-blind Study: 17 pts. were placed on a high polyunsaturated fat, low saturated fat diet and supplemented with MaxEPA 10 capsules (1.8 gm EPA) daily, while 20 controls received a typical American diet and placebo capsules. After 12 wks., the EPA gp. had significantly less morning stiffness (as stiffness had worsened only in the control gp.). Joints were also less tender and HGb improved, but these measures did not reach significance. A rapid deterioration with increased pain and stiffness was seen in treated pts. compared to controls upon cessation of the experimental diet (*Kremer JM et al. Effect of manipulation of dietary fatty acids on clinical manifestations of rheumatoid arthritis.* Lancet *1:184-7, 1985*).

- <u>Omega-6 Fatty Acids</u>:

> Example: <u>Evening Primrose Oil</u>: 1 gram four times daily (3 month trial)

Supplementation may be beneficial.

> **Negative Experimental Study:** 20 pts. with definite or classical RA were treated with evening primrose oil (Efamol) 1 gm 4 times daily combined with cofactors zinc, ascorbic acid, niacin and pyridoxine (Efavit) without significant changes in their condition after 12 wks. (*Hansen TM et al. Treatment of rheumatoid arthritis with prostaglandin E₁ precursors cis-linoleic acid and gamma-linolenic acid. Scand J Rheumatol 12:85-88, 1983*).

>> *Note: Since at least some of these pts. were on non-steroidal anti-inflammatory drugs (which were stopped 4 days prior to supplementation), it is unclear if the supplements were actually as effective as these medications.*

> **Animal Experimental Study:** Supplementation with evening primrose oil prior to adjuvant challenge resulted in a delay in onset and suppression of the polyarthritis (*Kunkel SL et al. Suppression of chronic inflammation by evening primrose oil. Prog Lipid Res 20:885-88, 1982*).

> **Review Article:** Early studies suggest:
> 1. Relatively ineffective in pts. receiving more than trivial doses of steroids or non-steroidal anti-inflammatory drugs, although it may permit their dosage to be reduced after 1-3 months.
> 2. The effects do not usually become apparent in less than 4-12 weeks.
> 3. Some of the pts. who show the best long-term response have a transient worsening in the first 1-2 weeks.
> 4. The course of the disease may actually be stopped in some patients.
> (*Horrobin DF. The importance of gamma-linolenic acid and prostaglandin E₁ in human nutrition and medicine. J Holistic Med 3:118-139, 1981*).

> **Experimental Study:** Several pts. were given 2.1 gm. primrose oil daily. After 3 mo. of treatment, results were seen which suggest that it may be effective (*McCormick JN et al. Immunosuppressive effect of linoleic acid. Lancet 2:508, 1977*).

<u>D.L Phenylalanine</u>:   750 mg 15-30 minutes before meals 3 times daily (2-21 days for results).
                                        Double the dose if ineffective for up to another 3 weeks.

Supplementation may be beneficial.

> **Case Report:** A 47 year-old woman with an 18-yr. history of RA had marked inflammation and swelling of the dorsum of her hands causing the MCP joints to become hidden. Seven days after starting DLPA her pain had faded and the swelling was so greatly reduced that the knuckles were visible. In addition there was dramatic improvement in joint flexibility (*Study reported in Hopkins P. Phenylalanine & relief of chronic pain. Anabolism (4)2, 1985*).

<u>Quercitin</u>:

RA is characterized by substantially increased numbers of mast cells in synovial membranes and fluids. Degranulation of these mast cells are believed to be a major factor in the tissue destruction. Quercetin, a bioflavonoid, is a potent inhibitor of mast cell degranulation.

<u>Saponin Extract</u> (from <u>Yucca</u>):

Administration may be beneficial.

> **Experimental Double-blind Study:** 149 arthritis pts., 41.1% with a positive RA fixation test, were randomly given either yucca saponin extract ("Desert Pride Herbal Food Tablets") 4 daily (range of 2 - 8) or placebo in periods ranging from 1 wk. to 15 mo. before re-evaluation. 61% noted less swelling, pain and stiffness versus 22% on placebo. Some improved in days, some in wks., and some in 3 mo. or longer (*Bingham R et al. Yucca plant saponin in the management of arthritis. J Appl Nutr 27:45-50, 1975*).

<u>Superoxide Dismutase</u>:

An enzyme that eliminates the highly reactive superoxide radical.

> *Note: Oral SOD has no effect on tissue levels, although it is conceivable (but unproven) that an enteric-coated pill could escape digestion (Zidenberg-Cherr S et al. Dietary superoxide dismutase does not affect tissue levels. <u>Am J Clin Nutr</u> 37:5, 1983).*

Activity is increased in the synovial fluid of the affected joints, suggesting that SOD activity is a manifestation of the acute inflammatory stage of RA (*Igari T et al. A remarkable increase of superoxide dismutase activity in synovial fluid of patients with rheumatoid arthritis. <u>Clin Orthop</u> (162):282-87, 1982*).

Parenteral supplementation may be beneficial.

> **Review Article:** Systemic treatment of RA by SOD has yielded disappointing results (*Flohë L. Superoxide dismutase for therpeutic use: clinical experience, dead ends and hopes. <u>Mol Cell Biochem</u> 84(2):123-31, 1988*).

> **Experimental Double-blind Study:** 30 pts. with active classical RA affecting the knee received intra-articular injections of bovine-derived Zn,Cu superoxide dismutase (Orgotein) 4 mg/wk or aspirin 4 mg for 6 weeks. After 12 wks., clinical and biochemical assessments showed that orgotein was superior to aspirin and resulted in significant improvement. Changes in synovial fluid suggest that the anti-inflammatory properties of orgotein may lie in its effect on proliferating synovia (*Goebel KM et al. Intrasynovial orgotein therapy in rheumatoid arthritis. <u>Lancet</u> 1:1015-17, 1981*).

<u>Tryptophan</u>:

Supplementation may be beneficial.

> **Animal Experimental Study:** Tryptophan had a marked effect in reducing the edema of adjuvant arthritis induced in rat paws (an animal model of rheumatoid arthritis) compared to controls (*Rand SA, Forst MB. Treatment of adjuvant arthritis with nonsteroidal agents: A comparative study. <u>J Am Podiatry Assoc</u> 70(2):65-70, 1980*).

> **Animal Experimental Study:** Both L- and D,L-tryptophan were effective in suppressing both acute inflammatory exudate formation and the proliferative phase of inflammation in an animal model using rats, with their efficacy equivalent to that of pheylbutazone (*Madan BR et al. Anti-inflammatory activity of L-tryptophan and DL-tryptophan. <u>Indian J Med Res</u> 68:708-13, 1978 *).

> **Experimental Study:** Pts. treated for depression with tryptophan had relief of rheumatoid arthritis (*Broadhurst AD. Tryptophan and rheumatic diseases. Letter. <u>Br Med J</u> 2(6084):456, 1977*).

- -

OTHER FACTORS

Rule out <u>food sensitivities</u>.

Rheumatoid arthritis was absent in prehistory, when cereals and dairy products were not consumed and prolonged cooking was not done. The frequency of gut mucosal lesions and excessive permeability of the intestinal wall found in RA patients today suggests that the enterocyte enzymes are not adapted for modern food in most patients (*Seignalet J. Diet, fasting, and rhematoid arthritis. Letter. <u>Lancet</u> 339:68-9, 1992; Seignalet J. Les associations entre HLA and polyarthrite rhumatoide. II. une théorie sur la pathogénie de la polyarthrite rhumatoide. <u>Rev Int Rhumatol</u> 19:155-70, 1989*).

Fasting and some elimination diets may produce improvement. When successful, subsequent food challenges may produce exacerbations.

> **Experimental Controlled Study:** 27 pts., after an initial 7-10 day subtotal fast, were put on an individually adjusted gluten-free vegan diet for 3-5 mo.; then the food was gradually changed to a lactovegetarian diet for the remainder of the study. If the introduction of a new food item was followed by an increase in pain, stiffness, or joint swelling within 2-48 hrs., this item was omitted for at least 7 days and then reintroduced. If symptoms were exacerbated again, it was excluded for the rest of the study period. A control gp. of 26 pts. ate an ordinary diet. After the initial 4 wks., the experimental gp. showed a significant improvement in number of tender joints,

Ritchie's articular index, number of swollen joints, pain score, duration of morning stiffness, grip strength, RBC sedimentation rate, C-reactive protein, WBC count, and a health assessment questionnaire score. In the control gp., only pain score improved significantly. The benefits in the diet gp. were still present after 1 yr., and evaluation of the whole course showed signficant advantages for the diet gp. in all measured scores (*Kjeldsen-Kragh J et al. Controlled trial of fasting and one-year vegetarian diet in rheumatoid arthritis. Lancet 338:899-902, 1991*).

> *Note: A criticism of this study is that patients were not randomly selected; thus bias was introduced. To participate, patients had to be willing to spend a year on a health farm. Evidence of self-selection includes the female-to-male sex ratio of 45 to 8, the high frequency of seronegativity (45%) and of "food allergy" (43%). Such patients would probably be highly susceptible to placebo effects (Abuzakouk M, O'Farrelly C. Diet, fasting and rheumatoid arthritis. Letter. Lancet 339:68, 1992). Moreover, the test group had intensive personal contacts with dieticians and others while they stayed on a health farm, while the controls were consigned to a convalescent home. These major differences in management may have influenced the results due to the possible effects of central nervous system influence on inflammatory processes (Panayi GS. Diet, fasting and rheumatoid arthritis. Letter. Lancet 339:68-9, 1992).*

Review Article: While purines, sodium nitrate, wheat, maize, beef and black walnut are some of the documented initiators of arthritis, there seems to be no one consistent cause. The antigens which could be responsible are not well characterized, and antigen absorption in the gut, which is difficult to study, is not well understood (*Merry P et al. Modification of rheumatic symptoms by diet and drugs. Proc Nutr Soc 48:363-69, 1989*).

Theoretical Discussion: It is plausible that nutritional modification might alter immune responsiveness and thereby affect manifestations of rheumatic diseases and/or that rheumatic disease may be a manifestation of food allergy or hypersensitivity (*Panush RS. Possible role of food sensitivity in arthritis. Abstract of presentation at the VI International Food Allergy Symposium, November 13-14, 1987. Immunol Allergy Pract 10(3):124-25, 1988*).

Experimental Double-blind Case Report: 52 year-old white female with an 11 yr.history of joint pain, tenderness, swelling and stiffness fulfilled the criteria for active RA and achieved only fair results from NSAIDs. She was placed on a baseline diet for 6 days, a 3-day mineral water fast and vanilla-flavored Vivonex (an elemental diet) for 2 days. She was then challenged with encapsulated lyophilized foods or D-xylose placebo. Within 24 hrs. of starting the water fast, there was noticable symptomatic relief which was sustained on Vivonex. There were no notable responses to 52 placebo challenges, but she responded with symptomatic deterioration and worsening of ESR and other peak responses to cow's milk challenge on 4 separate occasions. While no elevation of IgE antibodies to foods was noted, she did have mildly increased amts. of IgG anti-milk and large amts. of IgG4 anti-milk antibodies, and IgG- and milk-containing circulating immune complexes were marginally elevated 48 hrs. following one of the milk challenges (*Panush RS et al. Food-induced (allergic) arthritis. Arthritis Rheum 29(2):220-26, 1986*).

Experimental Single-blind Study: After 2 wks. in which all previous therapy was withdrawn and a normal diet consumed, 45 pts. were randomly divided into an immediate dietary gp. (Gp. B) and a control gp. which received placebo for 6 wks. prior to dietary therapy (Gp. C). Foods producing symptoms in Gp. B following a hypoallergenic dietary baseline were eliminated. When compared to the scores of Gp. C during their placebo period, Gp. B did better for all 13 subjective and objective variables measured for which the differences were significant, while Gp. C during its subsequent diet did better than during the placebo period for all 12 variables which showed significant differences. 33/45 (73%) of pts. considered their condition to be "better" or "much better" following dietary therapy (*Darlington LG et al. Placebo-controlled, blind study of dietary manipulation therapy in rheumatoid arthritis. Lancet 1:236-8, 1986*).

Experimental Double-blind Study: 11/26 pts. were placed on a diet free of additives, preservatives, fruit, red meat, herbs and dairy products, while 15/26 were placed on a "placebo diet" with random food exclusions. After 10 wks., there were no clinically important differences between groups. Two pts. on the experimental diet improved notably, elected to remain on it, have continued to improve, and noted exacerbations of disease upon challenges of certain of the excluded foods (*Panush RS et al. Diet therapy for rheumatoid arthritis. Arthritis Rheum 26:462-71, 1984*).

Experimental Crossover Study: 13 RA pts. were fasted for 7 days in comparison to a control regimen. During fasting, joint inflammation and ESR decreased while, during the control regimen, the joints were unchanged or worse and ESR was unchanged. Improvement in joint inflammation was associated with enchancement of neutrophil bactericidal capacity (*Uden AM et al. Neutrophil functions and clinical performance after total fasting in patients with rheumatoid arthritis. Ann Rheum Dis 42(1):45-51, 1983*).

Symptom provocation during food challenges may be due to the release of serotonin from platelets (*Little CH et al. Platelet serotonin release in rheumatoid arthritis: A study in food-intolerant patients. Lancet 2:297, 1983*).

Mast cell activation, which could result from a food reaction, may play a role in some patients with episodic joint swelling.

> **Animal Experimental Study:** IgE-dependent synovial mast cell degranulation was found to cause a transient, nondestructive arthritis in rats (*Malone DG, Metcalfe DD. Demonstration and characterization of a transient arthritis in rats following sensitization of synovial mast cells with antigen-specific IgE and parenteral challenge with specific antigen. Arthritis Rheum 31(8):1063-67, 1988*).

> **Experimental Studies:** There was a highly significant correlation between the number of synovial fluid mast cells and the inflammatory index of RA pts., and mast cells removed from synovial fluid degranulated when exposed *in vitro* to anti-human IgE antibody (*Dean Metcalfe, head of the Mast Cell Physiology Section, National Institutes of Allergy and Infectious Diseases, Bethesda, Md., USA - quoted in Allergy Observer 5(2):3-4, 1988*).

Intestinal permeability to food antigens may decrease during fasting.

> **Experimental Study:** 5 RA pts. underwent fasting and subsequently were placed on a lactovegetarian diet. During fasting, disease activity (measured by a clinical 6-joint score) decreased and both intestinal and non-intestinal permeability (using low-molecular weight polyethylence glycols as probe molecules) decreased. On the subsequent diet, disease activity and both intestinal and non-intestinal permeability increased again (*Sundquist T et al. Influence of fasting on intestinal permeability and disease activity in patients with rheumatoid arthritis. Scand J Rheumatol 11(1):33-8, 1982*

Food sensitivities may be promoted by the use of non-steroidal anti-inflammatory drugs.

> **Observational Study:** Pts. receiving non-steroidal anti-inflammatory medication excreted significantly more radioactively labeled EDTA, while untreated pts. did not differ from controls. This suggests that NSAIDs are associated with increased intestinal permeability to food antigens (*Bjarnason I et al. Intestinal permeability and inflammation in rheumatoid arthritis: Effects of non-steroidal anti-inflammatory drugs. Lancet 2:1171-74, 1984*).

Rule out <u>hydrochloric acid deficiency</u>.

> *Note: While gastric anacidity had been reported in the past to be a relatively common condition which was associated with acne rosacea and a number of other illnesses, the presence of achlorhydria is no longer accepted unless a potent parietal-cell stimulant (such as histamine) is employed in gastric analysis. More recent studies suggest that histamine-fast anacidity is uncommon before the fifth decade of life and, although it probably does not occur in a normal stomach, its presence is not necessarily associated with symptoms (Rappaport EM. Achlorhydria: Associated symptoms and response to hydrochloric acid. N Engl J Med 252(19):802-5, 1955).*

Observational Study: In a gp. of 35 female pts. (ave. age 41) 10 (28.6%) were achlorhydric, while 6 (17%) were hypochlorhydric. By comparison, 2 studies of normal females of similar ages reported an incidence of achlorhydria of 10.8% and 6.5% (*Hartung EF, Steinbrocker O. Gastric acidity in chronic arthritis. Ann Intern Med 9:252-7, 1935*).

<u>Beche-de-Mer</u> (<u>Sea Cucumber</u>):

Administration of an extract may be beneficial.

> **Experimental Double-blind Study:** 34 RA pts. randomly received either C-Cure (Pacif. Pharm., Ltd., Australia), an extract derived from sea cucumber, 1 cap twice daily, or placebo. There were initially no significant differences in articular index or in grip strength between the 2 groups. After 18 wks. and 24 wks., the articular index was significantly lower and the grip strength significantly higher in the experimental group. There were no side effects (*Ron A. Hazelton, Senior lecturer in medicine (rheumatology), U. of Queensland, Australia. C-Cure in rheumatoid arthritis. A six month placebo-controlled Study. Unpublished manuscript, 1988*).

> **Experimental Double-blind Study:** 30 pts. with various forms of arthritis received either C-Cure (Aldgate Grove Pty., Ltd., Australia) or placebo. After 3 mo., about half found the product to be of subjective benefit, while none found benefit from placebo. No side effects were reported (*MJE McPhillips, MacKay, Queensland, Australia. Unpublished manuscript, 1985*).

Perna canaliculus (Green-lipped mussel):

A rich source of glycosaminoglycans, although the explanation for its therapeutic benefits is unknown.

Administration of the extract may be beneficial.

Experimental Double-blind Study: 25 pts. (mean age 57 yrs.) with classical RA who had failed to respond to non-steroidal anti-inflammatory drugs for several months to several yrs. randomly received either an extract of Perna canaliculus (Seatone, McFarlane Labs, Auckland, NZ) 1050 mg daily or placebo in addition to their NSAIDs. After 3 mo., 10/15 (67%) of the treated pts. improved compared to 3/10 (30%) of the controls. Comparison of their pain as scored by visual analog scales, functional index, and the time taken to walk 50 ft. showed improvements in the treated gp. which were significant at the 95%, 90%, and 95% confidence levels, respectively, compared to controls. All pts. then received treatment with active extract. After an additional 3 mo., 60% of pts. switched from placebo to active treatment were improved. Side-effects were limited to rare nausea, flatulence, fluid retention and, in 2 pts., increased stiffness lasting 2-3 wks. (*Gibson RG et al. Green-lipped mussel extra.. in arthritis. Letter. Lancet 1:439, 1981; Gibson RG et al. Perna canaliculus in the treatment of arthritis. Practitioner 224:955-60, 1980*).

Experimental Study: 55 pts. received NZ Green Mussel Extract (Seatone, McFarlane, Aukland) for 6 mo. to 4 1/2 years. 67% benefited. Adverse side-effects were uncommon and generally mild (*Gibson RG et al. Perna canaliculus in the treatment of arthritis. Practitioner 224:955-60, 1980*).

Negative Double-blind Crossover Study: Five pts. received New Zealand Green Mussel Extract (Seatone, McFarlane, Auckland) and placebo for 6 wks. each in random order. Anti-inflammatory drugs were withdrawn 14 days prior to the study but maintenance gold or low dose steroids were continued. Paracetamol was used for analgesia. Pts. expressed no consistent preference for either Seatone or placebo. Joint tenderness was greater in 4 pts. on Seatone and in 1 on placebo. 4 pts. had improvement in joint swelling on Seatone while 1 had worsening. Grip strength was greater in 1 pt. on Seatone and less in 4, while morning stiffness was less in 3 and greater in 2. Pt. discomfort was less in 1, greater in 3 and unchanged in 1 on Seatone. There were fewer tender and swollen joints in 3 on Seatone and more in 2. Sed rate was higher and more paracetamol was taken by all 5 pts. on Seatone, while the time to walk 10 meters was greater in 2 and less in 2 (*Highton TC, McArthur AW. Pilot study on the effect of New Zealand Green Mussel on rheumatoid arthritis. N Z Med J March 12, 1975, pp.261-62*).

Wobenzyme®:

An enteric-coated tablet consisting of a mixture of pancreatin (beef) 100 mg, bromelain 45 mg, papain 60 mg, lipase 10 mg, amylase 10 mg, trypsin 24 mg and alpha-chymotrypsin 1 mg combined with rutin 50 mg.

Administration may be beneficial.

Experimental Study: 42 pts. with definite or classical RA were treated with 8 tablets of Wobenzyme® 4 times daily. After 6 wks., 26 (61.9%) improved, 13 (30.9%) were unchanged, and 3 (17.1%) were worse. Pts. who primarily showed no immune complexes (measured by C1q-solid phase RIA) or pts. who had immune complexes which became negative during treatment showed improvement more often than pts. who had immune complexes during the entire course of therapy (*Steffen C et al. Enzymtherapie im vergleich mit immunokomplex-bestimmungen bei chronischer polyarthritis. Z Rheumatol 44:51-56, 1985*).

SCLERODERMA

See Also: AUTO-IMMUNE DISORDERS (GENERAL)

VITAMINS

Vitamin E: 800 IU of D-alpha tocopheryl acetate daily 15 minutes before meals.
Increase to 1600 IU if needed; then decrease to minimal maintenance dosage.
Avoid taking iron at the same time.

An experimental progeria-like syndrome in rats with soft tissue calcifications can be prevented by concomitant administration of vitamin E along with the inciting agent.

    - with Methyltestosterone:

        Animal Experimental Study: A progeria-like syndrome in the rat induced by chronic intoxication with dihydrotachysterol was prevented by concurrent D-alpha-tocopherol and methyltestosterone treatment (*Tuchweber B et al. Effect of vitamin E and methyltestosterone upon the progeria-like syndrome produced by dihydrotachysterol. Am J Clin Nutr 13:238-42, 1963*).

Supplementation may be beneficial.

        Experimental Study: 3 pts. with systemic sclerosis improved following supplementation with vitamin E as did 3 pts. with localized scleroderma (morphea) (*Ayres S et al. Raynaud's phenomenon, scleroderma and calcinosis cutis: Response to vitamin E. Cutis 11:54-62, 1973*).

- -

OTHER NUTRITIONAL FACTORS

Omega-6 Fatty acids:

Supplementation may be beneficial.

        Experimental Study: 4 female pts. with systemic sclerosis for 5-13 yrs. duration received evening primrose oil (rich in gamma-linolenic acid) 1 gm 3 times daily. After 1 yr. clinical benefits included relief of pain in the extremities, improvement of telangiectasia and skin texture, and healing of ulcers. It is suggested that 6 gms daily may be of greater benefit (*Strong AMM et al. The effect of oral linoleic acid and gamma-linolenic acid (Efamol). Br J Clin Pract Nov/Dec 1985, p. 444*).

Para-amino benzoic acid: 12 gm daily of the potassium salt (Potaba, Glenwood)

        WARNING: Potential side-effects include skin rash, anorexia, nausea and fever (*Physicians' Desk Reference. Oradell, NJ, Med. Economics Co., Inc., 1989*) as well as vitiligo (*Hughes CG. Oral PABA and vitiligo. J Am Acad Dermatol 9:770, 1983*) and, rarely, liver toxicity (*Kantor GR, Ratz JL. Liver toxicity from potassium para-aminobenzoate. Letter. J Am Acad Dermatol 13(4):671-72, 1985; Zarafonetis CJD et al. Potassium para-amino-benzoate and liver function test findings. J Am Acad Dermatol 15(1):144-49, 1986*).

Supplementation may result in softening of the skin.

        Experimental Study: In a retrospective study, analyses were made of records of 390 pts. with clinical features of scleroderma without manifestations of other collagen disease. 90% of 224 pts. treated with Potaba experienced mild, moderate, or marked skin softening while, among a parallel gp. of 96 pts. who did not receive Potaba, <20% were noted to have mild or moderate skin improvement at the end of follow-up, a highly significant difference were noted to have mild or moderate skin improvement at the end of follow-up, a highly significant difference (p<0.0001) (*Zarafonetis CJD et al. Retrospective studies in scleroderma: Skin response to potassium para-aminobenzoate therapy.* Clin Exp Rheumatol *6:261-68, 1988*).

Experimental Double-blind Study: 12 pts. with diffuse skin involvement were treated with potassium para-aminobenzoate or placebo which contained the same amt. of potassium ion. After 6 mo., the 7 pts. in the experimental gp. demonstrated a significant increase in skin mobility (p<0.001) compared to pre-treatment values, while those receiving placebo were unchanged (*Bushnell WJ et al. The treatment of progressive systemic sclerosis: A comparison of para-aminobenzoate and placebo in a double-blind study. Abstract.* Arthritis Rheum *9:495, 1966*).

Experimental Study: Of 135 pts. with diffuse systemic sclerosis treated with potassium para-aminobenzoate (Potaba, Glenwood), every pt. except one demonstrated softening of the involved skin if treatment was continued for at least 3 months. The single exception was a pt. with an almost incredible total body rock-like sclerosis. Some pts. reached essentially complete clinical remission and treatment was discontinued. In addition, 17 pts. with morphea or linear scleroderma were treated as the lesions were so localized that further disfigurement or functional impairment may have resulted from pressure atrophy secondary to the sclerotic process. All of the pts. showed softening of the sclerotic component (*Zarafonetis CJD. Antifibrotic therapy with Potaba.* Am J Med Sci *November, 1964, pp. 550-61*).

Case Reports:
1. A 45 year-old female with a 10 yr. history of progressive disease despite a thoracic sympathectomy and most of the accepted therapies. After starting supplementation with potassium para-aminobenzoate (Potaba, Glenwood) 20 gm daily she noted a softening of the skin and a wider range of joint motion. This was the first improvement since the disease began. Dosage was reduced to 10 gm daily and continued indefinitely.
2. A 53 year-old female with a 6-mo. history of progressive disease. Steroids and physiotherapy were of no benefit, but she improved over 2 yrs. once started on potassium para-aminobenzoate (Potaba, Glenwood) 12 gm daily (*Grace WJ et al. Therapy of scleroderma and dermatomyositis.* N Y State J Med *63(1):140-44, 1963*).

Experimental Study: In a retrospective report of 104 consecutive, unselected cases, 97 showed moderate to considerable improvement of the involved skin. 5/7 pts. who failed to show significant improvement had received the drug for less than 3 months (*Zarafonetis CJD. The treatment of scleroderma: Results of potassium para-aminobenzoate therapy in 104 cases, in LC Mills & JH Moyer, Eds.* Inflammation and Diseases of Connective Tissue. *Philadelphia, W.B. Saunders Co., 1961:688-696*).

Supplementation may increase lifespan.

Experimental Study: In a retrospective study, 219 pts. were treated with potassium para-aminobenzoate (Potaba, Glenwood), usually 10-12.5 gm/day until maximal skin softening had occurred. Mean duration of treatment was 4.2 yrs., with a range of 3 mo. to 20 years. Compared to non-supplemented pts., pts. who received Potaba survived significantly longer, with a 88.5% 5 yr. survival and a 76.6% 10 yr. survival (*Zarafonetis CJD et al. Retrospective studies in scleroderma: Effect of potassium para-aminobenzoate on survival.* J Clin Epidemiol *41:193-204, 1988*).

SEBORRHEIC DERMATITIS

VITAMINS

<u>Folic Acid</u>:   2 mg. daily

Supplementation may be beneficial (<u>not</u> for seborrhea sicca).

> **Experimental Study:** Following folic acid supplementation (2.5 mg daily for infants, 5 mg daily for children, and 10 mg daily for adults), 3/5 cases of SD of infancy were much improved, while 17/20 cases of SD in adults responded (9/20 cases much improved, 8/20 improved) (*Callaghan TJ. The effect of folic acid on seborrheic dermatitis. <u>Cutis</u> 3:583-588, 1967*).

<u>Vitamin B$_6$</u>: ointment (50 mg/g) in water-soluble base

> *Note: Initial worsening is considered a positive sign.*

Topical application may be beneficial in seborrhea sicca ("dandruff" - greasy adherent scales on an erythematous base).

> **Experimental Study:** When a pyridoxine deficiency was produced by the use of pyridoxine antagonists, a seborrhea-like lesion developed about the eyes, nasolabial fold and mouth, with extension to the eyebrows and skin behind the ears. Many of these cases responded well to the local application of pyridoxine in an ointment base, while little effect was noted when the vitamin was given orally or parenterally (*Schreiner AW et al. Seborrheic dermatitis: A local metabolic defect involving pyridoxine. <u>J Lab Clin Med</u> 40:121-30, 1952*).

<u>Vitamin B$_{12}$</u>:   Intramuscular injections

Supplementation may be beneficial.

> **Experimental Study:** 37 pts. were treated with vitamin B$_{12}$ IM 10-30 mcg every wk. to every 3 weeks. Improvement was usually seen after 2 or 3 injections. 16/37 (43.5%) were greatly improved or apparently cured, 16/37 (43.5%) were improved, and 3/37 (8%) were slightly improved (*Andrews GC et al. Seborrheic dermatitis: Supplemental treatment with vitamin B$_{12}$. <u>N Y State Med J</u> 50:1921-25, 1950*).

<u>Vitamin E</u>:

Supplementation may be beneficial.

> **Experimental Study:** Following 150 mg vitamin E IM 2-3 times weekly in addition to 100-150 mg 3 times daily after meals, 5/8 pts. with dry, scaly skin (ichthyosis or seborrhea sicca) had excellent results and 3 had good results (*Block MT. Vitamin E in the treatment of diseases of the skin. <u>Clin Med</u> January 1953, pp. 31-34*).

- -

MINERALS

<u>Lithium</u>:

Topical application of lithium succinate ointment may be beneficial.

> - with <u>Vitamin E</u> and <u>Zinc</u>:

> > **Experimental Double-blind Crossover Study:** 11 men and 8 women pts. aged 15-64 randomly received an ointment containing lithium succinate 8%, zinc sulfate 0.05%, and D,L-α tocopherol in a lanolin base, and an

ointment containing only the lanolin base, in either order for 4 wks. each, to apply twice daily. Two pts. withdrew: one found the active treatment effective and did not wish the other treatment; the other found both treatments irritating to the skin. Of the remaining 17 pts., 14 improved with lithium ointment, 2 had no response to either treatment, and 1 responded to placebo. All assessments showed a significant improvement in mean severity score after 4 wks. when lithium was compared to baseline and when it was compared to placebo. The response to treatment generally occurred within the first 2 wks. (*Boyle J et al. Use of topical lithium succinate for seborrhoeic dermatitis. Br Med J 292:28, 1986*).

Selenium:

Topical application of selenium oxide has had inconsistent results (*Brenner S, Horwitz C. Possible nutrient mediators in psoriasis and seborrheic dermatitis. II. Nutrient mediators. Wld Rev Nutr Diet 55:165-82, 1988*).

- -

OTHER NUTRITIONAL FACTORS

Biotin:

May be deficient in infants. If so, supplementation may be beneficial.

Experimental Study: As biotin was unavailable, infants with extensive seborrheic dermatitis unresponsive to local treatment were fed liver and egg yolk (which have large amts. of biotin) early in the first month or two of life, with good clinical improvement. Those infants with more widespread involvement improved more rapidly when B complex injections (1 cc either once or repeated in 1 wk.) were added (*Nisenson A. Treatment of seborrheic dermatitis with biotin and vitamin B complex. Letter. J Pediatr 81:630-31, 1972*).

- -

OTHER FACTORS

Rule out hydrochloric acid deficiency.

Experimental Study: Of 68 subacute or chronic pts. whose condition had resisted all forms of local treatment, 15 (22%) had no HCl and only 9 (13%) had normal HCl levels. The severity of the condition seemed to correlate with the extent of the HCl deficiency and also seemed to be associated with signs of vitamin B complex deficiency. Improvement of the HCl deficient pts. followed treatment with supplemental HCl and vitamin B complex (*Allison JR. The relation of hydrochloric acid and vitamin B complex deficiency in certain skin diseases. South Med J 38:235-241, 1945*).

SPORTS INJURIES

See Also: WOUND HEALING

VITAMINS

Vitamin C:

Supplementation has <u>not</u> been shown to be beneficial.

> **Experimental Study:** For 286 male soldiers, supplementation with vitamin C 1000 mg in divided doses failed to affect the rate, severity or duration of athletic injuries (*Gey GO, Cooper KH, Bottenberg RA. Effect of ascorbic acid on endurance performance and athletic injury. <u>JAMA</u> 211(1):105, 1970*).

OTHER NUTRITIONAL FACTORS

Bioflavonoids:

Supplementation with citrus bioflavonoids may reduce recovery time.

> **Experimental Placebo-controlled Study:** The effects of citrus bioflavonoids, ascorbic acid, citrus bioflavonoids and ascorbic acid together, and placebo were compared regarding recovery from athletic injuries. The injury recovery rate in the bioflavonoid gps. was twice as rapid as the ascorbic acid and placebo controls (*Cragin RB. The use of bioflavonoids in the prevention and treatment of athletic injuries. <u>Med Times</u> 90:529-30, 1962*).

> **Experimental Double-blind Study:** Starting 10 days prior to their initial practice, football players received either citrus bioflavonoids 600 mg 3 times daily for the first wk., then 200 mg 3 times daily, or placebo. While the incidence of injury was similar for both gps., loss of playing time averaged 0.67 days for the treated gp. compared to 2.2 days for the controls (*Miller MJ. Injuries to athletes. <u>Med Times</u> 88:313-14, 1960*).

Topical application of an escin gel may reduce recovery time (*Arslanagïc I, Brkïc N. [Personal experience in the treatment of acute sports injuries with Essaven Gel.] <u>Med Arh</u> 36(4):205-8, 1982; Crielaard JM, Franchimont P. [Value of using Reparil-gel in sports traumatology.] <u>Acta Belg Med Phys</u> 9(4):287-98, 1986; Imparato FM, Gigliofiorito S. [Traumatic contusions of athletes.] <u>Clin Ter</u> 120(2):119-24, 1987*).

> *Note: Escin is a mixture of saponins occurring in the seed of the horse chestnut tree.*

Coenzyme Q_{10}: (ubiquinone)

May protect against exercise-induced muscle injury.

> **Animal Experimental Study:** Both treated and control rats were exercised by 90 min. of downhill treadmill running. A portion of both gps. was sacrificed immediately after exercise and the others were sacrificed after 40 hours. Immediately after exercise, serum creatine kinase and lactate dehydrogenase activities were elevated in controls but not in treated rats. However, after 40 hrs., enzyme levels of the treated rats increased to similar levels as those of controls. Treatment resulted in increased muscle CoQ_{10} levels. Results suggest that treatment protected skeletal muscles against injury caused by the exercise, but not aginast damage related to inflammatory processes after exercise (*Shimomura Y et al. Protective effect of coenzyme Q_{10} on exercise-induced muscular injury. <u>Biochem Biophys Res Commun</u> 176:349-55, 1991*).

Glucosamine sulfate:

Supplementation may speed healing of chondropathia patellae and thus prevent arthroses.

Experimental Study: 51 young male athletes (mean age 19.3 yrs. ± 6.6) and 17 young female athletes (mean age 18.9 yrs. ± 5.9) with a chondropathy of the first to third degree (Bentley) received glucosamine sulfate 500 mg 3 times daily for 40 days followed by 250 mg 3 times daily for 90-100 days. 52/68 (76%) had complete involution of their symptoms (pain at rest, walking, standing, sitting and during movement; with palpation: rubbing noise, pain at displacement, pain at pressure, medial or lateral side pain, apical pressure pain) and, after 4-5 mo., athletic training could be resumed at the initial intensity. Follow-up 12 mo. later showed no signs of recrudescence of patellar chondropathy. In 14/68 (21%), who had primarily third degree chondropathy, complete pain resolution required supplementary electrotherapy which was only begun if there failed to be decisive improvement after 2 mo. of supplementation. On the basis of analysis of synovial fluid, 20 pts. with marked accumulation of fluid could be classified into 6 cases of a mere disturbance of cartilage cell metabolism (chondropathia patellae) and 14 cases of an inflammatory/infectious process with the participation of synovia, leading to secondary cartilage injury. In the first case, glucosamine sulfate was administered alone while, in the second case, supplementary therapeutic measures had to be applied (*Böhmer D et al. Treatment of chondropathia patellae in young athletes with glucosamine sulfate, in N Bachl, L Prokop, R Suchert, Eds. Current Topics in Sports Medicine. Proc World Congress of Sports Med, Vienna, 1982. Urban & Schwarzenberg, 1984*).

ULCERATIVE COLITIS

See also: CROHN'S DISEASE

DIETARY FACTORS

GENERAL:

Theoretical Discussion: The rarity of UC and other noninfective large bowel diseases in black populations of sub-Saharan Africa contrasts with their high prevalences in white populations. While the reasons are unknown, this population still consumes a largely traditional diet. Insufficient exposure to environmental changes linked with urbanization and genetic factors are other possible causes (*Segal I et al. The rarity of ulcerative colitis in South African blacks. Am J Gastroenterol 74(4):332-36, 1980*).

Avoid refined carbohydrates.

Theoretical Discussion: A diet high in refined carbohydrate is implicated in the etiology of ulcerative colitis and certain other diseases of the colon. It is suggested that spasm of the smooth muscle is the common pathogenetic mechanism, and the strength of the spasm producing increased pressure in the colonic lumen or wall and the length of time for which the colon has been affected are believed to determine the type of disease resulting. A diet high in refined carbohydrate allows the intense muscle spasm to occur because the physical buffering effect of fecal bulk is considerably reduced (*Grimes DS. Refined carbohydrate, smooth-muscle spasm and disease of the colon. Lancet 1:395-97, 1976*).

High fiber diet.

Observational Study: 64 pts. in remission were studied for at least 6 months. 16/64 (28%) had a relapse in a mean period of 9 mo. after entering the study. Only 3 factors were useful predictors of relapse: a fiber-poor diet, >10 previous relapses, and the presence of extra-intestinal manifestations (*Leo S et al. Ulcerative colitis in remission: is it possible to predict the risk of relapse? Digestion 44(4):217-21, 1989*).

Review Article: Recently some preliminary studies have shown the possible correlation of low dietary fiber intake with a greater incidence of ulcerative colitis, but these studies are too limited in number and scope to allow any conclusion to be reached at this time (*Spiller GA, Freeman HJ. Recent advances in dietary fiber and colorectal diseases. Am J Clin Nutr 34(6):1145-52, 1981*).

- -

VITAMINS

Folic Acid:

May be deficient due to inadequate diet, malabsorption, or chronic sulfasalazine-induced low-grade hemolysis (*Baum CL et al. Antifolate actions of sulfasalazine on intact lymphocytes. J Lab Clin Med 97(6):779-84, 1981; Elsborg L, Larsen L. Folate deficiency in chronic inflammatory bowel disease. Scand J Gastroenterol 14:1019-24, 1979*).

Supplementation may reduce diarrhea (*Carruthers LB. Chronic diarrhea treated with folic acid. Lancet 1:849, 1946*).

Pantothenic Acid:

May fail to be converted into Coenzyme A in the colonic mucosa.

Observational Study: Colonic tissues of 29 pts. with chronic ulcerative and granulomatous colitis were assayed for pantothenic acid and coenzyme A activity and compared to normal colonic tissues from 31 controls. Compared to normal gut mucosa, CoA activity was markedly low in mucosa from pts. despite the presence of normal amts. of free and bound pantothenic acid, suggesting that there is a block in the conversion of bound pantothenic acid to CoA in diseased mucosa (*Ellestad-Sayed JJ et al. Pantothenic acid, coenzyme A, and human chronic ulcerative and granulomatous colitis. Am J Clin Nutr 29:1333-38, 1976*).

Vitamin A:

Absorption may be impaired (*Page RC, Bercovitz Z. The absorption of vitamin A in chronic ulcerative colitis. Am J Dig Dis 10:174-77, 1943*).

Vitamin D:

May be deficient (*Dibble JB et al. A survey of vitamin D deficiency in gastrointestinal and liver disorders. Quart J Med 53:119-34, 1984*).

Vitamin E:

Supplementation may be beneficial.

Negative Experimental Study: 8 pts. with active UC confined to the rectum and off of all drug treatment received alpha-tocopherol 1920 IU daily. Luminal concentrations of pro-inflammatory prostaglandin E_2 and leukotriene B_4 were significantly raised compared to normal controls prior to supplementation. Although, following supplementation, serum tocopherol showed a 3-fold increase, supplements caused no change in these levels either at day 4 or 15. In addition, disease activity was unaffected (*Lauritsen K et al. Does vitamin E supplementation modulate in vivo arachidonate metabolism in human inflammation? Pharmacol Toxicol 61(4):246-49, 1987*).

Experimental Study: 3 pts. with nonspecific UC failed to respond to a 12-wk. combined treatment program consisting of a low-carbohydrate, moderately high-protein and fat diet, removal of foods to which they may have been sensitive, nutritional supplementation, stress reduction and spinal manipulation. All therapeutic measures except for the low-carbohydrate, moderately high-protein and fat diet, wheat germ 4-6 tbsp/d and yeast 1 tbsp/d were discontinued, and alpha tocopherol pearls 40 IU/kg/d were added to the treatment program. Within 2 wks., all 3 pts. experienced a rapid decrease in amt. of blood lost per bowel action, and 2/3 pts. reported a substantial and rapid decrease in the amt. of mucous present with each evacuation. Tormina and tenesmus eased greatly and were almost gone within 4 weeks. All reported a marked lessening in the number of daily bowel movements and well-formed stools. Proctosigmoid examinations revealed less weeping of blood and less swelling in the rectal and sigmoid mucosa with a decrease in both the area and amt. of capillary seepage. After 8 wks., 2/3 pts. had no rectal capillary oozing, excessive mucous production, or inflammation. One pt. showed a small amt. of capillary bleeding but the area of hemotumescent rectal mucous membrane showed continued shrinkage. By the 12th wk., all pts. showed total healing of the rectal and sigmoid mucosa with no evidence of capillary bleeding or inflammation, and bowel actions had returned to normal (*Hood RP. Nonspecific ulcerative colitis: Successful treatment with D-alpha tocopherol. Digest of Chiropractic Economics Sept.-Oct., 1984*).

- as alpha-tocopherylquinone (with a low fat diet):

Case Report: The author had a 5-yr. history of severe, continuously active UC which had failed to respond adequately to medical treatment. Prednisone was beneficial, but symptoms became severe whenever its dosage was reduced below 30 mg/d. A very low fat diet (3% fat by weight) supplemented with vitamin E 3000 IU and ferrous gluconate 1.95 g along with sulphasalazine 1.5 g and intermittent naproxen 750 mg/d was found to reduce the symptoms sufficiently for corticosteroids to be discontinued, but symptoms of bloody diarrhea, arthritis, abdominal cramps and skin lesions remained. Colonoscopy revealed severe inflammation in the sigmoid and descending colon. As vitamin E alone or ferrous gluconate alone had no beneficial effect, the active substance was postulated to be a product of *in vivo* interaction of vitamin E and iron, most likely α-tocopherylquinone (α-TQ). Administration of α-TQ was started and the dosage was gradually increased to 50 mg/kg/d or greater. There was dramatic improvement until the only symptom was a mild facial rash. Colonoscopy revealed mild inflammation in the sigmoid and descending colon. Several times, α-TQ was discontinued for 1-2 days, and each time a recurrence of inflammation was noted until the current dosage of α-TQ was restored. There were no adverse side effects (*Bennet JD. Use of a-tocopherylquinone in the treatment of ulcerative colitis.* Gut *27:695-97, 1986*).

Vitamin K:

May be deficient (*Krasinski SD et al. The prevalence of vitamin K deficiency in chronic gastrointestinal disorders.* Am J Clin Nutr *41(3):639-43, 1985*).

If deficient, supplementation may normalize prothrombin levels.

Experimental Study: Abnormal prothrombin levels returned toward normal in vitamin K-deficient pts. treated with vitamin K (*Krasinski SD et al. The prevalence of vitamin K deficiency in chronic gastrointestinal disorders.* Am J Clin Nutr *41(3):639-43, 1985*).

- -

MINERALS

Calcium:

May be deficient due to loss of absorptive surfaces, steatorrhea, corticosteroid treatment, and vitamin D deficiency (*Rosenberg IH et al. Nutritional aspects of inflammatory bowel disease.* Annu Rev Nutr *5:463-84, 1985*).

Iron:

May be deficient due to chronic blood loss through the gut (*Rosenberg IH et al. Nutritional aspects of inflammatory bowel disease.* Annu Rev Nutr *5:463-84, 1985*).

Magnesium:

While serum levels are rarely decreased, intracellular magnesium levels are frequently low and may be associated with weakness, anorexia, hypotension, confusion, hyperirritability, tetany, convulsions, and EKG or EEG abnormalities (*Rosenberg IH et al. Nutritional aspects of inflammatory bowel disease.* Annu Rev Nutr *5:463-84, 1985*).

Review Article: Magnesium deficiency is a frequent complication of inflammatory bowel disease which occurs in 13-88% of pts. due primarily to decreased intake, malabsorption and increased intestinal losses. Parenteral magnesium requirements are at least 120 mg daily, and oral requirements may be as great as 700 mg daily (*Galland L. Magnesium and inflammatory bowel disease.* Magnesium *7(2):78-83, 1988*).

Zinc:

May be deficient.

Review Article: The prevalence of zinc deficiency ranges from 35-45% in stable outpatients with inflammatory bowel disease. Depressed serum zinc levels correlate with the degree of hypoalbuminemia and may be depressed in response to acute inflammation. Measurement of immune function, zinc-dependent proteins or enzymes and their response to a zinc supplement can help confirm zinc deficiency in borderline cases. Underlying mechanisms postulated as causing the deficiency include impaired intestinal absorption, increased endogenous losses, or low dietary intake due to anorexia (*Hendricks KM, Walker WA. Zinc deficiency in inflammatory bowel disease.* Nutr Rev *46(12):401-08, 1988*).

If deficient, supplementation may reverse the signs and symptoms of zinc deficiency.

Review Article: Case reports of severe zinc deficiency in inflammatory bowel disease have shown pts. to be rapidly responsive to oral supplements of 210-750 mg zinc sulfate per day. Little information exists, however, on which to make recommendations for mild to moderate zinc deficiency (*Hendricks KM, Walker WA. Zinc deficiency in inflammatory bowel disease.* Nutr Rev *46(12):401-08, 1988*).

Negative Experimental Double-blind Study: 51 pts. randomly received either zinc sulfate 220 mg 3 times daily or placebo. After 4 wks., improvement tended to be slightly greater in those receiving zinc than those given placebo; however, the differences were not significant (*Dronfield MW et al. Zinc in ulcerative colitis: A therapeutic trial and report on plasma levels. Gut 18(1):33-36, 1977*).

- -

OTHER NUTRITIONAL FACTORS

Fatty Acids:

Omega-3 Fatty Acids:

Cold-water fish are a rich source.

Administration of fish oils may be beneficial.

Experimental Study: 10 pts. with mild to moderate UC who had either failed (n=9) or refused (n=1) conventional therapy received 15 Max-EPA (fish oil) capsules containing a total of 2.7 g of EPA in 3 divided doses daily.   After 8 wks., 7/10 pts. had moderate to marked improvement; steroid dose could be reduced in 4/5 pts. on prednisone.   3/10 pts. had little or no improvement.   All pts. tolerated the fish oil and showed no alteration in routine blood studies (*Salomon P et al. Treatment of ulcerative colitis with fish oil in n-3-omega fatty acid: an open trial. J Clin Gastroenterol 12(2):157-61, 1990*).

Experimental Double-blind Crossover Study: 39 pts. with chronic inflammatory bowel disease randomly received either fish oil containing about 3.2 g n-3 fatty acids daily or placebo in either order for 7 months. At control, biopsies from inflamed mucosa contained higher levels of arachidonic acid than uninvolved mucosa.   Dietary n-3 fatty acids were incorporated into plasma and enteric mucosa phospholipids at the expense of n-6 fatty acids.   The arachidonic acid-derived prostanoid generation was reduced by fish oil and the extent and severity of macroscopic bowel involvement was moderately improved.   In pts. with ulcerative colitis, clinical disease activity fell during fish oil supplementation and thereafter; this was not significant, however (*Lorenz R et al. Supplementation with n-3 fatty acids from fish oil in chronic inflammatory bowel disease: a randomized, placebo-controlled, double-blind cross-over trial. J Intern Med Suppl 225(731):225-32, 1989*).

Short-chain Fatty Acids:

May be reduced.

Observational Study: Decreases in short-chain fatty acids, especially n-butyrate, were observed in 24-hr. fecal collections from pts. with severe UC (*Vernia P et al. Organic anions and the diarrhea of inflammatory bowel disease. Dig Dis Sci 33:1353-58, 1988*).

Local irrigation may be beneficial.

Experimental Placebo-controlled Study: 21 pts. with left-side UC treated themselves with a twice-daily enema of acetate, proprionate, and butyrate in a 100-ml saline solution, while a control gp. of 20 similar pts. used enemas with saline alone.   After 6 wks., 10/17 evaluable pts. in the treatment gp. had improved compared to 6/20 controls.   5 pts. in the treatment gp. had disease activity index scores that dropped below 4.0, the minimum score needed to enter the study, compared to none of the controls.   2 pts. in the treatment gp. experienced complete remission.   Some pts. in the treatment gp. had a worsening of the disease after treatment, but others have been followed for up to a yr. without relapse (*Richard Breuer, associate professor of medicine, Northwestern U., Chicago. Presentation at a Boston meeting of the Am. College of Gastroenterology - reported in Med World News December, 1991*).

Local irrigation may cure diversion colitis (which is microscopically indistinguishable from ulcerative colitis).

Experimental Study: After 4-6 wks., irrigation of excluded segments of the rectosigmoid exhibiting diversion colitis with sodium n-butyrate, sodium acetate and sodium propionate resulted in disappearance of symptoms and inflammatory changes, suggesting that the inflammation may have resulted from a nutritional deficiency (*Harig JM et al. Treatment of diversion colitis with short-chain-fatty acid irrigation. N Engl J Med 320:23-28, 1989*).

- <u>Butyric Acid</u>:

A short-chain fatty acid produced by the anaerobic bacteria of the colon through the degradation of fibers (cellulose and hemicellulose) and starch, butyric acid accounts for the major part of the energy needs of colonic epithelial cells and is a stimulus for their growth (*Roediger WE. Role of anaerobic bacteria in the metabolic welfare of the colonic mucosa in man. Gut 21:793-98, 1980*).

A cellular energy deficiency develops in the diseased colon in pts. with active disease due to decreased utilization of n-butyrate by colonocytes (*Roediger WE. The colonic epithelium in ulcerative colitis: An energy-deficiency disease? Lancet 2:712-15, 1980*).

Glycosaminoglycans:

Part of the ground substance of connective tissue.

Consist of long, unbranched chains made up of disaccharide repeating units, usually in combination with protein. Except for hyaluronic acid, they contain sulfate groups.

Their therapeutic effect is thought to be due to the anti-inflammatory effects of the chrondroitin sulfates, of which condroitin-4-sulfate is thought to be the most important.

Supplementation may be beneficial.

Experimental Study: 6 pts received sub-cut. injections of an activated acid-pepsin-digested calf tracheal cartilage preparation ("Catrix-S"). 5/6 had responded poorly to traditional treatments. 3/6 had an excellent response: 2 went into total remission but later had recurrences, while 1 showed progressive improvement. 2/6 had a good response: 1 who had been sensitive to sulfasalazine and developed massive edema on prednisone, and 1 who was spared a total colectomy but continued to have 6 movements daily. 1/6 had a fair response which was improved with the addition of prednisone. In an earlier series, oral Catrix powder capsules (3 gm 4 times daily) markedly improved sigmoidoscopic appearance but was unsatisfactory because the long-chain glycosaminoglycan molecule produced an osmotic diarrhea (*Prudden JF, Balassa LL. The biological activity of bovine cartilage preparations. Semin Arthritis Rheum 3(4):287-321, 1974*).

– –

OTHER FACTORS

Rule out <u>food sensitivities</u>.

GENERAL

Review Article: "No simple relationship between eating particular foods and disease activity . . . has emerged. . . . Patients with inflammatory bowel disease have enhanced immune responses against food antigens, but also against other antigens in the gut, particularly bacteria and bacterial products. . . . Expression of these immune responses may contribute to inflammation, and dietary alterations can induce remission. It seems just as likely that changes in faecal consistency and bacterial content are responsible for improvement, as that the withdrawal of a specific food antigen is responsible. Finally, however, there are striking geographical variations. . . . Epidemiological studies have shown that increasing westernisation leads to a higher incidence. . . . These emerging trends, as people of different races take up similar life-styles, point convincingly to environmental causes. While 'food allergy' remains the language of the enthusiast, a 'major influence of the constituents of the diet' seems likely to be an aetiological factor of greater significance" (*Hodgson HJF. Inflammatory bowel disease and food intolerance. J R Coll Physicians London 20(1):45-48, 1986*).

Observational Study: Compared to 100 controls, total serum IgE was not significantly different for 50 pts. matched for sex and age. However, in regard to RAST results with 10 selected foods, the percentage of positive reactions to specific IgE was significantly higher in patients. Results suggest a greater absorption of antigens through the diseased wall (*Brignola C et al. Dietary allergy evaluated by PRIST and RAST in inflammatory bowel disease. Hepatogastroenterology 33(3):128-30, 1986*).

Observational Study: Pts. with inflammatory bowel disease had significantly elevated serum levels of both IgG and IgM but normal levels of IgA. Serum IgE concentration, as well as the prevalence of pts. with "high IgE" were significantly increased. Among pts. with inflammatory bowel disease, those with Crohn's disease or those in relapse had the highest IgE levels (*Levo Y et al. Serum IgE levels in patients with inflammatory bowel disease. Ann Allergy 56(1):85-87, 1986*).

Experimental and Observational Study: Based on a symptom survey listing atopic allergic symptoms, 42/59 (71%) pts. were judged to be possibly allergic. In addition, over 50 pts. treated with inhalent allergy hyposensitization and dietary changes consisting of rotation and diversification of allergic foods were considerably improved in both their respiratory and abdominal symptoms, suggesting an allergic diathesis (*Siegel J. Inflammatory bowel disease: Another possible facet of the allergic diathesis. Ann Allergy 47:92-94, 1981*).

DAIRY PRODUCTS

Observational Study: Lactose intolerance was found in 25-35% of pts. with inflammatory bowel disease compared to 5-10% of the normal population, suggesting that a low lactose diet may be beneficial (*Meryn S. [Role of nutrition in acute and long-term therapy of chronic inflammatory bowel diseases.] Wien Klin Wochenschr 98(22):774-79, 1986*).

Observational Study: IgG and IgM antibodies to cow's milk proteins were found to be increased in pts. (*Jewell DP, Truelove SC. Circulating antibodies to cow's milk in ulcerative colitis. Gut 13:796, 1972*).

Experimental Controlled Study: After 1 year, 10/13 pts. on a dairy-free diet had remained symptom-free compared to 5/13 pts. on a "dummy" control diet (*Wright R, Truelove SC. A controlled therapeutic trial of various diets in ulcerative colitis. Br Med J 2:138, 1965*).

Lactobacillus Acidophilus: (may require weeks to months for beneficial effects)

Administration may be beneficial.

Experimental Study: Successful implantation of LA was followed by symptom relief in mucous colitis, irritable colon, idiopathic ulcerative colitis, and various other disorders causing constipation (*Rettger LF et al. Lactobacillus Acidophilus. Its Therapeutic Application. New Haven, Yale U. Press, 1935*).

ULCERS
(DUODENAL AND GASTRIC)

See Also: HEARTBURN

DIETARY FACTORS

High fiber diet.

Negative Observational Study: 78 pts. were compared to age- and sex-matched community controls. Relative risks for duodenal ulcer tended to be reduced with low refined sugar intake and high vegetable fiber intake. The relationship with low refined sugar intake persisted after being controlled for smoking, social class and relative weight; however, the relationship with a high vegetable fiber intake was reduced. Results suggest that, while a lack of cereal or total fiber intake plays no part in duodenal ulcer development, a low refined sugar intake may be a protective factor (*Katschinski BD et al. Duodenal ulcer and refined carbohydrate intake: a case-control study assessing dietary fibre and refined sugar intake. Gut 31(9):993-6, 1990*).

Observational Study: Compared to 40 healthy controls, dietary fiber intake was significantly lower in 38 pts. with peptic ulcer disease and in 40 pts. with non-ulcer dyspepsia (*Kearney J et al. Dietary intakes and adipose tissue levels of linoleic acid in peptic ulcer disease. Br J Nutr 62:699-706, 1989*).

Negative Experimental Placebo-controlled Study: 83 pts. with recently healed ulcers diagnosed by endoscopy randomly received apple pectin USP powder 10 gm twice daily, rantidine 150 mg at night, or rantidine-matching placebo at night. After 6 mo., recurrences occurred in 23/27 (85%) pts. on pectin, 6/28 (21%) pts. taking rantidine, and 20/28 (71%) pts. taking placebo. The ave. amt. of pectin taken was 12.7 gm/day in pts. who relapsed and 12.4 gm/day in whose who did not (*Kang JY et al. Dietary supplementation with pectin in the maintenance treatment of duodenal ulcer: A controlled study. Scand J Gastroenterol 23(1):95-99, 1988*).

Negative Experimental Controlled Study: 80 pts. were treated with 1 low-dose anacid tablet 4 times daily. In addition, they were randomly divided to receive either a fiber-rich or a fiber-poor diet. After 4 wks., the ulcer had healed in 67.5% of the fiber-rich and 60% of the fiber-poor gp. (p<0.5). Ulcer symptoms did not differ significantly between gps. during the treatment period. Constipation was seen in 27.5% of the low-fiber gp. and 10% of the high-fiber gp. (p<0.05) (*Rydning A, Berstad A. Fiber diet and antacids in the short-term treatment of duodenal ulcer. Scand J Gastroenterol 20(9):1078-82, 1985*).

Experimental Controlled Study: 73 people with recently healed duodenal ulcers were asked to change diets. On a random basis, 38 were told to eat lots of whole grain bread, porridge made from wheat, barley or oats, and lots of vegetables, while 35 were told to avoid these foods. After 6 mo., 28/35 (80%) in the low fiber gp. had suffered a relapse documented by endoscopy compared to 17/38 (45%) in the high fiber gp. (p=0.01). 14/15 who ate the least amt. of fiber developed new ulcers (*Rydning A et al. Prophylactic effect of dietary fiber in duodenal ulcer disease. Lancet 2:736-39, 1982*).

Experimental Controlled Study: 21 chronic duodenal ulcer pts. in a rice-eating area were put on an unrefined wheat diet and 21 continued on their previous rice diet. After 5 yrs., only 14% of the first gp. had had relapses compared to 81% of the controls. A similar 5-yr. relapse rate (80%) was obtained in a gp. of 30 pts. from another area with a more varied rice diet. This difference may be due to the increased mastication required by the unrefined wheat diet, which is associated with an increase in saliva, lower stomach acidity and reduced bile output (*Malhotra SL. A comparison of unrefined wheat and rice diets in the management of duodenal ulcer. Postgrad Med J 54:6-9, 1978*).

Eat dinner early.

An early dinner is associated with reduced gastric acidity.

>   **Experimental Study:** 23 healthy volunteers ate standarized meals at 7 am and 12 noon. They ate dinner at either 6 or 9 pm in random order, and the time of going to bed was standardized. With early dinner, nocturnal pH was higher than with late dinner (p<0.001) (*Duroux P et al. Early dinner reduces nocturnal gastric acidity. Gut 30(8):1063-67, 1989*).

Bland diets and strict dietary programs have not been proven effective in controlled studies (*Welsh JD. Diet therapy of peptic ulcer disease. Gastroenterology 72:740-45, 1977*).

>   **Experimental Study:** The ingestion of highly spiced meals by normal individuals was not associated with endoscopically demonstrable gastroduodenal mucosal damage (*Graham DY et al. Spicy food and the stomach: Evaluation by videoendoscopy. JAMA 260(23):3473-75, 1988*).

>   **Experimental Study:** When half of 50 duodenal ulcer pts. were given red chili powder 1 gm with each meal for 4 wks., the rate of ulcer healing (80%) was identical in both groups (*Kumar N et al. Br Med J 288:1803-04, 1984*).

Avoid alcohol.

>   Stimulates gastric acid secretion (*Lenz HJ et al. Wine and five percent ethanol are potent stimulants of gastric acid secretion in humans. Gastroenterology 85(5):1082-87, 1983*).

>   While moderate alcohol consumption does not appear to affect the incidence of peptic ulcer, continuous alcohol abuse seems to increase the prevalence of duodenal ulcer (*Holstege A. [Effects of nicotine, alcohol and caffeine on the incidence, healing and recurrence rate of peptic ulcer.] Z Gastroenterol 25 Suppl 3:33-40, 1987*).

Avoid caffeine.

>   While most studies show that caffeine does not cause ulcers, it may exacerbate preexisting conditions and increase ulcer symptoms (*Turnberg LA. Coffee and the gastrointestinal tract. Editorial. Gastroenterology 75(3):529-30, 1978*).

>   Stimulates gastric acid secretion (*McArthur K et al. Relative stimulatory effects of commonly ingested beverages on gastric acid secretion in humans. Gastroenterology 83:199-203, 1982*).

Avoid tea.

May increase gastric acid secretion.

>   **Experimental Study:** 36 pts. with duodenal ulcer and 56 normal controls drank a 200 ml cup of tea which resulted in an acid secretory response which was almost equal to that after a maximal dose (0.04 mg/kg) of histamine. This effect was mainly due to its local chemical action upon the gastric mucosa (*Dubey P et al. Effect of tea on gastric acid secretion. Dig Dis Sci 29(3):202-06, 1984*).

Avoid decaffeinated coffee.

>   Stimulates gastric acid secretion (*Marotta RB, Floch MH. Diet and nutrition in ulcer disease. Med Clin North Am 75(4):967-9, 1991*).

Avoid milk.

>   Milk has only a transient neutralizing effect on gastric acidity followed by a rise in acid secretion (*Ippoliti AF et al. The effect of various forms of milk on gastric-acid secretion. Ann Intern Med 84:286-89, 1976*).

>   **Experimental Controlled Study:** 65 pts. with endoscopy-confirmed duodenal ulcers under treatment with cimetidine were randomly assigned to either a normal hospital diet or one consisting exclusively of milk. Both gps. were allowed to add sugar and fruit as desired. After 4 wks., endoscopic examination showed that the proportion

of healed ulcers was significantly higher in the normal diet gp. (78%) than in those given milk (53%) (*Kumar N et al. Effect of milk on patients with duodenal ulcers. Br Med J 293:666, 1986*).

Avoid sugar.

May increase the risk of duodenal ulcer.

> **Observational Study:** 78 pts. were compared to age- and sex-matched community controls. Relative risks for duodenal ulcer tended to be reduced with low refined sugar intake and high vegetable fiber intake. The relationship with low refined sugar intake persisted after being controlled for smoking, social class and relative weight; however, the relationship with a high vegetable fiber intake was reduced. Results suggest that, while a lack of cereal or total fiber intake plays no part in duodenal ulcer development, a low refined sugar intake may be a protective factor (*Katschinski BD et al. Duodenal ulcer and refined carbohydrate intake: a case-control study assessing dietary fibre and refined sugar intake. Gut 31(9):993-6, 1990*).

May increase ulcer symptoms by increasing gastric acidity.

> **Experimental Crossover Study:** 41 pts. followed a low-carbohydrate diet (60-70 gm/day) for 3 mo. followed by a high-carbohydrate diet (the standard "gastric diet") for 3 months. 28/41 felt better on the low-carbohydrate diet, 11 noted no difference and only 2/41 felt better on the high-carbohydrate diet. In order to ascertain whether the reduction in dietary starch or sugar (sucrose) was the cause of symptomatic improvement from the low-carbohydrate diet, the gastric juice of 7 healthy young volunteers was examined following 2 wks. on a high-sugar diet in which dietary starch was reduced by the same amt. that dietary sugar was increased. A test meal before breakfast revealed a 20% increase in peak gastric activity and a 250% increase in peak pepsin activity (*Yudkin J. Eating and ulcers. Letter. Br Med J February 16, 1980, pp. 483-84*).

-- --

VITAMINS

Vitamin A: Adults: 100,000 IU A twice daily
             Children: 50,000 IU A twice daily

> WARNING: May cause serious side effects at these dosages.

Supplementation may combat the development of duodenal ulcers due to excessive gastric acid secretion (*Mahmood T et al. Prevention of duodenal ulcer formation in the rat by dietary vitamin A supplementation. JPEN J Parenter Enteral Nutr 10(1):74-7, 1986*).

Supplementation may aid in the healing of peptic ulcers.

> **Experimental Controlled Study:** 16 pts. with chronic gastric ulcers were randomly given anacids only (gp. 1), 18 were given antacids plus vitamin A 3x50,000 IU orally (gp. 2), and 22 were given anacids, vitamin A and cyproheptadine 3x4 mg. orally daily (gp. 3). After 4 wks., ulcers had completely healed in 3/16 (18%) in gp. 1, 7/18 (38%) in gp. 2 and 8/22 (36%) in gp. 3. While ulcer sizes were comparable prior to treatment, after 4 wks. they were significantly larger in gp. 1 than either those of gp. 2 or those of gp. 3 (*Patty E et al. Controlled trial of vitamin A in gastric ulcer. Letter. Lancet 2:876, 1982*).

Supplementation may prevent the development of stress ulcers.

> **Experimental Controlled Study:** 52 pts. who had had severe physiologic stresses (burns, organ injuries or post-op. organ disturbances) were randomly divided into treatment and control groups. Treatment consisted of water soluble vitamin A 100,000 IU twice daily for adults and 1/2 the dose for children. Additional vitamin A was given if serum vitamin A did not promptly normalize. 63% of the controls but only 18% of the treatment group showed evidence of stress ulcer, a significant difference. Since, in burn pts., serum vitamin A often falls from initially normal levels and returns to normal after pts. receive a high protein diet, the authors speculate that lack of retinol binding protein is responsible for the drop in vitamin A levels (*Chernow MS et al. Stress ulcer: A preventable disease. J Trauma 12:831, 1972*).

<u>Vitamin B₆</u>:

May be deficient in patients with gastric ulcers.

    Observational Study: In a gp. of 50 pts. with endoscopically confirmed active peptic ulceration, fasting serum pyridoxal was below normal in 28/30 (93%) in the gastric ulcer gp. compared to only 1/14 (7%) of the duodenal ulcer group. There were no significant differences in age, sex, drug or alcohol intake or diet between the 2 gps. (*Sanderson CR, Davis RE. Serum pyridoxal in patients with active peptic ulceration. <u>Gut</u> 16(3):177-80, 1975*).

Pyridoxal deficiency in peptic gastric ulcers may be a non-specific concomitant of gastric pathology.

    Observational Study: 44/52 pts. with dyspepsia and gastric pathology (gastritis, gastric carcinoma or benign polyps) had a low fasting serum pyridoxal (*Sanderson CR, Davis RE. Serum pyridoxal in patients with gastric pathology. <u>Gut</u> 17(5):371-4, 1976*).

Supplementation may promote the healing of peptic ulcers (*Lemeshko FP, Grebenshchikova VG. [Experience with treatment of gastric ulcer and duodenal ulcer with pyridoxine.] <u>Sov Med</u> 29(2):31-3, 1966*).

Supplementation may protect against stress ulcers.

    Animal Experimental Study: The injection of pyridoxine prior to immobilization stress protected mice from the development of ulcers of the gastric mucosa (*Lindenbaum ES, Mueller JJ. Effects of pyridoxine on mice after immobilization stress. <u>Nutr Metab</u> 17:368-74, 1974*).

<u>Vitamin C</u>:   0.5 gm. potassium ascorbate before meals and at bedtime.
                For gastric distress: 1.5 gm. in 2 oz. water.

Dietary analysis in patients with chronic peptic ulcer has shown an inadequate vitamin C intake to be common (*Riggs HE et al. <u>JAMA</u> 124:639, 1944*).

Blood and urine levels may be inversely related to the risk of peptic ulceration and bleeding.

    Observational Study: The plasma content of reduced ascorbic acid, the leukocyte ascorbic acid and the urinary excretion of ascorbic acid were significantly subnormal in 25 peptic ulcer pts., while dehydroascorbic acid was significantly higher, than in 10 controls (*Dubey SS et al. Ascorbic acid, dehydroascorbic acid, glutathione and histamine in peptic ulcer. <u>Indian J Med Res</u> 76:859-62, 1982*).

    Observational Study: 60 hospitalized patients with GI hemorrhage (2 with peptic ulcer) were compared to pts. with uncomplicated peptic ulcer and healthy controls. Ascorbic acid levels were significantly lower in the bleeders than in the pts. with uncomplicated peptic ulcers whose levels were significantly lower than those of the healthy controls. Only 6 of the bleeders had clinical evidence of scurvy (*Russell RL et al. Ascorbic acid levels in leucocytes of patients with gastrointestinal hemorrhage. <u>Lancet</u> 2:603-6, 1968*).

    Observational Study: A study of plasma ascorbic acid in pts. with active peptic ulcer showed both a low initial level and a flat saturation curve following a loading test. Pts. with hemorrhage had the lowest initial level and the poorest response to vitamin C loading. The difference between these pts. and normal controls was significant. Dietary histories reflected the laboratory findings, with the highest vitamin C intakes in the pts. who had a history of ulcers but were now asymptomatic (*Crescenzo VM, Cayer D. Plasma vitamin C levels in patients with peptic ulcer. Response to oral load of ascorbic acid. <u>Gastroenterology</u> 8:755-61, 1947*

Gastric aspirate level may be inversely related to the risk of peptic ulceration.

    Observational Study: In a study of 73 pts. underoing endoscopy, pts. with normal findings had significantly higher intragastric concentrations of vitamin C than those with gastric ulcer (p<0.01) or duodenal ulcer (p<0.05) (*O'Connor JH et al. Vitamin C in the human stomach: relation to gastric pH, gastroduodenal disease, and possible sources. <u>Gut</u> 30(4):436-42, 1989*).

Deficiency may be associated with an increased risk of peptic ulceration.

Animal Experimental Study: Guinea pigs fed a diet deficient in vitamin C developed peptic ulcerations (*Smith DT, McConkey M. Peptic ulcers (gastric, pyloric and duodenal) occurence in guinea-pigs fed on a diet deficient in vitamin C. Arch Intern Med 51:413-26, 1933*).

Supplementation may improve healing.

Experimental Study: 48 pts. with duodenal ulcer, 30 pts. with gastric ulcer and 2 pts. with post-operative ulcer, all verified by x-ray, received vitamin C 2 gm along with atropine 0.5 mg IV over 3-4 min. 3 times weekly for a total of 20 injecions. 34/80 (42.5%) had a good result and 39/80 (48.5%) an incomplete result, suggesting that treatment with vitamin C is at least as effective as the classic intravenous therapies (*Debray C et al. [Treatment of gastro-duodenal ulcers with large doses of ascorbic acid.] Semaine Therapeutique (Paris) 44:393-8, 1968*).

- with ferrous sulfate:

Experimental Controlled Study: While, in gastric ulcer pts., the healing index of the gp. given ascorbic acid and ferrous sulfate was significantly higher than that of controls, in duodenal ulcer pts., no significant difference was observed (*Miwa M et al. The therapeutics of peptic ulcers: Clinical evaluation of C-Fe therapy. Tokai J Exp Clin Med 5(1):41-44, 1980*).

Vitamin E:

Peptic ulcer disease is associated with a vitamin E deficit and an enhancement of lipid peroxidation (*Dalidovich KK et al. [Lipid peroxidation and antioxidants in duodenal ulcer.] Klin Med (Mosk) 66(10):109-12, 1988; Litinskaia EV et al. [The vitamin E concentration and lipid peroxidation status of patients with peptic ulcer undergoing laser therapy.] Vrach Delo (8):70-2, 1989*).

Volunteers on a vitamin-E deficient diet develop gastric ulcers (*Horwitt MK. Fed Proc 18:530, 1959; Horwitt MK. Fed Proc 17:245, 1958*).

Supplementation may protect against gastric ulceration.

Animal Experimental Study: Gastric mucosal injury induced by ischemia-reperfusion was more severe than that in vitamin E-nondeficient rats (*Yoshikawa T et al. Vitamin E ion gastric mucosal injury induced by ischemia-reperfusion. Am J Clin Nutr 53:210S-4S, 1991*).

Experimental Study: Laser therapy of peptic ulcer disease was found to be more effective when pts. were given alpha-tocopherol and cholinolytic agents (*Litinskaia EV et al. [The vitamin E concentration and lipid peroxidation status of patients with peptic ulcer undergoing laser therapy.] Vrach Delo (8):70-2, 1989*).

Animal Experimental Study: The effect of vitamin E on damage to the stomach lining produced by various ulcer-inducing agents (indomethacin, reserpine, hydrochloric acid, sodium chloride, alcohol and hypothermic re-straint) was studied. Pretreatment with vitamin E significantly decreased induced ulcer formation in the stomach (*Tariq M. Gastric anti-ulcer and cytoprotective effect of vitamin E in rats. Chem Pathol Pharmacol 60:87-96, 1988*).

Supplementation may aid in the healing of peptic ulcer (*Arutiniunian VM et al. [Use of alpha-tocopherol acetate (vitamin E) and sodium nucleinate in the treatment of patients with stomach and duodenal ulcer.] Klin Med (Mosk) 61(4):52-4, 1983; Toteva ET et al. [Use of alpha-tocopherol in the complex treatment of patients with peptic ulcer.] Vrach Delo (2):79-81, 1988*).

‒ ‒

MINERALS

Aluminum:

Aluminum salts may enhance the healing of chronic gastroduodenal ulcers.

WARNING: Aluminum is suspected of promoting the development of Alzheimer's dementia.

WARNING: While aluminum hydroxide is believed to be non-absorbable, it interferes with phosphorus absorption raising the possibility of osteomalacia and other adverse effects with chronic use (*Lotz M, Zisman E, Bartter FC. Evidence for a phosphorus-depletion syndrome in man. N Engl J Med 278(8):409-15, 1968*).

Experimental Double-blind Study: 91 duodenal ulcer pts. randomly received either aluminum phosphate or rantidine. At 4 wks., endoscopy showed a 60% healing rate in the aluminum phosphate gp. vs. 55% in the rantidine gp (n.s.). Results suggest that aluminum phosphate is an effective, safe and inexpensive treatment (*Poynard T et al. Randomized double-blind clinical trial of aluminum phosphate versus rantidine in the acute treatment of duodenal ulcer. Digestion 47(2):105-10, 1990*).

Bismuth: 120 mg 4 times daily 20 minutes before meals and at bedtime for 6-8 weeks

Inhibits the growth of Campylobacter pylori both *in vitro* and *in vivo* (*McNulty CAM et al. Susceptibility of clinical isolates of Campylobacter pyloridis to 11 antimicrobial agents. Antimicrob Agents Chemother 28:837-38, 1985*).

Experimental Study: 64 pts. with endoscopically proven duodenal ulcer randomly received either tri-potassium di-citrato bismuthate (120 mg elemental bismuth 4 times daily) or cimetidine 400 mg twice daily. After 6 wks., although healing rates were similar, pts. treated given bismuth showed a decreased incidence of C. pylori from 94% to 52%, while those taking cimetidine showed no change (p<0.001) (*McKenna D et al. Campylobacter pyloridis and histological gastritis in duodenal ulcer: A controlled prospective randomized trial. Gastroenterology 92:1528, 1987*).

Administration may be beneficial.

Review Article: In peptic ulcer disease, bismuth sulfate is as effective as the H_2-receptor antagonists, costs considerably less, and offers a lower rate of relapse. It suppresses, but does not eliminate, Helicobacter pylori. In combination with conventional antibiotics, however, H. pylori is eliminated and symptoms are ameliorated for periods longer than 1 year. Neurological toxicity has been rare with bismuth subsalicylate and colloidal bismuth subcitrate. However, recent studies have demonstrated intestinal absorption of bismuth and sequestration in multiple tissue sites even over a 6-wk. period, suggesting that treatment periods with any bismuth-containing compound should last no longer than 6-8 wks. followed by 8-wk. bismuth-free intervals (*Gorbach SL. Bismuth therapy in gastrointestinal diseases. Gastroenterology 99(3):863-75, 1990*).

Calcium: calcium carbonate 1-4 g one and three hours after meals and at bedtime

Calcium carbonate is a potent and inexpensive anacid which is converted to calcium chloride in the stomach. Its ingestion is following by stimulation of gastric acid secretion due primarily to the direct action of calcium in stimulating parietal cell secretion and, to a lesser extent, to calcium-mediated stimulation of gastrin release. In addition, regular ingestion may occasionally cause the milk-alkali syndrome which can be associated with renal calcinosis and progressive renal insufficiency. For these reasons, it is not recommended for the treatment of duodenal ulcer (*McGuigan JE. Peptic ulcer and gastritis, in JD Wilson et al, Eds. Harrison's Principles of Internal Medicine, Twelfth Edition. New York, McGraw-Hill Book Company, 1991*).

Magnesium: Example: magnesium hydroxide 30-60 ml (100-140 meq of neutralizing activity) given 1 and 3 h after each meal and at bedtime for six weeks.

WARNING: While magnesium hydroxide is believed to be non-absorbable, it interferes with phosphorus absorption raising the possibility of osteomalacia and other adverse effects with chronic use (*Lotz M, Zisman E, Bartter FC. Evidence for a phosphorus-depletion syndrome in man. N Engl J Med 278(8):409-15, 1968*).

Magnesium hydroxide is a potent anacid which is effective in the treatment of duodenal ulcer. It neutralizes hydrochloric acid to produce magnesium chloride. From 5-10% of magnesium hydroxide is abosrbed from the small intestine. As magnesium hydroxide may produce loosening of the stools, it is often combined with aluminum hydroxide which is constipating. Magnesium trisilicate is a slow-acting weak anacid (*McGuigan JE. Peptic ulcer and gastritis, in JD Wilson et al, Eds. Harrison's Principles of Internal Medicine, Twelfh Edition. New York, McGraw-Hill Book Company, 1991*).

Zinc: zinc sulfate 220 mg. three times daily

May inhibit stress-induced release of vasoactive agents from gastric mast cells, thus preventing the subsequent micro-circulatory changes known to produce mucosal ulceration.

Animal Experimental Study: Pretreatment with zinc sulfate prevented gastric ulcer formation in a dose related manner in rats exposed to immobilization and cold stress. It also prevented the stress-related decline in stomach wall mast cell counts and the increase in microcirculatory blood volume (*Oner G et al. The role of zinc ion in the development of gastric ulcers in rats.* Eur J Pharmacol *70:241, 1981*).

Animal Experimental Study: Injection of zinc sulfate reduced the incidence of stress ulcers and enhanced gastric mucus content in rats subjected to pyloric occlusion and stress 48 h later (*Cho CH, Ogle CW. Does increased gastric mucus play a role in the ulcer-protecting effects of zinc sulphate?* Experientia *34:90, 1978*).

Supplementation may be beneficial.

Review Article: Zinc acexamate (ZAC) is the first zinc compound developed and marketed for use in the therapy of peptic ulcer. In experimental models, it reduces acid and peptic secretion, increases mucus secretion, protects mucosa from disruption by aspirin and reverses the reduction of blood flow caused by noradrenaline. Clinically, ZAC has proven to be a useful drug in the healing of peptic ulcer. Reduction of inflammatory associated processes of peptic ulcer, which has not been seen with H_2-blockers, suggests that ZAC may be highly effective in preventing ulcer relapse (*Banos JE, Bulbena O. Zinc compounds as therapeutic agents in peptic ulcer.* Methods Find Exp Clin Pharmacol *11 Suppl 1:117-22, 1989*).

Experimental Double-blind Study: 15 pts. with gastric ulcers and normal zinc levels were treated randomly with either zinc sulfate 220 mg 3 times daily or placebo. After 3 wks., the absolute reduction in size of the ulcer crater was 3 times as great in the treated group (statistically significant). Zinc reduced pain markedly within 4 days in some patients. There were no side effects (*Frommer DJ. The healing of gastric ulcers by zinc sulphate.* Med J Aust *2:793-6, 1975*).

— —

OTHER NUTRITIONAL FACTORS

Glutamine: 400 mg. four times daily 1 hour before meals and before retiring

Supplementation may be beneficial.

Experimental Double-blind Study: 57 pts. were given either glutamine 400 mg 4 times daily or lactose in addition to standard treatment (antacids, antispasmodics, milk and a bland diet). 22/24 pts. receiving glutamine showed complete healing on x-ray within 4 weeks (*Shive W et al. Glutamine in treatment of peptic ulcer.* Texas State J Med *53:840-3, 1957*).

S-methylmethionine ("Vitamin U"):

Found in trace amounts in certain raw foods, particularly green vegetables.

Administration may be beneficial.

Animal Experimental Study: S-methylmethionine was found to protect dogs against experimental ulcers (*Szabo S, Vargha G. Unhtersuchung de Wirkungswiese des sogenannten "Vitamin U" mit histochemischen Reaktionen.* Arzneimittelforsch *10:23-8, 1960*) (*in German*)

Experimental Placebo-controlled Study: Pts. were treated with conventional milk diet therapy. In addition, 26 pts. were treated with concentrated cabbage juice, while 19 controls received a facsimile which contained no cabbage juice. After 3 wks., x-rays showed healing in 24/26 (92%) of treated pts. compared to 6/19 (32%) of controls (*Cheney G. Calif Med January, 1956*).

Omega-3 Fatty Acids:

Supplementation with fish oil (a source of eicosapentaenoic acid) may reduce gastric erosions and ulcers caused by the ingestion of ethanol, aspirin, acid or alkali by "stealing" glutathione available for leukotriene synthesis (*Rogers C et al. Role for leukotrienes in the pathogenesis of hemorrhagic mucosal lesions induced by ethanol or HCl in the rat. Gastroenterology 90:1797, 1986; Szabo S, Rogers C. Diet, ulcer disease, and fish oil. Letter. Lancet 1:119, 1988*).

Omega-6 Fatty Acids:

Theoretical Discussion: The incidence and virulence of peptic ulcer disease have been declining for the past few decades. Evidence is accumulating that the elaboration of prostaglandins, mainly of the E gp., is a major factor in the intrinsic defense against ulceration by the gastroduodenal mucosa. As the dietary availability of linoleic acid has increased by 200% since 1909, it is suggested that this change in dietary habits could account for part of the concomitant decrease in peptic ulcer disease (*Hollander D, Tarnawski A. Dietary essential fatty acids and the decline in p.,tic ulcer disease - a hypothesis. Gut 27:239-42, 1986*).

Theoretical Discussion: In addition to serving as prostaglandin precursors, omega-6 essential fatty acids may themselves have the ability to enhance ulcer healing and possess cytoprotective properties (*Das UN et al. Essential fatty acids and peptic ulcer disease. Letter. Gut 28(7):914-16, 1987*).

Linoleic acid concentration in tissues may be reduced, and dietary linoleic acid may be inadequate.

Observational Study: Compared to 35 matched controls, the mean percentage of linoleic acid in adipose tissue taken from the anterior abdominal wall was significantly lower in men with chronic duodenal ulcers. The adipose fatty acid profile closely reflected dietary intake. Results suggest that the diets of pts. with duodenal ulcers are deficient in linoleic acid and that this may be of etiologic significance (*Grant HW et al. Duodenal ulcer is associated with low dietary linoleic acid intake. Gut 31(9):997-8, 1990*).

Observational Study: Compared to 40 healthy controls, adipose tissue linoleic acid levels were significantly lower in 38 pts. with peptic ulcer disease and in 40 pts. with non-ulcer dyspepsia. A dietary history revealed a lower intake of linoleic acid in both gps. of pts. as compared to controls (*Kearney J et al. Dietary intakes and adipose tissue levels of linoleic acid in peptic ulcer disease. Br J Nutr 62(3):699-706, 1989*).

Supplementation may be beneficial.

Theoretical Discussion: Various lines of evidence indicated that the prostaglandins may play a physiological role in protecting the gastric mucosa, suggesting that supplementation with essential fatty acids that are efficient prostaglandin precursors (such as evening primrose oil as a soure of GLA) may have value in the prevention and treatment of gastric ulceration and gastritis (*McCarty MF. Nutritional modulation of mineralocorticoid and prostaglandin production: potential role in prevention and treatment of gastric pathology. Med Hypotheses 11(4):381-9, 1983*).

- -

OTHER FACTORS

Rule out food sensitivities.

Experimental Study: In 50 duodenal ulcer pts. and 50 non-ulcer dyspepsia pts. suffering from low to moderate epigastric pain, the intolerance of 39 foods was increased as compared to 50 healthy controls. Food intolerance was not different between the 2 pt. groups. Intolerance was related in the majority of foods to aversion and pain or to an increased incidence of aversion alone. In duodenal ulcer, coffee and fruit juice were associated with an elevated incidence of pain (*Kaess H, Kellermann M, Castro A. Food intolerance in duodenal ulcer patients, non ulcer dyspeptic patients and healthy subjects. A prospective study. Klin Wochenschr 66(5):208-11, 1988*).

Experimental Double-blind Study: 30 pts. with a history of food allergy which was confirmed with double-blind challenges and 20 controls had food allergens applied via an endoscope to the gastric mucosa. In all 30 pts., macroscopic reactions (swelling, erosions, bleedings) were observed along with elevated lymphocyte counts, tissue histamine concentrations and mast cell counts. Skin and RAST tests were positive in only 46.7% and 50%, respectively, of the food-allergic patients (*Reimann HJ, Ewin J. Gastric mucosal reactions in patients with food allergy. Am J Gastroenterol 83(11):1212-19, 1988*).

Theoretical Discussion: It is argued that all chronic gastroduodenal peptic ulcers result from localized increase in mucosal susceptibility to acid attack at the interface between a segment of gastroduodenitis and gastric fundus or duodenal mucosa. Destructive or stimulatory immune reactions could affect the gastrin-secreting G cells and other paracrine cells causing tropic and inflammatory reactions predisposing to peptic ulceration (*Kirk RM. Could chronic peptic ulcers be localised areas of acid susceptibility generated by autoimmunity? Lancet 1:772-4, 1986,*).

Observational Study: 70% of 241 pts. aged 16-65 with peptic ulcer manifested allergic reactions. 25% of pts. had food allergies, while 30% had drug allergies. Food allergy was more frequent among young pts. (aged 16-25), while drug allergies were more typical for pts. aged 50-65 years. About 1/3 manifested reactions to 2 or more allergen gps. (food, drug and others). The prevalence of different types of allergy increased with age. Of 173 pts. examined, immunoglobulin E was elevated in the blood of 47% (*Budagovskaia VN, Voïtko NE. [Allergic reactions in patients with peptic ulcer; incidence of food and drug allergy.] Vopr Pitan (3):30-3, 1984*).

Observational Study: Biopsies obtained from the edges of gastric and duodenal peptic ulcers demonstrate a marked increase of immunoglobulin E containing cells at the lesion edges, suggesting that mucosal anaphylaxis may be the cause of the lesions (*Andre C et al. Evidence for anaphylactic reactions in peptic ulcer and varioliform gastritis. Ann Allergy 51:325-7, 1983*).

Observational Study: 25 out of 43 (58%) allergic children with symptoms suggestive of duodenal ulceration had x-ray evidence of peptic duodenal ulcers (*Rebhun J. Duodenal ulceration in allergic children. Ann Allergy 34:145-49, 1975*).

Observational Study: 98% of pts. with x-ray evidence of peptic ulcer had coexisting upper and lower respiratory tract allergic disease (*Siegel J. Gastrointestinal ulcer - Arthus reaction! Ann Allergy 32:127-30, 1974*).

Experimental Study: Food reactions diminished peristalsis causing delayed gastric emptying time and caused severe hyperemia and edema of the stomach, mainly in the lower one-third (*Pollard HM, Stuart GJ. Experimental reproduction of gastric allergy in human beings with controlled observations on the mucosa. J Allergy 13:467-73, 1942*).

ULCERS (SKIN)

See Also: **ATHEROSCLEROSIS**
PERIPHERAL VASCULAR DISEASE
WOUND HEALING

DIETARY FACTORS

Pressure sores are often associated with malnutrition.

Observational Study: All pts. in a nursing home who had pressure sores were also severely malnourished (*Pinchcofsky-Devin GD, Kaminski MV. J Am J Geriatr Soc 43:435, 1986*).

- -

VITAMINS

Folic Acid:

Supplementation may be beneficial for the treatment of ulcers secondary to peripheral arteriosclerosis.

Review Article: Blood levels of the toxic amino acid homocysteine may be elevated in certain forms of vascular disease. As folic acid can lower elevated homocysteine levels, supplementation may help to prevent the forms of vascular disease related to the atherogenic amino acids (*Nutr Rev 47(8):247-9, 1989*).

Experimental Study: 3 men and 7 women (ave. age 61) with ulcers due to moderate to advanced peripheral atherosclerosis received 5 mg folic acid orally 3 times daily and 20 mg IM twice weekly. In 6-8 wks., complete healing was achieved in the pts. with smaller ulcers (1-3 cm in diameter), while larger ulcers healed by 12 wks. except for 1 pt. whose ulcer was reduced to 1/2 its former size. The author suggests that healing was due to the vasodilating property of the vitamin (*Kopjas TL. Effect of folic acid on collateral circulation in diffuse chronic arteriosclerosis. J Am Geriatr Soc 14(11):1187-92, 1966*).

- with Vitamin C:

Case Reports: A 57 year-old diabetic male smoker on sulfonylurea exhibited a nonhealing foot ulcer of 1 year's duration which had failed to respond to all conventional treatments. Due to continuous pain, he was unable to walk 100 yds. and amputation had been suggested. He responded dramatically to folic acid 80 mg daily along with ascorbic acid. After 3 mo., he was able to walk again. After 5 mo, he was able to dance and play golf. 8 other pts. aged 50-89 yrs. have had similar results. The author believes that healing was because folic acid is an extremely potent xanthine oxidase inhibitor (*Oster KA. The absorption and inhibition of xanthine oxidase. Am Lab October, 1976, pp. 47-49*).

Vitamin A:

Topical application may reverse the inhibitory effect of corticosteroids on healing.

Case Report: 18-year-old female receiving a corticosteroid for a skin disease banged her leg and developed an ulceration in the wound which continued to enlarge despite normal medical treatment until vitamin A ointment was applied to the wound 3 times daily. Within 3 days, the wound began to heal. 28 days later, it had completely healed (*Hunt TK et al. Effect of vitamin A on reversing the inhibitory effect of cortisone on healing of open wounds in animals and man. Ann Surg 170(4):633-41, 1969*).

Vitamin C:

Leukocyte level may be reduced (*Burr RG, Rajan KT. Leucocyte ascorbic acid and pressure sores in paraplegia. Br J Nutr 28:275-81, 1972*).

Supplementation may be beneficial.

> **Experimental Double-blind Study:** 10/20 pts. with pressure sores received ascorbic acid 500 mg twice daily while controls received placebo. After 1 month ulcers had decreased in size by an average of 84% in the supplemented gp. compared to 43% in the control group, a significant difference (p<0.005) (*Taylor TV et al. Ascorbic acid supplementation in the treatment of pressure sores. Lancet 2:544-6, 1974*).

> **Experimental Study:** 7 pts. with decubitus ulcers were given 500 mg ascorbic acid twice daily. After 3 days, biopsies showed enhanced collagen formation (*Burr RG, Rajan KT. Leucocyte ascorbic acid and pressure sores in paraplegia. Br J Nutr 28:275-81, 1972*).

Vitamin E:

Supplementation may be beneficial.

> **Experimental Controlled Study:** 20 pts. with chronic venous stasis ulceration received debridement and split-thickness skin graft coverage and were divided into 2 equal groups. Gp. I received vitamin E 400 IU daily, while Gp. II did not. After 18 mo., results of skin grafts showed that 9/10 in the treated gp. were stable, with one having a small, shallow recurrence. In the unsupplemented gp., all skin grafts were unstable (*Ramasastry SS et al. Biochemical evidence of lipoperoxidation in venous stasis ulcer. Vitamin E: Biochemistry and Health Implications 570:506-8, 1989*).

> - with topical vitamin E ointment:

> > **Clinical Observation and Case Report:** Bedsores, diabetic ulcers and ulcerated surgical incisions responded. A pt. who had previously been treated in 5 different hospitals and clinics without success for extensive ulceration over his lower body was treated with vitamin E 800 IU twice daily and topical applications of vitamin E ointment. The wounds healed completely within 4 months (*Fisher D. The Summary vol. 26, December, 1974*).

MINERALS

Copper:

Serum level may be elevated (*Agren MS et al. Selenium, zinc, iron and copper levels in serum of patients with arterial and venous leg ulcers. Acta Derm Venereol (Stockh) 66(3):237-40, 1986*).

Selenium:

Serum level may be reduced (*Agren MS et al. Selenium, zinc, iron and copper levels in serum of patients with arterial and venous leg ulcers. Acta Derm Venereol (Stockh) 66(3):237-40, 1986*).

Zinc:

Serum level may be reduced (*Agren MS et al. Selenium, zinc, iron and copper levels in serum of patients with arterial and venous leg ulcers. Acta Derm Venereol (Stockh) 66(3):237-40, 1986*).

If deficient, supplementation may be beneficial.

> **Experimental Study:** 15% of 20 pts. with crural varicose ulcers (mean duration 11 yrs.) had low plasma zinc and 10% had low RBC zinc (results n.s.). It was found that plasma zinc levels were important in predicting the efficacy of administering zinc-containing preparations (*Gasior-Chrzan B, Milian A. [Zinc in crural varicose ulcers.] Prezegl Dermatol 76(2):152-5, 1989*) (in Polish).

Case Report: Zinc supplementation is only successful in the treatment of leg ulcers if there is a primary zinc deficiency. This principle is illustrated by the case of a female pt. who developed an epithelialization rate of 2.31 cm^2/day during zinc treatment (*Leyh F. [Zinc- - a new therapeutic principle in dermatology?]* _Z Hautkr_ *62(14):1064, 1069-72, 1075, 1987*) (*in German*).

Experimental Controlled Study: 7 pts. with low serum zinc and 7 with normal serum zinc randomly received oral zinc sulphate 200 mg 3 times daily with meals, while 7 pts. pts. with low serum zinc and 9 with normal serum zinc served as controls. Within 1 yr., the ulcers were healed in all but 2 of the pts. with low initial serum zinc levels who were unsupplemented. Slowest healing was in the low serum zinc gp. without supplementation, and fastest healing was in the gp. with normal zinc levels receiving zinc (*Haeger K, Lanner E. Oral zinc sulphate and ischemic leg ulcers.* _Vasa_ *3(1):77-81, 1974*).

Experimental Double-blind Study: Zinc supplements significantly accelerated the rate of healing of venous leg ulcers, but only in zinc-deficient pts. (*Hallböök T, Lanner E. Serum zinc and healing of venous leg ulcers.* _Lancet_ *2:780-2, 1972*).

Copper/Zinc ratio:

May be elevated.

Observational Study: In a gp. of geriatric pts. with and without leg ulcers, the serum copper/zinc ratio was significantly higher in the leg ulcer gp. compared to the controls, and the serum copper/zinc ratio was raised in pts. with poor ulcer healing (*Agren MS et al. Selenium, zinc, iron and copper levels in serum of patients with arterial and venous leg ulcers.* _Acta Derm Venereol (Stockh)_ *66(3):237-40, 1986*).

- -

COMBINED NUTRITIONAL TREATMENT

Sugar:
Essential Amino Acids, and
Vitamin C:

Topical application may be beneficial.

Experimental Study: 30 pts. with treatment-resistent bedsores resulting from diabetes, varicose veins or burns were treated with a solution of simple and complex sugars, essential amino acids and vitamin C daily following wound debridement. Response began in 24-73 hrs. with full healing of the smaller ulcers and successful skin grafting of the larger ones (*Silvetti AN et al. Accelerated wound healing and infection control through the topical application of nutrients.* _Fed Proc_ *40(3) Part II p. 922, abstract no. 3929, March 1, 1981*).

- -

OTHER NUTRITIONAL FACTORS

Hydroxyethylrutosides:

Administration may be beneficial.

Experimental Study: 107 pts. with acute venous leg ulcers received either compression alone or compression and O-(beta-hydroxyethyl)-rutosides. While both objective and subjective parameters were improved in both gps., there was a statistically significant superiority with the combination in the cure of the ulcers (*Stegmann W et al. [Efficacy of O-(beta-hydroxyethyl)-rutosides in the treatment of venous leg ulcers.]* _Phlebologie_ *40(1):149-56, 1987*) (*in French*).

Omega-6 Fatty Acids:

Supplementation may be beneficial.

Experimental Study: Oral supplementation with evening primrose oil (Efamol) healed and/or greatly reduced the size of lower leg ulcers which had been indolent or slowly extending for years (*Simpson LO et al. Large leg ulcers, Efamol and hyperbaric oxygen.* _N Z Med J_ *99:552, 1986*).

URTICARIA (CHRONIC)

including ANGIOEDEMA

See Also: ALLERGY

VITAMINS

Beta Carotene:

Supplementation may be beneficial in <u>solar</u> urticaria (*Pollitt N. Beta-carotene and the photodermatoses. Br J Dermatol 93:721, 1975*).

Niacin:

Inhibits mast cell degradation and histamine release (*Bekier E, Maslinski CZ. Antihistaminic action of nicotinamide. Agents Actions 4(3):196, 1974*).

Vitamin B_{12}:   Intramuscular injections

Supplementation may be beneficial.

> **Experimental Study:** Over 100 pts. were treated with vitamin B_{12} 1000 µg weekly with relief obtained in the majority (*Simon SW, Edmonds P. Cyanocobalamin (B_{12}): Comparison of aqueous and repository preparations in urticaria: Possible mode of action. J Am Geriatr Soc 12:79-85, 1964*).

> **Experimental Study:** 9/10 pts. were greatly improved following vitamin B_{12} 1000 µg IM weekly for 4 weeks (*Simon SW. Vitamin B_{12} therapy in allergy and chronic dermatoses. J Allergy 22:183-85, 1951*).

Vitamin C:

May be deficient. If so, supplementation may be beneficial.

> **Case Reports:** 7 cases of chronic urticaria are described which were associated with poor dietary habits and deficient levels of blood vitamin C. All responded when citrus fruits were added to the diet (*Rosenberg W. Vitamin C deficiency as a cause of urticaria. Arch Dermatol Syphilol 37:1010-14, 1938*).

- -

MINERALS

Magnesium:

Blood levels may be reduced.

> **Observational Study:** Magnesium levels were studied in 42 pts. during an acute urticarial reaction and during remission. At the start of the reaction, magnesium levels were below the normal limit with a mean of 0.5 mmol/L. This value increased towards the normal limit during remission (*Muresan D et al. Investigations of magnesium, histamine and immunoglobulins dynamics in acute urticaria. Arch Roum Pathol Exp Microbiol 49(1):31, 1990*).

OTHER FACTORS

Rule out food and chemical sensitivities.

Experimental Double-blind Study: 81/132 pts. with the urticaria-angioedema syndrome obtained good results from a food elimination diet (p<0.001). Double-blind challenge testing was positive in 42; 29 of these pts. (22%) had food allergy and 13 (10%) had food intolerance (*Lunardi C et al. [Prevalence of food allergy in patients with urticaria-angioedema syndrome.] G Ital Dermatol Venereol 125(7-8):319-22, 1990) (in Italian).*

Review Article: "In patients with chronic urticaria, adverse reactions to food additives are worth looking for. Improvement on a diet free from the additives and a positive double-blind provocation test is today the only way to prove the diagnosis. The mechanism for such adverse reactions is still obscure" (*Juhlin L. Additives and chronic urticaria. Ann Allergy 59(5 Pt 2):119-23, 1987*).

Case Report: A 47 year-old male presented with treatment-resistant generalized chronic urticaria associated with weight loss, general malaise and subfebrility. Small bowel biopsy revealed total villous atrophy and a diffuse mononuclear infiltrate consistent with celiac disease. Anti-gliadin antibodies were positive for both IgG and IgA but negative for gliadin-specific IgM. He was placed on a gluten-free diet with disappearance of the urticaria by 3 mo. along with a 15 lb weight gain. Repeat small bowel biopsy showed partial regeneration of the intestinal villi (*Hautekeete ML et al. Chronic urticaria associated with coeliac disease. Lancet 2:1157-58, 1986*).

Experimental Double-blind Study: 43 children suffering from urticaria and/or angio-edema who had responded to an additive-free diet received double-blind challenges of a variety of artificial food additives. 24 reacted to one or more of the additives, while 18 had no reaction and remained well on reintroduction of the normal diet. One of the 24 was found to be aspirin-sensitive. Also tested were tartrazine, sunset yellow, amaranth, indigo carmine, carmoisine, sodium benzoate, monosodium glutamate and sodium metabisulphite (*Supramaniam G, Warner JO. Artificial food additive intolerance in patients with angio-oedema and urticaria. Lancet 2:907-909, 1986*).

Experimental Double-blind Study: 86/140 children with recurrent urticaria displayed significant improvement on a salicylate-free diet, and nearly 3/4 reacted to double-blind salicylate challenge. Reactions to many other compounds such as preservatives, azo-dyes and brewer's yeast were also observed (*Swain A et al. Salicylates, oligoantigenic diets, and behavior. Lancet 2:41-2, 1985*).

Rule out hydrochloric acid deficiency.

Note: While gastric anacidity had been reported in the past to be a relatively common condition which was associated with a number of illnesses, the presence of achlorhydria is no longer accepted unless a potent parietal-cell stimulant (such as histamine) is employed in gastric analysis. More recent studies suggest that histamine-fast anacidity is uncommon before the fifth decade of life and, although it probably does not occur in a normal stomach, its presence is not necessarily associated with symptoms (Rappaport EM. Achlorhydria: Associated symptoms and response to hydrochloric acid. N Engl J Med 252(19):802-5, 1955).

Experimental Study: Of 77 pts., 24 (31%) had no hydrochloric acid and only 12 (16%) had normal hydrochloric acid levels. Pts. with urticaria due to food poisoning, drug reactions or infections were excluded. Signs of vitamin B complex deficiency seemed to be correlated with the extent of the hydrochloric acid deficiency. Treatment of the 84% of patients who presented with diminished hydrochloric acid levels with vitamin B complex and hydrochloric acid gave "remarkable" results (*Allison JR. The relation of hydrochloric acid and vitamin B complex deficiency in certain skin diseases. South Med J 38:235-241, 1945*).

VASCULITIS

See Also: AUTO-IMMUNE DISORDERS (GENERAL)
CAPILLARY FRAGILITY

VITAMINS

Vitamin E:

Supplementation may be beneficial.

Case Reports: "We have successfully treated five patients with vasculitis-type eruptions, including erythema nodosum, pityriasis lichenoides chronica, and purpura annularis telangiectodes, and one patient with capillaritis of two years' duration involving the right thigh, possibly of drug-induced origin. Three of the patients remained clear over a two-year observation period, except on several occasions when flares occurred after medication was discontinued. The flares subsided when vitamin E intake was resumed" (*Ayres S, Mihan R. Is vitamin E involved in the autoimmune mechanism? Cutis 21:321-5, 1978*).

- -

MINERALS

Magnesium:

Deficiency may be associated with lower limb arteritis (*Debrand J. Deficit magneseque et agregabilite plaquettaire. These de Medicine, Bescancon, 1974*).

Selenium:

Supplementation may be beneficial.

- with Vitamin E:

Experimental Study: 16 pts. with vasculitis were found to have depressed values of glutathione peroxidase compared to normal controls (p<0.01) and 2/16 were treated with tablets containing 0.2 mg selenium as Na_2SeO_3 along with 10 mg tocopheryl succinate. The glutathione peroxidase levels increased slowly within 6-8 wks. and the clinical effect was encouraging (*Juhlin L et al. Blood glutathione-peroxidase levels in skin diseases: Effect of selenium and vitamin E treatment. Acta Derm Venereol (Stockh) 62(3):211-14, 1982*).

- -

OTHER FACTORS

Rule out food sensitivities (hypersensitivity vasculitis).

Observational Study: "Because previous studies have shown that mast cells can be activated by IgE-mediated mechanisms to release potent mediators which affect coronary blood flow, we measured serum IgE levels in 156 patients with coronary arterial diseae and in 53 healthy controls (27 men, 26 women, mean 54 years). . . . In a model including the factors that may affect the serum levels of IgE (namely, age, sex, cigarette smoking, parasites, and family and personal history of allergy), IgE levels were found to be significantly higher in the patients with unstable angina and acute myocardial infarction compared to the patients with stable angina pectoris and controls. These data indicate that IgE may play a role in the pathogenesis of unstable angina pectoris and acute myocardial infarction" (*Korkmaz ME et al. Levels of IgE in the serum of patients with coronary artery disease. Int J Cardiol 31(2):199-204, 1991*).

Case Report: A 60-year-old man on verapamil and digoxin for 5 yrs. developed asymptomatic, nonpalpable, purpuric macules on his legs which spread to his back, buttocks, and arms. While a biopsy showed no signs of vasculitis, direct immunofluroescence disclosed deposits of IgA in the dermal vessels, suggesting an immune-complex vasculitis. While on a food elimination diet, he noted purpuric lesions only after drinking wine or eating foods dressed with vinegar. Oral provocation with 250 ml of wine resulted in purpura on his legs in 2 hrs., wheras provocation with sodium metabisulfite (a wine preservative) and tannic acid failed to provoke a reaction. Severe purpura also developed 3 hrs. after ingesting 250 ml of 10% ethanol. A skin-prick test with 10% ethanol was negative. Oral challenge with 1 ml of 5% acetic acid and a skin-prick test with 1% acetic acid also failed to provoke a reaction. Since the pt. stopped drinking alcoholic beverages and using salad dressings containing vinegar, he has had no further purpura (*Alibrandi B et al. Purpura due to ethanol. Letter. N Engl J Med 322:702, 1990*).

Experimental Study: 10 consecutive pts. with non-specific small vessel vasculitis (petechiae, spontaneous bruising, vascular spasm and recurrent edema) were hospitalized in a unit designed to minimize environmental triggering agents. All medications were stopped. After pts. had reached a basal state free of signs and symptoms of vasculitis, they were challenged with up to 4 less chemically contaminated source foods every 24 hours. All pts. were cleared of evidence of vasculitis in 3-7 days and had their vasculitis reproduced on at least 3 separate occasions, usually within 5 min. after ingestion (*Rea WJ. Environmentally triggered small vessel vasculitis. Ann Allergy 38:245-51, 1977*).

Experimental Study: Pts. are described for whom exposure to tree pollen, foods and chemicals triggered small vessel vasculitis (*Theorell H et al. Demonstration of reactivity to airborn and food antigens in cutaneous vasculitis by variation in fibrino peptide and others, blood coagulation, fibrinolysis, and complement parameters. Thromb Haemost 36:593, 1976*).

Case Report: A 58 year-old white female presented with a 9-year history of recurrent dragging of her right foot. Physical exam revealed extensive noninflammatory purpura, eczema, petechiae, and spontaneous bruising. Her symptoms subsided following a 5-day fast in an environmentally-controlled hospital unit. Challenge testing with several foods was followed by headache within 5 min. following by severe right-sided pain and spontaneous bruising, culminating in wide-spread noninflammatory purpura. Angiography revealed spasm of the peripheral arteries (*Rea WJ et al. Environmentally triggered large vessel vasculitis, in H Johnson & JT Spencer, Eds. Allergy: Immunology and Medical Treatment. Chicago, Symposia Specialists, 1975:185-98*).

·VITILIGO

MINERALS

Copper:

Necessary for the activation of tyrosinase. Decreased tyrosinase activity will impede the conversion of tyrosine to the melanins, resulting in albinism and vitiligo (*Chorazak T, Rzempoluch E. Etiopathogenesis of vitiligo in the light of our studies. Pol Med J 7(2):494-500, 1968; Genov D et al. Copper pathochemistry in vitiligo. Clin Chim Acta 37:207-11, 1972; Lal S et al. Serum caeruloplasmin in vitiligo. Indian J Med Sci 24(10):678-79, 1970; Sen S. Caeruloplasmin, copper and disease. J Indian Med Assoc 52(4):182-84, 1969*).

Supplementation may be beneficial (*Bagaeva MI. [Treatment of vitiligo in children with copper sulfate.] Vestn Dermatol Vernerol (3):48-50, 1979 (in Russian)*)

- -

OTHER NUTRITIONAL FACTORS

Para Amino Benzoic Acid (PABA):

WARNING: Vitiligo has been reported as being <u>caused</u> by PABA (*Hughes CG. Oral PABA and vitiligo. Letter. J Am Acad Dermatol 9(5):770, 1983*). Other potential side-effects include skin rash, anorexia, nausea and fever (*Physicians' Desk Reference. Oradell, N.J., Med. Economics Co., Inc., 1986*) as well as liver toxicity (*Kantor GR, Ratz JL. Liver toxicity from potassium para-aminobenzoate. Letter. J Am Acad Dermatol 13(4):671-72, 1985*).

Supplementation may be beneficial.

- with <u>Vitamin B Complex</u>:

Experimental Study: 48 pts. (25 females, 23 males) were studied over 10 months. Most had a history of inadequate diet and symptoms of fatigue, irritability, emotional instability, constipation, headaches and joint pains were common. Pts. received PABA 100 mg 3-4 times daily in addition to vitamin B complex. Later, due to the slowness of the effect, parenteral monoethanolamine PABA 100 mg was added twice daily in order to maintain adequate blood levels. Results were slow, but were striking by 6-7 mo. of treatment (*Sieve BF. Further investigations in the treatment of vitiligo. Virginia Med Monthly January 1945, pp. 6-17*).

L-Phenylalanine   50 mg/kg

Precursor to tyrosine.

- and <u>Ultraviolet-A radiation</u>:

Experimental Study: 21 pts. were treated with oral L-phenylalanine 100 mg/kg and with UVA exposure. In addition, 10 of these pts. also applied a cream containing 10% phenylalanine to the vitiliginous areas, and this gp. had the best results. Neither gp. had side effects (*Antoniou C et al. Vitiligo therapy with oral and topical phenylalanine with UVA exposure. Int J Dermatol 28(8):545-7, 1989*).

Experimental Study: 13 children were supplemented with L-phenylalanine and treated with ultaviolet light (UVA) radiation. 3 experienced repigmentation of all vitiliginous areas, 6 showed 50-90% improvement, and 4 failed to respond. None experienced side effects (*Schulpis CH et al. Phenylalanine plus ultraviolet light: preliminary report of a promising treatment for childhood vitiligo. Pediatr Dermatol 6(4):332-5, 1989*).

Experimental Study: 20 pts. were treated with L-phenylalanine 50 mg/kg and UVA radiation. 85% had a follicular and partially confluent repigmentation, which did not exceed 50% of the vitiliginous area (*Thiele B, Steigleder GK. [Repigmentation treatment of vitiligo with L-phenylalanine and UVA radiation.* Z Hautkr *62(7):519-23, 1987)* (*in German*).

Experimental Study: Pts. were treated thrice weekly with L-phenylalanine 50 mg/kg and exposed to sunlight as a source of UVA. 81% responded; 43% responded within 3 months. One pt. was over-irradiated. The repigmentation was predominantly of the follicular pattern (*Kuiters GR et al. Oral phenylalanine loading and sunlight as source of UVA irradiation in vitiligo on the Caribbean island of Curacao NA.* J Trop Med Hyg *89(3):149-55, 1986).*

Experimental Study: Pts. received phenylalanine 50 mg/kg along with exposure to UVA light 30-45 min. after ingestion (the time of peak blood concentrations). After 4 mo. (32 treatments), "reasonable" repigmentation occurred. Apart from the repigmentation of hypo-pigmented macules, pts. became able to tolerate more sun than usual, especially at the vitiliginous lesion (*Cormane RH et al. Phenylalanine and UVA light for the treatment of vitiligo.* Arch Dermatol Res *277(2):126-30, 1985).*

- -

OTHER FACTORS

Arsenic:

Chronic arsenicism may be associated with vitiligo (*Binkley LK, Papa CM. Chronic arsenicism with vitiligo, hyperthyroidism, and cancer.* N J Med *86(5):377-80, 1989).*

Nickel:

Chronic skin contact may be associated with vitiligo.

Case Reports: 2 pts. showed "vitiligo-like depigmentations" where their skin had been in close contact with a metal spectacle frame made of nickel alloy. Both had nickel hypersensitivity; however, they showed clinical and histologic findings indicating that the depigmentation did not result from postinflammatory hypopigmentation but from chemical hypomelanosis. The mechanism is unexplained (*Kim HI et al. Two cases of nickel dermatitis showing vitiligo-like depigmentations.* Yonsei Med J *32(1):79-81, 1991).*

Rule out hydrochloric acid deficiency.

Observational Study: Gastric acid secretion was assessed in 102 consecutive pts. by means of the augmented histamine test. 20/102 (19.6%) were achlorhydric, and 19 of the 20 were female. 8 of the 20 (all females) were found to have pernicious anemia (*Howitz J., Schwartz M. Vitiligo, achlorhydria, and pernicious anemia.* Lancet *1:1331-35, 1971).*

Experimental and Observational Study: Of 29 pts., 10 (35%) had no HCl and only 3 (10%) had normal HCl levels. The severity of the condition seemed to correlate with the extent of the HCl deficiency and also seemed to be associated with signs of vitamin B complex deficiency. Good results were obtained following HCl and vitamin B complex supplementation where a definite hypochlorhydria was found (*Allison JR. The relation of HCl and vitamin B complex deficiency in certain skin diseases.* South Med J *38:235-241, 1945).*

Experimental Study: 4 pts. with vitiligo and achlorhydria experienced disappearance of the vitiligo by 2 yrs. after starting hydrochloric acid 15 cc with each meal (*Francis HW. Achlorhydria as an etiological factor in vitiligo, with report of four cases.* Nebraska Med J *16:25-26, 1931).*

WOUND HEALING

See Also: SPORTS INJURIES
ULCERS (SKIN)

DIETARY FACTORS

GENERAL

Malnutrition is common in the frail elderly and constitutes a major impairment to wound healing (*Morley JE. Am J Med 81:670, 1986*).

Clinical observations suggest that nutritional support during illness may help to counteract, even if it does not abolish, the response to injury. Such support may provide substrate when reserves are depleted from antecedent malnutrition or when they are used up more rapidly by the response to injury (*Nutrition and the metabolic response to injury. Editorial. Lancet 1:995-97, 1989*).

Low fat diet.

> When over 30% fat was provided in a total parenteral formula, the postsurgical results were very unsatisfactory, perhaps because fat inhibits the movement of leukocytes which are essential for the prevention of sepsis and the stimulation of scar tissue formation (*RS Sparkman, Ed. The Healing of Surgical Wounds: State of the Art in the Ninth Decade of the 20th Century. American Cyanamid Co., 1985:75-80, 119*) (*transcript of panel discussion*).

- -

VITAMINS

Pantothenic Acid:

> Supplementation may accelerate the normal healing process.

> > **Animal Experimental Study:** In a controlled study, pantothenic acid (20 mg/kg/day) was injected into rabbits and wound healing was observed over a 1 month postoperative period. Chronic pre- and postoperative supplementation significantly increased aponeurosis strength after surgery, slightly, but not significantly, improved skin strength, and increased the fibroblast content of the scar (*Aprahamian M et al. Am J Clin Nutr 578-89, 1985*).

Thiamine:

> Deficiency may interfere with collagen synthesis.

> > **Animal Experimental Study:** Granulation tissue in wounds of thiamine-deficient rats was 1/5 the mass of controls and was greatly deficient in hydroxyproline, confirming that collagen biosynthesis was severely disrupted (*Alvarez OM, Gilbreath RL. Thiamin influence on collagen during the granulation of skin wounds. J Surg Res 32:24-31, 1982*).

Vitamin A:

> May ensure that scar tissue is strong and resistent to tearing.

Animal Experimental Study: Rats were fed a vitamin A deficient diet for 2 weeks then divided into 2 groups. One received only a "basal" diet while the other also received additional vitamin A as beta-carotene, retinoic acid or retinyl acetate. After 5 days, the supplemental retinyl acetate and beta-carotene "resulted in increases of 35% and 70%, respectively, over the wound tensile strength of rats fed the basal level of vitamin A" (*Gerber LE, Erdman JW Jr. Wound healing in rats fed small supplements of retinyl acetate, beta-carotene or retinoic acid. Fed Proc March 1, 1981, #3453, p. 838*).

Animal Experimental Study: The impairment of wound healing noted in streptozotocin diabetic rats was prevented by supplementation with vitamin A (*Seifter E et al. Impaired wound healing in streptozotocin diabetes. Prevention by supplemental vitamin A. Ann Surg 194(1):42-50, 1981*).

Animal Experimental Study: Scars of wounds of rats given vitamin A supplements had greater tensile strength and less risk of breakage than those of controls (*Seitfer E et al. Influence of vitamin A on wound healing in rats with femoral fracture. Ann Surg 181(6):836-41, 1975*).

Vitamin C: 500 mg. with meals and at bedtime

Promotes collagen and elastin formation (*Chatterjee IB. Ascorbic acid metabolism. World Rev Nutr Diet 30:69-87, 1978*).

In vitro Experimental Study: When vitamin C was added to cultured human skin fibroblasts, collagen synthesis increased by 8 times (*Murad S et al. Regulation of collagen synthesis by ascorbic acid. Proc Natl Acad Sci U S A, 78(5):2879-82, 1981*).

Wound healing may be impaired if vitamin C nutriture is reduced (*Ingalls TH, Warren HA. Asymptomatic scurvy. Its relation to wound healing and its incidence in patients with peptic ulcer. N Engl J Med 217:443-6, 1937; Schwartz PL. Ascorbic acid in wound healing - A review. J Am Diet Assoc 56:497-503, 1970*).

Supplementation may be beneficial.

Experimental Controlled Study: Before surgery, 82 pts. with complicated cholecystitis had reduced blood levels of ascorbic acid compared to established norms. Following surgery, 50 pts. received ascorbic acid 4 mg/kg (200-250 mg) in a 10% glucose solution IV while 32 pts. served as controls. In the experimental gp., blood ascorbate levels reached the normal range within 6-7 days after surgery; in the control gp., the ascorbate blood levels gradually rose, but failed to reach the normal range by the time they had recovered clinically from surgery. Pts. in the experimental gp. were discharged 1-2 days earlier than usual and were able to return to work more quickly (*Fishchenko Ala et al. [Vitamin C correction in patients with complicated cholecystitis.] Vrach Delo (11):21-23, 1988*) (*in Russian*).

Experimental Controlled Study: A plug of gingival tissue was removed from two subjects and permitted to heal. The procedure was then repeated while the subjects were receiving 250 mg. vitamin C at meals and at bedtime, and again with 500 mg. vitamin C. Compared to the control condition, wound healing was 40% faster at the lower dosage and 50% faster at the higher dosage (*Ringsdorf WM Jr, Cheraskin E. Vitamin C and human wound healing. Oral Surg 53(3):231-36, 1982*).

Experimental Double-blind Study: 20 patients with bedsores were randomly given either vitamin C 500 mg. twice daily or placebo. After one month, the bedsores of the treated group had decreased an average of 84% in size compared to only a 43% decrease in the placebo group (p<0.005). Six pressure sores were completely healed in the experimental gp. compared to 3 in the controls (*Taylor TV et al. Ascorbic acid supplementation in the treatment of pressure-sores. Lancet 2:544-46, 1974*).

- and Pantothenic Acid:

Supplementation may be beneficial.

In vitro Experimental Study: The effects of ascorbic and pantothenic acids upon the growth of fibroblasts obtained from fetal human skin or foreskin were studied. The rate of cell growth was unchanged when PA or AA were added to the culture medium. PA, but not AA, increased the basal incorporation of 14C proline into precipitated material. However, when cultures were incubated with PA and AA, the release of intracellular protein into the culture medium increased. These results suggest that the combined use of these 2 vitamins may be of interest in postsurgical therapy and in wound healing (*Lacroix B et al. Role of pantothenic and ascorbic acid in wound healing processes: In vitro study on fibroblasts. Int J Vitam Nutr Res 58(4):407-13, 1988*).

Vitamin E:

Supplementation may be beneficial.

Animal Experimental Study: 3 gps. of rats received a total of 30, 60 or 120 IU vitamin E injected into the abdominal cavity over 6 days, followed by local radiation and subsequent surgical incisions. Radiation exposure significantly reduced the ave. breaking strength of wounds. The breaking strength of wounds exposed to pre-operative radiation increased with increasing levels of vitamin E administration, suggesting that vitamin E may reduce the detrimental effects of radiation on the breaking strength of wounds (*Taren DL et al. Increasing the breaking strength of wounds exposed to pre-operative irradiation using vitamin E supplementation. Int J Vitam Nutr Res 57:133-37, 1987*).

Animal Experimental Study: Gingival wounds in rats healed faster in supplemented rats compared to controls (*Kim JE, Shklar G. The effect of vitamin E on the healing of gingival wounds in rats. J Periodontol 54:305, 1983*).

- with topical application of vitamin E ointment:

Clinical Observations: Bedsores, diabetic ulcers and ulcerated surgical incisions responded. A pt. who had previously been treated in 5 different hospitals and clinics without success for extensive ulceration over his lower body was treated with vitamin E 800 IU twice daily and topical applications of vitamin E ointment. The wounds healed completely within 4 months (*Fisher D. The Summary vol. 26, December, 1974.*)

Treatment with vitamin E may facilitate healing of skin grafts.

In vitro Animal Experimental Study: Skin tissue removed from rats was treated with vitamin E or served as controls. After 12 hrs., untreated grafts showed lipid peroxide levels >1340 nmol/g, while vitamin E-treated grafts showed only modest elevations of peroxides of 196 nmol/g. The elevation in free radicals was associated with decreased glutathione levels, which was not prevented by vitamin E supplementation. Results show that vitamin E helps prevent excessive free radical oxidation to damaged tissues, thus reducing secondary damage and improving the healing process (*Goldstein R et al. Effect of vitamin E and allopurinol on lipid peroxide and glutathione level in acute skin grafts. J Inves Dermatol 95:470, 1990*).

MINERALS

Copper:

Co-factor for the action of lysyl amine oxidase in the aldehyde reactions which generate strong covalent bonds in collagen (*Miller EJ. Chemistry, structure and function of collagen, in L Manaker, Ed. Biologic Basis of Wound Healing. New York, Harper and Row, 1975:164-9*).

Manganese:

Necessary for the glycosylation of hydroxyproline residues in the formation of collagen (*Miller EJ. Chemistry, structure and function of collagen, in L Manaker, Ed. Biologic Basis of Wound Healing. New York, Harper and Row, 1975:164-9*).

Zinc:

After surgery, accidental trauma, or thermal injury, serum zinc generally decreases, while urinary zinc excretion increases (*Boosalis MG et al. Serum zinc response to thermal injury. J Am Coll Nutr 7(1):69-76, 1988; Fell GS et al. Urinary zinc levels as an indication of muscle catabolism. Lancet 1:280-82, 1973; Hallbook T, Hedelin H. Zinc metabolism and surgical traumas. Br J Surg 64:271-73, 1977; Tengrup I, Samuelsson H. Changes in serum zinc during and after surgical procedures. Acta Chir Scand 143:195-99, 1977*).

If deficient, supplementation may be beneficial.

> **Review Articles:** A number of studies have found zinc supplementation to have a beneficial effect upon wound healing, while a number of other studies have had negative results. It appears from animal studies that zinc supplementation is only beneficial when deficient; however, zinc nutriture is difficult to evaluate in man as serum zinc concentration may not accurately reflect the total bodily status of zinc metabolism (*Haley JV. Zinc sulfate and wound healing. J Surg Res 27(3):168-74, 1979; Henkin RI. Zinc in wound healing. Editorial. N Engl J Med 291(13):675-76, 1974*).

> **Experimental Study:** Supplemental zinc stimulated wound healing, but only in pts. who were zinc-deficient (*Fulghum DD. Ascorbic acid revisited. Arch Dermatol 113(1):91-92, 1977*)

- -

OTHER NUTRITIONAL FACTORS

Arginine:

May minimize immediate post-injury weight loss and accelerate wound healing.

> **Review Article:** Arginine is a consitutent of wound proteins and is the penultimate substrate for polyamine synthesis that signals scar tissue proliferation. It also influences wound healing by relaxing vascular smooth muscle, thereby causing fluids and some cells to accumulate in wound sites (*Seifter E et al. Supplemental arginine: Endocrine, autocrine, and paracrine effects on wound healing. Abstract. J Am Coll Nutr 8(5):437, 1989*).

Essential Fatty Acids:

> As fatty acids are essential for the transport of substances across cell membranes, a deficiency in essential fatty acids is associated with poor wound healing (*Dowling RJ et al. Use of fat emulsions, in M Deitel, Ed. Nutrition in Clinical Surgery. Baltimore, Williams and Wilkins, 1985:139-47*).

- -

COMBINED NUTRITIONAL SUPPLEMENTATION

Vitamin C,
Vitamin E,
Beta-carotene and
Glutathione:

Combined supplementation may improve the changes of skin flap survival.

> **Animal Experimental Study:** As recent studies suggest that tissue injury occurs during oxygen reperfusion of skin flaps due to free radical formation, the use of antioxidant vitamins C and E and beta-carotene as free radical scavengers and glutathione as a protector of cell membranes from lipid peroxidation was explored using an acute axial random skin flap model in rats. Combined supplementation resulted in significant improvement of skin flap survival as compared to controls (*Hayden RE et al. The effect of glutathione and vitamins A, C and E on acute skin flap survival. Laryngoscope 97:1176-79, 1987*).

TOPICAL TREATMENTS

Glycosaminoglycans:

Topical application may accelerate wound healing.

Experimental Controlled Study: 15 volunteers received small paired skin incisions in precisely corresponding anatomical sites. One wound was treated with a fine-grind acid-pepsin digested calf tracheal cartilage powder while the other wound served as the control. Closure was identical. After 7-14 days, the wounds were excised with a margin and the resulting defects closed. In 12/15 wound pairs, the tensile strength of the treated wound was greater. The overall percentage increase in tensile strength resulting from the treatment was 42% (highly significant) (*Prudden JF, Allen J. The clinical acceleration of healing with a cartilage preparation; a controlled study. JAMA 192:352-56, 1965*).

Animal Experimental Study: Topical application of heterologous cartilage powder slightly but significantly accelerated the closure of open granulating wounds in rats (*Sabo JC et al. Acceleration of open wound healing by cartilage. Arch Surg 90:414-17, 1965*).

Sugar:

Within wounds, sugar pastes reduce the available water and thus inhibit bacterial growth; however, they still allow granulation tissue to form and epithelialization to take place at a rate similar to control wounds (*Archer HG et al. A controlled model of moist wound healing: comparison between semi-permeable film, antiseptics and sugar paste. J Exp Pathol 71:155-70, 1990*).

Topical application may be beneficial.

WARNING: A patient developed acute renal failure after the use of granulated sugar in a deep infected wound in the right chest following irrigation with gentamicin. After 4 days of therapy, the serum level of sucrose was 48 mmol/l (*Debure A et al. Acute renal failure after use of granulated sugar in deep infected wound. Letter. Lancet 1:1034-35, 1987*).

Note: In the presence of sucrose-induced osmotic nephrosis, it has been questioned why the concentration of gentamicin in the serum was not reported and why gentamicin toxicity was thought unlikely (Archer H et al. Toxicity of topical sugar. Lancet 1:1485-86, 1987).

Clinical Observations: "We have found that packing cavity wounds, such as infected malodorous bed sores (decubitus ulcers) with thick sugar paste has been especially helpful. Not only does the foul odour of anerobic bacterial growth disappear after several days but necrotic tissue is safely debrided. Regular packing twice daily, with bandages to hold the sugar paste in place, has led to considerable success in healing such bed sores in bed-bound semi-paralytic patients. When granulation tissue is established, however, and the wound is shrinking, application of sugar paste will cause bleeding and it should be replaced. . ." (*Seal DV, Middleton K. Healing of cavity wound with sugar. Letter. Lancet 338:571-2, 1991*).

Experimental Study: The open wounds of 150 pts. were treated with a sugar paste which consisted of icing caster sugar, polyethyleneglycol 400, and hydrogen peroxide. Based on results, the authors recommend this therapy for infected wounds and pressure sores. They note that the pastes have osmotic and antibacterial effects which reduce and clear infected slough and can be packed into deep wounds without causing pain. They appear not to delay granulation tissue formation and are apparently non-toxic to tissue. While they avoid its use in pts. with renal failure, they have not experienced any toxicity from the absorption of sucrose (*Archer H et al. Toxicity of topical sugar. Lancet 1:1485-86, 1987*).

Experimental Study: 19 critically ill adults with acute mediastinitis after cardiac surgery, 8 of whom had failed to respond to continuous irrigation, were treated by packing the mediastinal cavity with granulated sugar every 3-4 hours. Mediastinal tissue cultures were positive in 18 patients. There was near-complete debridement of the wounds with rapid formation of granulation tissue in all pts. and sterilization of the wounds after an ave. of 7.6 days (*Trouillet JL et al. Use of granulated sugar in treatment of open mediastinitis after cardiac surgery. Lancet 2:180-84, 1985*).

<u>Vitamin A</u>:

Topical application may reverse the inhibitory effect of corticosteroids on the healing of open wounds.

> **Case Report:** An 18 year-old female receiving a corticosteroid for a skin disease banged her leg and developed an ulceration in the wound which continued to enlarge despite normal medical treatment until vitamin A ointment was applied to the wound 3 times daily. Within 3 days, the wound began to heal. 28 days later, it had completely healed (*Hunt TK et al. Effect of vitamin A on reversing the inhibitory effect of cortisone on healing of open wounds in animals and man. Ann Surg 170(2):203-6, 1969*).

> **Animal Experimental Study:** Wounds of rabbits receiving cortisone healed normally when they received topical applications of vitamin E (*Hunt TK et al. Effect of vitamin A on reversing the inhibitory effect of cortisone on healing of open wounds in animals and man. Ann Surg 170(2):203-6, 1969*).

<u>Zinc</u>:

Topical application may assist the healing of open wounds (*Williams KW et al. The effect of topically applied zinc on the healing of open wounds. J Surg Res 27:62-67, 1979*).

PART TWO

APPENDICES

Appendix A

COMMON NUTRITIONAL DEFICIENCIES

GENERAL

Hospitalized patients are frequently nutritionally deficient.

Note: Albumin and other negative acute-phase proteins fall after any episode resulting in a rise in release of cytokines; they may therefore be inappropriate as a measure of malnutrition for acutely ill patients (Fleck A, Smith G. Assessment of malnutrition in elderly patients. Letter. Lancet 337:793, 1991).

Observational Study: In a 30 mo. study of records of 800 pts. admitted to two American hospitals with pneumonia, hip fracture, or inflammatory bowel disease, or in order to have hip, bowel or abdominal surgery, some degree of malnutrition was found in 55% of all pts. (based on: serum albumin below 3.4 g/dl; weight <90% of ideal body weight; total lymphocyte count <1400/mm^3; history of recent weight loss). Among the nonsurgical gps., malnourished pts. stayed in the hospital an ave. of 2 days longer than well-nourished pts. while, among the surgical gps., malnourished pts. stayed 5 days longer (*Nutritional therapy saves lives, costs. Med World News February 24, 1986, p. 99*).

Observational Study: 583/15,876 pts. (3.67%) were suffering from malnutrition or had nutritional risk factors (NRFs) (cancer, nothing by mouth for 3 or more days, loss of appetite, difficulty chewing or swallowing, persistent fever, cancer chemotherapy or radiation therapy) upon admission. 182/583 received nutritional support and were excluded from the study. After 3 wks., the remaining pts. were reassessed and had significant decreases in nutritional parameters: 622 pts. with deficits in one parameter on admission had a significant decrease in all parameters (p<0.001) and there was a deterioration in nutritional status in those pts. entering the hospital with NRFs only or with one low parameter (*Pinchcofsky GD, Kaminski MV Jr. Increasing malnutrition during hospitalization: Documentation by a nutritional screening program. J Am Coll Nutr 4(4):471-79, 1985*).

Observational Study: In a study of 3172 hospitalized American pts., 58% were malnourished according to at least one of the following indicators: serum albumin, total lymphocyte count, hemoglobin values, and weight-for-height measurement (*S Kamath - reported in Am Med News May 24/31, 1985*).

Hospital diets may be nutritionally deficient.

Observational Study: Dietary registration was undertaken in 56 consecutive pts. admitted to a department of general medicine ward for an ave. of 10.2 days. In 40 pts. (71.4%) the energy intake was less than the corresponding energy requirement as assessed from the the ave. requirement for sick adults (*Stellfeld M, Gyldendorf B. [Dietary investigation in a general medical ward: The energy, protein and zinc intakes of 56 patients during a period of hospitalization.] Ugeskr Laeger 150(25):1537-40, 1988*).

Observational Study: The daily intake of energy, protein, iron and vitamins of pts. on different wards of an English hospital was found to be less than those recommended for healthy adults (*Todd EA et al. What do patients eat in hospital. Hum Nutr Appl Nutr 38A:294-97, 1984*).

Nursing home patients are frequently nutritionally deficient.

Observational Study: In a study of male residents in a 400 bed VA nursing home, protein-calorie undernutrition was found in 30% of residents requiring partial or total assistance. Mortality rates rose from 10% to 60% per year with each decrement in body weight as % of ideal from 100% to 70%. The prevalence of protein-calorie undernutrition increased in direct proportion to degree of functional impairment, and to frequency of intercurrent infection.

Serum cholesterol and hemoglobin were the most sensitive nutritional indicators (*Rudman D. Nutritional status of nursing home men. Abstract. J Am Coll Nutr 6(5):420, 1987*).

Parenteral nutrition (TPN) often causes nutritional deficiencies. Within the first wk., there are severe deficiencies of phosphorus, potassium, sodium, magnesium and essential fatty acids, while long-term TPN often leads to depletion of vitamins A and E, folic acid, biotin and pyridoxine as well as zinc, copper, chromium and selenium (*Chipponi J. Total parenteral nutrition (TPN) often causes nutrient deficiencies. Am J Clin Nutr 35:1112-16, 1982*).

Pregnant women are frequently nutritionally deficient.

Observational Study: Of 76 healthy pregnant American women, 78% had one or more glaring vitamin deficiencies (*Dostaolova L. Dev Pharmacol Ther 4 (Suppl 1):45, 1982*).

Observational Study: In a gp. of 174 pregnant women taking supplements, deficiencies in folic acid, niacin and vitamins A, B6, B12, and C were common (*Baker H et al. Am J Clin Nutr 28:56, 1975*).

The elderly frequently fail to ingest adequate amounts of certain nutrients.

Observational Study: 403 elderly europeans residing at home were interviewed in regard to their vitamin and mineral intake. Compared to the Recommended Dietary Allowances, the Joint Nordic Recommendations and the Absolute Minimal Necessary Amounts, folacin intake was low in 100%, cholecalciferol in 62%, pyridoxine in 83%, and zinc in 87% (although the risk of zinc deficiency was only present in 0.5%). Intakes of the other major vitamins and minerals were sufficient. In conclusion, the diet of the elderly, possibly with the exception of folacin, is well above their absolute minimal requirements, but the margin towards malnutrition is small (*Elsborg L et al. The intake of vitamins and minerals by the elderly at home. Int J Vitam Nutr Res 53(3):321-29, 1983*).

Observational Study: The nutrient content of meals planned for elderly Americans in 14 nursing homes were deficient in energy, niacin, magnesium, zinc, vitamin B6, and total folate. Their actual intakes were low, not only for these nutrients, but also for 9 others. Approx. 30% consumed fewer than 1,200 Kcal (*Sempos CT et al. A dietary survey of 14 Wisconsin nursing homes. J Am Diet Assoc 81(1):35-40, 1982*).

The elderly are frequently nutritionally deficient.

Review Article: Protein-calorie malnutrition of the nursing-home elderly is widespread, with substandard body weight, midarm muscle circumference, and serum albumin levels in 30-50% (*Arora VD, Rudman D. Protein-calorie undernutrition in the nursing home. Geriatr Med Today 7(7):66, 1988*).

Observational Study: Status of vitamins B1, B2, B6 and C in 19 hospitalized pts. ages 65-89 were compared to 10 healthy controls. Both thiamine and ascorbic acid deficiencies were common in both gps., while only the pts. were frequently deficient in pyridoxine. Only 1 person in each gp. was deficient in vitamin B2. These deficiencies were not manifested clinically as classic vitamin deficiency syndromes; thus biochemical assays are necessary for their detection (*Keatinge AMB et al. Vitamin B1, B2, B6 and C status in the elderly. Ir Med J 76:488-90, 1983*).

- -

NUTRIENTS

Amino Acids:

Plasma levels of essential amino acids may be suboptimal in the elderly.

Observational Study: The fasting plasma amino acid profile in 22 healthy young men aged 25-35 was compared to the profile in 21 healthy independent elderly men aged 65-85, in 23 orally-fed nursing home men with dementia aged 65-92, and in 17 tube-fed nursing home men with dementia aged 65-88. Compared to the young men, all 3 gps. of elderly men had significantly (p<0.05) lower levels of methionine and branched-chain amino acids than the healthy young men and the ratio of essential to nonessential amino acids was significantly lower. Methionine was significantly lower in the elderly men with dementia than in the elderly men without dementia (*Rudman D et al. Fasting plasma amino acids in elderly men. Am J Clin Nutr 49:559-66, 1989*).

Calcium: 1.5 gm. daily for postmenopausal women
            (1 gm. daily for premenopausal women over 35)

Women who ingest less than the above amounts are in negative calcium balance (*Heaney RP et al. Menopausal changes in calcium balance performance. J Lab Clin Med 92(6):953-63, 1978*).

> **Observational Study:** Daily calcium intakes based on 3-day dietary records from the USDA's 1977-8 Nationwide Food Consumption Survey were below the Recommended Dietary Allowance for the majority of the U.S. population, particularly for adult women (*Morgan KJ et al. Magnesium and calcium dietary intakes of the U.S. population. J Am Coll Nutr 4:195, 1985*).

> **NIH Consensus Conference:** Calcium intake is commonly insufficient and insufficient intake is associated with decreased bone mineral density. The typical American diet supplies about 450-550 mg daily, well below the RDA. "It seems likely that an increase in calcium intake to 1,000 to 1,500 mg/day beginning well before the menopause will reduce the incidence of osteoporosis in postmenopausal women. Increased calcium intake may prevent age-related bone loss in men as well" (*NIH Consensus Conference: Osteoporosis. JAMA 252(6):799-802, 1984*).

Calcium is the only mineral whose requirement doubles during pregnancy (*Truswell AS. Nutrition for pregnancy. Br Med J July, 1985*).

Intake by the elderly is often inadequate (*Chapuy M et al. Calcium and vitamin D supplements: Effect on calcium metabolism in elderly people. Am J Clin Nutr 46:324-28, 1987*).

Chromium:

Marginal deficiency is common in Western diets due to the high consumption of refined foods and sugars (*Anderson RA, Kozlovsky AS. Chromium intake, absorption and excretion of subjects consuming self-selected diets. Am J Clin Nutr 41:1177-83, 1985; Kumpulainen JT. J Agric Food Chem 27(3), 1979; Schroeder HA. The role of chromium in mammalian nutrition. Am J Clin Nutr 21(3):230-44, 1968*).

Copper:

The average daily intake by individuals consuming typical Western diets (1.0-1.5 mg) is lower than the 2-3 mg recommended to be safe and adequate (*Schoenemann HM et al. Consequences of severe copper deficiency are independent of dietary carbohydrate in young pigs. Am J Clin Nutr 52:147-54, 1990*).

Pregnant women may be in negative copper balance unless supplemented.

> **Experimental and Observational Study:** 24 women in their second trimester were found to ingest less than the US RDA of copper. Copper retention was -0.02 mg/day until they were supplemented with copper which raised copper retention to 0.89 mg/day (*Taper L et al. Am J Clin Nutr 41:1184-1192, 1985*).

Folic acid:

Intake may be inadequate.

> **Observational Study:** Analysis of dietary data taken from a survey of US adults aged 19-74 (NHANES II) found mean daily folate intake to be 242 ± 2.8 mg for all adults, compared to the US RDA of 400 mg/d (*Subar AF et al. Folate intake and food sources in the US population. Am J Clin Nutr 50:508-16, 1989*).

Often deficient in the elderly (*Baker H et al. Severe impairment of dietary folate utilization in the elderly. J Am Geriatr Soc 26(5):218-221, 1978*) even despite adequate food intake and daily oral supplementation (*Frank O et al. Superiority of periodic intramuscular vitamins over daily oral vitamins in maintaining normal vitamin titers in a geriatric population. Am J Clin Nutr 30:630, 1977*).

Often reduced in <u>adolescent females</u>.

> **Observational Study:** The folacin status of 103 adolescent females aged 12, 14, and 16 yrs. was evaulated. 11.7% and 47.6% had serum and RBC folate levels <3 ng/ml (6.8 nmol/l) and 140 ng/ml (317 nmol/l), respectively. Folacin status was unrelated to per capita income (*Clark AJ et al. Folacin status in adolescent females. Am J Clin Nutr 46:302-06, 1987*).

May be deficient in the absence of a megaloblastic anemia (*Matthews J et al. Effect of therapy with vitamin B₁₂ and folic acid on elderly patients with low concentrations of serum vitamin B₁₂ or erythrocyte folate but not normal blood counts. Acta Haematologica 79:84-87, 1988*).

The only vitamin whose requirement doubles in <u>pregnancy</u>. Serum and RBC folate levels decline during pregnancy and some degree of megaloblastic change can be found in substantial minorities of women in late pregnancy (*Truswell AS. Nutrition for pregnancy. Br Med J July, 1985*).

Iodine:

Severe iodine deficiency is common in many countries (*Hetzel BS. Iodine-deficiency disorders. Lancet 1:1386-87, 1988*).

Iron:

Deficiency is believed to be the most prevalent worldwide nutritional deficiency and the most frequent cause of anemia (*Bernat I. Iron deficiency, in Iron Metabolism. New York, Plenum Press, 1983:215-74; Stoskman JA. Iron deficiency anemia: Have we come far enough? JAMA 258:1645-47, 1987*).

The most common nutrient deficiency in American <u>children</u> (*Worthington-Roberts B. Suboptimal nutrition and behavior in children, in Contemporary Developments in Nutrition. St. Louis, Mo., CV Mosby, 1981:524-62*).

Frequently deficient in <u>adolescents</u> (*Armstrong PL. Iron deficiency in adolescents. Br Med J 298:499, 1989*).

Dietary need is known to be increased during <u>pregnancy</u> and increased iron absorption may not be adequate to make up for the extra demands if storage iron is low (*Wallenburg HCS et al. Effect of oral iron supplementation during pregnancy on maternal and fetal iron status. J Perinat Med 12(1):7-12, 1984*).

Magnesium:

Dietary intake is often inadequate.

> **Review Article:** Among elderly Americans, there is decreased availability of magnesium in the food supply, lower magnesium intake and widespread use of supplementation (*Costello RB, Moser-Veillon PB. A review of magnesium intake in the elderly. A cause for concern? Magnes Res 5(1):61-7, 1992*).

> **Observational Study:** In a survey of over 27,000 Americans, only 25% had a dietary intake of magnesium that equalled or exceeded the RDA (*Wester PO. Magnesium. Am J Clin Nutr 45(5 Suppl):1305-12, 1987*).

> **Observational Study:** Daily magnesium intakes based on 3-day dietary records from the USDA's 1977-8 Nationwide Food Consumption Survey were below the Recommended Dietary Allowance for all age and sex classes, with the exception of children younger than 5 years. Magnesium consumption was particularly low among adolescent females, adult females, and elderly males; 75-85% of individuals in these gps. ingested less than the RDA (*Morgan KJ et al. Magnesium and calcium dietary intakes of the U.S. population. J Am Coll Nutr 4:195, 1985*).

> **Review Article:** While the typical American diet provides only 1/2 - 2/3 of the RDA (400 mg), it raises the magnesium requirement to 500-800 mg due to its high content of certain nutritional factors (*Seelig M. Magnesium Deficiency in the Pathogenesis of Disease. New York, Plenum Press, 1980*).

<u>Pregnant women</u> often have an inadequate intake (*Franz KB. Magnesium intake during pregnancy. Magnesium 6:18-27, 1987*).

Frequently deficient in <u>hospitalized patients</u>, especially in those who are acutely medically ill.

Review Article: Magnesium deficiency and its clinical manifestations are common in pts. presenting to the emergency department. Since serum magnesium is the only readily available clinical test and may not be accurate in predicting intracellular magnesium, empiric magnesium therapy should be considered in high-risk pts. (*Reinhart RA. Magnesium deficiency: recognition and treatment in the emergency room setting. <u>Am J Emerg Med</u> 10(1):78-83, 1992*).

Observational Study: The frequency and prevalence of hypomagnesemia in the acute and chronic divisions of a medical center was studied. (The acute facility handles acute medical and all surgical cases, while the chronic facility handles primarily psychiatric cases.) In the acute population, the frequency was 41.4% (222/536 determinations) and the prevalence 26.1% (92/353 pts.) compared to 12.5% (50/399 determinations) and 3.5% (9/258 pts.), respectively, in the chronic population. In the acute care facility, the most common diagnoses associated with hypomagnesemia were coronary artery disease, malignancy, coronary artery bypass surgery, chronic obstructive pulmonary disease and alcoholism, while in the chronic care facility, alcoholism, liver disease and carcinoma were the most frequent diagnoses associated with hypomagnesemia (*Lum G. Hypomagnesemia in acute and chronic care patient populations. <u>Am J Clin Pathol</u> 97(6):827-30, 1992*).

Occasionally deficient in <u>the elderly</u> (*Touitou Y et al. Prevalence of magnesium and potassium deficiencies in the elderly. <u>Clin Chem</u> 33:518-23, 1987*).

Niacin:

Often deficient in <u>the elderly</u>, even despite adequate dietary intake and oral supplementation (*Baker H et al. Vitamin profiles in elderly persons living at home or in nursing homes, versus profiles in healthy subjects. <u>J Am Geriatr Soc</u> 27:444, 1979; Frank O et al. Superiority of periodic intramuscular vitamins over daily oral vitamins in maintaining normal vitamin titers in a geriatric population. <u>Am J Clin Nutr</u> 30:630, 1977*).

Pantothenic Acid:

The average American nursing home resident surveyed consumed only 3.75 mg of pantothenic acid (unless supplemented with beverages and snacks), while the US RDA is 4-7 mg (*Walsh J H et al. Pantothenic acid content of a nursing home diet. <u>Ann Nutr Metab</u> 25:(3)178,-81 1981*).

Potassium:

Intake is frequently inadequate in <u>the elderly</u> (*Abdulla M et al. Dietary intake of potassium in the elderly. Letter. <u>Lancet</u> 2:562, 1975*).

Occasionally deficient in <u>the elderly</u> (*Touitou Y et al. Prevalence of magnesium and potassium deficiencies in the elderly. <u>Clin Chem</u> 33:518-23, 1987*).

Often deficient in <u>hospitalized patients</u> (*Surawicz B et al. Clinical manifestations of hypopotassemia. <u>Am J Med Sci</u> 233:603, 1957*).

Riboflavin:

Intake may be inadequate in <u>the elderly</u> (*Elsborg L et al. The intake of vitamins and minerals by the elderly at home. <u>Int J Vitam Nutr Res</u> 53:321-29, 1983*).

Frequently marginally deficient in <u>the elderly</u> (*Powers H, Thornham D. <u>Br J Nutr</u> 46:257, 1981*).

Frequently marginally deficient in <u>the poor</u> (*Lopez R et al. Riboflavin deficiency in an adolescent population in New York City. <u>Am J Clin Nutr</u> 33:1283-86, 1980*).

Selenium:

Frequently inadequate in <u>Western diets</u>.

Review Article: In the early 1980's, it became evident that selenium intake in the Nordic countries was lower than the "safe and adequate" intake of 50-200 µg proposed by the US National Academy of Sciences. In Finland, it averaged 20-30 µg, in Denmark 45 µg, in Sweden 30 µg, and in Norway 50-70 µg (*Tolonen M. Finnish studies on antioxidants with special reference to cancer, cardiovascular diseaes and ageing. Int Clin Nutr Rev 9(2):68-75, 1989*).

Deficiency states have been demonstrated for inhabitants of regions where selenium supply is limited, in protein-energy malnutrition, and in pts. on total parenteral nutrition without selenium supplementation (*Neve J et al. Selenium deficiency. Clin Endocrinol Metab 14(3):629-56, 1985*).

It has been estimated that the typical selenium consumption in the U.S. is about 100 µg, while 250-300 µg daily can prevent most cancers (*Gerhard Schrauzer, professor of chemistry, U. of California, San Diego - 1981*).

Thiamine:

Often deficient in the elderly (*Keatinge AMB et al. Vitamin B1, B2, B6 and C status in the elderly. Irish Med J 76:488-90, 1983; Bowman BB, Rosenberg IH. Am J Clin Nutr 35:1142-51, 1982*), sometimes even when dietary intake appears to be adequate.

Vitamin A:

It is estimated that 1 million people develop vitamin A deficiency each year (*Bauernfeind JC. The Safe Use Of Vitamin A: A Report of the International Vitamin A Consultative Group. Washington, DC: The Nutrition Foundation, 1980*).

In two major American nutrition surveys (NHANES I, 1971-74; USDA Nationwide Food Consumption Survey (1977-78), vitamin A was found to be a problem nutrient, i.e., one in which ≥20% of the population surveyed was obtaining <70% of the Recommended Dietary Allowance. The data were confirmed more recently (NHANES II) (*Bendich A, Langseth L. Safety of vitamin A. Am J Clin Nutr 49:358-71, 1989*).

Intake may be inadequate among the elderly (*Elsborg L et al. The intake of vitamins and minerals by the elderly at home. Int J Vitam Nutr Res 53:321-9, 1983*).

Vitamin B6:

Intake is commonly below the US Recommended Daily Allowance.

> **Observational Study:** Based on the the Second National US Health and Nutrition Examination Survey (NHANES II) of 11,658 adults aged 19-74 yrs., 71% of males and 90% of females consumed less than the 1980 US RDA of vitamin B6 (*Kant AK, Block G. Dietary vitamin B-6 intake and food sources in the US population: NHANES II, 1976-1980. Am J Clin Nutr 52:707-16, 1990*).

Marginally deficient in about 50% of pregnant women, and studies have shown that supplementation with 20 mg pyridoxine daily may be necessary to keep the laboratory measurements of pyridoxine in the normal range (*Heller S et al. Vitamin B6 status in pregnancy. Am J Clin Nutr 26(12):1339-48, 1973*).

Often deficient in the elderly, even despite adequate dietary intake and oral supplementation (*Frank O et al. Superiority of periodic intramuscular vitamins over daily oral vitamins in maintaining normal vitamin titers in a geriatric population. Am J Clin Nutr 30:630, 1977*).

> **Observational Study:** In a study of 198 free-living, low-income, elderly persons (aged ≥60) in the U.S., vitamin B6 status was low (PLP<32 nmol/L) in 32% and could be attributed to low dietary intakes and/or the presence of health problems reported to alter vitamin B6 status (*Manore MM et al. Plasma pyridoxal 5^1-phosphate concentration and dietary B-6 intake in free-living, low-income elderly people. Am J Clin Nutr 50:339-45, 1989*).

Vitamin B12:

Often deficient in the elderly, even despite adequate dietary intake and oral supplementation (*Frank O et al. Superiority of periodic intramuscular vitamins over daily oral vitamins in maintaining normal vitamin titers in a geriatric population. Am J Clin Nutr 30:630, 1977; Elsborg L et al. Serum vitamin B12 levels in the aged. Acta Med Scand 200:309-14, 1976).*

Note: Food cobalamin malabsorption occurs frequently in patients with unexplained low serum cobalamin levels (Carmel R et al. Food cobalamin malabsorption occurs frequently in patients with unexplained low serum cobalamin levels. Arch Intern Med 148(8):1715-9, 1988).

Observational Study: Serum samples were obtained from 152 hospital out-pts. aged 65-99. Vitamin B12 levels were low in 8.5% of pts. and were moderately low in 16.5%. Marked elevations of methylmalonic acid and homocysteine, vitamin B12 metabolites, were seen in 62% of those with very low serum B12 levels and in 56% of those with moderately low serum B12 levels (*Pennypacker C et al. High prevalence of cobalamin (CBL, vitamin B-12) deficiency in elderly outpatients. J Am Gerontol Soc 8:A9, 1990*).

May be deficient in the absence of a megaloblastic anemia.

Observational Study: 3/17 elderly pts. with low concentrations of serum vitamin B12 or RBC folate but normal blood counts had bone marrow suppression, and 2 of the 3 also had megaloblastic changes in the marrow, suggesting that the low concentrations of serum B12 or RBC folate found in about 1/4 of elderly pts. might indicate actual tissue deficiencies even when blood counts were normal (*Matthews J et al. Effect of therapy with vitamin B12 and folic acid on elderly patients with low concentrations of serum vitamin B12 or erythrocyte folate but not normal blood counts. Acta Haematologica 79:84-87, 1988*).

If deficient, supplementation may be beneficial.

Experimental Study: 14 hospital out-pts. aged 65-99 with marked elevations of methylmalonic acid acid and homocysteine, vitamin B12 metabolites, received vitamin B12 therapy. At the end of 8 wks., all 14 pts. had normal B12 metabolite levels (*Pennypacker C et al. High prevalence of cobalamin (CBL, vitamin B-12) deficiency in elderly outpatients. J Am Gerontol Soc 8:A9, 1990*).

Experimental Study: 19 pts. aged 57-98 attending a medical out-patient clinic who had serum vitamin B12 levels <200 pg/ml were supplemented with vitamin B12. 52.6% benefited. Hematologic abnormalities were corrected in 5/7; neurologic abnormalities were corrected in 3/7; and mental status improved in 2/11 pts. with dementia (*Timiras M. Vitamin B12 deficiency in geriatric clinic patients. J Am Geriatr Soc 3898:A47, 1990*).

Vitamin C:

Intake is commonly below the Dutch RDAs in Holland.

Observational Study: The Dutch RDAs are based on the goal of tissue vitamin C saturation. In a survey of 5898 subjects, most population gps. studied had a median vitamin C intake below the RDA. The lowest intake (median as percentage of RDA) was seen among boys (78%) and girls (75%) aged 13-15. Frank vitamin C deficiency is unlikely for most of the nonsmoking independently living population, but many of the Dutch population may not have tissue vitamin C saturation (*Löwik MRH et al. Assessment of the adequacy of vitamin C intake in the Netherlands. Abstract. J Am Coll Nutr 10(5):544, 1991*).

Among American women, 20-50% have a vitamin C intake below 70% of the RDA of 60 milligrams daily (*US Dept. of Agriculture*).

Intake is often inadequate in the chronically sick elderly (*Newton HM et al. The cause and correction of low blood vitamin C concentrations in the elderly. Am J Clin Nutr 42(4):656-59, 1985*).

Intake may occasionally be inadequate in the healthy elderly (*Elsborg L et al. The intake of vitamins and minerals by the elderly at home. Int J Vitam Nutr Res 53:321-29, 1983*).

Serum levels may be low in the healthy elderly (*Garry PH et al. Am J Clin Nutr 36:332, 1982; VanderJagt DJ et al. Am J Clin Nutr 46:290, 1987*).

Other groups at high risk for vitamin C deficiency are men who live alone, individuals who avoid "acid"-containing foods due to dyspepsia or reflux esophagitis, food fadists, patients undergoing peritoneal dialysis and hemodialysis, and alcoholics (*Reuler JB et al. Adult scurvy. JAMA 253(6):805-7, 1985*).

Vitamin D:

Lack of sunshine (ultraviolet light is necessary for endogenous vitamin D production) can cause vitamin D deficiency.

> **Observational Study:** Vitamin D levels of 23 older people were measured every 3 mo. for 16 months. In July, their levels were normal. By November, levels had dropped 19%. By February, levels had dropped 65% to a range where 9 had levels consistent with the development of disease. The May measurement was 62% below the initial measurement, which was equalled again in the next July measurement (*Lawson DE et al. Relative contributions of diet and sunlight to vitamin D state in the elderly. Br Med J 2:303-5, August 4, 1979*).

It is recommended that the elderly receive a total supply of 600-800 IU (15-20 mg) daily of vitamin D (*Parfitt AM et al Vitamin D and bone health in the elderly. Am J Clin Nutr 36(5 Suppl.):1014-31, 1982*).

Dietary intake below the U.S. Recommended Daily Allowance (200 IU) is common among the elderly (*Elsborg L et al. The intake of vitamins and minerals by the elderly at home. Int J Vitam Nutr Res 53:321-29, 1983; Omdahl JL et al. Nutritional status in a healthy elderly population: vitamin D. Am J Clin Nutr 36:1225-33, 1982*).

Vitamin E:

Median intakes may be considerably below the U.S. RDA (*Murphy SP et al. Vitamin E intakes and sources in the United States. Am J Clin Nutr 52:361-67, 1990*).

The ratio of vitamin E to polyunsaturated fatty acids may be low.

> **Observational Study:** Based on 24-hr. recall data from 11,658 adults interviewed in the US Second National Health and Nutrition Examination Survey (NHANES II), if a ratio of vitamin E to PUFAs of ≥0.4 is considered desirable, 23% of men and 15% of women had diets with low ratios (*Murphy SP et al. Vitamin E intakes and sources in the United States. Am J Clin Nutr 52:361-67, 1990*).

Vitamin K:

Sub-clinical deficiency during pregnancy and in the newborn is common (*Block CA et al. Mother-infant prothrombin precursor status at birth. J Pediatr Gastroenterol Nutr 3(1):101-03, 1984*).

Zinc:

Commonly inadequate in the Western diet (*Prasad AS. Role of zinc in human health. Contemp Nutr 16(5), 1991; Singh A et al. Magnesium, zinc, and copper status of US Navy SEAL trainees. Am J Clin Nutr 49:695-700, 1989*).

Children and teenagers are especially susceptible to zinc deficiency due to their increased requirements for growth and development (*Sanstead HH. Am J Clin Nutr 26:1251-60, 1973*).

Zinc nutriture is often inadequate during pregnancy (*Hambridge KM et al. Zinc nutritional status during pregnancy: A longitudinal study. Am J Clin Nutr 37:429-42, 1983; Truswell AS. Nutrition for pregnancy. Br Med J July, 1985*).

The elderly are especially susceptible to zinc deficiency due to:
1. lower zinc consumption than younger individuals.
2. poor bioavailability of their dietary zinc.
3. the presence of certain disease states.
4. the use of various medications which affect zinc nutriture.
(*Greger JL. Prevalence and significance of zinc deficiency in the elderly. Geriatr Med Today 3(1):24-30, 1984; J Am Diet Assoc 82:148-53, 1983*).

Severe zinc deficiency can occur with total parenteral nutrition unless supplementation is given (*Goldwasser B et al. Isr J Med Sci 17:1155-57, 1981*).

<u>Hospital diets</u> may be inadequate in zinc.

Observational Study: Dietary registration was undertaken in 56 consecutive pts. admitted to a department of general medicine ward for an ave. of 10.2 days. Only 1/56 (1.8%) received zinc in the quantity recommended for healthy adults (*Stellfeld M, Gyldendorf B. [Dietary investigation in a internal medical ward: The energy, protein and zinc intakes of 56 pts. during hospitalization.] Ugeskr Laeger 150(25):1537-40, 1988*).

Observational Study: The mean daily level of zinc intake in hospital diets in the U.S. was 9.4 mg compared to the 13 mg thought to be required daily by adults (*Klevay LM et al. Evidence of dietary copper and zinc deficiencies. JAMA 241:1916-18, 1979*).

Appendix B

DANGERS OF SUPPLEMENTATION

NOTE: Drug interactions should also be considered

<u>Beta-Carotene:</u>

Stored in fatty deposits in the body, especially the liver. Hypercarotenemia is associated with <u>orange discoloration of the skin</u> (especially palms, soles and naso-labial folds) (*Vakil DV et al. Hypercarotenaemia: A case report and review of the literature. <u>Nutr Res</u> 5:911-17, 1985*).

Experimental Placebo-controlled Study: 5 men randomly received carotenoid supplementation either as 30 mg purified beta-carotene, 12 mg beta-carotene, 272 g cooked carrots, 300 g cooked broccoli, 180 g tomato juice or placebo. Definite carotenodermia was first noted between 25-42 days and persisted 14 to >42 days posttreatment. It was only observed after plasma total carotenoid levels exceeded 4.0 mg/L (*Micozzi MS et al. Carotenodermia in men with elevated carotenoid intake from foods and beta-carotene supplements. <u>Am J Clin Nutr</u> 48:1061-64, 1988*).

Hypercarotenemia is associated with reversible <u>leukopenia</u>, <u>weakness</u>, <u>enlarged liver</u>, <u>low blood pressure</u> and <u>weight loss</u> (*Vakil DV et al. Hypercarotenaemia: A case report and review of the literature. <u>Nutr Res</u> 5:911-17, 1985*).

Note: Reports of carotenoid-associated toxicity were the result of the consumption of foods containing carotenoids rather than a pure product; thus other components of these foods are likely to be the major cause of the reported adverse effects. This pro-vitamin has been taken by many individuals at doses between 30 and 180 mg/d over a 15 year period without any adverse effects being noted (Bendich A. The safety of beta-carotene. <u>Nutr Cancer</u> 11:207-14, 1988).

<u>Bioflavonoids:</u>

Cianidanol may induce intravascular or extravascular immune hemolysis and fever (*Jaeger A et al. Side effects of flavonoids in medical practice. <u>Prog Clin Biol Res</u> 280:379-94, 1988*).

<u>Bismuth:</u>

Adverse side-effects appear limited to mild dizziness, headache and diarrhea. Anacids or milk should not be taken within 30 minutes before or after ingestion. Bismuth compounds should not be given to patients with renal or hepatic impairment. Due to lack of safety data, they should not be given during pregnancy (*Wagstaff AJ et al. Colloidal bismuth subcitrate: A review of its pharmacodynamic and pharmacokinetic properties, and its therapeutic use in peptic ulcer disease. <u>Drugs</u> 36:132-57, 1988*).

<u>Calcium:</u>

Usually no adverse effects at customary supplemental doses.

A calcium to phosphorus ratio above 2:1 due to excess calcium results in <u>reduced bone strength</u> and interferes with vitamin K synthesis and/or absorption, which could theoretically cause <u>internal bleeding</u> (*Calcium: How much is too much? <u>Nutr Rev</u> 43(11):345, 1985*).

Primary <u>hyperparathyroidism</u> may be caused by a daily calcium intake of over 2 grams (*Shaker JL, Krawczyc KW, Finding JW. Primary hyperparathyroidism and severe hypercalcaemia with low circulating 1,25-dihydroxyvitamin D levels. <u>J Clin Endocrinol Metab</u> 62:1305-08, 1986*).

Carnitine:

Supplementation with D,L-carnitine 900-1200 mg daily (but not with L-carnitine) has been associated with a myasthenia-like syndrome in patients with renal impairment (*McCarty MF. A note on 'orthomolecular' aids for dieting - myasthenic syndrome due to DL-carnitine. Med Hypotheses December, 1982, pp. 661-2; Bazzato G et al. Myasthenia-like syndrome after DL - but not L - carnitine. Lancet 2:1209, 1981*).

In clinical studies of L-carnitine, 41% of patients developed GI side-effects and 11% developed a body odor. In no patient was it discontinued due to these side-effects, and a decrease in dosage reduced or eliminated them (*FDA Drug Bulletin, June, 1986*).

Copper:

Elevated levels (often due to contaminated drinking water) can be toxic, causing profound mental and physical fatigue, poor memory, severe depression and insomnia (*Nolan KB. Nutr Rev 41:318-20, 1983*).

Evening Primrose Oil:

May exacerbate temporal lobe epilepsy (*Holman CP, Bell AFJ. A trial of evening primrose oil in the treatment of chronic schizophrenia. J Orthomol Psychiatry 12:302-04, 1983; Vaddadi KS. The use of gamma-linolenic acid and linoleic acid to differentiate between temporal lobe epilepsy and schizophrenia. Prostaglandins Med 6:375-79, 1981*).

May exacerbate mania (*Horrobin DF. The regulation of prostaglandin biosynthesis by the manipulation of essential fatty acid metabolism. Rev Pure Appl Pharmacol 4:339-83, 1983*).

Fluoride:

In experimental animals, administration inhibits the enzyme phosphatase which is critically important for the assimilation of calcium and other minerals (*Yanick P. Solving problematic tinnitus. A clinical scientific approach. Townsend Letter for Doctors. February - March, 1985, p. 31*).

Damages the surface of the gastric mucosa at therapeutic dosages (*Spak C-J et al. Tissue response of gastric mucosa after ingestion of fluoride. Br Med J 298:1686-87, 1989*).

May increase the risk of osteosarcoma (*National Center for Toxicological Research, US Food and Drug Administration - noted in FDA Consumer May, 1991*).

Folic Acid:

Daily oral supplements of 5-10 mg appear to be well-tolerated and without toxicity in normal non-pregnant subjects; some studies suggest ensuring adequate zinc intake if folate supplements are used during pregnancy (*Butterworth CE Jr, Tamura T. Folic acid safety and toxicity: A brief review. Am J Clin Nutr 50:353-58, 1989*).

Adverse effects may be seen at higher dosages.

Case Reports: 2 pts. are described who showed exacerbation of psychotic behavior during treatment with folic acid for folate deficiency which was associated with elevated RBC folate levels (*Prakash R, Petrie WM. Psychiatric changes associated with an excess of folic acid. Am J Psychiatry. 139(9):1192-93, 1982*).

Experimental Study: 14 normal subjects received folic acid 15 mg daily. By 1 mo., 60% had developed GI side-effects (abdominal distension, flatulence, nausea, anorexia), sleep disturbances with vivid dreams, malaise and irritability (*Hunter R et al. Toxicity of folic acid given in pharmacological doses to healthy volunteers. Lancet 1:61-63, 1970*).

Supplementation should be used with caution in drug-controlled epileptics as occasionally seizure activity may be induced (*Butterworth CE Jr, Tamura T. Folic acid safety and toxicity: A brief review. Am J Clin Nutr 50:353-58, 1989*).

Supplementation in the presence of pernicious anemia due to vitamin B12 deficiency will cure the anemia but fail to prevent progression of the neuropathology (*Davidson LSP, Girdwood RH. Folic acid as a therapeutic agent. Br Med J 1:587-91, 1947*).

High dose therapy may decrease vitamin B12 levels; thus B12 supplementation or regular monitoring is indicated (*Hunter R et al. Effect of folic-acid supplement on serum-vitamin-B12 levels in patients on anticonvulsants. Lancet 2:50, 1969*).

Gamma-hydroxybutyrate:

At doses ranging from 1/4 tsp to 4 tbsp, adverse effects have included coma and tonic-clonic seizure-like activity. Acute effects resolve within 7 hrs. (*Dyer JE. gamma-Hydroxybutyrate: a health-food product producing coma and seizurelike activity. Am J Emerg Med 9(4):321-4, 1991*). Other reported acute symptoms are abrupt drowsiness, dizziness, a "high," headache, and nausea and vomiting. Following discontinuation of the supplement, there is full recovery. No clear dose-response effect has been observed (*Chin MY, Kreutzer RA, Dyer JE. Acute poisoning from gamma-hydroxybutyrate in California. West J Med 156(4):380-4, 1992*).

Germanium:

Long-term ingestion of germanium dioxide may be nephrotoxic.

> **Review Article:** Acute renal failure or renal dysfunction associated with germanium-induced nephrotoxicity has been reported in 18 pts. since 1982. In 17/18 cases, biopsies showed vacuolar degeneration in renal tubular epithelial cells in the absence of glomerular changes, without proteinuria or hematuria. Although the mechanism for germanium-induced nephrotoxicity is unknown, the inorganic germanium salts, such as germanium dioxide, are the suspected cause. While sufficient evidence for a role of organogermanium compounds, such as carboxyethyl germanium sesquioxide ("Ge 132") or citrate-lactate germanate, is lacking, the introduction of germanium "nutritional" supplements increases the risk of additional cases of germanium-induced nephrotoxicity, especially if appreciable levels of inorganic germanium salts are present and consumed for longer than 3 mo. at levels above the ave. daily estimated intake for germanium (*Schauss AG. Nephrotoxicity in humans by the ultratrace element germanium. Ren Fail 13(1):1-4, 1991*).

> **Case Reports:** Ingestion of germanium dioxide 50-250 mg daily for at least several mo. was associated with the development of renal failure in 2 patients. Renal function gradually improved after discontinuation of the germanium, but never recovered completely. 8 other cases of germanium dioxide-induced nephropathy have been reported in the Japanese medical literature (*Matsusaka T et al. Germanium-induced nephropathy: Report of 2 cases and review of the literature. Clin Nephrol 30:341-5, 1988*).

L-Glutamine:

Megadoses (at least 1 gm/d) may cause mania (*Mebane AH. L-Glutamine and Mania. Letter. Am J Psychiatry 141(10), October, 1984*).

Guar Gum:

May adversely affect food absorption (*Meyer JH, Doty JE. Transit and absorption of solid food: Multiple effects of guar. Am J Clin Nutr 267-73, 1988*).

L-5-Hydroxytryptophan:

Gastrointestinal side effects (nausea, vomiting, diarrhea) are the only side effects of practical importance and are dose-dependent. They can be minimized by raising the dosage gradually and taking the supplement at mealtimes (*van Praag HM, Westenberg HGM. The treatment of depressions with l-5-hydroxytryptophan. Adv Biol Psychiatry 10:94-128, 1983*).

Iron:

Only supplement if deficient - otherwise supplementation can cause subclinical iron excess which may contribute to a wide variety of diseases (*Gordeuk V et al. Iron overload: causes and consequences. Annu Rev Nutr 7:485-508, 1987;*

Halliday J, Powell L. Iron overload. Sem Hematol 19:42-53, 1982), including cancer and infection (*Bergeron RJ et al. Influence of iron on in vivo proliferation and lethality of L1210 cells. J Nutr 115:369-74, 1985; Weinberg ED. Iron withholding: A defense against infection and neoplasia. Physiol Rev 64:65-102, 1984*).

Gastrointestinal side effects (ex. nausea, vomiting, epigastric discomfort) are commonly reported after iron supplementation (*Passmore R, Eastwood MA. Davidson and Passmore: Human Nutrition and Dietetics. Edinburgh, Churchill Livingstone, 1986, p. 463*) that may turn the stools black.

L-Lysine:

May increase cholesterol and triglyceride levels (*Schmeisser DD et al. Effect of excess dietary lysine on plasma lipids of the chick. J Nutr 113(9):1777-83, 1983*).

Manganese:

Supplementation may occasionally elevate blood pressure in people over 40 or cause hypertensive headaches (*Pfeiffer CC, LaMola S. Zinc and manganese in the schizophrenias. J Orthomol Psychiatry 12:215-234, 1983*).

Chronic manganese intoxication may cause potentially irreversible movement and other neurologic disorders (*Donaldson J, Barbeau A. Manganese neurotoxicity: Possible clues to the etiology of human brain disorders, in S Gabay et al, Eds. Metal Ions in Neurology and Psychiatry. New York, Alan R. Liss, 1985:259-85; Weiner WJ et al. Regional brain manganese levels in an animal model of tardive dyskinesia, in WE Fann et al, Eds. Tardive Dyskinesia: Research and Treatment. New York, SP Medical and Scientific Books, 1980:159-163*).

Niacin:

Note: "The principal side effects of nicotinic acid . . . must be attributable to the high doses necessary to achieve a therapeutic effect, and can as a rule be prevented or alleviated by the use of nicotinic acid derivatives" (Hotz W. Nicotinic acid and its derivatives: A short survey. Adv Lipid Res 20:195-217, 1983).

1. Histamine flush: Common side-effect due to histamine release from mast cells. Starts in 20 minutes and can last 1-1 1/2 hours. Usually lessened after 3 days and may disappear at higher doses. Can be minimized by taking niacin with meals and raising the dosage gradually. ASA 300 mg. 15-30 minutes before ingestion may prevent or ameliorate it.

2. Hyperuricemia due to its competition with uric acid for renal excretion is common, although exacerbation of gout or uric acid stone formation is rare (*Buist RA. Editorial: Vitamin toxicities, side effects and contraindications. Int Clin Nutr Rev 4(4):159-71, 1984; Pfeiffer CC. Mental and Elemental Nutrients. New Canaan, Conn., Keats Publishing, 1975, p. 121*).

3. Deterioration of oral glucose tolerance is a relatively common side effect (*Balasse EO, Neef A. Metabolism 22:1193, 1973; Gaut QN et al, in KF Gey & LA Carlson, Eds. Metabolic Effects Of Nicotinic Acid and Its Derivatives. Bern, Huber, 1971, p. 923; Mosher LR. Am J Psychiatry 126:1290, 1970*).

4. Hepatic toxicity A rare complication which usually occurs with ingestion of over 3 gm daily (perform baseline liver function studies and every 6-8 mo.) (*Mullin GE et al. Fulminant hepatic failure after ingestion of sustained-release nicotinic acid. Ann Intern Med 111(3):253-55, 1989; Patterson DJ et al. Niacin hepatitis. South Med J 76(2):239-41, 1983*).

Note: Hepatotoxicity is more likely from sustained-release niacin (Christensen NA et al. Nicotinic acid treatment of hypercholesterolemia, comparison of plain and sustained action preparations, and report of two cases of jaundice. JAMA 177:546-50, 1961; Henkin Y et al. Rechallenge with crystalline niacin after drug-induced hepatitis from sustained-relaease niacin. JAMA 264(2):241-43, 1990 Mullin GE et al. Fulminant hepatic failure after ingestion of sustained-release nicotinic acid. Ann Intern Med 111(3):253-55, 1989).

Long-term ingestion of sustained-release niacin may cause prolonged bleeding with a prolonged thrombin time (*Dearing B et al. Coagulopathy induced by sustained-release niacin. Abstract. Clin Res 39:A159, 1991*).

Long-term ingestion of sustained-release niacin may cause lactic acidosis with nausea and vomiting (*Earthman T, Odom L, Mullins C. Lactic acidosis associated with high-dose niacin therapy. South Med J 84:496-7, 1991*).

Other side-effects: Pruritis, hyperpigmentation, rash, acanthosis nigricans, nausea, diarrhea, aggravation of peptic ulcers, hypotension, and atrial fibrillation (*Coronary Drug Project Research Group: Clofibrate and niacin in coronary heart disease. JAMA 231:360-81, 1975*).

Niacinamide (nicotinamide):

Common side effect: sedation

Large doses may cause hepatic toxicity (*Winter SL, Boyer JL. Hepatic toxicity from large doses of vitamin B3 (nicotinamide). N Engl J Med 289(22):1180-2, 1973*)

Omega-3 Fatty Acids:

Supplementation may require additional vitamin E intake to prevent increased membrane peroxidation and immune suppression (*Kramer TR et al. Increased vitamin E intake restores fish oil-induced suppressed blastogenesis of mitogen-stimulated T lymphocytes. Am J Clin Nutr 54:896-902, 1991; Meydani M et al. Effect of long-term fish oil supplementation on vitamin E status and lipid peroxidation in women. J Nutr 121:484-91, 1991*).

Supplementation may cause a temporary thrombocytopenia (*Goodnight S. The antithrombotic effects of fish oil, in AP Simopoulos et al, Eds. Health Effects of Polyunsaturated Fatty Acids in Seafoods. New York, Academic Press, 1986:135-48*).

In type I (insulin-dependent) diabetics, supplementation may increase total cholesterol with increases in both HDL_2 and LDL fractions (*Vandongen R et al. Hypercholesterolaemic effect of fish oil in insulin-dependent diabetic patients. Med J Aust 148:141-43, 1988*).

Supplementation may increase fasting plasma glucose and triacylglycerol levels and decrease insulin activity (*Bhathena SJ et al. Effects of ω3 fatty acids and vitamin E on hormones involved in carbohydrate and lipid metabolism in men. Am J Clin Nutr 54:684-8, 1991*).

In type II (non-insulin-dependent) diabetics, supplementation may cause reversible metabolic deterioration (*Glauber H et al. Adverse metabolic effect of omega-3 fatty acids in non-insulin-dependent diabetes mellitus. Ann Intern Med 108(5):663-68, 1988*).

Supplementation may decrease several indices of cell-mediated immunity (*Meydani S et al. Effect of low-fat, low cholesterol (LF-FCHL) diet enriched in N-3 fatty acids (FA) on the immune response of humans. FASEB J 5:1449A, 1991*).

Para-amino Benzoic Acid:

Potential side-effects include skin rash, anorexia, nausea and fever (*Physicians' Desk Reference. Oradell, N.J., Med. Economics Co., Inc., 1986*) as well as vitiligo (*Hughes CG. Oral PABA and vitiligo. J Am Acad Dermatol 9:770, 1983*) and liver toxicity (*Kantor GR, Ratz JL. Liver toxicity from potassium para-aminobenzoate. Letter. J Am Acad Dermatol 13(4):671-72, 1985*).

Phenylalanine:

Supplementation may cause anxiety, headache and hypertension and should be avoided by phenylketourics and women who are pregnant or lactating.

Quercitin:

Review Article: Has been shown to be mutagenic to mammalian cells *in vitro*; however all but one *in vivo* study of carcinogenicity have been negative, and numerous researchers have been unable to confirm the results of that study despite using markedly greater dosages. In addition, the one positive study found an increase in bladder cancer in a strain of rat known to have an extremely high rate of spontaneous bladder cancer. More recent research seems to support quecitin as a suppressor of tumor formation (*Murray MT. "Disinformation" concerning quercetin. Letter. Townsend Letter for Doctors 53:377-78, 1987*).

Selenium:

Toxicity may be associated with hair loss, thickened, fragile fingernails, muscle discomfort, dermatitis, nausea, garlic breath odor, fatigue and suppression of phagocytic and natural killer cell function.

Selenite has been shown in a Japanese study to interact with glutathione in the presence of oxygen to generate free radicals. Since glutathione is found in all cells, this form of selenium may be unsuitable for human use (*Schrauzer GN. Benefits of nutritional selenium. Report of presentation from the Fourth International Symposium on Selenium in Biology and Medicine, Tubingen U., W. Germany, July, 1988. Anabolism 7(4):5, 1988*).

Sodium selenate in high dosage is less likely to be toxic as it is more rapidly excreted in the urine than selenite (*Thompson CD, Robinson MF. Urinary and fecal excretions and absorption of a large supplement of selenium: Superiority of selenate over selenite. Am J Clin Nutr 44:659-63, 1986*).

Thiamine:

Toxic side-effects have mostly occurred after IM or parenteral injections and have included generalized urticaria, facial edema, dyspnea, cyanosis, wheezing and anaphylactic shock.

Oral supplementation has very rarely produced side-effects, although nervousness, itching, flushing, shortness of breath, tachycardia, a sensation of heat and perfuse perspiration have been reported. (*Buist RA. Editorial: Vitamin toxicities, side effects and contraindications. Int Clin Nutr Rev 4(4):159-71, 1984*)

L-Tryptophan:

In recent years, the ingestion of tryptophan supplements has been associated with the eosinophilia-myalgia syndrome (*Martin RW et al. The clinical spectrum of the eosinophilia-myalgia syndrome associated with L-tryptophan ingestion. Ann Intern Med 113:124-34, 1990*). While most cases are now known to be due to a contaminant introduced during the manufacturing process by one manufacturer (*Mayeno AN et al. Characterization of 'peak E' a novel amino acid associated with exposure of tryptophan from a single manufacturer. JAMA 264:213-17, 1990*), tryptophan has been removed from the market in many countries until its safety is better proven.

It has been suggested (*Soukes TL. Toxicology of serotonin precursors. Adv Biol Psychiatry 10:160-75, 1983*) that the following groups not receive large, chronic doses of tryptophan:

1. Patients with cancer or a history of it
2. Patients with any source of irritation of the urinary bladder
3. Children and pregnant women
4. Diabetics and patients with a family history of diabetes
5. Patients with a history of any scleroderma-like condition
6. Patients with large flora high in the intestinal tract (e.g. those with achlorhydria)

High doses are frequently associated with nausea (*Greenwood MW et al. The acute effects of oral tryptophan in human subjects. Br J Clin Pharmacol 2:165-72, 1975*).

Supplementation may aggravate bronchial asthma (*Urge G et al. Effect of dietary tryptophan restrictions on clinical symptoms in patients with endogenous asthma. Allergy 38:211-2, 1983*).

Lupus patients are said to have decreased serotonin levels, perhaps due to deficient conversion of tryptophan to serotonin. The tryptophan breakdown products may lead to auto-antibody production (*Cardin de'Stefani E, Costa C. [Changes in the metabolism of tryptophan in erythematosus.] Boll Soc Ital Biol Sper 60(8):1535-40, 1984; McCormick JP et al. Characterization of a cell-lethal product from the photooxidation of tryptophan: Hydrogen peroxide. Science 191:468-9, 1976*).

Supplementation may be harmful during pregnancy (*Meier AH, Wilson JM. Tryptophan feeding adversely influences pregnancy. Life Sci. 32:1193, 1983*).

Supplementation may promote <u>bladder cancer</u> in patients who are <u>vitamin B6-deficient</u> (*Birt DF et al. Effect of L-tryptophan excess and vitamin B6 deficiency on rat urinary bladder cancer promotion. Cancer Res 47:1244-50, 1987*).

Supplementation may be toxic to patients with <u>adrenal insufficiency</u> (*Trulson ME et al. Low doses of L-tryptophan are lethal in rats with adrenal insufficiency. Life Sci 41:349-53, 1987*).

Supplementation may reduce the efficacy of <u>morphine analgesia</u> (*Franklin KB et al. Tryptophan-morphine interactions and postoperative pain. Pharmacol Biochem Behav 35(1):157-63, 1990*).

Vitamin A:

Hypervitaminosis A is by far the most common cause of vitamin toxicity. The dosage required to produce toxicity is highly variable. While it is possible to receive as much as 1 million IU daily for 5 years without developing toxicity (*Hruban Z et al. Am J Pathol 76:451-61, 1974*), doses of ≥100,000 IU/d for days to weeks, or doses as low as 25,000-50,000 IU/d for several months or longer can produce toxic effects, especially in persons with liver function compromised by drugs, viral hepatitis, or protein-energy malnutrition. Reports of toxicity in adults with supplemental intakes <50,000 IU/d mainly involve persons with unusually high dietary intakes or with confounding medical conditions (*Hathcock JN et al. Evaluation of vitamin A toxicity. Am J Clin Nutr 52:183-202, 1990*).

Worldwide, the incidence of vitamin A excess, or hypervitaminosis A, is estimated to be only 200 cases annually (*Bauernfeind JC. The Safe Use Of Vitamin A: A Report of the International Vitamin A Consultative Group. Washington, DC, The Nutrition Foundation, 1980*). Over the last 50 years, the number of reported cases has remained relatively constant despite the significant growth in production and use of vitamin A supplements (*Bendich A, Langseth L. Safety of vitamin A. Am J Clin Nutr 49:358-71, 1989*).

When vitamin A toxicity has developed following administration under medical supervision, so that the level of reported intake is likely to be more accurate, manifestations of hypervitaminosis A were abstract or slight (*Bauernfeind JC. The Safe Use Of Vitamin A: A Report of the International Vitamin A Consultative Group. Washington, DC, The Nutrition Foundation, 1980*).

Reported manifestations of chronic toxicity include <u>fatigue, malaise and lethargy</u>, <u>headaches</u>, <u>abdominal discomfort</u>, <u>constipation</u>, <u>insomnia</u> and <u>restlessness</u>. Later, <u>night sweats</u>, <u>alopecia</u>, <u>brittle nails</u>, <u>irregular menses</u>, <u>emotional lability</u>, <u>mouth fissures</u>, <u>dry, scaly, rough, yellowish skin</u>, <u>superficial retinal hemorrhages</u>, <u>exophthalmos</u>, <u>peripheral edema</u> and <u>increased intracranial pressure</u> with headaches, nausea and vomiting may develop (*Buist RA. Editorial: Vitamin toxicities, side effects and contraindications. Int Clin Nutr Rev 4(4):159-71, 1984*).

May cause <u>abnormal bone growth</u> in young children due to premature epiphyseal closing and thickening of the cortical regions (*Buist RA. Editorial: Vitamin toxicities, side effects and contraindications. Int Clin Nutr Rev 4(4):159-71, 1984*).

Very high doses of vitamin A have been shown to produce more than 70 types of <u>congenital abnormalities</u> in experimental animals, and 5 cases of human birth defects have been reported where unusually high doses of vitamin A had been taken during pregnancy; however, no clear cause-and-effect relationship was demonstrated in any of these cases (*Bauernfeind JC. The Safe Use Of Vitamin A: A Report of the International Vitamin A Consultative Group. Washington, DC, The Nutrition Foundation, 1980*).

Hypervitaminosis A is often associated with <u>hypercalcemia</u> and <u>hypercalciuria</u> and calcium deposition in soft tissues may occur (*Buist RA. Editorial: Vitamin toxicities, side effects and contraindications. Int Clin Nutr Rev 4(4):159-71, 1984*).

<u>Hyperplasia of both liver and spleen</u> may occur with megadosages with elevation of AST. Liver biopsies reveal hepatic fibrosis, fat deposition, obstruction of portal blood flow with portal hypertension and sclerosis of vessels (*Buist RA. Editorial: Vitamin toxicities, side effects and contraindications. Int Clin Nutr Rev 4(4):159-71, 1984; Krasinski SD et al. Relationship of vitamin A and vitamin E intake to fasting plasma retinol, retinol-binding protein, retinyl esters, carotene, α-tocopherol, and cholesterol among elderly people and young adults: increased plasma retinyl esters among vitamin A-supplement users. Am J Clin Nutr 49:112-20, 1989*).

Elevated retinol levels may play an important role in the development of some attacks of gouty arthritis (*Marson AR. Letter. Lancet 1:1181, 1984*).

In most cases, when vitamin A intake is discontinued, many symptoms are relieved within a few days or a week, and full recovery usually follows within weeks or months. Irreversible effects include bone changes and cirrhosis (*Bauernfeind JC. The Safe Use Of Vitamin A: A Report of the International Vitamin A Consultative Group. Washington, DC, The Nutrition Foundation, 1980*).

Despite its potential for side effects, megadoses of vitamin A appear to be reasonably safe for the treatment of cancer (*Infante M et al. Laboratory evaluation during high-dose vitamin A administration: A randomized study on lung cancer patients after surgical resection. J Cancer Res 117:156-62, 1991*).

Vitamin B₆:

Supplementation may cause a sensory neuropathy in doses as low as 200 mg daily over 3 years (usually 2-5 gm daily). The neurotoxicity is believed to be due to exceeding the liver's ability to phosphorylate pyridoxine to the active coenzyme, pyridoxal phosphate. The resulting high pyridoxine blood level could be directly neurotoxic or may compete for binding sites with pyridoxal phosphate resulting in a relative deficiency of the active metabolite (*Parry GJ, Bredesen DE. Sensory neuropathy with low-dose pyridoxine. Neurology 35:1466-68, 1985; Waterston JA, Gilligan BS. Pyridoxine neuropathy. Med J Aust 146:640-42, 1987*). Supplementation in the form of pyridoxal phosphate should thus avoid this danger.

> **Experimental and Observational Study:** 103/172 (60%) women with premenstrual syndrome who had elevated blood pyridoxine levels complained of neurological symptoms (paresthesias, hyperesthesia, bone pain, muscle weakness, numbness, fasciculations). On average, their daily dose had been 117 mg for 2.9 years. 3 mo. after stopping B₆ supplements (and following a program of PMS treatment), 55% reported partial or complete symptom relief. After 6 mo., all women were asymptomatic. 7 pts. who failed to stop B₆ continued to have symptoms (*Dalton K, Dalton MJT. Characteristics of pyridoxine overdose neuropathy syndrome. Acta Neurol Scand 76:8, 1987*).

> *Note: Vague neurological complaints are common among PMS sufferers and may be due to numerous causes. This uncontrolled study on patients who were simultaneously in active multi-faceted treatment program fails to demonstrate that symptom relief was due to stopping pyridoxine supplements. The patients who failed to improve and also failed to stop pyridoxine may well have been treatment failures because of their failure to comply with other aspects of the treatment program (Gaby AR. Editorial: Vitamin B₆ toxicity: How much is too much? Townsend Letter for Doctors, May, 1988, p. 184).*

Supplementation with 100 mg or more daily may impair memorization (*Molimard R et al. Impairment of memorization by high doses of pyridoxine in man. Biomedicine 32:88-92, 1980*).

Supplementation may cause an acniform eruption or worsening of acne vulgaris (*Braun-Falco O, Lincke H. [The problem of vitamin B₆/B₁₂ acne. A contribution on acne medicamentosa. MMW 118(6):155-60, 1976*).

Vitamin B₁₂:

Supplementation may cause an acniform eruption or worsening of acne vulgaris (*Braun-Falco O, Lincke H. [The problem of vitamin B₆/B₁₂ acne. A contribution on acne medicamentosa. MMW 118(6):155-60, 1976*).

Vitamin C:

Diarrhea is the major side-effect of large doses.

Megadoses (over 6 gm daily) may increase urinary oxalate excretion which may be contraindicated in renal insufficiency and in calcium oxalate stone-formers.

> **Review Article:** Urinary oxalate excretion generally does not increase significantly for both normal subjects and stone-formers with ascorbic acid supplementation unless doses exceed 6 gm daily; however, oxalate excretion even at those high doses is still usually in the range achievable by dietary influences alone. The exceptions derive from anecdotal reports of a small number of cases and from one poorly-controlled trial with unstated methodology

and questionable assay techniques (*Piesse JW. Nutritional factors in calcium containing kidney stones with particular emphasis on vitamin C. Int Clin Nutr Rev 5(3):110-129, 1985*).

Contraindicated in cases of <u>iron overload</u> due to its enhancement of iron absorption (*Nienhuis A. N Engl J Med 304(3):170-71, 1981*).

Sudden discontinuation of large doses can cause <u>rebound scurvy</u> (*New roles for vitamin C. New Scientist 11:23, 1985; Jakovlieu N. Lanachrunestorschune 3:446, 1958*); thus supplementation should be gradually tapered over several days or weeks.

Enhances aluminum absorption; therefore should not be taken with aluminum-containing substances, especially when the patient has renal insufficiency (*Domingo JL et al. Effect of ascorbic acid on gastrointestinal aluminum absorption. Letter. Lancet 338:1467, 1991*).

Vitamin D:

Excessive intake may cause <u>hypercalcemia</u> due to increased intestinal absorption of calcium which can quickly lead to reduction of kidney function (due to nephocalcinosis from deposition of calcium phosphate) and soft tissue calcifications, especially in the joints, blood vessels, stomach, lungs and heart (*Buist RA. Editorial: Vitamin toxicities, side effects and contraindications. Int Clin Nutr Rev 4(4):159-71, 1984*).

Vitamin E:

In reviewing over 10,000 cases of subjects consuming 200-3000 IU/d for up to 11 years, the incidence of nonspecific side effects was 0.8%, a level expected in untreated populations (*Salkald RM. Safety and tolerance of high-dose vitamin E administration in man: A review of the literature. Fed Register (US) 44:16172, 1979*).

Reports of adverse symptoms from large supplemental doses are largely subjective and based on limited observations. In fact, doses as high as 3200 mg/d have not been found to induce adverse side effects. However, vitamin E supplementation has been shown to exacerbate the effects of vitamin K deficiency (*Bendich A, Machlin LJ. Safety of oral intake of vitamin E. Am J Clin Nutr 48:612-19, 1988*).

The most common complaint following large supplemental doses is transient <u>GI disturbances</u> (nausea, flatulence, or diarrhea) (*Bieri JG. Medical uses of vitamin E. N Engl J Med 308(18):1063-71, 1983*).

Supplementation may exacerbate <u>hypertension</u>. When the oily form is used, this effect is accompanied by an increase in the serum triglycerides:vitamin E ratio; thus the water miscible form is preferred for patients with <u>cardiovascular disorders</u> and <u>diabetes mellitus</u> (*Buist RA. Editorial: Vitamin toxicities, side effects and contraindications. Int Clin Nutr Rev 4(4):159-71, 1984*).

As Vitamin E may reduce the insulin requirement, <u>diabetics on insulin</u> should be started on 100 IU or less daily and the dosage raised showly with adjustment of the insulin dose (*Vogelsang A. Vitamin E in the treatment of diabetes mellitus. Ann N Y Acad Sci 52:406, 1949*).

Daily doses of 40,000 IU or more during <u>pregnancy</u> may be teratogenic (*Martinez-Frias ML, Salvador J. Megadose vitamin A and teratogenicity. Letter. Lancet 1:236, 1988*), while doses lower than 10,000 IU appear to be safe (*Smithell RW. Spina bifida and vitamins. Br Med J 286:388-89, 1983*).

Reports of megadoses of vitamin E causing a <u>decrease in thyroid hormone</u> (*Roberts HJ. Thrombophlebitis associated with vitamin E therapy with commentary on other medical side effects. Angiology 30:169-76, 1979; Tsai AC et al. Study on the effect of megavitamin E supplementation in man. Am J Clin Nutr 31:831-37, 1978*) were not confirmed in a double-blind study (*Brin MF et al. Relationship between dose of vitamin E administered and blood level. Ann N Y Acad Sci, 1989*).

Zinc:

Pharmacologic doses of zinc (≈100-300 mg daily) for several weeks can impair immune responses (*Chandra RK. Excessive intake of zinc impairs immune responses. JAMA 252(11):1443-46, 1984*).

Pharmacologic doses of zinc (≈100-300 mg daily) for several months can produce a severe copper deficiency causing hypocupremia, anemia, leukopenia and neutropenia (*Copper deficiency induced by megadoses of zinc. Nutr Rev 43(5):148-49, 1985; Broun RE et al. Excessive zinc ingestion: a reversible cause of sideroblastic anemia and bone marrow depression. JAMA 264:1441-3, 1990; Forman WB et al. Zinc abuse: an unsuspected cause of sideroblastic anemia. West J Med 152:190-2, 1990; Hoffman HN II et al. Zinc-induced copper deficiency. Gastroenterology 94:508-12, 1988; Prasad AS et al. Hypocupremia induced by zinc deficiency in adults. JAMA 240:2166-8, 1978*).

Similarly, the lowering of copper levels in response to high doses of zinc (>150 mg daily) may be responsible for causing a marked decrease in HDL cholesterol (*Hooper PL et al. Zinc lowers high-density lipoprotein-cholesterol levels. JAMA 244:1960, 1980; Klevey LM. Interactions of copper and zinc in cardiovascular disease. Ann N Y Acad Sci 355:140-51, 1980; Fischer P et al. The effect of dietary copper and zinc on cholesterol metabolism. Am J Clin Nutr 33:1019-25, 1980*).
Concurrent supplementation with 1.0 mg daily of copper will prevent copper deficiency due to zinc supplementation; also copper status can be easily monitored by following serum ceruloplasmin levels (*Yuzbasiyan-Gurkan V, Brewer GJ. The therapeutic use of zinc in macular degeneration. Letter. Arch Ophthalmol 107:1723, 1989*).

Other possible side-effects of pharmacologic dosages are occasional nausea, increased sweating, alcohol intolerance and transient worsening of depression or hallucinations. In addition, zinc supplementation may increase grand mal seizures in epileptics, possibly due to a reduction in blood manganese levels; thus, for epileptics, manganese supplementation should be started prior to zinc supplementation (*Pfeiffer CC, LaMola S. Zinc and manganese in the schizophrenias. J Orthomol Psychiatry 12:215-234, 1983*).

LABORATORY METHODS FOR NUTRITIONAL EVALUATION

Note: Tests are presented in the rough order of preference, with tests that appear superior listed first.

GENERAL: (Protein Energy Malnutrition)

Laboratory indicators (*Wright RA. Commentary: Nutritional assessment. JAMA 244(6),1980*):

1. decreased serum albumin concentration in the absence of liver disease (< 3.4 g/dL).
2. decreased serum transferrin (seen in starvation earlier than decreased serum albumin).
3. decreased total lymphocyte count (< 1500/mm^3).
4. decreased 24-hour urine creatinine (roughly proportional to skeletal muscle mass).

Aluminum:

Hair analysis, when properly performed, is a reliable measure of tissue levels (*Yokel RA. Clin Chem 28(4):662-5, 1982; Jenkins DW. Toxic Metals in Mammalian Hair and Nails. EPA Report 600/4-79-049 August, 1979 - available through the U.S. Natl Technical Information Service*). As yet, it cannot be concluded whether aluminum concentrations in hair give a better representation of the body burden than serum aluminum levels do (*De Groot HJ et al. Determination by flameless atomic absorption of aluminum in serum and hair by toxicological monitoring of patients on chronic intermittent haemodialysis. Pharm Weekbl [Sci] 6(1):11-15, 1984*).

Arsenic:

Hair analysis, when properly performed, is a reliable measure of tissue levels (*Jenkins DW. Toxic Metals in Mammalian Hair and Nails. EPA Report 600/4-79-049 August, 1979 - available through the U.S. Natl Technical Information Service*).

Urine arsenic levels, like hair levels, increase as intake increases. Blood arsenic levels, however, do not increase until chronic toxicity is reached and give variable results for lower levels of exposure (*Valentine JL et al. Arsenic levels in human blood, urine, and hair in response to exposure via drinking water. Environ Res 20:24-32, 1979*).

Biotin:

There are no sensitive chemical methods for biotin assay, but the flagellate Ochromonas danica, which has a specific and ultrasensitive biotin requirement, has provided a suitable microbiological assay for measuring biotin in blood, serum, urine, brain and liver (*Baker H. Assessment of biotin status: Clinical implications. Ann N Y Acad Sci. 447:129-32, 1985*).

The two principal criteria of biotin status are blood and urine levels. Blood levels can show extremely wide variation between individuals, so the significance of low plasma levels is uncertain, especially since biotin deficiency seems rare. In children, however, blood and urine levels are more helpful. For example, levels are lower than normal in infants with seborrheic dermatitis and Leiner's Disease who respond to biotin injections (*Whitehead CC. The assessment of biotin status in man and animals. Proc Nutr Sci 40:165-72, 1981*).

Cadmium:

Hair analysis, when properly performed, is a reliable measure of tissue levels (*Jenkins DW. Toxic Metals in Mammalian Hair and Nails. EPA Report 600/4-79-049 August, 1979 - available through the U.S. Natl Technical Information Service*) and is superior to blood in reflecting long term cadmium exposure (*Thatcher RW et al. Effects of low levels of cadmium and lead on cognitive functioning in children. Arch Environ Health 37:159-65, 1982*).

Blood levels are a poor measure of cadmium toxicity as the metal remains in the blood for only a very brief period of time and thus the levels are always extremely low (*Petering HG et al. Trace element content of hair: Cadmium and lead of human hair. Arch Environ Health 27:327-30, 1973*).

Calcium:

Ionized calcium, a measure of unbound serum calcium, is perhaps the most useful measure of calcium balance at present when it is low, but values can be normal in the presence of a negative calcium balance (*Albanese A. Bone Loss: Causes, Detection and Therapy. New York, Alan R. Liss, Inc., 1977*). Total serum calcium is subjected to such close homeostatic regulation that it fails to reflect body calcium status.

Hair analysis is of some value, but its results are limited by the fact that a negative calcium balance may by accompanied by elevated hair levels, and by the lack of norms for grey hair which is naturally lower in calcium (*Cranton EM. Update on hair element analysis in clinical medicine. J Holistic Med 7(2):120-134, 1985*).

Carnitine:

Plasma and RBC levels may vary independently.

> **Observational Study:** Healthy adult blood was sampled for carnitine content. It appeared that carnitine pools may exist in at least 2 different compartments: plasma and RBC. One may be high and the other low, with different effects seen for each deficiency (*Borum PR et al. Am J Clin Nutr 46:437, 1987*).

Chromium:

The most dependable criterion for the diagnosis of chromium deficiency may be the correction of impaired glucose tolerance in response to chromium supplementation, but it requires strict control of dietary intake over an extended period (*Glinsmann WH et al. Plasma chromium after glucose administration. Science 152:1243-45, 1966*).

Although evaluation is hindered by the extremely low levels involved, urinary chromium is a reasonable measure of chromium absorption as the majority of absorbed chromium is excreted in the urine (*Anderson RA, Kozlovsky AS. Chromium intake, absorption and excretion of subjects consuming self-selected diets. Am J Clin Nutr 41:1177-83, 1985*). Repeating urinary chromium after an oral glucose load, according to some authors, may be useful - as the lack of an increase suggests exhaustion of biologically important chromium stores (*Mertz W. Effects and metabolism of glucose tolerance factor, in Present Knowledge in Nutrition. Fourth Edition. Washington, D.C., The Nutrition Foundation, Inc., 1976*). However, urinary chromium excretion may be unaffected by chromium supplementation (*Anderson RA et al. Urinary chromium excretion of human subjects: Effects of chromium supplementation and glucose loading. Am J Clin Nutr 36, 1982*).

Hair analysis cannot distinguish between contamination by the hexavalent, toxic chromium and the trivalent, nutritional chromium (*Passwater, RA, Cranton EM. Trace Elements, Hair Analysis and Nutrition. New Canaan, Conn., Keats Publishing, Inc., 1983:195*). Moreover, because of the low levels involved, hair chromium content has been considered to be too insensitive to identify any but the most severe deficiencies (*Richman S. Chromium, an overview. Anabolism 1-2:5,12, 1984; Hambridge KM. Chromium nutrition in man. Am J Clin Nutr 27:505-14, 1974*). At least one study, however, suggests that hair chromium levels may be a useful index of chromium status (*Hunt AE et al. Effect of chromium supplementation on hair chromium concentration and diabetic status. Nutr Res 5:131-40, 1985*).

In response to a standard glucose load, serum chromium levels may drop one hour later in subjects with presumably inadequate chromium storage. An improvement in the ratio of the serum chromium level one hour after glucose loading to the baseline level (the "relative chromium response") after chromium supplementation may thus be a measure of improved chromium status (*Lui VJK, Morris S. Relative chromium response as an indicator of chromium status. Am J Clin Nutr 31:972-76, 1978*).

A reliable range for serum chromium is lacking (*Sauberlich HE et al. Laboratory Tests For The Assessment Of Nutritional Status. Florida, CRC Press, 1984*). Chromium supplementation may not affect serum levels (*Polansky MM et al. Serum chromium as an indicator of chromium status of humans. Fed Proc 43, 1984*), and serum chromium is not in equilibrium with tissue stores (*Underwood EJ. Trace Elements in Human and Animal Nutrition. New York, Academic Press, 1977*). Likewise, whole blood chromium has not been shown to reflect tissue stores (*Mertz W. Physiol Rev 49:163-239, 1969*).

Copper:

RBC superoxide dismutase is probably the best index of copper status (*Hill G, Edes TE. Diabetes and carbohydrates: The copper connection. JAMA 257(19):2593, 1987*).

Confirmation of an elevated body copper burden can be provided by the D-penicillamine challenge test. D-penicillamine 250 mg is given orally every 6 hours away from meals and the urine test is performed on the third day of treatment. Copper urinary excretion usually increases 10-20 fold. In normals, it will be in the range of 500 µg/24h while, in patients with Wilson's Disease, it will be at least 1,000 µg/24h or even above 2,000 µg/24h (*Walshe JM. The discovery of the therapeutic use of D-penicillamine. J Rheumatol (Suppl 7) 8:3-8, 1981*).

Total RBC copper concentration is widely available. 60% of RBC copper is in superoxide dismutase, while the remainder is in both a readily diffusable pool and a non-dialyzed protein-bound pool (*Halloran SP, in DF Williams, Ed. Copper In Systemic Aspects Of Biocompatability, Vol. 1. Boca Raton FL, CDC Press, 1981:211*).

Whole blood copper levels are a combination of approximately equal quantities of copper in the cells and plasma (*Kiem J et al. Sampling and sample preparation of platelets for trace element analysis in nuclear activation techniques in the life sciences, 1978. IAEA, Vienna, 1979:143*); thus, when whole blood copper is depressed, it suggests a deficiency in cells, plasma or both. Normal or elevated whole blood copper may be reflecting an elevation in one blood fraction while another fraction may be normal or even depressed.

90-95% of serum copper is tightly bound to ceruloplasmin which may make it an insensitive test for marginal deficiencies (*Fisher G. Function and homeostasis of Cu and Zn in mammals. Sci Total Environ 4:373, 1975*). In addition, ceruloplasmin is an acute-phase reactant protein, and thus its levels may vary without regard to copper nutriture (*Hill G, Edes TE. Diabetes and carbohydrates: The copper connection. JAMA 257(19):2593, 1987*).

Hair copper correlates well with copper levels in other organs, although errors from external contamination of hair (copper-containing fungicides in swimming pools, contaminated water supplies, hair treatments) may occur, and levels are unreliable in the presence of copper-loading liver diseases (*Cranton EM. Update on hair element analysis in clinical medicine. J Holistic Med 7(2):120-134, 1985; Jacob RA. Hair as a biopsy material v. hair metal as an index of hepatic metal in rats: Copper and zinc. Am J Clin Nutr 31:477-80, 1978*). In addition, hair copper may be normal despite gross copper deficiency (*Bradfield RB et al. Preliminary communication: hair copper in copper deficiency. Lancet 2:343-44, 1980*).

Folic Acid:

While serum folate tends to reflect recent dietary intake and folate balance, RBC folate concentration is less sensitive to short-term variations in folate balance. Thus, as a better measure of body folate stores, it is more reliable for indicating risk of development of folate deficiency and can be used as an index of folate depletion (*Anderson SA, Talbot JM. A Review Of Folate Intake, Methodology And Status. Bethesda, MD, Federation of American Societies for Experimental Biology, 1981; Herbert V. Making sense of laboratory test of folate status: folate requirements to sustain normality. Am J Hematol 26:199-207, 1987*).

However, folate depletion in erythrocytes occurs only in the later stages of folic acid deficiency and is usually accompanied by megaloblastic anemia; thus patients with both acquired and inherited folate deficiency may remain moderately deficient for months or years, taking in just enough folate to prevent low RBC folate concentrations and frank anemia (*Botez MI et al. Neurologic disorders responsive to folic acid therapy. Can Med Assoc J 115:217-22, 1976; Herbert V. Experimental nutritional folate deficiency in man. Trans Assoc Am Physicians 75:307, 1962*). Therefore, both RBC and serum folate studies should be done to evaluate for folate deficiency.

Microbiological assays remain the standard procedure for measuring total folic acid activity in serum, blood, tissues, and foods. Although a number of commercial radioassay kits are available for measuring folic acid levels in serum and erythrocytes, some uncertanties exist about the validity of the folate values obtained (*Sauberlich HE. Newer laboratory methods for assessing nutriture of selected B-complex vitamins. Annu Rev Nutr 4:377-407, 1984*).

> *Note: A recent study found that, when chronically ill elderly pts. were compared to healthy young controls, radioimmunoassays showed normal serum and RBC folate concentrations in all elderly patients and all but one of the controls, while microbiological assays showed below normal values of serum folate in 6.8% of the elderly patients and 12.2% of the controls, and below normal values of RBC folate in 1.8% of patients and 4.8% of controls, suggesting that radioimmunoassay procedures are superior (Grinblat J et al. Folate and vitamin B$_{12}$ levels in an urban elderly population with chronic diseases. J Am Geriatr Soc 34:627-32, 1986).*

Serum folate is highly correlated with CSF folate and better correlated with CSF folate than is RBC folate. However, it is not known in man whether a low CSF folate is necessarily accompanied by a fall in brain folate level, but experimental studies have suggested that the latter falls last, when stores elsewhere are severely depleted (*Reynolds EH. Interrelationships between the neurology of folate and vitamin B$_{12}$ deficiency, in MI Botez, EH Reynolds, Eds. Folic Acid in Neurology, Psychiatry, and Internal Medicine. New York, Raven Press, 1979*).

In folate deficiency, the urine formiminoglutamic acid (FIGLU) level rises. High FIGLU excretion also occurs, however, in vitamin B$_{12}$ deficiency and in liver disease; thus it is not specific for folate deficiency (*Herbert V. Experimental nutritional folate deficiency in man. Trans Assoc Am Phys 75:307-20, 1962*).

The determination of hypersegmentation of neutrophils is a useful measure of folate deficiency, although it is unreliable during pregnancy and fails to distinguish folate and vitamin B$_{12}$ deficiciencies (*Sauberlich HE. Newer laboratory methods for assessing nutriture of selected B-complex vitamins. Annu Rev Nutr 4:377-407, 1984*):

$$\text{hypersegmentation index} = \frac{\text{neutrophils with 5 or more "lobes"}}{\text{neutrophils with 4 "lobes"}} \times 100$$

Normal (serum folate 3.5-16 mg/ml): hypersegmentation index of 2-30% (mean: 10.3%)
Abnormal: hypersegmentation index of 31.5-116% (mean: 62.4%)

(*Bills T, Spatz L. Neutrophilic hypersegmentation as an indication of incipient folic acid deficiency. Am J Clin Pathol 68(2):263, 1977*).

> *Note: Supplementation of 5 mg folate daily will usually bring the index to 0%, but higher amounts are sometimes necessary (rule out vitamin B$_{12}$ deficiency and uremia) (Wright J. The neutrophilic hypersegmentation index ("NHI"): an inexpensive, underutilized test of folate nutrition. Int Clin Nutr Rev 10(4):435-37, 1990).*

Iron:

Bone marrow aspiration is the procedure of choice, while serum ferritin, an iron storage protein, is a reasonably good indicator of total body iron storage. Serum iron is a poor measure of iron nutriture as iron may be deficient despite the lack of anemia and normal serum iron levels. Like transferrin saturation, it may only become abnormal after iron stores have been completely exhausted (*Finch CA. Editorial: Evaluation of iron status. JAMA 251(15):2004, 1984; Frank P, Wang S. Serum iron and total iron binding capacity compared with serum ferritin in assessment of iron deficiency. Clin Chem 27(2):276-79, 1981; Cook JD et al. Serum ferritin as a measure of iron stores in normal subjects. Am J Clin Nutr 27:681-7, 1974*).

In children, transferrin saturation, hemoglobin and a peripheral blood smear must be done in conjunction with serum ferritin, as ferritin may be normal despite iron deficiency (*Madanat F et al. Serum ferritin in evaluation of iron status in children. Acta Haematol 71:111, 1984*).

An iron tolerance test may be useful in determining iron deficiency:

> **Observational Study:** Men with normal iron stores showed little change in plasma iron after ingesting 5, 10 or 20 mg of ferrous sulfate or ferrous fumarate, while plasma iron levels rose significantly when men with a mild

iron deficiency took similar doses of iron (*Crosby WH, O'Neill-Cutting MA. A small dose iron tolerance test as an indicator of mild iron deficiency. JAMA 251(15):1986-87, 1984*).

The automated blood cell count, when it includes the red cell distribution width (RDW), is an inexpensive yet adequate screening test for iron deficiency, but only in healthy patients (*Bessman JD, McClure S. Detection of iron deficiency anemia. Letter. JAMA 266(12):1649, 1991*).

Hair iron has no known relationship to tissue levels.

Lead:

Hair analysis, when properly performed, is a reliable measure of tissue levels and the method of choice for diagnosing lead poisoning, although confirmatory studies are necessary (*Passwater, RA, Cranton EM. Trace Elements, Hair Analysis and Nutrition. New Canaan, Conn., Keats Publishing, Inc., 1983; Jenkins DW. Toxic Metals in Mammalian Hair and Nails. EPA Report 600/4-79-049 August, 1979 - available through the U.S. Natl Technical Information Service; Rabinowitz M et al. Delayed appearance of tracer lead in facial hair. Arch Environ Health July/Aug., 1976, pp. 220-23*).

Zinc protoporphyrin content is a second choice for diagnosing lead poisoning, while blood lead levels are inadequate as blood rapidly deposits lead into the skeletal tissues and hair (*Passwater, RA, Cranton EM. Trace Elements, Hair Analysis and Nutrition. New Canaan, Conn., Keats Publishing, Inc., 1983:195*).

Magnesium:

A magnesium challenge test is the best method of ascertaining body stores (*Fourth Internat. Sympos. on Magnesium. J Am Coll Nutr 4:303, 1985*) as serum and RBC magnesium levels remain normal unless magnesium depletion is severe (*Rea WJ et al. Magnesium deficiency in patients with chemical sensitivity. Clin Ecology 4(1):17-20, 1986*):

While on a stable intake of magnesium, a baseline urine is obtained and magnesium chloride or magnesium sulfate 0.2 meq/kg IV is given over a 4 hour period. A second urine is began at challenge and continued over a 24 hour period. Deficiency is defined as <80% excretion of the amt. of challenged magnesium (*Jones JE et al. Magnesium requirements in adults. Med J Clin Nutr 20:632-35, 1967*).

24-hour urinary excretion of magnesium is a sensitive index of magnesium status (*Galland L. Magnesium and inflammatory bowel disease. Magnesium 7(2):78-83, 1988*). A finding of <25 mg/day suggests magnesium depletion (*Lauler DP. Introduction: Magnesium - Coming of age. Am J Cardiol 63(14):1G, 1989*).

Leukocyte and lymphocyte magnesium levels are better correlated with tissue magnesium levels than are serum levels (*Peter WF et al. Leucocyte magnesium concentration as an indicator of myocardial magnesium. Nutr Rep Int 26:105, July 1982; Juan D. Clinical review: The clinical importance of hypomagnesemia. Surgery 5:510-16, 1982*).

RBC magnesium is less reliable than WBC magnesium as magnesium concentrations are 3-4 times as high in reticulocytes as in mature cells and they decline with the age of cells (*Watson WS et al. Magnesium metabolism in blood and the whole body in man using [28]magnesium. Metabolism 28:90-5, 1979*). Moreover, RBC magnesium does not correlated with the magnesium content of other cell types (*Alfrey AC, Miller NL, Butkus D. Evaluation of body magnesium stores. J Lab Clin Med 84:153-62, 1974; Elin RJ, Hosseini JM. Magnesium content of mononuclear blood cells. Clin Chem 31:377-80, 1985*) and is at least partly genetically determined (*Henrotte JB. Genetic regulation of red blood cell magnesium content and major histocampatibility complex. Magnesium 5:317-27, 1982*).

Blood magnesium parameters (plasma, serum, RBC, mononuclear blood cells) may fail to correlate with one another (*Ralston MA et al. Magnesium content of serum, circulating mononuclear cells, skeletal muscle, and myocardium in congestive heart failure. Circulation 80(3):573-80, 1989; Yang XY et al. Blood and urine magnesium parameters compared. Abstract. J Am Coll Nutr 8(5):462, 1989*).

Skeletal and myocardial magnesium levels may fail to correlate with one another as well as with blood magnesium parameters (serum and circulating mononuclear cells) (*Ralston MA et al. Magnesium content of serum, circulating mononuclear cells, skeletal muscle, and myocardium in congestive heart failure. Circulation 80(3):573-80, 1989*).

Blood magnesium parameters fail to correlate with urine excretion and clearance of magnesium (*Yang XY et al. Blood and urine magnesium parameters compared. Abstract. J Am Coll Nutr 8(5):462, 1989*).

Serum magnesium may fail to reflect tissue magnesium levels (*L'Estrange JL, Axford R. Study of magnesium and calcium metabolism in lactating ewes fed semi-purified diet low in magnesium. J Agric Sci 62, 1964; Richardson JA, Welt LG. Hypomagnesemia of vitamin D administration. Proc Soc Exp Biol Med 118, 1965*).

Hair magnesium levels are not always reliable as they tend to be elevated when magnesium is is being lost from bones and are lower in grey hair (*Cranton EM. Update on hair element analysis in clinical medicine. J Holistic Med 7(2):120-134, 1985*).

Manganese:

Whole blood manganese is considered to be a valid indicator of body manganese and soft tissue levels (*Keen CL et al. Whole blood manganese as an indicator of body manganese. N Engl J Med 308:1230, 1983*).

Lymphocyte manganese has been shown to be a reliable indicator of manganese nutriture (*Matsuda A et al. Quantifying manganese in lymphocytes to assess manganese nutritional status. Clin Chem 35(9):1939-41, 1989*).

Serum and sweat manganese levels correlate well with the activation of isocitrate dehydrogenase, a simple and inexpensive functional test of manganese nutriture, suggesting that all 3 measures are valid indicators (*Hunnisett A et al. A new functional test of manganese status. J Nutr Med 1:209-15, 1990*).

Hair manganese may be a reliable indicator of body manganese status (*Cranton EM. Update on hair element analysis in clinical medicine. J Holistic Med 7(2):120-134, 1985*), although greying hair has a lower concentration than black hair (*Guillard O et al. Manganese concentration in the hair of greying ("salt and pepper") men reconsidered. Clin Chem 31(7):1251, 1985*).

Mercury:

The amount of hair mercury reflects the body burden of mercury (*Airey D. Mercury in human hair due to environment and diet: A review. Environ Health Perspect 52:303-16, 1983*).

Blood mercury is useful for assessing recent methyl mercury exposure (*Berglund F et al. [Methyl mercury in fish, a toxologic-epidemiologic evaluation of risks: Report from an expert group.] Nord Hyg T Suppl. 4, 1971 - published in Nord Hyg T Suppl. 3, 1970*), but not for assessing exposure to inorganic mercurials (*Friberg L, Nordberg GF. Inorganic mercury: Relation between exposure and effects, in L Friberg, L, J Vostal, Eds. Mercury in the Environment. Cleveland, Ohio, Chemical Rubber Co. Press, 1972:113-39*).

Urinary mercury measurements are unreliable as an indication of mercury poisoning (*Ladd AD et al. Absorption and exretion of mercury in man. II. Urinary mercury in relation to duration of exposure. Arch Environ Health 6:480-3, 1963*).

Niacin:

Attempts to diagnose deficiency by measuring nicotinic acid in body fluids have proved disappointing; measurements of metabolites have been more meaningful. In general, plasma niacin metabolites are generally less reliable than urinary metabolites (*Jacob RA et al. Biochemical markers for asessment of niacin status in young men: urinary and blood levels of niacin metabolites. J Nutr 119(4):591-8, 1989*).

The urinary excretion of N^1-methylnicotinamide (NMN) and of 2-pyr are reasonably good measures of niacin status (*Jacob RA et al. Biochemical markers for asessment of niacin status in young men: urinary and blood levels of niacin metabolites. J Nutr 119(4):591-8, 1989*). The excretion ratio of 2-pyr to NMN was formerly considered the most reliable indicator (*Sauberlich HE et al. Laboratory Tests for the Assessment of Nutritional Status. Boca Raton, Florida, CRC Press, 1974:70-4*). However, in a recent study, it was less useful than individual measurements of the 2 metabolites (*Jacob RA et al. Biochemical markers for asessment of niacin status in young men: urinary and blood levels of niacin metabolites. J Nutr 119(4):591-8, 1989*).

Erythrocyte nicotinamide adenine nucleotide (NAD) also appears to be a sensitive indicator of niacin nutriture, and a ratio of RBC NAD to RBC nicotinamide nucleotide phosphate (NADP) below 1.0 may identify subjects at risk of developing a niacin deficiency (*Fu CS et al. Biochemical markers for assessment of niacin status in young men: levels of erythrocyte niacin coenzymes and plasma tryptophan. J Nutr 119(12):1949-55, 1989*).

Nickel:

Hair analysis, when properly performed, is a reliable measure of tissue levels when nickel levels are elevated; low hair nickel has no known clinical significance. Due to the possibility of external contamination, blood or urine studies should be performed for confirmation (*Passwater, RA, Cranton EM. Trace Elements, Hair Analysis and Nutrition. New Canaan, Conn., Keats Publishing, Inc., 1983; Jenkins DW. Toxic Metals in Mammalian Hair and Nails. EPA Report 600/4-79-049 August, 1979 - available through the U.S. Natl Technical Information Service*).

Pantothenic Acid:

Blood pantothenic acid responds less readily to intake than urinary pantothenic acid although, in general, blood pantothenic acid levels decrease in subjects given a pantothenic acid deficient diet (*Fry PC, Fox HM, Tao HG. Metabolic response to a pantothenic acid deficient diet in humans. J Nutr Sci Vitaminol 22:339-46, 1976*).

Phosphorus:

Plasma phosphate is mainly controlled by renal excretion.

Hair phosphorus has little or no relationship to phosphorus metabolism in the body or to dietary phosphorus intake (*Passwater RA, Cranton EM. Trace Elements, Hair Analysis and Nutrition. New Canaan, Connecticut, Keats Publishing, 1983:61*).

Potassium:

Red blood cell potassium (or whole blood potassium) is superior to serum potassium level as an index of cellular potassium stores (*Bahemuka M, Hodkinson HM. Red-blood-cell potassium as a practical index of potassium status in elderly patients. Age Ageing 5:24, 1976; Sangiori GB et al. Serum potassium levels, red-blood-cell potassium and alterations of the repolarization phase of electrocardiography in old subjects. Age Ageing 13:309, 1984*).

Serum potassium levels are slightly higher than plasma levels (*Hyman D, Kaplan NM. The difference between serum and plasma potassium. Letter. N Engl J Med September 5, 1985, p. 642*).

Plasma potassium may be falsely increased by up to 1.0 mmol/l by fist-clenching to make the veins more prominent for venipuncture (*Brown JJ et al. Falsely high plasma potassium values in patients with hyperaldosteronism. Br Med J 2:18-20, 1970*), and anxiety over venipuncture may produce enough hyperventilation-induced respiratory alkalosis to lower the level by that much or more (*Edwards R et al. Acute hypocapneic hypokalemia: An iatrogenic anesthetic complication. Anesth Analg 56:786-92, 1977*).

Hair potassium levels do not reflect dietary intake or body stores (*Passwater RA, Cranton EM. Trace Elements, Hair Analysis and Nutrition. New Canaan, Connecticut, Keats Publishing, 1983:85*).

Riboflavin:

The procedure most commonly used to evaluate riboflavin nutriture is the measurement of RBC glutathione reductase (EGR) activity and the stimulation of this activity by flavin adenine dinucleotide (FAD) added *in vitro*. The EGR activity is commonly expressed in terms of "activity coefficient" or in terms of percent stimulation, both of which are derived from the stimulating effect of FAD added *in vitro* to the enzyme reaction. Some animal studies suggest that certain deficiencies, such as thiamine, nicotinic acid and pyridoxine, may reduce the apo-enzyme level (*Sharada D, Bamji MS. Erythrocyte glutathione reductase activity and riboflavin concentration in experimental deficiency of some water soluble vitamins. Int J Vitam Nutr Res 42:43-49, 1972*). Both the age of the subject and the age of the red cell may also influence EGR activity, and the assay may not be valid in subjects with low RBC glucose-6-phosphate dehydrogenase activity (*Sauberlich HE. Newer laboratory methods for assessing nutriture of selected B-complex vitamins. Annu Rev Nutr 4:377-407, 1984*).

Blood riboflavin levels are not necessarily good measures of riboflavin status because of the difficulty in achieving accurate measurements (*Bamjii MS et al. Relationship between biochemical and clinical indices of B-vitamin deficiency. A study in rural school boys. Br J Nutr 41:431-41, 1979*), although new analytical procedures for measure blood and urinary riboflavin may prove to be useful (*Sauberlich HE. Newer laboratory methods for assessing nutriture of selected B-complex vitamins. Annu Rev Nutr 4:377-407, 1984*).

Urinary riboflavin excretion depends upon nitrogen balance, kidney function and recent intake (*Heller S et al. Riboflavin status in pregnancy. Am J Clin Nutr 27:1225-30, 1974*).

Selenium:

The only true evidence of selenium deficiency lies in a positive response to selenium therapy (*Neve J et al. Selenium deficiency. Clin Endocrinol Metab 14(3):629-56, 1985*).

The level of blood glutathione peroxidase has been shown to be a sensitive index of its selenium content in animals and man (*Ganther HE et al. Selenium and glutathione peroxidase in health and disease - a review, in AS Prasad, D Overleas, Eds. Trace Elements in Human Health and Disease, Volume II. New York, Academic Press, 1976:165*).

Hair selenium is significantly correlated with selenium concentrations in the liver, lung and renal cortex (p<0.01) (*Cheng YD et al. Study of correlation of Se content in human hair and internal organs by INAA. Biol Trace Elem Res 28:737-41 1990*). It also correlates well with selenium intake, and may be superior to whole blood selenium if organic selenium (L-selenomethionine) is the source of selenium (*Gallagher ML et al. Selenium levels in new growth hair and in whole blood during injection of a selenium supplement for six weeks. Nutr Res 4:577-82, 1984; Valentine, JL et al. Selenium levels in human blood, urine and hair in response to exposure via drinking water. Environ Res 17:347-55, 1978*). When additional dietary selenium comes from an inorganic source (selenate or selenite), however, hair selenium rises while muscle selenium levels are relatively unchanged (*Salbe AD, Levander OA. Hair and nails as indicators of selenium status in rats fed elevated dietary levels of selenium as L-selenomethionine (SeMet) or sodium selenate (Na2SeO4). Fed Proc 46(4), March 5, 1987*). In addition, selenium-containing shampoos will falsely elevate hair selenium levels.

The value of blood selenium levels as an indicator of selenium nutriture is limited as it may fail to correlate with selenium intake except at the extremes (*Lane HW et al. Blood selenium and glutathione peroxidase levels and dietary selenium of free living and institutionalized elderly subjects. Proc Soc Exp Biol Med 173(1):87-95, 1985*). Also, once adequate selenium intake is achieved, the blood selenium level may not continue to rise with increases in dietary selenium until toxic levels of intake are reached (*Valentine JL et al. Selenium levels in human blood, urine and hair in response to exposure via drinking water. Environ Res 17:347-55, 1978*).

Toenail selenium reflects blood selenium levels for up to one year (*Kok FJ et al. Decreased selenium levels in myocardial infarction. JAMA 261(8):1161-64, 1989*).

Urinary selenium is an inadequate indicator of tissue nutriture (*Neve J et al. Selenium deficiency. Clin Endocrinol Metab 14(3):629-56, 1985*) but may be useful to confirm the findings when blood selenium is being measured (*Valentine JL et al. Selenium levels in human blood, urine and hair in response to exposure via drinking water. Environ Res 17:347-55, 1978*).

Sodium:

Serum sodium levels are commonly used as a measure of sodium nutriture. The principal cation of the extracellular fluid, any change in serum sodium is associated with a fluid shift into or out of the cell. Serum levels, however, do not reflect total body sodium content (*Webb WL, Gehi M. Psychosomatics 22(3):199-203, 1981*).

Hair sodium levels do not reflect dietary intake or body stores (*Passwater RA, Cranton EM. Trace Elements, Hair Analysis and Nutrition. New Canaan, Connecticut, Keats Publishing, 1983:85*).

Sulfur:

Hair sulfur is a useful diagnostic screen for the evaluation of hair disorders (*Kutner M et al. A critique: Hair sulfur analysis for evaulation of normal and abnormal hair, in AC Brown, Ed. First Human Hair Symposium, Medcom Press*). While low hair sulfur does not appear to correlate with hair loss, and supplementation with sulfur when hair sulfur is low does not appear to stimulate hair growth, alopecia resulting from dietary inadequacies may be reflected by low hair sulfur. In these cases, upon correction of the diet, hair growth is restored and hair sulfur increases (*Brown H, Klauder JV. Sulphur content of hair and of nails in abnormal states. Arch Derm Syphilol 27:584, 1933*).

Taurine:

Because plasma and whole-blood taurine are not correlated, assessment of both provides the most accurate estimate of taurine status. Short of that, whole-blood taurine would appear to be the best single measure (*Trautwein EA, Hayes KC. Taurine concentrations in plasma and whole blood in humans: estimation of error from intra- and interindividual variation and sampling technique. Am J Clin Nutr 52:758-64, 1990*).

Thiamine:

The most commonly used procedure for assessing thiamine nutriture has been the measurement of RBC transketolase activity and its stimulation *in vitro* by the addition of thiamine pyrophosphate (TPP effect). Some disease conditions may influence RBC transketolase activity independent of thiamine status. For example, patients in negative nitrogen balance will have diminished RBC transketolase activity due to insufficient apoenzyme to activate transketolase. In addition, low transketolase in diabetes mellitus and polyneuritis does not reflect a thiamine deficit, while patients with pernicious anemia may have elevated transketolase levels unrelated to thiamine status (*Sauberlich HE. Newer laboratory methods for assessing nutriture of selected B-complex vitamins. Annu Rev Nutr 4:377-407, 1984*).

> Note: *"Frequently, no transketolase effect is observable in patients with neuropathies, liver diseases and other ailments even in severe thiamine deficiency"* (*Baker H et al. B-Complex vitamin analyses and their clinical value. J Appl Nutr 41(1):3-12, 1989*).

RBC thiamine diphosphate levels may be superior to RBC transketolase activity as thiamine diphosphate is more stable in frozen red blood cells, is easier to standardize, and is not subject to the variables present in the transketolase assay (*Baines M, Davies G. The evaluation of erythrocyte thiamine diphosphate as an indicator of thiamine status in man, and its comparison with erythrocyte transketolase activity measurements. Ann Clin Biochem 25:698-705, 1988*).

Several studies have demonstrated a relationship between RBC transketolase activity and urinary thiamine excretion (*Sauberlich HE. Newer laboratory methods for assessing nutriture of selected B-complex vitamins. Annu Rev Nutr 4:377-407, 1984*).

On a thiamine-deficient diet, a decrease in the blood thiamine level is the earliest sign of a thiamine deficiency (*Baker H. Analysis of vitamin status. J Med Soc N J 80:633-6, 1983*). However, blood thiamine determinations have not been satisfactory primarily because of limitations in methodology, as the decreases in blood thiamine during deficiency are not great (*Sauberlich HE. Newer laboratory methods for assessing nutriture of selected B-complex vitamins. Annu Rev Nutr 4:377-407, 1984*).

Vitamin A:

A liver biopsy is by far the most accurate method of assessing vitamin A status (*Pitt GAJ. The assessment of vitamin A status. Proc Nutr Sci 40:173, 1981*).

Isotope dilution assay with tetradeuterated vitamin A can validly estimate total body reserves in both the marginal and satisfactory ranges (*Furr HC et al. Vitamin A concentrations in liver determined by isotope dilution assay with tetradeuterated vitamin A and by biopsy in generally healthy adult humans. Am J Clin Nutr 49:713-16, 1989*).

Plasma retinol is commonly measured to assess vitamin A status. It should be noted, however, that when insufficient RBP is available, toxicity due to hypervitaminosis A can occur despite a low concentration of plasma retinol; thus, in addition to plasma retinol concentration, it is important that retinol-binding protein also be measured (*Nutr Rev 40(10), October, 1982*). Although determination of plasma retinol as the retinol-RBP (retinol-binding protein) complex would appear to be a promising method, the major limitation on its value is that plasma retinol concentration is kept reasonably constant to supply vitamin A to the tissues. While there is some relationship between plasma values and liver content, the plasma content only falls substantially if the liver reserves of retinyl esters are effectively exhausted (*Pitt GAJ. The assessment of vitamin A status. Proc Nutr Sci 40:173, 1981*).

In addition, other factors besides vitamin A nutriture can influence plasma retinol levels. If dietary protein is inadequate, or if various diseases are present, insufficient RBP is synthesized by the liver, and the plasma retinol concentration will fall. Estrogens and oral contraceptives can increase plasma retinol-RBP concentrations. Poor growth depresses, and accelerated growth increases, the plasma retinol concentration, and giving retinoids other than retinol can paradoxically depress plasma retinol concentration as a consequence of diminishing tissue demand for retinol (*Pitt GAJ. The assessment of vitamin A status. Proc Nutr Sci 40:173, 1981*).

Vitamin B6:

Pyridoxal-5^1-phosphate (PLP) and pyridoxal (PL), its hydrolysis product and the ultimate transport form of B6, are the predominant B6 vitamers in the circulation. The measurement of erythrocyte PLP and/or PL may be more informative about vitamin B6 status than is plasma PLP as a number of physiologic conditions may change the dynamic equilibrium between the various B6 vitamers in the plasma. Also, in acute myocardial infarction, extracellular PLP may be redistributed to the intracellular compartment (*Vermaak WJH et al. Vitamin B-6 nutrition status and cigarette smoking. Am J Clin Nutr 51:1958-61, 1990*).

There are certain difficulties with using vitamin B6-dependent enzyme activities as a measure of B6 status:
1. Some B6-deficient pts., such as those with liver disease, have high pyridoxal-dependent RBC transaminase levels despite low blood pyridoxine (*Sauberlich HE. Newer laboratory methods for assessing nutriture of selected B-complex vitamins. Annu Rev Nutr 4:377-407, 1984*).
2. The activity of the RBC aminotransferases also increase in thiamine, riboflavin and pantothenate deficiencies and in various disease states (*Baker H. Analysis of vitamin status. J Med Soc N J 80:633-6, 1983*).
3. Finally, RBC glutamate-pyruvate transaminase (alanine aminotransaminase) activity differs significantly among 3 phenotypes despite similar plasma pyridoxal-5^1-phosphate levels; thus E-GPT activity can only be used to assess vitamin B6 nutritional status if the GPT phenotype is accounted for (*Ubbink JB et al. Genetic polymorphism of glutamate-pyruvate transaminase (alanine aminotransaminase): Influence on erythrocyte activity as a marker of vitamin B-6 nutritional status. Am J Clin Nutr 50:1420-8, 1989*).

Xanthurenic acid and kyurenine excretion after a tryptophan load most likely represents an aberrant reaction to the load and has no documented clinical significance. In addition, pregnancy and contraceptive pills may render the test abnormal due to inhibition of kynureninase by estrogens (*Baker H. Analysis of vitamin status. J Med Soc N J 80:633-6, 1983; Sauberlich HE. Newer laboratory methods for assessing nutriture of selected B-complex vitamins. Annu Rev Nutr 4:377-407, 1984*).

Vitamin B12:

With its excellent sensitivity and specificity, urinary methylmalonic acid assay using gas chromatography-mass spectometry may be the preferred test for vitamin B12 deficiency.

> *Note: MMA excretion may be elevated in other conditions such as benign methylmalonic aciduria (Ledley FD et al. Benign methylmalonic aciduria. N Engl J Med 311:1015-1018, 1984), and carnitine supplementation may cause MMA levels to decrease (Roe CR et al. Metabolic response to carnitine in methylmalonic aciduria. Arch Dis Child 58:916-20, 1983).*

Observational Study: 75 pts. with low serum B12 levels and 68 normal controls were studied. Of 96 evaluable pts., 7 had clinical deficiency; all had urinary methylmalonic acid levels >5 µg/mg creatinine (sensitivity, 100%). Of the 89 pts. who were not clinically deficient, 88 had urinary methylmalonic acid levels <5 µg/mg creatinine (specificity 99%) (*Matchar DB et al. Isotope-dilution assay for urinary methylmalonic acid in the diagnosis of vitamin B12 deficiency. A prospective clinical evaluation. Ann Intern Med 106(5):707-10, 1987*).

While microbiological serum assays are reliable (*Baker H et al. Vitamin analyses in medicine, in RS Goodhart, ME Shils, Eds. Modern Nutrition in Health and Disease. Sixth Edition. Philadelphia, Lea & Febiger, 1980:611*), RIA serum assays are unreliable because they also measure inactive cobalamin analogues (*Cohen KL, Donaldson, Jr RM. Unreliability of radiodilution assays as screening tests for cobalamin (vitamin B12) deficiency. JAMA October 24, 1980, pp. 1942-5; Kolhouse JF et al. Cobalamin analogues are present in human plasma and can mask cobalamin deficiency because current radioisotope dilution assays are not specific for true cobalamin. N Engl J Med 299:787, 1978*).

Serum B$_{12}$ levels are frequently normal despite depressed levels in the cerebrospinal fluid (*van Tiggelen CJM et al. Vitamin B$_{12}$ levels of cerebrospinal fluid in patients with organic mental disorder. J Orthomol Psychiatry 12:305-311, 1983*); thus the CNS concentration of vitamin B$_{12}$ is a better marker of B$_{12}$ deficiency with regard to brain function than serum concentrations (*Gottfries CG, president of the European College of Neuropsychopharmacology - reported in Clin Psychiatry News, September, 1989*).

Even in the absence of hematological and neurological evidence of pernicious anemia, serum B$_{12}$ levels may be deficient (*Karnaze DS, Carmel R. Neurologic and evoked potential abnormalities in subtle cobalamin deficiency states, including deficiency without anemia and with normal absorption of free cobalamin. Arch Neurol 47(9):1008-12, 1990*).

The Schilling test is a popular test of B$_{12}$ absorption (*Zuckier LS, Chervu LR. J Nucl Med 25:1032, 1984*). Its newer version, the dual-isotope variation, is independent of urine volume and renal function, and is thus the test of choice in the elderly patient (*Lum MC, Mooradian AD. Vitamin B$_{12}$ deficiency: The sepulveda GRECC method. No. 14. Geriatr Med Today 5(10):93-97, 1986*).

The determination of hypersegmentation of neutrophils is a useful measure of vitamin B$_{12}$ deficiency, although it is unreliable during pregnancy and fails to distinguish between vitamin B$_{12}$ and folate deficiencies (*Sauberlich HE. Newer laboratory methods for assessing nutriture of selected B-complex vitamins. Annu Rev Nutr 4:377-407, 1984*).

Vitamin C:

There is to date no satisfactory assay technique for ascorbic acid status. Once collected, AA readily oxidizes to dehydroascorbic acid and then to diketogulonic acid. The latter step is irreversible but the former may be prevented by acidification of the specimen immediately upon collection. Many factors influence the levels present at any particular time (physiologic status, drug ingestion, etc.) (*Lee W et al. Ascorbic acid status: Biochemical and clinical considerations. Am J Clin Nutr 48:286-90, 1988*).

The leukocyte ascorbic acid concentration tends to respond less readily than does the serum level to recent dietary intake and may be more closely related to tissue stores than are serum levels (*Burr ML et al. Plasma and leukocyte ascorbic acid levels in the elderly. Am J Clin Nutr 27:144, 1974*), although it may be normal despite other evidence of vitamin C deficiency (*Thomas AJ et al. Is leucocyte ascorbic acid an unreliable estimate of vitamin C deficiency? Age Ageing 13(4):243-47, 1984*). Factors such as infection, suppressed immunity, myocardial infarction and hyperglycemia may lower these levels, as may such drugs as aspirin, oral contraceptives and hydrocortisone (*Lee W et al. Ascorbic acid status: Biochemical and clinical considerations. Am J Clin Nutr 48:286-90, 1988*).

While serum and plasma ascorbate levels may not always fully reflect vitamin C intakes or the state of tissue ascorbate reserves, within a limited range, serum ascorbate levels show a linear relationship with vitamin C intake and low serum levels indicate low or inadequate intake with probably only partial reserves present (*Sauberlich HE. Vitamin C status: Methods and findings. Ann N Y Acad Sci 258:438-49, 1975*).

>   *Note: Except for high-performance liquid chromatography (HPLC), commonly used analytic procedures for plasma or serum vitamin C cannot distinguish between ascorbic acid and its isomer, erythorbic acid, which is widely used as a food additive, especially in processed meats. Therefore, unless the HPLC-amperometric method is used, plasma or serum vitamin C analyses should be conducted on overnight fasting blood specimens (Sauberlich HE et al. Influence of dietary intakes of erythorbic acid on plasma vitamina C analyses. Am J Clin Nutr 54:1319S-22S, 1991).*

Erythrocyte and whole-blood ascorbic acid levels appear to be less sensitive indicators of vitamin C deficiency than are serum levels (*Sauberlich HE. Vitamin C status: Methods and findings. Ann N Y Acad Sci 258:438-49, 1975*).

Urinary excretion of ascorbic acid declines to undetectable levels in vitamin C depletion and thus could be used to corroborate other findings (*Hodges RE et al. Clinical manifestations of ascorbic acid deficiency in man. Am J Clin Nutr 24:432, 1971*).

The ascorbic acid saturation test must be carefully conducted and interpreted with caution, but the results can conclusively exclude scurvy as a diagnosis (*Sauberlich HE. Vitamin C status: Methods and findings. Ann N Y Acad Sci 258:438-49, 1975; Dutra De Oliveira JE et al. Clinical usefulness of the oral ascorbic acid tolerance test in scurvy. Am J Clin Nutr 7:630, 1959*).

Results of the lingual ascorbic acid test are not related to changes in ascorbic acid intake and are not consistent with plasma or leukocyte ascorbate concentrations (*Leggott PJ et al. Response of lingual ascorbic acid test and salivary ascorbate levels to changes in ascorbic acid intake. J Dent Res 65(2):131-34, 1986; Ascorbic acid intake and salivary ascorbate levels. Nutr Rev 44(10):328-30, 1986*).

Vitamin D:

Cholecalciferol (vitamin D_3) is the natural vitamin, while ergocalciferol (vitamin D_2) is obtained exclusively from the diet. Each is biologically inert until it undergoes successive enzymatic hydroxylations, at C-25 in the liver and at C-1 in the kidney, to produce 1,25-dihydroxyvitamin D. While intracellular 25-hydroxyvitamin D may serve a specific function, it is unproved and can be regarded as part of the body stores of vitamin D. Measurement of plasma 25-hydroxyvitamin D provides an index of the the bodily reserve of the pro-hormone, and measurement of plasma 1,25-dihydroxyvitamin D an index of prevailing biological action, although the level of 1,25-dihydroxyvitamin D can only be interpreted with reference to the subject's mineral nutrition and the prevailing physiological state (*Stanbury SW. Vitamin D: metamorphosis from nutrient to hormonal system. Proc Nutr Soc 40:179-86, 1981*).

Vitamin E:

Platelet tocopherol levels appear to be the best blood measure of the dietary intake of vitamin E (*Lehmann J et al. Vitamin E and relationships among tocopherols in human plasma, platelets, lymphocytes, and red blood cells. Am J Clin Nutr 47:470-74, 1988*).

Since plasma and serum vitamin E levels are closely correlated with total serum triglycerides (*Farrell PM, Biere JG. Am J Clin Nutr 28:1381, 1975*), tocopherol to triglyceride serum ratios should be calculated in assessing tocopherol status when plasma or serum vitamin E is being measured. The normal range of this ratio is 35-120 (*Bland J, Prestbo E. Vitamin E: Comparative absorption studies. Int Clin Nutr Rev 4(2):82-86, 1984*).

> *Note: Plasma vitamin E levels are also significantly correlated (p<0.001) with total cholesterol and total lipid (Vandewoude MF, Vandewoude MG. Vitamin E status in an normal population: The influence of age. J Am Coll Nutr 6(4):307-11, 1987).*

Vitamin K:

While prothrombin time and clotting time are commonly used to assess vitamin K, subclinical deficiency is better assessed by methods which quantify the fraction of hepatic prothrombin which fails to become carboxylated in the hepatic reticulum under the influence of vitamin K (*Abnormal plasma prothrombin in the diagnosis of subclinical vitamin K deficiency. Nutr Rev 40(10):298-300, 1982*).

Alternative methods are the indirect ratio approach (*Corrigan JJ Jr et al. J Pediatr 99:254-57, 1981*) and direct measurement of both native prothrombin and the abnormal species with RIA procedures (*Blanchard RA et al. N Engl J Med 305:242-48, 1981*).

Zinc:

The most reliable method of diagnosing zinc deficiency is a therapeutic trial (*Editorial: Another look at zinc. Br Med J 282:1098-99, 1981*).

Since serum, salivary urinary and hair zinc levels may fail to correspond (*Capel ID et al. The assessment of zinc status by the zinc tolerance test in various groups of patients. Clin Biochem 15(5):257-60, 1982*), the zinc tolerance test is perhaps the best available method of determining body zinc nutriture. After a fast, a baseline plasma level is drawn, and an oral loading dose of zinc sulfate 220 mg (50 mg elemental zinc) is given. Two hours later, plasma zinc is redrawn. A two or threefold increase in plasma zinc is indicative of zinc inadequacy (*Capel ID et al. The assessment of zinc status by the zinc tolerance test in various groups of patients. Clin Biochem 15(5):257-60, 1982; Sullivan JF et al. A zinc tolerance test. J Lab Clin Med 93(3):485-92, 1979*).

Neutrophil zinc and alkaline phosphatase activity in neutrophils may be the preferred assays for the diagnosis of zinc deficiency (*Prasad AS. Laboratory diagnosis of zinc deficiency. J Am Coll Nutr 4(6):591-98, 1985*)

<u>Leukocyte zinc</u> is a useful index of body stores which has been shown to correlate with muscle zinc levels (*Jones RB et al. The relationship between leukocyte and muscle zinc in health and disease. <u>Clin Sci</u> 60:237-39, 1981*).

<u>Sweat zinc</u> is a useful and sensitive index of zinc status which is more reliable than either hair or serum zinc (*Davies S. Assessment of zinc status. <u>Int Clin Nutr Rev</u> 4(3):122-9, 1984; Howard JMH. Serum, leukocyte, sweat and hair zinc levels - a correlational study. <u>J Nutr Med</u> 1:119-26, 1990*).

Depressed <u>hair zinc levels</u> reliably indicate depletion, but normal or even high values do not rule out low body stores (*Davies S. Assessment of zinc status. <u>Int Clin Nutr Rev</u> 4(3):122-29, 1984; Pekarek RS et al. Abnormal cellular immune responses during acquired zinc deficiency. <u>Am J Clin Nutr</u> 32:1466-71, 1979; Hambridge KM et al. Low levels of zinc in hair, anorexia, poor growth and hypogeusia in children. <u>Pediatr Res</u> 6:808-74, 1971*). In addition, because standard washing procedures are unable to remove exogenous zinc without reducing endogenous zinc levels, hair levels are unreliable when external zinc contamination is likely to have occurred (*Buckley RA, Dreosti I. <u>Am J Clin Nutr</u> 40:840-6, 1984*), and hair zinc may fail to reflect increases in dietary zinc in subjects whose initial zinc status is adequate (*Medeiros DM et al. Failure of oral zinc supplementation to alter hair zinc levels among healthy human volunteers. <u>Nutr Res</u> 7:1109-15, 1987*).

<u>Plasma zinc</u>, which is decreased in moderate to severe zinc deficency (*Prasad AS. Zinc in growth and development and spectrum of human zinc deficiency. <u>J Am Coll Nutr</u> 7(5):377-84, 1988*) is a poor measure of total body zinc stores (*Solomons NW. On the assessment of zinc and copper nutriture in man. <u>Am J Clin Nutr</u> 32:856-71, 1979*). A moderately low plasma level may simply reflect mobilization of zinc from plasma to the liver and other tissues as part of the normal response to infection or stress (*Wagner PA. Zinc nutriture in the elderly. <u>Geriatrics</u> 40:111-13,117-8, 124-5, 1985*). In addition, plasma zinc concentrations depend upon albumin concentration (*Ainley CC et al. Zinc state in anorexia nervosa. <u>Br Med. J.</u> Vol. 293, October 18, 1986*). Therefore, plasma zinc determinations should be complemented with zinc determinations in a nucleated tissue, such as liver, muscle or bone (*Abdulla M. How adequate is plasma zinc as an indicator of zinc status? <u>Prog Clin Biol Res</u> 129:171-83, 1983*).

<u>Serum zinc</u> is a poor measure of total body zinc stores (*Solomons NW. On the assessment of zinc and copper nutriture in man. <u>Am J Clin Nutr</u> 32:856-71, 1979*). Combining measurement of the serum zinc concentration with <u>urinary zinc excretion</u> will provide a more accurate assessment; however, any bodily process that involves the breakdown or rapid turnover of cells (including decreased food intake and starvation) is associated with increased urinary zinc excretion, which may or may not be reflected in serum zinc. Also, stress from any source, including surgery, may cause a redistribution of bodily zinc, and a transient urinary zinc loss may be evident for a few days (*Henkin RI. Zinc in Wound Healing. Editorial. <u>N Engl J Med</u> 291(13):675-6, 1974*).

<u>Red cell zinc</u>, while sometimes low in zinc deficiency, is unreliable as RBC zinc levels are substantially influenced by factors controlling the partitioning of zinc across red cell membranes (*Davies S. Assessment of zinc status. <u>Int Clin Nutr Rev</u> 4(3):122-9, 1984*). In addition, as erythrocytes turn over slowly, their zinc levels do not reflect recent changes in zinc status (*Prasad AS. Laboratory diagnosis of zinc deficiency. <u>J Am Coll Nutr</u> 4(6):591-8, 1985*).

A simple <u>zinc taste test</u> which suggests that there will be a favorable response to zinc supplementation uses a test solution made by dissolving zinc sulfate 1 gm in 1 liter of distilled water (0.1% solution). If the subject tasting 5 -10 ml notes either no taste or a dry and furry taste developing after a few minutes, zinc supplementation is suggested. Adequate zinc nutriture is suggested by an immediate taste which may be strong and unpleasant (*Bryce-Smith D, Simpson RID. Anorexia, depression, and zinc deficiency. <u>Lancet</u> 2:1162, 1984*). This test, however, has not been well-validated.

NUTRIENT BIOAVAILABILITY
AND INTERACTIONS

NOTE: Drug interactions should also be considered.

<u>Biotin</u>:

  - and <u>Ethanol</u>:

    Inhibits the intestinal transport of biotin and is associated with a significant decrease in plasma biotin concentrations (*Said HM et al. Chronic ethanol feeding and acute ethanol exposure in vitro: effect on intestinal transport of biotin. <u>Am J Clin Nutr</u> 52:1083-6, 1990*).

<u>Calcium</u>:

Calcium retention is not necessarily enhanced by supplementation.

    Experimental Study: The ingestion of milk or calcium supplements may not increase calcium retention in healthy young men due to depression of calcium absorption in the gut and fractional tubular absorption in the kidneys; whether the same is true for healthy young women is uncertain (*Lewis NM et al. Calcium supplements and milk: effects on acid-base balance and on retention of calcium, magnesium, and phosphorus. <u>Am J Clin Nutr</u> 49:527-33, 1989*).

    Experimental Study: "Our data suggest that many women may respond to calcium supplementation by increasing urinary calcium excretion moderately; however, a significant number may exhibit hypercalciuria or no response to calcium supplementation. Therefore, monitoring urinary calcium levels in response to short-term supplementation might be a quick way to assess which women should be evaluated further because calcium supplementation may induce hypercalciuria and related problems" (*Storey ML et al. Urinary calcium and magnesium excretion by women in response to short-term calcium supplementation. <u>Nutr Res</u> 8:617-24, 1988*).

Calcium is better absorbed when taken with a <u>light meal</u> than when taken alone (*Heaney RP et al. Meal effects on calcium absorption. <u>Am J Clin Nutr</u> 49:372-76, 1989*).

Results of studies of normal subjects have suggested that <u>calcium citrate</u> may be more bioavailable than other calcium salts (*Harvey JA et al. Superior calcium absorption from calcium citrate than calcium carbonate using external forearm counting. <u>J Am Coll Nutr</u> 9(6):583-7, 1990; Nicar MJ, Pak CY. Calcium bioavailability from calcium carbonate and calcium citrate. <u>J Clin Endocrinol Metab</u> 61(2):391-93, 1985; Schutte SA, Knowles JB. Intestinal absorption of Ca(H2PO4)2 and Ca citrate compared by two methods. <u>Am J Clin Nutr</u> 47(5):884-88, 1988*). <u>Calcium citrate-mala</u>te may even be superior as it has about 6 times the solubility of either calcium citrate or calcium malate (*Smith KT et al. Calcium absorption from a new calcium delivery system (CCM). <u>Calcif Tissue Int</u> 41:351-2, 1987*).

    Note: Alkali citrate may <u>inhibit</u> calcium absorption, perhaps due to complexation of calcium by citrate (Rumenapf G, Schwille PO. The influence of oral alkali citrate on intestinal calcium absorption in healthy man. <u>Clin Science</u> 73:117-21, 1987).

Calcium absorption from food is not impaired by achlorhydria (*Knox TA et al. Effect of high fiber diet and gastric acidity on calcium absorption in the elderly by the whole-body counter method. Abstract. <u>J Am Coll Nutr</u> 8(5):450, 1989*); however calcium from calcium carbonate may be less efficiently utilized in individuals with low gastric acid production (*Allen LH. Calcium and osteoporosis. Nutr Today 21(3):6-10, 1986*). In achlorhydric subjects, calcium citrate is ten times as well absorbed as is calcium carbonate (*Recker RR. Calcium absorption and achlorhydria. N Engl J Med 313(2):70-73, 1985*).

Calcium is over 5 times better absorbed from milk than from spinach (mean of 27.6% vs. 5.1%), since the calcium in spinach is bound to oxalate (*Heaney RP et al. Calcium absorbability from spinach. Am J Clin Nutr 47:707-09, 1988*).

- and Caffeine:

    May increase urinary calcium excretion (*Yeh JK et al. Influence of injected caffeine on the metabolism of calcium and the retention and excretion of sodium, potassium, phosphorus, magnesium, zinc and copper in rats. J Nutr 116(2):273-80, 1986*).

- and Fatty Acids:

    May decrease calcium absorption due to the formation of calcium soaps in the GI tract (*Weiser NM, in NW Solomons, IH Rosenberg, Eds. Absorption and Malabsorption of Mineral Nutrients. New York, Alan R. Liss, 1984:15*).

- and Fiber:

    May decrease intestinal calcium absorption (*Heaney RP et al. Calcium nutrition and bone health in the elderly. Am J Clin Nutr 36(5 Suppl):986-1013, 1982*).

    Negative Experimental Study: Under conditions that mimic those in the intestines, the binding of calcium to soluble fibers (pectin, alginate, carrageenan, guar gum) is extremely weak. If calcium is bound to fiber in the duodenum, it will be released again as it enters the jejunum and ileum, where it can still be effectively absorbed (*Schlemmer U. Studies of the binding of copper, zinc, and calcium to pectin, alginate, carrageenan, and guar gum in HCO3-CO2 buffer. Food Chem 32:223-34, 1989*).

- and Iron:

    May enhance calcium absorption (*Roth-Bassell HA, Clydesdale FM. The influence of zinc, magnesium, and iron on calcium uptake in brush border membrane vesicles. J Am Coll Nutr 10(1):44-9, 1991*).

- and Lactose:

    May enhance calcium absorption, but the evidence is controversial (*Allen LH. Calcium and osteoporosis. Nutr Today 21(3):6-10, 1986*).

- and Magnesium:

    May reduce calcium absorption (*Roth-Bassell HA, Clydesdale FM. The influence of zinc, magnesium, and iron on calcium uptake in brush border membrane vesicles. J Am Coll Nutr 10(1):44-9, 1991*).

    Chronic magnesium deficiency is associated with hypocalcemia (*Leicht E, Biro G. Mechanisms of hypocalcaemia in the clinical form of severe magnesium deficit in the human. Magnes Res 5(1):47-44, 1992*).

    Magnesium regulates the neuromuscular activity of the Ca^{++} ion and a deficiency enhances the availability of ionic calcium; thus magnesium is a natural calcium-channel blocker (*Iseri LT, French JH. Magnesium: Nature's calcium blocker. Am Heart J July, 1984, p. 188*).

- and Oxalates:

    High in certain leafy green vegetables which are also high in calcium such as spinach, but not in Brassica oleracea (broccoli, turnip greens, collard greens, mustard greens).

    May inhibit the absorption of calcium contained in its food source, but not the absorption of calcium from other foods simultaneously ingested (*Allen LH. Calcium and osteoporosis. Nutr Today 21(3):6-10, 1986*).

- and <u>Phosphorus</u>:

The ideal calcium to phosphorus ratio is 1:1 (*Linkswiler HM, Zemel MB. Calcium to phosphorus ratios. <u>Contemp Nutr</u> 4(5), May, 1979*).

High phosphorus intakes (meat, grains, potatoes and soft drinks) promote calcium loss through the induction of "nutritional hyperparathyroidism" in order to maintain normal serum calcium levels in the face of decreased Ca/P ratios (*Jowsey J. Osteoporosis. <u>Postgrad Med</u> 60:75-9, 1976*).

> *Note: A phosphorus intake of up to 2000 mg/d does not have adverse effects on calcium metabolism; however the type of phosphate contained in carbonated beverages may not behave in the same manner (Spencer H et al. Do protein and phosphorus cause calcium loss? <u>J Nutr</u> 118:657-660, 1988).*

Fecal phosphorus appears to bind calcium and reduce its intestinal absorption (*Franz KB. Influence of dietary phosphorus on absorption of dietary calcium and magnesium in humans. Abstract. <u>J Am Coll Nutr</u> 6(5):444, 1987*).

- and <u>Phytates</u>:

Found in the bran layer of <u>cereal grains</u>.

May decrease intestinal calcium absorption (*Goodhart RS, Shils ME. <u>Modern Nutrition in Health and Disease</u>. 6th Edition. Philadelphia, Lee & Febiger, 1980*).

- and <u>Protein</u>:

May increase urinary calcium excretion (*Allen LH. Calcium and osteoporosis. <u>Nutr Today</u> 21(3):6-10, 1986*).

> **Negative Review Article:** Controlled human studies show that commonly used complex dietary proteins, which have a high phosphorus content, do not cause calcium loss in adult humans. In contrast, a diet low in protein and phosphorus may have adverse effects on calcium balance in the elderly (*Spencer H et al. Do protein and phosphorus cause calcium loss? <u>J Nutr</u> 118:657-60, 1988*).

- and <u>Sodium</u>:

May increase urinary calcium excretion (*Heaney RP. Calcium bioavailability. <u>Contemp Nutr</u> 11(8), 1986*).

- and <u>Sodium Bicarbonate</u>:

May improve urinary calcium retention in protein-induced hypercalciuria (*Lutz J. Calcium balance and acid-base status of women as affected by increased protein intake and by sodium bicarbonate ingestion. <u>Am J Clin Nutr</u> 39:281-88, 1984*).

- and <u>Sugar</u>:

Glucose may increase calcium absorption (*Wood RJ et al. Effects of glucose and glucose polymers on calcium absorption in healthy subjects. <u>Am J Clin Nutr</u> 46(4):699-701, 1987*).

May increase urinary calcium concentration (*Holl M, Allen L. Sucrose ingestion, insulin response and mineral metabolism. <u>J Nutr</u> 117:1229-33, 1987; Thom JA et al. The influence of refined carbohydrate on urinary calcium excretion. <u>Br J Urology</u> 50:459-64, 1978*).

- and <u>Uronic Acid</u>:

(found in the hemi-cellulose fiber component of <u>fruit</u> and <u>vegetables</u>.)

May inhibit intestinal calcium absorption (*Allen LH. Calcium and osteoporosis. <u>Nutr Today</u> 21(3):6-10, 1986*).

- and <u>Vitamin D</u>:

   May promote calcium absorption and mobilize calcium from bone (*Passmore R, Eastwood MA. <u>Davidson and Passmore: Human Nutrition and Dietetics</u>. Eighth Edition. London, Churchill Livingstone, 1986:139*).

- and <u>Zinc</u>:

   May decrease calcium absorption when a high level of daily zinc supplementation (140 mg) is given along with a low daily dietary calcium intake (200 mg) but not with a normal calcium intake (800 mg) (*Roth-Bassell HA, Clydesdale FM. The influence of zinc, magnesium, and iron on calcium uptake in brush border membrane vesicles. <u>J Am Coll Nutr</u> 10(1):44-9, 1991; Spencer H et al. Effect of zinc supplements on the intestinal absorption of calcium. <u>J Am Coll Nutr</u> 6(1):47-51, 1987*).

Carnitine:

- and <u>Vitamin C</u>:

   May increase urinary excretion (*Davies HEF et al. Ascorbic acid and carnitine in man. <u>Nutr Rep Int</u> 36:941, 1987*).

Chromium:

- and <u>Calcium Carbonate</u>:

   May reduce chromium absorption (*Seaborn C, Stoecker B. Effects of antacid or ascorbic acid on tissue accumulation and urinary excretion of chromium. <u>Nutr Res</u> 10:1401-7, 1990*).

- and <u>Sugar</u>:

   May increase urinary chromium loss (*Kozlovsky AS et al. Effects of diets high in simple sugars on urinary chromium losses. <u>Metabolism</u> 35:515, 1986*).

Copper:

- and <u>Alcohol</u>:

   May aggravate copper deficiency (*Fields M, Lewis C. Alcohol consumption aggravates copper deficiency. <u>Metabolism</u> 39:610-13, 1990*).

- and <u>Egg</u>:

   Egg yolk forms an insoluble copper sulfide with free copper in the digestive tract (*Schultze MO et al. Further studies on the avialability of copper from various sources as a supplement to iron in hemoglobin formation. <u>J Biol Chem</u> 115:453-7, 1936*).

- and <u>Fructose</u>:

   The fructose moiety of sucrose may contribute to copper deficiency when used as a major source of dietary carbohydrate (*Reiser S et al. Indices of copper status in humans consuming a typical American diet containing either fructose or starch. <u>Am J Clin Nutr</u> 42:242-251, 1985*).

- and <u>Iron</u>:

   May decrease GI absorption of copper (*Haschke F e tla. Effect of iron fortification of infant formula on trace mineral absorption. <u>J Pediatr Gastroenterol Nutr</u> 5:768-73, 1986*).

- and <u>Molybdenum</u>:

May increase copper excretion (*Doesthale YG, Gopalan C. The effect of molybdenum levels in sorghum (Sorghum Vulgare Pers.) on uric acid and copper excretion in man. Br J Nutr 31:351-5, 1974*).

- and <u>Phytates</u>:

May reduce copper absorption and retention (*Davies NT, Nightingale R. The effects of phytate on intestinal absorption and secretion of zinc and whole-body retention of zinc, copper, iron and manganese by rats. Br J Nutr 34:243-58, 1975; Turnlund JR et al. A stable isotope study of copper absorption in young men: effect of phytate and α-cellulose. Am J Clin Nutr 42:18-23, 1985*).

- and <u>Vitamin B6</u>:

Deficiency may decrease GI absorption (*Keyes W et al. Copper, iron, and zinc absorption, retention, and status of young women fed vitamin B6 deficient diets. FASEB J 5:A556, 1991*).

- and <u>Vitamin C</u>:

High levels of supplementation may decrease GI absorption of copper (*Milne DB et al. Effects of ascorbic acid supplements and a diet marginal in copper on indices of copper nutriture in women. Nutr Res 8:865-73, 1988; Van Campen DR, Gross E. Influences of ascorbic acid on the absorption of copper in rats. J Nutr 95:617-22, 1968*).

Ascorbate also has a postabsorption role in the transfer of copper ions into cells. It reacts with ceruloplasmin, a serum copper protein, labilizing the bound copper atoms and facilitating their cross-membrane transport, thus stimulating tissue copper utilization. Also, at physiological levels and above, ascorbate impedes the intracellular binding of copper to Cu,Zn superoxide dismutase - which may or may not have physiological significance (*Harris ED, Percival SS. A role for ascorbic acid in copper transport. Am J Clin Nutr 54:1193S-7S, 1991*).

- and <u>Zinc</u>:

May decrease copper absorption.

Case Report: A 35-year-old Caucasian woman ingested 110-165 mg elemental zinc as zinc sulfate for 10 months. She developed a slowly worsening microcytic-hypochromic anemia found to be due to copper deficiency. Zinc supplementation was eliminated and she was supplemented with 2 mg copper daily. After 2 mo., her anemia was unchanged. She received 10 mg copper chloride IV over a period of 5 days, and responded (*Hoffman HN 2nd et al. Zinc-induced copper deficiency. Gastroenterology 94:508-12, 1988*).

Negative Experimental Study: Healthy men and women consumed either 50 mg zinc 3 times daily or placebo. After 3 mo., there were no adverse effects on plasma copper levels (*Samman S, Roberts D. The effect of zinc supplements on plasma zinc and copper levels and the reported symptoms in healthy volunteers. Med J Aust 146:246-47, 1987*).

Review Article: It appears that tissues must be loaded with zinc before an effect on copper absorption is observed (*Brewer GJ et al. Biological roles of ionic zinc. Prog Clin Biol Res 129:35-51, 1983*).

<u>Essential Fatty Acids</u>:

Omega-6 fatty acids cannot accumulate normally in cell membranes if the supply of omega-3 fatty acids is too low (*Bjerve KS et al. α-linolenic acid and long-chain ω-3 fatty acid deficiency: effect on lymphocyte function, plasma and red cell lipids, and prostanoid formation. Am J Clin Nutr 49:290-300, 1989*).

- and <u>Vitamin E</u>:

Vitamin E prevents the peroxidation of polyunsaturated fatty acids and thus is recommended whenever they are heavily supplemented (*Chow CK. Nutritional influences on cellular antioxidant defense systems. Am J Clin Nutr 32:1066-1081, 1979*).

Folic Acid:

  - and Pancreatic Enzymes:

    Bind with folic acid to form insoluble complexes, thus decreasing folate absorption (*Russell RM et al. Impairment of folic acid absorption by oral pancreatic extracts. Dig Dis Sci 25(5):369, 1980*).

  - and Vitamin B$_{12}$:

    Regulates folic acid metabolism (*Chanarin I et al. Vitamin B$_{12}$ regulates folate metabolism by the supply of formate. Lancet 2:505-7, 1980*).

    Deficiency may induce a functional folate deficiency (*Shane B, Stokstad EL. Vitamin B$_{12}$-folate interrelationships. Annu Rev Nutr 5:115-41, 1985*).

  - and Zinc:

    Review Article: "Although high concentrations of folate may interfere with the intestinal absorption of zinc in experimental animals, the weight of current evidence indicates that daily oral supplements of 5-15 mg folate do not adversely affect zinc balance in normal humans over periods of 6 mo. to 4 yrs." (*Butterworth CE Jr, Tamura T. Folic acid safety and toxicity: A brief review. Am J Clin Nutr 50:353-58, 1989*).

Iron:

  If deficient, oral supplementation is preferred (*Fairbanks VF, Bentler E. Iron deficiency, in Hematology. McGraw Hill, 1983:466-89*).

  Oral supplementation is best absorbed on an empty stomach (*Martinez-Torres C, Layrisse M. Nutritional factors in iron deficiency: Food iron absorption. Clin Haematol 2(2):339-52, 1973*).

  Ferrous iron is 1 1/2 to 15 times better absorbed than ferric iron (*Hahn PF et al. The relative absorption and utilization of ferrous and ferric iron in anemia as determined with the radioactive isotope. Am J Physiol 143:191, 1945; Moore CV et al. Absorption of ferrous and ferric radioactive iron by human subjects and dogs. J Clin Invest 23:755, 1944*).

  Iron in meat (heme iron) is much better absorbed than iron in plant foodstuffs (non-heme iron) (*Hallberg L, Rossander L. Effect of soy protein on nonheme iron absorption in man. Am J Clin Nutr 36:514, 1982*).

  - and Calcium:

    Excessive supplementation may decrease iron absorption in a dose-defined manner leading to iron deficiency anemia. Perhaps 23% of those ingesting more than 2 gm daily are at risk (*Cook JD et al. Calcium supplementation: effect on iron absorption. Am J Clin Nutr 53:106-11, 1991; Hallberg L et al. Calcium: effect of different amounts on nonheme- and heme-iron absorption in humans. Am J Clin Nutr 53:112-19, 1991 ;Read MH et al. Mineral supplementation practices of adults in seven western states. Nutr Res 6:375-83, 1986*).

  - and Cobalt:

    Competes with iron for absorption (*Pollack S et al. The absorption of nonferrous metals in iron deficiency. J Clin Invest 44:1470, 1965*).

  - and Coffee:

    May decrease iron absorption (*Morck TA et al. Inhibition of food iron absorption by coffee. Am J Clin Nutr 37(3):416-20, 1983*).

- and Hydrochloric Acid:

If deficient, iron absorption may be impaired (*Rabinowich IM. Achlorhydria and its clinical significance in diabetes mellitus. Am J Dig Dis 16:322-32, 1949*).

- and Manganese:

May inhibit iron absorption (*Hurley LS, Keen CL. Manganese, in E Underwood and W Mertz, Eds. Trace Elements in Human Health and Animal Nutrition. New York, Academic Press, 1987:185-223; Rossander-Hultén L et al. Competitive inhibition of iron absorption by manganese and zinc in humans. Am J Clin Nutr 54:152-6, 1991*).

- and Milk:

May inhibit iron absorption (*Deehr MS et al. Effects of different calcium sources on iron absorption in postmenopausal women. Am J Clin Nutr 51:95-9, 1990*).

- and Phenolics:

Usually tannins or polyphenols, these compounds are present in tea, coffee, certain spices, fruits and vegetables.

Powerfully inhibit nonheme-iron absorption (*Tuntawiroon M et al. Dose-dependent inhibitory effect of phenolic compounds in foods on nonheme-iron absorption in men. Am J Clin Nutr 53:554-7, 1991*).

- and Phytates:

Present in cereals, certain vegetables, roots, nuts, etc.

The main cause of the inhibitory effect of bran on iron absorption (*Hallberg L et al. Phytates and the inhibitory effect of bran on iron absorption in man. Am J Clin Nutr 45:988-96, 1987*).

- and Protein:

Beef, lamb, chicken, pork and fish enhance iron absorption, while soy decreases it (*Kane AP, Miller DD. In vitro estimation of the effects of selected proteins on iron bioavailability. Am J Clin Nutr 393-401, 1984*) as do the two major milk proteins (*Hurrell RF et al. Iron absorption in humans as influenced by bovine milk proteins. Am J Clin Nutr 49:546-52, 1989*).

- and Riboflavin:

Iron absorption, the mobilization of intracellular iron, and the retention of absorbed iron are all sensitive to changes in riboflavin status (*Bates CJ et al. Vitamins, iron, and physical work. Lancet 2:313-14, 1989*).

- and Tea:

May decrease absorption (*Morck TA et al. Inhibition of food iron absorption by coffee. Am J Clin Nutr 37(3):416-20, 1983*).

> *Note: Tannins in tea are one of many types of phenolic compounds in foods. Phenolics usually polymerize to large complex molecules (polyphenols), some of which bind iron which inhibits its absorption (Hallberg L. Search for nutritional confounding factors in the relationship between iron deficiency and brain function. Am J Clin Nutr 50:598-606, 1989).*

- and Vitamin A:

Deficiency impairs mobilization of iron stores and decreases iron utilization for hemoglobin formation (*Bloem MW et al. Vitamin A intervention: short-term effects of a single, oral, massive dose on iron metabolism. Am J Clin Nutr 51:76-9, 1990*).

- and <u>Vitamin B6</u>:

Deficiency may decrease iron status without reducing GI absorption (*Keyes W et al. Copper, iron, and zinc absorption, retention, and status of young women fed vitamin B6 deficient diets. FASEB J 5:A556, 1991*).

- and <u>Vitamin C</u>:

When given concurrently with iron, markedly enhances non-heme iron absorption by keeping iron in the reduced (ferrous) state to prevent or delay the formation of insoluble or undissociated ferric compounds, thus keeping it soluble and available for absorption at the alkaline pH of the duodenum (*Brise H, Hallberg L. Effect of ascorbic acid on iron absorption. Acta Med Scand Suppl 376, 171:51, 1962; Conrad ME, Schade SG. Ascorbic acid chelates in iron absorption: A role for hydrochloric acid and bile. Gastroenterology 55:35, 1968; Monsen ER. Ascorbic acid: An enhancing factor in iron absorption, in Nutritional Bioavailability of Iron. American Chemical Society, 1982:85-95*).

Ferritin regulates the bioavailability of iron within cells. It keeps iron in a relatively accessible form while providing storage capacity to reduce the threat of iron-catalyzed oxidant damage. By contrast, iron stored in hemosiderin is inaccessible. Ascorbate increases the proportion of iron stored in ferritin, which increases iron availability in the cell (*Hoffman KE, Yanellki K, Bridges KR. Ascorbic acid and iron metabolism: alterations in lysomal function. Am J Clin Nutr 54:1188S-92S, 1991*).

Counteracts the inhibition of iron absorption by phenols and phytates, suggesting that, in diets with a high phenol or phytate content, the desired levels of ascorbic acid should also be high (*Hallberg L et al. Iron absorption in man: ascorbic acid and dose-dependent inhibition by phytate. Am J Clin Nutr 49:140-4, 1989; Siegenberg D et al. Ascorbic acid prevents the dose-dependent inhibitory effects of polyphenols and phytates on nonheme-iron absorption. Am J Clin Nutr 53:537-41, 1991*).

- and <u>Vitamin D</u>:

By enhancing the absorption of calcium (which competes with iron for absorption), may decrease iron absorption (*Pollack S et al. The absorption of nonferrous metals in iron deficiency. J Clin Invest 44, 1965*).

- and <u>Zinc</u>:

Supplementation may impair the intestinal absorption of iron (*Crofton RW et al. Inorganic zinc and the intestinal absorption of ferrous iron. Am J Clin Nutr 50:141-44, 1989; Meadows NJ et al. Oral iron and the bioavailability of zinc. Br Med J 287:1013-4, 1983*).

Note: Instead of competitive inhibition, an intraluminal reaction may occur - as a fivefold excess of zinc to iron reduced iron absorption by 56% when given in a water solution but not when given with a hamberger meal (Rossander-Hultén L et al. Competitive inhibition of iron absorption by manganese and zinc in humans. Am J Clin Nutr 54:152-6, 1991).

Supplementation may impair iron status (*Yadrick MK et al. Iron, copper, and zinc status: response to supplementation with zinc or zinc and iron in adult females. Am J Clin Nutr 49:145-50, 1989*).

<u>Magnesium</u>:

Oral magnesium supplementation may restore magnesium depots in patients with magnesium deficiency in six weeks (*Gullestad L et al. Oral versus intravenous magnesium supplementation in patients with magnesium deficiency. Magnes Trace Elem 10(1):11-16, 1991-92*).

Intestinal absorption of magnesium appears to be the same from various preparations so long as it is free and in the ionized form (*Leonhard S et al. Transport of magnesium across an isolated preparation of sheep rumen: A comparison of magnesium chloride, magnesium aspartate, magnesium picolinate, and Mg-EDTA. Magnes Trace Elem 9(5):265-71, 1990-91*).

<u>Magnesium citrate</u> is more soluble and bioavailable than <u>magnesium oxide</u> (*Lindberg JS et al. Magnesium bioavailability from magnesium citrate and magnesium oxide. J Am Coll Nutr 9(1):48-55, 1990*).

Magnesium chloride is more soluble than magnesium oxide, gluconate, citrate, hydroxide or sulfate) (*Lange NA. Handbook of Chemistry, Edition 10. San Francisco, McGraw-Hill, 1967:282-5*) and does not require stomach acid for solubility (*Laban E, Charbon GA. Magnesium and cardiac arrhythmias: Nutrient or drug? J Am Coll Nutr 5:521-32, 1986*) but its use is limited due to its hygroscopic properties (*Robins TL et al. Magnesium lactate bioavailability in dogs is not impaired by decreased gastric acidity. Abstract. J Am Coll Nutr 8(5):462, 1989*).

In studies in dogs, magnesium lactate tolerance and bioavailability compares favorably to that of enteric-coated magnesium chloride, and gastric acidity does not impair its availability (*Robins TL et al. Magnesium lactate bioavailability in dogs is not impaired by decreased gastric acidity. Abstract. J Am Coll Nutr 8(5):462, 1989*).

Magnesium citrate/lactate with or without magnesium hydroxide, magnesium hydroxide alone and magnesium chloride alone may all be equally bioavailable (*Bohmer T et a. Bioavailability of oral magnesium supplementation in female students evaluation from eleimination of mangesium in 24-hour urine. Magnes Trace Elem 9(5):272-8, 1990(1991)*).

Magnesium absorption may be enhanced by the addition of a glucose polymer solution (example: Frodex-15, Ross) (*Bei L et al. Glucose polymer increases jejunal calcium, magnesium, and zinc absorption in humans. Am J Clin Nutr 44(2):244-7, 1986*).

- and Alcohol:

    Increases urinary magnesium excretion (*Lindeman RD et al. Magnesium in Health and Disease. Jamaica, N.Y., SP Medical and Scientific Books, 1980:236-45*).

- and Caffeine:

    Increases urinary magnesium excretion (*Yeh JK et al. Influence of injected caffeine on the metabolism of calcium and the retention and excretion of sodium, potassium, phosphorus, magnesium, zinc and copper in rats. J Nutr 116(2):273-80, 1986*).

- and Calcium:

    Impairs absorption of magnesium, probably due to competition for a common transport system (*O'Donnell JM, Smith DW. Uptake of calcium and magnesium by rat duodenal mucosa analyzed by means of competing metals. J Physiol 229:733, 1973*).

- and Fat:

    High levels of fat in the intestinal lumen interfere with magnesium absorption because soaps that are formed from fat and divalent cations like magnesium are not absorbed (*Seelig MS. Magnesium requirements in human nutrition. Magnesium Bull 3(Suppl 1a):26-47, 1981*).

- and Fiber:

    "The results of metabolic balance studies suggest that fiber causes loss of minerals, including magnesium" (*Seelig MS. Magnesium requirements in human nutrition. Magnesium Bull 3(Suppl 1a):26-47, 1981*).

- and Folic Acid:

    May increase the metabolic need for magnesium by increasing the activity of glycolytic enzymes that require it (*Hodges RE, Ed. Human Nutrition: A Comprehensive Treatise. New York, Plenum Press, 1979*).

- and Iron:

    May decrease magnesium absorption (*Watts DL. The nutritional relationships of magnesium. J Orthomol Med 3(4):197-201, 1988*).

- and <u>Manganese</u>:

May decrease magnesium absorption; however, it can take the place of magnesium in some enzyme systmes that require magnesium (*Watts DL. The nutritional relationships of magnesium. J Orthomol Med 3(4):197-201, 1988*).

- and <u>Phosphorus</u>:

Fecal phosphorus appears to bind magnesium and reduce its intestinal absorption (*Franz KB. Influence of dietary phosphorus on absorption of dietary calcium and magnesium in humans. Abstract. J Am Coll Nutr 6(5):444, 1987*).

- and <u>Potassium</u>:

Potassium supplementation may increase urinary magnesium excretion (*Saito N, Kuchiba A. The changes of magnesium under high salt diets and by administration of antihypertensive diuretics. Magnesium Bull 9:53, 1987*).

- and <u>Protein</u>:

"During protein-synthesis and formation of new tissue by growing and developing children, by athletes-in-training, by pregnant or lactating women, and by those recovering from starvation or wasting illness, high-protein diets increase magnesium needs" (*Seelig MS. Magnesium requirements in human nutrition. Magnesium Bull 3(Suppl 1a):26-47, 1981*).

- and <u>Riboflavin</u>:

High-dosage riboflavin may increase the risk of magnesium deficiency (*Seelig MS. Magnesium requirements in human nutrition. Magnesium Bull 3(Suppl 1a):26-47, 1981*).

- and <u>Sodium</u>:

Greater sodium loads, such as are provided when saline is used to expand the extracellular volume, decrease serum magnesium levels and increase urinary magnesium excretion. Magnesium deficiency is associated with sodium and water retention, while repletion produces sodium and water loss (*Seelig MS. Magnesium requirements in human nutrition. Magnes Bull 3(Suppl 1a):26-47, 1981*).

- and <u>Sugar</u>:

High intake of sugar increases the need for magnesium (*Durlach J. Le Diabete 19:99-113, 1971*) and increases urinary magnesium excretion (*Lindeman RB et al, in Magnesium in Health and Disease. Jamaica, N.Y., SP Medical and Scientific Books, 1980:236-45; Lindeman RB. Influence of various nutrients and hormones on urinary divalent cation excretion. Ann N Y Acad Sci 162:802-09, 1969*).

- and <u>Vitamin B6</u>:

Magnesium and vitamin B6 deficiency produce comparable clinical disorders, and treatment with either or both has been found effective in several clinical conditions in which one or the other has been investigated (*Seelig MS. Magnesium requirements in human nutrition. Magnesium Bull 3(Suppl 1a):26-47, 1981*).

Increases cell membrane transfer and utilization of magnesium (*Aikawa JK. Proc Soc Exp Biol Med 104:461-63, 1960; Durlach J. Donnees Actuelles Sur les mecanismes de Synergie entre Vitamin B6 et Magnesium. J Medicine de Besancon 5:349, 1969*) to increase tissue magnesium levels (*Majumdar P, Boylan M. Alteration of tissue magnesium levels in rats by dietary vitamin B6 supplementation. Int J Vitam Nutr Res 59:300-3, 1989*).

Supplementation may normalize deficient intracellular magnesium levels (*Abraham GE et al. Effect of vitamin B6 plasma red blood cell magnesium levels in premenopausal women. Ann Clin Lab Sci 11(4):333-36, 1981*).

- and <u>Vitamin D</u>:

Stimulates intestinal magnesium absorption (*Nordin BEC. Plasma calcium and plasma magnesium homeostasis, in BEC Nordin, Ed. Calcium, Phosphorus and Magnesium Metabolism. New York, Churchill Livingstone, 1976).* It may enhance magnesium deficiency, however, as it increases calcium absorption more than it increases magnesium absorption; thus tissue calcium accumulation may displace magnesium (*Magnesium in Human Nutrition. US Department of Agriculture Home Econ. Res. Report No. 19, 1962*).

- and <u>Vitamin E</u>:

Deficiency may lower tissue magnesium levels (*Seelig MS. Magnesium requirements in human nutrition. Magnesium Bull 3(Suppl 1a):26-47, 1981*).

Manganese:

- and <u>Calcium</u>:

May block plasma uptake (*Freeland-Graves JH, Lin P-H. Plasma uptake of manganese as affected by oral loads of manganese, calcium, milk, phosphorus, copper, and zinc. J Am Coll Nutr 10(1):38-43, 1991*).

- and <u>Copper</u>:

May impair plasma uptake (*Freeland-Graves JH, Lin P-H. Plasma uptake of manganese as affected by oral loads of manganese, calcium, milk, phosphorus, copper, and zinc. J Am Coll Nutr 10(1):38-43, 1991*).

- and <u>Iron</u>:

May accelerate the development of manganese deficiency (*Hurley LS, Keen CL. Manganese, in E Underwood and W Mertz, Eds. Trace Elements in Human Health and Animal Nutrition. New York, Academic Press, 1987:185-223*) and impairs manganese utilization (*Thomson ABR et al. Interrelation of intestinal transport system for manganese and iron. J Lab Clin Med 73:6422, 1971*).

- and <u>Zinc</u>:

May increase plasma manganese levels (*Freeland-Graves JH, Lin P-H. Plasma uptake of manganese as affected by oral loads of manganese, calcium, milk, phosphorus, copper, and zinc. J Am Coll Nutr 10(1):38-43, 1991*).

Phosphorus:

- and <u>Caffeine</u>:

May increase urinary excretion of inorganic phosphate and may cause a negative balance (*Yeh JK et al. Influence of injected caffeine on the metabolism of calcium and the retention and excretion of sodium, potassium, phosphorus, magnesium, zinc and copper in rats. J Nutr 116(2):273-80, 1986*).

- and <u>Calcium</u>:

Increases fecal phosphorus excretion by binding primarily dietary but also endogenous phosphorus (*Schiller LR et al. Effect of the time of administration of calcium acetate on phosphorus binding. N Engl J Med 320:1110-13, 1989*).

A calcium to phosphorus ratio above 2:1 due to excess calcium results in reduced bone strength and interferes with vitamin K synthesis and/or absorption, causing internal bleeding (*Calcium: How much is too much? Nutr Rev 43(11):345, 1985*).

- and <u>Vitamin D</u>:

Facilitates phosphate absorption (*Passmore R, Eastwood MA. Davidson and Passmore: Human Nutrition and Dietetics. Eighth Edition. London, Churchill Livingstone, 1986:139*).

Potassium:

 - and Caffeine:

   Increases urinary potassium excretion and may cause a negative balance (*Yeh JK et al. Influence of injected caffeine on the metabolism of calcium and the retention and excretion of sodium, potassium, phosphorus, magnesium, zinc and copper in rats. J Nutr 116(2):273-80, 1986*).

 - and Magnesium:

   Potassium deficiency may be refractory in the presence of magnesium depletion (*Rude RK. Physiology of magnesium metabolism and the important role of magnesium in postassium deficiency. Am J Cardiol 63(14):31G-34G, 1989; Whang R et al. Magnesium depletion as a cause of refractory potassium repletion. Arch Intern Med 145(9):1686-9, 1985*) which has been found in 42% of patients with hypokalemia (*Whang R et al. Predictors of clinical hypomagnesemia. Hypokalemia, hypophosphatemia, hyponatremia, and hypocalcemia. Arch Intern Med 144(9):1794-6, 1984*).

Selenium:

Organic selenium (L-selenomethionine) is rapidly and completely absorbed, while inorganic selenium (selenite and selenate) is less well absorbed and retained (*Swanson CA et al. Human [^{74}Se]selenomethionine metabolism: a kinetic model. Am J Clin Nutr 54:917-26, 1991*). Similarly, inorganic selenium, in contrast to organic selenium, has been found to be nearly ineffective in various *in vitro* experiments against selenium deficiency in several species, starting with the study of Schwartz and Fultz (*J Biol Chem 233:245-51, 1958*) and reconfirmed repeatedly. In addition, selenite has been shown in a Japanese study to interact with glutathione in the presence of oxygen to generate free radicals. Since glutathione is found in all cells, this form of selenium may be unsuitable for human use (*Schrauzer GN. Benefits of nutritional selenium. Report of presentation from the Fourth International Symposium on Selenium in Biology and Medicine, Tubingen U., W. Germany, July, 1988. Anabolism 7(4):5, 1988*). Also, ingestion of selenomethionine (which is plant-derived) will produce higher blood and tissue selenium levels than ingestion of selenocysteine (which is animal-derived) as animals treat selenomethionine as methionine. They thus incorporate it into proteins in place of methionine and, when catabolized, it becomes nutritionally available for incorporation into glutathione peroxidase. Selenocysteine, by contrast, is only incorporated into selenoproteins such as glutathione peroxidase and is excreted once the enzyme reaches control levels. Thus selenium levels merely reflect differences in the plant and animal components of the diet (*Burk RF. Letter. JAMA 262(6):775, 1989*).

 - and Vitamin C:

   An adequate ascorbic acid status is important in the maintenance of body selenium metabolism (*Martin RF et al. Ascorbic acid-selenite interactions in humans studied with a oral dose of ^{74}SeO$_3$$^{2-}$. Am J Clin Nutr 49:862-69, 1989*).

   Sodium selenide is reduced by vitamin C *in vitro* to the ineffective elemental selenium, a reaction which is the basis for the analytical measurement of selenium (*Newberry & Christian, IOAC, 48:322, 1965*). *In vivo* confirmation has been provided by a study showing that the cancer-protective action of selenium in experimental animals is significantly reduced by simultaneous vitamin C supplementation (*Jacobs & Griffin, Biol Trace Element Res 1:1, 1979*).

 - and Vitamin E:

   Deficiency syndromes of both vitamin E and selenium overlap and most can be treated successfully with either nutrient due to their closely-related mechanisms of action (*Combs GF. Assessment of vitamin E status in animals and man. Proc Nutr Soc 40:187-94, 1981*).

Sodium:

- and Caffeine:

Increases urinary sodium excretion and may cause a negative balance (*Yeh JK et al. Influence of injected caffeine on the metabolism of calcium and the retention and excretion of sodium, potassium, phosphorus, magnesium, zinc and copper in rats. J Nutr 116(2):273-80, 1986*).

Thiamine:

- and Magnesium:

Necessary for the conversion of thiamine into thiamine pyrophosphate, its biologically active form (*Seelig MS. Nutritional status and requirements of magnesium with consideration of individual differences and prevention of cardiovascular disease. Magnesium Bull 8:170-84, 1986*).

L-Tryptophan:

- and Niacinamide:

The rationale for the addition of niacinamide is that the high rate of catabolism of tryptophan by the liver suggested by animal work can be inhibited with niacinamide (*Young SN, Sourkes TL. The antidepressant effect of tryptophan. Lancet 2:897-8, 1974*). Recent data, however, indicate that niacinamide will not inhibit breakdown of tryptophan in humans at clinical doses following an acute loading (*Green AR et al. Metabolism of an oral tryptophan load: Effect of pretreatment with the putative tryptophan pyrollase inhibitors nicotinamide or allopurinol. Br J Clin Pharmacol 10:611-15, 1980*). In addition, in pts. receiving up to 6 gm tryptophan daily along with niacinamide, tryptophan metabolism was still highly variable; thus it is unlikely that niacinamide is a useful adjunct (*Chouinard G et al. Tryptophan in the treatment of depression and mania. Adv Biol Psychiatry 10:47-66, 1983*).

- and Protein:

Effects protentiated by avoiding protein for 90 minutes before or afterwards (*Fernstrom JD et al. Diurnal variations in plasma concentrations of tryptophan, tyrosine, and other neutral amino acids: Effects of dietary protein intake. Am J Clin Nutr 32:1912-22, 1979*).

- and Sugar:

Effects potentiated by ingesting tryptophan along with carbohydrate to stimulate insulin release which takes up the other amino acids into the tissues, thus improving brain tryptophan intake (*Fernstrom JD. Effects of the diet on brain neurotransmitters. Metabolism 26:207-33, 1977*).

- and Vitamin B6:

May increase brain tryptophan levels by reducing levels of kynurenine which competes with tryptophan for transport.

Review Articles: Kynurenine is derived from tryptophan by the action of tryptophan pyrrolase in the liver and is taken up in the brain and transferred by the same transport carrier as tryptophan where it has a competitively inhibitory effect upon tryptophan equal to that of the competing amino acids (*Möller SE et al. Tryptophan availability in endogenous depression - relation to efficacy of L-tryptophan treatment. Adv Biol Psychiatry 10:30-46, 1983*). Supplementation with tryptophan increases the plasma concentration of kynurenine in proportion to the dose given and, after longer-term administration, there is a marked increase in basal kynurenine with a further substantial increase following a further dose of tryptophan. This large increase in kynurenine concentration might reflect a relative saturation of the kynurenine pathway, possibly because of vitamin B6 depletion since many of the degradative enzymes down the pathway are B6-dependent. Consistent with this hypothesis are findings that, when tryptophan is given for 7 days with pyridoxine, the basal plasma kynurenine is half that seen in subjects given tryptophan alone, and the peak kynurenine concentration following a single load is the same after long-term pre-treatment with tryptophan plus pyridoxine as after no pre-treatment and only half that seen in subjects who have taken longer-term tryptophan without pyridoxine (*Green AR, Aronson JK. The pharmacokinetics of oral L-tryptophan: Effects of dose and concomitant pyridoxine, allopurinol or nicotinamide administration. Adv Biol Psychiatry 10:67-81, 1983*).

Vitamin A:

- and Vitamin E:

Vitamin A absorption may be markedly impaired in vitamin E deficiency (*Ames SR. Factors affecting absorption, transport and storage of vitamin A. Am J Clin Nutr 22:934, 1969*).

Vitamin E protects vitamin A from oxidation in both the intestinal lumen and in the tissues, and by joining with it within the membranous parts of cells in performing its functions (*Tappel AL. Nutrition Today July-August 1973*). It is therefore suggested that vitamin E be added whenever megadoses of vitamin A are desirable.

- and Zinc:

Deficiency impairs vitamin A metabolism as it is crucial in the enzyme alcohol dehydrogenase - which converts retinol (the ingested form of vitamin A) into retinaldehyde, the first usable breakdown product (*Rogers S. AAEM Newsletter, Winter, 1988; Smith JC, in OA Levander, L Cheng, Eds. Vitamins, Minerals and Hazardous Elements. Vol. 355. New York, N Y Academy of Sciences, 198:.62*).

Deficiency impairs the synthesis of retinol-binding protein which is necessary to release vitamin A into the blood (*Smith JC Jr et al. Zinc: a trace element essential in vitamin A metabolism. Science 181:954-5, 1973; Smith JE et al. The effect of zinc deficiency on the metabolism of retinol-binding protein in the rat. J Lab Clin Med 84:692-7, 1974*).

Vitamin B6:

- and Magnesium:

Magnesium and vitamin B6 deficiency produce comparable clinical disorders, and treatment with either magnesium or B6, or both, have been found effective in several clinical conditions in which one or the other has been investigated (*Seelig MS. Magnesium requirements in human nutrition. Magnesium Bull 3(Suppl 1a):26-47, 1981*).

Vitamin B12:

Oral or sublingual administration of B12 results in negligible blood levels compared to IM injection (*Sohler A et al. Effectiveness and route of administration of vitamin B12. Int Clin Nutr Rev 9(2):64-65, 1989*).

Vitamin B12 from plant foods may not be bioavailable (*Pagnelie PC et al. Vitamin B-12 from algae appears not to be bioavailable. Am J Clin Nutr 53:695-7, 1991*).

- and Folic Acid:

High doses of folic acid may decrease vitamin B12 levels (*Hunter R et al. Effect of folic-acid supplement on serum-vitamin B12 levels in patients on anti-convulsants. Lancet 2:50, 1969*).

Vitamin C:

35% better absorbed in a natural citrus extract containing bioflavonoids, proteins, and carbohydrates than as synthetic ascorbic acid alone (*Vinson JA, Bose P. Comparative bioavailability to humans of ascorbic acid alone or in a citrus extract. Am J Clin Nutr 48:601-04, 1988*).

- and Bioflavonoids:

Results of both human and guinea pig studies suggest that vitamin C mixed with citrus bioflavonoids is more readily absorbed and remains in the body longer than equivalent quantities of vitamin C alone (*Vinson JA, Bose P. Bioavailability of synthetic ascorbic acid and a citrus extract. Ann N Y Acad Sci 498:525-6, 1987*).

Vitamin D:

Supplementation with 25-hydroxyvitamin D₃ 25 µg/day may be effective for maintaining vitamin D nutriture in the elderly with insufficient exposure to sunlight (*Shany S et al. Vitamin D-deficiency in the elderly: Treatment with ergocalciferol and hydroxylated analogues of vitamin D₃. First J Med Sci 24:160, 1988*).

- and Phosphorus:

Phosphorus intake strongly influences vitamin D metabolism (*Portale AA et al. Dietary intake of phosphorus modulates the circadian rhythm in serum concentration of phosphorus. J Clin Invest 80:1147-54, 1987; Portale A. Oral intake of phosphorus can determine the serum concentration of 1,25-dihydroxyvitamin D by determining its production rate in humans. J Clin Invest 77:7-12, 1986*).

- and Vitamin E:

Deficiency inhibits vitamin D metabolism in the liver and kidneys (*Sergeev IN, Arkhapchev YP, Spirichev VB. The role of vitamin E in the metabolism and reception of vitamin D. Biochimiya-Engl Tr 55:1483-7, 1990*).

Vitamin E:

Vitamin E succinate may be more effective in preventing free radical damage than alpha tocopherol (*Fariss M. Oxygen toxicity: Unique cytoprotective properties of vitamin E succinate in hepatocytes. Free Rad Biol Med 9:333-43, 1990*).

- and inorganic (ferric) Iron:

Oxidizes vitamin E in the intestines, causing its inactivation.

> *Note: Ferrous iron, which is the form of iron commonly used for supplementation, does not oxidize vitamin E.*

- and Selenium:

Deficiency syndromes of both vitamin E and selenium overlap and most can be treated successfully with either nutrient due to their closely-related mechanisms of action (*Combs GF. Assessment of vitamin E status in animals and man. Proc Nutr Soc 40:187-94, 1981*).

- and Zinc:

Deficiency may worsen the effects of vitamin E deficiency (*Bunk MJ et al. Dietary zinc deficiency decreases plasma concentrations of vitamin E. Proc Soc Exp Biol Med 190:379-84, 1989; Harding AJ et al. Teratogenic effect of vitamin E and zinc deficiency in the 11 day rat embryo. Nutr Rep Int 36:473-82, 1987*).

Vitamin K:

- and Calcium:

Excessive doses of calcium or a calcium to phosphorus ratio above 2:1 due to excess calcium interferes with vitamin K synthesis and/or absorption, causing internal bleeding (*Calcium: How much is too much? Nutr Rev 43(11):345, 1985*).

- and Vitamin E:

A large intake may reduce intestinal absorption of vitamin K and antagonize the effect of vitamin K on coagulation at the level of prothrombin formation (*Bieri JG et al. Medical uses of vitamin E. N Engl J Med 308(18):1063-71, 1983*).

Zinc:

Supplementation is best taken away from meals, as eggs, milk, and cereal (as well as possibly other foods) will decrease its bioavailability (*Moser PB, Gunderson CJ. Changes in plasma zinc following the ingestion of a zinc multivitamin-mineral supplement with and without breakfast. Nutr Res 3:279-84, 1983; Oelshlegel FS Jr, Brewer GJ. Absorption of pharmacological doses of zinc, in GJ Brewer, AS Prasad, Eds. Zinc Metabolism: Current Aspects in Health and Disease. New York, Alan R. Liss, Inc., 1977:299-311*).

Absorption from foods may be less than the 40% assumed for the US RDA (*Johnson P et al. Zinc availability from beef served with various carbohydrates or beverages. Nutr Res 10:155-62, 1990*).

Zinc picolinate is significantly better absorbed than zinc gluconate or zinc citrate (*Barrie SA et al. Comparative absorption of zinc picolinate, zinc citrate and zinc gluconate in humans. Agents Actions 21(1-2):223-8, 1987*).

In comparing the rate of increase of zinc levels in serum, plasma and urine for a group of patients with anorexia nervosa and low zinc levels, citrate >gluconate >orotate >sulfate (results not significant) (*Ward NI. Assessment of zinc status and oral supplementation in anorexia nervosa. J Nutr Med 1:171-7, 1990*).

Zinc sulfate may produce gastric irritation and is less well tolerated than zinc acetate or gluconate (*Prasad AS. Clinical, biochemical and pharmacological role of zinc. Ann Rev Pharmacol Toxicol 19:393-426, 1979*).

Zinc absorption may be enhanced by the addition of a glucose polymer solution (example: Frodex-15, Ross) (*Bei L et al. Glucose polymer increases jejunal calcium, magnesium, and zinc absorption in humans. Am J Clin Nutr 44(2):244-7, 1986*).

- and Calcium

May decrease zinc absorption in the presence of phytates (*Solomons NW. Mineral interactions in the diet. Contemp Nutr 7(7), July, 1982*).

- and Copper:

May decrease zinc absorption (*Castillo-Durán C et al. Oral copper supplementation: effect on copper and zinc balance during acute gastroenteritis in infants. Am J Clin Nutr 51:1088-92, 1990*).

Negative Experimental Study: In a study of healthy adult male humans, high doses of oral copper had no effect on zinc absorption (*Valberg LS et al. Effects of iron, tin, and copper on zinc absorption in humans. Am J Clin Nutr 40:536-51, 1984*).

- and Folic Acid:

May decrease zinc absorption (*Simmer K et al. Are iron-folate supplements harmful? Am J Clin Nutr 45(1):122-5, 1987*).

Negative Experimental Blinded Study: Plasma zinc concentration was not significantly different following supplementation with folic acid 10 mg/d for up to 4 mo. (*Butterworth CE et al. Zinc concentration in plasma and erythrocytes of subjects receiving folic acid supplementation. Am J Clin Nutr 47:484-6, 1988*).

- and Iron:

Iron supplementation may exacerbate subclinical zinc depletion by competitively inhibiting intestinal absorption when iron to zinc ratios are greater than 2:1 (*Meadows NJ et al. Lancet 2:1135, 1981; Solomons NW, Jacob RA. Studies on the bioavailability of zinc in humans. Effects of heme and non-heme iron on the absorption of zinc. Am J Clin Nutr 34:475-82, 1981*).

When deficient, zinc absorption is enhanced (*Pollack S et al. The absorption of nonferrous metals in iron deficiency. J Clin Invest 44:1470, 1965*).

- and <u>Phytates</u>:

Diets high in vegetable fiber may be associated with poor bioavailability of zinc due to the presence of phytic acid, a zinc-binding compound, in high concentrations (*Navert B et al. A reduction of the phytate content of bran by leavening in bread and its effect on zinc absorption in man. Br J Nutr 53:47-53, 1985*).

- and <u>Vitamin A</u>:

May facilitate zinc absorption (*Berzin NI, Bauman VK. Vitamin-A-dependent zinc-binding protein and intestinal absorption of Zn in chicks. Br J Nutr 57(2):255-68, 1987*).

- and <u>Vitamin B$_6$</u>:

Deficiency may increase zinc absorption while decreasing serum zinc concentrations, suggesting that zinc is less available for metabolic processes (*Keyes W et al. Copper, iron, and zinc absorption, retention, and status of young women fed vitamin B$_6$ deficient diets. FASEB J 5:A556, 1991*).

Supplementation may increase zinc absorption (*Evans GW. Normal and abnormal zinc absorption in man and animals: The tryptophan connection. Nutr Rev 38:137, 1980*).

- and <u>Vitamin E</u>:

Deficiency may reduce plasma zinc concentration, possibly due to a redistribution of zinc for antioxidant function, membrane stabilization or prostaglandin production (*Goode HF et al. The effect of dietary vitamin E deficiency on plasma zinc and copper concentrations. Clin Nutr 10:233-5, 1991*).

Deficiency may worsen the effects of zinc deficiency, possibly due to the effect of each upon reducing lipid peroxidation (*Harding AJ et al. Teratogenic effect of vitamin E and zinc deficiency in the 11 day rat embryo. Nutr Rep Int 36:473-82, 1987*).

SIGNS AND SYMPTOMS OF ABNORMAL TISSUE NUTRIENT LEVELS

Biotin:

Deficiency associated with:

Alopecia
Anemia
Anorexia & Nausea
Depression
Fatigue
Hypercholesterolemia
Hyperglycemia
Insomnia
Muscle Pain
Muscle Weakness
Dry, Greyish Skin
Pale, Smooth Tongue

Calcium:

Deficiency associated with:

Agitation
Brittle Fingernails
Cognitive Impairment
Delusions
Depression
Eczema
Hyperactivity
Hypertension
Insomnia
Irritability
Limb Numbness
Muscle Cramps
Nervousness
Neuromuscular Excitability
Osteomalacia
Osteoporosis
Palpitations
Paresthesias
Periodontal Disease
Rickets
Stunted Growth
Tetany

Tooth Decay

Toxicity associated with:

Anorexia
Aphasia (transient)
Ataxia
Depressed Deep Tenson Reflexes
Depression
Irritability
Memory Impairment
Muscle Weakness
Psychosis

Choline:

Deficiency associated with:

Cardiac Symptoms
Fat Intolerance
Gastric Ulcers
Growth Retardation
Hypertension
Kidney Impairment
Liver Impairment

Chromium:

Deficiency associated with:

Anxiety
Fatigue
Glucose Intolerance
Growth Impairment
Hypercholesterolemia

Toxicity associated with:

Dermatitis
GI Ulcers
Kidney Impairment
Liver Impairment

Copper:

Deficiency associated with:

Alopecia
Anemia (hypochromic, microcytic)
Depression
Dermatoses
Diarrhea
Emphysema
Fatigue
Hypercholesterolemia
Infections
Leukopenia
Myocardial Degeneration
Neutropenia
Osteoporosis
Weakness

Toxicity associated with:

Depression
Irritability
Joint Pain
Muscle Pain
Nervousness

Essential Fatty Acids:

See also: Linoleic Acid
          Linolenic Acid

Deficiency associated with:

Acne
Alopecia
Diarrhea
Eczema
Atrophy of Exocrine Glands
Dry, Brittle Hair
Endocrine Dysfunction
Fatty Degeneration of Liver
Gallstones
Growth Impairment
Immunologic Dysfunction
Impaired Wound Healing
Kidney Dysfunction
Reproductive Failure
Xerosis

Folic Acid:

Deficiency associated with:

Anemia (megaloblastic)

Ankle Jerks Depressed
Anorexia
Apathy
Constipation
Digestive Disturbances
Dyspnea
Fatigue
Glossitis
Growth Impairment
Headaches
Hypoesthesia (Stocking-Type)
Insomnia
Memory Impairment
Paranoid Ideation
Restless Legs
Vibratory Sensation in Legs Diminished
Weakness

Toxicity associated with:

Euphoria
Excitability
Hyperactivity

Inositol:

Deficiency associated with:

Alopecia
Constipation
Eczema
Hypercholesterolemia

Iodine:

Deficiency associated with:

Fatigue
Cretinism
Weight Gain

Iron:

Deficiency associated with:

Anemia (hypochromic, microcytic)
Angular Stomatitis
Anorexia
Bones Fragile
Cold Sensitivity
Confusion
Constipation
Depression
Digestive Disturbances
Dizziness

Dysphagia
Exertional Palpitations
Fatigue
Growth Impairment
Headaches
Irritability
Nails Brittle
Tongue Inflammed

Toxicity associated with:

Anorexia
Dizziness
Fatigue
Headaches

Linoleic Acid:

Deficiency associated with:

Alopecia
Arthritis
Behavioral Disturbances
Cardiovascular Disease
Eczemoid Eruptions
Growth Retardation
Hepatic Degeneration
Infections
Kidney Degeneration
Miscarriages (females)
Sterility (males)
Thirst
Wound Healing Poor

Linolenic Acid:

Deficiency associated with:

Behavioral Disturbances
Growth Retardation
Incoordination
Learning Disability
Parethesias
Visual Impairment
Weakness

Magnesium:

Deficiency associated with:

Agitation
Anemia (hemolytic)
Anorexia
Anxiety
Ataxia

Cardiac Arrhythmias
Confusion
Depression
Disorientation
Eclampsia
Edema
Fasciculations
Hallucinations
Hands and Feet Cold
Hyperactivity
Hypertension
Hypotension
Hypothermia
Insomnia
Irritability
Kidney Stones
Muscle Pains
Muscle Tremor (coarse)
Muscular Weakness
Nausea & Vomiting
Nervousness
Nystagmus
Neuromuscular Irritability
Organic Brain Syndrome
Paresthesias
Pronounced Startle Response
Restlessness
Seizures
Sonophobia
Tachycardia
Vertigo

Toxicity associated with:

Bradydysrhythmias
Fatigue
Flushing
Hypotension
Mouth Dry
Muscle Weakness
Nausea & Vomiting
Respiratory Insufficiency
Thirst

Manganese:

Deficiency associated with:

Bone Fragility
Dermatitis
Disturbed Carbohydrate Metabolism
Hypocholesterolemia
Nausea
Ovarian/Testicular Degeneration
Weight Loss

Toxicity associated with:

    Anorexia
    Hallucinations
    Judgement and Memory Impairments
    Insomnia
    Muscle Pains
    Parkinsonian-like Neurologic Disorder

Niacin:

Deficiency associated with:

    Anorexia & Nausea
    Canker Sores
    Confusion
    Depression
    Dermatitis
        localized scaly, dark,
        pigmented lesions
    Diarrhea
    Emotional Lability
    Fatigue
    Halitosis
    Headaches
    Indigestion
    Insomnia
    Irritability
    Limb Pains
    Memory Impairment
    Muscular Weakness
    Skin Eruptions
    Skin Inflammation

Pantothenic Acid:

Deficiency associated with:

    Abdominal Pains
    Alopecia
    Anorexia
    Burning Feet
    Coordination Impairment
    Depression
    Eczema
    Faintness
    Fatigue
    Hypotension
    Infections
    Insomnia
    Irritability
    Muscle Spasms
    Nausea & Vomiting
    Nervousness

    Paresthesias
    Tachycardia
    Weakness

Para Aminobenzoic Acid (PABA):

Deficiency associated with:

    Constipation
    Depression
    Digestive Disorders
    Fatigue
    Greying Hair
    Headaches
    Irritability

Phosphorus:

Deficiency associated with:

    Anorexia
    Anxiety
    Apprehension
    Bone Pain
    Breathing Irregular
    Fatigue
    Irritability
    Numbness
    Paresthesias
    Tremulousness
    Weakness
    Weight Changes

Potassium:

Deficiency associated with:

    Acne
    Cognitive Impairment
    Constipation
    Depression
    Edema
    Fatigue
    Glucose Intolerance
    Growth Impairment
    Hypercholesterolemia
    Hyporeflexia
    Hypotension
    Insomnia
    Muscle Weakness
    Nervousness
    Polydypsia
    Proteinuria
    Respiratory Distress
    Salt Retention

Slow, Irregular Heartbeat
Xerosis

Toxicity associated with:

Cognitive Impairment
Dysarthria
Dysphasia
Weakness

Riboflavin:

Deficiency associated with:

Alopecia
Cataracts
Cheilosis
Depression
Dermatitis
    dryness with
    greasy scaling
Dizziness
Eyes Red, Itching, Burning
Glossitis
Growth Impairment
Photophobia
Vision Blurred

Selenium:

Deficiency associated with:

Growth Impairment
Hypercholesterolemia
Pancreatic Insufficiency
Infections
Liver Impairment
Sterility (in males)

Toxicity associated with:

Alopecia
Arthritis
Atrophic, Brittle Nails
Diabetes Mellitus
Fatigue
Garlic Breath Odor
GI Disorders
Immune Suppression
Irritability
Kidney Impairment
Lassitude
Liver Impairment
Metallic Taste
Muscle Discomfort

Pallor
Skin Eruptions
Yellowish Skin

Sodium:

Deficiency associated with:

Abdominal Cramps
Anorexia, Nausea & Vomiting
Ataxia
Confusion
Depression
Dermatoses
Dizziness
Emotional Lability
Fatigue
Flatulence
Hallucinations
Headache
Hypotension
Illusions
Infections
Lethargy
Memory Impairment
Muscular Weakness
Seizures
Taste Impairment
Weight Loss

Toxicity associated with:

Anorexia
Cognitive Dysfunction
Congestive Heart Failure
Edema
Hyperactive Deep Tendon Reflexes
Hyperactiviy
Hypertension
Hypertonia
Irritability
Polydypsia
Polyuria
Renal Failure
Seizures
Tremors
Weight Gain

Thiamine:

Deficiency associated with:

Anorexia
Confusion
Constipation

Coordination Impairment
Depression
Digestive Disturbances
Fatigue
Irritability
Memory Loss
Muscle Atrophy
Nervousness
Numbness of Hands and Feet
Pain Sensitivity
Shortness of Breath
Sonophobia
Weakness

Vitamin A:

Deficiency associated with:

Acne
Anosmia
Dry Hair
Fatigue
Growth Impairment
Insomnia
Hyperkeratosis
Infections
Night Blindness
Weight Loss
Xeropthalmia
Xerosis

Toxicity associated with:

Abdominal Pain
Alopecia
Amenorrhea
Bone Pain & Tenderness
Cheilosis
Fatigue
GI Disturbances
Headache
Hepatomegaly
Hydrocephalus
Irritability
Joint Pain
Nausea & Vomiting
Pruritis
Skin Itchy & Dry
Splenomegaly
Weakness
Weight Loss

Vitamin B6:

Deficiency associated with:

Acne
Alopecia
Anemia
Anorexia & Nausea
Arthritis
Cheilosis
Conjunctivitis
Depression
Dizziness
Facial Oiliness
Fatigue
Glossitis
Impaired Wound Healing
Irritability
Nervousness
Neurologic Symptoms
    numbness
    paresthesias
    "electric shock" sensations
Seizures
Sleepiness
Stomatitis
Stunted Growth
Weakness

Vitamin B12:

Deficiency associated with:

Achlorhydria (pathogenetic)
Anemia (macrocytic)
Constipation
Depression
Dizziness
Fatigue
GI Disturbances
Glossitis
Headaches
Irritabiliy
Labored Breathing
Moodiness
Numbness
Palpitations
Psychosis
Spinal Cord Degeneration

Vitamin C:

Deficiency associated with:

Bleeding Gums
Depression
Easy Bruising
Irritability

Joint Pains
Malaise
Teeth Loose
Tiredness
Wound Healing Impairment

Hypogonadism
Impotence
Infections
Infertility (male)
Irritability
Lethargy
Memory Impairment
Night Blindness
Paranoia
Sterility
White Spots on Nails
Wound Healing Impairment

Vitamin D:

Deficiency associated with:

Burning (mouth & throat)
Diaphoresis of scalp
Diarrhea
Insomnia
Myopia
Nervousness
Osteomalacia
Rickets

Vitamin E:

Deficiency associated with:

Neuromuscular Impairment
    areflexia
    gait disturbance
    ophthalmoplegia
    diminished proprioception
    diminished vibratory sense
Shortened RBC Half-life

Vitamin K:

Deficiency associated with:

Hemorrhaging

Zinc:

Deficiency associated with:

Acne
Alopecia
Amnesia
Anorexia
Apathy
Brittle Nails
Delayed Sexual Maturity
Depression
Diarrhea
Eczema
Fatigue
Growth Impairment
Hypercholesterolemia
Hypogeusia

Appendix F

SIGNS AND SYMPTOMS OF HEAVY METAL TOXICITY

Aluminum:

    Anorexia
    Ataxia
    Colic
    Dementia
    Dyspnea
    Esophagitis
    Gastroenteritis
    Hepatic Dysfunction
    Nephritis
    Pain in Muscles
    Psychosis
    Weakness

Cadmium:

    Alopecia
    Anemia (iron-deficiency)
    Anorexia
    Anosmia
    Emphysema
    Fatigue
    Hepatic Dysfunction
    Hypertension
    Joint Soreness
    Nephrocalcinosis
    Osteoporosis
    Pain in Back and Legs
    Skin Dry and Scaly
    Teeth Yellow

Lead:

    Anemia (iron-deficiency)
    Anorexia
    Anxiety
    Concentration Impairment
    Confusion
    Constipation
    Depression
    Dizziness
    Drowsiness

    Fatigue
    Headaches
    Hypertension
    Incoordination
    Indigestion
    Irritability
    Memory Impairment
    Pain in Abdomen
    Pain in Bones
    Pain in Muscles
    Restlessness
    Tremors

Mercury:

    Anemia
    Anorexia
    Ataxia
    Colitis
    Depression
    Dermatitis
    Dizziness
    Drowsiness
    Emotional Instability
    Erethism
    Fatigue
    Headaches
    Hearing Impairment
    Hypertension
    Incoordination
    Insomnia
    Irritability
    Kidney Dysfunction
    Memory Impairment
    Metallic Taste
    Numbness
    Paresthesias
    Psychosis
    Stomatitis
    Tremors
    Vision Impairment
    Weakness

<u>Nickel</u>:

Apathy
Cyanosis
Diarrhea
Dyspnea
Fever
Headaches
Insomnia
Nausea & Vomiting
Tachypnea

Appendix G

HOW TO RULE OUT FOOD SENSITIVITIES

When ingestion of a food is promptly followed by symptoms, the diagnosis is obvious. Often, however, the diagnosis is more elusive, as ingestion of inciting foods fails to elicit immediate symptoms. This occurs most often when inciting foods are eaten frequently, and is thought to be the result of the development of a chronic maladaptive state.

An elimination diet is the direct method for diagnosing food sensitivities; if the eliminated foods contributed to the illness, clinical improvement will occur. Foods must be eliminated for a minimum of five days to allow for the removal of their remains from the gastrointestinal tract and to provide time for the effects of their systemic absorption to dissipate. As some of these effects may be protracted, a longer period of food exclusion, ranging from two to six weeks, is more diagnostically definitive.

The nature of the elimination diet depends upon the history and clinical presentation, as well as upon individual motivation. Foods selected to remain in the diet should be those which are least suspected of causing symptoms. Most definitive, but most severe and potentially unhealthful, is a five-day water-only fast. An elemental diet, consisting of a liquid mixture in which as few of the ingredients as possible are food-derived, provides basic nourishment but is difficult to tolerate. A two-food diet, such as the lamb and pear diet, consists of one protein- and fat-rich food and one carbohydrate-rich food. People on such limited diets for diagnostic purposes should be in reasonably good health and should be followed medically.

A common food elimination diet is often the most practical. In this diet, only foods which are normally eaten more often than twice a week are eliminated. This diet commonly provides a wide enough variety of foods to ensure nutritional adequacy and minimizes the inconvenience to the patient. To be done correctly, patients must restrict themselves to foods whose exact composition they know. Unless the food sources of all their ingredients are known, medications, nutritional supplements and toothpaste may be sources of eliminated foods which could possibly reduce the diagnostic value of the diet. Of course, medications should not be discontinued without

the physician's approval. (Baking soda can be substituted for toothpaste.)

Sometimes only one food, or a few foods, need be eliminated. Occasionally specific foods have been linked to certain illnesses, such as gluten (which is found in wheat, oats, rye and barley) in schizophrenia. While unproven, unusually strong craving for a particular food is believed to suggest sensitivity to that food. Since eliminating only suspicious foods is the easiest elimination diet to follow, it can be tried first, and a more extensive elimination can be tried later if symptoms fail to improve.

Some patients will initially feel worse, usually starting 12-24 hours after beginning the diet. Their symptoms may worsen, or they may experience new symptoms, such as headache or a flu-like syndrome. Assuming that symptom production is not a nocebo (negative placebo) effect, this development is a preliminary indication that they are indeed sensitive to one or more of the eliminated foods, and that improvement should be expected with continued adherence to the diet.

If a food elimination diet results in improvement, eliminated foods are systematically reintroduced one at a time in order to identify the specific foods to which the person is sensitive. Nocebo effects can be eliminated if foods and a placebo are dispensed in capsules, each with a coded label.

Ideally, since reactions can be delayed as long as 72 hours, one food should be introduced every three days. When many foods have been eliminated, these food challenges may take a month or longer. They can be done more closely together, daily for example, but sometimes identification of inciting foods becomes difficult when delayed reactions overlap, and it may take several days before the patient returns to the baseline state.

During the elimination period, and especially during provocative testing, patients should keep a food diary. One column can be used to record the time each food was ingested, while another column can record changes in signs and symptoms. A particular symptom can be rated on a scale, and ratings at the end of each day can be averaged to provide a comparison over time.

Individualized elimination diets can be based on the results of blood testing. Several types of blood tests for food sensitivities are available. They may evaluate cellular damage when blood cells are exposed to a food (cytotoxic tests) or immune reactions to a food (IgE or IgG RAST; IgG immune complexes). Much of their appeal is due to their convenience, which is counterbalanced by their cost.

Despite improvements in recent years, different types of blood testing done on the same patient will yield different results; some even yield quite different results when repeated on the same patient. At best, blood tests for food sensitivities only indicate an abnormal response to a food; they are unable to tell whether that food is contributing to the illness, or even whether that food will eventually produce symptoms if it continues to be consumed.

Despite their limitations, elimination diets based on blood testing may be effective in reducing symptoms. When, however, such a diet has proven ineffective, a standard elimination diet should still be considered.

Skin testing is another diagnostic method. Prick and scratch tests, which only test for atopic (IgE-mediated) allergic reactions, are of very limited value for diagnosing food sensitivities. In provocative testing, various dilutions of each food are placed into or under the skin, or under the tongue, and both the patient and the clinician look for changes in signs or symptoms within the next 10 minutes. The attraction of provocative testing is that it is not only diagnostic, but it may also be therapeutic. However, while experienced clinicians report excellent results with this method, its efficacy is highly controversial.

FOR FURTHER INFORMATION

PROFESSIONAL BOOKS

Breneman JC. Basics of Food Allergy. Springfield, Illinois, Charles C. Thomas, 1978

J Brostoff, SJ Challacombe, Eds. Food Allergy and Intolerance. London, Baillière Tindall, 1987

JW Gerrard, Ed. Food Allergy: New Perspectives. Springfield, Illinois, Charles C. Thomas, 1980

POPULAR BOOKS

Brostoff J, Gamlin L. The Complete Guide to Food Allergy and Intolerance. London, Bloomsbury Publishing Ltd., 1989

Faelten S. The Allergy Self-Help Book. Emmaus, Penn., Rodale Press, 1983

Levin AS, Zellerbach M. The Type 1/Type 2 Allergy Relief Program. Los Angeles, Jeremy P. Tarcher, 1983

INDEX

INDEX

ORDERING INFORMATION

The following books by Melvyn R. Werbach, M.D. are available by mail directly from *Third Line Press*:

(USE THE HANDY ORDER FORM ON THE NEXT PAGE.)

1. Nutritional Influences on Illness. *Second* Edition

700 pages   8 1/2" x 11"   1993   hard cover   *Price:* **$64.95**

> *"I cannot imagine a health care provider who would not gain from appropriating the information in this book . . . ."*

> James Heffley, Ph.D.
> Editor, **Journal of Applied Nutrition**

2. Nutritional Influences on Mental Illness

360 pages   7" x 10"   1991   hard cover   *Price:* **$34.95**

The companion volume to **Nutritional Influences on Illness, Second Edition**: *Aggressive Behavior, Alcoholism, Anxiety, Attention-deficit Hyperactivity Disorder, Autism, Bipolar Disorder, Dementia, Depression, Eating Disorders, Fatigue, Insomnia, Learning Disabilities, Organic Mental Disorders, Premenstrual Syndrome, Schizophrenia, Tardive Dyskinesia*

> *"A worthy companion to . . . Nutritional Influences on Illness, considered by many a classic for its clarity, breadth and editorial care. . . . This is a book that deserves to be on every professional's shelf within easy reach."*

> Russell M. Jaffe, M.D., Ph.D.
> **International Clinical Nutritional Review**

3. Healing Through Nutrition. Published by *Harper/Collins (US)*

443 pages   6 1/2" x 9 1/2"   1993   hard cover   *Price:* **$25.00**

> *"In this informative volume, designed as a reference for medical offices, libraries and - most of all - for families, Dr. Werbach, widely regarded as the expert on the subject of nutritional influences on illness and wellness, shows how nutrition can be both the cause and the cure for our most common illnesses."*

> **Let's Live**

4. Third Line Medicine: Modern Treatment for Persistent Symptoms

215 pages   5" x 7 1/2"   1986   soft cover   *Price:* **$10.95**

An answer for patients who fail to benefit from mainstream treatments.

> *"For this clear exposition of what has happened and where we are going, all doctors . . . ought to be grateful."*

> Abram Hoffer, M.D., Ph.D.
> Editor-in-Chief, **Journal of Orthomolecular Medicine**

(over)

THIRD LINE PRESS

4751 Viviana Drive, Suite 102
Tarzana, California 91356
USA

Phone: (800) 916-0076
[In CA: (818) 996-0076]
FAX: (818) 774-1575

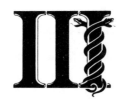

Please send:

_____ copies of **Nutritional Influences on Illness.** *Second* **Edition** @ $64.95 $ _____

_____ copies of **Nutritional Influences on Mental Illness**   @ $34.95 $ _____

_____ copies of **Healing Through Nutrition**   @ $25.00 $ _____

(This book is unavailable for orders going to the United Kingdom and Commonwealth countries.)

_____ copies of **Third Line Medicine: Modern Treatment**
for Persistent Symptoms   @ $10.95 $ _____

SHIPPING CHARGES
(add $3.00 for orders outside the US)
1 book $6.00
2 books: $7.00
3 books: $8.50
4-6 books: $10.00

Subtotal $ _____

8.25% tax (California only) $ _____

Shipping $ _____

QUANTITY PRICES ON REQUEST

TOTAL ENCLOSED $ _____

Outside of the United States:

* Beyond North America, shipping charges are for surface shipping (up to 3 months).
* Air mail rates are available on request.
* Payment may be made by Visa or MasterCard *(fill in the information below)*;
otherwise payment must be in US dollars by a check drawn on a US bank.

Please charge my: Visa _____   MasterCard _____

Card   #: _____ - _____ - _____ - _____ **Expiring:** _____

Signature: _____

NAME: _____

ADDRESS: _____

_____

_____

_____

TELEPHONE: _____   FAX: _____